Family Medicine

Obstetrics

Third Edition

Family Medicine

Obstetrics

Third Edition

Stephen D. Ratcliffe, MD, MSPH
Program Director
Department of Family and Community Medicine
Lancaster General Hospital
Lancaster, Pennsylvania

Elizabeth G. Baxley, MD
Professor and Chair
Department of Family and Preventive Medicine
University of South Carolina School of Medicine
Columbia, South Carolina

Matthew K. Cline, MD
Professor of Family Medicine
South Carolina AHEC
Medical University of South Carolina
Charleston, South Carolina;
Associate Residency Director
Family Medicine Residency
AnMed Health
Anderson, South Carolina

Ellen L. Sakornbut, MD
Private Practice
Family Health Center
Waterloo, Iowa

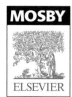

MOSBY

ELSEVIER

1600 John F. Kennedy Blvd.
Ste 1800
Philadelphia, PA 19103-2899

FAMILY MEDICINE OBSTETRICS, THIRD EDITION   ISBN: 978-0-323-04306-9

Notice

Knowledge and best practice in this field are constantly changing. As new research and experience broaden our knowledge, changes in practice, treatment, and drug therapy may become necessary or appropriate. Readers are advised to check the most current information provided (i) on procedures featured or (ii) by the manufacturer of each product to be administered, to verify the recommended dose or formula, the method and duration of administration, and contraindications. It is the responsibility of the practitioner, relying on their own experience and knowledge of the patient, to make diagnoses, to determine dosages and the best treatment for each individual patient, and to take all appropriate safety precautions. To the fullest extent of the law, neither the Publisher nor the Editors assume any liability for any injury and/or damage to persons or property arising out of or related to any use of the material contained in this book.

The Publisher

Library of Congress Cataloging-in-Publication Data
Family medicine obstetrics / [edited by] Stephen D. Ratcliffe ... [et al.].—3rd ed.
   p. ; cm.
     Rev. ed. of: Family practice obstetrics.
     Includes bibliographical references and index.
     ISBN 978-0-323-04306-9
  1. Obstetrics—Handbooks, manuals, etc. 2. Family medicine—Handbooks, manuals, etc. I. Ratcliffe, Stephen D., 1952- II. Family practice obstetrics.
     [DNLM: 1. Obstetrics—Handbooks. 2. Family Practice—Handbooks. WQ
   39 F1976 2008]
   RG531.F36 2008
   618.2—dc22

2007022572

Acquisitions Editor: Rolla Couchman
Developmental Editor: John Ingram
Project Manager: Bryan Hayward
Design Direction: Steve Stave

Printed in the United States of America

Last digit is the print number: 9 8 7 6 5 4 3 2 1

Contributors

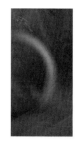

Patricia Adam, MD, MSPH
Assistant Professor
    Department of Family Medicine & Community
      Health
    University of Minnesota
    Minneapolis, Minnesota
    Chapter 19: The First Month of Life

Janice M. Anderson, MD, FAAFP
    Forbes Family Medicine Residency Program
    Department of Family Medicine
    Western Pennsylvania Hospital Forbes Regional
      Campus
    Pittsburgh, Pennsylvania
    Chapter 16: Intrapartum Complications

Thad J. Barkdull, MD
Fellow
    Primary Care Sports Medicine
    Tri-Services National Capital Consortium
    Dewitt Army Community Hospital
    Fort Belvoir, Virginia
    Chapter 4: Patient and Family Education

Wendy Brooks Barr, MD, MPH, MSCE
Research Director and Co-Maternity Care
  Coordinator
    Beth Israel Residency in Urban Family Practice
    Institute for Urban Family Health
    New York, New York;
Assistant Professor of Family and Social Medicine
    Department of Family and Social Medicine
    Albert Einstein College of Medicine, Yeshiva
      University
    New York, New York;

Research Director
    Department of Family Medicine
    Beth Israel Medical Center
    New York, New York
    Chapter 15: Management of Labor Abnormalities

Elizabeth G. Baxley, MD
Professor and Chair
    Department of Family and Preventive Medicine
    University of South Carolina School of
      Medicine
    Columbia, South Carolina
    Chapter 4: Patient and Family Education
    Chapter 5: Pregnancy Interventions
    *Chapter 13: Birth Crisis: Caring for the Family
      Experiencing Perinatal Death or the Birth
      of a Child with Medical Complications*
    Chapter 17: Malpresentation and Malpositions
    *Chapter 20: Postpartum Biomedical Concerns:
      Breastfeeding*

V. Leigh Beasley, MD, FAAFP
    Palmetto Health Clinic
    Palmetto Health Baptist Easley
    Easley, South Carolina
    Chapter 5: Pregnancy Interventions

Kevin J. Bennett, BS, MS, PhD
Assistant Professor
    Department of Family and Preventive Medicine
    University of South Carolina School of
      Medicine
    Columbia, South Carolina;

Adjunct Professor
    Health Services Policy & Management
    University of South Carolina Arnold School
      of Public Health
    Columbia, South Carolina
    Chapter 5: Pregnancy Interventions

Richard Beukema, MD
Physician
    Family Health Centers
    Okanogan, Washington;
Physician
    Mid Valley Hospital
    Omak, Washington
    Chapter 7: Complications of Pregnancy

Rachel Setzler Brown, MD
Assistant Professor
    Department of Family and Preventive Medicine
    University of South Carolina School
      of Medicine
    Columbia, South Carolina
    Chapter 4: Patient and Family Education

Charles Carter, MD
Assistant Professor
    Department of Family and Preventive Medicine
    University of South Carolina School
      of Medicine
    Columbia, South Carolina;
Residency Program Director
    Department of Family Medicine
    Palmetto Health Richland Hospital
    Columbia, South Carolina;
Assistant Editor
    American Family Physician
    American Academy of Family Physicians
    Leawood, Kansas
    Chapter 20: Postpartum Biomedical Concerns:
      Breastfeeding

Laura Chambers-Kersh, MD
Resident
    Department of Family Medicine
    University of Minnesota, North Memorial
    Minneapolis, Minnesota;
Medical Officer, Indian Health Service
    Department of Family Medicine
    Northern Navajo Medical Center
    Shiprock, New Mexico
    Chapter 19: The First Month of Life

Beth Choby, MD
Clinical Assistant Professor
    Department of Family and Community
      Medicine
    Baylor College of Medicine
    Houston, Texas;
Assistant Professor
    San Jacinto Methodist Family Medicine
      Residency
    The Methodist Hospital System Houston, Texas
    Baytown, Texas
    Chapter 3: Content of Prenatal Care

Matthew K. Cline, MD
Professor of Family Medicine
    South Carolina AHEC
    Medical University of South Carolina
    Charleston, South Carolina;
Associate Residency Director
    Family Medicine Residency
    AnMed Health
    Anderson, South Carolina
    Chapter 3: Content of Prenatal Care
    Chapter 8: Chronic Medical Conditions
      in Pregnancy
    Chapter 14: Management of Labor
    Chapter 15: Management of Labor Abnormalities

Andrew Coco, MD, MS
Associate Director of the Family Medicine
    Residency Program
    Department of Family and Community
      Medicine
    Lancaster General Hospital
    Lancaster, Pennsylvania
    Chapter 9: Commonly Encountered Medical
    Problems in Pregnancy

Donna Cohen, MD, MSc
Associate Director, Family Practice Residency Program
    Department of Family and Community
      Medicine
    Lancaster General Hospital
    Lancaster, Pennsylvania
    Chapter 9: Commonly Encountered Medical
    Problems in Pregnancy

James R. Damos, MD
Clinical Professor and Program Director
    Family Medicine
    University of Wisconsin and St. Mary's/Dean
      Ventures
    Baraboo, Wisconsin;
Physician
    Department of Family Medicine
    St. Clare Hospital
    Baraboo, Wisconsin
    Chapter 18: Intrapartum Procedures

Mark Deutchman, MD
Professor
    Department of Family Medicine
    University of Colorado Health Sciences Center
    Aurora, Colorado;
Professor
    Department of Family Medicine
    University of Colorado Hospital
    Aurora, Colorado
    Chapter 3: Content of Prenatal Care
    Chapter 6: Diagnosis and Management of First-
      Trimester Complications
    Chapter 9: Commonly Encountered Medical
      Problems in Pregnancy
    Chapter 18: Intrapartum Procedures

Lee T. Dresang, MD
Associate Professor
    Family Medicine
    University of Wisconsin School of Medicine
      and Public Health
    Madison, Wisconsin;
    Department of Family Medicine
    St. Mary's Hospital; Meriter Hospital;
      University of Wisconsin Hospital
    Madison, Wisconsin;
Advisory Board Member
    Chapter 16: Intrapartum Complications

Sherri Fong, BS
Community Program Assistant
    Department of Family Medicine & Community
      Health
    University of Minnesota, Twin Cities
    Minneapolis, Minnesota
    Chapter 19: The First Month of Life

Patricia Fontaine, MD, MS
Associate Professor
    Department of Family Medicine & Community
      Health
    University of Minnesota School of Medicine
    Minneapolis, Minnesota
    Chapter 19: The First Month of Life

Josephine R. Fowler, MD, MS, FAAFP
VP of Academic Affairs/Chief Academic Officer
    Department of Academic Affairs
    John Peter Smith Health Network
    Fort Worth, Texas;
VP of Academic Affairs/Chief Academic Officer
    Family Medicine & Academic Affairs
    John Peter Smith Health Network
    Fort Worth, Texas
    Chapter 2: Preconception Care: Improving Birth
      Outcomes through Care before Pregnancy

Karen Jankowski Fruechte, MD
Resident Physician
    Department of Family Medicine
    University of Minnesota
    Minneapolis, Minnesota;
Resident Physician
    Family Medicine
    North Memorial Medical Center
    Robbinsdale, Minnesota
    Chapter 19: The First Month of Life

Thomas J. Gates, MD
Associate Director
    Department of Family & Community Medicine
    Lancaster General Hospital
    Lancaster, Pennsylvania
    Chapter 7: Complications of Pregnancy

Dwenda K. Gjerdingen, MD, MS
Professor
    Department of Family Medicine & Community
      Health
    University of Minnesota
    Minneapolis, Minnesota;
Active Staff
    Family Medicine
    St. Joseph's Hospital
    St. Paul, Minnesota
    Chapter 21: Postpartum Psychosocial Concerns

Robert W. Gobbo, MD
Clinical Associate Professor of Family Medicine
    Department of Family Medicine
    Oregon Health Science University School
      of Medicine
    Portland, Oregon;
Clinical Associate Professor
    Providence Family Medicine Residency
    Milwaukie, Oregon
    Chapter 18: Intrapartum Procedures

Rachel Elizabeth Hall, MD, FAAFP
Assistant Professor
    Department of Family and Preventive Medicine
    University of South Carolina School
      of Medicine
    Columbia, South Carolina;
Attending Physician
    Family Medicine
    Palmetto Health–Richland
    Columbia, South Carolina
    *Chapter 9: Commonly Encountered Medical
      Problems in Pregnancy*
    Chapter 18: Intrapartum Procedures

John C. Houchins, MD
Assistant Professor
    Department of Family and Preventive Medicine
    University of Utah
    Salt Lake City, Utah
    Chapter 7: Complications of Pregnancy
    Chapter 16: Intrapartum Complications

Richard Hudspeth, MD
Faculty
    Department of Family Medicine
    Henderson Family Medicine Residency
      Program,
    Mountain Area Health Education Center
    University of North Carolina–Chapel Hill
    Hendersonville, North Carolina;
Clinical Assistant Professor
    Hendersonville Family Medicine Residency
    University of North Carolina–Chapel Hill
    Hendersonville, North Carolina;

Medical Director
    Access II Care
    Asheville, North Carolina
    *Chapter 9: Commonly Encountered Medical
      Problems in Pregnancy*
    *Chapter 11: Antenatal Testing for Fetal
      Surveillance and Management of the Postterm
      Pregnancy*

Brian W. Jack, MD
Associate Professor and Vice Chair
    Department of Family Medicine
    Boston University School of Medicine–Boston
      Medical Center
    Boston, Massachusetts
    *Chapter 2: Preconception Care: Improving Birth
      Outcomes through Care before Pregnancy*

Elizabeth A. Joy, MD
Clinical Associate Professor
    Department of Family and Preventive Medicine
    University of Utah
    Salt Lake City, Utah
    Chapter 4: Patient and Family Education

Jacqueline E. Julius, MD
Family Medicine Resident
    Lancaster General Hospital Family Medicine
      Residency Program
    Lancaster General Hospital
    Lancaster, Pennsylvania
    *Chapter 8: Chronic Medical Conditions
      in Pregnancy*

Barbara F. Kelly, MD
Assistant Professor
    Department of Family Medicine
    University of Colorado at Denver and Health
      Sciences Center
    Denver, Colorado;
Active Medical Staff
    Family Medicine
    University Hospital
    Aurora, Colorado
    Chapter 7: Complications of Pregnancy

Cynthia Kilbourn, MD
Associate Director
    Department of Family & Community Medicine
    Lancaster General Hospital
    Lancaster, Pennsylvania
    Chapter 3: Content of Prenatal Care

Valerie J. King, MD, MPH
Associate Professor
    Department of Family Medicine
    Oregon Health and Science University
    Portland, Oregon
    Chapter 7: Complications of Pregnancy
    Chapter 14: Management of Labor

Jeffrey T. Kirchner, DO, FAAFP
Associate Director–Family Medicine Residency
  Program
    Family and Community Medicine
    Lancaster General Hospital
    Lancaster, Pennsylvania
    Chapter 8: Chronic Medical Conditions
      in Pregnancy

Walter L. Larimore, MD
Clinical Assistant Professor
    Department of Family Medicine
    University of Colorado Health Sciences Center
    Denver, Colorado;
Visiting Faculty and Clinical Instructor
    Family Medicine Residency Program
    In His Image
    Tulsa, Oklahoma
    Chapter 14: Management of Labor

Lawrence Leeman, MD, MPH
Associate Professor
    Family and Community Medicine, Obstetrics
      and Gynecology
    University of New Mexico
    Albuquerque, New Mexico;
Co-Medical Director Mother–Baby Unity
    Family and Community Medicine, Obstetrics
      and Gynecology
    University Hospital
    Albuquerque, New Mexico
    Chapter 8: Chronic Medical Conditions
      in Pregnancy
    Chapter 16: Intrapartum Complications
    Chapter 18: Intrapartum Procedures

Jamee H. Lucas, MD, AAFP
Associate Professor
    Department of Family and Preventive Medicine
    University of South Carolina School
      of Medicine
    Columbia, South Carolina
    Chapter 4: Patient and Family Education
    Chapter 17: Malpresentation and Malpositions

Jose Matthew Mata, MD, MS
Staff Physician
    Family Medicine
    Cascade Valley Hospital
    Arlington, Washington;
Staff Physician
    Medicine
    SeaMar Community Health Center
    Marysville, Washington
    Chapter 16: Intrapartum Complications

Neil J. Murphy, MD
Clinical Instructor
    Department of Family Medicine
    University of Washington School of Medicine
    Seattle, Washington;
Chief Clinical Consultant, OB/GYN
    Women's Health Service–Southcentral
      Foundation
    Alaska Native Medical Center
    Anchorage, Alaska;
Chief Clinical Consultant
    Obstetrics and Gynecology
    Indian Health Service
    Rockville, Maryland
    Chapter 18: Intrapartum Procedures

James M. Nicholson, MD, MSCE
Assistant Professor
    Department of Family Medicine & Community
      Health
    University of Pennsylvania Health System
    Philadelphia, Pennsylvania
    Chapter 15: Management of Labor Abnormalities

Stephen T. Olin, MD
Clinical Assistant Professor of Community
  Medicine
    Temple University School of Medicine
    Philadelphia, Pennsylvania;
Clinical Assistant Professor of Family
  and Community Medicine
    Pennsylvania State University College
      of Medicine
    Hershey, Pennsylvania;
Associate Director
    Family and Community Medicine Residency
      Program
    Lancaster General Hospital
    Lancaster, Pennsylvania
    Chapter 9: Commonly Encountered Medical
      Problems in Pregnancy

Patricia Ann Payne, BSN, CNM, MPH
Nurse Midwife
Nurse Midwifery Service
Department of OB/GYN, Division
of Maternal–Fetal Medicine
Duke University Medical Center
Durham, North Carolina
Chapter 4: Patient and Family Education
Chapter 20: Postpartum Biomedical Concerns:
Breastfeeding

Kent Petrie, MD
Assistant Clinical Professor
Department of Family Medicine
University of Colorado Health Sciences Center
Denver, Colorado;
Private Practice
Colorado Mountain Medical, P.C.
Vail, Colorado
Chapter 3: Content of Prenatal Care
Chapter 14: Management of Labor
Chapter 16: Intrapartum Complications
Chapter 17: Malpresentation and Malpositions
Appendix E: Drugs for Common Conditions in
Pregnancy

Narayana Rao V. Pula, MD
Family Medicine Resident
Forbes Family Medicine Residency Program
Western Pennsylvania Hospital–Forbes
Regional Campus
Monroeville, Pennsylvania
Chapter 16: Intrapartum Complications

Jeffrey D. Quinlan, MD
Assistant Professor
Family Medicine
Uniformed Services University of Health
Sciences
Bethesda, Maryland;
Program Director
Family Medicine Residency Program
Naval Hospital Jacksonville
Jacksonville, Florida;
Chair
Advanced Life Support in Obstetrics Advisory
Board
American Academy of Family Physicians
Leawood, Kansas
Chapter 3: Content of Prenatal Care

Miranda Raiche, MD
Attending
Family Medicine
Mid-Valley Hospital
Omak, Washington
Chapter 7: Complications of Pregnancy

Mark L. Rast, MD
Associate Residency Director of the Family
Medicine Residency
Department of Family and Community
Medicine
Lancaster General Hospital
Lancaster, Pennsylvania;
Clinical Assistant Professor
Temple University School of Medicine
Pennsylvania State University School
of Medicine
Hershey, Pennsylvania
Chapter 7: Complications of Pregnancy

Stephen D. Ratcliffe, MD, MSPH
Program Director
Department of Family and Community
Medicine
Lancaster General Hospital
Lancaster, Pennsylvania
Chapter 9: Commonly Encountered Medical
Problems in Pregnancy
Chapter 11: Antenatal Testing for Fetal
Surveillance and Management of the Postterm
Pregnancy
Chapter 12: Preterm Labor
Chapter 16: Intrapartum Complications
Chapter 17: Malpresentation and Malpositions
Chapter 18: Intrapartum Procedures

Amity Rubeor, DO
Assistant Clinical Professor
Department of Family Medicine
Memorial Hospital of Rhode Island
Pawtucket, Rhode Island;
Assistant Clinical Professor
Department of Family Medicine
Brown Medical School
Pawtucket, Rhode Island
Chapter 9: Commonly Encountered Medical
Problems in Pregnancy

Ellen L. Sakornbut, MD
Private Practice
    Family Health Center
    Waterloo, Iowa
    Chapter 3: Content of Prenatal Care
    Chapter 7: Complications of Pregnancy
    Chapter 8: Chronic Medical Conditions
        in Pregnancy
    Chapter 9: Commonly Encountered Medical
        Problems in Pregnancy
    Chapter 10: Treatment of Psychiatric Disorders
        in Pregnancy
    Chapter 17: Malpresentation and Malpositions
    Chapter 18: Intrapartum Procedures

Osman N. Sanyer, MD
Assistant Professor
    Department of Family and Preventive Medicine
    University of Utah
    Salt Lake City, Utah
    Chapter 16: Intrapartum Complications

William Gosnell Sayres, Jr., MD
Clinical Chief
    Group Health Cooperative
    Spokane, Washington;
Clinical Instructor
    Department of Family Medicine
    University of Washington School of Medicine
    Seattle, Washington;
Family Practice
    Sacred Heart Medical Center
    Spokane, Washington
    Chapter 12: Preterm Labor

Ted R. Schultz, MD
Staff Physician
    Family Medicine
    University of Utah Hospital
    Salt Lake City, Utah;
Staff Physician
    Family Medicine
    LDS Hospital
    Salt Lake City, Utah;
Staff Physician
    Community Health Center
    Stephen D. Ratcliffe Clinic
    Salt Lake City, Utah
    Chapter 8: Chronic Medical Conditions
        in Pregnancy

Elizabeth Ann Shaw, BSc, MD, FCFP
Postgraduate Program Director
    Department of Family Medicine
    McMaster University
    Hamilton, Ontario, Canada;
Active Staff
    Family Medicine and Service of Family
        Medicine Obstetrics
    St. Joseph's Healthcare
    Hamilton, Ontario, Canada;
Courtesy Staff
    Family Medicine
    Hamilton Health Sciences Corporation
    Hamilton, Ontario, Canada
    Chapter 21: Postpartum Psychosocial Concerns

Christine Stabler, MD, FAAFP
Assistant Professor
    Department of Family Medicine
    Temple University School of Medicine
    Philadelphia, Pennsylvania;
Active Staff
    Family and Community Medicine
    Lancaster General Hospital
    Lancaster, Pennsylvania
    Chapter 20: Postpartum Biomedical Concerns:
        Breastfeeding

Harry A. Taylor, MD, MPH
Executive Officer
    U.S. Naval Hospital Sigonella
    Sicily, Italy
    Chapter 1: Improving Safety and Quality
        in Maternity Care

Kathryn J. Trotter, RN, MSN, CNM, FNP
Assistant Clinical Professor
    School of Nursing
    Duke University
    Durham, North Carolina;
Nurse Practitioner
    Department of Surgery, Breast Clinic
    Duke University
    Durham, North Carolina
    Chapter 5: Pregnancy Interventions

Mary Rose Tully, MPH, IBCLC
Faculty
    Center for Infant and Young Child Feeding
      and Care
    Maternal Child Health, School of Public Health
    University of North Carolina at Chapel Hill
    Chapel Hill, North Carolina;
Director
    Lactation Services
    NC Women's & Children's Hospitals, UNC
      Healthcare
    Chapel Hill, North Carolina
    Chapter 4: Patient and Family Education
    Chapter 20: Postpartum Biomedical Concerns:
      Breastfeeding

Ann Tumblin, BA
Perinatal Education Specialist
    Birth and Parent Education
    Wake Med
    Raleigh, North Carolina;
Doula Trainer, Education Committee
    DONA International
    Jasper, Indiana;
Program Trainer, Education Council
    Lamaze International
    Washington, DC
    Chapter 4: Patient and Family Education

David Turok, MD, MPH
Assistant Clinical Professor
    Obstetrics & Gynecology and Family
      and Preventive Medicine
    University of Utah
    Salt Lake City, Utah;
Staff Physician
    Obstetrics & Gynecology
    Community Health Centers, Inc.
    Salt Lake City, Utah
    Chapter 6: Diagnosis and Management
      of First-Trimester Complications
    Chapter 7: Complications of Pregnancy
    Chapter 8: Chronic Medical Conditions
      in Pregnancy
    Chapter 16: Intrapartum Complications

Sharon S.-L. Wong, PhD, RD
Assistant Professor
    School of Nutrition
    Ryerson University
    Toronto, Ontario, Canada
    Chapter 21: Postpartum Psychosocial Concerns

Preface to the Third Edition

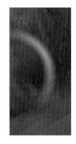

The past decade has seen major changes in the provision of maternity care to women in the United States. The most striking change has been the rapidly escalating rate of cesarean section intervention that has seen the national cesarean section rate climb from 20.7% in 1996 to 30% in 2006. With the publication of the Institute of Medicine's *Crossing the Quality Chasm: A New Health System* and *To Err Is Human: Building a Safer Health System*, the emphasis on improving communication and medical team function in maternity care has grown immensely. During the past 5 years, Family Medicine has been actively involved in reinventing itself with the Future of Family Medicine Project. This ambitious project has affirmed the essential role that family physicians play in the provision of maternity care for women in the United States.

In this challenging and exciting environment we are honored to have this opportunity to produce a third edition of *Family Medicine Obstetrics*. This edition remains anchored in the philosophy of providing woman- and family-centered care. We have continued our reliance of basing diagnostic and treatment recommendations on the highest level of evidence.

Our editorial team has enjoyed stability while undergoing some change. With this edition we saw the retirement of Janis Byrd, MD, who played a strong visionary role with the first two editions. We also welcome Matthew Cline, MD, to the role of Associate Editor. We have greatly expanded our group of writers from 32 to 65 contributors from the second to the third edition. Our writers include family medicine physicians, fellows, residents, midwives, childbirth educators, and behavioral scientists. We believe the result of this collaboration will be a beneficial one for maternity care providers!

Although much of the content of the third edition remains the same, we have encouraged our writers to go into greater depth and to produce summary recommendations based on level A evidence at the end of most sections.

Additional new content in the third edition includes:

- A chapter that summarizes practical applications of how to incorporate continuous quality improvement and enhanced medical safety into the maternity care setting
- A section that provides guidance as to which immunizations can be used during pregnancy
- A section that describes a new model of care, Group Prenatal Care: Centering Pregnancy
- A section that examines the proliferation of tests available to screen for fetal aneuploidy
- A section that provides a comprehensive and international view of vaginal birth after cesarean section

Stephen D. Ratcliffe, MD, MSPH
Elizabeth G. Baxley, MD
Matthew K. Cline, MD
Ellen L. Sakornbut, MD

Preface to the Second Edition

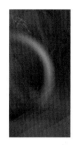

The basic tenets of the first edition provide the foundation of the second edition. This book is intended for family physicians and other practitioners who strive to provide maternity services in a *patient-* and *family-centered* manner. We have continued to emphasize the use of the *best evidence* to guide our practices. We aim to present a balanced approach to disease prevention and health promotion with an ability to anticipate and respond to obstetric urgencies and emergencies.

What is new in the second edition? In terms of content, we have added new sections that address alternative medicine and prenatal care (Chapter 2, Section F), exercise in pregnancy (Chapter 3, Section G), persistent occiput posterior (Chapter 16, Section G), evaluation and management of infection in the newborn (Chapter 18, Section E), and return to work issues (Chapter 20, Section G). We have added an entire new chapter on commonly encountered mental health problems in pregnancy. The original content has been updated and expanded in its depth, although we have maintained a succinct format to allow quick access to key clinical information.

Our intention was to present the highest level of medical evidence in the form of randomized controlled trials to support recommendations throughout this text. We have once again extensively drawn upon the Cochrane Library for much of the evidence. The reader is directed to Appendix D where an in-depth explanation of clinical effectiveness as measured by "number needed to treat" is presented. This concept is emphasized throughout the book.

Finally, we have doubled the number of authors who have contributed to the second edition, including three nurse midwives. We hope that our collective effort will contribute to the safety and well-being of our patients and will increase the satisfaction and enjoyment of providing maternity care.

Stephen D. Ratcliffe, MD, MSPH
Elizabeth G. Baxley, MD
Janis E. Byrd, MD
Ellen L. Sakornbut, MD

Acknowledgments

The creation of the third edition of *Family Medicine Obstetrics* has been a "labor of love and devotion" to the safe, respectful process of providing maternal and infant care. We thank our team of 65 writers and their loved ones who made tremendous sacrifices of time and energy to produce their contributions to this book. As editors and writers, we could not have sustained our focus and vision to complete this effort without the patience and support of our families as well.

We acknowledge and thank the ongoing, substantive contributions of Barbara Flory and Donna Roop at in the Department of Family and Community Medicine at Lancaster General Hospital in Lancaster, Pennsylvania. Rolla Couchman of Elsevier has been an excellent supporter and partner during the design and writing phase of the project. John Ingram of Elsevier has provided splendid assistance in the production phase of assembling the work of our writing team.

Our newest and youngest editor, Matt Cline, acknowledges and credits his wife, Jennifer, who lived out and involved him in the extraordinary process that is family-centered birthing in a personal way with the birth of their two sons. Her spirit, determination, and energy exemplify the power that women bring to this signature event in their lives and to which clinicians and families are blessed to be a part.

We dedicate this book to all family physicians who have incorporated maternity care into their practices either in the past, present, or future.

Contents

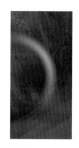

CHAPTER **1**

*Improving Safety and Quality
in Maternity Care*   1
Harry A. Taylor, MD, MPH

CHAPTER **2**

*Preconception Care: Improving
Birth Outcomes through Care
before Pregnancy*   10
Josephine R. Fowler, MD, MS, FAAFP,
and Brian W. Jack, MD

CHAPTER **3**

Content of Prenatal Care   21

SECTION A History of Prenatal Care   21
Beth Choby, MD

SECTION B Diagnosis and Dating
of Pregnancy   22
Beth Choby, MD

SECTION C Prenatal Visits   24
Beth Choby, MD

SECTION D Initial Assessment   28
Beth Choby, MD

SECTION E Monitoring the Progress
of Pregnancy   33
Jeffrey D. Quinlan, MD

SECTION F Screening in Pregnancy
and Predictive Value   34
Jeffrey D. Quinlan, MD,
and Matthew K. Cline, MD

SECTION G Medications
in Pregnancy   43
Kent Petrie, MD

SECTION H Immunizations
in Pregnancy   47
Cynthia Kilbourn, MD

SECTION I Complementary and
Alternative Medicine in Maternity Care   51
Kent Petrie, MD

SECTION J Diagnostic Ultrasound
in Pregnancy   59
Ellen L. Sakornbut, MD,
and Mark Deutchman, MD

CHAPTER **4**

Patient and Family Education   66

SECTION A Nutrition in Pregnancy
and Lactation   66
Elizabeth G. Baxley, MD,
and Rachel Setzler Brown, MD

SECTION B Educational Preparation
for Childbirth, Parenting, and Newborn
Care   73
Ann Tumblin, BA,
and Patricia Ann Payne, BSN, CNM, MPH

SECTION C Preparation
for Parenting and Family Issues   78
Elizabeth G. Baxley, MD,
and Jamee H. Lucas, MD, AAFP

SECTION D Breastfeeding Promotion   79
Patricia Ann Payne, BSN, CNM, MPH,
and Mary Rose Tully, MPH, IBCLC

SECTION E Physiologic Changes
and Common Discomforts of Pregnancy   86
Elizabeth G. Baxley, MD

SECTION F   Exercise and Pregnancy   95
Elizabeth A. Joy, MD,
and Thad J. Barkdull, MD

CHAPTER 5

Pregnancy Interventions   102

SECTION A   Psychosocial
Interventions   102
Elizabeth G. Baxley, MD,
and Kevin J. Bennett, BS, MS, PhD

SECTION B   Adolescent Pregnancy
Interventions   107
V. Leigh Beasley, MD, FAAFP

SECTION C   Substance Abuse
in Pregnancy   112
V. Leigh Beasley, MD, FAAFP

SECTION D   Smoking in Pregnancy   120
Elizabeth G. Baxley, MD

SECTION E   Group Prenatal Care:
CenteringPregnancy®   127
Kathryn J. Trotter, RN, MSN, CNM, FNP

CHAPTER 6

*Diagnosis and Management
of First-Trimester Complications*   130

SECTION A   Diagnosis   130
Mark Deutchman, MD

SECTION B   Management of Ectopic
Pregnancy   140
Mark Deutchman, MD

SECTION C   Management
of Miscarriage   144
David Turok, MD, MPH

CHAPTER 7

Complications of Pregnancy   151

SECTION A   Gestational Diabetes
Mellitus   151
Richard Beukema, MD,
Miranda Raiche, MD,
and David Turok, MD, MPH

SECTION B   Multiple Gestation   161
Ellen L. Sakornbut, MD

SECTION C   Vaginal Bleeding
in the Second and Third Trimesters   165
John C. Houchins, MD

SECTION D   Vaginal Birth
after Cesarean   169
Valerie J. King, MD, MPH

SECTION E   Small-for-Dates
Pregnancy   179
Ellen L. Sakornbut, MD

SECTION F   Large-for-Dates
Pregnancy Including Macrosomia   186
Thomas J. Gates, MD

SECTION G   Disorders of Amniotic
Fluid Including Oligohydramnios
and Polyhydramnios   189
Mark L. Rast, MD

SECTION H   Possible Indicators
of Fetal Abnormalities   192
Barbara F. Kelly, MD

CHAPTER 8

*Chronic Medical Conditions
in Pregnancy*   202

SECTION A   Pulmonary Problems
in Pregnancy   202
Matthew K. Cline, MD

SECTION B   Cardiovascular
Conditions   213
Ellen L. Sakornbut, MD

SECTION C   Chronic Hypertension   219
Lawrence Leeman, MD, MPH

SECTION D   Thromboembolic
Disease and Chronic Anticoagulation   223
Jeffrey T. Kirchner, DO, FAAFP

SECTION E   Hematologic
Conditions in Pregnancy   227
Jacqueline E. Julius, MD,
and Jeffrey T. Kirchner, DO, FAAFP

SECTION F   Gastrointestinal
Conditions   232
Ellen L. Sakornbut, MD

SECTION G   Neurologic Conditions   234
Ellen L. Sakornbut, MD

SECTION H   Renal Disease   241
Ellen L. Sakornbut, MD

SECTION I   Endocrine Conditions   243
David Turok, MD, MPH,
and Ted R. Schultz, MD

SECTION J   Autoimmune Conditions   254
Ellen L. Sakornbut, MD

CHAPTER **9**
Commonly Encountered Medical Problems in Pregnancy   258

SECTION A   Infections in Pregnancy   258
Stephen D. Ratcliffe, MD, MSPH,
Rachel Elizabeth Hall, MD, FAAFP,
Amity Rubeor, DO,
Andrew Coco, MD, MS,
and Donna Cohen, MD, MSc

SECTION B   Abdominal Pain and Gastrointestinal Illness   306
Ellen L. Sakornbut, MD

SECTION C   Trauma in Pregnancy   311
Mark Deutchman, MD

SECTION D   Dermatoses of Pregnancy   317
Stephen T. Olin, MD

SECTION E   Acute Neurologic Conditions   321
Ellen L. Sakornbut, MD

SECTION F   Cervical Cytology in Pregnancy   323
Richard Hudspeth, MD

CHAPTER **10**
Treatment of Psychiatric Disorders in Pregnancy   330

Ellen L. Sakornbut, MD

SECTION A   Affective Disorders   330
SECTION B   Anxiety Disorders   336
SECTION C   Schizophrenia   337

CHAPTER **11**
Antenatal Testing for Fetal Surveillance and Management of the Postterm Pregnancy   339

SECTION A   Overview of Antenatal Testing   339
Stephen D. Ratcliffe, MD, MSPH

SECTION B   Types of Antenatal Testing   341
Stephen D. Ratcliffe, MD, MSPH

SECTION C   Management of the Postterm Pregnancy   348
Richard Hudspeth, MD

CHAPTER **12**
Preterm Labor   352

SECTION A   Risk Factors for Preterm Delivery   352
William Gosnell Sayres, Jr., MD

SECTION B   Antenatal Interventions for Prevention of Preterm Delivery   356
William Gosnell Sayres, Jr., MD

SECTION C   Diagnosis of Preterm Labor   358
William Gosnell Sayres, Jr., MD

SECTION D   Pharmacologic Management of Preterm Labor   361
William Gosnell Sayres, Jr., MD

SECTION E   Incompetent Cervix   366
William Gosnell Sayres, Jr., MD

SECTION F   Management of Preterm Delivery   368
William Gosnell Sayres, Jr., MD

SECTION G   Programs Aimed at Identifying Patients at Risk for Preterm Labor and Subsequent Patient Care   369
Stephen D. Ratcliffe, MD, MSPH

SECTION H   Preterm Premature Rupture of the Membranes   371
William Gosnell Sayres, Jr., MD

SECTION I   Conclusion   374
William Gosnell Sayres, Jr., MD

CHAPTER **13**

Birth Crisis: Caring for the Family Experiencing Perinatal Death or the Birth of a Child with Medical Complications   375
Elizabeth G. Baxley, MD

CHAPTER **14**

Management of Labor   382
Kent Petrie, MD,
and Walter L. Larimore, MD

S E C T I O N   A   Normal Labor   383
Kent Petrie, MD,
and Walter L. Larimore, MD

S E C T I O N   B   Ambulation and Positions in Labor   395
Kent Petrie, MD,
and Walter L. Larimore, MD

S E C T I O N   C   Intrapartum Pain Management   398
Kent Petrie, MD,
and Walter L. Larimore, MD

S E C T I O N   D   Support in Labor   406
Kent Petrie, MD,
and Walter L. Larimore, MD

S E C T I O N   E   Intrapartum Fetal Heart Rate Monitoring   409
Kent Petrie, MD,
and Walter L. Larimore, MD

S E C T I O N   F   Normal Delivery and Birthing Positions   413
Kent Petrie, MD,
and Walter L. Larimore, MD

S E C T I O N   G   Management of the Second Stage   419
Matthew K. Cline, MD

S E C T I O N   H   Management of the Perineum   423
Valerie J. King, MD, MPH

S E C T I O N   I   Management of Third-Stage Labor   430
Kent Petrie, MD,
and Walter L. Larimore, MD

CHAPTER **15**

Management of Labor Abnormalities   435

S E C T I O N   A   Dystocia in the Nulliparous Patient   435
Matthew K. Cline, MD

S E C T I O N   B   Term Premature Rupture of the Membranes   442
Wendy Brooks Barr, MD, MPH, MSCE

S E C T I O N   C   Induction of Labor   445
James M. Nicholson, MD, MSCE

CHAPTER **16**

Intrapartum Complications   454

S E C T I O N   A   Fetal Intolerance of Labor   454
Kent Petrie, MD

S E C T I O N   B   Shoulder Dystocia   465
Osman N. Sanyer, MD

S E C T I O N   C   Chorioamnionitis   471
Stephen D. Ratcliffe, MD, MSPH

S E C T I O N   D   Intrapartum Bleeding   475
John C. Houchins, MD

S E C T I O N   E   Postpartum Hemorrhage   479
Janice M. Anderson, MD, FAAFP,
and Narayana Rao V. Pula, MD

S E C T I O N   F   Retained Placenta   488
Jose Matthew Mata, MD, MS,
and David Turok, MD, MPH

S E C T I O N   G   Preeclampsia and Eclampsia   491
Lawrence Leeman, MD, MPH

S E C T I O N   H   Medical Emergencies in Pregnancy   495
Lee T. Dresang, MD

CHAPTER **17**

Malpresentation and Malpositions   500

S E C T I O N   A   Diagnosis   500
Jamee H. Lucas, MD, AAFP,
and Elizabeth G. Baxley, MD

S E C T I O N   B   Face Presentation   502
Elizabeth G. Baxley, MD,
and Jamee H. Lucas, MD, AAFP

SECTION C Brow Presentation 504
Elizabeth G. Baxley, MD,
and Jamee H. Lucas, MD, AAFP

SECTION D Transverse Lie 505
Elizabeth G. Baxley, MD,
and Jamee H. Lucas, MD, AAFP

SECTION E Transverse Arrest 506
Stephen D. Ratcliffe, MD, MSPH

SECTION F Occiput Posterior
Position 507
Stephen D. Ratcliffe, MD, MSPH

SECTION G Breech Presentation 510
Stephen D. Ratcliffe, MD, MSPH

SECTION H External Cephalic
Version 516
Kent Petrie, MD

SECTION I Twin Gestation 521
Ellen L. Sakornbut, MD

CHAPTER **18**
Intrapartum Procedures 523

SECTION A Use of Ultrasound
in Labor and Delivery 523
Ellen L. Sakornbut, MD

SECTION B Pudendal
and Paracervical Blocks 529
Rachel Elizabeth Hall, MD, FAAFP

SECTION C Amnioinfusion
and Use of Intrauterine Pressure Catheter 532
Stephen D. Ratcliffe, MD, MSPH

SECTION D Assisted Deliveries 534
Stephen D. Ratcliffe, MD, MSPH,
and James R. Damos, MD

SECTION E Episiotomy and Repair
of Perineal Lacerations and Episiotomies 542
Robert W. Gobbo, MD,
and Lawrence Leeman, MD, MPH

SECTION F Amniocentesis during
the Third Trimester of Pregnancy 555
Mark Deutchman, MD

SECTION G Cesarean Delivery 560
Mark Deutchman, MD,
and Neil J. Murphy, MD

CHAPTER **19**
The First Month of Life 572

SECTION A Initial Management
of the Normal Newborn 572
Patricia Fontaine, MD, MS

SECTION B Neonatal Resuscitation 580
Patricia Adam, MD, MSPH,
and Patricia Fontaine, MD, MS

SECTION C Neonatal Circumcision 588
Patricia Fontaine, MD, MS

SECTION D Neonatal Jaundice 594
Karen Jankowski Fruechte, MD,
and Patricia Fontaine, MD, MS

SECTION E Evaluation and
Management of Infection in the
Newborn 602
Laura Chambers-Kersh, MD,
and Patricia Fontaine, MD, MS

SECTION F Infant Feeding
and Nutrition 609
Patricia Fontaine, MD, MS

SECTION G Bonding and Family
Adaptation 612
Patricia Fontaine, MD, MS

SECTION H General Care
of the Neonate 615
Patricia Fontaine, MD, MS,
and Sherri Fong, BS

CHAPTER **20**
Postpartum Biomedical Concerns:
Breastfeeding 618

SECTION A Delayed Postpartum
Hemorrhage 618
Charles Carter, MD,
and Elizabeth G. Baxley, MD

SECTION B Postpartum Endometritis 619
Elizabeth G. Baxley, MD,
and Charles Carter, MD

SECTION C Breastfeeding 623
Mary Rose Tully, MPH, IBCLC,
and Patricia Ann Payne, BSN, CNM, MPH

SECTION D Mastitis   633
Charles Carter, MD,
and Elizabeth G. Baxley, MD

SECTION E Postpartum Thyroiditis   635
Charles Carter, MD,
and Elizabeth G. Baxley, MD

SECTION F Septic Pelvic
Thrombophlebitis   637
Charles Carter, MD

SECTION G Postpartum
Contraception   639
Christine Stabler, MD, FAAFP

CHAPTER **21**
Postpartum Psychosocial Concerns   645
Dwenda K. Gjerdingen, MD, MS,
Elizabeth Ann Shaw, BSc, MD, FCFP,
and Sharon S.-L. Wong, PhD, RD

SECTION A Maternal Adjustment   645
SECTION B Paternal Adjustment   654
SECTION C Marital Adjustment   655
SECTION D Sibling Adjustment   657
SECTION E Specific Family Situations   657
SECTION F Return to Work   660

APPENDIX **A**
Interpretation of Summary Tables   664

APPENDIX **B**
Analysis of Screening Tests   665

APPENDIX **C**
Immunization during Pregnancy   667

APPENDIX **D**
*Measuring Clinical Effectiveness
by Calculating the Number Needed
to Treat*   674

APPENDIX **E**
*Drugs for Common Conditions
in Pregnancy*   676
Kent Petrie, MD

INDEX   685

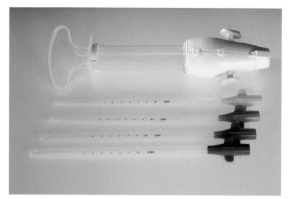

FIGURE 6-17. Manual vacuum aspirator (MVA) with suction cannulae. (Courtesy IPAS, Carrboro, NC.) (See page 146.)

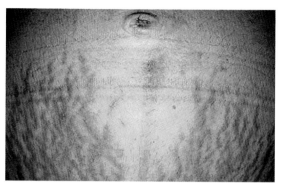

FIGURE 9-4. Pruritic urticarial papules/plaques of pregnancy (PUPPP). (See page 319.)

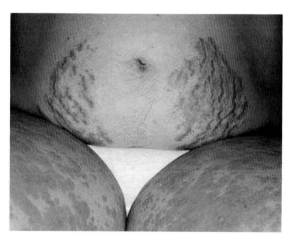

FIGURE 9-2. Pemphigoid gestationis. (See page 319.)

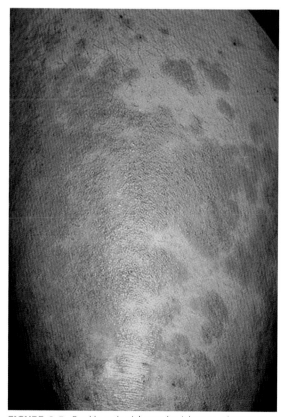

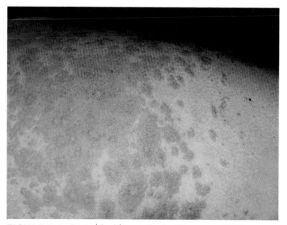

FIGURE 9-3. Pemphigoid gestationis. (See page 319.)

FIGURE 9-5. Pruritic urticarial papules/plaques of pregnancy (PUPPP). (See page 320.)

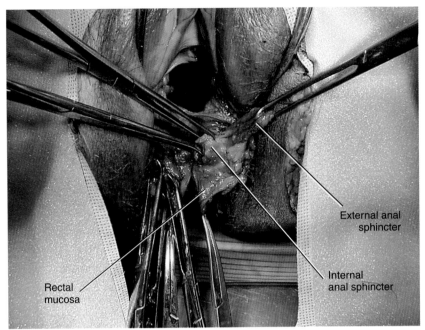

FIGURE 18-11. Anal sphincter complex (cadaver dissection). (See page 544.)

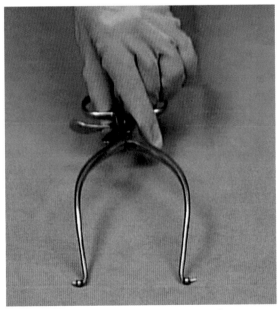

FIGURE 18-14. A Gelpi retractor. (See page 547.)

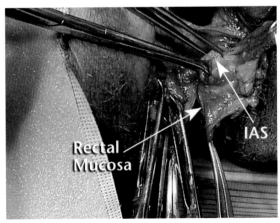

FIGURE 18-16. Rectal mucosa and internal anal sphincter (IAS). (See page 549.)

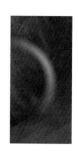

CHAPTER 1

Improving Safety and Quality in Maternity Care

Harry A. Taylor, MD, MPH

The 2001 Institute of Medicine report titled "Crossing the Quality Chasm: A New Health System for the 21st Century"[1] presents a bold vision of health care in the future. In this report, the Institute of Medicine identified six areas of our current health-care system for improvement, beginning with patient safety and the effectiveness, patient centeredness, timeliness, efficiency, and equitability of the care we deliver to patients. Furthermore, in *To Err Is Human: Building a Safer Health System,* the Institute of Medicine concludes that up to 40,000 to 100,000 patients may die each year as a result of their medical care, not necessarily because of their underlying disease.[2]

This chapter provides an overview of the nature of errors in medicine and also strategies to mitigate harm to patients. The principles of a high-reliability organization are discussed, and the application of those principles will be extended to the provision of safe maternity care. Finally, an overview of continuous quality improvement and the evidence on modifying clinician behaviors prepares the reader to use the information in the remainder of this book to improve the safety, effectiveness, patient centeredness, timeliness, efficiency, and equitability of their own practice and the perinatal system within their organization.

I. IMPROVING PATIENT SAFETY

Health care, especially care occurring within the hospital, can be viewed as a high-hazard industry, not unlike the aviation industry, nuclear power industry, or the military. High-hazard industries are simply those industries where there is great potential to harm employees, customers/clients, or the general public. Researchers in the area of organizational safety have focused on the role of organizations and systems in preventing or generating accidents, particularly in high-hazard industries.

Over time, two predominant theories of organizational safety have emerged from the study of these high-hazard industries: Normal Accidents Theory and High Reliability Organizations Theory.

A. Normal Accidents Theory

Normal Accidents Theory was described by sociologist Charles Perrow.[3] It focuses on two system features: the level of complexity and how tightly the interactions are between components in the system. In Normal Accidents Theory, the roots of any error are embedded in the organizational system; they are latent until the right combination of factors is present to allow the error to occur. This is often described as the "Swiss Cheese Model of Accidents," where a variety of organizational, technical, and or procedural barriers stand between naturally occurring errors and an accident. Each barrier is semipermeable with holes that vary in size and number. When a problem cascade begins and all the holes in the barriers line up, an accident occurs. Seen through the prism of Normal Accidents Theory, accidents are an inevitable part of complex, tightly coupled systems such as providing care for a laboring patient in the modern hospital setting.

B. High Reliability Organizations Theory

The other dominant theory of organizational safety is High Reliability Organizations Theory described by researchers at University of California Berkeley.[3] High Reliability Organizations Theory postulates that proper organization of people, technology, and processes can handle complex and hazardous activities at acceptable levels of performance. Because one can never eliminate accidents completely, this "acceptability" is really the comparison of the benefits derived from any activity and the estimated absolute risk for failure.

Naval aviation safety provides dramatic, if only observational, evidence for the effectiveness of applying Normal Accidents Theory and High Reliability Organizations Theory to improve organizational safety in high-hazard areas. In 1954, the U.S. Navy lost 776 aircraft and had a Class A mishap rate (serious mishaps resulting in loss of life and/or aircraft) of more than 50 per 100,000 flight hours. By 1996, the rate of Class A mishaps was down to 2.39 per 100,000 flight hours, and only 39 aircraft were destroyed.[4] This dramatic improvement in naval aviation safety over time resulted from a combination of factors, including structural changes, organization changes, improved training for aviators, and meticulous attention to human factors.

1. Structural changes

    An example of a structural change is angling the aircraft carrier's flight deck, thereby ensuring that aircraft were not landing and taking off in the same space.

2. Organizational changes

    Examples of organizational changes include setting up a Naval Aviation Safety Center and implementing a squadron safety program.

3. Improved training for aviators

    For example, aviators who were new to or returning to a specific aircraft type were assigned to the Replacement Air Group for that specific aircraft type to obtain competency in its operation before being permanently assigned to an operational squadron.

4. Meticulous attention to human factors

    This occurred through the implementation of Aviation Crew Training (ACT) for all air crews and the use of human factor boards to expeditiously identify and manage "at-risk" aviators.

II. STRATEGIES TO IMPROVE PATIENT SAFETY

Many errors in medicine are directly linked to characteristics of human cognition and occur with a predictable rate for risk. Furthermore, systems can be engineered to help prevent errors from harming patients. In this section, basic principles of safety engineering are presented. The foremost goal is to prevent medical errors from harming patients. The premise of Normal Accidents Theory is that medical errors are an inevitable and predictable part of working in a complex health-care system. This theory assumes that systems and a culture can be developed to significantly reduce the risk for an accident, defined as an error that harms a patient.

Four strategies to improve patient safety arise from the goal of preventing harm to patients: provide evidence-based health care, prevent errors where possible, make errors visible, and mitigate the effects of errors that occur.

A. Provide Evidence-Based Health Care

Sackett and colleagues[5] define evidence-based medicine as "the conscientious and judicious use of current best evidence from clinical care research in the management of individual patients." In addition, Slawson and Shaughnessy[6] describe patient-oriented evidence that matters (POEMS) as compelling outcomes-based evidence that should change individual or group practice either by incorporating new proven diagnostic or therapeutic interventions or by discontinuing practice that is harmful or of unproven value. It follows that individual clinicians and health-care systems that consistently offer only those interventions that do more good than harm at a reasonable cost to the right patients while ensuring that that care is delivered at a high standard demonstrate a proactive evidence-based strategy to increase the good-to-harm ratio.[7]

B. Prevent Errors Where Possible

To prevent errors, clinicians and organizations need to look at the underlying factors that influence the rate of errors in their own unique system. It is not enough to look for the proximate cause of an error; rather, we need to explore the "blunt end" of the system, "the institutional context, organization and management, work environment, care team, individual team member, the task performed and patient."[3] Human errors occur at predictable rates, and the rate increases with the number of steps in any given process.

1. Complexity

   Complexity is common in most medical settings with many processes of care having 50 to 100 different elements or steps. Tables 1-1 and 1-2 illustrate the problems inherent in a complex medical system.[8] As shown in Table 1-2, errors become the norm (error rates of 0.39-0.99) rather than the exception in complex systems (those with 50-100 steps) that rely on human cognition (base error rate at each step, 0.05-0.01) to safeguard against harm. Complexity causes errors. As shown in Table 1-2, once a process gets beyond 25 steps, the chance of an error occurring is significant at the level of

safety provided by human cognition. One way to reduce the chance of error is to simplify the number of steps in the processes. Not infrequently, additional steps have been added to processes in response to a breakdown in an earlier process. Rather than adding additional checks and balances, it is more productive to evaluate the entire care process, looking for critical steps that are tightly coupled and concentrating efforts on ensuring safety around those critical few steps.

2. Eliminating unnecessary variation

   Eliminating unnecessary variation in clinical practice because of personal preference is another target for reducing complexity. Lucian Leape's work reminds us of the opportunities for error posed by nontherapeutic differences in drug dosages or times of administration, different locations for resuscitation equipment on different units, and different methods for the same surgical dressing.[3] An Institute for Healthcare Improvement (IHI) Collaborative on Improving Patient Safety in High-Hazard Areas demonstrated that complexity is reduced, and outcomes are improved, by eliminating delays (e.g., 30-minute cesarean section drills), ensuring availability of accurate and complete data (e.g., comprehensive mother and baby records), and reducing other defects in operations (e.g., protocols for managing magnesium sulfate).[9]

C. Make Errors Visible

To focus attention on the blunt end of the system, we must work hard to uncover and explore not only the "sentinel events," but also near misses—that is, errors that do result in little or no harm to patients but are symptoms of underlying system problems.[10] Some experts use the analogy of an iceberg to describe the relation among accidents, incidents, near misses, and underlying unsafe conditions. In this analogy, accidents (sentinel events and near misses) represent the small fraction of the iceberg visible above the surface of the water, with unsafe conditions making up the larger volume of the iceberg of risk that lies hidden below.

The Joint Commission (TJC) mandates healthcare organizations make use of two powerful tools, root cause analysis (RCA) and failure mode and effects analysis (FMEA), to identify and correct underlying conditions that may affect the safety of patients. TJC requires organizations to conduct an RCA whenever a sentinel event, such as wrong site surgery, patient elopement, or an unanticipated death occurs within their facility. RCA is a retrospective analysis

TABLE 1-1 Sample Human Error Rates

Activity	Probability of Error
Error of commission (misreading a label)	0.003
Error of omission (no reminders present)	0.01
Simple arithmetic errors	0.03
General error under high stress levels	0.25

Adapted from Nolan TW: System changes to improve patient safety, *BMJ* 320:771-773, 2000, with permission.

TABLE 1-2 Error Rates for Processes with Multiple Steps

Number of Steps	Base Error Rate at Each Step			
	0.05	0.01	0.001	0.0001
1	0.05	0.01	0.001	0.0001
5	0.33	0.05	0.005	0.002
25	0.72	0.22	0.02	0.003
50	0.92	0.39	0.05	0.005
100	0.99	0.63	0.1	0.01

Adapted from Nolan TW: System changes to improve patient safety, *BMJ* 320:771-773, 2000, with permission.

that determines the sequence of events leading up to a sentinel event, defining causal factors, analyzing each causal factor's root causes, identifying the generic cause for each root cause, and finally developing, evaluating, implementing, and monitoring corrective actions.[11] FMEA is a proactive analysis of a high-risk process to identify failure modes where variation or deviation in the process could lead to significant negative outcomes for patients. RCA of potential variation at each failure mode is accomplished followed by process redesign and testing, once process implementation and monitoring of the process changes throughout the organization.

D. Mitigate the Effects of Errors that Occur

Methods to mitigate the effects of errors must be developed when they do occur. There must be processes in place to quickly reverse or stop the harm caused to the patient by the error. An example of mitigation would be keeping calcium gluconate readily available on the labor and delivery ward to reverse the effects of magnesium sulfate toxicity.[12]

Human factors play a large role in errors within all settings,[13] and attention to this area is especially important in reducing errors in high-hazard areas. Nowhere is this truer than in the setting of a clinical emergency. In an emergency, the clinician, usually operating as a team leader, is faced with the need to make rapid decisions and perform complex tasks under pressure. It is not unusual for the performance of the team leader to be "impaired" by fatigue, hunger, or other physical or psychological condition, which can lead to loss of situational awareness.

At the same time, each team member faces similar challenges, and the whole team faces the challenge of communicating and coordinating competing and sometimes conflicting actions. Not infrequently, information is not available when needed by the team and team leader. Finally, these activities occur in the presence of conflicting occupational cultures where there is often a reluctance to question those in positions of authority or seniority. Table 1-3 demonstrates that the human error rate under these circumstances can be as high as 25%, and the performance of the team is directly linked to the performance of the team leader.

Military Aviation estimates that "human factors" play a critical role in more than 70% of aircraft mishaps. As a result, the U.S. Navy developed ACT to aid crewmembers in identifying and eliminating human factors that lead to mishaps. Clinical team training,

not unlike ACT, is a promising intervention to enable clinical teams to improve functioning and reduce errors caused by human factors.[14]

III. CHARACTERISTICS OF HIGH-RELIABILITY ORGANIZATIONS

A. High-Reliability Organizations

High-reliability organizations are those that operate technologically complex systems essentially without error over a long period. Examples include the Aviation and Nuclear Power industries. Behavioral scientists note that these organizations have common characteristics, including[15]:

1. Safety is recognized as the hallmark of organizational culture.
2. Operation of the system is a team rather than an individual function. Communication is highly valued and rewarded.
3. Emergencies are rehearsed, and the unexpected is practiced.
4. Successful outcomes are paradoxically viewed as potentially dangerous "normalization of deviance."

It is reasonable to evaluate perinatal care as a high-reliability organization because the care system is complex with a large network of different providers and a tremendous amount of technology. In addition, the perinatal system is expected to operate without preventable neonatal or maternal harm (accident analog) over a long period. Finally, because the outcome for most normal pregnancies is good, perinatal care is a system prone to normalizing deviance.

Knox and co-workers[15] note significant variation in the rates of obstetrical lawsuits within a large malpractice database that included 10 years of obstetrical malpractice claims data involving more than 250 U.S. hospitals. Some units experienced a disproportionate number of lawsuits, whereas others had none or only a few nuisance type lawsuits. Observational analysis, by these risk management experts, of those centers experiencing none or few law suits over the 10-year period identified organizational structures similar to that found in other high-reliability organizations. These investigators also identify five common recurring clinical problems accounting for the majority of fetal or neonatal injuries. The authors surmise that the ability to form high-reliability perinatal units around the five issues listed next was essential to the performance of the

TABLE 1-3 Opportunities for Improvement

Eliminate Waste	Look for ways of eliminating any activity or resource in the organization that does not add value to an external customer.
Improve Work Flow	Improving the flow of work in processes is an important way to improve the quality of the goods and services produced by those processes.
Optimize Inventory	Inventory of all types is a possible source of waste in organizations. Understanding where inventory is stored in the system is the first step in finding opportunities for improvement.
Change the Work Environment	Changing the work environment itself can be a high-leverage opportunity for making all other process changes more effective.
Producer/Customer Interface	To benefit from improvements in quality of products and services, the customer must recognize and appreciate the improvements.
Manage Time	An organization can gain a competitive advantage by reducing the time to develop new products, waiting time for services, lead times for orders and deliveries, and cycle times for all functions in the organization.
Focus on Variation	Reducing variation improves the predictability of outcomes and helps reduce the frequency of poor results.
Error Proofing	Organizations can reduce errors by redesigning the system to make it less likely for people in the system to make errors. One way to error-proof a system is to make the information necessary to perform a task available in the external world, and not just in one's memory, by writing it down or actually making it inherent in the product or process.
Focus on the Product or Service	Although many organizations focus on ways to improve the processes, it is also important to address improvement of products and services.

Adapted from the Institute for Health Care Improvement website at http://www.ihi.org/IHI/Topics/Improvement/ImprovementMethods/Measures, 2007, with permission.

units experiencing no or little litigation. These key issues include:

1. Inability to recognize and/or respond to fetal distress
2. Inability to effect a timely cesarean delivery (30 minutes from decision to incision) when indicated
3. Inability to appropriately resuscitate a depressed infant
4. Inappropriate use of oxytocin
5. Inappropriate use of forceps and/or vacuum extraction

B. Characteristics of High-Reliability Perinatal Units[5]

1. Clearly stated purpose: Among the array of competing values, *patient safety* ranks at the top.
2. Plans for the unexpected are in place.
3. Procedures are in place to ensure timely transfer of patients to facilities that can care for all potential problems.
4. Thirty-minute decision-to-incision drills are practiced.

5. There is ready availability of surgical support.
6. Resuscitation teams are present for all births where there is a question of fetal distress.

C. Clear Language: Fetal Well-being

1. Definition of fetal well-being is mutually agreed on and understood by *ALL* clinicians and nurses.
2. Every evaluation of the pregnant patient includes an assessment of fetal well-being.
3. The presence of fetal well-being is a necessary condition for maternal discharge, maternal medication, epidural analgesia, and the use of oxytocin.
4. The absence of fetal well-being necessitates direct physician evaluation.

D. Clear Organization: Teamwork

1. Hierarchies between nurses and physicians are minimized.
2. Everyone has an obligation and a duty to speak up if an issue arises regarding patient safety.

3. Questions regarding patient safety are encouraged.
4. Professional relationships are collegial.
5. Communication is in real time, consistent, and constant.

E. Simplification: Minimum Number of Unit Policies

1. An inverse relation exists between the number of unit policies and reliable function on the unit.
2. One policy is present consistently in these high-reliability units: A physician will come to the unit when requested by a nurse.

F. Clear Operating Style: Adherence to Agreed-upon Protocols and Guidelines

When organizations adhere to agreed-upon protocols, there is minimal intervention in the context of a well-designed safety net.

IV. CLINICAL PROCESS IMPROVEMENT

The IHI uses a model for improvement developed by Associates in Process Improvement.[16] This model is composed of two parts.

A. Three Key Questions (Can Be Addressed in any Order)

1. What are we trying to accomplish?
   This question focuses attention on time-specific and measurable goals for a specific population of patients.
2. How will we know that a change is an improvement?

Only by developing quantitative measures can one track the impact of any changes made in a system.
3. What changes can we make that will result in improvement?
   Not all changes result in improvement. The change in clinical care should derive from the best available science and may result in a package of bundled clinical process improvements.[17]

B. The Plan-Do-Study-Act Cycle

The Plan-Do-Study-Act (PDSA) cycle is used to test and implement changes in real work settings. In the IHI model for improvement, changes are tested on a small scale, multiple times learning from each test and refining the change through several PDSA cycles before a change is implemented on a broader scale.[18]

The IHI has an excellent website (www.ihi.org) that fully outlines their model for improvement, provides clinical process improvement tools, and shares success stories of organizations. In addition to the opportunities that Knox and co-workers[15] identified in creating a high-reliability perinatal unit, IHI has identified nine general areas for organizational improvement (see Table 1-3) that, if addressed, would improve the delivery of quality care. One caveat, however, is that many health-care professionals mistake the PDSA cycle of process improvement for the rigorous methodology mandated by clinical investigational studies such as randomized controlled trials. Table 1-4 briefly outlines the differences between the two methodologies.

It is best to remember that clinical process improvement involves both the "what" and the "how" of care delivery. The "what" should derive from the best available science and may result in a package of bundled clinical process improvements. In other words, the wise clinician uses the tools of evidence-based practice to

TABLE 1-4 Difference in Measurement between Research and Process Improvement

	Measurement for Research	*Measurement for Learning and Process Improvement*
Purpose	To discover new knowledge	To bring new knowledge into daily practice
Tests	One large "blind" test	Many sequential observable tests
Biases	Control for as many biases as possible	Stabilize the biases from test to test
Data	Gather as much data as possible, "just in case"	Gather "just enough" data to learn and complete another cycle
Duration	Can take long periods to obtain results	"Small tests of significant changes" accelerates the rate of improvement

Adapted from the Institute for Health Care Improvement website at http://www.ihi.org/IHI/Topics/Improvement/ImprovementMethods/Measures, 2007, with permission.

determine the "what" of their clinical process improvement. The "how" is the method by which evidence-based care is delivered, and it is the "how" that is subjected to small tests of change using the PDSA cycle. To quote from the IHI white paper on Idealized Design of Perinatal Care, "To improve safety and reliability, *what* we do and *how* we do it must come together as the *way* we provide effective perinatal care."[17]

V. CHANGING CLINICIAN'S PRACTICE

The current evidence base on changing clinician behavior is incomplete. However, a comprehensive review of the systematic review literature on changing provider behavior identified 41 reviews and demonstrated these general results.[19] Passive approaches, such as guideline dissemination and classic lecture format teaching, are not effective and are unlikely to change clinician behavior. Most active interventions such as participatory small-group education, audit and feedback, use of automated reminders, clinical opinion leaders, and academic detailing are effective under some conditions, but none is effective under all conditions. Table 1-5 provides a short, annotated outline of available interventions to change clinical behaviors.[20]

Successful efforts to implement any change in clinical practice should begin with a diagnostic analysis to identify factors likely to influence implementation of the proposed change.[12] Force-field analysis (Figure 1-1) has been used effectively by one organization to identify the various driving and restraining forces that affect clinical practice guideline implementation.[21] By analyzing the forces acting to drive change and, more importantly, those factors working to resist change within the system, you can target interventions to increase the likelihood of successful change. Organizational change, as classically described, involves three phases: unfreezing old behaviors or practices, implementation of the change, and then refreezing to embed the change within the organization.[22] Multifaceted approaches targeting different barriers to change are more likely to be effective than a single intervention.[23]

VI. CONCLUSION

Armed with an understanding of the basics of patient safety theory, a proven model for implementing clinical process improvement, and an understanding of the literature on changing clinician behaviors, the careful reader of this text will be prepared to examine and improve their own maternity care practice and become an agent for change within their local healthcare system.

TABLE 1-5 **Interventions to Change Clinician Behavior**

Intervention	Comments
Clinical decision support	Summaries, reminders, and pocket cards Most important to clinicians
Classic (lecture format) education	Raises awareness but not effective in changing behavior
Small-group and individual education	Effective in changing clinician behaviors if participatory
Feedback	Active feedback on performance Individual feedback is more effective than group feedback
Academic detailing	One-on-one planned conversations targeted to specific educational and behavioral goals
Clinical opinion leaders	Target academic detailing to these key people Influence other clinicians at teachable moments
Patient-specific decision support	Patient-specific data such as registries and patient-specific computer prompts
Patient-centered strategies	Shared decision making, interactive video or computer tools, group visits, etc.
Clinical process redesign	Changes in roles, facilities, equipment, methods, and processes
Administrative or regulatory	Policies and rules are effective but may be resented by clinicians

Adapted from Grimshaw JM, Shirran L, Thomas R et al: Changing provider behavior: an overview of systematic reviews of interventions, *Med Care* 39(8 suppl 2):II2-II45, 2001; and Handley MR, Stuart M, Hennessy CJ: *Evidence-based medicine and clinical practice guidelines syllabus.* Seattle, WA, 1999, Group Health Cooperative of Puget Sound.

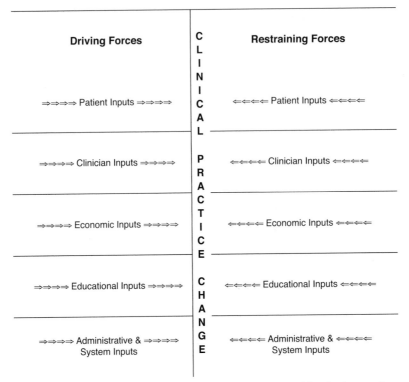

FIGURE 1-1. The five classic influences as a force field affecting guideline implementation.

VII. SOR A RECOMMENDATIONS

RECOMMENDATIONS	REFERENCES
Passive interventions, such as guideline dissemination and lecture format teaching, are ineffective and unlikely to change clinician behaviors.	19, 23
Active interventions, such as participatory small-group education, audit and feedback, use of automated reminders, clinical opinion leaders, and academic detailing are effective in changing clinician behavior under some conditions, but none is effective under all conditions.	19, 23
Multifaceted approaches targeting different barriers to change are more likely to be effective than a single intervention in changing clinician behaviors.	19, 23

REFERENCES

1. *Crossing the quality chasm: a new health system for the 21st century,* Washington, DC, 2001, Committee on Quality Healthcare in America, Institute of Medicine, National Academy Press.
2. Kohn L, Corrigan J, Donaldson M: *To err is human: building a safer health system.* Washington, DC, 1999, National Academy Press.
3. Gaba DM: Structural and organizational issues in patient safety: a comparison of health care to other high-hazard industries, *Calif Manage Rev* 43:83-102, 2000.
4. Naval Safety Center: *Human factor analysis and classification system presentation preview.* Available at: http://www.safetycenter.navy.mil/presentations/aviation/hfacs.htm. Accessed August 15, 2007.
5. Sackett DL, Rosenberg WMC, Gray JA et al: Evidence based medicine: what it is and what it isn't, *BMJ* 312:71-72, 1996.
6. Slawson DC, Shaughnessy AF: Becoming an information master: using POEMs to change practice with confidence, *J Fam Pract* 49(1):63-67, 2000.
7. Gray JAM: *Evidence-based healthcare; how to make health policy and management decisions,* London, 2001, Churchill Livingstone.
8. Nolan TW: System changes to improve patient safety, *BMJ* 320:771-773, 2000.

9. Andrea Kabcenell, RN, MPH, Executive Director for Pursuing Perfection, Institute for Healthcare Improvement, personal communication regarding a Department of Defense and Department of Veterans Affairs Collaborative with the Institute for Healthcare Improvement to Improve Patient Safety in High Risk Areas, December 2006.

10. Barach P, Small SD: Reporting and preventing medical mishaps: lessons from non-medical near miss reporting systems, *BMJ* 320:759-763, 2000.

11. Paradies M, Unger L: *TapRoot® the system for root cause analysis, problem investigation, and proactive improvement,* Knoxville, TN, 2000, System Improvements Inc.

12. Nolan TW: System changes to improve patient safety, *BMJ* 320:771-773, 2000.

13. Stripe SC, Best LG, Cole-Harding S et al: Aviation model cognitive risk factors applied to medical malpractice cases, *J Am Board Fam Med* 19:627-632, 2006.

14. Mann S, Marcus R, Sachs B: Lessons from the cockpit: how team training can reduce errors on L&D, *Contemporary OB/GYN* 34-45, January 2006.

15. Knox GE, Rice Simpson K, Garite TJ: High reliability perinatal units: an approach to the prevention of patient injury and medical malpractice claims, *J Healthc Risk Manag* 19(2):24-32, 1999.

16. Langley GL, Nolan KM, Nolan TW et al: *The improvement guide: a practical approach to enhancing performance.* Available at: http://www.ihi.org/IHI/Topics/Improvement/ImprovementMethods/HowToImprove. Accessed August 15, 2007.

17. Cherouny PH, Federico FA, Haraden C et al: *Idealized design of perinatal care. IHI innovation series white paper,* Cambridge, MA, 2005, Institute for Healthcare Improvement.

18. Deming WE: *The new economics for industry, government, education,* ed 2, Cambridge, MA, 2000, The MIT Press.

19. Grimshaw JM, Shirran L, Thomas R et al: Changing provider behavior: an overview of systematic reviews of interventions, *Med Care* 39(8 suppl 2): II2-II45, 2001.

20. Handley MR, Stuart M, Hennessy CJ: *Evidence-based medicine and clinical practice guidelines syllabus,* Seattle, WA, 1999, Group Health Cooperative of Puget Sound.

21. Stuart M: *Effective implementation of evidence-based clinical improvements. Directions in health care: evidence-based medicine,* Seattle, WA, May 12, 2000, Group Health Cooperative of Puget Sound.

22. Lewin K: Field theory and learning. In Carthwright D, editor: *Field theory in social science: select theoretical papers,* New York, 1951, Harper Collins.

23. Grimshaw J, Shirran E, Thomas R et al: Effective health care bulletin: getting evidence into practice, NHS Centre for reviews and dissemination, *Royal Society of Medicine Press* 5(1), 1999.

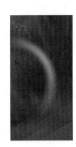

CHAPTER 2

Preconception Care: Improving Birth Outcomes through Care before Pregnancy

Josephine R. Fowler, MD, MS, FAAFP, and Brian W. Jack, MD

Preconception care is widely recognized as an important component of health care for women of reproductive age.[1-4] The overarching goal of preconception care is to provide health promotion, screening, and interventions to women of reproductive age to reduce risk factors that may affect future pregnancies.[5,6] Preconception guidelines should incorporate practical tools to address contraception and birth spacing, health education literacy and promotion, nutrition and weight management, tobacco and substance abuse, environmental exposures, medication benefits and risks, risky sexual behaviors, infection risks, optimal management of medical problems, stress reduction, and identification of skilled, trained health-care teams to address issues before considering pregnancy.

I. RATIONALE FOR PRECONCEPTION CARE

Preconception care is important because, for some conditions, treatment before pregnancy is essential to improvement in outcomes.

A. Impact of Preconception Intervention

1. Folic acid supplementation
   Folic acid supplementation reduces the risk for neural tube defects by 50% to 75%.[7,8]
   Motivated women may benefit from education surrounding the benefits of taking folate.

2. Glycemic control in women with diabetes
   Women with normal glycemic control and glycosylated hemoglobin (HgbA1C) levels less than 8.5% before pregnancy and during organogenesis have lower risk for congenital anomalies and spontaneous abortions when compared with women with HgbA1C levels greater than 8.5%.[9,10]
   The relative risk for cardiac anomalies is four times greater in women with poor glycemic control when compared with women with normal glycemic control.[11]

II. COMPONENTS OF PRECONCEPTION CARE

Preconception care includes the provision of health education individualized to a woman's or couple's needs (health promotion), a thorough and systematic identification of risks (risk assessment), and the initiation of actions to address those risks (interventions).

III. PRECONCEPTION HEALTH PROMOTION

Health promotion for women of childbearing age and their partners is an important component of preconception care and consists of counseling and education to support healthful behavior about pregnancy and parenting. In family practice, education about pregnancy, birth, and parenting occurs throughout the parenting years. The preconception visit is an opportunity for more intensive involvement.

IV. PREGNANCY READINESS

An objective of preconception care is to assess a woman's readiness for pregnancy. Unwanted and unintended pregnancy is a major problem in the United States. Unintended pregnancy is associated with delays in the initiation of prenatal care and with behaviors that increase the risk for adverse birth outcomes.[8] Interventions to prevent unwanted pregnancy obviously must occur before conception.

A. Preconception Promotion of Pregnancy Readiness

Preconception efforts to promote pregnancy readiness include the following tools:
1. Counseling about benefits of pregnancy planning
2. Education about the importance of birth spacing
3. Contraception counseling
4. Counseling about the availability of social programs, including vocational training

V. FAMILY PLANNING

Family planning and pregnancy prevention education should be considered part of preconception care. Because approximately half of the pregnancies in the United States are unintended, many authors have suggested that health risks and behaviors need to be addressed at all encounters with the health-care system.[12,13]

The post-partum stage is an appropriate period to present organized contraceptive education before a subsequent pregnancy if not done before the index pregnancy. Patients receiving physician instruction and education have high levels of satisfaction with counseling.[14]

Counseling to promote and support healthful behavior should foster the idea that women can choose healthy behaviors. Examples include a discussion of exercise programs, dietary habits, and optimal weight.

Health promotion topics include:
1. Smoking cessation
2. Alcohol and drug use prevention education
3. Avoidance of teratogenic medications
4. Avoidance of occupational hazards: Working mothers can be counseled about workplace hazards,

legal rights of pregnant workers, and childcare options
5. Avoidance of environmental toxins
6. Sexually transmitted disease (STD) prevention
   Counseling about safe sexual practices and ways to prevent STDs, including human immunodeficiency virus (HIV), are important before pregnancy.

VI. PROMOTE EARLY PRENATAL CARE AND ONGOING PRIMARY CARE

Preconception care should stress the value of early enrollment for prenatal care. Knowledge about publicly funded prenatal programs, eligibility requirements, and application processes may help women with low incomes plan for risk reduction visits before and during pregnancy. Women should be encouraged to maintain an accurate menstruation calendar together with a record of the discontinuation of oral contraceptives and any nonmenstrual bleeding. This promotes more accurate dating of conception, which can better identify those women who are truly postdates and require intervention, and can reduce the number of women erroneously considered postmature.

VII. PRECONCEPTION RISK ASSESSMENT

Preconception risk assessment identifies potential risk and addresses those risks before conception. Risk assessment includes inquiring about general health status of both potential parents.

A. Guidelines for Risk Assessment

Guidelines for risk assessment are as follows:
1. Inquire about maternal health and social well-being.
2. Assess for paternal health and social well-being.
3. Obtain a family history.
4. Know the family structure.
5. Compile a three-generation family history.
6. Obtain a social history.
7. Obtain a mental health history.
8. Develop an immunization plan.
9. Determine infectious, environmental, and occupational exposures before, during, and after pregnancy.

VIII. MEDICAL CONDITIONS

Several medical conditions could have an adverse effect on pregnancy outcomes, leading to pregnancy loss, infant death, birth defects, or other complications for mothers and infants, and for which evidence exists that the effect could be impacted by preconception care. For example, in 2002, 6.1% of women of reproductive age had asthma, 5% were obese, 3.4% had cardiac disease, 3% had hypertension, 9.3% had diabetes, and 1.4% had thyroid disorder.[15]

A. Diabetes (see Chapter 8, Section I)

One percent of women of childbearing age have diabetes. Uncontrolled diabetes is associated with many adverse effects during the perinatal period. These include both maternal and fetal morbidities.

1. Maternal complications
   a. Congenital anomalies
   b. Fetal loss
   c. Macrosomia
2. Fetal complications
   a. Abnormalities of the spine and skeleton
   b. Cardiovascular system
   c. Renal system
      Every woman of childbearing age should be counseled on the effects of poorly controlled diabetes to herself and the unborn child. Counseling should include importance of diabetes control before considering pregnancy.
3. History
   a. Age at diagnosis
   b. Severity of disease
   c. Baseline HgbA1C
   d. Comorbid conditions
   e. Medication regimen
4. Important counseling topics
   a. Maintaining optimal weight control
   b. Maximizing diabetes control including glucose self-monitoring
   c. Maintaining a regular exercise program
   d. Smoking cessation
   e. Alcohol and drug cessation
   f. Social support to assist during the pregnancy
      Women with diabetes are rarely discouraged from becoming pregnant, except those with renal complications, heart problems, or vision complications associated with their uncontrolled diabetes.

B. Hypertension (see Chapter 8, Section C)

Hypertension in pregnancy is associated with many adverse outcomes for both mother and fetus. Twenty percent of women of childbearing age have a diagnosis of chronic hypertension. Women with controlled chronic hypertension tend to have better outcomes than women with preeclampsia. However, superimposed preeclampsia in women with hypertension and renal hypertension are both associated with significant adverse perinatal outcomes.[16] Women with chronic hypertension should be advised on needed medication changes before conception (discontinuation of diuretics and ACE inhibitors) and the risks associated with hypertension in pregnancy for both mother and infant.

Before pregnancy, providers should assess:

1. Medication regimen
2. Evidence of comorbid conditions, such as diabetes and heart disease, and renal function
3. Baseline laboratory studies
   Baseline proteinuria and uric acid levels are important because changes in pregnancy may indicate worsening disease. Hyperuricemia and proteinuria in gestational hypertension are significantly associated with maternal complications and lower-birth-weight babies when compared with women with normal plasma uric acid levels.[17] Therefore, knowing baseline laboratory studies in these areas is important information for management in late pregnancy for those with superimposed preeclampsia.

C. Systemic Lupus Erythematosus (see Chapter 8, Section J)

Women with systemic lupus erythematosus (SLE) may seek information regarding pregnancy planning. The perinatal outcome will depend on the stability of the disease. They should be counseled that 50% of patients with lupus will have a normal pregnancy, 25% will experience preterm delivery, and the remaining 25% will result in spontaneous abortion. However, all lupus pregnancies should be considered high risk and managed with involvement of a high-risk perinatal team. Women should wait at least 6 months after remission before conceiving. This "wait interval" will decrease the risk for flaring during pregnancy. Concerns about medication use should be reviewed. Most medications taken by patients with lupus are safe during pregnancy. Cytoxan should be avoided during pregnancy, especially during the first trimester. The greatest risk is that of prematurity and the sequelae that come with preterm delivery. Approximately 10% of women with lupus and anti-Ro antibodies have a baby with neonatal lupus. Parents should be told this is not SLE and the baby can have a normal life. Women with anti-Ro/SSA and anti-La/SSB antibodies should consider preconception counseling to discuss the risk for congenital heart block in the newborn and perinatal management before becoming pregnant.

D. Epilepsy (see Chapter 8, Section G)

Preconception counseling is important in women with seizure disorders. Complications associated with seizure disorder include an increased frequency of seizure, fetal malformations associated with medication use, miscarriage, and perinatal death. Medications have been associated with cleft lip and palate, cardiac anomalies, facial abnormalities, intrauterine growth restriction (IUGR), skeletal abnormalities, and low intelligence quotient (IQ). The patient and her partner should be counseled on the opportune time for conception. The best time to conceive is after being seizure free and not taking antiseizure medications for 2 years. However, women who are taking medications should not discontinue their medication without consulting a physician. Physicians may consider a trial without medication for women with a normal electroencephalogram who have not had a seizure in several years. For those with active seizure history, the least toxic anticonvulsant medication should be initiated before pregnancy and the medication adjusted frequently to keep serum levels in the lowest effective range.[18,19]

E. Anemia (see Chapter 8, Section E)

Anemia in pregnancy is associated with poor fetal growth, preterm delivery, and low birth weight. Iron deficiency anemia is associated with a greater risk for preeclampsia during pregnancy. Women planning pregnancy should be counseled on eating foods rich in vitamin C, iron, folate, and vitamin B_{12}. Providers should recommend a well-balanced diet rich in fruits, lean meats, leafy green vegetables and legumes, wheat bread, and other iron-rich foods.

1. Iron deficiency
   The U.S. Preventive Services Task Force (USPSTF) has found little evidence to support recommending iron supplementation to nonanemic pregnant women. In addition, limited evidence exists that iron supplementation improves perinatal outcomes for mother or infant. The daily requirement of iron in pregnancy is 30 to 50 mg.

2. Folate deficiency
   The benefit of a diet rich in folic acid is well proven. Folic acid supplementation should be offered to all women of reproduction age. Folic acid 0.4 mg daily reduces neural tube defects by 66%, and 4 mg daily for those women with a prior delivery of a child with neural tube defect reduces the risk by 77%. Folic acid is suggested to prevent occurrence of neural tube defect and decrease severity of neural tube defects.[20]

3. Hemoglobinopathies
   Hemoglobinopathies are generally limited to populations at risk.
   a. Sickle cell disease: The incidence of the SS gene in the African American population is 1 in 12, with the theoretical incidence 1 in 576 births. The gene is also prevalent in many Southeast Asian populations. Sickle cell is an autosomal recessive disorder; each parent must have the gene for the infant to have the disease. In infants with sickle cell disease, the fetal hemoglobin disappears by 3 to 6 months of age and symptoms of sickling begin.
   b. Thalassemia: Populations at risk include people of Mediterranean descent and some Southeast Asians. These diseases also are autosomal recessive and require each parent to carry the gene for the infant to be affected. There are different types of sickle cell disease and thalassemia, and they vary in severity and even in penetrance; thus, it is difficult to prognosticate to concerned parents in an office visit. All parents with abnormal hemoglobin results should consider genetic counseling before conception.
   c. The following actions should be done for patients with risk factors for hemoglobinopathies:
       i. Review old records for verification.
      ii. Check complete blood cell count, hemoglobin electrophoresis, and smear if homozygous disease.
     iii. Request old records from hematologist.
      iv. Check status of hemoglobin of the father of the infant.
       v. Schedule an appointment with genetic counseling or discuss risk associated with pregnancy.
      vi. Discuss team approach to pregnancy including high-risk specialist and hematology

oncology department input if homozygous disease.

vii. Encourage good nutrition and hydration.

viii. Make sure patient is up to date on immunizations, especially the pneumococcal vaccine.

ix. Discuss risk for asymptomatic bacteruria in pregnancy if sickle trait.

x. Discuss possible need for transfusions (discuss with consultants) during pregnancy if severely anemic.

IX. NUTRITION

Maintaining optimal weight before pregnancy is expected to result in health benefits yet to be proven. Maternal obesity has been linked to increase risk for cesarean delivery, increased maternal complications in pregnancy, and subsequent childhood obesity for the offspring. Maternal underweight is associated with having a low-birth-weight infant.

X. PARENTAL SOCIAL BEHAVIOR

Several maternal and paternal behaviors adversely affect perinatal outcomes, and evidence suggests that many of these effects can be impacted by preconception care. A substantial proportion of women who become pregnant engage in high-risk behaviors proven to contribute to adverse pregnancy outcomes. In 2003, 10.7% of pregnant women smoked during pregnancy, a risk factor for low birth weight, whereas in 2002, 10.1% of pregnant women and 54.9% of women at risk for getting pregnant consumed alcohol, which may cause fetal alcohol syndrome.[21] Although a smaller proportion of women use illicit drugs, they are at extremely high risk for adverse outcomes.

XI. TOBACCO (SEE CHAPTER 5, SECTION D)

Smoking is a major contributor of poor perinatal outcomes accounting for one third of low-birth-weight babies, a known indicator for infant morbidity and mortality.[22,23] Of the 120 million women who continue in pregnancy, 11% to 12% report smoking, with the greatest percentage among women in their late teens.[24]

A. Fetal Effects of Smoking

Fetal effects of smoking during pregnancy include[25]:

1. IUGR

2. Prematurity

3. Low birth weight (relative risk [RR], 1.28; 95% confidence interval [CI], 1.04-1.58)

B. Secondary Exposure Associations

Secondary exposure associations of smoking during pregnancy include:

1. Respiratory illnesses such as asthma and bronchitis (RR, 2.25; 95% CI, 1.58-3.19)

2. Ear infections

3. Sudden infant death syndrome

C. Maternal Complications of Smoking

Maternal complications of smoking include[26]:

1. Placental abruption (RR, 1.6; 95% CI, 1.3-1.8; increases 40% with each pack per day)

2. Preterm labor

Families desiring pregnancy should be counseled on the benefits of not smoking before, during, and after the pregnancy, and should be educated about the risks of secondhand smoke on each person living in the household.[27]

XII. ALCOHOL (SEE CHAPTER 5, SECTION C)

Fetal alcohol syndrome is the most common cause of preventable mental retardation. Every couple should be given accurate information about alcohol and its effect on pregnancy. Alcohol consumption during pregnancy causes fetal wastage, growth retardation, organ anomalies, neurosensory problems, and mental retardation. Currently, we are unable to say this is a dose-dependent relation. Therefore, avoiding alcohol during pregnancy is the best instruction. Preconception instructions include review of associated risk, identification of programs that would help in cessation and long-term abstinence, and offering support during the treatment program.

XIII. COCAINE

Substance use during pregnancy is associated with morbidity to both mother and infant. Cocaine use is associated with preterm delivery, placental abruption, low birth weight, poor growth, poor feeding, developmental delay, cerebral infarction, poor bonding, and sudden infant death syndrome. Parents should be counseled on the risks and offered information on programs that support abstinence and rehabilitation.

XIV. HEROIN

Heroin use during pregnancy is associated with similar outcomes as women who use cocaine. Heroin use increases risk for preterm delivery, miscarriage, IUGR, placenta abruption, stillbirth, and neonatal withdrawal syndromes. Women should be directed to a program that can offer weaning from heroin use. They should not stop abruptly. The provider should recommend delaying pregnancy until completely drug free.

XV. GENETICS

Birth defects are the number one cause of infant deaths in the United States. One in 28 infants will have a birth defect. Several inherited disorders are commonly associated with chronic debilitating diseases such as sickle cell anemia, cystic fibrosis, Tay–Sachs disease, and thalassemia. Providers should take every available opportunity to assess, screen, refer for genetic counseling, and treat families with genetic disorders. Because screening tests identify only 10% to 20% of genetic defects, those at risk should be offered referral to a trained genetic counselor to discuss risks for having a child with birth defects.

Risk factors that may prompt a visit to the genetic counselor include:

1. Strong family history of genetic disorders
2. Advanced maternal and/or paternal age
3. Previous child with neural tube defect
4. Presence of balanced chromosomal translocation in either parent
5. Use of teratogenic medications
6. Family history of congenital anomaly or mental retardation
7. History of intrauterine fetal demise or recurrent miscarriages
8. Known specific disease or positive screening test
   Women and men at risk for delivering a child with a birth defect may choose not to become pregnant rather than consider an abortion later.

XVI. INFECTIOUS DISEASES (SEE CHAPTER 9, SECTION A)

Several infectious diseases adversely affect perinatal outcomes, and evidence exists that many of these effects can be impacted by preconception care.

A. Hepatitis B

Hepatitis B is predominantly a sexually transmitted disease in the United States.[28] Causes of hepatitis B transmission include blood transfusions and lower transmissions through semen, infected wounds, and vaginal secretions. Other populations at high risk for hepatitis B include men who have sex with men, intravenous (IV) drug users, and those with multiple sex partners.

Preconception prevention of transmission begins in childhood at birth or at the time of complete vaccination.

1. Vaccination is recommended for all children aged 0 to 18 years.
2. Children between the ages of 0 and 18 years who have not been vaccinated and adults who engage in high-risk behavior should be offered vaccination during routine office visits before conception and during the peripartum period.
3. The USPSTF does not recommend routine screening of the general population for hepatitis B.
4. All pregnant women should be screened for hepatitis B. Routine screening for hepatitis B surface antigen is protocol for prenatal care. If a woman is negative for hepatitis B and she is considered high risk because of her occupation, sexual partner, or lifestyle practices, she should be offered vaccination. Vaccination is safe during both pregnancy and the breastfeeding period.
5. Reduction of long-term sequelae to hepatitis B is prevented by administration of immunoprophylaxis at birth to infants with seropositive mothers. However, infants exposed to acute infection in utero have additional risks, including low birth weight[29] and prematurity.[30]
6. All men and women who have hepatitis B should be told the risks for transmission to the mother and subsequent risk to the infant if infected. Almost 25% of sexual contacts of a seropositive partner will become infected. The risks for neonatal transmission range from 10% in the first trimester to 90% in the third trimester if the woman acquires an acute hepatitis B infection during pregnancy.[31] Chronic infection occurs in more than 90% of infected infants. Chronic infection poses a risk for cirrhosis and hepatocellular carcinoma. Women who are chronic carriers are counseled on the importance of informing the pediatrician or family physician at birth.

B. Hepatitis C

Hepatitis C is the silent epidemic in the United States. Many patients are unaware that they are carriers. Nearly 4 million Americans are infected with hepatitis C. Hepatitis C is transmitted through contaminated blood and blood products. Methods of transmission include blood transfusion, use of infected instruments during surgical procedures or body piercing, perinatal transmission during childbirth, hemodialysis, sharing of infected instruments in barber shops or nail salons, sharing straws for snorting among cocaine users, and IV drug use.

1. Partners that are at high risk should be screened before conception.
2. The number of women testing positive for anti-HCV antibody in pregnancy ranges from 0.1% to 4.5%.[32-34] Women testing positive should be counseled on the risk for transmission to others and possible risk to the newborn.
3. Women with hepatitis C can breastfeed. The neonatal transmission rate in pregnancy is about 5%. Hepatitis C is not transmitted through breastfeeding. The risk increases in HIV-positive women and in proportion to the maternal viral load. In the United States, the majority of neonatal transmission cases are mild.

Currently, treatments for mother or infant or means to decrease perinatal transmission are not available; therefore, routine preconception screening is not recommended.[35] Women who are positive for hepatitis C and desire pregnancy should be counseled regarding uncertain infectivity, the link between viral load and neonatal transmission, the importance of avoiding hepatotoxic drugs, and the risk for chronic liver disease.

C. Varicella

Varicella is a highly contagious disease. The advisory committee on immunization practices currently recommends vaccination for nonpregnant women of childbearing age.[36] Because varicella vaccination is becoming widely implemented, women receiving the vaccine should be counseled not to become pregnant for at least 1 month after being vaccinated. Women with active disease during the first trimester or early second trimester are at risk for delivering an infant with limb atrophy, scarring of the skin of the extremities, central nervous system abnormalities, and eye problems. The risk for congenital varicella from perinatal transmission during the first and second trimester ranges from 0.4% to 2.0%. In addition, the maternal risk for severe infection, including varicella pneumonia, is high.[37] The risk for congenital disease from vaccination is very low.

D. Rubella

Preventing congenital rubella is important because it can affect all organ systems. Deafness is the most common sequela of congenital rubella syndrome. Parents should be counseled on the importance of immunization. Routine screening should be offered to all women of reproductive age who have not been vaccinated. Women should be counseled not to become pregnant for 3 months after receiving vaccination because of a theoretical risk for transmission. A woman who does become pregnant can be reassured that no documented cases of congenital rubella as a result of vaccination have been reported. A woman with rubella in early gestation is at risk for prematurity, spontaneous abortion, and fetal death. Neonatal infections are rare when maternal infection occurs after 20 weeks. However, in women who are infected in the first trimester, 85% will have an infected fetus or infant. Women should be counseled that infants with congenital rubella are highly contagious and caretakers who are not immunized are at risk for infection.

E. Tuberculosis

Worldwide, tuberculosis (TB) is the number one infectious disease killer. The Centers for Disease Control and Prevention (CDC) reported more than 15,000 cases of TB in 2001 and 10 to 15 million latent infections. TB affects all parts of the body, including the pulmonary, skeletal, gastrointestinal, genitourinary, and cutaneous systems. The case fatality rate approaches 50% in untreated patients, areas of multidrug resistance, and infants with congenital disease. TB in pregnancy is a risk factor for low birth weight and subsequently poor perinatal outcomes. Screening for TB before pregnancy allows for prophylaxis completion and the opportunity to reduce these risks.

TB reduction includes first identifying those at risk for disease. High-risk groups include individuals with active TB within 2 years, those with personal contact to someone with active TB, illicit drug users, foreign-born persons from high-risk countries who are in the United States less than 5 years, older adults, children younger than 4 exposed to high-risk adults, and individuals with chronic medical conditions such as HIV, diabetes, organ transplant, end-stage renal disease, cancer, chronic steroid use, underweight, health-care workers, incarcerated individuals, and those working in correctional institutions.[38] The opportunity to screen for TB is available at routine visits and annual examinations for any woman stating a desire to become pregnant in the future and for any person included among the high-risk groups listed above.

F. Sexually Transmitted Infections

Some women engage in high-risk sexual behavior, potentially exposing themselves to STDs and HIV.[39] Men and women being treated for STDs should be counseled on the risk for infertility imposed by having STDs. Untreated STDs can affect all parts of the reproductive tract for men and women.

1. Human immunodeficiency virus
   Worldwide, there are more than 1900 infant lives lost to HIV daily and more than 700,000 lost annually. Perinatal HIV transmission still accounts for more than 90% of pediatric acquired immune deficiency syndrome (AIDS) cases in the United States. In addition, 40% of these infants are born to mothers who are unaware of their HIV status. Preconception prevention of perinatal HIV transmission requires a multifaceted approach. Primary prevention includes:
   a. Couples should be counseled that transmission can occur during pregnancy, during labor, and after birth through breastfeeding.
   b. Encourage men and women to know their HIV status before pregnancy.
   c. Reduce barriers to screening.
   d. Institute global education about risk and HIV transmission, treatment options, and effective follow-up strategies for HIV-positive women, and discuss further risk reduction in treated HIV-positive women.
   e. Women with HIV should be counseled to seek prenatal care as soon as they suspect they are pregnant.
   Women who receive antiretrovirals beginning in the first trimester through the labor period followed by treatment of the infant for 6 months reduces transmission from 25% to 4 to 10%.[40] Studies confirm that treating HIV-positive mothers with antiretrovirals can reduce perinatal transmission to 2% or less in those women with a low viral load who do not breastfeed.[41]

The CDC recommends HIV screening to all women who are pregnant. Evaluation of two programs, the opt-in and opt-out approaches, assesses the frequency of HIV testing. The opt-in approach included informing women of their risk for HIV transmission to their newborn and offering them the HIV test. The opt-out approach included informing women that HIV testing was part of the standard laboratory testing unless they declined being tested. Women given the opt-out approach tend to test more often, implying reduced perinatal transmission.[42] For women of reproductive age, knowing their HIV status before pregnancy allows for treatment and reduction of viral load, therefore decreasing transmission.

2. Gonorrhea
   According to the CDC, gonorrhea occurs in about 125 per 100,000 people. It is the most common cause of pelvic inflammatory disease (PID). Women with PID are at risk for internal infections, chronic pelvic pain, and damage to fallopian tubes. In men, gonorrhea can block tubes that carry sperm. If a woman has gonorrhea when she delivers, she can pass the infection to her baby, causing blindness, joint infections, or blood infections. Women should be counseled on the importance of treatment for gonorrhea as soon as it is evident.

3. Chlamydia
   Chlamydia has similar effects as gonorrhea in untreated women and men. An untreated pregnant woman is at increased risk for preterm delivery and can pass the infection to her baby during vaginal delivery, leading to conjunctivitis or pneumonia. Early treatment and repeat testing are important in infected women.

4. Syphilis[43-45]
   The World Health Organization estimates 12 million new cases of syphilis annually. In 2002, the CDC reported 32,000 cases of syphilis. Syphilis has declined in both women and neonates. Women planning pregnancy should inquire thoroughly about sexual practices in their partner because the incidence of syphilis is increasing in men having sex with men, and overall the rate of disease in men is 3.5 times that of women. Preconception screening for syphilis in high-risk populations is an important step in reduction of neonatal syphilis. Individuals at risk for syphilis include men having sex with men, individuals in correctional facilities, commercial sex workers,

those who trade sex for money, those having sex with high-risk partners, and individuals diagnosed with other STDs. In addition, the USPSTF recommends screening all pregnant women for syphilis in the first trimester. Understanding the importance of avoiding syphilis transmission, many states require syphilis screening as a part of their premarital screening.

Syphilis can be cured if treated in its early stages. However, treatment does not prevent reinfection. Even if adequate treatment is established, repeat testing should occur before pregnancy and during pregnancy in the first and third trimesters. A woman with syphilis should be counseled about the risk to the unborn if untreated. Studies show that the majority of stillbirths occur around 30 weeks of gestation. Therefore, even in unplanned pregnancies, treatment of syphilis immediately might decrease risk for stillbirth and other perinatal morbidities. Perinatal morbidity and mortality are as high as 40% in women who are untreated. Additional risks include prematurity, neonatal death, developmental delay, blindness, deafness, bone and teeth abnormalities, and seizures.

5. Herpes

Genital herpes is common in the United States. Women with herpes should be counseled on the risk to the fetus and newborn child. It is important to teach couples about the appearance of herpetic lesions because they may be asymptomatic. Women with active lesions at delivery should be offered cesarean section to avoid perinatal transmission.

XVII. TOXICITIES

A. Lead

Lead is most commonly found in lead-based paint, through occupational exposure, and in contaminated soil. Mothers exposed to high levels of lead or have known high lead levels should be counseled on the risk of lead to the pregnancy and the unborn child. If suspected lead exposure is known, testing for serum lead level might be indicated. Fetal exposure as early as 12 weeks of gestation can pose a risk to the fetus. Lead levels of 10 to 15 mcg/dl may lead to central nervous system damage, hydroceles, skin tags, hemangiomas, lymphangiomas, undescended testicles in male individuals, miscarriage, and stillbirth. Women with lead exposure should be counseled on risk and offered opportunity to screen before pregnancy.

B. Mercury

Mercury is another element found in the workplace, and women should be counseled on risk of exposure. Mercury exposure is associated with stillbirth, birth defects, and spontaneous abortions. Preconception counseling includes directing women in high-risk areas to discuss workplace safety with their employers.

C. Organic Solvents

Occupational exposure to solvents may be the most difficult to avoid. Women of reproductive age exposed to solvents should wear protective garments, gloves, and masks. Women working in areas with exposure should be counseled that risk for neurodevelopmental delay in language and behavioral skills increases with duration and dose of exposure.

XVIII. PSYCHOSOCIAL RISKS (SEE CHAPTER 5, SECTION A)

Psychosocial determinants of women's health also play a role in pregnancy outcome. The health status of poor and minority women contributes to persistent, and sometimes increasing, disparities in birth outcomes. Lower physical functioning, emotional health, and overall health status of women with low incomes in the month before pregnancy has been associated with an increased risk for preterm labor.[46] However, a study by Goldenberg and colleagues[47] suggests that medical, psychosocial, and behavioral risks may not account for the increased low birth weight among black women. Socioeconomic status directly and indirectly influences three major determinants of health: access to health care, environmental exposure, and health behavior.[48] Racial inequalities and unequal treatment likewise influence these determinants.[49]

XIX. DOMESTIC VIOLENCE

One study recently reported a greater incidence of low birth weight, placental abruption, and adverse outcomes in a small cohort of women reporting verbal and physical abuse during pregnancy and in a group of women with suspected abuse but not willing to report.[50] Although additional studies may be necessary to confirm causation, couples should be questioned about risk of abuse and offered information on safety to prevent harm to both parent and child.

XX. MENTAL HEALTH AND PERINATAL OUTCOMES (SEE CHAPTER 10)

XXI. CONCLUSION

Today, the greatest opportunities for further improvement in pregnancy outcomes—in improving the health of women, children, and families—lie in prevention strategies that must be implemented before conception to be effective, that is, through preconception care.

The context for these recommendations is that preconception care is not a single visit but rather a process of care designed to meet the needs of a woman during the different stages of her reproductive life. The purpose is to promote health throughout the life span for women, children, and families. Preconception care offers health services that allow couples to maintain optimal health for themselves, choose the number and spacing of their pregnancies, and, when desired, to prepare for a healthy baby.

XXII. SOR A RECOMMENDATIONS

RECOMMENDATIONS	REFERENCES
Women with preexisting diabetes should achieve euglycemic control before conception and maintain near euglycemic control (<1% above normal range) during organogenesis to decrease risk for congenital malformations.	*9-11*
Preconception HIV screening of women and men of reproductive age allows for early counseling and treatment of HIV-positive women before and during pregnancy, reducing viral load and the risk for neonatal transmission.	*39, 40*
Women in high-risk populations of reproductive age should be screened and treated for active syphilis before and during pregnancy. Untreated syphilis could result in neonatal syphilis, stillbirth, and other perinatal morbidities.	*43-45*
Women and men who are planning pregnancy should be offered tobacco cessation counseling together with adjunct therapy such as nicotine patch and gum.	*24*

REFERENCES

1. Institute of Medicine, Committee to Study the Prevention of Low Birth Weight: *Preventing low birth weight,* Washington, DC, 1985, National Academy Press.
2. Moos MK, Cefalo RC: Preconceptual health promotion: a focus for obstetric care, *Am J Perinatol* 47:63-67, 1987.
3. Public Health Service: Caring for our future: the content of prenatal care—a report of the Public Health Service Expert Panel on the Content of Prenatal Care. Washington, DC, 1989, US Department of Health and Human Services, Public Health Service.
4. Jack BW, Culpepper L: Preconception care: risk reduction and health promotion in preparation for pregnancy, *JAMA* 264:1147-1149, 1990.
5. Fowler JR, Jack BS: Preconception care. In Taylor RB, David AK, Fields SA et al, editors: *Family medicine principles and practice,* ed 6, New York, 2003, Springer, pp 85-94.
6. Jack BW, Culpepper L: Preconception care, *J Fam Pract* 32:306-315, 1991.
7. Czeizel AE, Dudas I, Metneki J: Prevention of the first occurrence of neural-tube defects by periconceptional vitamin supplementation, *N Engl J Med* 327:1832-1835, 1992.
8. Lumley J, Watson L, Watson M et al: Periconceptional supplementation with folate and/or multivitamins for preventing neural tube defects, *Cochrane Database Syst Rev* (3): CD001056, 2001.
9. Kitzmiller JL, Buchanan TA, Kjos S et al: Preconception care of diabetes, congenital malformations, and spontaneous abortions, *Diabetes Care* 19:514-541, 1996.
10. American Diabetes Association: Preconception care of women with diabetes, *Diabetes Care* 27:S76-S78, 2004.
11. Kucera J: Rate and type of congenital anomalies among offspring of diabetic women, *J Reprod Med* 7(2):73-82, 1971.
12. Institute of Medicine: *Best intentions. Unintended pregnancy and the well-being of children and families,* Washington, DC, 1995, National Academy Press.
13. Henshaw SK: Unintended pregnancy in the United States, *Fam Plann Perspect* 30:24-32, 1998.
14. Proctor A, Jenkins TR, Loeb T et al: Patient satisfaction with 3 methods of postpartum contraceptive counseling, *J Reprod Med* 51:377-382, 2006.
15. U.S. Department of Health and Human Services, Health Resources and Services Administration, Maternal and Child Health Bureau: *Women's health USA 2002,* Rockville, MD, 2002, US Department of Health and Human Services.
16. Brown MA, Buddle M: Hypertension in pregnancy: maternal and fetal outcomes according to laboratory and clinical features, *Med J Aust* 165:360-365, 1996.
17. Roberts JM, Bodnar LM, Lain KM et al: Uric acid is as important as proteinuria in fetal risk in women with gestational hypertension, *Hypertension* 46:1263-1269, 2005.
18. Taysi K: Preconceptional counseling, *Obstet Gynecol Clin North Am* 15:167-178, 1988.
19. Delgado-Escueta AV, Janz D: Consensus guideline: preconception counseling, management, and care of the pregnant women with epilepsy, *Neurology* 42:149-160, 1992.
20. Bol KA, Collins JS, Kirby RS, for the National Birth Defects Prevention Network: Survival of infants with neural tube defects in the presence of folic acid fortification, *Pediatrics* 117:803-813, 2006.
21. Centers for Disease Control and Prevention: Alcohol consumption among women who are pregnant or who might

become pregnant—United States, 2002, *MMWR Morb Mortal Wkly Rep* 53(50):1178-1181, 2004.

22. American College of Obstetricians and Gynecologists (ACOG) educational bulletin: Smoking cessation during pregnancy. Number 260, September 2000. American College of Obstetricians and Gynecologists, *Int J Gynaecol Obstet* 75:345-348, 2001.

23. U.S. Preventive Services Task Force: *November 2003. Counseling: tobacco use. Guide to preventive services: periodic updates,* ed 3. Available at http://www.ahrq.gov/clinic/3rduspstf/tobacccoun/tobcounrs.pdf. Accessed December 2003.

24. Martin JA, Hamilton BE, Sutton PD et al: Births: final data for 2002, *Natl Vital Stat Rep* 52(10):1-113, 2003.

25. Gold DR, Burge HA, Carey V et al: Predictors of repeated wheeze in the first year of life. The relative roles of cockroach, birth weight, acute lower respiratory illness, and maternal smoking, *Am J Respir Crit Care Med* 160:227-236, 1999.

26. *The health consequences of smoking a report of the Surgeon General,* Washington, DC, 2004, U.S. Department of Health and Human Services, Centers for Disease Control and Prevention, National Center for Chronic Disease and Promotion, Office of Smoking and Health.

27. Hopkins DP, Briss PA, Ricard CJ et al; Task Force on Community Preventive Services: Reviews of evidence regarding interventions to reduce tobacco use and exposure to environmental tobacco smoke, *Am J Prev Med* 20:16-66, 2001.

28. Centers for Disease Control and Prevention: Sexually transmitted diseases treatment guidelines—2002, *MMWR Recomm Rep* 51(RR-6):1-78, 2002.

29. Shepard TH: *Catalog of teratogenic agents,* ed 9, Baltimore, 1998, Johns Hopkins University Press.

30. Hieber JP, Dalton D, Shorey J et al: Hepatitis and pregnancy, *J Pediatr* 91(4):545-549, 1977.

31. ACOG educational bulletin. Viral hepatitis in pregnancy. Number 248, July 1998. American College of Obstetricians and Gynecologists, *Int J Gynaecol Obstet* 63:195-202, 1998.

32. Reinus JF, Leikin EL, Alter HJ et al: Failure to detect vertical transmission of hepatitis C virus, *Ann Intern Med* 117:881-886, 1992.

33. Moriya T, Sasaki F, Mizui M: Transmission of hepatitis C virus from mothers to infants: its frequency and risk factors revisited, *Biomed Pharmacother* 49:59-64, 1995.

34. Bohman VR, Stettler W, Little BB et al: Seroprevalence and risk factors for hepatitis C virus antibody in pregnancy, *Obstet Gynecol* 80:609-613, 1992.

35. Zanetti AR, Tanzi E, Newell ML: Mother-to-infant transmission of hepatitis C virus, *J Hepatol* 31(suppl 1):96-100, 1999.

36. Prevention of varicella. Updated recommendations of the Advisory Committee on Immunization Practices (ACIP), *MMWR Recomm Rep* 48(RR-6):1-5, 1999.

37. Paryani S, Arvin A: Intrauterine infection with varicella-zoster virus after maternal varicella, *N Engl J Med* 314:1542-1546, 1986 (abstract).

38. Jerant JF, Bannon M, Rittenhouse S: Identification and management of tuberculosis, *Am Fam Physician* 61:2667-2678, 2681-2682, 2000.

39. Centers for Disease Control and Prevention: Revised guidelines for HIV counseling, testing, and referral. Revised recommendations for HIV screening of pregnant women, *MMWR Recomm Rep* 50(RR-19):1-14, 2001.

40. Public Health Service Task Force: Recommendations for use of antiretroviral drugs in pregnant HIV-1-infected women for maternal health and interventions to reduce perinatal HIV-1 transmission in the United States. Available at http://aidsinfo.nih.gov/contentfiles/PerinatalGL.pdf. Accessed October 2006.

41. Ioannidis JP, Abrams EJ, Ammann A et al: Perinatal transmission of human immunodeficiency virus type 1 by pregnant women with RNA virus loads <1000 copies/ml, *J Infect Dis* 183:539-545, 2001.

42. Centers for Disease Control and Prevention (CDC): HIV testing among pregnant women—United States and Canada, 1998–2001, *MMWR Morb Mortal Wkly Rep* 51(45):1013-1016, 2002.

43. American Academy of Pediatrics: *Guidelines for perinatal care,* ed 5, Elk Grove Village, IL, 2002, American College of Obstetricians and Gynecologists.

44. Nelson HD, Glass N, Huffman L et al: *Screening for syphilis: a brief update for the U.S. Preventive Services Task Force,* Rockville, MD, 2004, Agency for Healthcare Research and Quality.

45. U.S. Preventive Services Task Force: *Screening for syphilis,* Washington, DC, 2004, Office of Disease Prevention and Health Promotion.

46. Kramer MS: Intrauterine growth and gestational duration determinants, *Pediatrics* 80:502-511, 1987.

47. Goldenberg RL, Cliver SP, Mulvihill FX, et al: Medical, psychosocial, and behavioral risk factors do not explain the increased risk for LBW among black women, *Am J Obstet Gynecol* 175:1317-1324, 1996.

48. Adler NE, Newman K: Socioeconomic disparities in health: pathways and policies, *Health Affairs* 21(2):60-76, 2002.

49. Misra D: *The women's health data book: a profile of women's health in the United States,* ed 3, Washington, DC, 2001, Jacobs Institute of Women's Health and the Henry J. Kaiser Family Foundation.

50. Yost NP, Bloom SL, McIntire DD, Leveno KJ: A prospective observational study of domestic violence during pregnancy, *Obstet Gynecol* 106(1):61-65, 2005.

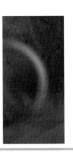

CHAPTER 3

Content of Prenatal Care

SECTION A History of Prenatal Care

Beth Choby, MD

Antenatal care is the evaluation of generally healthy pregnant women with the goal of detecting and preventing adverse maternal and neonatal outcomes. The first organized programs of prenatal care were introduced in the United States during the early twentieth century. During the 1930s, increased emphasis was placed on educating health-care providers who provided maternity care. Women were encouraged to receive care while pregnant and to give birth in the hospital rather than at home. Antenatal programs were credited with significant reductions in maternal and neonatal mortality, and were also assumed to be cost-effective. In 1985, the Institute of Medicine emphasized prenatal care as a national policy issue, resulting in Congress enacting legislation that expanded Medicaid coverage to pregnant women.[1] The percentage of women receiving prenatal care has increased since the early 1980s, as has earlier entry into prenatal care.[2]

Public spending for prenatal care in recent years is justified primarily by the cost-saving argument. Prenatal care purportedly decreases the adverse outcomes and complications associated with low birth weight, thus "paying for itself" over time. The evidence for the effectiveness of prenatal care is not as clear-cut. With a highly sophisticated health-care system and highest per capita health-care spending in the world, the United States ranks 28th among developed countries for infant mortality. This runs counterintuitive to the fact that the number of women receiving prenatal care has increased, whereas rates of preterm and low-birth-weight delivery have worsened over the past decades.

Historically, proving whether prenatal care is effective is difficult for several reasons. In early cross-sectional studies, selection bias skewed results. Random assignment to "no prenatal care" control groups is neither feasible nor ethical, and in many studies, women self-selected into study groups. Women who choose routine prenatal care or early care are likely different from women who do not receive care. This hinders generalization of whether improved outcomes from prenatal care are real or due to selection bias. Factors such as socioeconomic level, education, stress, baseline health, and family dynamics all influence why women do or do not seek care. These factors are difficult to randomize, making it difficult to conclusively link improved pregnancy outcomes with prenatal care, or conversely, poor obstetric outcomes with lack of care.

More recent studies suggest that prenatal care is associated with improved birth outcomes. A large prospective population study shows that women with inadequate prenatal care have two to three times greater risk for having a preterm delivery.[3] Two other retrospective population samples examine the influence of antenatal care among different racial groups. Prenatal care is associated with fewer preterm births in both the presence and absence of high-risk conditions for both African American and white women. African American women who lack prenatal care have preterm birth rates of 34.9%, compared with 15.1% among women with care. White women without prenatal care have preterm delivery rates of 21.9%, compared with 8.3% of women who seek care.[4] Lack of prenatal care is also a risk factor for neonatal death in both African American and white women, especially in gestations complicated by pregnancy-induced hypertension, small for gestation infants, postdates, or intrapartum fever.[5]

Additional research identifies characteristics of women who deliver with no prenatal care. These women are more likely to be multiparous, living with a child, less educated, uninsured, and smokers and have a history of substance use/abuse.[6] Risk factors for inadequate prenatal care include age younger than 20, low educational achievement, high parity, and being unmarried. Ensuring that women receive prenatal care actually may involve more than simply funding the care. A recent study of women covered by either private insurance or Medicaid finds that low-income women with unintended/unwanted pregnancies, no regular healthcare provider before conception, and less than a high school education are significantly less likely to get timely prenatal care compared with other women with low incomes with similar insurance coverage.[7] Other barriers include a limited number of providers to care for low-income women, lack of transportation and child care availability, difficulty with enrollment in public programs, and cultural/language barriers.

Future research must examine whether certain groups of women benefit from alternative types of prenatal care. Identifying women at high risk for adverse pregnancy outcomes, especially the young, the uninsured, and women with cultural/language barriers, may allow for provision of extended prenatal care. This care will likely be more intensive and expensive than routine prenatal care for women considered to be low risk. The expense may be justified if the end result is a decrease in the rate of low-birth-weight infants. With the huge financial costs of caring for severely preterm infants, alternative means of prenatal care may end up being more cost-effective than less expensive traditional care.

Even if prenatal care is not cost-effective, it may have less straightforward benefits. Prenatal visits introduce expectant mothers into the health-care system, possibly improving maternal health and increasing the chance that infants receive recommended care after birth. The relationship between prenatal care and the adoption of healthy behaviors is receiving increased attention. Research into whether the content and delivery of prenatal care is associated with other preconception planning—that is, pregnancy planning, contraceptive use, preconception visits, exercise and nutrition, and tobacco/substance use—may provide further insight into the role of prenatal care.[8]

REFERENCES

1. Guyer B: Medicaid and prenatal care. Necessary but not sufficient, *JAMA* 264:2264-2265, 1990.
2. Kogan MD, Martin JA, Alexander GR et al: The changing pattern of prenatal care utilization in the United States, 1981-1995 using different prenatal care indices, *JAMA* 279(20):1623-1628, 1998.
3. Krueger PM, Scholl TO: Adequacy of prenatal care and pregnancy outcome, *J Am Osteopath Assoc* 100(8):485-491, 2000.
4. Vintzileos AM, Ananth CV, Smulian JC et al: The impact of prenatal care in the United States on preterm births in the presence and absence of antenatal high-risk conditions, *Am J Obstet Gynecol* 187:1254-1257, 2002.
5. Vintzileos AM, Ananth CV, Smulian JC et al: The impact of prenatal care on postneonatal deaths in the presence and absence of antenatal high-risk conditions, *Am J Obstet Gynecol* 187:1258-1262, 2002.
6. Maupin R, Lyman R, Fatsis J et al: Characteristics of women who deliver with no prenatal care, *J Matern Fetal Neonatal Med* 16(1):45-50, 2004.
7. Braveman D, Marchi K, Egerter S et al: Barriers to timely prenatal care among women with insurance: the importance of pre-pregnancy factors, *Obstet Gynecol* 95:874-880, 2000.
8. Alexander GR, Kotelchuk M: Assessing the role and effectiveness of prenatal care: history, challenges, and directions for future research, *Public Health Reports* 116:306-316, 2001.

SECTION B Diagnosis and Dating of Pregnancy

Beth Choby, MD

I. BACKGROUND

Women often seek medical attention after a first missed menses. Many report a variety of symptoms associated with early pregnancy. Because historical factors do not always reliably predict pregnancy, the clinical evaluation includes a confirmation of the diagnosis of pregnancy and an estimation of gestational age. Useful adjuncts include the medical history, physical examination, laboratory testing, and ultrasound.

II. SIGNS AND SYMPTOMS OF PREGNANCY

Common symptoms of early pregnancy include fatigue, amenorrhea, nausea, and breast tenderness. Several studies examine the usefulness of these symptoms for predicting pregnancy. Fatigue results from increased progesterone levels in the first trimester.

Amenorrhea in a sexually active female is presumed to be due to pregnancy until proved otherwise. It has a sensitivity of 63% to 68% and a specificity of 40% to 60% when used to predict pregnancy.[1,2] Nausea gravidarum (morning sickness) is 39% sensitive and 86% specific for diagnosing pregnancy. About 36% to 72% of women reporting breast tenderness and amenorrhea are pregnant.[3]

Several signs of pregnancy involve the skin and mucous membranes. Hegar's sign refers to the softening of the cervical and uterine tissue, which results in a globular shape of the uterus. Chadwick's sign occurs because of pelvic organ vascular engorgement, resulting in a bluish appearance of the vulva, vagina, and cervix in early pregnancy. Vaginal changes have low sensitivity (18%) for diagnosing pregnancy but are fairly specific (94%).[4] Skin changes include the linea nigra and chloasma, or the "pregnancy mask."

III. DIAGNOSIS OF PREGNANCY

Important clinical information includes the menstrual history, the usual pattern of cycles, and a description of the previous period in terms of timing, length, and flow. The first day of the last menstrual period (LMP) is the date generally used for calculating the day of delivery (280 days later based on Näegele's rule). This dating is most useful in women with normal 28-day cycles followed by abrupt cessation of menses. Only 15% of women have regular 28-day cycles, however.[5] Irregular menses, an atypical LMP, or the recent use of hormonal contraceptives confuses the diagnosis and dating of pregnancy. Some recent studies question the validity of Näegele's rule, estimating that the mode and median of time between the first day of a certain LMP and delivery date may be up to 282 days.[6]

Pregnancy tests are usually based on monoclonal antibodies raised against the β subunit of human chorionic gonadotrophin (β-hCG). These tests, including most home pregnancy tests, detect β-hCG concentrations in urine from 25 to 50 mIU/ml. Pregnancy may be diagnosed as early as 3 to 4 days after implantation, with positive results in 98% of women by 1 week after implantation (the time of missed menses).[7] Inaccurate readings occur as a result of not following the test instructions or misinterpreting the results. Serum radioimmunoassay testing detects β-hCG concentrations in the range of 2 to 10 mIU/ml.

Mean serum β-hCG levels correlate closely with gestational age during early pregnancy. Serum levels increase linearly during the first 6 weeks, doubling every 1.3 to 2 days in healthy gestations. Levels peak at 9 to 10 weeks, with the average β-hCG concentration around 50,000 mIU/ml. Women with levels less than 5000 mIU/ml are generally no further than 6 weeks of gestation.

IV. ESTABLISHING THE ESTIMATED DATE OF CONFINEMENT

Bimanual palpation of uterine size is necessary in the first 8 to 10 weeks because the fundus is not palpable transabdominally. In one prospective, blinded study, bimanual examinations done by faculty and residents were found to agree with ultrasound (±2 weeks) in 92% and 75% of examinations, respectively.[8] By 12 weeks, the fundus is palpable above the symphysis pubis, and fetal heart tones can be heard. Quickening, the subjective sensation of fetal movement, occurs between 16 and 18 weeks in multiparous women and between 19 and 20 weeks in primiparas. The fundus is at the umbilicus at 20 weeks; gestational age roughly corresponds to the centimeters between the symphysis pubis and fundus between 20 and 30 weeks.

Transvaginal ultrasound is a most accurate way of confirming intrauterine pregnancy and determining gestational age during the first trimester. It is particularly useful in women with an unknown LMP, irregular cycles, or in women taking oral contraceptives. In general, the earlier in pregnancy that the ultrasound is done, the less variability there is in the final due date. Earlier scans, therefore, provide more accurate estimates of gestational age. First-trimester scans can confirm gestational age within ±4 days. Transabdominal surveys done at 18 weeks confirm dating within ±1.5 weeks and usually include an anatomic screen for fetal anomalies.

No evidence directly correlates routine ultrasound screening with improved fetal outcomes. Routine ultrasound before 24 weeks allows for improved assessment of gestational age and decreased need for labor induction for postterm pregnancies. It allows for earlier detection of multifetal gestations and identification of fetal malformations at a time when termination is an option. No significant differences exist in clinical outcomes such as perinatal mortality.[9]

Nonmedical use of ultrasound has gained popularity, especially with the advent of three- and four-dimensional resolution scans. Both the American

Institute of Ultrasound in Medicine and the American College of Obstetricians and Gynecologists (ACOG) have endorsed policies against this practice. They strongly discourage the nonmedical use of ultrasound for entertainment purposes such as creating keepsake photos or videos. The use of ultrasound to view the fetus, to take photographs, or determine the sex without a medical indication is considered "contrary to responsible medical practice."[10] Nonmedical scans for entertainment purposes may falsely reassure women that the gestation is healthy when, in fact, a full anatomic survey is not done. Although these scans are marketed as nonmedical, abnormalities found may be unable to be addressed in this setting. This raises concerns expressed by both academies about adequate follow-up in the case of abnormal imaging.

V. SOR A RECOMMENDATION

RECOMMENDATION	REFERENCE
Routine ultrasound before 24 weeks allows for improved assessment of gestational age and decreased need for postterm induction. It allows for earlier detection of multifetal gestations and identification of fetal malformations at a time when termination is an option. No significant differences exist in clinical outcomes such as perinatal mortality.	*11*

REFERENCES

1. Robinson ET, Barber JH: Early diagnosis of pregnancy in general practice, *J R Coll Gen Pract* 27:335-338, 1977.
2. Zabin LS, Emerson MR, Ringers PA et al: Adolescents with negative pregnancy test results: an accessible at-risk group, *JAMA* 275:113-117, 1996.
3. Paul M, Schaff E, Nichols M: The roles of clinical assessment, human chorionic gonadotropin assays and ultrasonography in medical abortion practice, *Am J Obstet Gynecol* 183(2):S34-S43, 2000.
4. Krueger PM, Scholl TO: Adequacy of prenatal care and pregnancy outcome, *J Am Osteopath Assoc* 100(8):485-491, 2000.
5. Speroff L, Glass RH, Kase NG: *Clinical gynecologic endocrinology and infertility,* ed 6, Baltimore, 1999, Lippincott Williams & Wilkins.
6. Taipale P, Hiilesmaa V: Predicting delivery date by ultrasound and last menstrual period in early gestation, *Obstet Gynecol* 97:189-194, 2001.
7. Chard T: Pregnancy tests: a review, *Hum Reprod* 7:701-710, 1992.
8. Nichols M, Morgan E, Jensen JT: Comparing bimanual pelvic examination to ultrasound measurement for assessment of gestational age in the first trimester of pregnancy, *J Reprod Med* 47(10):825-828, 2002.
9. Neilson JP: Ultrasound for fetal assessment in early pregnancy, *Cochrane Database Syst Rev* (2):CD000182, 2000.
10. ACOG Committee on Ethics: ACOG Committee Opinion. Number 297, August 2004. Nonmedical use of obstetric ultrasonography, *Obstet Gynecol* 104(2):423-424, 2004.
11. Alexander GR, Kotelchuk M: Assessing the role and effectiveness of prenatal care: history, challenges, and directions for future research, *Public Health Rep* 116:306-316, 2001.

S E C T I O N   C   Prenatal Visits

Beth Choby, MD

I. PRECONCEPTION CARE

Preconception care involves the prevention of maternal–fetal morbidity and mortality through early detection and reduction of modifiable risks. Encompassing health promotion, risk assessment, and ntervention, it is a crucial encounter for addressing reproductive risk. Despite its usefulness in modifying risks from birth defects and adverse pregnancy outcomes, few women in the United States receive preconception care (see Chapter 2).

Why preconception care is underutilized is multifaceted. In the United States, planned pregnancies are the exception, as 50% of pregnancies in adults and 95% of pregnancies among teenagers are unplanned.[1] In a survey of health-care providers, 88% knew about the concept of preconception care, 93% considered it a part of their job responsibilities, and 91% planned to provide more of this care in the future. Still, 53% indicated that they lacked sufficient knowledge to provide adequate advice to prospective parents.[2] Factors hindering the provision of preconception care include resource constraints, lack of training, inadequate practice policies/procedures, and difficulty in identifying women planning to become pregnant. Further research is needed to explore these roadblocks.

All women of reproductive age should be considered at risk for pregnancy and be advised about anticipatory issues that are important in preconception. Ideal situations include office visits for contraception or negative pregnancy tests, well-woman examinations/Pap screening, and follow-up examinations for women with spontaneous pregnancy loss. Women with chronic medical problems such as diabetes, epilepsy, or heart disease benefit from addressing preconception issues at routine medical visits.

II. TOPICS OF INTEREST IN PRECONCEPTION CARE

A. Folic Acid

Annually, about 3000 pregnancies in the United States are affected by neural tube defects.[3] Periconceptual use of the B vitamin folic acid reduces the incidence of neural tube defects by 50% to 70%. Mothers with previous children with neural tube defects reduce their chance of having another affected pregnancy 72% by taking 4 mg folic acid daily in the preconception period and during the first trimester.[4] Women in their childbearing years should consume 400 μg folic acid daily through supplements, fortified foods, and a diet of folate-rich foods.

A recent national study found that only 40% of surveyed women reported routine use of vitamins with folic acid.[5] Nonwhite, young, and less educated women were least likely to report daily folic acid vitamin consumption. Twenty-four percent of women realized that folic acid prevents birth defects, whereas a mere 12% knew that folic acid provides maximum protection only when consumed before conception.

B. Diabetes

The worldwide prevalence of diabetes and impaired glucose tolerance in women of childbearing age is increasing, especially in young minority groups. In many areas of the world, pregnancies complicated by adult-onset diabetes are more common than type 1 diabetic gestations. The exact prevalence of diabetes in pregnancy is not well defined because large population studies are not available.[6]

Diabetes is associated with decreased fertility, spontaneous abortion, and congenital anomalies. Major congenital malformations are found in 4% to 10% of infants of mothers with diabetes compared with 1.2% to 2.1% of infants in the general population.[7] High levels of hemoglobin A1c (HgA1c) during organogenesis may cause malformations, with anomalies of the cardiac, skeletal, and nervous systems generally occurring before 8 weeks of gestation. Whether the association between HgA1c and malformations is linear or results when a certain glycemic threshold is reached is unknown.

Preconception care of the patient with diabetes emphasizes strict glycemic control before conception. The target for HgA1c is less than 6%, with fasting blood glucose levels between 4 and 7 mmol/L. Women should be counseled regarding risks for malformations, obstetric complications, effects of the pregnancy on maternal diabetes, and management options. A recent metaanalysis compared the risk for major congenital anomalies in women with pregestational diabetes who received preconception care verses those who did not. The 16 studies included both inpatient and outpatient glycemic manipulation. HgA1c values were significantly lower in the women who received preconception care. The crude pooled rate for major and minor anomalies was 2.4% in the women with preconception care compared with 7.7% in the noncare group.[8] Preconception care is likely cost-effective in women with diabetes, with estimates suggesting savings of $34,000 per patient.[9]

C. Epilepsy

Women with epilepsy have increased risks for infertility, spontaneous pregnancy loss, and fetuses with congenital anomalies. It is unknown whether anomalies result from the disease itself or the drugs used to manage it. One study compared three groups of pregnant women: women taking antiepileptic medication, women with epilepsy who were not taking medications, and a control group. The rate of major and minor malformations among the medicated group was 20.6%, compared with around 9% in the control and nonmedicated epileptic groups.[10] Congenital anomalies are more strongly linked to older antiepileptic medications including carbamazepine, valproic acid, and phenytoin. Polytherapy further increases risk. Newer medications such as gabapentin and lamotrigine may be safer, but insufficient data are currently available. Taking an increased dose of folic acid (1-4 mg daily) is recommended for women with epilepsy.

Preconception care benefits women with epilepsy. In a recent cohort study, women seen in a preconception epilepsy clinic were compared with women who received care after becoming pregnant. Women with preconception care were started on folic acid, shifted to monotherapy when possible, and 6% were able to completely discontinue antiepileptic medications. The group of women with preconception care had no major fetal anomalies, compared with 18% in the control group.[11]

D. Immunizations

Vaccines recommended for routine administration include inactivated influenza virus and tetanus/diphtheria toxoid.

1. Influenza

   Influenza vaccine is made from inactivated viruses and is safe at any stage of pregnancy. Vaccination is recommended in pregnancy because immune system down-regulation may increase the risk for influenza complications such as pneumonia. Risk is greatest during the third trimester and in women with underlying pulmonary pathology (e.g., asthma). All pregnant women who will be in the second or third trimester during flu season should be offered the influenza vaccine. Pregnant women with underlying health conditions should be immunized regardless of the stage of pregnancy.[12] Contraindications to influenza immunization include hypersensitivity to eggs (avidin) or to the preservatives used to manufacture the vaccine.

2. Diphtheria/tetanus

   Immunization with the diphtheria and tetanus toxoid vaccine 6 weeks before delivery protects the neonate against tetanus neonatorum via maternal IgG antibodies that cross the placenta. Women are similarly protected against puerperal tetanus. If there is no documentation of a diphtheria and tetanus booster within the past decade, one should be provided. Contraindications include a previous severe reaction to diphtheria and tetanus such as anaphylaxis, angioedema, or generalized urticaria. In pregnant women who have never received the initial tetanus series, the first dose should be followed by a second dose given 1 month later and a third dose given at 1 year.

E. Occupational and Environmental Issues

Because the majority of pregnant women work outside the home, workplace issues are important to address at the preconception visit. Many women ask their physicians about special work restrictions or precautions. Preterm delivery, low birth weight, fetal malformations, and prenatal mortality are not increased among employed women. Although employment does not increase risk, certain working conditions are associated with adverse pregnancy outcome. These include working more than 36 hours weekly or 10 hours daily, prolonged standing of more than 6 hours per shift, heavy lifting, excessive noise, and high fatigue score (more than 4 hours standing per shift, mental stress, and work environments with cold temperature or high noise levels).[13]

Counseling women to avoid toxic exposures is worthwhile during a preconception visit. Certain agents influence not only fertility but early gestation. Exposure to solvents (e.g., toluene, xylene, paint strippers, and thinners) or chemotherapeutic agents may increase rates of miscarriage and birth defects. Waste anesthetic gas may reduce fertility. Heavy metals (lead, mercury, and cadmium) adversely affect fetal neurologic development. Women anticipating becoming pregnant should avoid hyperthermia, known environmental toxins, and ionizing radiation. Microwaves, ultrasound, and radio waves are nonionizing and considered safe.

Significant amounts of information on occupational exposure are available, but quality varies because much of the literature is not evidence based. Because randomized controlled trials of pregnant women are not appropriate for ethical reasons, current guidance comes mostly from case series, expert opinion, and animal research.

III. SCHEDULE OF PRENATAL VISITS

Obstetric visits traditionally begin at 6 to 8 weeks of gestation, with return visits occurring monthly until 28 weeks of gestation. Visits are scheduled every 2 weeks from 28 to 36 weeks of gestation, with weekly visits thereafter until delivery. The schedule is more tradition based than evidenced based. A recent meta-analysis concludes that the traditional visit schedule can be abbreviated without increasing adverse maternal or perinatal outcomes. Although the abbreviated schedule is less expensive than the traditional schedule, women may be less satisfied with the reduced number of visits.[14] Still, one-third of women prefer an alternative visit schedule. Women with a history of stillbirth, miscarriage, or negative birth outcome may desire more visits, whereas multiparas and women older than 35 prefer an abbreviated course.[15]

Continuity of care during pregnancy by a single provider or team benefits women. Women with a continuity provider are more likely to discuss antenatal and postnatal concerns, attend prenatal education, require less analgesia during labor, and feel well prepared for the delivery and care of an infant.[16] Care provided by family physicians, midwives, and obstetricians is equally effective, although women may be more satisfied with care from family physicians and midwives.[17]

Women are sometimes given their own "case notes" detailing their prenatal care. Benefits include increased availability of records during hospitalization and increased maternal control and satisfaction. A Cochrane review noted that women carrying case notes have more operative deliveries, but that there is insufficient evidence of additional effects.[18]

IV. DOCUMENTATION OF CARE

Information collected during prenatal visits serves several purposes, the most important of which is identification of maternal or fetal risk factors that necessitate a higher acuity of care. Records are vehicles for quality assurance and medicolegal documentation, as well as for communication with other providers. A recent randomized controlled trial compared three methods of obtaining a prenatal history. Unstructured written histories were compared with structured written history (a paper checklist) and an interactive computer questionnaire. Whereas structured written notes provided better information and risk factor stratification than unstructured ones, computerized systems offered no benefit over structured written prenatal forms.[19]

V. SOR A RECOMMENDATIONS

RECOMMENDATIONS	REFERENCES
Women in their childbearing years should consume 400 μg folic acid daily through supplements, fortified foods, and a diet of folate-rich foods.	*20, 21*
The traditional visit schedule can be abbreviated without increasing adverse maternal or perinatal outcomes. Although the abbreviated schedule is less expensive than the traditional schedule, women may be less satisfied with the reduced number of visits.	*22*
Women with a continuity provider are more likely to discuss antenatal and postnatal concerns, attend prenatal education, require less analgesia during labor, and feel well prepared for the delivery and care of an infant.	*23*

REFERENCES

1. Henshaw S: Unintended pregnancy in the United States, *Fam Plann Perspect* 30:24-29, 1998.
2. Gaytant MA, Cikot RJ, Braspenning JC et al: Preconception counseling in family practice: a survey of 100 family physicians, *Ned Tijdschr Geneeskd* 142(21):1206-1210, 1998.
3. Centers for Disease Control: Spina bifida and anencephaly before and after folic acid mandate—United States, 1995-1996 and 1999-2000, *MMWR Morb Mortal Wkly Rep* 53:362-365, 2004.
4. Medical Research Council Vitamin Study Research Group: Prevention of neural tube defects: results of the Medical Research Council Vitamin Study, *Lancet* 338:131-137, 1991.
5. Center for Disease Control: Use of vitamins containing folic acid among women of childbearing age—United States, 2004, *MMWR Morb Mortal Wkly Rep* 53:847-850, 2004.
6. Lapolla A, Dalfra MG, Lencioni C et al: Epidemiology of diabetes in pregnancy: a review of Italian data, *Diabetes Nutr Metab* 17(6):358-367, 2004.
7. Muchowski K, Palandine H: An ounce of prevention: the evidence supporting periconception health care, *J Fam Pract* 53(2):126-133, 2004.
8. Ray JG, O'Brien TE, Chan WS: Preconception care and the risk of congenital anomalies in the offspring of women with diabetes mellitus: a meta-analysis, *QJM* 94(8):435-444, 2001.
9. Herman WH, Janz NK, Becker MP et al: Diabetes and pregnancy preconception care, pregnancy outcomes, resource utilization and costs, *J Reprod Med* 44:33-38, 1999.
10. Holmes LB, Harvey EA, Coull BA et al: The teratogenicity of anticonvulsant drugs, *N Engl J Med* 344:1132-1138, 2001.
11. Betts T, Fox C: Proactive pre-conception counseling for women with epilepsy—is it effective? *Seizure* 8:322-327, 1999.
12. Prevention and control of influenza: recommendations of the Advisory Committee on Immunization Practices, *MMWR Recomm Rep* 48(RR-4):1-28, 1999.
13. Institute for Clinical Systems Improvement: *Routine prenatal care.* Retrieved from www.icsi.org/guidelines_and_moreguidelines_order_sets_protocols_womens_health/prenatal_care_4/prenatal_care_routine_3.html. Accessed September 1, 2005.
14. Villar J, Carroli G, Khan-Neelofur D et al: Patterns of routine antenatal care for low-risk pregnancy, *Cochrane Database Syst Rev* (4):CD000934, 2001.
15. Hildingsson I, Waldenstrom U, Radestad I: Women's expectations on antenatal care as assessed in early pregnancy: number of visits, continuity of caregiver and general content, *Acta Obstet Gynecol Scand* 81(2):118-125, 2002.
16. Hodnett ED: Continuity of caregivers for care during pregnancy and childbirth, *Cochrane Database Syst Rev* (2):CD000062, 2000.
17. Vintzileos AM, Ananth CV, Smulian JC et al: The impact of prenatal care on postneonatal deaths in the presence and absence of antenatal high-risk conditions, *Am J Obstet Gynecol* 187:1258-1262, 2002.
18. Brown HC, Smith HJ: Giving women their own case notes to carry during pregnancy, *Cochrane Database Syst Rev* (2): CD002856, 2004.
19. Lilford RJ, Kelly M, Baines A et al: Effect of using protocols on medical care: randomized trial of three methods of taking an antenatal history, *Br Med J* 39:54-57, 1992.
20. Vintzileos AM, Ananth CV, Smulian JC et al: The impact of prenatal care in the United States on preterm births in the presence and absence of antenatal high-risk conditions, *Am J Obstet Gynecol* 187:1254-1257, 2002.
21. Braveman D, Marchi K, Egerter S et al: Barriers to timely prenatal care among women with insurance: the importance of pre-pregnancy factors, *Obstet Gynecol* 95:874-880, 2000.
22. Chard T: Pregnancy tests: a review, *Hum Reprod* 7:701-710, 1992.
23. Neilson JP: Ultrasound for fetal assessment in early pregnancy, *Cochrane Database Syst Rev* (2):CD000182, 2000.

Section D **Initial Assessment**

Beth Choby, MD

The first prenatal visit is comprehensive, with significant time dedicated to the medical and obstetric history and the initial physical examination. The appointment ideally occurs during the first trimester and sometimes requires an additional visit to cover all pertinent information. Needs of the pregnant patient are assessed during this appointment, with attention to identifying women at increased risk for adverse maternal–fetal outcomes. The visit also serves as a counseling session, particularly for women who lack preconception care.

I. INITIAL PRENATAL VISIT HISTORY

A. Medical and Surgical History

A thorough obstetric, medical, surgical, and family history should be obtained. Documentation of gravidity, parity, spontaneous pregnancy loss/induced abortion, and living children should be recorded. Parity is easily remembered using the mnemonic TPAL (term deliveries, preterm deliveries, abortions: spontaneous or induced, and total living children). Previous poor obstetric outcomes should be explored, especially preterm delivery and stillbirth. Women with a history of gestational diabetes, type 2 diabetes, gestational hypertension, multiple gestation, or isoimmunization need to be identified and triaged to an appropriate level of care. Surgical history of importance includes any procedures involving the uterus, fallopian tubes, cervix, or vagina. Cervical insufficiency (incompetence) sometimes occurs after loop electrosurgical excision procedure (LEEP). A prior cesarean delivery increases the risk for uterine rupture. Scar type and indication for surgery should be documented. Careful risk stratification is essential for any woman contemplating a trial of labor after cesarean.

B. Family and Genetic History

The ethnicity of both parents should be determined to allow for discussion of risk assessment and genetic counseling. Family history of interest includes any birth defects, mental retardation, or genetic conditions on the maternal or paternal sides. Genetic testing and informed consent are discussed in the following section.

C. Social History/Use of Substances

1. Maternal alcohol use
   Maternal alcohol use is the leading cause of birth defects and mental retardation in the United States. Fetal alcohol syndrome (FAS) is more prevalent than spina bifida or Down syndrome. Risk for FAS is related to the gestational age at the time of alcohol exposure and the amount and frequency of consumption. Women who binge drink or drink heavily are at increased risk for FAS. Episodic binge drinking (defined as greater than five drinks on a single day) is more dangerous to fetal neurologic development than nonbinge consumption.[1] Whether there is a safe amount of alcohol use in pregnancy has yet to be elucidated. Women have historically been advised not to drink any alcohol while pregnant. Certain guidelines suggest that women limit alcohol consumption to no more than one serving of alcohol daily (one regular shot, one small glass wine, or one half pint of beer).[2] Because current information on alcohol consumption during pregnancy is inconsistent, most physicians continue to recommend that women not consume alcohol when pregnant.

2. Smoking
   Smoking is a major modifiable cause of adverse pregnancy outcomes; the dangers of smoking during pregnancy are widely publicized. Vasoconstriction of placental blood flow restricts the delivery of oxygen and nutrients to the fetus. Carbon monoxide diffuses across the placenta and displaces oxygen needed by the fetus. Meta-analyses demonstrate significant associations between maternal smoking and increased perinatal mortality, placental abruption, preterm premature rupture of membranes, placenta previa, preterm delivery, miscarriage and ectopic pregnancy, low birth weight, sudden infant death syndrome, and cleft lip/palate in offspring of smokers.[3] The incidence of preeclampsia may be decreased in a dose-effect manner in women who smoke, although this finding must be taken in context with the numerous harmful risks caused by smoking during pregnancy.[4]
   Approximately 11.5% of pregnant women in the United States smoke while pregnant. These statistics are improved from 1990, when 18.4% of pregnant women reported smoking (38% decrease).[5] The percentage of women in the United States

who smoke during pregnancy is greatest in white women (15.6%), moderate in African American women (9.1%), and lowest in Hispanic women (3.5%).[6] The percentage of teenagers who smoke during pregnancy has also declined.

Neonatal health-care expenditures attributed to maternal smoking cost $366 million annually in the United States.[7] Smoking cessation programs may be a crucial means for preventing adverse obstetric outcomes and decreasing the financial and social costs of pregnancy care. A Cochrane review finds a significant reduction in smoking during late pregnancy in women who attend smoking cessation programs versus those who do not.[8] Studies show a reduction in preterm birth and an increase in mean birth weight of 28 g in women who receive intervention, although no difference is noted in very low-birth-weight or perinatal mortality. Another review shows that antenatal smoking cessation programs significantly increase the percentage of expectant women who quit smoking.[9] Even a reduction in the number of cigarettes smoked confers a benefit on the fetus secondary to increased birth weight.

3. Use of illicit drugs

Approximately 5% of women in the United States use illicit substances during pregnancy. Of women who use illicit drugs, half are in their childbearing years (age, 15-44 years). Marijuana and cocaine are the most frequently used drugs, although ecstasy, amphetamines (crystal meth), heroin, and prescription narcotics are also abused. Women using illicit drugs during pregnancy are at increased risk for adverse pregnancy outcome, including sexually transmitted disease, hepatitis, abruption, and psychiatric morbidity. Infants are at risk for preterm delivery, low birth weight, and possible long-term behavioral problems. Women should be counseled about the risks of illicit substance use in pregnancy and offered treatment.

II. INITIAL CLINICAL EXAMINATION

A. Key Elements of the General Examination

The initial prenatal visit involves a complete physical examination. The head and neck examination includes evaluation of the thyroid and dentition. Periodontitis in pregnancy is associated with an increased risk for preterm delivery. A recent randomized controlled trial demonstrated that the aggressive prenatal management of periodontal disease did not reduce the incidence of preterm delivery.[10] Cardiac auscultation reveals increased splitting of the first and second heart sounds by the end of the first trimester. A systolic flow murmur along the left sternal border is often heard. The abdominal examination should include documentation of any scars and a comparison with the previous surgical history. A brief neurologic examination includes patellar and ankle reflexes. Because preeclampsia often presents with changes in reflexes, the initial examination can be used for later comparison when needed.

Clinical components of routine prenatal visits are not universally agreed on. Although most guidelines recommend routine measurement of fundal height, blood pressure, maternal weight, and fetal heart tones, the evidence supporting the recommendations varies. Specific issues for which direct evidence is available are discussed later.

B. Weight Gain

The normal range of weight gain in pregnancy varies for each woman. Recommended weight gain during pregnancy depends on the prepregnancy body mass index (BMI) (Table 3-1).

Maternal weight and height should be measured and BMI calculated during the initial examination.[11] Although a correlation exists between maternal weight gain and infant birth weight, this is not a reliable screening method for predicting low-birth-weight deliveries. Historically, maternal weight is measured at each prenatal visit. Some recent guidelines question whether routine weights should be abandoned because the information may not change clinical management and creates undue anxiety.[3] Women in whom nutrition is of concern (i.e., initial BMI <19.8 or >29) may benefit from routine weights.

C. Measurement of Blood Pressure

Most clinical guidelines recommend blood pressure monitoring. The Institute for Clinical Systems Improvement (ICSI), Veteran's Health Administration, and National Collaborating Centre for Women's and Children's Health all recommend routine blood pressure measurement at the initial and return visits.[12-14] The Korotkoff 5 sound, or the disappearance of sound, is used for determining the diastolic blood pressure.

TABLE 3-1 **Recommended Weight Gain during Pregnancy**

Maternal Classification	Weight Gain (kg)		Weight Gain (lb)	
	Total (kg)	Rate (kg/4 wk)*	Total (lb)	Rate (lb/4 wk)*
Prepregnant BMI†				
Underweight (<19.8)	12.7-18.2	2.3	28-40	5.0
Normal weight (19.8-28.0)	11.4-15.9	1.8	25-35	4.0
Overweight (28.1-29.0)	6.8-11.4	1.2	16-25	2.6
Obese (>29.0)	6.8	0.9	15	2.0
Twin gestation	15.9-20.4	2.7	35-45	6.0

*Rate applies to the second and third trimesters.
†Body mass index (BMI) is derived from metric units.
Adapted from National Academy of Sciences: *Nutrition during pregnancy,* Washington, DC, 1990, National Academy Press.

D. Breast Examination

The breast examination is done at the first visit to look for flat or inverted nipples or, less commonly, signs of breast disease such as fibrocystic changes or cancer. Traditionally, women with flat or inverted nipples were prescribed either breast shields or nipple exercises. Two randomized controlled trials find no clear evidence that either treatment improves success in breastfeeding and recommend that routine examination of the nipples be discontinued.[15,16] Although not recommended for the promotion of breastfeeding, routine breast examination during the initial visit may be useful in diagnosing occult breast disease.

E. Pelvic Examination

The initial pelvic examination is useful for detecting anatomic abnormalities of the reproductive tract and screening for sexually transmitted diseases and cervical dysplasia. Pelvimetry and bimanual examination of the uterus and cervix are traditional components.

The cervical examination includes documentation of the cervical length, effacement, and dilation. Comparison with the initial examination is important in case preterm labor or cervical insufficiency develop later in the gestation. Routine cervical examination (at every prenatal visit) is not an effective method of predicting preterm birth and should be discouraged.[12] Medically indicated cervical examinations, that is, gravid women with abdominal pain, are

recommended. Screening recommendations for cervical cancer and sexually transmitted disease are covered in Section E.

Clinical pelvimetry is considered by many physicians to be a routine part of the initial examination. Information is used both for an estimate of pelvic adequacy and as a predictor for cesarean delivery. In several recent studies, however, the prognostic value of pelvimetry in cephalic presentations is unclear.[17] Limited evidence exists of interobserver agreement with pelvimetry, and x-ray pelvimetry, presumed to be more accurate, is not a successful predictor of need for cesarean delivery.[18] Because most women are offered a trial of labor, pelvimetry may be less likely to alter labor management. A Cochrane review of x-ray pelvimetry similarly finds insufficient evidence to support its use in pregnant women with fetuses in cephalic presentation.[19] Three national guidelines recommend discontinuing routine pelvimetry (clinical or radiographic) in routine prenatal care secondary to concerns of its inability to predict actual cephalopelvic disproportion and the association with increased cesarean rates.[11,12,20]

F. Fundal Height and Fetal Heart Tones

If the patient presents for care in the second or third trimester, measurement of the symphysis-fundal height provides a good estimate of uterine size and gestational age. Sequential measurements allow for monitoring of fetal growth over time. Currently, not enough evidence is available to evaluate the use of fundal height in routine antenatal care. Considering that it is inexpensive and requires minimal resources and training to provide, it is not recommended that it be discontinued unless better research becomes available. Whether fundal height measurements are of clinical use after 36 weeks of gestation has yet to be determined.[2]

Auscultation of the fetal heart is an anticipated part of standard prenatal visits for many expectant parents. Although hearing the fetal heart confirms that the fetus is alive, fetal well-being is difficult to evaluate, because decelerations or variability are rarely noted with Doppler. This part of the examination is likely reassuring for pregnant women and physicians, although research has not been done to this end. Guidelines differ regarding the use of routine fetal heart rate auscultation. Both ICSI and the VA recommend assessing fetal heart tones at each prenatal visit beginning at 10 to 12 weeks; the recommendations are based on expert opinion. National Institute for Clinical Excellence (NICE) guidelines state that routine auscultation cannot be recommended using currently available studies. However, when requested by the mother, fetal heart auscultation is believed to be reassuring. Further large randomized controlled trials are necessary to clarify the role and effect of fetal heart rate monitoring.

III. COUNSELING AT THE FIRST PRENATAL VISIT

Time should be provided at the initial visit for counseling on nutrition and exercise, lifestyle changes, and infectious exposures.

A. Dietary and Nutritional Needs

Pregnant women have an additional caloric requirement of 150 calories per day in the first trimester and 300 to 500 extra calories per day in the last two trimesters. Average daily caloric intake is 1900 to 2800 calories for most gravid women.

Women should be provided information about the benefits of a varied diet during pregnancy. Fifty to sixty percent of the diet should be carbohydrate based because the fetus uses glucose as an energy source and carbohydrate depletion can affect fetal growth. Fats comprise 30% of the diet. An additional 30 g protein is needed daily in pregnancy. This is best obtained through dairy sources such as milk, cheese, and yogurt. Recent Cochrane reviews on protein supplementation for pregnant women did not find adequate evidence to recommend extra protein supplements.[21,22]

B. Dietary Restrictions and Safety Issues

Pregnant women are at risk for certain food-borne diseases, including listeriosis. Listeriosis is a bacterial infection associated with preterm delivery, chorioamnionitis, and fetal demise. Transmission is food-borne, and pregnant women should avoid milk, fruit juice, cheese, or dairy products that are not pasteurized. Soft mold-ripened cheese, such as Camembert and Brie, and all varieties of pâté are best avoided. Recent outbreaks of listeriosis have been linked to certain delicatessen cold cuts.

Additional foods that present a risk during pregnancy include undercooked meat, raw shellfish, and certain varieties of fish. Consuming undercooked beef can result in *Escherichia coli* food poisoning. Pregnant women should be counseled to eat beef that is cooked well-done. *Vibrio parahemolyticus,* hepatitis A, *Vibrio cholerae,* shigatoxin, and certain parasites are found in raw shellfish such as oysters and some types of sushi. Mercury exposure is possible with consumption of tilefish, monkfish, swordfish, shark, and king mackerel. Because mercury may adversely affect fetal neurologic function, the U.S. Food and Drug Administration (FDA) advises women not to consume more than 12 ounces of tuna per week if they are pregnant.[23]

Caffeine intake of less than 300 mg a day does not increase the risk for miscarriage or low birth weight. Caffeine crosses the placenta and affects the fetus. Artificial sweeteners such as aspartame and Splenda are unlikely to cause fetal toxicity. Because the major breakdown product of aspartame is phenylalanine, women with phenylketonuria should avoid this product. Serum levels that cause mental retardation in fetuses of women with phenylketonuria are generally far greater than those levels found with average intake of aspartame.

C. Exercise in Pregnancy

Historically, physical activity during pregnancy has been discouraged because of theoretical concerns of hyperthermia, exercise-induced injury, fetal hypoxia, and the risk for preterm labor (see Chapter 4, Section F). Only recently has good evidence demonstrated that exercise in pregnancy is safe and beneficial. Numerous studies since 1985 show no adverse fetal effects in women who participate in mild-to-moderate exercise. ACOG recently modified its guidelines, stating that pregnancy is an excellent time for behavior modification, and that evidence no longer supports the idea that pregnancy requires a sedentary lifestyle. In the absence of medical complications, ACOG now recommends 30 minutes of mild-to-moderate physical activity during most days of the week. Women with medical problems are encouraged to have a medical evaluation before beginning an exercise program. Additional research suggests that exercise plays a role in the prevention and management of gestational diabetes.[24]

Regular exercise improves maternal fitness and well-being, moderates maternal weight gain, and reduces many musculoskeletal complaints. Pregnant women should be offered individualized exercise programs based on their prepregnancy fitness level.

D. Seat Belt Use

Motor vehicle accidents are a leading cause of death and disability in pregnant women. Although the effectiveness of restraints in reducing morbidity is well established, compliance with seatbelt use is less than ideal. In one study of restraint use, 98% of women claimed to wear a seatbelt when in the front seat. About 68% of backseat passengers reported seat belt use. Less than 50% of respondents could correctly identify how to wear a seatbelt while pregnant. Only one-third of women reported being counseled on the importance of using restraints.[25] Pregnant women should be counseled to wear three-point restraints either when driving or as passenger. The belt should fit snugly, with the lap belt positioned under the uterus and across the hips and the shoulder belt above the fundus and between the breasts. Belts should never be worn over the uterus or atop the fundus.

E. Sexual Intercourse during Pregnancy

Large cohort studies report an inverse relation between the frequency of intercourse and the risk for preterm delivery. Pregnant women should be counseled that sexual intercourse is not known to be associated with adverse pregnancy outcomes.

IV. SOR A RECOMMENDATIONS

RECOMMENDATIONS	REFERENCES
Pregnant women should be counseled on the adverse effects of smoking during pregnancy such as low birth weight and preterm delivery. Benefits of quitting exist at all stages of pregnancy. Women unable to quit should be encouraged to reduce smoking.	26, 27
Interventions useful in reducing smoking in pregnancy include physician advice, group sessions, and behavioral modification.	20
Pregnant women should be offered fundal height measurement at each antenatal appointment to detect small- or large-for-gestational-age fetuses.	20
Healthy, pregnant women are encouraged to participate in mild-to-moderate exercise three or more times weekly.	28, 29
Pregnant women should be informed that sexual intercourse during pregnancy is not associated with any untoward effects.	3

REFERENCES

1. Maier SE, West JR: Drinking patterns and alcohol-related birth defects, *Alcohol Res Health* 25:168-174, 2001.
2. Vintzileos AM, Ananth CV, Smulian JC et al: The impact of prenatal care in the United States on preterm births in the presence and absence of antenatal high-risk conditions, *Am J Obstet Gynecol* 187:1254-1257, 2002.
3. National Collaborating Centre for Women's and Children's Health: Antenatal care routine care for the healthy prenatal woman. Clinical Guideline October 2003. Royal College of Obstetricians and Gynecologists. Retrieved from www.rcog.org.uk/index.asp?pageID=693. Accessed August 19, 2007.
4. Hammoud AO, Bujold E, Sorokin Y et al: Smoking in pregnancy revisited: findings from a large population-based study. *Am J Obstet Gynecol* 192:1856-1863, 2005.
5. Centers for Disease Control: MMWR weekly reporter; smoking during pregnancy—1990-2002, *MMWR Morb Mortal Wkly Rep* 53(39):511-519, 2004.
6. MacDorman MF, Minino AM, Strobino DM et al: Annual summary of vital statistics—2001, *Pediatrics* 110:1037-1052, 2002.
7. U.S. Department of Health and Human Services, Public Health Service: *Women and smoking: a report of the Surgeon General.* Washington, DC, 2001, Office of the Surgeon General.
8. Lumley J, Oliver S, Walter E: Interventions for promoting smoking cessation during pregnancy, *Cochrane Database Syst Rev* (4):CD001055, 2004.

9. Law M, Tang JL: An analysis of the effectiveness of interventions intended to help people stop smoking, *Arch Int Med* 155:1933-1941, 1995.

10. Michalowicz BS, Hodges JS, DiAngelis AJ et al: Treatment of periodontal disease and the risk of preterm birth, *N Engl J Med* 355:1885-1894, 2006.

11. Krueger PM, Scholl TO: Adequacy of prenatal care and pregnancy outcome, *JAOA* 100(8):485-491, 2000.

12. Guyer B: Medicaid and prenatal care. Necessary but not sufficient, *JAMA* 264:2264-2265, 1990.

13. Institute for Clinical Systems Improvement (ICSI): *Routine prenatal care,* Bloomington, MN, 2004, Institute for Clinical Systems Improvement (ICSI).

14. Veterans Health Administration, Department of Defense: *DoD/VA clinical practice guideline for the management of uncomplicated pregnancy,* Washington, DC, 2002, Department of Veteran Affairs.

15. Alexander JM, Grant AM, Campbell MJ: Randomized controlled trial of breast shells and Hoffman's exercises for inverted and non-protractile nipples, *BMJ* 304(6833):1030-1032, 1992.

16. Preparing for breastfeeding: treatment of non-protractile and inverted nipples in pregnancy. The MAIN Trial Collaborative Group, *Midwifery* 10(4):200-214, 1994.

17. Van Loon AJ, Mantingh A, Serlier EK et al: Randomized controlled trial of magnetic-resonance pelvimetry in breech presentation at term, *Lancet* 350:1799-1804, 1997.

18. Blackadar CS, Viera AJ: A retrospective review of performance and utility of routine clinical pelvimetry, *Fam Med* 36(7):505-507, 2004.

19. Pattinson RC: Pelvimetry for fetal cephalic presentations at term, *Cochrane Database Syst Rev* CD000161, 2003.

20. Kogan MD, Martin JA, Alexander GR et al: The changing pattern of prenatal care utilization in the United States, 1981-1995 using different prenatal care indices, *JAMA* 279(20):1623-1628, 1998.

21. Kramer MS: High protein supplementation in pregnancy, *Cochrane Database Syst Rev* CD000105, 2000.

22. Kramer MS: Isocaloric balanced protein supplementation in pregnancy, *Cochrane Database Syst Rev* CD000118, 2000.

23. March of Dimes: *Food safety.* Available at: http://www.marchofdimes.com/pnhec/159_826.asp. Accessed August 28, 2005.

24. Artal R, O'Toole M: Guidelines of the American College of Obstetricians and Gynecologists for exercise during pregnancy and the postpartum period, *Br J Sports Med* 37:6-12, 2003.

25. Tyroch AH, Kaups KL, Rohan J et al: Pregnant women and car restraints: beliefs and practices, *J Trauma Infect Cri Care* 46(2):241-245, 1999.

26. Maupin R, Lyman R, Fatsis J et al: Characteristics of women who deliver with no prenatal care, *J Matern Fetal Neonatal Med* 16:45-50, 2004.

27. Braveman D, Marchi K, Egerter S et al: Barriers to timely prenatal care among women with insurance: the importance of pre-pregnancy factors, *Obstet Gynecol* 95:874-880, 2000.

28. Speroff L, Glass RH, Kase NG: *Clinical gynecologic endocrinology and infertility,* ed 6, Baltimore, 1999, Lippincott Williams & Wilkins.

29. Medical Research Council Vitamin Study Research Group: Prevention of neural tube defects: results of the Medical Research Council Vitamin Study, *Lancet* 338:131-137, 1991.

S E C T I O N E Monitoring
the Progress of Pregnancy

Jeffrey D. Quinlan, MD

I. ONGOING RISK ASSESSMENT

History taking after the initial complete evaluation should focus on continuous risk assessment. If during the initial evaluation, high-risk conditions, such as substance abuse (including tobacco and alcohol), poor nutrition, teratogen exposure, or social problems (including domestic abuse), have been identified, ongoing surveillance and appropriate treatment should occur. If referrals were made based on these findings, determination of patient compliance should be documented. If referrals or counseling have not been completed, the patient should be encouraged to do so. Ongoing risk assessment is important due to the dynamic and changing nature of pregnancy; unfortunately, risk scoring systems have not been shown to replace this ongoing assessment by prenatal care providers because of their low positive predictive value.[1]

A. Important Signs and Symptoms

Nausea, vaginal bleeding, discharge or leaking of fluid, contractions, and dysuria are commonly encountered in pregnancy. Because each may indicate potential complications with the pregnancy, assessment for them should be made at each visit.

B. Preterm Labor

In the middle of the second trimester, patients should be educated about the common signs of preterm labor and should be questioned about the presence of clinical signs of preterm labor at each visit between 20 and 36 weeks. Scoring systems that have been published for stratifying risk for preterm labor or delivery have been evaluated in a systematic review[2] and were found to vary widely by their ability to accurately predict preterm delivery.

C. Fetal Movement

Fetal movement has been demonstrated to be a sign of fetal well-being (see Chapter 11, Section B). Because 98% of infants have been shown to move by the 75th minute of evaluation beginning at 24 weeks of gestation,[3] women should be educated in the late second trimester to evaluate for fetal movement on a daily basis. History at each antenatal visit should then address the woman's ability to determine movement. However, fetal movement counting is best viewed as a long-term assessment of placental sufficiency and, if abnormal, should prompt additional testing such as a nonstress test or biophysical profile, depending on the setting.[4]

D. Symptoms Suggestive of Hypertensive Disorders

In the third trimester, evaluation for symptoms of hypertensive disorders of pregnancy should be made, including determining the presence of headache, visual disturbance, and/or abdominal pain.

II. PHYSICAL EXAMINATION

Physical examination during the second and third trimesters should include auscultation of fetal heart tones, measurement of fundal height, and screening for hypertensive disorders and inappropriate weight gain. If the patient's blood pressure or history indicates possible hypertensive disorders of pregnancy, further neurologic examination should be completed, including examination for deep tendon reflexes and presence of clonus.

By 34 to 36 weeks, determination of fetal presentation should be made. This can be done with Leopold's maneuvers, cervical examination, or ultrasound. Routine cervical examination for the determination of preterm labor is not recommended. Likewise, although routine evaluation for edema, as a sign of hypertensive disorder of pregnancy, was previously commonplace, the presence of dependent edema is too common to be beneficial.

III. LABORATORY TESTING

The evidence and rationale for routine and selective laboratory testing in pregnancy are presented in the following section (see Section F).

IV. HEALTH PROMOTION ACTIVITIES

Health promotion efforts should be directed at educating the woman and her family about physiologic changes of pregnancy, sexuality, and common discomforts that most women experience, together with corresponding comfort measures. Exercise and fitness

and the benefits of breastfeeding should be encouraged beginning early and continuing throughout normal pregnancy. Advice on seatbelts and travel precautions should be given. In the third trimester, more information on fetal development, anticipated family adjustments, childbirth (normal and possible complications), parenting classes, and postpartum family planning should be covered. All patient education should be documented in the record.[5] Kirkham and colleagues[6] have written an excellent evidence-based review of patient counseling issues during pregnancy (review is available online at: http://www.aafp.org/afp/20050401/1307.pdf).

REFERENCES

1. Wall EM: Assessing obstetric risk. A review of obstetric risk-scoring systems, *J Fam Pract* 27:153-163, 1988.
2. Honest H, Bachmann LM, Sundaram R et al: The accuracy of risk scores in predicting preterm birth: a systematic review, *J Obstet Gynaecol* 24:343-359, 2004.
3. Rayburn WF: Monitoring fetal body movement, *Clin Obstet Gynecol* 30:899-911, 1987.
4. Christensen FC, Rayburn WF: Fetal movement counts, *Obstet Gynecol Clin North Am* 26(4):607-621, 1999.
5. Cline MK, Baxley EG, Noller KL: *Updated version: Normal pregnancy reference guide,* ed 8, Lexington, KY, 2003, American Board of Family Practice.
6. Kirkham C, Harris S, Grzybowski S: Evidence-based prenatal care: part 1. General prenatal care and counseling issues, *Am Fam Physician* 71:1307-1316, 2005.

SECTION F Screening in Pregnancy and Predictive Value

Jeffrey D. Quinlan, MD, and Matthew K. Cline, MD

I. APPROPRIATE SETTINGS AND CRITERIA FOR SCREENING TESTS

For screening of medical conditions in pregnancy to be of value, the condition and the screening test have to satisfy several criteria:

1. The condition has a significant impact on care or outcomes.

2. The incidence of the problem is sufficient to support the costs of screening.
3. Acceptable treatment exists.
4. An asymptomatic window exists during which the screening test can detect the condition.
5. Treatment during the asymptomatic phase yields superior results.
6. The screening test needs to be:
   a. Available
   b. Acceptable to patients
   c. Accurate (sensitive and specific)
   d. Affordable

One test that meets these criteria is the screening of all prenatal patients for syphilis at the first prenatal visit. Congenital syphilis can have a significant impact on prenatal outcomes because it may cause stillbirth, miscarriage, or newborn disease, as well as cardiac or neurologic infection in the mother. The incidence, although low, has been increasing slowly in the United States. Injectable penicillin is an effective and acceptable treatment, and treatment during early pregnancy can cure the mother and prevent neonatal complications. The screening test is widely available, has good accuracy except in very early or late disease, is generally acceptable to patients in that it is a simple blood test, and is affordable. With all of these factors, cost analysis has shown that prenatal screening for syphilis is cost-effective when the prevalence of disease is as low as 1 in 20,000 patients (0.005%).[1]

II. USE OF THE NUMBER NEEDED TO DIAGNOSE

The evaluation of screening tests is affected by the varying prevalence in different populations. This variation leads to changing positive and negative predictive value depending on the disease prevalence of the screened population. Positive predictive value is the likelihood that a positive test result reflects the presence of the target condition or disease, whereas negative predictive value is the likelihood that a negative test result reflects the absence of a target condition or disease.

Evidence-based medicine has led to widespread use of the concept of *number needed to treat* (NNT). One method of evaluating screening tests that is less dependent on population details is the *number needed to diagnose* (NND), which is defined as the number of patients with the condition in question who need to be screened to detect a single case.[2] In this construct, a perfect test would have a NND of 1.00, whereas

TABLE 3-2 Diagnosis of Asymptomatic Bacteriuria

Test	Sensitivity	Specificity	Number Needed to Diagnose
Leukocyte esterase	85%	73%	1.72
Nitrites	60%	96%	1.78
Microscopic evaluation	83%	59%	2.38

most screening tests vary from NNDs of just greater than 1.00 to 1.5. The larger the NND, the greater the number of patients (with the target condition) who would have to be screened to detect a single case. The NND would allow each clinician to determine the usefulness of any screening test in a local population based on local prevalence of a known condition.

As an example of the use of the NND, consider the alternatives to urine culture for diagnosis of asymptomatic bacteriuria (ASB; see Section J in following section): dipstick tests (presence of leukocyte esterase or nitrite) or microscopic evaluation of the sediment for white blood cells and bacteria. For each of these alternative tests, the average sensitivity, specificity, and NND are shown in Table 3-2.[3]

Given this information, the dipstick tests would be viewed as superior to a microscopic evaluation of the urinary sediment as a screening test for ASB, with the leukocyte esterase having a slightly better NND. With a NND greater than 1.5, however, none of these tests would serve as a good screening test because they require 1.72 to 2.38 patients with ASB to be screened to detect 1 patient with the condition. Because of these limitations, culture remains the recommended screening test for ASB.

III. SPECIFIC SCREENING TESTS

A. Hepatitis B Surface Antigen

An estimated 22,000 infants are born in the United States each year to women who have chronic hepatitis B infection. The incidence of acute infection in pregnancy is 1 to 2 per 1000 pregnancies, and the prevalence of chronic infection is 5 to 15 per 1000 pregnancies. Women who are positive for the hepatitis B antigen at the time of delivery have a 70% to 90% risk of infecting their offspring. Vaccination plus a single dose of hepatitis B immunoglobulin given within 12 hours of birth is at least 75% effective in preventing hepatitis B infection in the newborn.[4]

Risk factors for maternal hepatitis B infection include multiple sexual partners and intravenous drug abuse, but population studies have failed to find a known risk factor in greater than 30% of cases.[5] Targeted screening in urban and minority populations has been able to detect only 35% to 65% of pregnant women who are positive for hepatitis B surface antigen. The U.S. Preventive Services Task Force states that universal screening at the first prenatal visit is a level A recommendation,[6] indicating that all pregnant women should be screened at the initial prenatal visit with a hepatitis B surface antigen assay.

Presence of hepatitis B surface antigen is detected by an immunoassay that has a reported sensitivity and specificity exceeding 98%.[7] Using 0.98 for each, the NND for this test is 1.04, which is excellent (i.e., to detect 1 patient with the presence of hepatitis B surface antigen using this immunoassay would require screening 1.04 patients who actually have this condition).

In groups with a greater prevalence of hepatitis B infection (Southeast Asians, Pacific Islanders, Alaskan Native Americans, drug addicts, transfusion recipients, women on dialysis, and those who have had recent tattoos), consideration should be given to re-screening for hepatitis B in the late second trimester or early third trimester (SOR C, Expert Opinion).[8]

B. Syphilis

Congenital syphilis is spread in a transplacental fashion during pregnancy from an infected mother to the fetus and is associated with significant morbidity and mortality for the newborn. Congenital syphilis infection results in fetal or perinatal death in 40% of affected pregnancies,[9] as well as disease complications in surviving newborns, including central nervous system abnormalities, deafness, multiple skin, bone, and joint deformities, and hematologic disorders.[10] Although rates of syphilis decreased steadily in the 1990s, in 2001, rates increased for the first time in a decade. In 2002, the rate of congenital syphilis infection nationwide was 11.1 per 100,000 live births, with state incident rates ranging from 0 to 31.1 per 100,000 live births.[11]

Early detection allows use of antibiotics that can cure infection and prevent future sequelae or congenital infection of the newborn. Cost-effectiveness studies show benefit for prenatal screening when the prevalence of disease is 1 in 20,000 births (0.005%).[12] The U.S. Preventive Services Task Force recommends (level A) routine serologic testing of all pregnant women for syphilis at the onset of prenatal care,[13] and the Centers for Disease Control and Prevention (CDC) suggests repeat serologic testing in the third trimester for patients at high risk, such as those with multiple sexual partners or intravenous drug users.[14]

Testing for syphilis is done using a serologic (nontreponemal test) such as the rapid plasma reagin (RPR) or Venereal Disease Research Laboratory (VDRL). These tests are sensitive to the anticardiolipin antibody that occurs during the primary stage of syphilis. Sensitivity of the RPR and VDRL tests are estimated to be 78% to 86% for detecting primary syphilis infection, 100% for detecting secondary syphilis infection, and 95% to 98% for detecting latent syphilis infection. Specificity ranges from 85% to 99%. False-positive results are common because similar antibodies can occur during other conditions such as collagen vascular disease, pregnancy, intravenous drug use, advanced malignancy, tuberculosis, malaria, and viral and rickettsial diseases. Because of this lower specificity, a positive serologic test always should be confirmed by a specific treponemal test, such as the fluorescent treponemal antibody absorption or microhemagglutination-*Treponema pallidum*. These tests have a specificity of about 96% but remain positive for life (as compared with serologic tests, which decline in titer or revert to negative with successful treatment).[15]

With the aforementioned sensitivity and specificity, serologic tests of syphilis have a range of NND based on the stage of the illness. For early primary and late tertiary syphilis, the NND is 2.1 to 2.7. For late primary and secondary syphilis, the NND is 1.18 to 1.33.

C. Chlamydia

Chlamydia is the most common nonviral sexually transmitted disease in the United States, with more than 2.4 million cases reported annually. More than 70% of women are asymptomatic. The prevalence of chlamydial infection in pregnant women ranges between 10.1% and 17.1%[16,17]; and about 155,000 mothers each year are infected at the time of delivery, and more than half of their offspring experience development of infection (either a conjunctivitis or pneumonitis).

Detection early in pregnancy allows for treatment with oral antibiotics, such as erythromycin or azithromycin. This treatment has been linked with significantly lower rates of preterm delivery, preterm rupture of membranes, and low birth weight compared with infected women who are not treated. The incidence in pregnant populations is considerably lower in women older than 25 and women who are married, however, leading the U.S. Preventive Services Task Force to recommend only targeted screening (level B). Pregnant women at high risk for infection, including those younger than 25, should be tested. Universal screening in pregnancy carries a recommendation with level C evidence.[18]

Although culture has been quoted as the gold standard for detection of chlamydia, it requires special handling, is expensive, and has a lower sensitivity than other methods of detection (with a NND of 1.11-1.42).[19] Advances in recent years have provided for accurate alternatives. Antigen detection using a swab sample has a reported 80% to 95% sensitivity compared with culture. Genetic probe, using the same sampling technique, has a sensitivity and specificity of at least 95%, giving it a maximum NND of 1.11. Nucleic acid amplification tests (NAATs) that use polymerase or ligase chain reaction technology have resulted in sensitivities and specificities that exceed 95%. Although rapid, this technology is expensive. Urine testing is now possible to detect *Chlamydia trachomatis*. Urine testing allows screening when pelvic examination cannot be performed immediately. The sensitivity of NAATs using urine to detect *Chlamydia trachomatis*, of 95% to 99%, is similar to endocervical swab sampling methods, and the specificity is greater than 99%. This results in a NND of 1.01 to 1.06.

D. Human Immunodeficiency Virus

A demonstrated decreased perinatal transmission from a transmission rate of 25.5% to 8.3%[20] occurs when antiretroviral therapy is given during the third trimester and throughout labor. Therefore, prenatal human immunodeficiency virus (HIV) screening can offer benefit to the fetus and the mother and care team.[21] Risk factors for HIV infection include use of intravenous drugs, receipt of a blood transfusion between 1978 and 1985, and high-risk sexual practices or sexual partners with high-risk behaviors. Pregnant women infected with HIV who have CD4 counts less than 200 are appropriate candidates for prophylaxis against *Pneumocystis* and other infections (see Chapter 9, Section A).

Studies have indicated that counseling and testing strategies that offer testing only to those women who report risk fail to identify up to 50% to 70% of HIV-infected women. Although the U.S. Public Health Service and American Academy of Pediatrics/ACOG recommend universal screening, the U.S. Preventive Services Task Force rates HIV testing for all pregnant women as a level C recommendation. Screening of patients who are at increased risk or who come from a community where the prevalence of seropositive newborns is greater than 1 per 1000 should occur at the beginning of prenatal care (level A).[22]

Testing is done using an enzyme immunoassay (EIA) for specific antibodies against HIV. These occur 3 weeks to 6 months after infection, leaving a window period during which the patient can be infected and transmit the disease but have a negative test. Outside this window period, sensitivity approaches 100%, and specificity is 99.7% or better (NND, 1.003).[23] False-positive results are rare, even in low-risk settings; however, false-positive results can occur with immunologic disease (such as lupus or rheumatoid arthritis) and have been reported to occur after many routine vaccinations.[24] Because of these false-positive results, each positive EIA is followed by a Western blot for confirmation, which has a sensitivity greater than 98% and a specificity of nearly 100%. The NND of the Western blot is 1.031, which is greater than that of the EIA because of the decreased sensitivity and supports the use of EIA rather than Western blot for population screening. Indeterminate results may occur slightly more commonly in parous and pregnant women; however, the diagnostic accuracy of standard HIV testing is thought to be similar for men and pregnant and nonpregnant women.[25] Additional FDA-approved rapid screening tests also are highly accurate and may increase patients' acceptance of testing. Compared with standard HIV testing, the reported sensitivities of rapid tests on blood specimens range from 96% to 100%, with specificities greater than 99.9%, and may be used to assess HIV status during labor.[26] Both urine and oral fluid tests are also available. Reported sensitivities and specificities of oral fluid HIV tests also are high (>99%).[27] The diagnostic accuracy of urine tests appear to be lower than that of standard testing.[28] Finally, the FDA has approved a home collection kit that uses a fingerstick blood spot sample. One study found it to be highly accurate compared with standard testing.[29]

E. Maternal Rubella Serology

Rubella infection in the first 16 weeks of pregnancy can result in miscarriage, abortion, stillbirth, and congenital rubella syndrome (CRS). CRS is a constellation of findings in newborns including hearing loss, developmental delay, and ocular and cardiac defects. Approximately 20% of infants born to women with infection during the first 16 weeks of pregnancy will show signs of CRS.[30] The incidence has declined dramatically since the introduction of rubella vaccination in 1969. The CDC reported in March 2005 that there have been fewer than 25 cases per year in the United States since 1991.[31]

Detection of lack of immunity during preconceptual visits can allow for appropriate immunization before pregnancy because vaccination provides long-lasting immunity in greater than 90% of healthy recipients. The vaccine is contraindicated during pregnancy because of possible concerns over teratogenicity but can be given at least 3 months before conception or during the postpartum period.[32]

Testing for immunity to rubella is done using EIA or latex agglutination testing. Sensitivity is 92% to 100% and specificity is 71% to 100%, giving a NND of 1.00 to 1.58. Testing has its shortcomings. In 1990, when the records of mothers with 21 cases of CRS were evaluated, 71% had a previous positive serologic test for immunity.[33]

F. Maternal Blood Type, Rh, and Antibody Screening

Since the introduction of anti-D (RhoGAM) immunoglobulin injections during and after pregnancy in women who are negative for D antigen, the incidence of isoimmunization has decreased from 10 to 1.3 cases per 1000 live births. Currently, the U.S. Preventive Services Task Force recommends blood type, Rh, and antibody screen at the first prenatal visit (level A). A repeat antibody screen at 24 to 28 weeks, followed by a full dose of RhoGAM to help prevent sensitization from small hemorrhages that can occur in the third trimester, carries a level B recommendation.[34] A full dose of 300 mg RhoGAM is to be given to all D-antigen–negative women who deliver a D-antigen–positive infant (level A).

G. Hemoglobinopathy Screening

Sickle cell disease occurs in 1 in 375 African Americans and 1 in 3000 Native Americans. α-Thalassemias are common in Southeast Asians, with 1% having the 3 gene deletion of the α-hemoglobin gene known as *hemoglobin H* associated with significant anemia. The U.S. Preventive Services Task Force recommends offering screening for hemoglobinopathy to all pregnant women at the first prenatal visit (level B). Maternal carriers identified through screening should have the father tested and should receive information on the availability of prenatal diagnosis if the father also is a carrier and the fetus is at risk for a clinically significant hemoglobinopathy.[35] Preconceptual screening can play an important role in appropriate counseling of patients at risk for having a child with a hemoglobinopathy.

Screening for sickle cell anemia is usually done with a sickle cell prep or slide, or a purchased kit such as a Sickledex. Each of these tests patients' red blood cells to low oxygen tension or high osmolality solutions to determine whether they will deform. As such, they are sensitive for many different abnormal hemoglobins but are not specific for hemoglobin S (as they also can detect the carrier state). Different tests are used by different laboratories, and their sensitivity, although high, depends on the test. Confirmation of a positive screening test is done with a hemoglobin electrophoresis utilizing thin-layer isoelectric focusing, which has a sensitivity of 96%, a specificity of nearly 100%, and a NND of 1.05 for the presence of sickle cell disease. The positive predictive value of this test is 73%, but the negative predictive value exceeds 99.9%.[36]

H. Cystic Fibrosis Screening

Cystic fibrosis is the most common autosomal recessive genetic disease in whites, with a frequency of 1 in 3300, and a carrier state of 1 in 29.[37] Other races are affected at significantly lower rates (Table 3-3). Currently, the American College of Medical Genetics (ACMG), ACOG, and National Institutes of Health (NIH) all recommend counseling and subsequent testing; however, these recommendations are based on expert opinion. When using the core panel of 25 mutations, the detection rate is 80%.

TABLE 3-3 Cystic Fibrosis Carrier Rates

Whites	1/29
Asian Americans	1/90
African Americans	1/65
Hispanic Americans	1/46

I. Amniocentesis or Chorionic Villus Sampling for Advanced Maternal Age

Risk for specific genetic abnormalities of the fetus increases with maternal age, including trisomy 21 (Down syndrome). When a mother reaches the age of 35, the risk for genetic defect in the offspring reaches 1 in 204 (with a risk for Down syndrome of 1/385). Because of this increased risk, the U.S. Preventive Services Task Force recommends offering amniocentesis at 15 to 18 weeks to women of advanced maternal age (level B).[38] Other organizations, including ACOG, the Canadian Task Force, and the ACMG, also recommend amniocentesis for advanced maternal age or presence of other risk factors (positive family history) that would increase suspicion for a genetic defect.

Because cytogenetic analysis requires growth of fetal cells (or placental cells, in the case of chorionic villus sampling [CVS]) in culture, the possibility for an inaccurate diagnosis based on genetic mosaicism or through contamination with maternal cell lines exists. Despite these shortcomings, amniocentesis has a sensitivity for trisomy 21 (and similar genetic translocations) of 97%, with specificity of 100%, giving it a NND of 1.03.

When evaluating these tests as part of the screening tests of pregnancy, an important aspect should be considered: risk to the fetus caused by the test itself. The generally reported risk for miscarriage after amniocentesis is 0.5% and after CVS is 1% to 1.5%. CVS has a currently reported risk of transverse limb defects of 0.03% to 0.1%, with the risk being greater before 10 weeks. After 10 weeks, most of the limb defects associated with CVS have been limited to the digits.[39] Table 3-4 compares CVS and amniocentesis.

J. Urine Culture at 12 to 16 Weeks for Asymptomatic Bacteriuria

Asymptomatic bacteriuria (ASB) occurs in 2% to 7% of all pregnant women. If untreated, 13% to 27% of these patients experience development of pyelonephritis, which is associated with a 1.5- to 2-fold increase in the risk for preterm labor and delivery. The gold standard for diagnosis is culture, with growth of 100,000 organisms per milliliter or greater of a single species on a clean-catch specimen considered a positive result. A single culture at 12 to 16 weeks identifies 80% of patients who have ASB during the pregnancy, with repeated monthly screening adding only about 2% more per month. Screening with a single culture in early pregnancy is cost-effective as long as the prevalence of ASB is greater than 2%.[40] Treatment of ASB reduces the risk for maternal pyelonephritis (NNT=7), preterm delivery, and/or low-birth-weight infants (NNT=21).[41]

Despite its accuracy for ASB and urinary tract infection, culture has its drawbacks. It is labor intensive, is more expensive than rapid tests, and involves some delay before the results are known.

TABLE 3-4 Comparison of Chorionic Villus Sampling and Amniocentesis

Characteristics	Chorionic Villus Sampling	Amniocentesis
Technique	Transabdominal or transcervical biopsy of placental cells	Transabdominal removal of amniotic fluid
Gestational age	10-12 weeks	15-18 weeks
Abnormalities	Fetal aneuploidy	Fetal aneuploidy (studies done)
	DNA-based diagnosis of certain genetic conditions	DNA-based diagnosis of genetic conditions
	Cannot detect NTD	AFP testing for NTD
Advantages	Earlier detection of genetic abnormalities than amniocentesis	Ability to test amniotic fluid for AFP and acetylcholinesterase
Risks	Miscarriage: 0.5-1.0%	Miscarriage 0.25-0.50%
	Limb deficiency: 0.03-0.10%	

AFP, α-fetoprotein; NTD, neural tube defects.
From Centers for Disease Control and Prevention: Chorionic villus sampling and amniocentesis: recommendations for prenatal counseling, *MMWR Morbid Mortal Wkly Rep* 44(RR-9):1-12, 1995.

Alternatives that have been evaluated include dipstick tests for leukocyte esterase or nitrites and microscopic examination of urinary sediment. When compared with culture, leukocyte esterase has sensitivity of 72% to 97%, with specificity 64% to 82%, giving a NND of 1.27 to 2.78. A positive nitrite on the dipstick test has a lower sensitivity of 35% to 85% but a higher specificity of 92% to 100%, yielding a NND of 1.17 to 3.70. During pregnancy, microscopic evaluation of the urinary sediment for bacteriuria or pyuria had a sensitivity of 83% but a specificity of 59%,[42] resulting in a NND of 2.38. As noted earlier, these tests are not accurate enough to fit the criteria of a good screening test, especially with a NND greater than 1.5. The U.S. Preventive Services Task Force recommends routine urine culture at the first visit in all patients (level A), with routine screening using dipstick testing to be avoided (level D).[43]

K. Serum α-Fetoprotein Screening

Neural tube defects occur in about 7.2 to 15.6 cases per 10,000 live births, and vary from small asymptomatic cases of spina bifida to open myelomeningoceles to anencephaly (which is incompatible with prolonged life after birth). Maternal serum α-fetoprotein (MSAFP) levels are increased in greater than 80% of pregnancies in which the fetus has an open neural tube defect; other anomalies, such as open ventral wall defects of the abdomen, also can lead to increased levels. MSAFP levels are, on average, almost four times greater in cases of open spina bifida (3.8 vs 1.0 multiples of the median [MoM]) and about seven times greater in cases of anencephaly (7.0 vs 1.0 MoM) compared with unaffected infants.[44]

Folate supplementation of at least 0.4 mg started at least 4 weeks before conception and continued through the first 6 weeks of pregnancy is associated with a decreased incidence of neural tube defects. Larger doses (4 mg) are associated with a lower incidence of recurrence among mothers with a previous infant affected by a neural tube defect.

An increased MSAFP level generally is defined as greater than 2.5 MoM. At 2.5 MoM or greater, the false-positive rate is approximately 1.5%, and the detection rate for open spina bifida is 80% and for anencephaly is 90%. In one study, sensitivity of MSAFP was reported as 85%, with specificity of 96%, positive predictive value of 4.8%, and negative predictive value of 99.9%; these numbers result in a NND of 1.23.

Increased MSAFP values can be caused by factors other than a neural tube defect. Inaccurate gestational age is the most common cause of a falsely increased result, but this also can occur with multiple gestation, intrauterine growth restriction (IUGR), or fetal demise. An ultrasound can be used to differentiate these possibilities. In high-risk prenatal populations and centers with special expertise, ultrasound has been shown to have a sensitivity of 79% to 96% and a specificity of 90% to 100% at detecting open neural tube defects; this results in a NND of 1.04 to 1.45.[45]

Patients who have an unexplained increase after ultrasound are offered an amniocentesis, by which an amniotic fluid α-fetoprotein (AFP) and amniotic fluid acetylcholinesterase can be determined. Even if the amniocentesis studies are normal, an unexplained increased MSAFP level has been associated with an increased risk for stillbirth, congenital anomalies, and low birth weight.

L. Multiple Marker Testing for Down Syndrome

In women at high risk (e.g., those >35 years old or who have had a prior pregnancy complicated by chromosomal abnormalities), the definitive test for chromosomal abnormalities is CVS or amniocentesis with karyotype determination because the possibility of genetic abnormality is thought to exceed the potential risk for fetal loss (Table 3-5). In patients at low risk, the risk for miscarriage resulting

TABLE 3-5 Age-Specific Rates of Trisomy 21 and Chromosomal Abnormalities

Maternal Age (yr)	Risk for Trisomy 21	Risk for Any Chromosomal Abnormalities
20	1/1667	1/526
25	1/1259	1/476
30	1/952	1/384
35	1/385	1/204
40	1/106	1/65
45	1/30	1/20

Adapted from Gabbe SG, Niebyl JR, Simpson JL, editors: *Obstetrics: normal and problem pregnancies,* ed 3, New York, 1996, Churchill Livingstone.

from amniocentesis is significantly greater than the chance of detecting a chromosomal abnormality. This has led to the development of multiple marker testing (MMT).

MMT should be offered to all pregnant women but should not be considered as mandatory. Pretest counseling and patient education are essential to provide women an understanding of the limitations and high false-positive rate, in addition to the need for possible invasive testing based on the screen results. Similar to MSAFP testing, MMT can be falsely abnormal with inaccurate gestational age, twin gestation, and IUGR, necessitating an ultrasound for determination of accurate dates and other information as part of the evaluation of an abnormal test. Should the ultrasound confirm gestational age in an apparently normal singleton pregnancy, amniocentesis should be considered for karyotyping.

The combination of AFP, human chorionic gonadotropin (hCG), and unconjugated estriol (uE$_3$) with maternal age, commonly referred to as the *Triple Screen test,* detects 55% to 60% of fetal trisomy 21 cases in the second trimester with a false-positive rate of 5% in women younger than 35 years. Reported sensitivity varies from 48% to 91%, with specificity of 96% (positive predictive value of 1.2-1.8% and negative predictive value of 99.9%). This gives a range of NND from 1.15 to 2.27. This test is now commonplace in clinical practice. The addition of dimeric inhibin A to the above three maternal analytes, referred to as the Quad test, has further improved the detection rate to 70% to 75% at a similar false-positive rate.[46,47]

The current trend is to find screening tools that provide earlier and more accurate diagnosis. One such test includes the combination of two maternal serum biochemical markers, pregnancy-associated plasma protein A and the free β subunit of hCG (free β-hCG), both measured in the first trimester. This has shown to detect 60% of trisomy 21 cases at a false-positive rate of 5%.[48] In addition, the Fetal Medicine Foundation and others have shown that by combining first-trimester maternal serum analytes with sonographic measurement of the nuchal translucency, 80% to 90% of Down syndrome fetuses can be detected.[49] Some investigators have proposed a combination of first- and second-trimester screening to enhance the benefits of each technique (see Chapter 7, Section H).[50]

One alternative is the use of MMT to decrease the need for widespread amniocentesis or CVS in patients older than age 35. In one cohort study of 5385 women older than 35 with no other risk factors, all patients had MMT together with amniocentesis for karyotyping. If the MMT testing cutoff of 1 in 200 had been used as the level for amniocentesis, 75% of the amnioceteses could have been avoided while missing 11% of the fetuses with Down syndrome.[51] Offering MMT with follow-up ultrasound and possible amniocentesis is a level B recommendation by the U.S. Preventive Services Task Force.

IV. SOR A RECOMMENDATIONS

RECOMMENDATIONS	REFERENCES
All pregnant women should be tested for hepatitis B infection in the first trimester.	6
All pregnant women should be screened for syphilis in the first trimester.	9
Women at high risk should be tested for chlamydia in the first trimester.	18
Women at high risk should be tested for HIV in the first trimester.	22
All women should be screened for blood type and Rh in the first trimester.	34
All women should be screened with urine culture for ASB during the first trimester.	43
All women should be screened in the second trimester with MSAFP for the presence of neural tube defects.	45

REFERENCES

1. Williams K: Screening for syphilis in pregnancy: an assessment of the costs and benefits, *Commun Med* 7:37-42, 1985.
2. How good is that test? II. *Bandolier* (on-line version), 27-2, May 1996. Available at: http://www.jr2.ox.ac.uk/bandolier/band27/b27-2.html.
3. Kogan MD, Martin JA, Alexander GR et al: The changing pattern of prenatal care utilization in the United States, 1981-1995 using different prenatal care indices, *JAMA* 279(20):1623-1628, 1998.
4. Lo K-J, Tsai Y-T, Lee S-D et al: Immunoprophylaxis of infection with hepatitis B virus in infants born to hepatitis B surface antigen-positive carrier mothers, *J Infect Dis* 152:817-822, 1985.
5. Margolis HS, Alter MJ, Hadler SC: Hepatitis B: evolving epidemiology and implications for control, *Semin Liver Dis* 11:84-92, 1991.

6. U. S. Preventive Services Task Force: Screening for hepatitis B virus infection. *Guide to clinical preventive services,* ed 2, Washington, DC, 1996, Office of Disease Prevention and Health Promotion.

7. McCready JA, Morens D, Fields HA et al: Evaluation of enzyme immunoassay (EIA) as a screening method for hepatitis B markers in an open population, *Epidemiol Infect* 107:673-684, 1991.

8. Duff P: Hepatitis in pregnancy, *Semin Perinatol* 22(4):277-283, 1998.

9. U.S. Preventive Services Task Force: Screening for syphilis. *Guide to clinical preventive services,* ed 2, Washington, DC, 1996, Office of Disease Prevention and Health Promotion.

10. Walker DG, Walker GJ: Forgotten but not gone: the continuing scourge of congenital syphilis, *Lancet Infect Dis* 2:432-436, 2002.

11. Centers for Disease Control and Prevention: *Sexually transmitted disease surveillance, 2002 supplement, Syphilis Surveillance Report,* Atlanta, GA; January 2004. U.S. Department of Health and Human Services, Center for Disease Control and Prevention.

12. Guyer B: Medicaid and prenatal care. Necessary but not sufficient, *JAMA* 264:2264-2265, 1990.

13. U.S. Preventive Services Task Force: Screening for syphilis. *Guide to clinical preventive services,* ed 2, Baltimore, 1996, Williams & Wilkins.

14. Centers for Disease Control and Prevention: 1998 guidelines for treatment of sexually transmitted diseases, *MMWR Morb Mortal Wkly Rep* 47(RR-1):40-41, 1998.

15. Golden MR, Marra CM, Holmes KK: Update on syphilis: resurgence of an old problem, *JAMA* 290:1510-1514, 2003.

16. Wilson TE, Minkoff H, McCall S et al: The relationship between pregnancy and sexual risk taking, *Am J Obstet Gynecol* 174:1033-1036, 1996.

17. Campos-Outcalt D, Ryan K: Prevalence of sexually transmitted diseases in Mexican-American pregnant women by country of birth and length of time in the United States, *Sex Transm Dis* 22:78-82, 1995.

18. U. S. Preventive Services Task Force: Screening for chlamydial infection, including ocular prophylaxis in newborns. *Guide to clinical preventive services,* ed 2, Washington, DC, 1996, Office of Disease Prevention and Health Promotion.

19. Zenilman J: Genital *Chlamydia trachomatis* infections in women. In: Rose BD, editor. *UpToDate.* Wellesley, MA, 2004, UpToDate.

20. Connor EM, Sperling RS, Gelber R et al: Reduction of maternal-infant transmission of human immunodeficiency virus type 1 with zidovudine treatment. Pediatric AIDS Clinical Trials Group Protocol 076 Study Group, *N Engl J Med* 331(18):1173-1180, 1994.

21. Connor EM, Sperling RS, Gelbar R et al: Reduction of maternal-infant transmission of HIV-1 with zidovudine treatment, *N Engl J Med* 331:1173-1180, 1994.

22. U.S. Preventive Services Task Force: Screening for human immunodeficiency virus infection. *Guide to clinical preventive services,* ed 2, Washington, DC, 1996, Office of Disease Prevention and Health Promotion.

23. Centers for Disease Control and Prevention: Update: serologic testing for HIV-1 antibody—United States, 1988 and 1989, *MMWR Morb Mortal Wkly Rep* 39:380-383, 1990.

24. Kleinman S, Busch MP, Hall L, et al: False-positive HIV-1 test results in a low-risk screening setting of voluntary blood donation. Retrovirus Epidemiology Donor Study, *JAMA* 280:1080-1085, 1998.

25. Celum CL, Coombs RW, Jones M et al: Risk factors for repeatedly reactive HIV-1 EIA and indeterminate western blots, *Arch Intern Med* 154:1129–1137, 1994.

26. Butlerys M, Jamieson DJ, O'Sullivan MJ et al: Rapid HIV-1 testing during labor: a multicenter study, *JAMA* 292:219-223, 2004.

27. Gallo D, George JR, Fitchen JH et al: Evaluation of a system using oral mucosal transudate for HIV-1 antibody screening and confirmatory testing [published correction appears in JAMA 1997;227:792]. OrasSure HIV Clinical Trials Group, *JAMA* 277(3):254-258, 1997.

28. Martinez PM, Torres AR, de Lejarazu R et al: Human immunodeficiency virus antibody testing by enzyme-linked fluorescent and Western blot assays using serum, gingival-crevicular transudate, and urine samples, *J Clin Microbiol* 37:1100-1106, 1999.

29. Frank AP, Wandell MG, Headings MD et al: Anonymous HIV testing using home collection and telemedicine counseling. A multicenter evaluation, *Arch Intern Med* 157:309-314, 1997.

30. McElhaney RD Jr, Ringer M, DeHart DJ et al: Rubella immunity in a cohort of pregnant women, *Infect Control Hosp Epidemiol* 20(1):64-66, 1999.

31. Elimination of rubella and congenital rubella syndrome—United States, 1969–2004, *MMWR Morb Mortal Wkly Rep* 54:279-282, 2005.

32. American Academy of Pediatrics: Rubella. In Peter G, editor: *1997 red book: report of the Committee on Infectious Diseases,* ed 24, Elk Grove Village, IL, 1997, American Academy of Pediatrics.

33. Lee SH, Ewert DP, Frederick PD et al: Resurgence of congenital rubella syndrome in the 1990s: report on missed opportunities and failed prevention policies among women of childbearing age, *JAMA* 267:2616-2620, 1992.

34. *USPSTF Screening for Rh (D) Incompatibility. February 2004 update.* Available at: www.ahrq.gov/clinic/uspstf/uspsdrhi.htm. Accessed August 23, 2007.

35. U.S. Preventive Services Task Force: Screening for hemoglobinopathies. *Guide to clinical preventive services,* ed 2, Washington, DC, 1996, Office of Disease Prevention and Health Promotion.

36. Githens JH, Lane PA, McCurdy RS et al: Newborn screening in Colorado: the first ten years, *Am J Dis Child* 144:466-470, 1990.

37. American College of Obstetricians and Gynecologists (ACOG) and American College of Medical Geneticists (ACMG): Preconception and prenatal carrier screening for cystic fibrosis. Clinical and laboratory guideline, Washington, DC, October 2001, ACOG.

38. U.S. Preventive Services Task Force: Screening for Down syndrome. *Guide to clinical preventive services,* ed 2, Washington, DC, 1996, Office of Disease Prevention and Health Promotion.

39. Vintzileos AM, Ananth CV, Smulian JC et al: The impact of prenatal care on postneonatal deaths in the presence and absence of antenatal high-risk conditions, *Am J Obstet Gynecol* 187:1258-1262, 2002.

40. Wadland WC, Plante DA: Screening for asymptomatic bacteriuria in pregnancy. A decision and cost analysis, *J Fam Pract* 29:372-376, 1989.

41. Smaill F: Antibiotics for asymptomatic bacteriuria in pregnancy, *Cochrane Database Syst Rev* (2):CD000490, 2001.

42. Bachman JW, Heise RH, Naessens JM et al: A study of various tests to detect asymptomatic urinary tract infection in an obstetric population, *JAMA* 270:1971-1974, 1993.
43. U.S. Preventive Services Task Force: Screening for asymptomatic bacteriuria. *Guide to clinical preventive services,* ed 2, Washington, DC, 1996, Office of Disease Prevention and Health Promotion.
44. Knight GJ, Palomaki GE: Maternal serum alpha-fetoprotein and the detection of open neural tube defects. In Elias S, Simpson JL, editors: *Maternal serum screening for fetal genetic disorders,* New York, 1992, Churchill Livingstone.
45. U.S. Preventive Services Task Force: Screening for neural tube defects, including folic acid/folate prophylaxis. *Guide to clinical preventive services,* ed 2, Washington, DC, 1996, Office of Disease Prevention and Health Promotion.
46. Aitken D, Wallace E, Crossley J et al: Dimeric inhibin A as a marker for Down's syndrome in early pregnancy, *N Engl J Med* 334:1231-1236, 1996.
47. Wenstrom KD, Owen J, Chu DC et al: Elevated second-trimester dimeric inhibin A levels identify Down syndrome pregnancies, *Am J Obstet Gynecol* 177:992-996, 1997.
48. Cuckle H, vanLith J: Appropriate biochemical parameters in first-trimester screening for Down syndrome, *Prenat Diagn* 19:505-512, 1999.
49. Wapner R, Thom E, Simpson JL, et al, For the first trimester Maternal Serum Biochemistry and Fetal Nuchal Translucency Screening (BUN) Study Group: First-trimester screening for trisomies 21 and 18, *N Engl J Med* 349:1405-1413, 2003.
50. Wald N, Watt H, Hackshaw A: Integrated screening for Down's syndrome based on tests performed during the first and second trimesters, *N Engl J Med* 341:461-467, 1999.
51. Haddow JE, Palomaki GE, Knight GJ et al: Reducing the need for amniocentesis in women 35 years of age or older with serum markers for screening, *N Engl J Med* 330:1114-1118, 1994.
52. Paul M, Schaff E, Nichols M: The roles of clinical assessment, human chorionic gonadotropin assays and ultrasonography in medical abortion practice, *Am J Obstet Gynecol* 183(2): S34-S43, 2000.
53. Neilson JP: Ultrasound for fetal assessment in early pregnancy, *Cochrane Database Syst Rev* (2):CD000182, 2000.
54. Centers for Disease Control and Prevention (CDC): Spina bifida and anencephaly before and after folic acid mandate—United States, 1995-1996 and 1999-2000, *MMWR Morb Mortal Wkly Rep* 53:362-365, 2004.
55. Hildingsson I, Waldenstrom U, Radestad I: Women's expectations on antenatal care as assessed in early pregnancy: number of visits, continuity of caregiver and general content, *Acta Obstet Gynecol Scand* 81(2):118-125, 2002.
56. MacDorman MF, Minino AM, Strobino DM et al: Annual summary of vital statistics—2001, *Pediatrics* 110:1037-1052, 2002.
57. Lumley J, Oliver S, Walter E: Interventions for promoting smoking cessation during pregnancy, *Cochrane Database Syst Rev* 18(4):CD001055, 2004.

SECTION G Medications in Pregnancy

Kent Petrie, MD

I. HISTORY

Until the beginning of the twentieth century, most physicians believed that the uterus provided a protective environment for the fetus and served as a barricade against harm from the external environment. The fetal anomalies caused by thalidomide use in the 1960s shattered this concept, bringing increased public awareness to the potential harmful effects of medications on the developing fetus. Administered as an antianxiety and antinausea agent in the first trimester, thalidomide caused limb-reduction defects in one third of infants exposed. The drug had been determined safe in animal studies, so it took several years and many thousands of grossly malformed infants before the cause–effect relation was recognized. The thalidomide tragedy prompted the first drug regulations in the United States, requiring a drug to be proved safe and effective for the conditions of use prescribed in its labeling.[1]

II. MEDICATION USE IN PREGNANCY

A. Extent of Medication Use in Pregnancy

Six million pregnancies occur annually in the United States.[2,3] In a landmark World Health Organization survey, 86% of pregnant women used medications (excluding vitamins and minerals), with 30% using more than four drugs. Since 1980, the average number of drugs used during pregnancy has increased from 1.7 to 2.9. Six of the top 10 drugs used were over-the-counter products.[4-6]

B. Drug Exposure in Early Pregnancy

At least half of the pregnancies in North America are unplanned, placing hundreds of thousands of fetuses at risk for exposure to drugs before the pregnancy is known.[7]

C. Use of Medically Indicated Medications

Women may require drug therapy during pregnancy for chronic conditions diagnosed before pregnancy (e.g., epilepsy, asthma), pregnancy-induced conditions (e.g., hypertension, gestational diabetes), or acute conditions that develop during pregnancy (e.g., infections, nausea and vomiting).

D. Prescribing Imperatives during Pregnancy

The two imperatives for the family physician prescribing medications in pregnancy are to alleviate maternal suffering and illness while causing no harm to the fetus. Unfortunately, the thalidomide tragedy has had other consequences:

1. Women of childbearing age and their physicians may greatly overestimate the likelihood that drugs cause birth defects.
2. Pregnant women may be treated inappropriately or not treated at all for serious medical conditions.
3. Women may decide to terminate their pregnancy because of the misguided belief that the medication they took will cause birth defects.
4. Physicians and pharmaceutical companies may encourage pregnancy termination because of unrealistic perceptions of risk or because of fear of litigation.[4,8,9]

III. TERATOGENS

A. Classic Teratogens

Thalidomide was the classic teratogen, and it had its effect in the *classic teratogenic period*. If one considers a 280-day gestation, this teratogenic period is 31 to 71 days from the last menstrual period (or about the 5th to 10th week of gestation). This is the period during which maternal-fetal transport of substances is established and organogenesis occurs. During this time, chemicals can affect target organs at their time of greatest development.[10]

B. Broadened Definition of Teratogen

In the past, a teratogen was simply considered to be an agent that caused a physical malformation. The definition of teratogen has been extended to include a broader range of abnormal development, including complete pregnancy loss, structural anomalies, abnormal growth in utero, and long-term functional defects.[10]

C. Latency Period

It now is recognized that drug effects can be subtle, unexpected, and delayed (i.e., manifest changes after a latency period). Diethylstilbestrol is the classic example of the long latency period that can exist between fetal exposure and drug effect. Between 1940 and 1971, 6 million mothers and their fetuses were exposed to this estrogenic hormone to prevent a variety of reproductive problems ranging from miscarriage to premature delivery. By the late 1960s, it became apparent that, as adults, these exposed offspring were at significant increased risk for adenocarcinoma of the cervix and vagina and male reproductive anomalies.[1]

D. Background Incidence of Malformations and Structural Abnormalities

The risk for drug or chemical exposures in pregnancy must be assessed against the background incidence of malformations.[10] If congenital malformations or anomalies are defined as structural abnormalities of prenatal origin that are present at birth and interfere with viability or physical well-being, the incidence rates of such malformations are as follows:

1. Major malformations = 3%
(e.g., cleft palate, congenital heart defect)
2. Minor malformations = 4%
(e.g., accessory digit, external ear tag)

E. Causes of Congenital Malformations

Drugs account for only 3% of congenital malformations. Infections and maternal diseases account for 7%, and genetic causes account for 20%. Most congenital malformations (70%) have no known cause.

IV. CLASSIFICATION OF MEDICATIONS IN PREGNANCY

A. Known Teratogens

Although there are more than 1000 chemicals that are known teratogens in animals, the number of medications proven to pose teratogenic risk in humans is relatively small (Table 3-6).

B. Methods of Identifying Teratogens

1. Animal studies
   Animal studies may fail or may not be helpful in predicting human teratogenicity.[1]
   a. Interspecies variation: Thalidomide was shown to be safe in rats and mice but later was reported to cause anomalies in monkeys and rabbits.

TABLE 3-6 Medications with Known Teratogenic Risk

Alcohol

Androgens

Angiotensin-converting enzyme inhibitors

Angiotensin II receptor blockers

Anticonvulsants (trimethadione, valproic acid, phenytoin, carbamazepine)

Chemotherapeutic agents (antimetabolites and alkylating agents)

Iodides

Isotretinoin

Lithium

Tetracyclines

Thalidomide and diethylstilbestrol (of historic interest)

Warfarin

TABLE 3-7 U.S. Food and Drug Administration Medication Use-in-Pregnancy Classification

Category	Description of Risk
A	**Controlled studies show no risk**
	Well-controlled human studies have failed to demonstrate risk to the fetus.
B	**No evidence of risk in humans**
	Either animal studies show no fetal risk and no human data are available, or animal studies show a risk but human studies do not show fetal risk.
C	**Risk cannot be ruled out**
	Either animal studies indicate a fetal risk and there are no controlled studies in humans, or there are no available studies in humans or animals.
D	**Positive human evidence of fetal risk**
	Studies show fetal risk in humans, but potential benefits may outweigh the potential risk in certain situations.
X	**Contraindicated in pregnancy**
	Studies in animals or humans, or based on human experience, show definite fetal risk.

b. Animal defect data: These data may be so conclusive that warnings are issued before FDA approval. For example, isotretinoin (Accutane) animal studies showed craniofacial, cardiac, and central nervous system anomalies, prompting a category X rating and strict product labeling before release, and physician education and certification before prescribing (the iPLEDGE program).

2. Case reports
   Case reports identify rare events, often implicating drugs as teratogens that are exonerated by further studies. For example, Bendectin (pyridoxine 10 mg plus doxylamine 10 mg) was useful in the 1970s for treatment of morning sickness. Implication of associated anomalies was never proved in careful epidemiologic studies. Excessive litigation, however, prompted Merrill-Dow to remove the drug voluntarily from the U.S. marketplace in 1982.[1]

3. Epidemiologic studies
   Epidemiologic studies are the best but most difficult means of linking drugs to birth defects. Case–control and cohort studies require prohibitively large numbers to be statistically significant.

C. Food and Drug Administration Classification of Drugs in Pregnancy

1. Pregnancy precaution categories
   Based on animal and human data, since 1975 the FDA has placed all drugs into five pregnancy precaution categories: A, B, C, D, and X (Table 3-7). The safest drugs are those in category A, in which no fetal risk has been shown in well-controlled human studies. The relative risk of teratogenic effects increases through categories B, C, D, and X. Drugs in category X are known teratogens and should be avoided during pregnancy.[11]

2. Proposed FDA drug classification system
   The FDA has been criticized for the ambiguous statements used in the current classification system and for not modifying ratings when new data are made available. The Teratology Society has proposed that the FDA abandon the system in favor of a more evidence-based classification. In an attempt to address these concerns, the FDA's Reproductive Health Drugs Advisory Committee has proposed a new system of pregnancy labeling.[12] The new format will include a clinical management statement, a summary risk statement, and a section discussing the available data for each drug (Table 3-8).

TABLE 3-8 Proposed U.S. Food and Drug Administration Pregnancy Labeling System

1. Clinical Management (discussion of clinical use of medication in pregnancy)
2. Summary Risk Assessment (review of risks of drug use in pregnancy)
3. Discussion of Data (review of animal and human data)

V. PATIENT COUNSELING

Every day in practice the family physician is faced with the important task of counseling patients during their preconception and prenatal periods; therefore, family physicians must be prepared to address several questions.[2]

1. "Is this medication safe to take during my pregnancy?"

   Patients need to know that using medications during pregnancy entails acceptance of some small degree of risk. Failure to treat illness may jeopardize the health of the mother and fetus. Patients should be informed of known indications, risks, and benefits of any drug therapy and be involved in decisions regarding medications as much as possible. In doing so, both patients and physicians must assess their own risk tolerance and need for certainty.

2. "Since I took this drug before I knew I was pregnant, will my baby be born with a birth defect?"

   The clinician should gather as much information as possible to share with patients regarding risks of drug exposures. High-resolution ultrasound to detect major anomalies before 20 weeks may be offered to those for whom termination of pregnancy is an option or to prepare the parents for the birth of an infant with special needs.

3. "Did any of the medication I took cause this birth defect?"

   When faced with a baby born with a birth defect, open and direct discussion is important, showing an understanding of the patient's disbelief, anger, and guilt. The physician should describe basic teratology and the small window of vulnerability of the fetus, emphasizing that second- and third-trimester exposure is unlikely to cause a major defect. Consultation with a specialist in dysmor-phology may give insight into the problem. Autopsy is helpful in the case of intrauterine fetal death. Family counseling is essential in the event of loss or the challenge of raising a child with special needs.

VI. WHERE IN THE WORLD (WIDE WEB) CAN I FIND INFORMATION?

The following online sources provide information regarding medication use during pregnancy:

1. The REPRORISK system, which is available from Micromedex, contains four teratogen information databases: REPROTEXT, REPROTOX (www.reprotox.org), Shepard's Catalog of Teratogenic Agents, and Teratogen Information System (TERIS). These periodically updated, scientifically reviewed resources critically evaluate the literature regarding drug exposures in human and animal pregnancies.

2. Multidisciplinary teratogen information services include OTIS (Organization of Teratogen Information Services, www.otispregnancy.org), Motherisk (www.motherisk.org), and Focus Information Technology (www.perinatology.com).

3. Family Practice Notebook (www.fpnotebook.com) provides an excellent list of medications in pregnancy, listed by category and current FDA classification.

VII. TABLE OF COMMON MEDICATIONS IN PREGNANCY

Most drugs fall into FDA category C, and descriptions of drugs that appear in the *Physicians' Desk Reference* and similar sources often contain statements such as "Use in pregnancy is not recommended unless the potential benefits justify the potential risks to the fetus." Such disclaimers, although understandable from a medicolegal standpoint, are of little help to the practicing physician.

To provide a useful tool for the busy family physician, Appendix E lists common medications used in pregnancy and classifies them *acceptable,* to be used with *caution,* or to *avoid.* The table is compiled based on the best available data from large cohort studies or metaanalyses and the FDA ratings as published in the literature.[1,13-16] Where they exist, current controversies are listed under "Comments."

REFERENCES

1. Briggs GG, Freeman RL, Yaffe SJ: *Drugs in pregnancy and lactation,* ed 7, Baltimore, 2005, Lippincott Williams & Wilkins.
2. Larimore WL, Petrie KA: Drug use during pregnancy and lactation. In Larimore WL, editor: *Primary care clinics in office practice: update in maternity care,* Philadelphia, 2000, WB Saunders.
3. Martin JA, Hamilton BE, Sutton PD et al: Births: final data for 2004, *Natl Vital Stat Rep* 55(1):1-100, 2006.
4. Black RA, Hill DA: Over-the-counter medications in pregnancy, *Am Fam Physician* 67:2517-2524, 2003.
5. Collaborative Group on Drug Use in Pregnancy: An international survey on drug utilization during pregnancy, *Int J Risk Safety* 1:1, 1991.
6. Mitchell AA, Hernandez-Diaz S, Louik C et al: Medication uses in pregnancy: 1976-2000, *Pharmacoepidemiol Drug Saf* 10:S146, 2001.
7. Koren G, Pastuszak A, Ito S: Drugs in pregnancy, *N Engl J Med* 338:1128-1137, 1998.
8. Pole M, Einarson A, Pairaudeay N et al: Drug labeling and risk perceptions of teratogenicity: a survey of pregnant Canadian women and their health professionals, *J Clin Pharmacol* 40:573-577, 2000.
9. Uhl K, Kennedy DL, Kweder SL: Information on medication use in pregnancy, *Am Fam Physician* 67(12): 2476-2478, 2003.
10. American College of Obstetrics and Gynecology: Teratology, *ACOG Educational Bulletin,* 236, April 1997.
11. Teratology Society Public Affairs Committee: FDA classification of drugs for teratogenic risk, *Teratology* 49:446-447, 1994.
12. Kweder SL, Kennedy DL, Rodriquez E: Turning the wheels of change: FDA and pregnancy labeling. International Society for Pharmacoepidemiology, *Scribe Newsletter* 3:2-4, 10, 2000.
13. Koren G: *The complete guide to everyday risks in pregnancy and breastfeeding,* Toronto, 2004, Robert Rose, Inc.
14. Munoz FM, Englund JA: Vaccines in pregnancy, *Inf Dis Clin North Am* 15:1-15, 2001.
15. Niebyl JR: Drugs in pregnancy and lactation. In Gabbe SG, Simpson JL, Niebyl JR et al, editors: *Obstetrics. Normal and problem pregnancies,* ed 4, New York, 2007, Churchill Livingstone.
16. *Physicians' desk reference.* Montvale, NJ, 2005, Medical Economics Company, Inc.

SECTION   H

Immunizations in Pregnancy

Cynthia Kilbourn, MD

I. OVERVIEW

The benefits of immunization to the pregnant woman usually outweigh the theoretical risks for adverse effects.[1] Vaccination during pregnancy can protect the mother from dangerous infection and provide the infant with passive antibodies for the first 6 months of life. Vaccinating pregnant women with inactivated viral/bacterial vaccines or toxoids poses no known maternal or fetal risks.[2] Routine vaccines that generally are safe to administer during pregnancy include diphtheria, tetanus, influenza, and hepatitis B. Vaccines with more specific indications not altered by pregnancy include hepatitis A, meningococcus, pneumococcus, rabies, typhoid, anthrax, and inactivated polio. *Live* virus vaccines are generally contraindicated during pregnancy because of the potential risk for transmitting the virus to the developing fetus.[2] It is advised that these vaccines not be administered to pregnant women, and that women be counseled to avoid pregnancy for 4 weeks after vaccination. Vaccines containing live attenuated virus include measles, mumps, and rubella (MMR), varicella, bacilli Calmette–Guérin, smallpox, and yellow fever. Updates on safety of immunization can be found at the CDC website (www.cdc.gov/nip). Preconception immunization of women to prevent neonatal disease is preferred, and vaccination of women during the postpartum period, especially for rubella and varicella, is advised. No vaccines, inactivated nor live, are contraindicated during breastfeeding. Neither pregnancy nor breastfeeding adversely affects immunization response.[3]

II. SPECIFIC CONDITIONS

A. Diphtheria-Tetanus
1. Natural history[1]
   The maternal mortality rate from tetanus infection is 30% and from diphtheria is 10%. These rates are not altered by pregnancy. The neonatal tetanus mortality rate is 60% and 6 months of neonatal protection is provided by passive placental transfer of maternal antibody.
2. Booster doses
   A booster dose of diphtheria-tetanus (dT) toxoid is routinely indicated for pregnant women who were previously vaccinated but have not received a booster dose within the past 10 years. The booster dose should be given in the presence of a potentially contaminated wound if 5 years have elapsed from the previous dose. Although no evidence exists that these toxoids are teratogenic, waiting until the second trimester of pregnancy to administer dT is a reasonable precaution.[4]
3. Completion of booster series
   Pregnant women who are not immunized or only partially immunized should receive the complete primary series as follows: two doses intramuscularly

at 1- to 2-month intervals with a third dose 6 to 12 months after the second dose.

4. New vaccine: Adacel

Adacel is the new combination dTAP vaccination licensed for adolescents and adults. Despite the lack of data on safety and immunogenicity when women are given dTAP during pregnancy, the most recent Advisory Committee on Immunization Practice (ACIP) guidelines do not consider pregnancy a contraindication for use of dTAP.

dTAP may be preferred to Td alone in groups where the risk of pertussis is increased. These include adolescents, health-care personnel, and child care providers. If the vaccine is administered during pregnancy, the second or third trimester is preferred, and providers are encouraged to report administration to the appropriate manufacturer's pregnancy registry: for Boostrix to GlaxoSmithKline Biologicals at 1-888-825-5249, or for Adacel to sanofi pasteur at 1-800-822-2463.

B. Influenza

1. Natural history

Influenza is an annual seasonal infection that is generally self-limited. However, because of physiologic changes (decreased lung capacity; changes in immunologic function; and increases in heart rate, stroke volume, and oxygen consumption), pregnant women are at increased risk for influenza-related morbidity and mortality. Risks are greatest in the third trimester, when the hospitalization rate of pregnant women with influenza infection (250/100,000) is comparable to nonpregnant women with high-risk medical conditions.[5]

2. Current recommendations

All women who are pregnant during the flu season (October to March) should be given the inactivated influenza vaccination. This represents a 2004 ACIP modification of practice to include women in their first trimester of pregnancy in addition to those in their second and third trimesters.[6] Good evidence exists of no deleterious effect of inactivated influenza vaccine on the course of pregnancy or on the fetus, as a study of 2000 pregnant women demonstrated no adverse fetal effects associated with the influenza vaccine.[5]

C. Hepatitis B

1. Natural history

Hepatitis B infection during pregnancy results in a prolonged viremia persisting for weeks to months, providing time for vertical transmission of the virus to the neonate. Five to 10% of adults with acute infection will become chronic carriers and 25% of these will develop chronic active hepatitis. Infants infected by perinatal transmission have a 90% risk for chronic infection and up to 25% will die of chronic liver disease as adults.[6]

2. Vaccination during pregnancy

a. From limited experience, the hepatitis B vaccine (HBV) results in no risk for adverse effects to the developing fetus. Pregnancy is therefore not a contraindication to HBV vaccination and, in fact, may be an ideal time because prenatal care itself provides an excellent opportunity to complete the entire series of immunizations.

b. Pregnant women who are hepatitis B surface antigen seronegative but meet any of the following high-risk criteria should receive the vaccination series:

i. Persons with occupational risks—health-care workers or public service workers

ii. Persons with lifestyle risk—heterosexuals with multiple partners, heterosexuals with recent diagnosis of any sexually transmitted disease, intravenous drug users

iii. Persons with environmental risk—household and sexual contacts of HBV carriers, prison inmates, institutionalized persons and their staff, immigrants and refugees, travelers to HBV endemic areas

iv. Persons with hemophilia or undergoing hemodialysis

c. The vaccine is given as a series of three injections (at 0, 1, and 6 months).

d. Infants born to mothers who are known to be infected should be given the vaccine within the first 12 hours of life together with hepatitis B immunoglobulin and complete the three-injection primary series.[5]

D. Hepatitis A

1. Natural history

Hepatitis A infects approximately 100,000 persons each year in the United States, and 100 of these infections are fatal. Transmission of hepatitis A from an acutely infected woman to her fetus has never been documented. The absence of a carrier state and the short viremic phase of this infection are responsible for the lack of perinatal transmission.[5]

2. Safety of hepatitis A vaccine
   The safety of hepatitis A vaccine in pregnancy has not been studied. However, because it is produced from formalin-inactivated virus, the risk to the fetus is expected to be low.[2] Risks of administration should therefore be weighed against risks for infection. The vaccine is administered in a two-dose schedule, 6 months apart.
3. Indications for vaccination during pregnancy
   Vaccination should be considered in pregnant women with the following risks for exposure to hepatitis A:
   a. Living with an infected household member
   b. Working in close physical contact with infected persons or persons with poor toilet habits (e.g., daycare facilities, and institutions for the mentally retarded)
   c. Traveling to areas where hepatitis A is endemic
4. Exposure to hepatitis A during pregnancy
   Pregnant women exposed to the hepatitis A virus should receive 0.02 mg/kg immunoglobulin intramuscularly, and hepatitis A virus vaccine is recommended as postexposure prophylaxis. This is more than 85% effective in preventing acute infection. A second dose of vaccine should then be given in 6 months.

E. Pneumococcal Infection

1. Natural history[2,5]
   Streptococcus pneumoniae is a major cause of pneumonia, meningitis, and bacteremia, and the prevalence of multidrug resistance has increased the mortality associated with the disease.
2. Current vaccine
   The current vaccine includes purified capsular polysaccharide from the 23 most common types of *S. pneumoniae,* and it is recommended by the CDC for use in adults with underlying chronic medical conditions placing them at greater risk for the disease.
3. Indication for vaccine
   The indications for receiving the vaccine are not altered by pregnancy. Therefore, pregnant women with any of the following conditions should be appropriately immunized: diabetes, cardiovascular disease, pulmonary disease except for asthma, chronic renal or liver disease, asplenia, sickle cell anemia, alcoholism, or immunosuppression.[2]
4. Administration
   The vaccine is administered as a single injection. Administration during the second or third trimester of pregnancy is preferred.[4] Consideration

may be given to repeating the dose 5 years later in women at high risk.

F. Meningococcal Infection

1. Natural history[2]
   In the United States, meningococcal disease is the leading cause of bacterial meningitis in children ages 2 though 18 years, and approximately 10% of these infections are fatal. However, more than 25% of the cases of meningococcus occur in adults older than 20 years.
2. Meningococcal vaccine
   The meningococcal vaccine MPSV4 contains the purified polysaccharide of four serogroups of *Neisseria meningitides,* A, C, Y, and W-135. It is administered as a single subcutaneous dose.[2] The newer conjugated meningococcal vaccine MCV4 has similar efficacy but a longer duration of protection in adolescents and adults.[4]
3. Indications
   MCV4 is recommended for persons with specific indications including military recruits, persons with anatomic or functional asplenia, travelers to countries where the disease is endemic or epidemic, and adults with complement component deficiencies. Routine vaccination of preadolescents age 11-12 and of college freshmen living in dormitories has recently been recommended.[4]
4. Safety in pregnancy
   Studies have shown MPSV4 to be safe and effective when given to pregnant women, and pregnancy does not alter the indications outlined above. In contrast, the newer conjugated meningococcal vaccine MCV4 is not recommended during pregnancy because there is no information on its safety.[4]

G. Varicella

1. Natural history
   The varicella-zoster virus causes chickenpox and, more rarely, encephalitis and pneumonia. The incidence of these serious complications increases with age.[2] Pregnant women who develop primary varicella have a higher risk of serious complications than same-age nonpregnant women.[5]
2. Maternal exposure during pregnancy
   Congenital varicella occurs in 2% of fetuses infected during the second trimester. Therefore, susceptible women who are exposed to varicella zoster should be given varicella zoster immunoglobulin (VZIG) within 96 hours to prevent or modify the illness. In addition, infants born to mothers who develop varicella within 4 days

before or 2 days after delivery should receive VZIG to decrease the chance of serious or even fatal neonatal infection.[1]

3. Use of varicella vaccine during pregnancy
The varicella vaccine is an attenuated live virus that is contraindicated in pregnancy because the effects on the fetus are unknown. Inadvertent vaccinations during pregnancy have occurred, with more than 600 cases reported, and no increased adverse effects to mother or fetus noted.[5] The CDC and vaccine manufacturer have created a registry to report immunization during pregnancy (VARIVAX Pregnancy Registry 1-800-986-8999).[2] Still, women should be advised to avoid pregnancy for 1 month after each injection of varicella vaccine. Of note, household members of pregnant patients may safely be given Varivax.

4. Use of varicella vaccine outside of pregnancy
Susceptible persons older than 13 years should receive two doses of vaccine, with the second dose given 4 to 8 weeks after the first. Vaccination of susceptible women should be strongly considered in the postpartum period. Therefore, it is logical to clarify immune status during pregnancy, simplifying postexposure procedure and postpartum vaccination.

H. Measles, Mumps, and Rubella

1. Natural history[7]
Rubella infection was once a common childhood illness and was self-limited in most cases. However, the virus does have significant teratogenic potential, and fetal abnormalities are linked closely to gestational age. The risk for CRS, which may include cardiac, ophthalmologic, auditory, and neurologic abnormalities, is 90% when infection occurs in the first trimester. The fetal risk slowly decreases through the first 20 weeks of pregnancy such that after that gestational age, the fetal risk is minimal. Measles infection during pregnancy increases the risk for premature labor and spontaneous abortions, whereas mumps infection may cause an increase in spontaneous abortion rate with infection in the first trimester.

2. Eradication of CRS
Eradication of CRS can be accomplished only when rubella immunity is documented among all women of reproductive age. During pregnancy, routine prenatal screening for rubella immunity is standard of care. However, the MMR vaccine is live and contraindicated during

pregnancy; therefore, it is during the postpartum period that vaccination must occur. Unfortunately, a minority of hospitals has a postpartum rubella vaccination program in place.[8]

3. Inadvertent administration of rubella vaccine during pregnancy The CDC has maintained a registry of women inadvertently immunized with MMR during early pregnancy from 1971 through 1989. There have been no documented cases of CRS; therefore, vaccination with MMR during early pregnancy should not be considered a reason for termination of pregnancy.[4]

I. Poliomyelitis

1. Natural history[1]
Poliovirus is an enterovirus that can cause fetal loss during pregnancy and congenital paralytic infection during late pregnancy. Mortality is 50% in neonatal disease.

2. Vaccination during pregnancy
No adverse effects have been documented from either the oral polio vaccine or the inactivated polio vaccine (IPV), but it is advised that both vaccines be routinely avoided during pregnancy on theoretical grounds.[2]

3. Indications for use
Susceptible pregnant women traveling in endemic areas who have completed a primary series of polio vaccinations more than 10 years earlier should receive a single, one-time booster of IPV more than 4 weeks before possible exposure.[1]

III. SUMMARY

The importance of appropriate maternal immunization cannot be underestimated. In our efforts to provide the highest quality prenatal care to our patients, these simple interventions should not be forgotten. As recommendations change with some regularity, referencing the CDC website can be of great assistance.

A. Vaccines Specifically Indicated in Pregnancy

The influenza vaccine is specifically indicated in pregnancy.

B. Vaccines Used for Standard Indications in Pregnancy

1. Diphtheria/Tetanus
2. Pneumococcal
3. Meningococcal (MPSV4)

C. Vaccines to Be Avoided in Pregnancy

1. Varicella
2. MMR

D. Vaccines to Consider in Pregnancy in High-Risk Groups

1. Hepatitis A
2. Hepatitis B

REFERENCES

1. ACOG Committee Opinion—immunization during pregnancy. 282, January 2003.
2. Sur D, Wallis D, O'Connell T: Vaccinations in pregnancy, *Am Fam Physician* 68:299-304, 2003.
3. General recommendations on immunization—recommendations of the ACIP and AAFP, *MMWR* 51(RR-2):28-29, 2002.
4. *Guidelines for vaccinating pregnant women.* Updated May 2007. Abstracted from recommendations of the ACIP (Advisory Council on Immunization Practices). Available at: www.cdc.gov. Accessed August 26, 2007.
5. Gall S: Maternal immunization, *Obstet Gynecol Clin North Am* 30:623-636, 2003.
6. Zimmerman RK, Middleton DB: Vaccines for persons at high risk due to medical conditions, occupation, environment, or lifestyle, *J Fam Pract* 54:S27-S36, 2005.
7. Gonik B, Fasano N: The obstetrician-gynecologist's role in adult immunizations, *Am J Obstet Gynecol* 187:984-988, 2002.

SECTION I

Complementary and Alternative Medicine in Maternity Care

Kent Petrie, MD

Family physicians are confronted daily with questions from their patients about complementary and alternative medicine (CAM). When maternity care patients seek information about such therapies, careful attention must be paid to issues of safety and efficacy for the mother and her unborn child.

I. COMPLEMENTARY AND ALTERNATIVE MEDICINE USE IN THE UNITED STATES

The growth of alternative medicine in the United States was striking in the 1990s. In a landmark study[1] and a follow-up report,[2] Eisenberg and co-workers investigated the prevalence and costs of alternative medicine use between 1990 and 1997. Americans' annual use of at least one form of alternative medicine grew from 34% to 42% during that time. Visits to alternative therapists increased from 427 million to 629 million per year, exceeding annual visits to all primary care physicians. Although greater than 80% of patients using alternative medicine also sought treatment for the same condition from a physician, only 39% informed their physician they were doing so. By 1997, Americans spent $21.2 billion on this care, $12.2 billion of which was out-of-pocket expense. Subsequent national surveys indicate continued growth of alternative care in the United States.[3]

II. CATEGORIES OF COMPLEMENTARY AND ALTERNATIVE MEDICINE

In response to growing consumer interest in and use of alternative medicines, in 1992, the NIH established the National Center for Complementary and Alternative Medicine (NCCAM) as a clearinghouse to investigate the safety and efficacy of such therapies. For purposes of further study, NCCAM groups CAM practices into four domains, as well as "Whole Medical Systems," which may cut across all domains (see Table 3-9).[3-5] Many of the NCCAM categories are familiar and have been accepted into

---

TABLE 3-9 Complementary and Alternative Medicine Practice Domains

Biologically based practices use substances found in nature, such as herbs, special diets, or vitamins (in doses outside those used in conventional medicine).

Energy medicine involves the use of energy fields, such as magnetic fields or biofields (energy fields that some believe surround and penetrate the human body).

Manipulative and body-based practices are based on manipulation or movement of one or more body parts.

Mind–body medicine uses a variety of techniques designed to enhance the mind's ability to affect bodily function and symptoms.

Whole medical systems are built on complete systems of theory and practice. Often, these systems have evolved apart from and earlier than the conventional medical approach used in the United States.

TABLE 3-10 Complementary and Alternative Medicine Therapies Included in the 2002 National Health Information Survey

Acupuncture*
Ayurveda*
Biofeedback*
Chelation therapy*
Chiropractic care*
Deep breathing exercises
Diet-based therapies
   Vegetarian diet
   Macrobiotic diet
   Atkins diet
   Pritikin diet
   Ornish diet
   Zone diet
Energy healing therapy*
Folk medicine*
Guided imagery
Homeopathic treatment
Hypnosis*
Massage*
Meditation
Megavitamin therapy
Natural products (e.g., nonvitamin and nonmineral, such as herbs and other products from plants, enzymes)
Naturopathy*
Prayer for health reasons
   Prayed for own health
   Others ever prayed for your health
   Participate in prayer group
   Healing ritual for self
Progressive relaxation
Qigong
Reiki*
Tai chi
Yoga

For definitions of any of these therapies, see the full report or contact the *NCCAM Clearinghouse* (http://nccam.nih.gov).
*Practitioner-based therapy.

mainstream practice by primary care physicians (Table 3-10).

III. SELECTED COMPLEMENTARY AND ALTERNATIVE MEDICINE THERAPIES AND THEIR APPLICATIONS IN MATERNITY CARE

Many alternative medicine therapies have found application in the care of the maternity patient. Alternative therapies with the most evidence-based literature supporting their use include acupuncture, herbal medicine, and chiropractic and other manipulative therapies. Although not supported by a significant body of evidence, homeopathy also is growing in popularity and is discussed.

A. Acupuncture and Traditional Chinese Medicine

1. Acupuncture overview

Acupuncture (derived from Latin, *acus* = needle, *punctura* = puncture) involves the insertion of hair-thin needles into specific points in the body to prevent or treat disease. It is one component of the system of Traditional Chinese Medicine that has been in use for more than 2000 years.[6]

Acupuncture stimulates channels of energy, *Qi* (pronounced *chee* in Chinese, *key* in Japanese), that are said to flow through 12 major meridians under the surface of the skin, each of which is connected to a specific organ.[6] Classic acupuncture describes 365 points along these meridians. Over time, this number of points has increased to more than 2000, as a result of localized versions of acupuncture of the ear and hand.[7] Each point is given a number and often a name (e.g., P6/Neiguan). Chinese acupuncture points also may be stimulated by firm finger or mechanical pressure (acupressure), electric stimulation, or smoldering cones of the herb artemisia vulgaris or mugwort (moxibustion).[6] Acupuncture points commonly used in maternity care are diagrammed in Figure 3-1.

Complications of acupuncture are rare. There have been only 10 case reports of injury to internal organs since 1965 in the United States, and disposable needles have reduced the risk for infection.[8] Acupuncture and acupressure are safe in pregnancy.[7] In early pregnancy, it is recommended to avoid stimulation of points associated with uterine contractions (e.g., S6 and LI 4).[9]

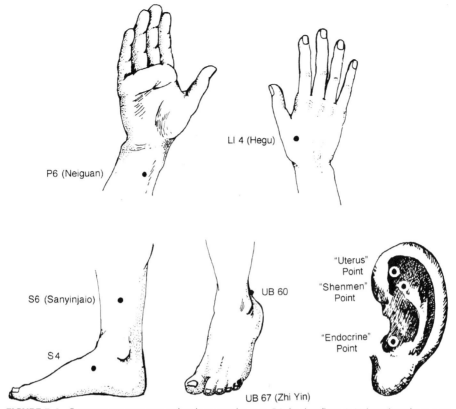

FIGURE 3-1. Common acupuncture points in maternity care. P6 (pericardium 6, Neiguan): reduces nausea and vomiting. LI4 (large intestine 4, Hegu): stimulates labor and reduces pain. S6 (spleen 6, Sanyinjaio): stimulates labor and reduces pain. S4 (spleen 4): reduces premature labor. UB 60 (urinary bladder 60): reduces low back pain. UB 67 (urinary bladder 67, Zhi Yin): facilitates version of breech. Uterus ear point: reduces labor pain and promotes relaxation. Shenmen ear point: reduces labor pain and promotes relaxation. Endocrine ear point: stimulates labor. (Courtesy Charmayne Bernhardt, Vail, CO.)

2. Acupuncture applications in maternity care
   a. Nausea and vomiting in pregnancy: Stimulation of P6, or Neiguan point (three fingerbreadths proximal to the distal wrist crease and between the two central flexor tendons of the forearm), by acupuncture needles, acupressure (purposeful stimulation for 5 minutes every 4 hours while awake), or continuous pressure with seasickness wrist bands has been shown in multiple trials[10,11] to be effective in reducing nausea and vomiting.
   b. Version of the breech presentation: Moxibustion has been studied when applied at acupuncture point UB 67 on the lateral aspect of the fifth toe. When performed bilaterally for 15 minutes each day beginning at 33 weeks of gestation, a 75% version rate by 35 weeks was shown compared with 47% in matched control subjects.[12] It is postulated that this stimulation causes increased maternal adrenocortical activity, increasing uterine tone and fetal activity, which stimulates spontaneous version.
   c. Premature labor: Acupuncture point Spleen 4 (S4), located at the base of the first metatarsal, has been reported in nonrandomized trials to treat premature labor successfully. Bilateral stimulation daily for 1 week at the onset of premature labor and then weekly thereafter has been demonstrated to delay the onset of labor.[13]

d. Induction and augmentation of labor: Although a recent Cochrane review suggests results are equivocal,[14] two small nonrandomized studies of multiple-point acupuncture have shown significant increases in contraction onset, frequency, and intensity.[13,15] Acupuncture points most commonly used to stimulate contractions are LI 4 (Hegu), on the back of the hand in the web space between the thumb and index finger, and S6 (Sanyinjiao), four fingerbreadths above the medial malleolus of the ankle. Acupressure may be applied to these points in six or more equal on/off cycles of 10 to 60 seconds, repeated as needed. Such stimulation has been suggested for outpatient cervical ripening.[7] Transcutaneous electrical nerve stimulation of these points has been reported to induce labor successfully in a series of postterm pregnancies.[9] The ear acupuncture point Endocrine also may be stimulated to increase contraction strength.[7] No cases of acupuncture causing uterine hyperstimulation have been reported in the literature.[7]

e. Pain relief in labor: Stimulation of points LI 4 and S6 has been shown to relieve pain and stimulate labor.[16,17] Acupressure may be applied to these points for 10 to 60 seconds, repeated as needed.[16,17] Two ear acupuncture points, Uterus and Shenmen, may be stimulated to reduce pain and promote general relaxation during labor.[7] Self-adhesive acupressure beads may be applied to one or both of these points and periodically pressed during labor by the patient or her birth attendant.

B. Herbal Medicine

1. Overview
   Late twentieth century dissatisfaction with the cost and side effects of synthetic pharmaceuticals has fostered a renewed interest in herbal remedies.[18] In 1997, U.S. sales of herbal products reached $3.24 billion, and herbal remedies were the top pharmacy growth category in drugstores.[18,19]
   Various forms of herbal medicines are available. Teas, steeped from delicate fresh or dried leaves or flowers, can be taken as hot or cold liquids. Tinctures or extracts are concentrated solutions, which can be taken by drops or teaspoon. Capsules or tablets are prepared from powdered herbs. Essential oils are highly concentrated oils naturally present in a plant. They have distinct aromas and are used for massage and aromatherapy.

Safety and efficacy testing of herbal preparations is not as strictly controlled as for testing of pharmaceuticals.[18] Under the FDA Dietary Supplement Health and Education Act of 1994, herbal products are considered *nutritional supplements,* not drugs. Although the FDA has forbidden placement of therapeutic information on labels, they are now tightening the restrictions on herbal remedy claims.[2] The English translation of the *German Commission E Monographs*[20] documents the European experience and has increased greatly the availability of credible information regarding herbal remedies. The *Physicians Drug Reference for Herbal Medicine* was first published in 1998 and is updated regularly.[21] Controlled trials of many remedies are being sponsored by the NIH, and more evidence-based articles on herbal remedies are beginning to appear in the primary care literature.[22] Often, however, patients think, "If it's natural, it must be safe." Herbs are potent chemicals. Many are emmenagogues (stimulate menses), and others stimulate uterine contractions. Table 3-11 lists current information on the use of herbal remedies in pregnancy.

2. Applications of herbal medicine in maternity care
   a. Nausea and vomiting
      i. Powdered gingerroot capsules (Zingiber officinale): Gingerroot at an oral dose of 250 to 500 mg four times a day has been shown to reduce nausea and emesis significantly in outpatients and in patients hospitalized with hyperemesis gravidarum.[23] The efficacy of ginger is believed to be due to its antispasmodic properties, as well as enhancing salivary secretions and increasing gastric motility.[24] A systematic review of the literature,[25] however, has cast some doubt on its absolute safety in pregnancy. Concerns have been raised because of ginger's effect on thromboxane synthetase activity and testosterone binding, which theoretically could increase bleeding in early pregnancy. The author concludes that ginger should be used with caution in pregnancy and should be avoided if the patient has a history of bleeding disorders or miscarriage.[26]

TABLE 3-11 Safety of Common Herbal Remedies in Pregnancy

Herbal Name	Common Use	Fetal Safety	Remarks
Alfalfa	High cholesterol Menopause	Probably safe when used as food	Restrict to dietary use
Aloe Vera	Infections, inflammation, laxative	UNSAFE	Induces abortions in animals
Black Cohosh	Premenstrual syndrome, dysmenorrhea, menopause	UNSAFE	Binds to estrogen receptors Induces uterine contractions Uterine hyperstimulation reported
Blue Cohosh	Dysmenorrhea, laxative, labor stimulant	UNSAFE	Teratogenicity in animals and fetal and newborn toxicity reported
Burdock	Water retention, constipation, fever, infections	UNSAFE	May stimulate uterine contractions
Calendula	Gastritis, ulcers	UNSAFE	Orally, may be an emmenagogue
Capsicum	Pain	Safe when used as food or topically	In high doses may stimulate uterine contractions
Chamomile	Gastrointestinal discomfort	UNSAFE	Was used traditionally to induce abortion
Cascara Sagrada	Constipation	Possibly safe	A stimulant laxative; bulk-forming agents or stool softeners are preferred in pregnancy
Chaste Tree	Premenstrual syndrome, menopause, insufficient lactation	UNSAFE	Orally, may be an emmenagogue
Cranberry	Urinary tract infection	Safe when used as a food	Restrict to dietary use
Dandelion Root	Liver conditions, diuretic, dyspepsia, appetite stimulant	Probably safe at low dose	
Devil's Claw	Joint inflammation, indigestion	Safety unknown	
Dong Quai	Menopause, dysmenorrhea, amenorrhea	UNSAFE	Traditional emmenagogue and abortifacient
Echinacea	Upper respiratory tract infections	Probably safe	
Evening Primrose	Eczema, premenstrual syndrome, menopause, endometritis, psychiatric conditions	Probably safe	<4 g/day
Feverfew	Migraine prevention	UNSAFE	Traditional emmenagogue and abortifacient
Garlic	Infections, hyperlipidemia	Probably safe	
Ginger	Nausea and vomiting	Probably safe	Avoid in patients with first-trimester bleeding
Ginkgo Biloba	Dementia, memory impairment	Unknown/unclear	
Goldenseal	Upper respiratory infections, urinary infections	UNSAFE	Stimulates uterine contractions

Continued

TABLE 3-11 Safety of Common Herbal Remedies in Pregnancy—cont'd

Herbal Name	Common Use	Fetal Safety	Remarks
Hops	Sleeplessness, agitation, dyspepsia, irritable bowel syndrome	UNSAFE	Contains hormone-like substances that relax myometrium
Juniper	Urinary infections, joint inflammation, indigestion	UNSAFE	Traditional emmenagogue and abortifacient
Kava	Anxiety, headache	Unknown/unclear	
Licorice	Gastric and duodenal ulcers, oral herpes, aphthous ulcers	UNSAFE	Traditional emmenagogue and abortifacient
Ma Huang	Weight loss, asthma	UNSAFE	Stimulates uterine contractions
Passion Flower	Sleeplessness, anxiety	UNSAFE	Stimulates uterine contractions
Peppermint	Gastrointestinal discomfort	UNSAFE	Traditional emmenagogue and abortifacient
Slippery Elm	Orally: gastritis, cough Topically: wound healing	UNSAFE	Traditional abortifacient
St. John's Wort	Depression	Probably safe	
Tea Tree Oil	Fungal infections	Unknown/unclear	
Uva-Ursi	Urinary tract infections	Unknown/unclear	
Valerian	Sleeplessness, anxiety	Probably safe	

Adapted from Koren G: *The complete guide to everyday risks in pregnancy and breastfeeding,* Toronto, 2004, Robert Rose Publishing (From the Motherisk Program).

ii. Vitamin B_6 (pyridoxine): Studies of pyridoxine in pregnancy show safety and efficacy in oral doses of 25 mg two to three times per day.[19] Because high doses of vitamin B_6 have been associated with neurologic problems in nonpregnant adults, questions have been raised about what constitutes excessive dosing for a developing embryo. Until further information is available, it is recommended that doses in pregnancy not exceed 75 mg/day.[11,26]

b. Induction and augmentation of labor
  i. Blue cohosh *(Caulophyllum thalictroides):* Blue cohosh tincture taken orally has been anecdotally reported to ripen the cervix and induce and augment labor.[24] Also known as squaw root and papoose root, blue cohosh is a traditional Native American herb used by various tribes to facilitate childbirth.[24] It contains steroidal saponins, which are known to stimulate the uterus. Recent animal data and human case reports suggest teratogenicity and potential fetal and newborn toxicity.[26] Despite its popularity among certain cultures, its use cannot be recommended.

  ii. Oil of evening primrose *(Oenothera biennis):* Oil of evening primrose by mouth or by placement of a capsule on the cervix has been reported for labor augmentation. The component of oil of evening primrose thought to stimulate uterine activity is the essential fatty acid gamma-linoleic acid, a precursor of prostaglandin E_1.[24]

c. Lactation suppression and prevention of engorgement
  i. Jasmine flowers: Jasmine flowers taped to the breast have been shown to be as effective as bromocriptine mesylate in suppression of lactation.[27]

    ii. Sage and parsley: Sage and parsley capsules taken by mouth have been reported to decrease the flow of milk.[7]

    iii. Cabbage leaves: Application of cold cabbage leaves, with holes cut to allow the nipples to remain dry, has been shown in randomized trials to prevent engorgement and has been associated with greater long-term breastfeeding success.[28]

  d. Increased breast milk production: Fenugreek, fennel seed, nettle, blessed thistle, and raspberry leaf have been described to increase milk flow when taken individually as capsules or combined in a tea.[7]

C. Homeopathy

1. Overview

Dr. Samuel Hahnemann (1755-1843) of Germany founded the practice of homeopathy (derived from Greek, *homois* = similar, *pathos* = suffering).[8] In the fifth century BC, Hippocrates claimed that there were two ways of healing, by *opposites* and *similars*.[8] Hahnemann founded homeopathy on the "law of similars" (i.e., "like cures like"); for example, for diarrhea, a dilute medicine is given that in high doses could cause diarrhea. Orthodox medicine, which Hahnemann named *allopathy* (derived from Greek, *allo* = other, different), focuses on opposites; for example, for constipation, a medicine is given that could cause diarrhea.

In addition to the law of similars, the principles of homeopathy include "potentiation by dilution and succussion" (vigorous shaking). This claim, that homeopathic remedies become stronger by successive dilution, has caused much skepticism among allopathic physicians, who claim that homeopathic remedies work by placebo effect only.[8] Potency scales of homeopathic remedies are noted as follows:

- Decimal scale (i.e., 6X = 6 dilutions of 10 [1:9])
- Centesimal scale (i.e., 30C = 30 dilutions of 100 [1:99])
- M scale (i.e., 50M or LM = 50 dilutions of 1000 [1:999])

Homeopathic remedies generally are considered safe for administration during pregnancy because of their minimal concentrations.[7]

Randomized controlled trials of homeopathic remedies for a variety of illnesses are beginning to appear in the literature to investigate their safety and efficacy.[8] Significant criticism has been presented of both the randomized controlled trials and the metaanalyses of these studies, however.[29]

2. Applications of homeopathy in maternity care

  a. Nausea and vomiting: Case reports of homeopathic remedies that purport to be effective include 30X to 30C dilutions of nux vomica (poison nut), *Pulsatilla* (windflower), *Cephaelis ipecacuanha* (ipecac), *Silicea* (silica), *Sepia* (cuttlefish), *Colchicum* (yellow saffron), and *Symphoricarpos racemosa* (snowberry).[7]

  b. Stimulation of labor: Homeopathic remedies have been studied prospectively to prepare the uterus for labor. A study group given *Pulsatilla nigrans, Secale cornutum, Caulophyllum thalictroides, Aceta racemosa,* and *Arnica montana* daily for 1 to 2 weeks before their due date had less false labor, fewer protracted first stages, and less postpartum blood loss than a control group.[30] Homeopathy remedies given during labor to stimulate progress include *Caulophyllum* (blue cohosh) and *Pulsatilla* (windflower) 30C administered hourly.[7] A recent Cochrane review found insufficient evidence to recommend homeopathy as a method of induction but reported no adverse effects.[31]

  c. Perineal care: The homeopathic remedy frequently used in the postpartum period is *Arnica montana* 30C every 2 to 4 hours as a liquid or tablet. It is reported to reduce bruising of the perineum, to prevent bleeding, and to reduce pain.[7,32] Witch hazel cleansings and lavender oil baths are reported to reduce perineal infection and pain.[7]

D. Chiropractic and Other Manipulative Medicine

1. Manipulative therapy overview

Chiropractic and osteopathy are two systems of manipulation that differ in theory and practice. In the simplest terms, osteopaths use arms and legs as fulcrums for bending and twisting the body (long-lever manipulation), whereas chiropractors generally manipulate only the protruding parts of the spinal vertebrae (short-lever manipulation).[8] In the twentieth century, osteopathy has evolved in the direction of conventional medicine and is no longer considered alternative. Chiropractic has continued its focus on spinal manipulation, and today chiropractors provide 94% of all manipulative therapy in the United States[33]; however, many primary care physicians (MD and DO trained) now are learning and applying techniques of spinal manipulation and mobilization in their practices.[34] Chiropractic care and other forms of spinal manipulation and mobilization are safe in pregnancy if treatments avoid direct pressure on the abdomen and uterus, and avoid prolonged supine positioning.[7] Manipulative therapy should be delivered gently, respecting the increased laxity of spinal and pelvic ligaments during pregnancy.

2. Applications of manipulative therapy in maternity care

   a. Back pain: During pregnancy, the hormone relaxin causes laxity of the anterior and posterior longitudinal ligaments of the spine, as well as the symphysis pubis and sacroiliac joints.[35] These changes, together with the body's altered center of gravity, contribute to back pain.[7] Chiropractic care and more traditional physical therapy have been proved effective in treatment of acute low back pain and can be administered safely during pregnancy.[7,36,37]

   b. Pain in labor: Counterpressure techniques applied during contractions and any time pain develops have been shown to reduce pain in the lumbar and sacroiliac areas effectively.[29] Techniques described in the literature include:

      i. Back counterpressure[38]: Steady direct manual pressure applied to the low back while the patient is standing, kneeling, sitting, or side-lying

      ii. Knee counterpressure[38]: Longitudinal pressure applied along the axis of the femur with hip and knee flexed while the patient is sitting in a chair or a birthing bed

      iii. Hip squeeze[38]: Firm pressure applied to both hips

   A variety of massage techniques has been shown to be safe and effective during labor.[39,40] It is important to encourage patient feedback on which of many massage techniques are helpful.

IV. INCORPORATING ALTERNATIVE MEDICINE INTO MATERNITY CARE

Incorporating alternative medicine into family practice maternity care is a challenge for the busy family physician. Table 3-12 lists reliable references for an

TABLE 3-12 An Office Library in Complementary and Alternative Medicine

Koren G: *The complete guide to everyday risks in pregnancy and breastfeeding,* Toronto, 2004, Robert Rose Publishing (From the Motherisk Program).

Larimore WL, O'Mathuna D: *Alternative medicine,* Grand Rapids, MI, 2001, Zondervan.

Physicians desk reference for nonprescription drugs, dietary supplements and herbs, Montvale, NJ, 2006, Thompson/Medical Economics Company.

Simkin P, Ancheta R: *The labor progress handbook,* Oxford, United Kingdom, 2000, Blackwell Science Ltd.

Tiran D, Mack S: *Complementary therapies for pregnancy and childbirth,* ed 2, London, 2000, Bailliere Tindall.

office library. Ongoing research information can be obtained from the NIH NCCAM at their website (http://nccam.nih.gov). Adding alternative medicines to maternity care requires that physicians adopt a *low-tech* approach in a *high-tech* world. Evidence is accumulating, however, on the safety, efficacy, and improved outcomes when low-tech and alternative therapies are applied to the care of the maternity patient.

V. SOR A RECOMMENDATIONS

RECOMMENDATIONS	REFERENCES
Ginger and vitamin B_6 are effective therapies for nausea and vomiting in early pregnancy.	10
Acupuncture, chiropractic manipulation, and physical therapy are effective therapies for the relief of pelvic and back pain in pregnancy.	36

REFERENCES

1. Eisenberg DM, Kessler RC, Foster C et al: Unconventional medicine in the United States. Prevalence, costs, and patterns of use, *N Engl J Med* 328:246-252, 1993.
2. Eisenberg DM, Davis RB, Ettner SL et al: Trends in alternative medicine use in the United States, 1990–1997. Results of a follow-up national survey, *JAMA* 280:1569-1575, 1998.
3. Barnes P, Powell-Griner E, McFann K et al: Complementary and alternative medicine use among adults: United States, 2002, *Adv Data* (343):1-19.

4. Alternative Medicine: expanding Medical Horizons: a report to the National Institutes of Health on Alternative Medical Systems and Practices in the United States, Washington, DC, 1994, U.S. Government Printing Office.

5. Practice and Policy Guidelines Panel, NIH Office of Alternative Medicine: Clinical practice guidelines in complementary and alternative medicine, *Arch Fam Med* 6:149-154, 1997.

6. Macipocia G: *The foundations of Chinese medicine,* Edinburgh, 1998, Churchill Livingstone.

7. Tiran D, Mack S: *Complementary therapies for pregnancy and childbirth,* ed 2, London, 2000, Bailliere Tindall, 2000.

8. Fugh-Berman A: *Alternative medicine: what works,* Baltimore, 1997, Williams & Wilkins.

9. Dunn DA, Rogers D, Halford K: Transcutaneous electrical nerve stimulation at acupuncture points in the induction of uterine contractions, *Obstet Gynecol* 73:286-290, 1989.

10. Jewell D, Young G: Interventions for nausea and vomiting in early pregnancy, *Cochrane Database Syst Rev* (4):CD000145, 2003.

11. Murphy PA: Alternative therapies for nausea and vomiting of pregnancy, *Obstet Gynecol* 91:149-155, 1998.

12. Cardini F, Weixin H: Moxibustion for correction of breech presentation: a randomized controlled trial, *JAMA* 280:1580-1584, 1998.

13. Tsuei JJ, Lai Y-F, Sharma SD: The influence of acupuncture stimulation during pregnancy: the induction and inhibition of labor, *Obstet Gynecol* 50:479-488, 1997.

14. Smith CA, Crowther CA: Acupuncture for induction of labour, *Cochrane Database Syst Rev* (1):CD002962, 2004.

15. Kudista E, Kucera H, Muller-Tyl E: Initiation contractions of the gravid uterus through electroacupuncture, *Am J Chin Med* 3:343-346, 1975.

16. Jimenez SLM: Acupuncture: pain relief at your fingertips, *Int J Childbirth Educ* 10:7-10, 1995.

17. Smith CA, Collins CT, Cyna AM et al: Complementary and alternative therapies for pain management in labour, *Cochrane Database Syst Rev* (1), 2004.

18. Bartels CL, Miller SJ: Herbal and related remedies, *Nutr Clin Pract* 12:5-19, 1998.

19. O'Hara MA, Kiefer D, Farrell K et al: A review of 12 commonly used medicinal herbs, *Arch Fam Med* 7:523-536, 1998.

20. Blumenthal M, Gruenwald J, Hall T et al: *German Commission E monographs: medicinal plants for human use,* Austin, TX, 1998, American Botanical Council.

21. LaGow B, Murray L: *Physicians drug reference for herbal medicine,* Monvale, NJ, 2004, Thomson PDR.

22. Shaughnessy AF: Weeds and seeds: the evidence behind natural products, *FP Recert* 19:53-56, 1997.

23. Fischer-Rasmussen W, Kjaer SK, Dahl C et al: Ginger treatment of hyperemesis gravidarum, *Eur J Obstet Gynaecol Reprod Biol* 38:19-24, 1990.

24. Chevallier A: *The encyclopedia of medicinal plants,* New York, 1996, DK Publishing.

25. Udani J, Hardy M: Ginger for motion sickness, hyperemesis gravidarum, chemotherapy, and anesthesia, *Altern Med Alert* 1:133–137, 1988.

26. Briggs GG, Freeman RK, Yaffe SJ: *Drugs in pregnancy and lactation,* ed 7, Philadelphia, 2005, Lippincott Williams & Wilkins.

27. Shrivastav P, George K, Balasubramanium N et al: Suppression of puerperal lactation using jasmine flowers (jasminum sambac), *Aust N Z J Obstet Gynaecol* 28:68-72, 1998.

28. Nikodem VC, Danziger D, Gebka N et al: Do cabbage leaves prevent breast engorgement? A randomized controlled study, *Birth* 20:61-64, 1993.

29. Kleijnen J, Knipschild P, terRiet G: Clinical trials of homeopathy, *BMJ* 302:316-323, 1992.

30. Ventoslovsky BM, Popov AV: Homeopathy as a practical alternative to traditional obstetric methods, *Br Homeopath J* 79:201-205, 1990.

31. Smith CA: Homeopathy for induction of labour, *Cochrane Database Syst Rev* (4), 2003.

32. Hofmeyr GJ, Piccioni V, Blauhof P: Postpartum homeopathic arnica montana: a potency-finding pilot study, *Br J Clin Pract* 44:619-621, 1990.

33. Shekelle PG, Brook RH: A community based study of the use of chiropractic services, *Am J Public Health* 81:439-442, 1991.

34. Gordon JS: Alternative medicine and the family physician, *Am Fam Physician* 54:2205-2212, 1996.

35. Kristiansson K, Svardsudd K, von Schoultz B: Serum relaxin, symphyseal pain, and back pain during pregnancy, *Am J Obstet Gynecol* 175:1342-1347, 1996.

36. Young G, Jewell D: Interventions for preventing and treating pelvic and back pain in pregnancy, *Cochrane Database Syst Rev* (1):CD001139, 2002.

37. Simkin P: Reducing pain and enhancing progress in labor: a guide to non-pharmacologic methods for maternity caregivers, *Birth* 22:161-171, 1995.

38. Simkin P: *Simkin's ratings of comfort measures for childbirth,* Waco, TX, 1997, Childbirth Graphics.

39. Simkin P: Psychological and other non-pharmacologic techniques. *Principles and practice of obstetric analgesia and anesthesia,* ed 2, Baltimore, 1995, Williams & Wilkins.

40. Elder H, Ladfors L, Olsen MF et al: Effects of acupuncture and stabilizing exercises as adjunct to standard treatment in pregnant women with pelvic girdle pain: randomized single blind controlled trial, *BMJ* 330:671, 2005.

SECTION J Diagnostic Ultrasound in Pregnancy

Ellen L. Sakornbut, MD,
and Mark Deutchman, MD

Diagnostic ultrasound is a major tool in modern pregnancy diagnosis and management. It is also a much-requested procedure by pregnant women. In many countries, pregnant women routinely receive one or more ultrasound scans. It is therefore important for physicians to understand the uses and limitations of ultrasound.

I. COMMON INDICATIONS

A 1984 NIH consensus panel identified 28 medical indications for ultrasonography in pregnancy. This list has withstood the test of time (Table 3-13).[1]

TABLE 3-13 National Institutes of Health Indications for Ultrasonography in Pregnancy

Gestational age assessment in cases of uncertain dates, termination of pregnancy, need for induction of labor, or repeat cesarean section before the onset of labor

Evaluation of fetal growth

Vaginal bleeding, rule out placenta previa

Determination of fetal presentation

Suspected multiple gestation

Adjunct to amniocentesis

Size-dates discrepancy

Maternal pelvic masses found clinically

Suspected hydatidiform mole

Adjunct to cervical cerclage placement or cervical length in cerclage patients

Suspected ectopic pregnancy

Adjunct to special procedures such as chorionic villus sampling

Suspected fetal death

Suspected uterine abnormality and evaluation of a cervical scar

Intrauterine contraceptive device localization

Ovarian follicle development surveillance

Biophysical evaluation for fetal well-being

Intrapartum events: to aid version of the second twin; guidance of manual placenta removal

Suspected polyhydramnios or oligohydramnios

Suspected placental abruption

Adjunct to external version from breech to vertex presentation

Fetal evaluation and weight estimation in cases of premature labor and premature rupture of the membranes

Investigation of abnormal serum α-fetoprotein

Follow-up observation of identified fetal anomaly

Repeat evaluation of placental location

History of a previous infant with a congenital anomaly

Serial evaluation of fetal growth in multiple gestation

Evaluation of the fetal age and condition when prenatal care has been started late or has not been sought before the onset of labor

From National Institutes of Health: Consensus conference: "The use of diagnostic ultrasound imaging during pregnancy," Bethesda, MD, 1984, Office of Medical Applications of Research, National Institutes of Health.

II. CLINICAL STANDARDS FOR OBSTETRIC ULTRASOUND EXAMINATIONS

A. Content of the Standard Examination

The American Institute of Ultrasound in Medicine, American College of Radiology, and ACOG are in agreement regarding the content of the standard ultrasound examination.[2] This agreement replaces concepts regarding level 1 and 2 examinations, previously developed by the British MSAFP screening program.

1. First-trimester scan
   a. Location of gestational sac, identification of embryo, and measurement of crown-rump length
   b. Documentation of fetal life
   c. Documentation of fetal number
   d. Evaluation of uterus, cervix, and adnexa
2. Second- or third-trimester scan
   a. Fetal cardiac activity, fetal presentation, and fetal number
   b. Qualitative or semiquantitative evaluation of amniotic fluid volume
   c. Placental location, appearance, and relation to internal cervical os; umbilical cord and number of vessels
   d. Biometric measurements to assess gestational age and fetal weight, biparietal diameter, head circumference, abdominal circumference, and femur length are measured for gestational age assessment. Abdominal diameters or circumferences are more reflective of the nutritional status of the fetus in the third trimester. Gestational age determination is less accurate in the third trimester (+3 weeks), but fetal weight determination may be of clinical value. Whenever possible, appropriateness of interval change from other measurements should be recorded. Biometric measurements should be recorded as actual measurements and not solely as the corresponding average gestational age on a chart.
   e. Evaluation of the maternal uterus and adnexa
   f. Fetal anatomic survey: Fetal anatomy can usually be assessed after 18 weeks, although fetal size, position, movement, and maternal conditions may obscure some features. When the

fetal anatomic survey is incomplete, this should be reported and a follow-up examination may be indicated.

h. Anatomy
   i. Head and neck: cerebellum, choroid plexus, cisterna magna, lateral cerebral ventricles, midline falx, cavum septi pellucidi
   ii. Chest: four-chamber view of the fetal heart and, if possible, an evaluation of the outflow tracts.
   iii. Abdomen: stomach (presence, size, and situs), kidneys, bladder, umbilical cord insertion site and number of vessels in the cord
   iv. Spine: cervical, thoracic, lumbar, and sacral spine
   v. Extremities: presence or absence of legs and arms
   vi. Sex determination: medically indicated in low-risk pregnancies only for evaluation of multifetal pregnancies

B. Role of Limited Ultrasound

Limited examinations may be indicated, particularly when a specific question requires an urgent answer such as determination of fetal presentation during labor, inability to hear the fetal heartbeat, or for assessment of amniotic fluid quantity. In most cases, the patient should also have a complete examination on record.

C. Specialized Scans

When a standard examination suggests a possible abnormality, more extensive examinations of the fetus may be indicated. Examples include Doppler studies and fetal echocardiograms.

III. CLINICAL APPLICATIONS

A. Routine Screening

Routine screening of all pregnant women with ultrasound has been the subject of many studies. These studies are complicated by the fact that many women, even the majority of women, will have one or more medical indications for ultrasound. Metaanalysis of this subject has concluded that routine ultrasound before 24 weeks provides better gestational age assessment, earlier detection of multifetal pregnancies, and earlier detection of otherwise unsuspected fetal anomalies at a time when termination of pregnancy is possible.[3] However, routine screening after 24 weeks has not been found to provide benefits.[4]

B. Gestational Age Assessment

Ultrasound is the most reliable method of assessing gestational age when the patient's last menses are unknown, unsure, or when she seeks care late in pregnancy.

1. First-trimester scans
   First-trimester transabdominal scans can establish the gestational age of a pregnancy within 3 to 5 days using the crown-rump length. Transvaginal scanning uses a higher frequency transducer with improvement of resolution, enabling small structures to be seen earlier. A fetal pole can be measured by approximately 6 weeks menstrual age (42 days) by transvaginal scanning, whereas it is not visualized until 7 to 8 weeks by transabdominal scanning. Measurement of a gestational sac before appearance of an embryo produces less certain results with respect to dating of pregnancy. Crown-rump length measurements after 12 weeks are unreliable because of fetal spine flexion.

2. Second-trimester scans
   Ultrasound scanning before 22 weeks of gestation is probably the most useful for confirmation of dates for patients with average-risk status. Multiple-parameter dating, including biparietal diameter, head and abdominal circumference, and femur length, produces an accurate gestational age within ±1.4 weeks. Fetal anatomy should also be evaluated at this time.

3. Late pregnancy scanning
   Second- and third-trimester ultrasounds are increasingly inaccurate in establishing gestational age, with a variance of 2.6 to 3 weeks in patients who have technically satisfactory scans. Generally, gestational age established by reliable ultrasound or ultrasound plus clinical data in early pregnancy (before 22 weeks of gestation) should not be altered by sonographic findings in the third trimester.

C. Growth Assessment

Intrauterine growth restriction (IUGR) is divided into two types (see Chapter 7, Section E): Symmetric IUGR comprises 30% and asymmetric IUGR comprises 70% of fetuses with inadequate growth.

1. Symmetric IUGR

   Symmetric IUGR occurs in fetuses with intrauterine infection or trisomy, and it can be most reliably diagnosed with serial ultrasound examinations. Only if menstrual dates are unequivocal and a follow-up scan shows abnormal growth velocity can a single scan establish this diagnosis.

2. Asymmetric IUGR

   Asymmetric IUGR can be suspected on a single ultrasound scan that shows a proportionately small abdominal circumference relative to head and long-bone measurements. This appearance occurs most commonly late in the second trimester or in the third trimester. A patient thought to be at risk for IUGR should have gestational age established firmly before 20 weeks of gestation. Screening for IUGR can be pursued with follow-up scans between 32 and 34 weeks of gestation, or sooner if there is poor fundal height progression or suggested compromise to uterine blood flow (e.g., preeclampsia).

3. Fetal macrosomia

   Fetal macrosomia may be diagnosed sonographically if the gestational age has been established previously. Fetal weight estimates in the early third trimester can be plotted on a growth curve to obtain a percentile rank. If the estimated fetal weight is above the 90th percentile, the diagnosis of macrosomia is suspected. Fetal weight estimates close to term are no more accurate than ±10% to 15%, limiting the use of this information in management decisions. Ultrasound assessment of macrosomia is most beneficial in conjunction with assessment of the patient with diabetes. (For further information regarding the use of ultrasound at term in patients with suspected macrosomia, see Chapter 7, Section F.)

D. Assessment of Bleeding

1. First-trimester bleeding is discussed more fully in Chapter 6. Ultrasound can be used to determine fetal viability and the presence or absence of an intrauterine pregnancy to rule out ectopic pregnancy.

2. Later in pregnancy, ultrasound is helpful to assess for placenta previa and abruption (see Chapter 16, Section D). Placenta previa, marginal previa, and low-lying placenta are frequent incidental findings during early dating scans (1:20). The accuracy of establishing the exact relation of the placenta to the cervical os is better with transvaginal ultrasound than with transabdominal ultrasound. Two choices of management are acceptable:

   a. Repeat scanning: Because approximately 9 of 10 patients with suspected placenta previa (by ultrasound done at <20 weeks of gestation) do not have a placenta previa in late pregnancy, a scan may be repeated after 30 weeks. Patients who have a placenta previa may present before this time, however, with vaginal bleeding.

   b. Transvaginal confirmation: Patients with suspected placenta previa may be evaluated at the time of the initial diagnostic scan with transvaginal ultrasound to eliminate the possibility of placenta covering the internal cervical os. In one series of patients evaluated by transabdominal scanning and transvaginal scanning for low-lying or suspected placenta previa, a change in diagnosis was established by transvaginal scanning in approximately 25% of cases.[5] In another study of more than 3600 patients, the placenta extended to or over the internal cervical os in 1.5% of women evaluated by transabdominal and transvaginal ultrasound scans. Use of a cutoff of placental extension 15 mm or more over the internal os leads to 19% positive predictive value for placenta previa at delivery with 100% sensitivity.[6] This finding occurred in only 0.7% of women. Although the positive predictive value of this finding was low, follow-up ultrasound examinations were needed in only a small percentage of women scanned. Use of this strategy should reduce the need for follow-up scans by fivefold (1:20 scans, or 5% reduced to <1%).

E. Assessment of the Cervical Length to Predict Preterm Birth

Typical risk factors for preterm birth include one or more previous preterm births, uterine anomalies, two or more voluntary terminations, diethylstilbestrol exposure, previous cone biopsy, twin or triplet pregnancies, preterm labor, and preterm prematurely ruptured membranes. The length of the cervix can be measured sonographically and the transvaginal scan route is particularly useful and is more reliable than digital examination. Results of studies on cervical length show the following charactertics[7]:

1. In women at risk for preterm birth:

   a. Cervical length of 25 mm is commonly considered the lower limit of "normal."

  b. The *negative* predictive value for preterm birth of a cervical length of 25 mm or greater is quite high: 75% to 90%.
  c. The *positive* predictive value for preterm birth of a cervical length of less than 25 mm varies widely between studies: 20% to 75%.
2. In women with actual symptoms of preterm labor
  a. Cervical length of 25 to 35 mm is commonly considered the lower limit of "normal."
  b. The *negative* predictive value for preterm birth of a cervical length of 25 mm or greater is quite high: 80% to 100%.
  c. The *positive* predictive value for preterm birth of a cervical length of less than 25 mm varies widely between studies: 50% to 89%.
3. In women with twin pregnancy
  a. Cervical length of 25 mm is commonly considered the lower limit of "normal."
  b. The *negative* predictive value for preterm birth of a cervical length of 25 mm or greater is quite high: 75% to 97%.
  c. The *positive* predictive value for preterm birth of a cervical length of less than 25 mm varies widely between studies: 31% to 67%.
4. Reasonable conclusions suggested by these results are as follows:
  a. Transvaginal cervical length measurements are better at identifying women who will not deliver prematurely than those who will.
  b. Cervical length of 25 mm or more may be a useful marker to *avoid* interventions for preterm delivery.

F. Assessment of Fetal Well-being

Examination of fetal circulatory parameters with Doppler ultrasound improves a number of obstetric care outcomes and appears promising in helping to reducing perinatal deaths in complicated pregnancies[8] but not in otherwise normal pregnancies (see Chapter 11, Section B).[9]

G. Assessment for Possible Fetal Structural or Chromosomal Abnormality

1. The value of ultrasound for detecting major fetal structural abnormalities such as anencephaly is undisputed. Sonographic diagnosis of a huge range of other major and minor abnormalities is possible depending on gestational age, maternal factors, equipment, and operator skill. Adherence to standard examination guidelines[2] maximizes the chances of identifying most major abnormalities. Controversy exists about which abnormalities should be diagnosed during a standard examination when the fetus is not at increased risk for any particular abnormality and about the clinical significance of detecting structural abnormalities. The Routine Antenatal Diagnostic Imaging with Ultrasound (RADIUS) study[10] failed to show clinical benefit associated with *routine* ultrasound and failed to detect a change in outcome associated with the diagnosis of congenital malformations, despite a greater than threefold increase in detection of malformations between the screened and control groups.[11] European trials addressing the issue of routine ultrasound found that perinatal mortality rates were reduced because of more frequent pregnancy terminations when serious malformations were diagnosed before 24 weeks of gestation.[12,13] Criticisms of the RADIUS trial include a relatively low rate of malformations detected before 24 weeks, but this rate appears to be consistent with another large trial with a similar number of patients. Notably, in the RADIUS study, approximately 60% of pregnant women were excluded from randomization to routine ultrasound or the control group because they had a medical indication for an ultrasound scan.
2. Screening for fetal aneuploidy, particularly trisomy 21, with the aim of decreasing need for genetic amniocentesis has been the target of many investigations. Screening strategies that include both maternal serum screening (MSAFP, unconjugated estriol, hCG, and inhibin A) and sonography have the greatest predictive value (see Chapter 7, Section H). Combining ultrasound with maternal serum screening helps refine knowledge of the patient's risk for aneuploidy in several ways[14]:
  a. In the first trimester, the maternal serum marker pregnancy-associated plasma protein A can be combined with a sonographic search for a thickened fetal nuchal translucency to identify fetuses with an increased risk for trisomy 21.[15]
  b. Accurate knowledge of gestational age, as assessed by ultrasound, is necessary to interpret the maternal serum screen values.
  c. Major structural anomalies occur in about 20% of second-trimester fetuses with trisomy 21 and other chromosomal abnormalities. Discovery of a major anomaly significantly increases the likelihood of aneuploidy and is usually followed by

offering the woman amniocentesis for definitive chromosome analysis. Major anomalies include heart defects, duodenal atresia, cerebral ventriculomegaly, flat facies with maxillary hypoplasia, enlarged tongue, brachycephaly, hydrops, and clubfoot.

   d. A large number of minor sonographic "markers" are seen more commonly in trisomy 21 than in unaffected fetuses. These include echogenic bowel, cerebral ventriculomegaly, renal pyelectasis, echogenic intracardiac focus, choroid plexus cyst, two-vessel cord, clinodactyly, sandal gap toe, wide pelvic angle, and others. Likelihood of trisomy 21 increases when more of these "markers" are present.

3. The presence of major structural anomalies and other "markers" can be combined with maternal serum screening results to modify the patient's risk for trisomy 21. Typical resulting accuracy is a sensitivity of 69% and a false-positive rate of 8%.[16]

4. When the patient's maternal serum screen is abnormal, but no structural abnormalities are found on ultrasound, her risk for carrying a fetus with trisomy 21, as reported from the maternal serum screen results, is typically reduced by about half.[17] This information may help the patient decide whether to undergo amniocentesis.

IV. TERMINOLOGY AND ABBREVIATIONS

Table 3-14 lists terminology and abbreviations pertinent to ultrasound scanning.

V. SOR A RECOMMENDATIONS

RECOMMENDATIONS	REFERENCES
Routine ultrasound in early pregnancy (before 24 weeks of gestation) appears to enable better gestational age assessment, earlier detection of multiple pregnancies, and earlier detection of clinically unsuspected fetal malformation at a time when termination of pregnancy is possible. However, the benefits for other substantive outcomes are less clear.	*3*
Routine late pregnancy ultrasound (after 24 weeks) in low-risk or unselected populations does not confer benefit on mother or baby.	*4*
The use of Doppler ultrasound in high-risk pregnancies appears to improve a number of obstetric care outcomes and appears promising in helping to reduce perinatal deaths.	*8*
Routine Doppler ultrasound in low-risk or unselected populations does not confer benefit on mother or baby.	*9*
When second-trimester ultrasound reveals fetal structural abnormalities, the likelihood of trisomy 21 is increased.	*16*

TABLE 3-14 Terminology and Abbreviations Used in Diagnostic Ultrasound

---

FL/BPD—femur length/biparietal diameter ratio, used to determine limb abnormalities, microcephaly, and other cranial abnormalities

GS—gestational sac

HC—head circumference

HC/AC—head/abdomen ratio, also used in growth assessment

MSD—mean sac diameter

Placental grade—using a system that includes the presence of echogenic densities, lobulation, and other characteristics; the placenta may be graded from 0 to 3; although grade 3 placentas are characterized as mature, they do not correlate fully with fetal lung maturity; many patients reach term without demonstration of a grade 3 placenta

TAD—transverse abdominal diameter

TAS—transabdominal scanning

TLU—translabial ultrasound (see intrapartum use)

TPS—transperineal scanning (same as TLU)

TTD—transverse trunk diameter

TVS—transvaginal scanning

YS—yolk sac

REFERENCES

1. National Institutes of Health: *Consensus conference: The use of diagnostic ultrasound imaging during pregnancy,* Bethesda, 1984, Office of Medical Applications of Research, National Institutes of Health.
2. *AIUM practice guideline for the performance of an antepartum obstetric ultrasound examination.* Available at: http://www.aium.org/publications/clinical/obstetrical.pdf. Accessed August 20, 2007.
3. Neilson JP: Ultrasound for fetal assessment in early pregnancy, *Cochrane Database Syst Rev* (2):CD000182, 2000.
4. Bricker L, Neilson JP: Routine ultrasound in late pregnancy (after 24 weeks gestation), *Cochrane Database Syst Rev* (3), 2006.

5. Smith R, Lauria M, Comstock C et al: Transvaginal ultrasonography for all placentas that appear to be low-lying or over the internal cervical os, *Ultrasound Obstet Gynecol* 9:22-24, 1997.
6. Taipale P, Hiilesmaa V, Ylostalo P: Transvaginal ultrasonography at 18–23 weeks in predicting placental previa at delivery, *Ultrasound Obstet Gynecol* 12:422-425, 1998.
7. Berghella V, Bega G, Tolosa JE et al: Ultrasound assessment of the cervix, *Clin Obstet Gynecol* 46(4):947-962, 2003.
8. Bricker L, Neilson JP: Routine Doppler ultrasound in pregnancy, *Cochrane Database Syst Rev* (2):CD001450, 2000.
9. Neilson JP, Alfirevic Z: Doppler ultrasound for fetal assessment in high-risk pregnancies, *Cochrane Database Syst Rev* (2):CD000073, 2000.
10. Lefevre M, Bain R, Ewigman B et al: A randomized trial of prenatal ultrasonographic screening: impact on maternal management and outcome. RADIUS (Routine Antenatal Diagnostic Imaging with Ultrasound) Study Group, *Am J Obstet Gynecol* 169:483-489, 1993.
11. Crane J, Lefevre M, Winborn R et al: A randomized trial of prenatal ultrasonographic screening: impact on the detection, management, and outcome of anomalous fetuses. The RADIUS Study Group, *Am J Obstet Gynecol* 171:392-399, 1994.
12. Saari-Kemppainen A, Karjalainen O, Ylostalo P et al: Ultrasound screening and perinatal mortality: controlled trial of systematic one-stage screening in pregnancy, *Lancet* 336:337–391, 1990.
13. Saari-Kemppainen A, Karjalainen O, Ylostalo P et al: Fetal anomalies in a controlled one-stage ultrasound screening trial: a report from the Helsinki Ultrasound Group, *J Perinat Med* 22:279-289. 1994.
14. Egan JF: The genetic sonogram in second trimester Down Syndrome screening, *Clin Obstet Gynecol* 46(4):897-908, 2003.
15. De Graaf I, Pajkrt E, Bilardo C et al: Early pregnancy screening for fetal aneuploidy with serum markers and nuchal translucency, *Prenat Diagn* 19:458-462, 1999.
16. Smith-Bindman R, Hosmer W, Feldstein VA et al: Second-trimester ultrasound to detect fetuses with Down syndrome: a meta-analysis, *JAMA* 285:1044-1055, 2001.
17. Vintzileos AM, Guzman ER, Smulian JC et al: Down syndrome risk estimation after normal genetic sonography, *Am J Obstet Gynecol* 187:1226-1229, 2002.

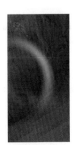

Patient and Family Education

SECTION A Nutrition in Pregnancy and Lactation

Elizabeth G. Baxley, MD,
and Rachel Setzler Brown, MD

During pregnancy, energy is necessary to support the physiologic, metabolic, and biochemical changes that occur in response to the growth and development of a healthy and appropriate-for-gestational-age-weight fetus. The pregnant woman's diet is the main source of this necessary energy.[1] One of the earliest purposes of prenatal care was to counsel patients regarding nutrition. Pregnant women may benefit from instruction on basic dietary adequacy and the additional nutritional requirements of pregnancy. Sound nutritional and weight gain advice by prenatal care providers, together with maternal compliance with these recommendations, has been shown in individual studies to have a positive effect on birth outcomes.[2] However, a published review of 7 randomized controlled trials (RCTs), 1 non-RCT, and 1 longitudinal, nonrandomized study of more than 4,000 women indicate that, although women may increase their intake of energy and protein to improve pregnancy outcomes, the evidence is insufficient to make the association between dietary changes and these positive outcomes.[3]

I. NUTRITIONAL STATUS

A. Nutritional Evaluation

1. History and dietary recall
   Assessment of nutritional adequacy may be achieved by use of a dietary recall that provides information about balance of food groupings and improper habits, such as fasting and meal skipping. Questions should be asked in a non-threatening manner and should cover several days of dietary recall. Weekly food charts have been recommended but may suffer from poor patient compliance.[1]
   The dietary history may alert the provider to patients at potential risk secondary to their nutritional habits, such as food faddists, women who practice pica, or women with low intake of dairy products. Women of high parity, women with previous low-birth-weight infants, or women with short interconceptual periods also are at risk and need special counseling and follow-up during their pregnancies. Beliefs and preferences regarding foods should be discussed, acknowledging the importance of ethnic, cultural, and family eating patterns. Financial stability and ability to purchase food should be determined, and women who lack financial resources to purchase sufficient amounts of nutritious foods should be referred to Women, Infants, and Children (WIC), a federal supplemental food program for pregnant women and their children.

2. Physical examination and laboratory evaluation
   Recommended weight gain can be estimated based on measurement of the body mass index (BMI) (Table 4-1). In the absence of other hematologic abnormalities, the hemoglobin is also a useful test of nutritional status.[1] Values of less than 11.0 g/dl in the first and third trimesters and less than 10.5 g/dl in the second trimester may indicate inadequate nutrition, and a ferritin level less than 20 mg/dl indicates deficient iron stores.

TABLE 4-1 Recommended Weight Gain during Pregnancy

Maternal Classification	Weight Gain (kg)		Weight Gain (lb)	
	Total (kg)	Rate (kg/4 wk)*	Total (lb)	Rate (lb/4 wk)*
Prepregnant BMI†				
Underweight (<19.8)	12.7-18.2	2.3	28-40	5.0
Normal weight (19.8-28.0)	11.4-15.9	1.8	25-35	4.0
Overweight (28.1-29.0)	6.8-11.4	1.2	16-25	2.6
Obese (>29.0)	6.8	0.9	15	2.0
Twin gestation	15.9-20.4	2.7	35-45	6.0

*Rate applies to the second and third trimesters.
†Body mass index (BMI) is derived from metric units.
Adapted from National Academy of Sciences: *Nutrition during pregnancy,* Washington, DC, 1990, National Academy Press.

B. Caloric Needs and Weight Gain

1. Calories

   The average pregnant woman should consume an average increase of 300 kcal/day depending on gestational age, with an additional 150 kcal/day needed during the first trimester and an additional 300 to 500 kcal/day during the second and third trimesters. An estimated total caloric intake for most pregnant women in the range of 1900 to 2750 kcal/day is recommended. Maternal weight gain is the best index for the adequacy of caloric intake.

2. Calorie sources

   Carbohydrates are necessary for normal energy production and provision of glucose for the fetus. A diet deficient in carbohydrates leads to decreased fetal growth and may contribute to neurologic defects.[4] Carbohydrates should comprise 50% to 60% of the total caloric intake, which may be achieved with a minimum of four servings of breads and cereals and two servings of fruits and vegetables. The best sources of carbohydrates include whole-grain foods, fresh fruits and vegetables, and milk.

   Protein is needed for fetal growth and development, placental growth, increased maternal blood volume, growth of the uterus and breasts, and colostrum production. Proteins should comprise 20% of the total calories of the pregnant woman's diet, with an additional 30 g/day required over nonpregnant needs (75-80 g/day). These enhanced requirements of pregnancy can be achieved by eating 8 ounces of a meat or meat substitute, plus three to four milk servings per day. Additional protein supplementation beyond this level has not been shown to improve pregnancy outcomes[5] and has been associated with increased risk for small for gestational age (SGA) births.

   High daily intake of total fat before pregnancy increases the risk for severe hyperemesis gravidarum.[6] However, fats are necessary for maternal energy production. They also provide fatty acids for myelination of fetal nerve cells and absorption of fat-soluble vitamins, and are stored for lactation. During pregnancy, fats should contribute no more than 30% of total daily calories in the diet.

3. Weight gain

   Maternal weight gain during pregnancy is a major determinant of birth weight and is a primary indicator of infant mortality and morbidity.[7] A linear relation exists between maternal weight gain and infant birth weight at all levels of prepregnancy body mass, age, parity, and mother's level of education.[2] The pattern of weight accumulation is an important factor in the overall evaluation of weight gain during pregnancy. The maternal component begins in the first trimester and is greatest during the first half of the pregnancy. Fetal growth is most rapid in the second half of pregnancy, with the fetus more than tripling its weight in the last trimester.[1] The remainder of weight gained represents interstitial fluid. The

TABLE 4-2 Components of Weight Gain in Normal Pregnancy

Organ, Tissue, or Fluid	Weight (g)
Maternal	
Uterus	970
Breasts	405
Blood	1250
Water	1680
Fat	3345
Subtotal	7650
Fetal	
Fetus	3400
Placenta	650
Amniotic fluid	800
Subtotal	4850
Total	12,500

Adapted from Hymen FE, Leitch L, editors: *The physiology of human pregnancy,* ed 2, Oxford, 1971, Blackwell Scientific Publications.

components of weight gain during pregnancy are listed in Table 4-2.

In addition to the BMI, recommendations for weight gain must consider other individual characteristics, such as maternal age (especially in adolescent pregnancies), parity, singleton versus multiple gestation, smoking, medical conditions, and special dietary needs.

  a. Normal prepregnancy weight: If a woman is at a desirable weight at the time of conception, a 25- to 35-lb weight gain for the pregnancy is recommended. Ideally, only 2 to 5 lb of this should be gained during the first trimester. For the second and third trimesters, an average gain of 0.5 to 1 lb/wk is desirable.

  b. Underweight women: Women at less than 90% of desired body weight at the beginning of pregnancy are at risk for delivering a low-birth-weight infant. When possible, women should be encouraged to gain weight before pregnancy. During pregnancy, a 30- to 35-lb weight gain is recommended for underweight women, with special attention placed on initial and ongoing dietary counseling and education to minimize the complications associated with low-birth-weight infants.

  c. Overweight women: Women at greater than 120% of their desirable body weight at the time

of conception have a greater risk for development of gestational diabetes, pregnancy-related hypertension, and thromboembolic complications. The impact of weight gain on the birth weight of the infant is diminished as compared with normal-weight or underweight women. Weight loss is not recommended, but lower rates of weight gains may be appropriate, with a weight gain of 18 to 20 lb recommended. Adherence to these parameters may reduce the rate of macrosomia and facilitate subsequent maternal weight loss after delivery.[2]

  d. Nonstandard weight gain patterns: Excessive weight gain is defined as greater than 6.5 lb/mo. In cases of excessive weight gain, the patient's diet should be reviewed for sources of excess calories. Medical complications should be excluded, including pregnancy-associated edema, diabetes, and preeclampsia. Weight loss should not be promoted, but slowing the rate of weight gain may be accomplished by reducing portion sizes and decreasing fat content. Energy/protein restriction of overweight pregnant women does appear to reduce weekly maternal weight gain and mean birth weight but has no effect on reducing potential pregnancy complications.[5] Excessive fat deposited during pregnancy contributes to chronic obesity, but fat stores can be reduced after parturition by breastfeeding.

Careful evaluation is needed for the pregnant woman who has gained less than 2.2 lb/mo at the end of the first trimester or less than 10 lb at 20 weeks of gestation. Risk factors for inadequate gain are low maternal prepregnancy weight, smoking during pregnancy, low family income, low educational level, unmarried status, and age younger than 20 or older than 35 years.[2] Vigorous nutritional intervention is indicated because low weight gain is associated with reduced expansion of plasma volume and development of intrauterine growth restriction (IUGR). Patients should be cautioned against dieting and meal skipping. Increasing the fat content in the diet and adding high-calorie dietary supplements three times per day should be recommended.

C. Vitamin and Mineral Needs

Blood levels for most vitamins and minerals are lower during pregnancy than at other times in a woman's life. All nutrients except for iron usually are supplied by a well-balanced diet, however. Routine multivitamin supplementation in women following a well-balanced diet may not be necessary but is common practice. Medical indications for supplementation include patient inability to eat the required diet or demonstration of high nutritional risk (Table 4-3).[1]

1. Iron

Requirements for iron are increased during pregnancy because of maternal blood volume expansion, fetal blood volume requirements, fetal iron storage, and blood loss during delivery. During the second trimester, red cell synthesis falls behind the expanding blood volume, resulting in the well-known physiologic anemia of pregnancy. Most often, these increased requirements can be met through dietary intake of iron-containing foods.

Although routine iron supplementation in healthy, well-nourished women may improve hematologic indexes, evidence-based reviews have failed to show that these changes translate into improved pregnancy outcomes.[8,9] In a long-term study of the effects of supplementation on subsequent childhood development, prenatal iron supplementation was shown to have no effect on the intelligence quotient of the offspring at 4 years of age.[10] High doses of iron are more likely to cause unpleasant maternal gastrointestinal side effects, including nausea and constipation, and have been associated with an increased risk for neonatal seizures in the first year of life. Selective supplementation for women with a hematocrit less than 30% before 33 weeks of gestation and less than 32% after 33 weeks of gestation is appropriate.[11]

Iron-rich foods include liver, legumes, dried fruits, whole-grain enriched breads, and iron-fortified cereals. When supplements are needed, 30 to 60 g elemental iron should be added to the diet. This level can be found in 150 mg ferrous sulfate, 300 mg ferrous gluconate, or 100 mg ferrous fumarate. Iron-related nausea can be minimized by waiting until the second trimester to begin supplementation and by taking iron after a meal, although this results in decreased absorption. Aluminum- and magnesium-containing antacids can

TABLE 4-3 Recommended Daily Allowances

Nutrient	Nonpregnant			Pregnant	Lactating (first 6 mo)
	15-18 yr	19-24 yr	25-50 yr		
Protein (g)	44	48	50	60	65
Calcium (mg)	1200	1200	800	1200	1200
Phosphorus (mg)	1200	1200	800	1200	1200
Magnesium (mg)	300	280	280	300	355
Iron (mg)	15	15	15	30	15
Zinc (mg)	12	12	12	15	19
Vitamin A (μg RE)	8000	800	800	800	1300
Vitamin D (μg)	10	10	5	10	10
Vitamin E (mg α-TE)	8	8	8	10	12
Vitamin C (mg)	80	80	60	70	95
Thiamine (mg)	1.1	1.1	1.1	1.5	1.6
Riboflavin (mg)	1.3	1.3	1.3	1.6	1.8
Niacin (mg NE)	15	15	15	17	20
Vitamin B_4 (mg)	1.5	1.6	1.8	2.2	2.1
Folic acid (μg)	180	180	180	400	280
Vitamin B_{12} (μg)	2	2	2	2.2	2.6

From National Academy of Sciences: *Recommended dietary allowances,* ed 10, Washington, DC, 1989, National Academy Press.

be used concomitantly without adversely affecting absorption. Increasing dietary fiber and fluid intake may reduce constipation. Supplementation should continue up to 3 months after birth, to replenish maternal stores.

2. Folic acid
   Folate supplementation before pregnancy and in the first 2 months of pregnancy is effective in protecting against neural tube defects (risk ratio [RR], 0.28; 95% confidence interval [CI], 0.13-0.58).[12,13] Women of reproductive age should be advised to take multivitamin supplements containing 0.4 mg folic acid daily. Most multivitamin preparations formulated for pregnancy contain 0.5 to 1.0 mg folic acid.

   In women who have previously had or aborted an infant with a neural tube defect, high-dose supplementation (4 mg/day) during the preconception period and during the first 4 to 6 weeks of pregnancy results in substantial reduction in the frequency of neural tube defects. Neural tube closure is complete by 4 weeks after conception; supplementation beyond this time is of no added value. Additional folate supplementation is necessary in women with multiple gestations, women who had used oral contraceptives before conception, and women who are taking anticonvulsant medication. Folate supplementation is also important in women who had a short interconceptual period (<2 years) and women whose diet was inadequate before pregnancy.[4] Good food sources of folic acid include dark green leafy vegetables, whole grains, and seeds.

3. Calcium
   For the developing fetal skeleton, 1200 mg calcium is needed daily, an increase of 400 mg over the allowance for the nonpregnant adult. Almost all of the skeletal accumulation occurs during the third trimester.[4] Calcium supplementation below this rate may result in maternal demineralization because fetal needs are met by taking from the mother. Three to four milk servings per day (equivalent to 1 quart of milk) are sufficient to achieve this additional need. In patients who are lactose intolerant, a supplement is needed. A Cochrane review demonstrated that the use of calcium supplementation (at least 1 g/day) for women at increased risk for hypertensive disorders and for women with baseline low calcium intake was associated with a decrease in the incidence of gestational hypertension and preeclampsia.[14]

4. Vitamin C
   The increased requirement for vitamin C during pregnancy is necessary for collagen synthesis. Low intake of vitamin C may be associated with pre-eclampsia, maternal anemia, and low-birth-weight infants. A Cochrane review of 5 trials involving 756 women concluded that evidence is lacking to conclude whether vitamin C supplementation, alone or in combination with other supplements, is beneficial during pregnancy.[15] In 3 of these studies (n = 583 women), preterm birth rates were greater with vitamin C supplementation (RR, 1.38; 95% CI, 1.04-1.82).

5. B vitamins
   Additional B vitamins are needed for fetal amino acid and protein synthesis, and can be derived from whole grains, nuts, seeds, beans, some meats, and fish. Vitamin B_6 is a water-soluble vitamin that helps with nervous system development and may play a role in the prevention of preeclampsia. A Cochrane review of 5 trials that included 1646 women showed a decrease in the risk for dental decay in pregnant women.[16] No differences were seen in the risk for eclampsia, preeclampsia, or low Apgar scores at 1 minute.

6. Vitamin D
   Vitamin D is obtained from the maternal diet and sun exposure on the skin. Unfortunately, it is found in few commonly consumed foods except for milk fortified with the vitamin. In some vegetarians, women who do not have adequate milk intake, and those who have little or no sun exposure, deficiency may occur. Substandard vitamin D intake during pregnancy has been associated with decreased birth weight,[17] though a Cochrane review indicates that insufficient evidence exists to evaluate the effect of routine vitamin D supplementation during pregnancy.[18] Vitamin D supplementation at the end of pregnancy should be considered in vulnerable groups, such as women taking the anticonvulsant phenytoin, women with a short interconceptual period, and women with low levels of sunlight exposure. The appropriate dose of vitamin D during pregnancy and lactation is unknown, although it appears to be greater than the current dietary reference intake of 200 to 400 IU/day (5-10 μg/day).[19]

7. Vitamin toxicity
   Vitamin excesses can result in fetal or neonatal abnormalities, and overuse of vitamin supplements should be observed for and cautioned

against in pregnant patients. Vitamin A in doses greater than 25,000 IU/day (700 μg) may be teratogenic, resulting in urogenital anomalies, ear malformations, cleft palate, and neural tube defects.[1,9] Megadose vitamin C (>5 g/day) has been known to cause infantile scurvy, a dependency withdrawal syndrome in neonates.[4] Vitamin D toxicity may result in infantile hypercalcemia syndrome, characterized by supraclavicular aortic stenosis, elfin facies, and mental retardation.[1]

D. Substances to Avoid

Both alcohol and caffeine should be avoided during pregnancy.

1. Alcohol
   Alcohol use during pregnancy has been associated with the development of fetal alcohol syndrome, whether with chronic or binge use (see Chapter 5, Section C). Safe levels of alcohol use during pregnancy have not been established, and it is best to recommend total avoidance. Alcohol depletes the body of zinc and magnesium, which are necessary for fetal development.

2. Caffeine
   The association between maternal caffeine use and pregnancy complications has been controversial, with some studies suggesting that excess intake increases the risk for IUGR, low birth weight, and spontaneous abortion.[4] One prospective cohort study reported that caffeine consumption of less than 300 mg/day (about three cups of coffee) did not increase the risk for spontaneous abortion, IUGR, or microcephaly.[20] A case–control study of caffeine consumption and fetal loss showed a significant twofold increase in the risk for spontaneous abortion associated with caffeine consumption of 163 mg/day during the first trimester.[21] The safety of low levels of caffeine intake (less than five cups of coffee per day) has been supported through measurement of maternal serum paraxanthine (a metabolite of caffeine) levels and correlation with rates of spontaneous abortion in women who were part of the National Collaborative Perinatal Project.[22] In this study, only high serum paraxanthine concentrations (equivalent to more than six cups per day) were associated with an increased abortion risk. Based on available evidence, it is safe to reassure women about low-to-moderate caffeine intake in the first trimester, as it relates to risk for spontaneous abortion.

II. SPECIAL CONDITIONS REQUIRING DIETARY MANAGEMENT

A. Diabetes

Pregnant women with diabetes, regardless of the classification, should follow an American Diabetes Association diet modified for the increased nutritional needs during pregnancy. The goal for these patients is adequate weight gain with normalization of blood glucose levels and absence of ketonuria. Caloric and nutrient requirements are the same as in the nondiabetic pregnancy, evenly distributed throughout the day with three meals and two to three snacks. Increasing the soluble fiber content (with fruits, vegetables, nuts, seeds, beans, and oat bran) and regular exercise help to improve glycemic control.

B. Vegetarianism

Plant proteins lack one or more amino acids needed for protein metabolism, but through a combination of different plant foods, pregnant women can achieve complete protein needs.[4] Lactoovovegetarians who eat vegetables, dairy products, and eggs need additional iron, zinc, and vitamin B_{12} but have no other nutritional problems during pregnancy. Lactovegetarians who eat only vegetables and dairy products need additional iron, zinc, iodine, and vitamin B_{12}. Strict vegans who eat no animal food, dairy products, or eggs may be deficient in protein, calcium, vitamin B_{12}, riboflavin, iron, iodine, and zinc. These latter two groups require special supplementation during pregnancy and lactation. With knowledge of these deficiencies, dietary counseling, and special care, the pregnant vegetarian can meet the recommended daily allowances for pregnancy.

C. Adolescent Pregnancy

Pregnant adolescents have unique needs related to the nutritional needs of pregnancy that are added to the demands of their own growth (see Chapter 5, Section B).[4] Weight gain during pregnancy in teenagers has less effect on infant birth weight of all women studied, likely resulting from a combination of the greater demands for growth and the poor quality of their nutrition. Adolescents often are concerned with their own body image, which may be in conflict with necessary weight gain to support the pregnancy. Providers should be alert to possible eating disorders when caring for pregnant teens.

Dietary recommendations should include a daily caloric intake of 2700 kcal.

D. Hyperemesis

Nausea and vomiting, particularly in early pregnancy, may necessitate specific dietary modifications. Eating dry carbohydrate, soft, low-fat foods and avoiding heavy seasonings and odors may lessen the nausea associated with pregnancy. Other helpful practices include increasing the frequency of meals, eating smaller portions, and avoiding drinking fluids with meals. If nausea and vomiting become severe (defined by dehydration, ketosis, hypochloremia, or hypocalcemia), intravenous fluids and occasionally parenteral nutrition are required to achieve adequate nutrition until symptoms abate. Medications that lessen the severity of pregnancy-related nausea and vomiting are discussed in Section E.

E. Lactose Intolerance

Lactose intolerance is a dose-dependent phenomenon, with 4 to 5 g of milk products or more causing symptoms of gastrointestinal pain and diarrhea. To achieve adequate calcium supplementation in women with lactose intolerance, a reduction in portion size, substitution with cheese or yogurt, or the addition of lactase enzyme tablets may be recommended.

F. Pica and Citta

Pica is the compulsive eating of nonnutritive substances, such as clay, starch, ice, and dirt. These substances bind iron, preventing its absorption. It is unclear whether pica predisposes to iron deficiency or vice versa, as it has been shown that some pica can be cured by iron supplementation. An additional risk for intestinal obstruction occurs in patients with this type of eating disorder.

Citta refers to unusual food cravings, which may occur during pregnancy. This condition is rarely problematic, unless women frequently substitute nonnutritious food in responding to their cravings.

G. Multiple Gestation

Nutritional needs in women with multiple gestations are greater because of the demands created by the increased blood volume and larger placental and fetal mass. A dietary consultation is advised when multiple gestation is recognized (see Chapter 7, Section B).

III. NUTRITIONAL REQUIREMENTS FOR LACTATION

The physiology of pregnancy prepares a woman's body to lactate and breastfeed. Preparation for breastfeeding begins during prenatal care and includes evaluation for nutritional risk factors, education, and counseling.

A. Caloric Needs

Production of breast milk requires an additional 640 kcal/day over nonpregnant needs so that optimal milk production requires a minimum of 1800 kcal/day.[1] Individual needs depend on the nutritional status of the mother and her weight gain during pregnancy. A weight gain of 22 to 28 lb provides maternal fat and energy stores to breastfeed for 3 months after delivery; for those nursing longer than 3 months, additional calories are needed. Neither increasing caloric intake above minimum requirements nor purposefully taking in excess fluid significantly increases milk production, and neither practice is recommended. A lactating mother of normal weight can expect to lose approximately 2 lb per month, whereas an obese mother may lose 4 lb per month. More rapid weight reduction is not recommended.

B. Components

Lactation requires a minimum of 20 g protein over nonpregnant needs, which can be gained by additional milk or meat added to the diet. Calcium needs during lactation are 400 mg/day more than the nonpregnant state, achieved through three to four milk servings per day or a calcium supplement.

C. Vitamins and Minerals

The increased daily food requirements necessary to support lactation usually are sufficient to meet minimum vitamin and mineral needs for maternal health and breast milk production. Neither vitamin nor mineral supplementation is required routinely. An associated loss of maternal iron occurs with breastfeeding, but it amounts to approximately half that of menses. The amenorrhea associated with lactation allows for replenishing of iron stores.

D. Substances to Avoid

Low levels of alcohol intake (one or two drinks per day) may not affect breast milk production, but breast milk levels of alcohol are similar to maternal serum concentrations. Caffeine also is expressed in breast milk. Two to three cups of coffee per day do not appear to affect infants, but more than three cups of coffee per day may result in an irritable, awake infant and decreased let-down reflex.[1]

IV. SOR A RECOMMENDATIONS

RECOMMENDATIONS	REFERENCES
Dietary supplementation with folic acid, before conception and up to 12 weeks of gestation, reduces the risk for neural tube defects. The recommended dose is 400 μg daily.	9, 12
Iron supplementation should not be offered routinely to all pregnant women. It does not benefit maternal or fetal health and may have unpleasant side effects.	8, 9
Vitamin D supplementation should not be offered routinely to pregnant women.	9
Pregnant women should be counseled to avoid excess vitamin A as levels greater than 700 μg daily may be teratogenic.	9

REFERENCES

1. American College of Obstetrics and Gynecology (ACOG): Nutrition during pregnancy, *Technical Bulletin* 179:1-7, 1993.
2. Seidman DS, Ever-Hadani P, Gale R: The effect of maternal weight gain in pregnancy on birth weight, *Obstet Gynecol* 74:240-246, 1989.
3. van Teijingen E, Wilson B, Barry N et al: *Effectiveness of interventions to promote healthy eating in pregnant women and women of childbearing age: a review,* London, 1998, Health Education Authority.
4. Campbell MK, Waller L, Andolsek KM: Maternal nutrition. In Andolsek KM, editor: *Obstetric care: standards of prenatal, intrapartum and postpartum management,* Philadelphia, 1990, Lea & Febiger.
5. Kramer MS, Kakuma R: Energy and protein intake in pregnancy, *Cochrane Database Syst Rev* (4):CD000032, 2003.
6. Signorello LB, Harlow BL, Wang S et al: Saturated fat intake and the risk of severe hyperemesis gravidarum, *Epidemiology* 9:636-640, 1998.
7. Anderson GD, Bliner IN, McClemont S et al: Determinants of size at birth in Canadian population, *Am J Obstet Gynecol* 150:236-244, 1984.
8. U.S. Preventive Services Task Force: Routine iron supplementation during pregnancy: policy statement, *JAMA* 270:2846-2848, 1993.
9. National Collaborating Centre for Women's and Children's Health: *Antenatal care: routine care for the healthy pregnant woman,* London: 2003, RCOG Press.
10. Zhou SJ, Gibson RA, Crowther CA et al: Effect of iron supplementation during pregnancy on the intelligence quotient and behavior of children at 4 y of age: long-term follow-up of a randomized controlled trial, *Am J Clin Nutr* 83(5):1112-1117, 2006.
11. Hemminki E, Merilainen J: Long-term follow-up of mothers and their infants in a randomized trial on iron prophylaxis during pregnancy, *Am J Obstet Gynecol* 173:205-209, 1995.
12. Lumley J, Watson L, Watson M et al: Periconceptual supplementation with folate and/or multivitamins for preventing neural tube defects, *Cochrane Database Syst Rev* (3):CD001056, 2001.
13. Locksmith GJ, Duff P: Preventing neural tube defects: the importance of periconceptual folic acid supplements, *Obstet Gynecol* 91:1027-1034, 1998.
14. Hofmeyr GJ, Atallah AN, Duley L: Calcium supplementation during pregnancy for preventing hypertensive disorders and related problems, *Cochrane Database Syst Rev* (3):CD001059, 2006.
15. Rumbold A, Crowther CA: Vitamin C supplementation in pregnancy, *Cochrane Database Syst Rev* (2):CD004072, 2005.
16. Thaver D, Saeed MA, Bhutta ZA: Pyridoxine (vitamin B6) supplementation in pregnancy, *Cochrane Database Syst Rev* (2):CD000179, 2006.
17. Mannion CA, Gray-Donald K, Koski K: Association of low intake of milk and vitamin D during pregnancy with decreased birth weight, *CMAJ* 174(9):1273-1277, 2006.
18. Mahomed K, Gulmezoglu AM: Vitamin D supplementation in pregnancy, *Cochrane Database Syst Rev* (2):CD000228, 2000.
19. Hollis BW, Wagner CL: Assessment of dietary vitamin D requirements during pregnancy and lactation, *CMAJ* 174(9): 1287-1290, 2006.
20. Mills JL, Holmes LB, Aarons JH et al: Moderate caffeine use and the risk of spontaneous abortion and intrauterine growth retardation, *JAMA* 269:593-597, 1993.
21. Infante-Rivard C, Fernandez A, Gauthier R et al: Fetal loss associated with caffeine intake before and during pregnancy, *JAMA* 270:2940-2943, 1993.
22. Klebanoff MA, Levine RJ, DerSimonian R: Maternal serum paraxanthine, a caffeine metabolite, and the risk of spontaneous abortion, *N Engl J Med* 341:1639-1644, 1999.

SECTION B **Educational Preparation for Childbirth, Parenting, and Newborn Care**

Ann Tumblin, BA, and Patricia Ann Payne, BSN, CNM, MPH

I. CURRENT TRENDS

Prepared childbirth classes are designed to provide information about pregnancy, labor and birth, non-pharmacologic forms of comfort for women in labor, care of the newborn, and to develop confidence in the woman's ability to birth her baby.[1,2] Empowerment and education are key components of family-centered care. Common marketing strategies promote the term *family-centered maternity care,* but little evidence exists to demonstrate institutional behaviors that empower and support women and families in the clinical setting. The most recent trend in childbirth classes is for hospitals to offer shorter classes, often teaching the entire series over one day or one weekend. No studies indicate that this approach to childbirth education is better or worse, but young couples with harried lives are drawn to a more condensed type of class. This shortened version of classes may not help a woman develop confidence in her body's ability to give birth, nor will it allow enough time for synthesis and processing information. Previously, most classes contained all-inclusive information on labor and birth, postpartum adjustment, newborn care, and breastfeeding. Currently, each of these topics is often offered as an à la carte menu of separate classes that women may choose to attend. Other current trends include watching contemporary television stories about birth or seeking information on the Internet rather than attending classes.

II. RESEARCH

A. Clinical Outcomes

Preparation for childbirth begins at an early age as preschoolers develop male and female behavior patterns. These perceptions of sexuality are influenced by parents, caregivers, and cultural attitudes. As women reach childbearing age, preconceptual education can encourage women to prepare physically and emotionally for a pregnancy. Formal childbirth education classes started with Grantley Dick Read in the 1950s. These classes evolved from a primary goal to reduce the fear and anxiety associated with the birth process to a model with much broader emphasis on empowerment and developing confidence in the woman's ability to trust her body to birth and developing confidence for both parents in their parenting roles.[1] Limited high-quality research about education to prepare women and their families for childbirth exists. Many of the studies are of poor methodology with diverse populations without controlling for the various types of classes, instructors, outcomes, class content, or cultural variations and expectations.[3]

In 2002, the Maternity Center Association conducted the First National U.S. Survey of Women's Childbearing Experiences, "Listening to Mothers." In the survey, women cite several reasons for attending childbirth preparation classes, including improved safety for mother and infant, more humanistic experience, better preparation, reduced fear, and shared childbirth with their partner.[4] Several questions in the survey included reference to childbirth education classes, but the results did not show mothers found a tremendous benefit from classes (Table 4-4). It is difficult to evaluate the responses related to childbirth education because the survey did not ask the length of the classes, content of classes, or certification/training

---

TABLE 4-4 Results of the Nationwide Listening to Mothers Survey

---

About 70% of first-time mothers took childbirth education classes, and only 19% of mothers who had given birth before did.

About 88% attended classes at a hospital site or in a physician's or midwife's office.

Mothers attending classes were more likely to use the techniques learned in class.

Attending classes did not generally impact the mother's experience of labor.

Almost two thirds of mothers used epidural analgesia but between 26% and 41% of mothers were unable to respond to questions about side effects associated with epidurals.

Mothers who took childbirth education classes were no more likely to feel calm, confident, or capable in labor.

Taking classes had no impact on mothers' feelings about whether birth was a natural process.

First-time mothers who took classes did report lower levels of postpartum mood disorders, but no difference was noted among experienced mothers.

Mothers wanted more information about informed consent.

From Maternity Center Association: *Listening to Mothers: report of the First National US Survey of Women's Childbearing Experiences execu-tive summary and recommendations issued by the Maternity Center Association,* New York, October 2002, Maternity Center Association.

of the instructor.[5] Further research needs to be done to determine what influence these variables may have on specific outcomes, such as use of pain medication, satisfaction, personal and cultural expectations, and what other interdependent factors that may produce outcomes measured (i.e., labor care providers, setting of birth, etc.).[6]

A number of variables including fear and anxiety, use of analgesia, length of labor, and parenting have been evaluated to determine whether any relation exists between prenatal education and clinical outcomes. Being informed about what to expect during the birth process decreases anxiety and dispels fear, resulting in increased relaxation. This information helps women to cope better with the pain of labor and increases maternal confidence significantly.[5] In studies of the relation of maternal confidence to pain perception, more than half of the variance in active labor pain may be explained by the mother's confidence in her ability to cope.[5] Acquiring knowledge about what to expect in labor and birth and how to put that knowledge to use is associated with women's desire for an active role during labor and delivery.[5,7] Prepared childbirth classes may work, in part, by empowering women and their support persons as well as relieving their anxiety, and allowing them to cope with the pain of labor with more nonpharmacologic techniques. This approach may reduce the need for analgesia during labor, a finding that has been shown in prospective studies.[5] During labor, anxiety can lead to increased plasma cortisol levels that, in turn, can increase the length of the first stage of labor. Anxiety also can lengthen the second stage of labor by increasing plasma epinephrine and decreasing uterine activity.[5] Prenatal preparation can allay this anxiety, potentially leading to shorter first and second stages of labor, although data are conflicting in this regard. Continuity of care by supportive laypersons, professional birth doulas or labor assistance providers, and nursing staff also has been associated with decreased length of labor, less use of drugs for pain relief in labor, and less need for resuscitation of newborns.[8]

Little evidence is available to evaluate a relation between parenting adaptive behaviors and prenatal education. A positive attitude toward the birth experience can be related to support and education. Couples receiving prenatal education about the transition into parenthood have less anxiety and an easier adjustment to parenthood. This situation may translate into an improved ability to deal with the many changes that occur when a new baby joins the family.

B. Future Directions

Studies of outcomes of prepared childbirth classes have been constrained by the question of whether the positive outcomes measured are related to childbirth education or to specific characteristics of the class attendees.[9] Some evidence exists that certain types of individuals feel attracted by birth preparation courses, whereas others (perhaps those less interested in education) may not attend childbirth classes.[3] Appropriate outcome measures may change over time and are unique to given populations. For example, the frequent use of epidural anesthesia in the United States may speak to a change in the outcomes that women perceive as beneficial. Looking at limited patient-oriented outcomes other than use of medication and satisfaction with the birth experience fails to recognize the potential benefit of empowerment for new parents. The attitudes and behaviors of caregivers will also have an impact on the woman's opinion of birth satisfaction regardless of the types of classes attended.[10]

Although the medical, midwifery, and nursing community have accepted the use of childbirth education, there has been insufficient evidence to guide them in how to best counsel women and families about how to navigate the options offered to them. Family physicians are in the unique position of providing recommendations to pregnant women as they sort through the menu of class options available in their community including childbirth, parenting, breastfeeding, sibling preparation, and cardiopulmonary resuscitation/child safety.

III. COMPONENTS OF CHILDBIRTH PREPARATION

A. Childbirth Classes

Providers of perinatal care should be aware of the benefits of prepared childbirth and their own ability to enhance this training or to render the teachings ineffective by not supporting them during the intrapartum and postpartum periods. (See Table 4-5 for suggestions of to create consistency within the community of childbirth education, hospital practices, and patient care.)

A variety of certifications are available for childbirth educators. Lamaze International has evolved from being a method of giving birth to being a

---

TABLE 4-5 Suggestions for Incorporation of Childbirth Preparation into Practice

---

Provide guidance to parents to assist in healthy sexual development before and during puberty.

Provide preconceptional counseling or classes

Adapt office environment to include pictures or poster portraying birth and breastfeeding as normal functions.

Provide families with evidenced-based information about the normalcy of birth.

Provide a birth ball in the waiting area and donate one to the hospital birthing unit.

Coordinate with hospital management to provide new obstetric nurses with a tour of your office/practice site.

Offer annual awards to hospital nurse who displays the most support of normal birth.

Encourage training for nurses to learn hands-on comfort measures.

Hire doula(s).

Consider Pregnancy Centering as model of care.

Encourage attendance at childbirth education classes that focus on the normalcy of birth and trust in the mother's ability to give birth.

Encourage mothers to write a birth plan that is directed at her concerns or fears.

---

philosophy that birth is normal, natural, and healthy. Therefore, today's Lamaze methods affirm the normalcy of birth, acknowledge women's inherent ability to birth their babies, and explore all the ways that women find strength and comfort during labor and birth.[1,2] Other types of certifications include International Childbirth Education Association, Birthing from Within, Bradley, a variety of preparations using hypnosis as a basis, and multiple eclectic institution-specific versions of classes. In the survey "Listening to Mothers," 88% of women attended classes in hospitals or physicians' offices.[4] The strength of each class depends on the strength and philosophy of the instructor and the restrictions put on the instructor.

In contrast with earlier childbirth preparation classes, today there is less emphasis on any one breathing technique and more information about the psychosocial and spiritual aspects of preparing women and their partners for birth.[1,9] Issues that may affect the childbirth experience, such as sexual abuse, relationship issues, and psychosocial issues, can be addressed in a safe environment by informed,

qualified individuals.[7,11] Many classes include the activity of developing a birth plan for women and their partners to share with providers during an office visit and nursing staff when they are in labor. Birth plans may be in the form of a checklist or may be directed at the individual woman's specific fears and concerns about giving birth, many of which may influence her ability to relax or feel safe. These birth plans often are used as a negotiating tool between patients and providers, with a focus on market demands rather than as an opportunity to explore underlying issues that may have a strong impact on the birth experience.

B. Preparation of Siblings for Birth

Childbirth affects the entire family. However, research that addresses the needs of a child preparing for the birth of a new sibling is lacking. When a new child enters the family unit, dynamics change. No matter how prepared a child is, he or she is likely to regress in his or her behavior and/or show some anger or aggressiveness as he or she adjusts to a new addition in the family. Sibling rivalry is expected and can start at any time. Rivalry is commonly exhibited by behaviors such as bed-wetting, thumb-sucking, temper tantrums, crying and/or quiet behavior, and aggressive behavior toward a parent or parents.[12] It is important to encourage parents to include their child in prenatal planning including prenatal visits. Many hospitals offer sibling classes with little or no evidence to suggest an improvement in behavior results because of this activity. Clinicians can provide parents with age-appropriate suggestions for siblings such as keeping a notebook of drawings that children make about becoming a new sibling, reading books about new babies, creating baby games to play, among others.

Children planning to participate in the birth of a sibling require a more intensive plan for this preparation, including an alternative plan should a child change his or her mind. Most facilities have a policy about including children at birth so that health-care providers should be aware of institutional policies before discussing with parents. Most children will tell their parents if they are interested in being present at the birth. If a child wants to be present at the birth, parents should identify a support person who is prepared to leave and/or take care of the child at any time. Parents should also share books and videos with their child about birth and describe what will happen during labor and birth. It is important that the child be prepared for what they might see (e.g., blood) and how women act in labor (e.g., noise, quiet, moving around). After the birth providers can encourage discussion and drawing about the experience, and talk with the child at a postpartum visit about his or her feelings related to the birth experience.

IV. ROLE OF FAMILY MEDICINE PHYSICIANS

Although outcome studies that attempt to measure the effects of prepared childbirth are difficult to interpret, one thing seems clear: Maternal satisfaction with the birth process affects women's perceptions of themselves[10,13] and enhances their abilities to provide nurturing care for their infants.[8] *Healthy People 2010* calls for an increase in the proportion of pregnant women who attend a series of prepared childbirth classes conducted by a certified childbirth educator[14] (Table 4-6). Pregnant women and partners/support persons often participate in childbirth classes based on recommendation of their care providers; the attitude of these providers may be the deciding factor whether women and their partners/support person attend childbirth education classes. Providers may assume that information in every childbirth education class is similar, but the philosophy and experience of the instructor can greatly affect the manner in which information is presented. Knowledge about the content and learning approach of the community childbirth classes and the degree to which adult learning principles and interactive teaching strategies are used will guide the provider in making appropriate recommendations. Women and their partners can use this information to sort through their options and identify the classes that best meet their needs. Therefore, as a piece of the family practice commitment to family-centered care, the provider has a responsibility to have the community resources needed to direct expectant mothers to excellent, confidence-building childbirth and parenting education.

TABLE 4-6 Components of a Comprehensive Childbirth Education Class

Basic information including the emotional and physical characteristics of normal labor and birth; interventions with benefits, trade-offs, and alternatives; preparation for the immediate postpartum period; breastfeeding; and infant care with focus on patient choice

A focus on normal birth with a variety of pain management strategies including both neurophysiologic and pharmacologic

Opportunities to practice positioning and neurophysiologic pain-management strategies

Opportunities for value clarification between pregnant woman and partner regarding personal choices during labor and birth

Communication skills to enhance relationship between partnership and provider

Focus on interactive teaching strategies, rather than didactic ones, using principles of adult education.

A class with these components can help a woman develop confidence in her body's ability to give birth.

REFERENCES

1. Lothian J, DeVries C: *The official lamaze guide: giving birth with confidence,* New York, 2005, Meadowbrook Press.
2. Adopted by Lamaze International Education Council Governing Board. Position Paper: Lamaze for the 21st century, Washington, DC, 2007, Lamaze International.
3. Gagnon AJ: Individual or group antenatal education for childbirth/parenthood, *Cochrane Database Syst Rev* (4):CD2869, 2000.
4. Maternity Center Association: *Listening to mothers: report of the First National US Survey of Women's Childbearing Experiences Executive Summary and Recommendations issued by the Maternity Center Association,* New York, October 2002, Maternity Center Association.
5. Lowe NK: The nature of labor pain, *Am J Obstet Gynecol* 186: S16-S24, 2002.
6. Koehn ML: Childbirth education outcomes: an integrative review of the literature, *J Perinatal Ed* 11(3):10-19, 2002.
7. Courtois CA, Riley CC: Pregnancy and childbirth as triggers for abuse memories: implications for care, *Birth* 19:222-223, 1997.
8. Hodnett ED, Gates S, Hofmeyr GJ et al: Continuous support for women during childbirth, *Cochrane Database Syst Rev* (3): CD003766, 2003.
9. Kane A: The biopsychosociospiritual approach to birth care, *Int J Childbirth Educ* 14:34-37, 1999.
10. Hodnett E: Pain and women's satisfaction with the experience of childbirth: a systematic review, *Am J Obstet Gynecol* 186: S160-S172, 2002.
11. Simkin P, Klau P: *When survivors give birth: understanding and healing the effects of early sexual abuse on childbearing women,* Seattle, WA, 2004, Classic Day Publishing.
12. Brazelton TB: *Touchpoints: birth to 3,* Cambridge, MA, 2006, Da Capo Press.
13. Simkin P: Just another day in a woman's life? Women's long-term perceptions of their first birth experience. Part 1, *Birth* 18:4, 1991.
14. Office of Disease Prevention and Health Promotion U.S. Department of Health and Human Services: Healthy People 2010, 2004.

Section C Preparation for Parenting and Family Issues

Elizabeth G. Baxley, MD,
and Jamee H. Lucas, MD, AAFP

I. PRENATAL COUNSELING

Prenatal counseling regarding parenting issues is a clinical practice that has been recommended widely for physicians who care for newborns.[1] Although most physicians do conduct prenatal counseling visits, they often do not discuss initial care and family impact of the newborn.[2,3] There are numerous reasons to discuss pediatric issues before the birth of a newborn. Doing so fosters an ongoing relationship with the expectant family and helps to build the foundation for a strong physician, parent, and child interaction, which, in turn, helps facilitate adequate health-care supervision for the family. Some evidence suggests that attending preparation for parenting classes may reduce postpartum depression in first-time mothers.[4] A Cochrane review claims that parenting classes can make a significant impact on the early adjustment of the new parents, although the long-term outcomes have not been well studied.[5]

II. PRENATAL PEDIATRIC VISIT

The term *prenatal pediatric visit* refers to a visit in which emphasis is placed on discussion of preparation for the birth and parenting of a newborn. In addition to reviewing pertinent aspects of the prenatal history, this visit allows the provider to identify psychosocial factors that may affect a family's adjustment to the newborn, answer parents' questions, relieve anxieties about the upcoming birth and hospital care, and discuss practical aspects of infant care. This visit also provides the physician with an opportunity to discuss issues of anticipatory guidance to promote child health and safety.[2]

A. Format

The ideal timing for the prenatal pediatric visit is in the latter part of the third trimester.[4] This visit should be scheduled with both parents present, and 30 to 45 minutes should be set aside for the session. A physician's private office may be a more desirable location to conduct this visit than an examination room. When time for scheduling and reimbursement systems are problematic, the provider may consider holding this type of visit with a group of parents in their third trimester, held in the evening so as not to interfere with busy office schedules and to allow more partners to attend. This approach has the advantage of group interaction among expectant couples, but it may hinder individuals or couples from sharing important psychosocial information. Another alternative to conserve time is to incorporate components of this visit into several routine prenatal visits.

B. Content

The provider should show concern for the entire family and a willingness to discuss psychosocial and parenting-readiness issues. Open-ended questions are best to encourage more open discussion by the parents. Questions should be encouraged and answered. An important goal of this visit is for the couple to leave feeling empowered in their new role as parents. This conversation should be patient centered, with an understanding of the differing needs of patients in relation to their support at home, their socioeconomic status, and their educational level.[6]

1. Psychosocial history
   The psychosocial history should include information about previous family function and experiences, including, when applicable, information about the new parents' families of origin. Feelings about this pregnancy should be ascertained: Was the pregnancy planned or unplanned? What has been the reaction of both partners to the pregnancy? Is the expected infant seen as a solution to marital turmoil? Has either parent experienced depression before or during the pregnancy? If this is not their first pregnancy, inquiring about prior parenting problems is appropriate, and a discussion of how these may be solved is appropriate.[5]
   Information about planned living arrangements should be ascertained, and expectant parents should identify support systems to call on after delivery. Discussion about the father's role is important, including identifying the occupational status of both parents and their individual plans for time out of work after the birth. Inquiring about psychosocial issues requires careful interviewing skills coupled with the ability to observe interactions between the parents or between parents and other children, if applicable.[2]

2. Hospital concerns

Newborn feeding plans should be inquired about and counseling regarding the benefits of breast-feeding is appropriate because most women make a decision about breastfeeding versus bottle-feeding in the third trimester. Questions about circumcision may be answered, and specific religious restrictions or preferences should be documented.[2] Rooming-in and sibling visitation protocols for the hospital may be discussed, and referral to hospital programs for siblings should be made when available.[7]

3. Home concerns

Issues of home safety, sleeping arrangements, and further questions about feeding may be discussed during this visit and in the hospital after delivery. The couple should identify, in advance, additional help for their first days at home, to provide the mother with opportunities for rest.[8]

4. Family adaptation

With the birth of a baby, a new family is formed, often with changes in the way that family members have responded to each other previously. This new situation typically requires some adaptation for new parents and any siblings who may be involved in the transformation. The physician should discuss expectations that parents may have about potential impact that the newborn may have on family function. When applicable, the involvement of a grandparent or other extended family members in newborn care should be discussed.

5. Schedule of infant well-child visits

At the conclusion of a prenatal pediatric visit, it is helpful to leave parents with a schedule for follow-up well-child visits and timing of immunizations. This visit can serve to review night-coverage arrangements and schedule of hospital visits, as well as fee arrangements for inpatient and outpatient care.

III. HOSPITAL CARE AND COUNSELING

The care of the mother and her newborn during their postpartum hospitalization allows new parents and their provider another chance to review pertinent aspects of newborn care and family adjustment, as well as to answer any questions that may have arisen since the prenatal visit. It is also an opportunity to review events that occurred during or surrounding the birth, to assess maternal satisfaction with the birth process, and to address any new problems or concerns related to the hospital course.

REFERENCES

1. Sprunger LW, Preece EW: Characteristics of prenatal interviews provided by pediatricians, *Clin Pediatr* 20:778-782, 1981.
2. Becker PG, Mendel SG: A family practice approach to the pediatric prenatal visit, *Am Fam Physician* 40:181-186, 1989.
3. Sprunger LW, Preece EW: Use of pediatric prenatal visits by family physicians, *J Fam Pract* 13:1007-1012, 1981.
4. Matthey S, Kavanagh DJ, Howie P et al: Prevention of postnatal distress or depression: an evaluation of an intervention at preparation for parenthood classes, *J Affect Disord* 79(1-3): 113-126, 2004.
5. Barlow J, Coren E: Parent-training programs for improving maternal psychosocial health, *Cochrane Database Syst Rev* (2): CD002020, 2001.
6. Sword W, Watt S: Learning the needs of postpartum women: does socioeconomic status matter? *Birth* 32:86-92, 2005.
7. Lieu TA, Wilder C, Capra AM et al: Clinical outcomes and maternal perceptions of an updated model of perinatal care, *Pediatrics* 102:1437-1444, 1998.
8. Gruis M: Beyond maternity: postpartum concerns of mothers, *MCN Am J Matern Child Nurs* 2:182-188, 1977.

S E C T I O N   D   Breastfeeding Promotion

Patricia Ann Payne, BSN, CNM, MPH, and Mary Rose Tully, MPH, IBCLC

Breastfeeding and the use of human milk is well recognized as optimal nutrition and immunologic protection for infants.[1-6] The benefits of lactating[7] and breastfeeding for mothers are also well documented.[1-6] However, breastfeeding is a health behavior that requires both promotion and support. It is often mistakenly portrayed as an optional benefit for the infant rather than the norm for infant feeding. Family physicians are in the ideal settings to promote and support breastfeeding from an early age.

I. BREASTFEEDING STATISTICS

Exclusive breastfeeding for the first 6 months of life is recommended[2,4,8] but may require creative suggestions and support from the mother's health-care provider. Breastfeeding goals established for the United States in the Surgeon General's *Healthy People 2010* documents are 75% initiation, 50% at 6 months, and 25% breastfeeding at a year.[7,9] The Centers for Disease Control and Prevention has tracked breastfeeding rates through the National Immunization survey. In 2004, they found that 14 states in the United States achieved a 75% initiation rate, but only 3 states achieved the objective at 6 months and 5 states achieved the objective at 1 year. Oregon and Utah were the only two states to meet all three objectives. Many other regions of the country fall far below the established goals, and health disparities continue to exist by race and socioeconomic strata.[10,11] The Special Supplemental Nutrition Program for Women, Infants, and Children (WIC) program continues to make great investments in breastfeeding promotion and in ongoing support. In some regions of the country, this effort is showing significant impact and breastfeeding initiation rates have increased, although duration remains a problem among vulnerable populations. In 10 states, the breastfeeding initiation rate increased from 57% in 1993 to 67.5% in 1998.[12] Notably, the initiation increased among vulnerable groups such as women with low incomes and black women, who are participants in WIC, and mothers of infants admitted to the neonatal intensive care unit. However, the percentage of women who initiated breastfeeding and were still predominantly breastfeeding at 10 weeks remained stable at about 58% between 1993 and 1998. More women in vulnerable populations initiated breastfeeding, but those from higher socioeconomic groups were more likely to continue.[12]

II. BENEFITS OF BREASTFEEDING: BREASTFEEDING IS AN IMPORTANT HEATH CHOICE

Infants who are not breastfed have more sick visits, more hospital admissions, and increased mortality in the first year of life, even in developed countries.[13-15] They have increased risk for upper respiratory infections, including ear infections, and more gastrointestinal infections.[2,4,6] The lifetime effects of not breastfeeding include certain childhood cancers,[2,4,16] increased risk for development of allergies, asthma, gastrointestinal conditions such as Crohn's disease and colitis, childhood obesity,[17] diabetes (types 1 or 2),[18,19] and heart disease. Women who breastfeed not only benefit by having healthier infants and children, evidence from case–control studies show a reduced risk for development of breast cancer,[20] certain types of ovarian cancer,[21] and osteoporosis.[22] It is important to recognize

the significance of colostrum and its unique role in the infant's adjustment to extrauterine life. Colostrum is concentrated nutrition, higher in protein than mature milk and lower in carbohydrates and fats. A large portion of the proteins in colostrum are IgA and SIgA. These proteins protect the infant from infection, including enteric infections and gut irritations, increased risk for allergy, and diabetes caused by exposure to human milk substitutes (formula).[5] Colostrum is present in the breasts from about the 16th week of gestation. If an infant appears not be receiving adequate feeding at the breast, it is important to assess the quality of milk transfer and work with the mother and infant to improve technique. Bottle-feeding in the hospital has been associated with lower breastfeeding satisfaction[16,23] and shorter duration.[24]

III. ENCOURAGING WOMEN TO CHOOSE BREASTFEEDING

A. Create a Breastfeeding–Friendly Environment

Most professionals are aware of the Baby Friendly Hospital Initiative by the World Health Organization and UNICEF to create positive environments in hospitals and clinical practice settings. The choice to breastfeed, however, may be influenced long before a mother is pregnant and has her baby. Breastfeeding preparation begins when both adults and children experience an environment that assumes babies will be breastfed. Thirty-four states in the United States have enacted legislation that protects the breastfeeding dyad and, in some cases, mandates support such as break time for breastfeeding mothers. The fact that laws are necessary to prohibit criminalization of breastfeeding as indecent exposure or immoral conduct speaks to the discomfort with nursing that continues to exist in our society. The health-care setting is another environment that may not specifically discourage breastfeeding but does not portray breastfeeding as the normal way to feed infants despite what clinicians may say. Accommodations for breastfeeding, artwork and posters that portray discreet breastfeeding, coloring pages and/or children's books that show nursing mothers, an absence of formula advertising (pens, note pads, name badge holders, etc.), and an absence of bottles and pacifiers as symbols of infancy are all strong, unspoken messages in the health-care setting. Children's books, for example, often portray a variety of mammals shown bottle-feeding as if that were reality. Why is it expected that children would then grow up and consider breastfeeding the norm? Books such as *We Like to Nurse* by Chia Martin are a good example of how to promote breastfeeding to young children, and it is available through many WIC programs in the United States.

B. Providing Information

Examination of the breasts, as part of routine care for nonpregnant women and as part of early prenatal care, provides an opportunity for exploring concerns/questions and explaining the physiology of milk production in simple terms. Often, a lack of open commitment to supporting breastfeeding or inappropriate advice given to patients is the key reason women give for not breastfeeding or for prematurely weaning. In fact, frequently women receive little, if any, breastfeeding information or encouragement from health-care workers if they initially express a preference for formula-feeding.

Several systematic reviews and other published research related to intervention programs promote breastfeeding.[25] The Oregon Health and Science University Evidence-Based Practice Center reported on a systematic review published in 2003 of studies of breastfeeding initiation and/or duration.[26] They examined RCTs and cohort studies in developed countries and identified 22 RCTs, 8 non-RCTs, and 5 systematic reviews to evaluate. They found 12 studies to be of fair quality, 2 of good quality, and 16 of poor quality. They found educational programs to be the single most effective intervention to promote breastfeeding up to 3 months. The number needed to treat is three to five that results in one woman who initiates breastfeeding and continues to breastfeed up to 3 months. They also found that the most significant differences in breastfeeding rates were among women in populations that had a breastfeeding rate of less than 50% before the intervention.

Dyson and colleagues[27] published a Cochrane review in 2005 that included five trials studying the use of health education to increase breastfeeding initiation and duration. These studies all targeted low-income women in the United States, and a meta-analysis of results showed a positive effect on both initiation and duration.

Not all women have the option to attend a breastfeeding class, and clinicians do not have the time to have lengthy discussions with women about their decision to breastfeed. However, most people have access to the media. A systematic review[28] of interventions to promote the initiation of breastfeeding found that the media is effective in changing attitudes about breastfeeding and increasing the number of women who initiate breastfeeding. The World Health Organization's countermarketing and the International Code on Marketing of Breast-milk Substitutes have made an attempt to counter the advertising campaigns for formula products and established standards for industry and health-care professionals' behavior regarding promotion of human milk substitutes to the public. Social marketing uses successful commercial marketing strategies to encourage healthy behaviors or support behavioral change. Two national social marketing campaigns have been used to address breastfeeding in the United States. *Babies Were Born to Be Breastfeed* is sponsored by the U.S. Department of Health and Human Services' Office on Women's Health and the Advertising Council, and *Loving Support Makes Breastfeeding Work* is sponsored by the U.S. Department of Agriculture's WIC Program created by Best Start Social Marketing. Best Start Social Marketing, Inc. developed a direct, simple three-step breastfeeding education/counseling strategy for use in a clinic or office setting during prenatal visits. Using this method, health-care workers ask patients at each prenatal visit what they think and/or know about breastfeeding; their response is acknowledged and validated, and then they are given small amounts of information targeted at their concerns/knowledge deficits. This technique has been effective in changing attitudes about breastfeeding. This approach uses open-ended questions that allow a woman to discuss her concerns, feelings, and attitudes. A significant component of the strategy is that whatever a woman says is acknowledged and validated before misinformation is corrected. This strategy can be used with pregnant and nonpregnant women to determine what concerns they have, affirm their concerns, and provide targeted education.

When a mother expresses concern or misconceptions about breastfeeding, clinicians need to be prepared to provide accurate information. The most common reasons women give for stopping breastfeeding prematurely include sore nipples and concern, usually unfounded, about insufficient milk supply.[29,30] No prenatal breast or nipple preparation has been found to be effective in preventing sore nipples, inverted nipples, or flat nipples. It is important to reassure women that each of these problems can be managed. The primary causes of sore nipples are the adjustment of the nipple tissue to being used and incorrect latch.[31-33] In the rare instance where no breast changes are noted, the woman is noted to have widely spaced, tuber-shaped breasts, or she has had breast surgery that could interrupt the milk ducts, it is prudent to discuss with the patient that there is a possibility that she will not lactate and/or may have some problems with milk volume, and it will be important to monitor her infant's early intake closely.[34,35] The patient can be reminded that there are supplemental feeding methods that may also assist her with nursing should the volume of milk be insufficient. Other than human immunodeficiency virus–positive status in a developed country or human t-lymphotropic virus (HTLV)-positive status, there are few contraindications to breastfeeding, except the rare instance where a mother is on chemotherapy or is addicted to illicit drugs.[36,37] Occasionally, a woman will need to interrupt contact with her infant for a few days, such as after radioisotope therapy, while initiating tuberculosis therapy (if she has not had contact with the infant), if she acquires chickenpox within 5 days of giving birth or 2 days after giving birth, has an active herpes lesion on the breast that cannot be covered during feeding, or is being treated for Chagas' disease.[6,38] In each of those situations, the mother's care is to facilitate pumping her breasts, ideally with a hospital-grade (multiple user) pump, every third hour to induce or maintain her milk supply. Except in the case of Chagas' disease, the milk can be fed to her infant.[16]

C. Support for Breastfeeding Mothers

1. Advice and help

    A positive attitude toward breastfeeding is important to help encourage women who are considering breastfeeding and to support mothers who are breastfeeding. Health-care providers should be knowledgeable about the health, nutritional, physiologic, and psychological aspects of breastfeeding, but they also should be familiar with the mechanics of breastfeeding and how best to support the normal physiologic process for mothers in a hospital or birth center as well as at home (see Chapter 20, Section C).

    Many health professionals lack accurate information about breastfeeding and human lactation, as well as optimal clinical management skills.[39] A new profession, that of the certified lactation consultant, has developed as an allied health profession to fill in this gap. Lactation consultants can provide support, information, and intensive consultations for mothers with breastfeeding problems (for more information, see the International Board of Lactation Consultant Examiners website: www.iblce.org). These professionals can assist the family physician who is working with families in hospitals and in community settings. Some physicians encourage individual staff members in an office/clinic to be trained and certified as international board-certified lactation consultants (IBCLCs), or network within their community and encourage classes provided by IBCLCs in their office settings.

2. Hospital routines

    Hospital routine procedures, even for healthy infants, can interfere with normal physical and psychological processes of the immediate postpartum period. This interference can decrease the likelihood of breastfeeding initiation and decrease duration.[6] Considerable published literature exists on how to provide support and address the most common problems and barriers that nursing mothers face. The International Lactation Consultant Association's *Clinical Guidelines for the Establishment of Exclusive Breastfeeding*[6] provides an evidence-based guide for clinical management of breastfeeding. It outlines strategies providers and institutions can use to support women during hospitalization and/or care of the newborn in the home. The Academy of Breastfeeding Medicine (www.bfmed.org) offers referenced model protocols for breastfeeding management. Each of these resources offers guidelines that can be tailored to individual patients and situations. These guides all have common themes related to early skin-to-skin contact and first feedings, rooming in, evaluation of milk transfer by trained clinicians, and early follow-up to monitor and treat both infant and mother for potential problems.

    a. First hours of life: Typically, neonates are very alert in the first hour or two after birth. Encouraging skin-to-skin contact between mother and neonate at this time and continuing contact until after the first feeding has been associated with enhanced an maternal–infant relationship, decreased nipple soreness and engorgement for the mother, decreased weight loss for the neonate, optimal blood sugar stability, and lower bilirubin levels for the neonate.[17] Oxytocin release occurs as a result of suckling and facilitates uterine contractions and the expulsion of the placenta during the third stage of labor. Early skin-to-skin contact is related to greater likelihood of prolonged breastfeeding, but no conclusive evidence exists.[6] Early contact may be a simple way of promoting breastfeeding for some mother–neonate pairs in the highly technologic hospital setting but may not be effective if contact does not continue and neonates spend most of their time in a newborn nursery.[27]

b. First days of life: In the early days after birth, it is important that all neonates are fed when they give hunger cues so they will learn that feeling hungry is best remedied by eating, not just by sucking. Keeping the neonate within easy reach of the mother 24 hours a day has been shown to increase the likelihood of successful breastfeeding.[6] Crying is a late cue for hunger.[4,6] Mothers who room-in are able to learn their neonate's early feeding cues, or early signs of hunger (sometimes called "demand feeding"), which can be missed if the neonate is not nearby. These cues include going into a light sleep with more general movement, rapid eye movement, sucking motions, hand-to-mouth movements, and cooing sounds. The term "cue-based feeding" may appeal more to parents who do not like the sound of "demand feeding." When mothers have unlimited access to their neonates, they feed whenever the neonate shows early feeding cues, feed more often, and use less supplementation.

c. Pacifier use: Studies have shown that infants using pacifiers are more likely to be weaned from the breast early.[41,42] However, it is difficult to determine whether infants are weaned because of lack of milk production because the pacifier substitutes for sucking at the breast, and thereby decreases the hormone releases necessary for increasing milk production, or whether pacifier use is a marker of an infant who has difficulty transferring milk and will soon be giving hunger cues that the mother (and possibly her care provider) will interpret as low milk supply. Pacifier use may prevent mothers from understanding their infant's feeding cues and from learning how to interpret cues for other needs.

d. Rooming in: Rooming in allows for closer contact with the father and other family members, whereas increasing staff availability for teaching because mothers care for their own infants. Mothers who room-in have been shown to have more self-confidence in the care of their infants and seek advice less often in the first postpartum month.[43] The risk for neonatal infection is also lower than in a closed nursery environment. Mothers do not necessarily sleep better if their babies are in the nursery at night.[44] Many women consider rooming in if it is discussed before delivery and not a decision made at the time of birth, when they are tired and may not appreciate the benefit of contact with their infant.

e. Factors that interfere with breastfeeding: Anesthesia, strong sedation, prolonged labor, surgical interventions, intravenous fluids during labor, and other sources of stress, discomfort, and fatigue for mothers and infants may impede the initiation of breastfeeding and even mature milk production. Central nervous system depressants given during labor can reduce a neonate's ability to suck or cause a disorganized suck for a few days. In the case of barbiturates, it may take 5 to 6 days for the effects to disappear.[45] Mothers giving birth by cesarean section usually have later first breastfeeding, but if the cultural and hospital environments generally promote breastfeeding, cesarean birth has little impact on breastfeeding outcome.[46] Milk production is not affected by postpartum surgical sterilization if done within the first 24 hours after birth, but establishment of mature milk production may be delayed if it is done on days 4 to 6 after birth, when it may interfere with regular breast emptying as lactogenesis is being established.

The distribution of formula sample diaper bags is common in the United States, although it directly violates the International Code of Marketing of Breast-milk Substitutes and has been shown to decrease breastfeeding duration.[46] The physician can create orders that eliminate distribution of this advertising, which implies both hospital and physician endorsement of the product, to his or her patients.

f. Medication use and breastfeeding: Few drugs are absolutely contraindicated for the breastfeeding mother because of their effect on the infant; however, a few other drugs can interfere with milk production, such as ergotamine tartrate for migraines, progesterone injections for birth control, and anything that dries mucous membranes. Radiopaque contrast agents and most antibiotics are not a problem. Having a thorough, quick reference, such as *Medications and Mothers' Milk* by Thomas W. Hale, PhD, is helpful.[37]

g. If breastfeeding is not possible: When mothers and/or their babies have special needs and nursing is not possible, mothers can choose to pump their milk and/or use milk from a donor milk bank. The Human Milk Banking Association of North America (HMBANA) publishes *Best Practice for Expressing, Storing, and Handling Human Milk in the Hospital, Home and Child Care Settings,* an evidence-based guide to assist the clinician in guiding mothers who are expressing milk for any reason. A list of non-profit donor milk banks and ordering information for HMBANA publications can be found at HMBANA's website (www.hmbana.org).

h. Posthospital support: With early hospital discharge (12-36 hours), breastfeeding and lactation are not well established, and it is important to schedule early follow-up. If a neonate is not feeding successfully and the discharge cannot be delayed, a feeding plan to protect the neonate and the milk supply need to be developed before discharge. Lactation consultants who make home visits can be invaluable in some situations, and phone support from lay breastfeeding support groups, such as the local La Leche League, can be helpful. It is important to know the community resources so the mother is referred to helpful resources. However, none of this support can replace early clinical follow-up to evaluate whether problems are resolving. Employment or returning to school is often considered barriers to continued breastfeeding. Refer women to lactation consultants or breastfeeding support groups for practical advice and information about pumps, pumping, or planning feeding times, if there is no one knowledgeable in the office.[22,47-49] Combining practical information and support with sensible hospital routines and postpartum follow-up will act as a powerful promoter of breastfeeding.

IV. FUTURE DIRECTIONS

Little attention has been paid to the reasons mothers give for stopping breastfeeding prematurely and to interventions that are effective in preventing untimely weaning. Studies about breastfeeding promotion vary in types of interventions and populations receiving interventions, making it difficult to determine what combination of factors is most effective. Further research may determine optimal clinical interventions, the significance of multiple social variables on breastfeeding initiation and duration, and how best to develop culturally sensitive breastfeeding promotion strategies targeted to specific populations.

V. ROLE OF FAMILY PHYSICIANS

Individual clinicians need to evaluate and continually update their breastfeeding knowledge base and identify personal feelings about breastfeeding. Women have clearly stated that firmly committed, knowledgeable providers who believe that breastfeeding is the normative method to feed a newborn are the most helpful to them.

VI. SOR A RECOMMENDATION

RECOMMENDATION	REFERENCE
Educational programs provide an effective intervention to promote breastfeeding up to 3 months.	26

REFERENCES

1. Academy of Breastfeeding Medicine: Mission statement; 2005, New Rochelle, NY. Available at: www.bfmed.org/index/asp. Accessed September 4, 2007.
2. American Academy of Family Physicians: *Breastfeeding policy and position statement,* Leawood, KS, 2001, American Academy of Family Physicians.
3. American Dietetic Association: Breaking the barriers to breastfeeding—position of ADA, *J Am Diet Assoc* 101:1213-1220, 2001.
4. Gartner L, Morton J, Lawrence R et al: Breastfeeding and the use of human milk, *Pediatrics* 115(2):496-506, 2005.
5. Hansen L: *Immunobiology of human milk: how breastfeeding protects babies,* Amarillo, TX, 2004, Pharmasoft Publishing.
6. International LCA: *Clinical guidelines for the establishment of exclusive breastfeeding,* Raleigh, NC, 2005, International Lactation Consultant Association.
7. U.S. Department of Health and Human Services: *Healthy people 2000,* Washington, DC, 1990, U.S. Department of Health and Human Services.

8. World Health Organization (WHO): *Expert consultation on the optimal duration of exclusive breastfeeding,* Geneva, 2001, WHO.

9. U.S. Department of Health and Human Services: *Healthy people 2010,* Washington, DC, 2000, U.S. Department of Health and Human Services.

10. Li R, Darling N, Maurice E et al: Breastfeeding rates in the United States by characteristics of the child, mother, or family: the 2002 National Immunization Survey, *Pediatrics* 115(1): e31-e37, 2005.

11. Li R, Zhao Z, Mokdad A et al: Prevalence of breastfeeding in the United States: the 2001 National Immunization Survey, *Pediatrics* 111(5 Part 2):1198-1201, 2003.

12. Ahluwalia I, Tessaro I, Grummer-Strawn LM et al: Georgia's breastfeeding promotion program for low-income women, *Pediatrics* 105(6):85-90, 2000.

13. Chen A, Rogan W: Breastfeeding and the risk of postneonatal death in the United States, *Pediatrics* 113(5):e435-e439, 2004.

14. Hoey C, Ware J: Economic advantages of breast-feeding in an HMO: setting a pilot study, *Am J Manag Care* 3(6):861-865, 1997.

15. Montgomery D, Splett P: Economic benefit of breast-feeding infants enrolled in WIC, *J Am Diet Assoc* 97(4):379-385, 1997.

16. Kearney M, Cronenwett L, Barrett J: Breast-feeding problems in the first week postpartum, *Nurs Res* 39(2):90-95, 1990.

17. Anderson G, Moore E, Hepworth J et al: Early skin-to-skin contact for mothers and their healthy newborn infants, *Cochrane Database Syst Rev* (2):CD003519, 2003.

18. Buinauskiene J, Baliutaviciene D, Zalinkevicius R: Glucose tolerance of 2- to 5-yr-old offspring of diabetic mothers, *Pediatr Diabetes* 5(3):143-146, 2004.

19. Sadauskaite-Kuehne V, Ludvigsson J, Padaiga Z et al: Longer breastfeeding is an independent protective factor against development of type 1 diabetes mellitus in childhood, *Diabetes Metab Res Rev* 20(2):150-157, 2004.

20. Freund C, Mirabel L, Annane K et al: Breastfeeding and breast cancer (review), *Gynecol Obstet Fertil* 33(10):739-744, 2005.

21. Tung K, Goodman M, Wu A et al: Reproductive factors and epithelial ovarian cancer risk by histologic type: a multiethnic case-control study, *Am J Epidemiol* 158(7):629-638, 2003.

22. Greenberg C, Smith K: Anticipatory guidance for the employed breast-feeding mother, *J Pediatr Health Care* 5(4): 204-209, 1991.

23. Kearney M, Cronenwett L, Reinhardt R: Cesarean delivery and breastfeeding outcomes, *Birth* 17(2):97-103, 1990.

24. Arenz S, Ruckerl R, Koletzko B et al: Breast-feeding and childhood obesity—a systematic review, *Int J Obes Relat Metab Disord* 28(10):1247-1256, 2004.

25. Shealy K, Li R, Benton-Davis S et al: *The CDC guide to breast-feeding interventions,* Atlanta, 2005, U.S. Department of Health and Human Services, Centers for Disease Control and Prevention.

26. Guise J, Palda V, Westhoff C et al: U.S. Preventive Services Task Force. The effectiveness of primary care-based interventions to promote breastfeeding: systematic evidence review and meta-analysis for the US Preventive Services Task Force 2003, *Ann Fam Med* 1(2):70-78, 2003.

27. Dyson L, McCormick F, Renfrew M: Interventions for promoting the initiation of breastfeeding, *Cochrane Database Syst Rev* (2):CD001688, 2005.

28. Fairbank L, O'Meara S, Renfrew M et al: A systematic review to evaluate the effectiveness of interventions to promote the initiation of breastfeeding, *Health Technol Assess* 4(25):1-171, 2000.

29. Loughlin H, Clapp C, Gehlbach S et al: Early termination of breast-feeding: identifying those at risk, *Pediatrics* 75(3): 508-513, 1985.

30. Yang Q, Wen S, Dubois L et al: Determinants of breast-feeding and weaning in Alberta, Canada, *J Obstet Gynaecol Can* 26(11):975-951, 2004.

31. Henderson A, Stamp G, Pincombe J: Postpartum positioning and attachment education for increasing breastfeeding: a randomized trial, *Birth* 28(4):236-242, 2001.

32. Ziemer M, Paone J, Schupay J et al: Methods to prevent and manage nipple pain in breastfeeding women, *West J Nurs Res* 12(6):732-744, 1990.

33. Ziemer M, Pigeon J: Skin changes and pain in the nipple during the 1st week of lactation, *J Obstet Gynecol Neonatal Nurs* 22(3):247-256, 1993.

34. Neifert M, DeMarzo S, Seacat J et al: The influence of breast surgery, breast appearance, and pregnancy-induced breast changes on lactation sufficiency as measured by infant weight gain, *Birth* 17(1):31-38, 1990.

35. Neifert M, Seacat J, Jobe W: Lactation failure due to insufficient glandular development of the breast, *Pediatrics* 76(5):823-828, 1985.

36. American Academy of Pediatrics: Transfer of drugs and other chemicals into human milk, *Pediatrics* 108:776-789, 2001.

37. Hale T: *Medications and mothers' milk,* ed 9, Amarillo, TX, 2004, Pharmasoft Publishing.

38. Lawrence RA, Lawrence RM: Breastfeeding: a guide for the medical profession, ed 5, St. Louis, MO, 1999, Mosby.

39. Freed GL, Jones TM, Fraley JK: Attitudes and education of pediatric house staff concerning breast-feeding, *South Med J* 85(5):483-485, 1992.

40. WHO/UNICEF: Protecting, promoting and supporting breastfeeding: the special role of maternity services. A joint WHO/UNICEF statement, *Int J Gynaecol Obstet* 31(suppl 1):171-183, 1990.

41. Victora CG, Barros FC, Olinto M: Use of pacifiers and breast-feeding duration, *Lancet* 341:404-406, 1993.

42. Victora C, Behague D, Barros F et al: Pacifier use and short breastfeeding duration: cause, consequence, or coincidence? *Pediatrics* 99(3):445-453, 1997.

43. Marchand L, Morrow MH: Infant feeding practices: understanding the decision-making process. *Fam Med* 26(5): 319-324, 1994.

44. Keefe M: The impact of infant rooming-in on maternal sleep at night, *J Obstet Gynecol Neonatal Nurs* 17(2):122-126, 1988.

45. Winikoff B, Baer E: The obstetrician's opportunity: translating "breast is best" from theory to practice, *Am J Obstet Gynecol* 138(1):105-117, 1980.

46. Donnelly A, Renfrew M, Woolridge M: Commercial hospital discharge packs for breastfeeding women (Cochrane Review). The Cochrane Library, 2001, Update Software(1).

47. Cohen R, Mrtek M: The impact of two corporate lactation programs on the incidence and duration of breast-feeding by employed mothers, *Am J Health Promot* 8(6):436-441, 1994.

48. Corbett-Dick P, Bezek S: Breastfeeding promotion for the employed mother, *J Pediatr Health Care* 11(1):12-19, 1997.

49. Tully M: Working and breastfeeding—helping new mothers figure it out, *AWHONN Lifelines* 9(3):198-203, 2005.

Section E Physiologic Changes and Common Discomforts of Pregnancy

Elizabeth G. Baxley, MD

Most pregnant women experience a variety of symptoms related to the normal physiologic changes of the pregnancy. Most symptoms are merely inconvenient, others may cause moderate discomfort, and some may represent real or potential danger. It is important for providers of prenatal care to be familiar with the common discomforts of pregnancy, to differentiate warning signs from benign conditions and to provide advice regarding comfort measures.

I. NAUSEA AND VOMITING

A. Prevalence and Epidemiology

Nausea is a nearly universal symptom of pregnancy, occurring in 70% to 85% of pregnancies.[1] Half of pregnant women experience vomiting, whereas 25% have nausea only.[2] Typically, these symptoms begin early, before 9 weeks of gestation, and continue until 13 to 16 weeks of gestation. Occasionally, nausea with or without vomiting may continue throughout the entire pregnancy. This condition is known to occur more commonly in primigravidas, younger women, women with less than 12 years' education, nonsmokers, and women weighing greater than 77 kg (170 lb). Although distressing, nausea and vomiting of pregnancy is usually self-limited and rarely prolonged or severe enough that nutrition suffers. However, the extreme of the spectrum, hyperemesis gravidarum, occurs in 0.5% to 2.0% of all pregnancies and is characterized by persistent vomiting unrelated to other causes, ketonuria, and weight loss. Electrolyte, thyroid, and liver function abnormalities may also be present.[2]

Nausea and vomiting are significant problems, however, in that 50% of employed women believe that their work efficiency is reduced because of these symptoms, and 24% report requiring time off from work because nausea and vomiting were disabling.[3] Women who experience nausea and vomiting are more likely to have recurrences in subsequent pregnancies than those who did not have symptoms in the first pregnancy.[4] Positive family history, history of motion sickness, and history of migraine headaches are also considered risk factors.

B. Causative Factors

Although data to support a clear cause are lacking, nausea and vomiting appear to occur more frequently in women with higher levels of circulating estrogen and human chorionic gonadotropin levels and/or estradiol levels, both of which have been associated with improved pregnancy outcome. It is most severe in women with increased placental mass, such as multiple gestation and hydatidiform mole.[2,5]

Emotional factors appear to play an important role but are thought to be contributory rather than causative. Concomitant thyroid disease should be ruled out when nausea and vomiting are persistent or severe because this may be an early manifestation of hyperthyroidism.

Though rare, significant morbidity may result from nausea and vomiting of pregnancy, including Wernicke's encephalopathy, splenic avulsion, esophageal rupture, pneumothorax, and acute tubular necrosis.[2] Pregnancy outcomes in women with uncomplicated nausea and vomiting are generally good, with only hyperemesis gravidarum associated with a greater risk for delivering a low-birth-weight infant.

C. Treatment

1. Dietary measures

    Symptoms often are alleviated by dietary measures, such as keeping food in the stomach with frequent, small meals. Other helpful dietary measures include avoidance of greasy and spicy foods, eating protein meals, and keeping dry crackers at the bedside to eat before rising in the morning.

2. Complementary or nonprescription options

    a. Ginger

    Beneficial effects have been demonstrated with the use of ginger therapy for nausea and vomiting during pregnancy. A systematic review of 6 double-blind RCTs involving 675 women and 1 prospective observation cohort study with 187 women showed that ginger was superior to placebo, and as effective as vitamin B_6, in relieving the severity of pregnancy-related nausea and vomiting.[6] No significant side effects or adverse effects on pregnancy outcomes were noted.

    b. Pyridoxine with or without doxylamine

    Pyridoxine (vitamin B_6), at a dose of 25 mg three times per day, has been shown to reduce the frequency and severity of nausea and vomiting.[1,2] Women with severe symptoms seem to experience a more beneficial response than those with only mild symptoms. When combined with 10 mg doxylamine, pyridoxine has been shown to result in a 70% reduction in nausea and vomiting. This combination has been found in studies involving more than 170,000 exposures to be safe with regard to fetal effects.[2]

c. Acupressure

Acupressure at the Neiguan, or P6, pressure point has been compared with a sham point and sensory afferent stimulation as a potential relief measure for pregnancy-related nausea and vomiting. The location of this acupressure point is on the volar surface of the forearm just above the wrist. Elastic bands (Sea-Bands) are often used to accomplish this, though self-applied pressure is equally as effective. In a systematic review of the literature that included six RCTs, acupressure significantly reduced the amount of nausea and vomiting associated with early pregnancy.[7] In women with ketonuria and symptoms severe enough to require hospitalization, a single RCT demonstrated that acupressure does not reduce the amount of antiemetic medication or intravenous fluid required or the overall length of stay.[8] Cochrane considers the results of 6 trials, including 1150 women, to be equivocal with respect to P6 acupressure.[1,9] All studies to date have shown that is well tolerated and not associated with an increase in perinatal morbidity or death.

3. Pharmacologic management

Antiemetics are needed occasionally when vomiting does not respond to conservative measures or when dehydration, ketosis, or electrolyte abnormalities are present. A Cochrane review, based on 12 trials, showed an overall reduction in nausea from antiemetic medication (odds ratio [OR], 0.16; 95% CI, 0.08-0.33).[1] Some evidence of adverse effects was reported, but little information was available from these RCTs regarding the effects on fetal outcomes. A number of prescription medications, particularly H1 antagonists and phenothiazine, are safe and effective for treatment of nausea and vomiting in pregnancy, though the comparative effectiveness of different agents is largely unknown.[10]

a. Antihistamines

Antihistamines can be used safely in the first trimester because they do not appear to increase the teratogenic potential.[11] Meclizine (Antivert, category B) is effective in relieving symptoms in doses of 12.5 to 25 mg every 8 hours as needed. Often, symptoms that are clustered in the morning respond to a single nightly dose of meclizine. Diphenhydramine (Benadryl, category B) also works well, but sedation is a bothersome side effect. A combination of an antihistamine and vitamin B_6 (debendox [Bendectin]) was previously widely used. It was withdrawn after its use was linked to limb defects in babies, but this was not confirmed by later research.[1]

b. Metoclopramide

Metoclopramide (Reglan, category B) is a dopamine receptor–blocking drug that is commonly used to treat nausea and vomiting during pregnancy. It can be used alone or in combination with pyridoxine, though combination therapy appears to be superior to monotherapy with either prochlorperazine or promethazine.[12] Metoclopramide use during the first trimester of pregnancy does not appear to be associated with an increased risk for malformations, spontaneous abortions, or decreased birth weight.[13,14]

c. Phenothiazines

Prospective studies have produced conflicting results regarding the use of phenothiazines (e.g., promethazine [Phenergan] and prochlorperazine [Compazine], both category C) during early pregnancy. Although a Cochrane review of observational studies suggests no evidence of teratogenicity from these agents,[1] use of this class of drugs is best reserved when nausea and vomiting threaten maternal nutrition.

d. Ondansetron

Ondansetron (Zofran, Category B) is a serotonin receptor antagonist that has been studied and used in the treatment of hyperemesis gravidarum.[15-17] This drug appears to be safe and effective but should be reserved for situations in which nutritional or hydration status of the mother is compromised. In these cases, a dose of 10 mg intravenously every 8 hours as needed has been used, although it has not been found to be superior to promethazine in controlling symptoms and costs considerably more.[15] In a prospective comparative observational study of 176 women, ondansetron does not appear to be associated with an increased risk for major malformations.[18]

II. HEARTBURN

A. Causative Factors

Reflux of gastric acid is common during pregnancy, causing the gravid woman to feel epigastric burning followed by a sense of fullness. The cause of this is twofold, with the primary contributor in the first trimester being progesterone-mediated reduced smooth muscle motility, including a reduction in lower esophageal sphincter pressure with resulting gastroesophageal reflux; alterations in gastric motor function associated with nausea and vomiting; and a decrease in the rate of small-bowel and colonic transit manifested primarily as abdominal bloating and constipation.[19] Later in pregnancy, typically during the third trimester, the expanding uterus displaces the stomach upward, compounding the reflux. Serious reflux complications during pregnancy are rare; hence, upper endoscopy and other diagnostic tests are needed infrequently.[20]

B. Treatment

1. Complementary or nonprescription options
   Reflux symptoms during pregnancy should be managed with a step-up algorithm beginning with lifestyle modifications and dietary changes.[20] Overeating and eating spicy foods exacerbate heartburn. Pregnant women should be advised to eat frequent small meals and to avoid lying recumbent soon after eating. Fried and gas-producing foods, such as cabbage, brussels sprouts, and onions, should be avoided. Sleeping on stacked pillows or raising the head of the bed on blocks may help prevent reflux.
2. Pharmacologic
   Antacids have been shown to relieve heartburn symptoms and are considered first-line drug therapy for reflux in pregnancy.[20,21] Calcium/magnesium-based antacids are recommended as the treatment of choice because of their good safety profile, whereas baking soda or antacids with a high sodium content, which can cause water retention and alkalosis, should be avoided. Aluminum-containing antacids may worsen constipation. In an open-label, multicenter, phase IV study in general practice and antenatal clinics in the United Kingdom and Republic of South Africa, a product that combined sodium alginate and potassium bicarbonate (Gaviscon Advance) was effective in producing a rapid response in managing heartburn during pregnancy, with no known significant safety concerns.[22] Sucralfate is an alternative first-line option.

If symptoms persist, any of the histamine2 receptor antagonists can be used safely.[20] Ranitidine is the best studied agent. Preliminary information indicates that use of proton pump inhibitors (PPIs) during pregnancy is safe, though RCTs are needed to examine their efficacy as compared with histamine2 receptor antagonists.[23] PPIs should be reserved for women with intractable symptoms or complicated reflux disease. All except omeprazole are U.S. Food and Drug Administration category B during pregnancy.

Most of these medications are excreted in breast milk. Only the histamine2 receptor antagonists, with the exception of nizatidine, are safe to use during lactation.[20]

III. CONSTIPATION

A. Causative Factors

Another common problem during both early and late pregnancy is constipation. Similar to heartburn, this physiologic discomfort is due to progesterone-mediated decreased bowel transit time during the first trimester, and is aggravated by displacement and compression of the intestine by the enlarging uterus in the third trimester. Iron supplementation may exacerbate constipation.

B. Treatment

1. Complementary or nonprescription options
   Liberal consumption of fluids and dietary supplements of bran or wheat fiber are likely to help women experiencing constipation in pregnancy.[24] Regular exercise provides additional benefit in the prevention and treatment of constipation.
2. Pharmacologic
   Mild laxatives, such as milk of magnesia, and stool softeners or bulk producers, such as methylcellulose or psyllium hydrophilic mucilloid, are safe and effective for use. In constipation, current data do not distinguish a hierarchy between polyethylene glycol (PEG)-based laxatives and other first-line treatments, although limitations are associated with stimulant- and bulk-forming laxatives. Where data are available, PEG is superior to lactulose in terms of efficacy.[21] Stimulant laxatives are more effective than bulk-forming laxatives (OR, 0.30; 95% CI, 0.14-0.61) but may cause more side effects.[24]

IV. HEMORRHOIDS

A. Causative Factors

Hemorrhoids are varicose veins of the rectum and are exacerbated by the increases in venous pressure that accompany advancing pregnancy. Symptoms are usually mild and transient, and include intermittent rectal bleeding and pain.[25] They are exacerbated by untreated constipation. Hemorrhoids typically regress after delivery, and conservative therapy is warranted during pregnancy. They are often worsened by a long second stage of labor and excessive pushing. Women should be advised to alert their provider if hemorrhoids become hard and tender, indicating potential thrombosis, or if they cause bleeding.

B. Treatment

1. Complementary or nonprescription options
   Prevention is aimed at avoidance of constipation and prolonged sitting. Kegel exercises improve muscle tone in the rectal area and should be routinely recommended. The herbal product 0-beta-hydroxyethyl-rutosides looks promising for symptom relief in treating hemorrhoids during pregnancy, but its use cannot be recommended until sufficient safety evidence is available.[25]
2. Pharmacologic/Surgical
   Commonly used therapies, such as Proctofoam, Anusol, and Preparation H, are safe and effective for use during pregnancy. Thrombosed external hemorrhoids may be able to be treated conservatively but often require incision and evacuation under local anesthesia.[3]

V. URINARY FREQUENCY AND INCONTINENCE

A. Causative Factors

Urinary frequency occurs most commonly during the first and third trimesters of pregnancy. In early gestation, the uterus places increased pressure on the bladder, limiting its ability to fill and resulting in urinary urgency. As the uterus rises out of the pelvis in the second trimester, symptoms may improve transiently, only to worsen again late in pregnancy when engagement of the presenting part exerts pressure on the urinary bladder. In addition, glomerular filtration rate is increased throughout pregnancy, contributing to urinary frequency.

Urinary incontinence during pregnancy is usually of the stress type, occurring when coughing, sneezing, or laughing increases pressure on the bladder. It is a common problem of late pregnancy and may be confused with premature rupture of membranes. Multigravidas, who often have reduced perineal muscle tone supporting the bladder, experience this symptom more often. Some degree of incontinence persists at 6 weeks after delivery in 11.36% of women, with the frequency of events declining over the postpartum year. In a prospective study of 523 women after delivery, postpartum incontinence was significantly associated with smoking (OR, 2.934; $p = 0.002$), incontinence during pregnancy (OR, 2.002; $p = 0.007$), length of breastfeeding (OR, 1.169; $p = 0.023$), vaginal delivery (OR, 2.360; $p = 0.002$), use of forceps (OR, 1.870; $p = 0.024$), frequency of urination (OR, 1.123; $p = <0.001$), and high BMI (OR, 1.055; $p = 0.005$).[26] Factors not associated with postpartum incontinence included age, race, education, episiotomy, number of vaginal deliveries, attendance at childbirth preparation classes, and performing pelvic floor muscle exercises during the postpartum period.

A pregnant woman who experiences burning or pain with urination should be evaluated to rule out urinary tract or vaginal infection, either of which may increase the risk for premature labor, fetal loss, or acute and chronic pyelonephritis.

B. Treatment

Decreasing fluid intake close to bedtime may help symptoms of frequency and urgency, although women should be cautioned not to restrict overall fluid intake. Kegel exercises may reduce or alleviate symptoms or urinary incontinence, although they may not resolve completely until after delivery.

VI. ABDOMINAL PAIN

A. Causative Factors

The most common abdominal pain experienced during pregnancy is the sharp pain caused by spasm of the round ligaments. As the uterus enlarges, more stretch is placed on these ligaments, which then become susceptible to strain. Often, this pain is associated with abrupt movements and is seen more often on the right side because of the normal dextrorotation of the uterus. Less commonly, uterine fibroids can undergo torsion or degeneration; the latter occurs most commonly at 12 to 18 weeks of gestation but can occur at any time during pregnancy. Women present with tenderness over the fibroid, which may be accompanied by nausea and low-grade fever. The condition is self-limited and is treated with rest and analgesics.

Abdominal pain in a pregnant woman in her second or third trimester should be evaluated to rule out premature contractions or other serious medical or obstetric complications. Providers should be alert to the possibility of abdominal problems unrelated to the pregnancy, such as gastroenteritis, appendicitis, pyelonephritis, and renal or biliary colic.

B. Treatment

Improved physical fitness and abdominal wall muscle toning provide added support for the uterus and helps reduce round ligament strain. Patients should be advised to rise and sit gradually, avoiding sudden movements. Rest, accompanied by local heat application (e.g., heating pad, warm bath), is the best treatment for this condition. Analgesia is occasionally necessary and can be achieved safely and effectively with acetaminophen.

VII. PELVIC/BACK AND LEG PAIN

A. Causative Factors

As the uterus enlarges during pregnancy, a woman's center of gravity is altered, and abdominal muscles are stretched. Her shoulders are shifted backward and her head is angled forward to maintain balance, causing a compensatory lumbar lordosis that predisposes to low back pain.[3] During the latter half of pregnancy, ligaments and joints of the back and pelvis are more lax, further promoting back injury or pain. Women with poor abdominal muscle tone or poor posture are more prone to back problems during pregnancy.

Many women also experience leg pain or cramps in pregnancy. They become more common as pregnancy progresses and are especially troublesome at night.

B. Treatment

1. Nonpharmacologic

Prevention is aimed at avoidance of excessive weight gain, improving posture, proper bending with a straight back, and wearing flat or low-heeled shoes. A firm bed mattress may help, and local heat, with or without massage, may relax back muscles.

Water aerobics has been shown to diminish pregnancy-related low back pain, as well as and

sick leave because of pregnancy-related low back pain, more than land-based physical exercise programs.[27] A Cochrane review of 3 trials, involving 376 women, demonstrated that water physical therapy, physiotherapy, acupuncture, and use of a specially shaped pillow, like a nest for the abdomen, help reduce back and pelvic pain.[28] Individually tailored programs are more effective than group programs.

Many patients with pregnancy-related pelvic girdle pain experience relief of pain when using a pelvic belt. In a small study of 25 women, sacroiliac joint laxity values and patient reports of pain decreased significantly during application of a pelvic belt, especially when placed just caudal to the anterior superior iliac spines rather than at the level of the pubic symphysis.[29]

If unilateral leg pain or weakness in one or both legs accompanies the back pain, patients should be evaluated for lumbar disk disease.

2. Pharmacologic

Acetaminophen is a safe analgesic throughout pregnancy for either back pain or leg cramps. Calcium and magnesium have been studied as potential treatments for leg cramps in pregnancy. A Cochrane review of 5 trials, involving 352 women, concluded that the evidence that calcium reduces cramps is weak and seems to depend on placebo effect.[30] The best evidence supports treatment with magnesium lactate or citrate, taken as a 5-mmol dose in the morning and 10-mmol dose in the evening, for troublesome leg cramps in pregnancy.

VIII. SHORTNESS OF BREATH

A. Causative Factors

In early pregnancy, increased circulating progesterone contributes to an increase in minute ventilation, often referred to as pregnancy-induced hyperventilation. Late in pregnancy, the growing uterus creates a mechanical limitation in the excursion of the diaphragm, bringing about a reduction in residual volume and functional residual capacity. These changes often cause a pregnant woman to experience dyspnea.

B. Treatment

Measures that may help improve or alleviate this dyspnea include having the patient stand, sit erect, or when lying, prop her shoulders and head up on one or more pillows. Women should be advised to breathe slowly and deeply, and to pace themselves to accommodate the added demand pregnancy places on pulmonary function.

IX. NASAL CONGESTION

A. Causative Factors

Increased perivascular edema and enlargement of the nasal turbinates occur in early pregnancy, mediated by estrogen, progesterone, and, possibly, placental growth hormone.[31] This often results in bothersome nasal stuffiness, known as pregnancy rhinitis, which affects one in five pregnant women, and may exacerbate preexisting allergy or sinus problems.[32] Smoking and sensitization to house dust mites are probable risk factors for this condition.[32] Nosebleeds also are common and can be reduced or prevented by application of petroleum jelly to the nasal mucosa with a cotton-tipped applicator.

B. Treatment

1. Nonpharmacologic
   Use of a room humidifier may alleviate some of the nasal congestion associated with pregnancy. Saline nose drops are safe and effective to use, as are topical nasal decongestants when indicated, as long as their use is limited to fewer than 3 days at a time to avoid rebound rhinitis medicamentosa.
2. Pharmacologic
   Nasal corticosteroids have not been shown to be effective for pregnancy rhinitis,[33] but they are safe to use when indicated for allergic rhinitis.[32,34] Cromolyn is the safest drug, although it requires multiple daily administration. Antihistamines should be considered as second-choice drugs, and their use is not recommended during the first 3 months of pregnancy.[35] It is not recommended to start specific immunotherapy in pregnancy, but it can be continued in patients who benefit from its use.

X. HEADACHES

A. Causative Factors

Headaches occur as commonly during pregnancy as in nonpregnant women. Some are related to sinus congestion from the rhinitis of pregnancy. Other common explanations cited for headaches during pregnancy include fatigue, tension, eyestrain, and migraines, although in most cases, no demonstrable cause is found. Providers should be alert to headaches that are accompanied by dizziness, blurred vision, or scotomata, and evaluate the patient for preeclampsia if these symptoms are reported.

B. Treatment

Relaxation and use of warm compresses may help with symptom relief. Acetaminophen may be necessary for analgesia and is safe to use throughout pregnancy.

XI. DIZZINESS AND SYNCOPE

A. Causative Factors

Venous pooling results from compression of lower extremity and pelvic veins that occurs with advancing uterine size. This pooling may cause pregnant women to experience dizziness or syncope. This problem is exacerbated in hot weather when peripheral vessels are dilated to dissipate body heat. In late pregnancy, women may experience similar symptoms on lying recumbent, secondary to pressure of the gravid uterus on the vena cava and resulting supine hypotension.

B. Treatment

Calf exercises and use of full-length support stockings may help prevent dizziness secondary to venous pooling of blood. Rest, with positioning in the left lateral tilt position, improves dizziness and helps women recover from vasovagal syncope.

XII. EDEMA AND VARICOSE VEINS

A. Causative Factors

Slowed venous return from uterine pressure on the vena cava contributes to lower extremity edema commonly seen in the third trimester. It can cause symptoms such as pain, feelings of heaviness, night cramps, and paraesthesias.[36] Patients and providers should be alert for edema that progresses rapidly or does not lessen overnight, particularly in the third trimester, when it may herald early preeclampsia. Increased venous pressure in the pelvis and lower extremities may also result in superficial varicosities of the legs and vulva, which, in turn, can add to leg fatigue and painful nighttime leg cramps. Varicose veins that become warm, hard, and painful suggest phlebitis and should be evaluated.

B. Treatment

Women should avoid sitting or standing for long periods and should perform daily leg exercises to prevent swelling. Uncomplicated pregnancy-associated lower extremity edema usually responds to rest and leg elevation. Support stockings are helpful in this situation, but tight waistbands or elastic leg bands may make the situation worse. External pneumatic compression appears to reduce ankle swelling.[36] Immersion in water for 50 minutes results in greater diuresis and decrease in blood pressure than the same amount of time at bedrest with leg elevation.

Rutosides, a mixture of natural or semisynthetic flavonoids that act primarily on the microvascular endothelium to reduce hyperpermeability, appear to relieve symptoms of venous insufficiency in late pregnancy. A Cochrane review of 3 trials, involving 115 women, showed that two thirds of women given rutoside capsules in the last 3 months of pregnancy noted an improvement in symptoms compared with only one third given placebo (OR, 0.30; 95% CI, 0.12-0.77).[36] This supplement has been used widely in Europe since the mid 1960s, as a treatment for edema, but it is difficult to find this supplement in North America, and its safety in pregnancy has not been established.

XIII. DENTAL PROBLEMS

A. Causative Factors

Gum hypertrophy and bleeding are common during pregnancy, when estrogen can cause the gums to become hyperemic and softened. Tooth decay and gum disease often progress more rapidly. Yet, data from the Centers for Disease Control and Prevention Pregnancy Risk Assessment Monitoring System survey indicates that the majority of women do not make a dental visit during pregnancy, even when experiencing oral symptoms.[37] Among those who do receive dental care, those with dental problems were more likely to have lower incomes and Medicaid coverage than those without dental problems.[38] A potential relation has recently emerged between the presence of maternal periodontal disease and delivery of preterm, low-birth-weight infants.[39]

B. Treatment

Adequate plaque control, using a soft toothbrush, mild toothpaste, and daily flossing, is recommended. Dental work can be done during pregnancy with local anesthesia, but general anesthesia should be avoided. Patients should be encouraged to schedule elective dental treatment during the second trimester but seek prompt care for acute dental problems.[40]

XIV. SKIN AND HAIR CHANGES

A. Causative Factors

Several characteristic skin changes occur during pregnancy, primarily relating to hormonally mediated stimulation of the melanocytes. The areolae of the breasts become darker, and a line of increased pigmentation develops from the xiphoid to the symphysis, termed the *linea nigra*. Moles that were present before pregnancy may darken. A reddish brown color over the bridge of the nose and under the eyes, called the *mask of pregnancy,* may be apparent. All of these changes are benign and reversible, and can be minimized initially by avoidance of direct sun and use of appropriate sunscreen.

Striae gravidarum (stretch marks) develop over the abdomen, breasts, and hips in 50% to 65% of pregnant women, and they are thought to be genetically predisposed.[41] In addition, women with higher body mass indexes and younger women are more prone to striae development.[42] Although striae typically remain after delivery, they usually fade to a pink or silver color.

B. Treatment

No evidence exists that any treatment removes striae once they have appeared, although in a small, prospective trial, women who applied tretinoin (retinoic acid) cream 0.1% daily for 3 months to abdominal stretch marks during pregnancy did note significant improvement in the clinical appearance of the striae.[44] Cocoa butter, vitamin E, and lotions may help with the itching that may accompany striae formation.

When systemic therapy is needed, aspirin appears be more effective than chlorpheniramine for relief of itching in pregnancy when no rash is present (OR, 2.39; 95% CI, 1.25-4.57). If a rash is present, chlorpheniramine may be more effective.[45]

XV. BREAST CHANGES

A. Causative Factors

Early in pregnancy, women normally experience breast tenderness. Pain may range from mild to severe and is usually transient, resolving by the end of the first trimester. Breast size also increases and breast tissue becomes more nodular during early pregnancy. Nipples become darker and more erectile. During the third trimester, colostrum may be produced.

B. Treatment

A good support bra should be worn throughout pregnancy and typically needs to be one cup size larger than that worn before pregnancy. When symptoms are severe, acetaminophen and cold compresses may help to alleviate pain.

XVI. LEUKORRHEA

A. Causative Factors

Vaginal discharge typically is increased in amount because of higher estrogen levels and greater vaginal blood flow. Whitish and variable in consistency, this leukorrhea of pregnancy is not indicative of a problem, unless the discharge is accompanied by itching, burning, foul odor, or labial swelling. A change in the quality or quantity of discharge in the third trimester should be differentiated from leaking or ruptured membranes, or from cervical dilation if accompanied by cramping or pressure.

B. Treatment

Patients should be advised to bathe daily and wear cotton underwear. Tub bathing is safe because water does not enter the vagina under normal conditions. Douching rarely is indicated and should be used only if advised by a physician. Use of a bulb syringe for douching is contraindicated because of the risk for air embolism.

XVII. SOR A RECOMMENDATIONS

RECOMMENDATIONS	REFERENCES
Most cases of nausea and vomiting in pregnancy will resolve spontaneously within 16 to 20 weeks of gestation, and nausea and vomiting usually are not associated with a poor pregnancy outcome. Nonpharmacologic interventions that appear to be effective in reducing symptoms include ginger, vitamin B_6, and acupressure. Pharmacologic agents that appear to be safe and effective include antihistamines and H1 antagonists.	*10, 11, 44*
Antacids may be offered to women whose heartburn does not respond to lifestyle and diet modification.	*44*
Liberal consumption of fluids and dietary supplements of bran or wheat fiber are likely to help women experiencing constipation in pregnancy.	*24*
Varicose veins are a common symptom of pregnancy that will not cause harm; compression stockings can improve the symptoms but will not prevent the varicose veins from emerging.	*44*
Women should be informed that exercising in water and massage therapy might help to ease back pain in pregnancy. Acupuncture and use of a specially shaped pillow also help reduce back and neck pain.	*27, 44*

REFERENCES

1. Young GL, Jewell D: Interventions for nausea and vomiting in early pregnancy, *Cochrane Database Syst Rev* (4):CD000145, 2003.
2. American College of Obstetrics and Gynecology: Nausea and vomiting of pregnancy, *ACOG Practice Bulletin Number* 52:103(4), 2004.
3. Vellacott ID, Cooke EJ, James CE: Nausea and vomiting in early pregnancy, *Int J Obstet Gynecol* 27:57-62, 1988.
4. Klebanoff MA, Koslowe PA, Kaslow R et al: Epidemiology of vomiting in early pregnancy, *Obstet Gynecol* 66:612-616, 1985.
5. Tierson FD, Olsen CL, Hook EB: Nausea and vomiting of pregnancy and association with pregnancy outcome, *Am J Obstet Gynecol* 155:1017-1022, 1986.
6. Borrelli F, Capasso R, Aviello G et al: Effectiveness and safety of ginger in the treatment of pregnancy-induced nausea and vomiting, *Obstet Gynecol* 105(4):849-856, 2005.
7. Freels DL, Coggins M: Acupressure at the Neiguan P6 point for treating nausea and vomiting in early pregnancy: an evaluation of the literature, *Mother Baby Journal* 5(3):17-22, 2000.
8. Heazell A, Thorneycroft J, Walton V et al: Acupressure for the in-patient treatment of nausea and vomiting in early pregnancy: a randomized control trial, *Am J Obstet Gynecol* 194(3):815-820, 2006.
9. Ezzo J, Streitberger K, Schneider A: Cochrane systematic reviews examine p6 acupuncture-point stimulation for nausea and vomiting, *J Altern Complement Med* 12(5):489-495, 2006.
10. Magee LA, Mazzotta P, Koren G: Evidence-based view of safety and effectiveness of pharmacologic therapy for nausea and vomiting of pregnancy (NVP), *Am J Obstet Gynecol* 186(5 Suppl Understanding):S256-261, 2002.
11. Seto A, Einarson T, Koren G: Pregnancy outcome following first trimester exposure to antihistamines: a meta-analysis, *Am J Perinatol* 14:119-124, 1997.
12. Bsat FA, Hoffman DE, Seubert DE: Comparison of three outpatient regimens in the management of nausea and vomiting in pregnancy, *J Perinatol* 23(7):531-535, 2003.
13. Berkovitch M, Mazzota P, Greenberg R et al: Metoclopramide for nausea and vomiting of pregnancy: a prospective multicenter international study, *Am J Perinatol* 19(6):311-316, 2002.
14. Sorensen HT, Nielsen GL, Christensen K et al: Birth outcome following maternal use of metoclopramide. The Euromap Study Group, *Br J Clin Pharmacol* 49(3):264-268, 2000.
15. Sullivan CA, Johnson CA, Roach H et al: A pilot study of intravenous ondansetron for hyperemesis gravidarum, *Am J Obstet Gynecol* 174:1565-1568, 1996.
16. Tincello DG, Johnstone MJ: Treatment of hyperemesis gravidarum with the 5-HT3 antagonist ondansetron (Zofran), *Postgrad Med J* 72:688-689, 1996.
17. World MJ: Ondansetron and hyperemesis gravidarum, *Lancet* 341:185-188, 1993.
18. Einarson A, Maltepe C, Navioz Y et al: The safety of ondansetron for nausea and vomiting of pregnancy: a prospective comparative study, *BJOG* 111(9):940-943, 2004.
19. Baron TH, Ramirez B, Richter JE: Gastrointestinal motility disorders during pregnancy, *Ann Intern Med* 118(5):366-375, 1993.
20. Richter JE: Review article: the management of heartburn in pregnancy, *Aliment Pharmacol Ther* 22(9):749-757, 2005.
21. Tytgat GN, Heading RC, Muller-Lissner S et al: Contemporary understanding and management of reflux and constipation in the general population and pregnancy: a consensus meeting, *Aliment Pharmacol Ther* 18(3):291-301, 2003.
22. Lindow SW, Regnell P, Sykes J et al: An open-label, multicentre study to assess the safety and efficacy of a novel reflux suppressant (Gaviscon Advance) in the treatment of heartburn during pregnancy, *Int J Clin Pract* 57(3):175-179, 2003.
23. Christopher L: The role of proton pump inhibitors in the treatment of heartburn during pregnancy, *J Am Acad Nurse Pract* 17(1):4-8, 2005.
24. Young GL, Jewell D: Interventions for treating constipation in pregnancy, *Cochrane Database Syst Rev* (2):CD001142, 2001.
25. Quijano CE, Abalos E: Conservative management of symptomatic and/or complicated haemorrhoids in pregnancy and the puerperium, *Cochrane Database Syst Rev* (3):CD004077, 2005.
26. Burgio KL, Zyczynski H, Locher JL et al: Urinary incontinence in the 12-month postpartum period, *Obstet Gynecol* 102(6):1291-1298, 2003.
27. Granath AB, Hellgren MS, Gunnarsson RK: Water aerobics reduces sick leave due to low back pain during pregnancy, *J Obstet Gynecol Neonatal Nurs* 35(4):465-471, 2006.
28. Young GL, Jewell D: Interventions for preventing and treating back pain in pregnancy, *Cochrane Database Syst Rev* (1): CD001139, 2002.
29. Mens JM, Damen L, Snijders CJ et al: The mechanical effect of a pelvic belt in patients with pregnancy-related pelvic pain, *Clin Biomech* 21(2):122-127, 2006.
30. Young GL, Jewell D: Interventions for leg cramps in pregnancy, *Cochrane Database Syst Rev* (1):CD000121, 2002.
31. Ellegard EK: Clinical and pathogenetic characteristics of pregnancy rhinitis, *Clin Rev Allergy Immunol* 26(3):149-159, 2004.
32. Ellegard EK: Pregnancy rhinitis, *Immunol Allergy Clin North Am* 26(1):119-135, 2006.
33. Ellegard EK, Hellgren M, Karlsson NG: Fluticasone propionate aqueous nasal spray in pregnancy rhinitis, *Clin Otolaryngol Allied Sci* 26(5):394-400, 2001.
34. Ellegard EK: The etiology and management of pregnancy rhinitis, *Am J Respir Med* 2(6):469-475, 2003.
35. Gani F, Braida A, Lombardi C et al: Rhinitis in pregnancy, *Allerg Immunol (Paris)* 35(8):306-313, 2003.
36. Young GL, Jewell D: Interventions for varicosities and leg oedema in pregnancy, *Cochrane Database Syst Rev* (1):CD001066, 2007.
37. Ressler-Maerlender J, Krishna R, Robison V: Oral health during pregnancy: current research, *J Womens Health (Larchmt)* 14(10):880-882, 2005.
38. Lydon-Rochelle MT, Krakowiak P, Hujoel PP et al: Dental care use and self-reported dental problems in relation to pregnancy, *Am J Public Health* 94(5):765-771, 2004.
39. Buduneli N, Baylas H, Buduneli E et al: Periodontal infections and pre-term low birth weight: a case-control study, *J Clin Periodontol* 32(2):174-181, 2005.
40. Mills LW, Moses DT: Oral health during pregnancy, *MCN Am J Matern Child Nurs* 27(5):275-280, 2002.
41. Chang AL, Agredano YZ, Kimball AB: Risk factors associated with striae gravidarum, *J Am Acad Dermatol* 51(6):881-885, 2004.
42. Thomas RG, Liston WA: Clinical associations of striae gravidarum, *J Obstet Gynaecol* 24(3):270-271, 2004.
43. Young GL, Jewell D: Creams for preventing stretch marks in pregnancy, *Cochrane Database Syst Rev* (2):CD000066, 2000.

44. Rangel O, Arias I, Garcia E et al: Topical tretinoin 0.1% for pregnancy-related abdominal striae: an open-label, multi-center, prospective study, *Adv Ther* 18(4):181-186, 2001.
45. Young GL, Jewell D: Antihistamines versus aspirin for itching in late pregnancy, *Cochrane* Database Syst Rev (2):CD000027, 2000.

SECTION F Exercise and Pregnancy

Elizabeth A. Joy, MD, and Thad J. Barkdull, MD

Physical activity and maintenance of physical fitness are essential to the health of women in their childbearing years. Pregnancy is a normal condition for women, and exercise can be part of a normal pregnancy. In the absence of medical or obstetric complications, women should be encouraged by their obstetric care provider to exercise regularly throughout pregnancy. Physicians and midwives need to be knowledgeable about the American College of Obstetricians and Gynecologists (ACOG) guidelines[1] for exercise during pregnancy and the postpartum period, as well as contraindications to exercise during pregnancy and the signals to stop exercising. Providers should be able to counsel women on the maternal and fetal benefits of regular exercise during pregnancy and know how to write an appropriate exercise prescription based on a woman's fitness level, interests, and exercise goals.

Nearly half of 10,000 women surveyed[2] reported exercising during pregnancy. Research to date supports the decision to continue or initiate an exercise program during pregnancy. The literature dealing with exercise during pregnancy has shown no deleterious effects of exercise on the mother or developing fetus.[3] Women are able not only to maintain but also to improve their fitness levels during pregnancy,[4,5] and a report suggests that infants of exercising mothers may be healthier than those of sedentary mothers.[6] Exercising women also report fewer discomforts of pregnancy than their sedentary counterparts.[7] For most pregnant women, exercise is not only safe but beneficial to the health of the mother and the infant.

I. GUIDELINES FOR EXERCISE DURING PREGNANCY

In 1985, the ACOG[1] published its first guidelines for exercise during pregnancy. These guidelines were based on limited scientific data and were criticized.[8,9] After numerous studies showed maternal benefits and no fetal or neonatal risks from regular maternal exercise, in 1994, the ACOG[10] revised and liberalized their guidelines for exercise during pregnancy and the postpartum period. Table 4-7 lists the guidelines from 1985 and 1994. The most striking changes from the earlier guidelines included *removal* of the recommendations not to exceed a heart rate of 140 beats/min or exercise beyond 15 minutes duration and the recommendation to avoid exercises employing the Valsalva maneuver (specifically weight lifting). These recommendations are only a *guide.* Each pregnant woman has a different experience with pregnancy and exercise. Exercise guidelines must be tailored to each individual woman.

II. CONTRAINDICATIONS TO EXERCISE DURING PREGNANCY

The ACOG guidelines apply to healthy women experiencing normal pregnancies. There are absolute and relative obstetric and medical contraindications to exercise during pregnancy.

A. Absolute Obstetric Contraindications

Absolute obstetric contraindications include pregnancy-induced hypertension, premature rupture of membranes, incompetent cervix or cerclage, persistent second- or third-trimester bleeding, and IUGR. The ACOG also lists preterm labor during the prior or current pregnancy, or both, as an absolute contraindication. One could argue that if a definitive cause for preterm labor (e.g., multiple gestations, pyelonephritis) in the prior pregnancy could be identified and was not evident in the present pregnancy, one could exercise safely.

B. Absolute Medical Contraindications

Absolute medical contraindications include hemodynamically significant heart disease, uncontrolled hypertension, uncontrolled renal disease, hemodynamically significant anemia, and uncontrolled diabetes mellitus.

TABLE 4-7 American College of Obstetricians and Gynecologists Guidelines for Exercise during Pregnancy and the Postpartum Period

1. Regular activity (three times/week) is preferable to intermittent activity.

2. Pregnant women who exercise in the first trimester should augment heat dissipation by ensuring adequate hydration, appropriate clothing, and optimal environmental surroundings.

3. Morphologic changes in pregnancy should serve as a relative contraindication to types of exercise in which balance could be detrimental to maternal or fetal well-being, especially in the third trimester. Any type of exercise involving the potential for mild abdominal trauma should be avoided.

4. Women should be aware of the decreased oxygen available for aerobic exercise during pregnancy. They should be encouraged to modify the intensity of exercise according to maternal symptoms. Pregnant women should stop exercising when fatigued and not exercise to exhaustion. Weight-bearing exercises may be continued under some circumstances at intensities similar to those before pregnancy throughout pregnancy. Non–weight-bearing exercises, such as cycling or swimming, minimize the risk for injury and facilitate the continuation of exercise during pregnancy.

5. Women should avoid exercise in the supine position after the first trimester. Such a position is associated with decreased cardiac output in most pregnant women. Prolonged periods of motionless standing also should be avoided.

6. Pregnancy requires an additional 300 kcal/day to maintain metabolic homeostasis. Women who exercise during pregnancy should be particularly careful to ensure adequate diet.

7. Many of the physiologic and morphologic changes of pregnancy persist 4 to 6 weeks after delivery. Prepregnancy exercise routines should be resumed gradually.

Data from American College of Obstetricians and Gynecologists (ACOG): Exercise during pregnancy and the postnatal period. *ACOG home exercise programs,* Washington, DC, 1985, ACOG; and ACOG: Exercise during pregnancy and the postpartum period, *ACOG Technical Bulletin No. 189,* Washington, DC, 1994, ACOG.

C. Relative Obstetric Contraindications

Relative obstetric contraindications include multiple gestation, breech position in the third trimester, and a history of precipitous labor and delivery. If any evidence suggests fetal compromise, maternal complication, or preterm labor, exercise activities would need to be changed or eliminated.

D. Relative Medical Contraindications

Relative medical contraindications may include but are not limited to malnutrition, certain cardiac arrhythmias, symptomatic anemia, active thyroid disease, and extreme obesity. Women with conditions such as these need to participate in a closely monitored exercise program.

III. BENEFITS OF EXERCISE DURING PREGNANCY

The many maternal benefits of exercise during pregnancy include improved cardiovascular fitness[5,11]; control of maternal weight gain[12]; reduction of some discomforts of pregnancy, such as swelling, leg cramps, fatigue, and shortness of breath[7]; and a positive influence on labor and delivery. Clapp[13] found that compared with women who discontinued exercise in the first trimester, women who exercised regularly at 50% of preconceptional levels throughout pregnancy had a lower incidence of vaginal or abdominal operative delivery, shorter active labor, and increased fetal tolerance of labor and delivery. Clinical evidence of fetal stress (e.g., meconium, fetal heart rate pattern, and Apgar score) was less frequent in the exercising group compared with the control group (Table 4-8).[13]

Regular exercise does not appear to negatively affect early pregnancy outcome. Clapp[14] prospectively followed 47 recreational runners, 40 aerobic dancers, and 28 physically active, fit controls. Spontaneous abortion occurred in 17% of the runners and 18% of the aerobic dancers compared with 25% in the control group. These results should be reassuring to obstetric care providers and their patients who exercise regularly.

The greatest benefits of exercise during pregnancy may be psychological. In one study, women reported that the chief benefits of exercise during pregnancy

TABLE 4-8 Course of Labor after Endurance Exercise during Pregnancy

	*Exercise Group (n = 87)**	*Control Group (n = 44)†*
Incidence rate of preterm labor	9%	9%
Length of gestation	277 days	282 days
Incidence rate of abdominal operative delivery	6%	30%
Incidence rate of vaginal operative delivery	6%	20%
Duration of labor	264 minutes	382 minutes
Clinical evidence of fetal stress‡	26%	50%

Study comprised 113 well-conditioned, recreational athletes.
*Women who continued regular exercise at 50% of their preconceptional level throughout pregnancy.
†Women who discontinued exercise before the end of the first trimester.
‡Evidence includes meconium, abnormal fetal heart rate pattern, and low Apgar score.
From Clapp JF: The course of labor after endurance exercise during pregnancy, *Am J Obstet Gynecol* 163:1799-1805, 1990.

were related to improved mental outlook, self-image, sense of control, and relief of tension.[12]

A considerable body of research has documented the role of regular physical activity in preventing gestational diabetes mellitus (GDM). Zhang and colleagues[15] prospectively followed 21,765 women in the Nurses Health Study II and found a significant inverse association between vigorous physical activity and the risk for GDM, after controlling for BMI, dietary factors, and other covariates. A recent Cochrane review found insufficient evidence to recommend exercise as a treatment intervention for GDM.[16]

There appear to be neonatal and childhood benefits to regular exercise during pregnancy as well. Clapp[17] reports on the offspring of 20 women who exercised and compared them with those of 20 physically active control subjects. The women and their offspring were matched for multiple prenatal and postnatal variables known to influence outcome. He found that at birth, head circumference and length were similar, but the offspring of exercising women weighed less (3400 vs. 3640 g) and had less body fat (10.5% vs. 15.1%). At 5 years of age, head circumference and length were similar, but the offspring of exercising women still weighed less (18.0 vs. 19.5 kg) and had a lower sum of five skin folds (37 vs. 44 mm). Motor, integrative, and academic readiness skills were evaluated by developmental psychologists blinded to maternal exercise status and were found to be similar in the two groups. However, the exercise offspring performed significantly better on Wechsler scales and tests of oral language skills.

IV. PHYSIOLOGIC ADAPTATIONS TO PREGNANCY AND THEIR INTERACTION WITH EXERCISE

A. Cardiovascular

Many cardiovascular adaptations throughout pregnancy influence and interact with a woman's ability to exercise. Cardiac output increases substantially during pregnancy as a result of increased venous return, which increases ventricular filling, and an increase in myocardial contractility. Heart rate is thought to increase as a result of decreased vagal tone or an increase in sympathetic drive to the sinoatrial node. During pregnancy, a woman's systemic vascular resistance decreases during aerobic exercise, resulting in larger increases in the cardiac output response to exercise.

Exercise and pregnancy have opposing effects on one another with respect to regional blood flow distribution. During exercise, splanchnic blood flow is diminished as blood flow is redistributed to skin and exercising muscles. During pregnancy, blood flow is shunted preferentially to uterine, renal, and cutaneous circulations. Increases in cardiac output, blood volume, and resting venous capacitance may negate any relative decline in uteroplacental blood flow during exercise, however. Placental adaptations to exercise may aid in fetal acquisition of oxygen and substrate. Clapp found that placental volumes were significantly greater in women who maintained a regular exercise regimen through the second trimester of pregnancy.[14]

It seems safe to conclude that this increase in placental volume would result in enhanced extraction of oxygen and substrate from the uteroplacental circulation and diminish further any relative decrease in uteroplacental circulation resulting from exercise.

B. Pulmonary

During pregnancy and exercise, minute ventilation and oxygen consumption increase. This increase results in an increase in arterial oxygen tension to 106 to 108 mmHg in the first trimester, declining to 101 to 106 mmHg in the third trimester.[10] Despite this increase in oxygen tension, the increased resting oxygen requirements of pregnancy and the increased work of breathing for any given workload result in decreased oxygen available for aerobic exercise. Most women appreciate a subjective increase in workload and a decline in maximal exercise performance.[10,18]

C. Thermoregulatory

Pregnancy and exercise result in an increase in maternal heat production. Exercise can result in significant increases in core temperature. During exercise, heat dissipation occurs as a result of increased blood flow to the skin, resulting in sweating. Fetal core temperature is approximately 0.5° to 1.0°C greater than maternal core temperature. This higher temperature normally is dissipated through umbilical and uterine circulations. Healthy, fit pregnant women tolerate thermal stress better than in the nonpregnant state as a result of maternal adaptations that eliminate the gradient between maternal and fetal circulation. Clapp[19] studied 18 recreational athletes before, during, and after 20 minutes of continuous exercise at 64% of maximum oxygen consumption. He found that peak rectal temperature reached during exercise decreased by 0.3°C at 8 weeks, then declined at a rate of 0.1°C per month through the 37th week. These changes were related to a decrease in rectal temperature at rest and a decrease in temperature when sweating occurred. The thermal stress for a given task is decreased by 20% in early pregnancy and 50% by the third trimester. No studies have shown fetal teratogenesis attributed to thermal stress in women participating in vigorous exercise during early pregnancy.[18]

D. Endocrine Response and Metabolism

Endocrine response and substrate use of pregnancy and exercise generally are in opposition to one another. This situation raises a concern that substrate may be diverted from the fetus to exercising muscles, resulting in lower fetal birth weights. In women who exercise at moderate levels, however, there appears to be no adverse effect on fetal birth weight.[20] Studies show lower blood glucose levels after a period of exercise in pregnant women.[21] It is prudent to remind women who exercise that they need to meet not only the extra energy demands of pregnancy, but also the energy demands of their exercise program. On average, a pregnant woman requires an extra 300 kcal of energy intake per day.[10] One can estimate safely that each 1 mile walked or run, every 3 miles on a bike, or 15 to 20 minutes of moderate-level aerobic dance requires an additional 100 kcal of energy.

Theoretic concerns regarding the conflicting endocrine responses during exercise and pregnancy relate primarily to whether the excess catecholamines and prostaglandins liberated during exercise result in uterine stimulation and subsequent preterm birth. No studies to date have shown any increase in the incidence of preterm delivery as a result of maternal exercise programs in otherwise healthy, normal pregnancies.[22]

V. EXERCISE PRESCRIPTION

The goal of exercise during pregnancy should be to maintain maternal fitness levels whereas minimizing risk to the developing fetus. Exercise guidelines should be tailored to each individual woman. The key to maintaining a safe, comfortable exercise program is flexibility of thought. As a woman's pregnancy changes, so must her exercise program. She should be prepared to stop or change her exercise regimen in response to changes in her pregnancy. When discussing or designing an exercise program, one must take into account a woman's fitness level, goals of exercise (maintain fitness, stress relief, weight management, competitive activities), work activities and job requirements, and gestational age. Exercise intensity, duration, and frequency should be kept at a level that does not result in excessive fatigue, pain, or extreme shortness of breath. For most women, over the course of their pregnancy, overall exercise performance decreases considerably as a result of pregnancy-related fatigue, nausea, vomiting, weight gain, and other morphologic changes.[10] Switching to non–weight-bearing forms of exercise, such as swimming or bicycling, may allow some women to continue with moderate to vigorous intensity exercise programs throughout their pregnancy.[23] Women whose job requires certain physical stresses (quiet standing, long hours, protracted ambulation, or heavy lifting) may be at increased risk for premature birth and low birth weight.[24] In addition to making appropriate changes in the work environment to avoid this risk, one must take these activities into account when discussing any exercise regimen.

Although there is no generally agreed on formula for determining an appropriate exercise prescription, one can recommend safely most exercise activities that women were doing before becoming pregnant. For women initiating an exercise program, there are many fitness activities that can be started safely during early pregnancy. Table 4-9 lists exercise modalities and their intensity, duration, and frequency appropriate for three levels of maternal fitness: previously sedentary women, recreational athletes and regular fitness exercisers, and elite athletes.

Women should be counseled regarding environmental conditions and their impact on maternal and fetal stress; this is especially true in regard to heat. Women should be cautioned to avoid exercise outdoors during the heat of the day. Women should dress appropriately to avoid excessive thermal stress and drink appropriate amounts of fluid before, during, and after exercise to counteract sweat losses. Recommendations regarding physical activity at altitude during pregnancy are based on few scientific studies, and providers should err on the side of caution when advising women facing short-term exposure to high altitude (>8000 feet above sea level) during pregnancy. Women who reside at higher altitudes and have higher levels of fitness tolerate altitude stress better than women who do not. Altitude in excess of 8000 feet should be avoided in the first 4 to 5 days of short-term exposure, and if exercise is to be performed at altitude, acclimatization should take place by exercising at lower altitudes for a few days.[25]

VI. SIGNALS TO STOP EXERCISING

Providers and patients need to be aware of the signals to stop exercising when pregnant. Table 4-10 lists symptoms that should elicit prompt evaluation and

TABLE 4-9 Guide to Exercise Prescription during Pregnancy

Sedentary Women

Mode	Walking, bicycling, stair climbing, aerobic dance, water aerobics, swimming
Intensity	65-75% maximum heart rate; perceived exertion = moderately hard
Duration	30 minutes
Frequency	Minimum of 3 times/wk

Recreational (athletes/regular fitness exercisers)

Mode	Same as above plus running/jogging, dance, tennis
Depending on skill level and gestational age: cross-country skiing, downhill skiing, water skiing (recommend wearing a wet suit), horseback riding	
Intensity	65-85% maximum heart rate; perceived exertion = moderately hard to hard
Duration	30-60 minutes
Frequency	3-5 times/wk

Elite Athletes

Mode	Same as above plus some competitive activities, depending on gestational age
Intensity	75-85% maximum heart rate; perceived exertion = hard
Duration	60-90 minutes
Frequency	4-6 times/wk

TABLE 4-10 Signals to Stop Exercising

Fatigue	Excessive nausea	Decreased fetal movement
Breathlessness	Chest pain or tightness	Uterine contractions
Dizziness	Palpitations or racing heart	Vaginal bleeding
Headache	Difficulty walking	Leakage of amniotic fluid
Muscle weakness	Significant swelling in feet or legs	Pain—back, hips, or pubic bone

From Paisley JE, Mellion MB: Exercise during pregnancy, *Am Fam Physician* 38:143-150, 1988.

appropriate modification in activity to avoid further risk to either mother or fetus.

VII. EXERCISES TO AVOID

Table 4-11 lists activities that women should, in most cases, avoid during pregnancy and activities that should prompt more frequent monitoring. Although there are no generally agreed on sports or activities that pregnant women can or cannot do, most practitioners take a commonsense approach in advising against activities that pose a threat of abdominal trauma. A woman's fitness level, skill level, and her own assumption of personal risk need to be taken into consideration when decisions are made regarding sports participation. Scuba diving during pregnancy is discouraged because the fetus is not protected from decompression problems and is at risk for malformation and gas embolism after decompression disease.[26] Maximal weight lifting has been shown to result in dramatic increases in blood pressure and probably should be avoided. Moderate strength training has not been shown to cause any deleterious effects among pregnant women, however.[5] The issue of high-intensity endurance training among elite athletes continues to be investigated. Some evidence exists that vigorous training performed throughout pregnancy results in lower birth weight infants, but there is no evidence of preterm birth.[26] Although there are no definitive guidelines for monitoring the high-intensity athlete during pregnancy, one should take a commonsense approach to this and look for signs of fetal stress. Maternal weight gain and fundal height measurements should be appropriate for gestational age regardless of maternal exercise levels. Contractions after moderate to vigorous intensity exercise are not uncommon and should resolve within 1 hour after the cessation of exercise.

VIII. CONCLUSION

Exercise during pregnancy has been found to be not only safe but beneficial in most cases to the mother and the developing fetus. Maternity care providers should encourage patients to continue or initiate exercise programs during pregnancy and work with them on a regular basis to modify exercise regimens in response to changes in the pregnancy.

TABLE 4-11 Exercises to Avoid during Pregnancy

Contact/collision sports
Boxing, field hockey, football, rugby, ice hockey, martial arts, rodeo, soccer, wrestling
High-risk activities
Deep-sea diving, hang gliding, parachute jumping, rock climbing, springboard diving, fencing, power weight lifting
Other at-risk activities*
Competitive distance running, competitive bodybuilding, professional dance, ballet

*Participation limited to women with high fitness and skill levels and under close medical supervision.

REFERENCES

1. American College of Obstetrics and Gynecology (ACOG): Exercise during pregnancy and the postnatal period. *ACOG home exercise programs*, Washington, DC, 1985, ACOG.
2. Zhang J, Savitz DA: Exercise during pregnancy among US women, *Ann Epidemiol* 6:53-59, 1996.
3. Sternfeld B: Physical activity and pregnancy outcome: review and recommendations, *Sports Med* 23:33-47, 1997.
4. Clapp JF, Capeless E: The VO_{2max} of recreational athletes before and after pregnancy, *Med Sci Sports Exerc* 23:1128-1133, 1991.
5. Kulpa PJ, White BM, Visscher R: Aerobic exercise in pregnancy, *Am J Obstet Gynecol* 156:139-143, 1987.

6. Clapp JF, Rizk KH: Effect of recreational exercise on midtrimester placental growth, *Am J Obstet Gynecol* 167:1518-1521, 1992.

7. Horns PN, Ratcliffe LP, Leggett JC et al: Pregnancy outcomes among active and sedentary primiparous women, *J Obstet Gynecol Neonat Nurs* 25:49-54, 1996.

8. Gauthier MM: Guidelines for exercise during pregnancy: too little or too much? *Phys Sportsmed* 14:162-169, 1986.

9. Monahan T: Should women go easy on exercise? *Phys Sportsmed* 14:188-197, 1986.

10. American College of Obstetrics and Gynecology (ACOG): Exercise during pregnancy and the postpartum period, *ACOG Technical Bulletin No. 189,* Washington, DC, 1994, ACOG.

11. Clapp JF, Capeless E: The VO$_{2max}$ of recreational athletes before and after pregnancy, *Med Sci Sports Exerc* 23:1128-1133, 1991.

12. Lee VC, Lutter JM: Exercise and pregnancy: choices, concerns, and recommendations. *Obstetric and gynecologic physical therapy,* New York, 1990, Churchill Livingstone.

13. Clapp JF: The course of labor after endurance exercise during pregnancy, *Am J Obstet Gynecol* 163:1799-1805, 1990.

14. Clapp JF: The effects of maternal exercise on early pregnancy outcome, *Am J Obstet Gynecol* 161:1453-1457, 1989.

15. Zhang C, Solomon CG, Manson JE et al: A prospective study of pregravid physical activity and sedentary behaviors in relation to the risk of gestational diabetes mellitus, *Arch Intern Med* 166(5):543-548, 2006.

16. Ceysens G, Rouiller D, Boulvain M: Exercise for diabetic pregnant women, *Cochrane Database Syst Rev* 3:CD004225, 2006.

17. Clapp JF: Morphometric and neurodevelopmental outcome at age five years of the offspring of women who continued to exercise regularly throughout pregnancy, *J Pediatr* 129:856-863, 1996.

18. Clapp JF: Exercise in pregnancy: a brief clinical review, *Fetal Med Rev* 2:89-101, 1990.

19. Clapp JF: The changing thermal response to endurance exercise during pregnancy, *Am J Obstet Gynecol* 165:1684-1689, 1991.

20. Pivarnik JM: Potential effects of maternal physical activity on birth weight: brief review, *Med Sci Sports Exerc* 30:400-406, 1998.

21. Soultanakis HN, Artal R, Wiswell RA: Prolonged exercise in pregnancy: glucose homeostasis, ventilatory and cardiovascular responses, *Semin Perinatol* 20:315-327, 1996.

22. Veille JC, Hohimer AR, Burry K et al: The effect of exercise on uterine activity in the last 8 weeks of pregnancy, *Am J Obstet Gynecol* 151:727-730, 1985.

23. Artal R, Masaki DI, Khodiquian N et al: Exercise prescription during pregnancy: weight-bearing versus non-weight-bearing exercise, *Am J Obstet Gynecol* 161:1464-1469, 1989.

24. Clapp JF: Pregnancy outcome: physical activities inside versus outside the workplace, *Semin Perinatol* 20:70-76, 1996.

25. Huch R: Physical activity at altitude in pregnancy, *Semin Perinatol* 20:303-314, 1996.

26. Hale RW, Milne L: The elite athlete and exercise in pregnancy, *Semin Perinatol* 20:277-284, 1996.

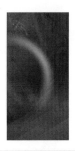

CHAPTER 5

Pregnancy Interventions

SECTION A **Psychosocial Interventions**

Elizabeth G. Baxley, MD,
and Kevin J. Bennett, BS, MS, PhD

I. PSYCHOSOCIAL INDICATORS AND ADVERSE PERINATAL OUTCOMES

Pregnancy is a time of significant life change for women and their partners. Changing roles, relationship difficulties, and negative life events may contribute to psychosocial consequences that impact the pregnancy. The relation between psychosocial risk factors and perinatal outcomes is well-established, and these risk factors disproportionately affect poor, minority women who lack social support.

A. Antenatal Complications

Adverse psychosocial conditions that are known to negatively affect pregnancy outcomes include poverty, single parenthood, teenage pregnancy, lack of social support, family dysfunction, substance abuse, and physical or sexual abuse. Greater rates of medical complications of pregnancy, particularly low birth weight (LBW) and preterm labor, are seen in women with these risk factors.[1-3]

Unplanned pregnancy or negative perception of the pregnancy has been associated with delay in seeking prenatal care or having no prenatal care. According to data collected by the Centers for Disease Control and Prevention in their ongoing Pregnancy Risk Assessment Monitoring System (PRAMS), the prevalence of an unintended pregnancy resulting in live birth ranges from 31.6% to 53.4%, depending on

geographic location of the women studied.[4,5] In most states, women who were younger, had less than a high-school education, were African American, lived in rural areas, and received Medicaid were more likely to report an unintended pregnancy and were less likely to seek prenatal care early in the pregnancy or at all.[6]

B. Postpartum Complications

Postpartum health and family function are also influenced by psychosocial indicators. A systematic review of the literature identifies 15 antenatal psychosocial risk factors; these factors are associated with poor postpartum outcomes, including woman abuse, child abuse, postpartum depression, marital/couple dysfunction, and increased physical illness.[7] These risk factors are grouped into the following general categories:

1. Family factors
   a. Poor marital adjustment or satisfaction
   b. Lack of social support
   c. Traditional, rigid sex-role expectations
   d. Recent stressful life events
2. Domestic violence
   a. Mother or her partner experienced or witnessed violence in childhood
   b. Current or past abuse of the woman by her partner
   c. Partner suspected of child abuse in the past or of harsh discipline of children
3. Maternal factors
   a. Poor relationship with parents
   b. Low self-esteem
   c. Past or present psychiatric disorder
   d. Unwanted pregnancy
   e. Antepartum depression
   f. Prenatal care not started until the third trimester

g. Refusal to take prenatal classes or dropping out of classes before completion

4. Substance abuse

a. Substance abuse by the mother or her partner

C. Intimate Partner Violence

Rates of intimate partner violence are greater during pregnancy and after delivery than at other times in women's lives. The prevalence rate of violence during pregnancy ranges from 0.9% to 20.1%, with variation depending on measures of violence and populations studied.[8] Between 4% and 8% of pregnant women are abused at least once during their pregnancy.[9] Despite this prevalence, a history of abuse is frequently not uncovered, either because providers may be uncomfortable in asking questions about violence or because some women are reluctant to discuss the abuse they suffer.

Greater rates of LBW, preterm delivery, operative delivery, maternal mortality, and infant mortality are associated with intimate partner violence.[10,11] Risk factors for intimate partner violence include having an unwanted pregnancy; increased parity; being younger, unmarried, and/or poor; substance abuse in the patient, partner, or other family members; minority race; and history of abuse in the patient's family of origin. Abused pregnant women often postpone prenatal care or have a complete lack of prenatal care.

Often, an increase in the number of incidents of abuse occurs in the postpartum period.[12,13] Child abuse and postpartum abuse of the mother by her partner have been strongly correlated with lack of social support, recent life stressors, psychiatric disturbance in the mother, and unwanted pregnancy.[14]

II. IDENTIFICATION

Identifying women who are vulnerable to adverse outcomes may contribute to better understanding of their experiences and would prompt intervention by health-care providers to prevent adverse outcomes. However, the majority of maternity care providers do not routinely integrate a comprehensive psychosocial assessment into prenatal care. Lack of time, training, evidence-based screening tools, and resources to manage identified problems are often cited as barriers to psychosocial assessment.

A variety of structured forms or guides has been developed to aid in collection of antenatal psychosocial data. Examples of these include:

A. The Prenatal Psychosocial Profile measures and scores women's stress, social support, and self-esteem.[15,16]

B. The Prenatal Social Environment Inventory determines the stress in women's lives.[17]

C. The Antenatal Psychosocial Health Assessment (ALPHA) is a practical and evidence-based tool that incorporates 15 risk factors identified in a systematic literature review as associated with 4 categories of poor postpartum outcomes: woman abuse, child abuse, postpartum depression, and couple dysfunction.[18,19]

D. Among women who answer "yes" to Questions 2, 3, or 4 of the Abuse Assessment Screen (Table 5-1) during prenatal visits, 1 in 6 (17%) reported abuse during pregnancy.[20] The findings from inquiring with these three clinical questions yielded similar results to those obtained with previously validated research instruments for identifying abuse, thus providing a simple clinical assessment screen for practice-based application.[20,21] However, with respect to intimate partner violence, insufficient evidence exists to recommend for or against routine screening.[22]

III. INTERVENTIONS

A. Psychosocial Support

It has been postulated that providing psychosocial services beyond basic prenatal care may ameliorate some of these adverse outcomes. Specific interventions aimed at providing social support, facilitating access to care, health education, and encouragement to verbalize feelings about problems have been shown to be significantly associated with the number of problems that pregnant African American women have been able to resolve during prenatal care.[1]

However, the benefit of interventions for psychosocial problems remains controversial. A Cochrane review of 18 trials, involving 12,658 women, compared social support during pregnancy with routine care for women at increased risk for delivering LBW newborns.[23] Psychosocial support could include some form of emotional support, such as counseling, reassurance, or sympathetic listening, and information or advice, or both, provided either in home visits or during clinic appointments. It also included tangible assistance, such as transportation to clinic appointments and assistance with the care of other children at home. Psychosocial support during at-risk pregnancy by

TABLE 5-1 Abuse Assessment Screen (AAS) for Use in Pregnancy

1. Have you ever been emotionally or physically abused by your partner or someone important to you?	Yes	No
2. Within the last year, have you been hit, slapped, kicked, or otherwise physically hurt by someone?	Yes	No

If Yes, by whom? (circle all that apply)

Husband   Ex-husband   Boyfriend   Stranger   Other   Multiple   —No. of times

3. Since you've been pregnant, have you been hit, slapped, kicked, or otherwise physically hurt by someone?	Yes	No

If Yes, by whom? (circle all that apply)

Husband   Ex-husband   Boyfriend   Stranger   Other   Multiple   —No. of times

Mark the area of injury on the body map (map included)

Score the most severe incident to the following scale:

    1 = Threats of abuse including use of weapon

    2 = Slapping, pushing; no. injuries and/or no. lasting pain

    3 = Punching, kicking, bruises, cuts, and/or continuing pain

    4 = Beaten up, severe contusions, burns, broken bones

    5 = Head, internal, and/or permanent injury

    6 = Use or weapon, wound from weapon

4. Within the past year, has anyone forced you to have sexual activities?	Yes	No

If yes, by whom? (circle all that apply)

Husband   Ex-husband   Boyfriend   Stranger   Other   Multiple   —No. of times

5. Are you afraid of your partner or anyone you listed above?	Yes	No

Responses are recorded on a data collection form, no other scoring information was provided.

From McFarlane J, Parker B, Soeken K, Bullock L: Assessing for abuse during pregnancy, *JAMA* 267:3176-3178, 1992.

either a professional (social worker, midwife, or nurse) or trained lay person, offered in the home, clinic, or over the phone, has not been shown to improve rates of LBW or other perinatal outcomes, although some improvements in immediate maternal psychosocial outcomes were found in individual trials.

Psychosocial interventions also do not appear to reduce the numbers of women who experience development of postpartum depression when compared with standard care (relative risk [RR], 0.81; 95% confidence interval [CI], 0.65-1.02).[24,25] One promising intervention appears to be the provision of intensive postpartum support provided by public health nurses or midwives (RR, 0.68; 95% CI, 0.55-0.84). Interventions with only a postpartum component appear to be more beneficial than interventions that also incorporate a prenatal component.

The U.S. Preventive Services Task Force reviewed evidence for the efficacy of interventions in reducing the harmful outcomes of intimate partner violence.[26] They found that nurse home visit programs during the prenatal and 2-year postpartum period improves short- and long-term outcomes of child abuse and neglect for low-income, first-time mothers. Two studies evaluating interventions to decrease intimate partner violence during pregnancy showed a trend toward women reporting decreased violence after brief counseling or outreach interventions.[27,28]

Counseling for women who are victims of intimate partner violence should be directed at providing the following:

1. Reassurance that they are not at fault and are not alone

2. Knowledge regarding the recurrent and progressive nature of abuse, including information about how repetitive patterns of abuse may affect families and children

3. Encouragement to find a safe living situation immediately, either with friends, relatives, or a local women's shelter

4. Encouragement to undergo counseling or join support groups of women in similar situations

B. Federal Funding for Prenatal Care

1. Medicaid

Federal funding for indigent women encourages states to support systems of comprehensive prenatal care. These programs provide reimbursement for physician services and have expanded eligibility for maternity services up to 185% of poverty level to provide coverage for the working poor and married women of low socioeconomic status. In many cases, this expanded eligibility has removed financial barriers to care, although in some settings, limited access still exists because of a limited number of providers who accept Medicaid.

Federal Medicaid law provides coverage for otherwise eligible undocumented immigrants for emergency services. The Personal Responsibility and Work Opportunity Reconciliation Act of 1996 fundamentally altered the legal structure for providing Medicaid and other public benefits to immigrants, by creating additional barriers to undocumented immigrants' eligibility for state and local benefits. No exceptions to these restrictions were made for pregnant women. As a result, many immigrants are ineligible for Medicaid coverage of prenatal care, although labor and delivery services remain Medicaid-reimbursable as an emergency medical service.

Medicaid programs for maternity care vary in their comprehensiveness. More expansive programs have been shown to increase the receipt of adequate prenatal care and to decrease the percentage of uninsured pregnant women, but the evidence is mixed, particularly for minority groups.[29-31] These expansions are at risk for reductions due to budgetary pressures experienced in the first half of the twenty-first century.[32] The bulk of the poor outcomes continue to occur in Medicaid-eligible women. Historical evaluations have suggested that Medicaid has produced some incremental improvement in outcome in those populations.[33,34]

In an effort to control costs, many states have implemented Medicaid Managed Care (MMC). Between 1991 and 2004, the number of MMC enrollees increased from less than 5% to more than 60% of all Medicaid recipients.[35] MMC has been associated with reduced preventable pregnancy complications in some states,[36,37] but its impact on other outcomes has been mixed.[38] The experience to date, however, does not indicate any negative impact of MMC on pregnancy outcomes.

2. Women, Infants and Children/Food stamps

Women, Infants and Children (WIC) is a supplemental feeding program that provides nutritional supplementation for women with low incomes and their children. It should be offered to all eligible pregnant women where available. The effectiveness of the program in improving pregnancy outcomes has been questioned, but some statewide programs have demonstrated improvement.[39-41] The financial incentive of the program has historically favored bottle-feeding over breastfeeding. However, new mothers can now receive supplemental WIC vouchers to ensure the adequacy of their own nutrition throughout breastfeeding, and the WIC program now actively promotes breast milk as the ideal nutrition for infants.

IV. SOR A RECOMMENDATIONS

RECOMMENDATIONS	REFERENCES
Psychosocial interventions do not reduce the numbers of women who experience development of postpartum depression. However, a promising intervention is the provision of intensive, professionally based postpartum support.	24
Programs that offer additional social support for at-risk pregnant women are not associated with improvements in perinatal outcomes. Some improvements in immediate maternal psychosocial outcomes have been found in individual trials.	23

REFERENCES

1. Gonzalez-Calvo J, Jackson J, Hansford C et al: Psychosocial factors and birth outcome: African American women in case management, *J Health Care Poor Underserved* 9(4):395-419, 1998.

2. Halbreich U: The association between pregnancy processes, preterm delivery, low birth weight, and postpartum depressions—the need for interdisciplinary integration, *Am J Obstet Gynecol* 193(4):1312-1322, 2005.

3. Hobel C, Culhane J: Role of psychosocial and nutritional stress on poor pregnancy outcome, *J Nutr* 133:1709S-1717S, 2003.

4. Colley Gilbert BJ, Johnson CH, Morrow B et al: Prevalence of selected maternal and infant characteristics, Pregnancy Risk Assessment Monitoring System (PRAMS), 1997, *MMWR CDC Surveill Summ* 48(5):1-37, 1999.

5. Clarke L, Bono C, Miller M et al: Prenatal care use in nonmetropolitan and metropolitan America: racial/ethnic differences, *J Health Care Poor Underserved* 6:410-433, 1995.

6. Tai-Seale M, LoSasso AT, Freund DA et al: Long-term effects of Medicaid managed care on obstetric care in three California Counties, *Health Serv Res* 36(4):751-771, 2001.

7. Wilson LM, Reid AJ, Midmer DK et al: Antenatal psychosocial risk factors associated with adverse postpartum family outcomes, *CMAJ* 155(6):785-799, 1996.

8. Gazamararian JA, Lazorick S, Spitz AM et al: Prevalence of violence against pregnant women, *JAMA* 275(24):1915-1920, 1996.

9. Gazmararian JA, Petersen R, Spitz AM et al: Violence and reproductive health: current knowledge and future research directions, *Matern Child Health J* 4(2):79-84, 2000.

10. Boy A, Salihu HM: Intimate partner violence and birth outcomes: a systematic review, *Int J Fertil Womens Med* 49(4):159-164, 2004.

11. Murphy CC, Schei B, Myhr TL et al: Abuse: a risk factor for low birth weight? A systematic review and meta-analysis, *CMAJ* 164(11):1578-1579, 2001.

12. Stewart DE: Incidence of postpartum abuse in women with a history of abuse during pregnancy, *CMAJ* 151(11):1601-1604, 1994.

13. Bowen E, Heron J, Waylen A et al: ALSPAC Study Team. Domestic violence risk during and after pregnancy: findings from a British longitudinal study, *BJOG* 112(8):1083-1089, 2005.

14. Campbell J, Poland M, Waller J et al: Correlates of battering during pregnancy, *Res Nurs Health* 15:219-226, 1992.

15. Curry MA, Burton D, Fields J: The Prenatal Psychosocial Profile: a research and clinical tool, *Res Nurs Health* 21(3):211-219, 1998.

16. Curry MA, Campbell RA, Christian M: Validity and reliability testing of the Prenatal Psychosocial Profile, *Res Nurs Health* 17(2):127-135, 1994.

17. Orr ST, James SA, Casper R: Psychosocial stressors and low birth weight: development of a questionnaire, *J Dev Behav Pediatr* 13(5):343-347, 1992.

18. Reid AJ, Biringer A, Carroll JD et al: Using the ALPHA form in practice to assess antenatal psychosocial health, *CMAJ* 159(6):677-684, 1998.

19. Carroll JC, Reid AJ, Biringer A et al: Effectiveness of the Antenatal Psychosocial Health Assessment (ALPHA) form in detecting psychosocial concerns: a randomized controlled trial, *CMAJ* 173(3):253-259, 2005.

20. McFarlane J, Parker B, Soeken K et al: Assessing for abuse during pregnancy. Severity and frequency of injuries and associated entry into prenatal care, *JAMA* 267(23):3176-3178, 1992.

21. McFarlane J, Parker B: *Abuse during pregnancy: a protocol for prevention and intervention*, White Plains, NY, 1994, The March of Dimes Birth Defects Foundation.

22. Wathen CN, MacMillan HL: Prevention of violence against women: recommendation statement from the Canadian Task Force on Preventive Health Care, *CMAJ* 169(16):582-584, 2003. Available at: http://www.guideline.gov/summary/summary.aspx?ss=15&doc_id=3657&nbr=2883. Accessed August 26, 2007.

23. Hodnett ED, Fredericks S: Support during pregnancy for women at increased risk of low birthweight babies, *Cochrane Database Syst Rev* (3):CD000198, 2003.

24. Dennis CL, Creedy D: Psychosocial and psychological interventions for preventing postpartum depression, *Cochrane Database Syst Rev* (4):CD001134, 2004.

25. Dennis CL: Psychosocial and psychological interventions for prevention of postnatal depression: a systematic review, *BMJ* 331(7507):15, 2005.

26. Screening for family and intimate partner violence: recommendation statement, *Ann Intern Med* 140(5):382-386, 2004. Available at: http://www.guideline.gov/summary/summary.aspx?view_id=1&doc_id=4427. Accessed August 26, 2007.

27. McFarlane J, Soeken K, Wiist W: An evaluation of interventions to decrease intimate partner violence to pregnant women, *Public Health Nurs* 17(6):443-451, 2000.

28. Parker B, McFarlane J, Soeken K et al: Testing an intervention to prevent further abuse to pregnant women, *Res Nurs Health* 22(1):59-66, 1999.

29. Dubay L, Joyce T, Kaestner R et al: Changes in prenatal care timing and low birth weight by race and socioeconomic status: implications for the Medicaid expansions for pregnant women, *Health Serv Res* 36:373-398, 2001.

30. Hessol NA, Vittinghoff E, Fuentes-Afflick E: Reduced risk of inadequate prenatal care in the era after Medicaid expansions in California, *Med Care* 42(5):416-422, 2004.

31. Howell E: The impact of the Medicaid explanations for pregnant women: a synthesis of the evidence, *Med Care Res Rev* 58:3-30, 2001.

32. Ross DC, Cox L: *In a time of growing need: state choices influence health coverage access for children and families*. Available at: http://www.kff.org/medicaid/7393.cfm. Accessed August 24, 2007.

33. Buescher PA, Smith C, Holliday JL et al: Source of prenatal care and infant birth weight: the case of a North Carolina county, *Am J Obstet Gynecol* 156:204-210, 1987.

34. Buescher PA, Ward NI: A comparison of low birth weight among Medicaid patients of public health departments and other providers of prenatal care in North Carolina and Kentucky, *Pub Health Rep* 107:54-59, 1992.

35. Centers for Medicare and Medicaid Services: *Medicaid: a brief summary, Centers for Medicare and Medicaid Services.* Available at: http://www.cms.hhs.gov/MedicaidManagCare. Accessed August 24, 2007.

36. Laditka SB, Laditka JN, Bennett KJ et al: Delivery complications associated with prenatal care access for Medicaid-insured mothers in rural and urban hospitals, *J Rural Health* 21(2):158-166, 2005.

37. Kenney G, Sommers AS, Dubay L: Moving to mandatory Medicaid managed care in Ohio: impacts on pregnant women and infants, *Med Care* 43(7):683-690, 2005.

38. Williams LM, Morrow B, Beck LF et al: *PRAMS 2000 surveillance report*, Atlanta, GA, 2005, Division of Reproductive Health, National Center for Chronic Disease Prevention and Health Promotion, Centers for Disease Control and Prevention.

39. Bitler MP, Currie J: Does WIC work? The effects of WIC on pregnancy and birth outcomes, *J Policy Anal Manage* 24(1):73-91, 2005.

40. Kotelchuck M, Schwartz JB, Anderka MT et al: WIC participation and pregnancy outcomes: Massachusetts statewide evaluation project, *Am J Public Health* 74:1086-1092, 1984.

41. Joyce T, Gibson D, Colman S: The changing association between prenatal participation in WIC and birth outcomes in New York City, *J Policy Anal Manage* 24(4):661-685, 2005.

SECTION B **Adolescent Pregnancy Interventions**

V. Leigh Beasley, MD, FAAFP

The pregnant adolescent often presents to her primary care provider with both psychosocial needs and biomedical risks. Although these needs are often formidable for the individual maternity care provider, family physicians are well suited to care for pregnant adolescents and assist them in preparation for parenthood. Coordinating adolescent prenatal care with social workers, drug and alcohol counselors, nutritionists, family counselors, child-birth educators, breastfeeding counselors, clergy, and the school system will assist the individual provider in caring for these challenging problems and optimize the outcome for both mother and child.

I. HISTORICAL PERSPECTIVE/ INCIDENCE

Historically, adolescent fertility rates have tended to follow trends in pregnancy rates for all women of childbearing age, except for young women 10 to 14 years old, a group for whom the fertility rate has been steadily increasing. Birth rates to all adolescents increased sharply in the late 1980s, but subsequently declined for U.S. teenagers from 1991 to 2005, decreasing to a low of 40.4 births/1000 female individuals aged 15 to 19 years. The U.S. rate of births to 15- to 19-year-old women in 2006 was a record low of 41.0 births/1000 female individuals in this age range—a 35% decrease from the 1991 high of 61.8 births/1000 female individuals aged 15 to 19 years.[1] Younger teen birth rates have seen a decrease of 50% from 1991 to 2005. The current rate is 0.7 birth/1000 female individuals aged 10 to 14 years.[1] Despite these decreases, pregnancy and birth rates for adolescents in the United States remain among the highest in industrialized countries.

A. Increasing Importance of Adolescent Pregnancy

Several factors explain why adolescent pregnancy is perceived to be an increasing problem.
1. Total birth rates
   Since the late 1980s, total birth rates have decreased much more than adolescent birth rates. Therefore, births to adolescents make up a larger proportion of all births.

TABLE 5-2 Birth Rates (per 1000) for Unmarried and Married Women Aged 15-19, 1940 to 1988

Year	Unmarried	Married
1940	7.4	—
1950	12.6	410
1960	15.1	530
1970	22.4	443
1980	27.5	350
1988	36.8	378

From U.S. Department Health Education and Welfare, Public Health Service, National Office of Vital Statistics: *Vital statistics of the U.S. 1990*, Vol 1, Washington, DC, 1994, Government Printing Office.

2. Teen marriage rates
   An increasing proportion of adolescent pregnancies has been occurring in unmarried girls, resulting in an increasing birth rate for single teens (Table 5-2). This coupled with a declining marriage rate (both preconception and postconception) for this age group makes teen pregnancy part of the larger social problem of single parenthood.[2]
3. Adoption
   Adoption rates have decreased since the late 1980s.
4. Teen employment rates
   Employment opportunities for adolescents are generally limited by the fact that more pregnant teenagers do not complete high school.
5. Economic costs
   Adolescent pregnancy costs the U.S. taxpayer approximately $6.9 billion each year in welfare benefits and food stamps. The medical costs for teenage mothers and their infants is $2.2 and $1.5 billion, respectively.[3]

B. Contributing Factors to Adolescent Pregnancy

Many single adolescents who are at risk for pregnancy may be identified in advance through a careful history (Table 5-3).

C. Pregnancy Interventions

Most adolescent sexual activity is not planned or anticipated. It is more the result of age-appropriate lack of anticipation of future consequences. Disappointingly, studies that review the effectiveness of

TABLE 5-3 Factors Associated with Adolescent Pregnancy

Personal Characteristics	Family Characteristics
Smoking	Divorced or single parent
Drinking alcohol	Alcoholic or substance-abusing parent
Using drugs	Other family dysfunction
Victim of physical or sexual abuse	Domestic violence
Few religious ties	History of sexual abuse
Regularly unsupervised after school	
Poor or no relationship with father	

primary prevention strategies to delay initiation of sexual intercourse, improve use of birth control, or reduce the number of teen pregnancies have shown most strategies to be ineffective.[4] In some cases, the pregnancy is actually planned, hoped for, or desired. In these situations, the single adolescent may have unrealistic expectations of what a baby will do for her (e.g., love her, get her out of a bad home situation, cause her boyfriend to marry her, make her feel good about herself). These young mothers-to-be often are not knowledgeable about the demands of parenthood or realistic about their ability to meet them.

The pregnant adolescent may also be cognitively ill-prepared to consider long-term consequences for herself and her child, a skill that is helpful in dealing with the challenges of pregnancy and parenthood. One intervention, known as previewing, helps pregnant teenagers to think about future events with their child and gives them an opportunity to "practice" their responses to certain situations. Use of this technique may assist the teenage parent and health-care provider in together identifying potential problems involving pregnancy and parenting, so that positive solutions can be developed.[5]

II. DEVELOPMENTAL CONCERNS

The pregnant adolescent must face the challenges of her own age-specific developmental tasks (e.g., individuation, autonomy, and vocational choices), while at the same time taking on the demands of parenting and guiding her child's development. As the age of menarche has become younger, there is a larger "gap" between the physical development of most teenagers and their cognitive and emotional development. Inquiring about the reason(s) a teenage patient gives for becoming pregnant may help identify some of her own developmental needs that have not been met. By identifying these needs, health-care professionals can design interventions that address patient-specific developmental needs.[6]

III. INCREASED RISKS FOR ADOLESCENT PREGNANCY

A. Adolescent

The incidence of sexually transmitted diseases (particularly among single adolescents), late onset of prenatal care, preterm labor, cephalopelvic disproportion, pregnancy-induced hypertension (especially in girls younger than 16, although this may be related to race and primigravid state rather than age), and eclampsia is increased in pregnant adolescents.

Pregnancy often results in curtailed educational achievement and poverty for many single teenage mothers. It also typically results in single parenthood for at least part of their childrearing years.

B. Infant/Child

Pregnant adolescents have greater rates of prematurity and deliver more LBW infants than older women. Many of their children grow up in poverty. Multiple factors converge to cause greater rates of poor school performance, child abuse and neglect, poor work history, single parenthood, and for boys in particular, criminal behavior among offspring of adolescent mothers.

IV. MANAGEMENT PRINCIPLES

A. Family Considerations

Adolescent pregnancy may represent a family crisis or may be considered a cultural norm, with variation in responses among different families. As such, it presents an opportunity for the physician to identify latent family problems that may have increased the likelihood of the pregnancy occurring. In doing so, attitudes of blame should be avoided because they hinder the necessary acceptance of responsibility and ability to change dysfunctional patterns.

B. Concurrent Psychosocial Risks

The presence of other psychosocial risk factors such as substance abuse and domestic violence should be assessed, with interventions as indicated. One in five pregnant adolescents reports physical or sexual abuse. Abused teenagers tend to enter prenatal care later, often in the third trimester. Abuse during pregnancy has been shown to be a significant risk factor for LBW, low maternal weight gain, first- or second-trimester bleeding, smoking, and the use of drugs and alcohol.[7]

Health-care providers need to be aware of the risk for increased interpersonal violence in the pregnant teenager's life and actively screen patients for this. Short abuse assessment screens are available (see Table 5-1). When issues of abuse are identified, the health-care provider must be familiar with referral sources, such as individual and family counselors and "safe houses."

C. Extended Family

Involvement of the extended family, especially grandparents, may be an essential contributor to the well-being of both the adolescent parent and child. Data suggest improved cognitive and health outcomes for infants of adolescent mothers if living with a grandmother.[8]

D. Social Isolation

Teenagers who are living alone or with friends typically have poor social support. Pregnant teenagers often face difficulty in locating appropriate housing and reliable transportation. Maternity care providers and other members of the health-care team should conduct ongoing assessments of patient support systems, and provide referral and individualized help as indicated. The Friends and Family Apgar (Table 5-4) is one validated tool that has been applied to a variety of ethnic groups and measures a woman's perception of support from her family and friends.[9,10]

E. Role of Education

All pregnant adolescents should be asked about their educational and vocational plans and should be encouraged to complete at least secondary education to enhance their employability in the future. Most pregnant teenagers recognize the importance of education and remaining in school. One study found school dropout rates to be more strongly related to sociocultural factors than individual characteristics (such as emotional support or psychological well-being). High school dropouts in this study tended to be white and had lower family incomes.[11] Many teenage parents are eligible to participate in night school or adult educational programs to earn their GED (general equivalency diploma) or high-school diploma.

Childbirth education, nutritional assessment, and counseling (particularly looking for evidence of eating disorders), parenting classes, and encouragement and education for breastfeeding are also important for both the pregnant adolescent and her partner.

F. Continuity of Care

Adolescents, in particular, benefit from continuity of prenatal care providers. Teenagers may not get early and continuous prenatal care for many reasons: fear of informing family members about the pregnancy, denial of the pregnancy itself, lack of knowledge about the availability and importance of prenatal care, economic concerns, or transportation problems. Pregnant teenagers typically experience a range of emotions during the course of prenatal care, including fear, denial, anger, and excitement.

Prenatal care of the teen must address medical, social, and emotional concerns. Scheduling appointments every 2 to 3 weeks instead of the traditional monthly visits may be beneficial in addressing all the various needs of the pregnant teenager and her family. Pregnant adolescents may also benefit from seeing one or two trusted providers who can better coordinate the variety of services the teenager may need. A team approach among the family physician and a social worker, registered nurse, or other allied health-care provider can be helpful in addressing *all* aspects of caring for the pregnant teenager. Programs such as Teen-Tot are comprehensive clinical programs involving teenage mothers and their children. Review of such programs report modest success in outcomes such as preventing repeat pregnancy, having the teenage mother complete her education, and improving the baby's health over 6 to 18 months.[12]

Teenage mothers should be followed closely in the immediate postpartum period. The traditional 6-week postpartum visit may be too late to address issues such as resumed sexual activity, the need for birth control, breastfeeding problems, postpartum stress or depression, and infant care. Ideally, teenagers should be seen within 2 weeks of delivery to address these concerns. Studies have shown improved

TABLE 5-4 Friends and Family Apgar Scoring System

Please fill out the following section to help us understand your family/friend support. "Family" means the person with whom you usually live. If you live alone, your "family" means the person whom you feel closest to emotionally. For each question, check only one box:

	Never	Hardly	Ever	Some of Time	Almost Always	Always
I am satisfied that I can turn to my family for help when something is troubling me.						
I am satisfied with the way that my family talks over things with me and shares problems with me.						
I am satisfied that my family accepts and supports my wishes to take on new activities and directions.						
I am satisfied with the way my family expresses affection and responds to my feelings, such as anger, sadness, and love.						
I am satisfied with the way my family and I share time together.						
I have a close friend to whom I can turn for help.						
I am satisfied with the support I receive from family and friends.						

From Smilkstein G, Ashworth C: Validity and reliability of the family APGAR as a test of family function, *J Fam Pract* 15:303-311, 1982; and Smilkstein G: The family APGAR: a proposal for a family function test and its use by physicians, *J Fam Pract* 6:1231-1239, 1978.

maternal and infant outcomes by using home health nursing visits during the immediate postpartum period.[13,14] An intensive early intervention program in which teenagers received 4 prenatal classes and approximately 17 home visits during the prenatal and postpartum period demonstrated a reduction in premature births to teenagers and a reduction in infant hospitalization during the first 6 weeks after birth.[14]

G. Decision Making

Adolescents have often made decisions regarding the fate of their pregnancy before seeking medical care. Nonetheless, many benefit from the opportunity to discuss their feelings about adoption, childrearing, or abortion. A sensitive and nonjudgmental approach is most appropriate when discussing short- and long-term consequences for the mother and her child. Providing a pregnant teenager with accurate information regarding all available medical options will help guide her decisions. To establish a trusting, therapeutic relationship, the physician should explain the confidential nature of any of their interactions.

Close follow-up is necessary regardless of the teenager's final decision regarding the pregnancy because she may face coercion, blame, or anger from her family or her partner. Counseling issues often cannot be adequately addressed in the constraints of prenatal office scheduling; referring the patient for more intensive supportive or crisis counseling in these situations is appropriate.

H. Parenting Skills

Family physicians should coordinate ongoing efforts (classes, one-on-one counseling) of the health-care team to help prepare the adolescent and her partner for the responsibilities of parenthood. These efforts should extend throughout the first several years after childbirth.

I. Breastfeeding

Breastfeeding should be encouraged for adolescents even though they are historically less inclined to breastfeed. Evidence exists of improved bonding between mother and child for breastfed infants. Breastfeeding also helps to teach and reinforce good nutritional concepts for the adolescent mother, causing her to focus on her own nutrition and that of her infant. Adolescent mothers who breastfeed may derive some personal developmental benefit from having successfully accomplished this task. This enhanced self-esteem and sense of competency may subsequently provide long-term benefits for the entire family unit.

Issues surrounding breastfeeding and returning to work or school are important to address. A teenage mother may need to schedule classes so she can have breaks to "pump" or feed her baby. Ensuring a comfortable and private place for nursing or pumping may be difficult for the teen; family physicians should advocate for young mothers with the local school system to support greater breastfeeding rates. Educating school administrators about the superiority of breastfeeding as a feeding choice will often help break down barriers that young mothers may face.

J. Role of the Father

It is essential to ascertain the current and intended level of involvement and commitment demonstrated by the father of the child. Although long-term benefits of involving the father in prenatal care and education have not been demonstrated, doing so is often beneficial in individual cases. Many young fathers are intimidated by the clinic or office setting and may not feel welcome. Fathers who desire involvement in prenatal visits should be strongly encouraged to do so. The opportunity to "hear the baby's heartbeat" using the Doppler and "see the baby" during an ultrasound examination may help the father to bond more closely with the unborn child. Pregnant adolescents should be asked if they are comfortable with the involvement of the baby's father in the examination room. During each visit, the adolescent should have time alone with a health-care provider when she can voice any concerns or problems relating to an abusive situation.

K. Labor Support

Labor support is important for the adolescent patient. Experienced supportive family members or friends, doulas, trained labor and delivery nurses, and the physician in attendance during the labor may all function in this role. Attendance at childbirth preparation classes will facilitate the teen mother's effective use of labor support persons.

L. Postpartum

During the postpartum period, caring for teen parents should include the following strategies:

1. Home visits
   Regular home visits by health professionals over a 2-year period have demonstrated improved child health and development outcomes.[13,14]
2. Follow-up
   Initiate follow-up 2 to 3 days after hospital discharge instead of the traditional 2-week infant visit or 6-week postpartum visit. Adolescents are at increased risk to discontinue breastfeeding prematurely and need increased levels of nursing and medical support to sustain this activity; also, screening for postpartum emotional disorders and possible child abuse should occur. This may take the form of home health-care nursing follow-up or a short office visit to check for jaundice, breastfeeding problems, and other complications.
3. Teens who select adoption
   For teen mothers who have selected adoption, there is increasing recognition of the grief process that accompanies this process. Many adoption agencies provide postadoption counseling to help deal with the grief response. Physicians should play an important role in facilitating this process.
4. Family planning
   The risks and benefits of abstinence and other methods of birth control must be fully explored with each patient, and every effort should be made to promote follow-up and compliance with the plan. From 1991 to 1997 there has been a 21% decrease in the rate of second births to teens. Discussion of future contraceptive use should be initiated during the prenatal visits so that the patient can be familiar with her options after delivery. Inquiring about past difficulty in remembering to take

prenatal vitamins may predict success or failure in using birth control pills and lead the patient and physician to consider other contraceptive methods. Newer methods of contraceptive delivery such is injections, dermal and vaginal delivery, may be explored with the patient as alternatives to a daily pill. Long-term contraceptive methods (intrauterine device [IUD], implantable contraception) may be appropriate for the adolescent mother.

5. Rapid repeat pregnancy

Rapid repeat pregnancy, defined as a pregnancy occurring within 12 to 24 months of the previous pregnancy, has been associated with physical or sexual abuse and greater rates of LBW infants among low-income adolescents.[15] Good evidence exists for an association between shortened interpregnancy intervals of less than 6 months and subsequent deliveries resulting in LBW newborns and preterm births.[16] Information gained from such studies emphasizes the need for close follow-up and continued care of the pregnant adolescent after delivery.

REFERENCES

1. Hamilton BE, Martin JA, Ventura SJ: *Births: preliminary data for 2005, Health E-Stats,* Hyattsville, MD, November 21, 2006, National Center for Health Statistics.
2. Fredrick I: Teenage pregnancy. Paper presented at the Scientific Assembly, New York State Academy of Family Physicians, Sarasota Springs, NY, May 1989.
3. Maynard R: *Kids having kids: economic costs and social consequences of teen pregnancy,* Washington, DC, 1996, Urban Institute Press.
4. DiCenso A, Guyatt G, Willan A et al: Interventions to reduce unintended pregnancies among adolescents: systemic review of randomized controlled trials, *BMJ* 324:1426, 2002.
5. Stevenson W, Maton KI, Teti DM: School importance and drop-out among pregnant adolescents, *J Adolesc Health* 22:376-382, 1998.
6. Poole C: Adolescent pregnancy and unfinished developmental tasks of childhood, *J Sch Health* 57:271-273, 1987.
7. Parker B, McFarlane J, Soeken K: Abuse during pregnancy: effects on maternal complications and birth weight in adult and teenage women, *Obstet Gynecol* 84(3):323-328, 1994.
8. Pope SK, Whiteside MS, Brooks-Gunn J et al: Low-birth-weight infants born to adolescent mothers: effects of coresidency with grandmother on child development, *JAMA* 269:1369-1400, 1993.
9. Smilkstein G, Ashworth C: Validity and reliability of the Family APGAR as a test of family function, *J Fam Pract* 15:303-311, 1982.
10. Smilkstein G: The family APGAR: a proposal for a family function test and its use by physicians, *J Fam Pract* 6:1231-1239, 1978.
11. O'Sullivan AL, Jacobson BS: A randomized trial of a health care program for first-time adolescent mothers and their infants, *Nurs Res* 41:210-215, 1992.
12. Akinbami L, Cheng T, Kornfeld D: A review of Teen-Tot programs: comprehensive clinical care for young parents and their children, *Adolescence* 36:381-393, 2001.
13. Kahn JR, Anderson KE: Intergenerational patterns of teenage fertility, *Demography* 29:39-57, 1992.
14. Koniak-Griffin D, Mathenge C, Anderson NL et al: An early intervention program for adolescent mothers: a nursing demonstration project, *J Obstet Gynecol Neonatal Nurs* 28:51-59, 1999.
15. Jacoby M, Gorenflo D, Black E et al: Rapid repeat pregnancy and experiences of interpersonal violence among low-income adolescents, *Am J Prev Med* 16:318-321, 1999.
16. Barr, Wendy, MD, MPH, MSCE: Shortened inter-pregnancy intervals, evidence-based review for the IMPLICIT FamMed Network, 2005, Unpublished manuscript.

SECTION C Substance Abuse in Pregnancy

V. Leigh Beasley, MD, FAAFP

Four major areas of substance abuse—cocaine, opiates, alcohol, and amphetamines (or methamphetamines)—are particularly problematic when encountered in pregnant women. Short- and long-term effects on both maternal and infant health are significant. Clinicians in all practice settings commonly encounter these problems, particularly if they screen for them regularly. According to a 2003 survey conducted by the Substance Abuse and Mental Health Services Administration, 4.3% of pregnant women aged 15 to 44 years reported using illicit drugs in the month before the interview and 4.1% reported binge alcohol use. Among pregnant women aged 15 to 25 years, the rate of illicit drug use was 8%.[1] Marijuana was the most commonly used illicit drug used during pregnancy, accounting for 76% of the reported illicit drug use. Cocaine and heroin accounted for 8% of those admitting to illicit drug use during pregnancy.[2] In May 2004, the American College of Obstetricians and Gynecologists (ACOG) Committee on Ethics published a committee opinion paper emphasizing the "ethical obligation of physicians to learn and use a protocol for universal screening questions, brief intervention and referral to treatment" to provide optimum patient care.[3] Effective strategies for intervention and treatment exist and should be offered to any pregnant woman who has a diagnosis of substance abuse.

I. CRACK AND COCAINE ABUSE IN PREGNANCY

A. Pharmacology

Cocaine (common slang names: bump, toot, C, flake, snow, coke, and candy) is available in two forms: cocaine hydrochloride and the more purified cocaine alkaloid, known as crack. The former is water soluble and is administered orally, intravenously, or nasally; the latter is not soluble in water and is smoked.[4] Cocaine exerts profound effects on the central and peripheral nervous systems by stimulating the adrenergic receptors thorough buildup of neurotransmitters at nerve synapses. Chronic use of cocaine results in a depletion of dopamine, which, in turn, leads to marked dysphoria and accompanying cravings.

B. Prevalence in Groups at Increased Risk

The estimated prevalence rate of cocaine use in pregnancy is between 10% and 15% among women in at-risk groups.[5] Although certain subgroups have greater usage rates, cocaine use among pregnant women occurs within *every* income and ethnic group. Of women delivering at a private suburban hospital, 6% tested positive for cocaine use by neonatal meconium analysis.[6] Statewide drug-abuse screening in public health clinics in Alabama failed to demonstrate any difference in the incidence of positive drug screenings between high- and low-risk populations.[7] A population-based prevalence study in Georgia in 1994 found at least 0.5% of all infants born in Georgia had perinatal exposure to cocaine.[8] Women with greater prevalence rates of cocaine use include those living in urban settings, particularly those of lower socioeconomic status.

C. Adverse Obstetric Outcomes

Numerous adverse outcomes are associated with maternal cocaine use. Causation is more difficult to ascertain because of multiple confounding factors, such as coexisting greater rates of smoking and poor nutritional status in substance-abusing mothers.[9]

1. Low-birth-weight infants
   Of 14 studies reviewed, 11 demonstrated a significant association between cocaine use in pregnancy and LBW outcomes.[10] Many of these LBW infants experienced much greater rates of morbidity and mortality.
   a. Prematurity: Some of the LBW outcomes are attributable to increased rates of preterm labor and delivery, particularly among cocaine-using women who receive little prenatal care. Many of these women also have concurrent conditions (e.g., sexually transmitted diseases and urinary tract infections) that have been associated with prematurity and LBW, and must be identified and treated effectively.
   b. Intrauterine growth restriction (IUGR): Multiple studies reviewed showed an independent association between cocaine use and IUGR, regardless of gestational age.[10,11]

2. Placental abruption
   Increased rates of placental abruption are associated with cocaine use, particularly if the use is continued throughout the pregnancy.[10]

3. Spontaneous abortion
   In a study of 400 pregnant women presenting to an emergency department in Philadelphia with spontaneous abortion, 29% tested positive for cocaine compared with 21% among 570 women who had ongoing pregnancies followed through 22 weeks of gestation. Based on risk estimate, cocaine use accounted for 8% of spontaneous abortions in this population.[12]

4. Physical and sexual abuse
   Pregnant women diagnosed with substance abuse are more often victims of violence compared with mothers who do not use drugs.[13] Studies also suggest that one third to half of substance-abusing women have experienced some sort of sexual abuse as a child.[14]

5. Comorbid mental health disorders
   Epidemiologic studies reveal that a majority of women with substance abuse issues have coexisting mental disorders, with depression being the most common codiagnosis.[14]

D. Adverse Neonatal Outcomes

The increased rate of LBW is the most significant medical complication of cocaine use in pregnancy when cost, morbidity, and mortality are considered. Additional adverse neonatal effects include the following:

1. Neonatal withdrawal
   Neonatal withdrawal symptoms may occur among infants whose mothers used cocaine. The withdrawal syndrome is characterized by irritability, hypertonicity, hyperactivity, tachypnea, decreased sleep, and loose stools.[9]

2. Teratogenic effects
   Microcephaly and deficiencies of cerebral midline neuronal development, such as optic atrophy, have

been associated with maternal cocaine use.[4] Genitourinary and renal anomalies secondary to cocaine ingestion have also been suggested by one large case–control study.

3. Central nervous system effects
Destructive effects to the fetal central nervous system, such as cerebral infarcts, may occur in utero as a result of vasospasm and hypoxemia related to placental insufficiency.[4]

E. Adverse Postneonatal Outcomes

1. Increased incidence of sudden infant death syndrome (SIDS)
The risk for SIDS may be somewhat increased in infants of mothers with substance abuse problems, but the association is not enough to justify home apnea monitoring of all of these infants. Parental neglect may, at times, play an associated role.[15] The role of cigarette smoking is also often a confounder.

2. Long-term effect on neurobehavioral development
Although suspected, an effect of substance abuse on subsequent neurobehavioral development has been difficult to determine because few instruments can assess subtle neurobehavioral differences. In addition, many confounding variables that often coexist with substance abuse have a deleterious effect on development (e.g., nutritional and environmental factors).[5,16] More recent reviews have found among children 6 years and younger, no convincing data exist that in utero cocaine exposure leads to more detrimental effects from that thought to be from other prenatal exposure (such as tobacco, marijuana, alcohol, or the quality of the child's environment).[17]

F. Diagnostic Options

1. Self-reporting
Self-reporting is the most commonly used method of assessing substance abuse in pregnant women. Underreporting of the true incidence of this problem occurs, however, because of patient reluctance to divulge sensitive information and clinician reluctance to inquire about substance abuse.

2. Administering a structured questionnaire
By administering a questionnaire that asked for detailed information about past or current substance abuse, Christmas and associates[18] identified twice as many substance-abusing women

than would have been identified with intermittent drug screenings alone.

3. Prenatal drug screening
Prenatal drug screening is most frequently accomplished by urine drug testing. However, because testing occurs sporadically, up to 47% of exposed infants are not detected.[4]

4. Neonatal drug screening
Neonatal urine testing identifies maternal cocaine use that occurred within the week before delivery. Testing of infant meconium for cocaine metabolites can document maternal use of cocaine that occurred up to 20 weeks before delivery.[19] Neonatal hair analysis may also be conducted to assess remote maternal cocaine use.[20] Dried blood spots from the heel-stick of newborns (routinely used to test for inborn errors of metabolism) were used in one study to screen for cocaine metabolites.[8] Waiting to test the neonate, instead of screening the mother before delivery, misses the opportunity to refer the drug-using mother for counseling and structured substance abuse treatment programs. This results in several more months of drug exposure for the fetus and potentially worse birth outcomes.

G. Ethical and Medicolegal Concerns

Although a thorough discussion of these issues is beyond the scope of this textbook, some of the more controversial issues include:

1. Involuntary versus voluntary screening and targeted versus universal screening
Voluntary consent for urine drug testing is preferred. Most successful prenatal substance abuse programs use voluntary screening, with consequences of a positive drug test explained to the patient before screening. Experience in a rural public health clinic in South Carolina shows that most patients consent to voluntary drug testing when screening and follow-up of positive drug screens is presented in a nonthreatening manner.[21] Targeted testing, determined by the physician or hospital staff, leads to the dilemma of introducing bias in the decision-making process of "whom to test." One argument for universal testing is that it is one way to eliminate the appearance of "social bias" in the criteria for testing.[22]

2. Maternal versus fetal rights
Little disagreement exists that drug use is harmful for both mother and fetus. What is often more

difficult is to determine whether a specific court, or state, will see maternal or fetal rights as primary, and at what gestational age. This issue has been decided in one state in favor of the rights of a viable fetus over the mother, in the case of *Whitner vs. State of South Carolina*. In the maternal use of illegal substance(s) the South Carolina Supreme Court wrote: "[D]uring her pregnancy after the fetus attained viability, Whitner enjoyed the same freedom to use cocaine that she enjoyed earlier in and predating her pregnancy—none whatsoever." The record goes on to say that the "issue of maternal rights [over the fetus] to use illegal substances is indeed not an issue" (*Whitner v. State of South Carolina*, p 38).[22a]

3. Involvement of law enforcement
Threat of criminal or civil sanctions with mandatory reporting is often applied inequitably to different socioeconomic or ethnic groups.[23] Sixteen states currently consider alcohol or drug use during pregnancy to be grounds for an investigation into possible child abuse or neglect, or both. Most state statutes involve testing the newborn for drugs after delivery and do not focus on the issue of child abuse and/or neglect in utero if a woman is using drugs while pregnant.[22] The focus of most state programs is on treatment for the substance-abusing pregnant mother, a belief that is shared by health-care providers, social-service agencies, and law enforcement.
The threat of losing custody of her child has been noted as a strong motivator for a pregnant woman to receive treatment.[24] Failing to screen during pregnancy may lead to a missed "window of opportunity" for the patient at a time when her motivation to seek help is typically greater.

4. Preservation of patient confidentiality[9]
The clinician and hospital face a major challenge in attempting to respect patient confidentiality while needing to adhere to state laws and trying to attain the best possible neonatal outcome.

H. Treatment

Maternity care providers must acknowledge that substance abuse occurs in every practice setting. Early screening and accurate diagnosis are essential. It is recommended that clinicians consider using both a detailed questionnaire and intermittent toxicology screenings to identify the substance-abusing pregnant patient. The risk for a cocaine-abusing pregnant patient having a premature infant has

been estimated to be reduced twofold to threefold if the patient remains in a system of adequate prenatal care.[25]

The following are important components of successful prenatal substance abuse treatment programs:
1. Coordination of care
Family physicians and their staff often need to coordinate the care of these women with government agencies (such as child protective services), high-risk prenatal care providers, substance abuse counselors, agencies, and in-hospital treatment programs.
2. Systems for identifying pregnant substance abusers
These systems are important so that intervention is started as early as possible in the pregnancy.
3. Intensive case management
Intensive care management is often a critical component of prenatal care to link pregnant women with substance abuse problems with the services they need, such as child care, job training, transportation, and housing.[24]

II. ABUSE OF OPIATES DURING PREGNANCY

A. Pathophysiology

Opiates are derived from naturally occurring opium alkaloids and chemically related derivatives. Opiates work within the central nervous system and affect mood, sensorium, pain tolerance, alertness, and many other factors. Physiologic addiction and tolerance, the need for ever-increasing amounts of drug ingestion, occur commonly.[16]

B. Prevalence

An estimated 10,000 infants per year are born to women who use opiates during pregnancy. Every family physician in urban, suburban, or rural settings can be expected to encounter opiate-addicted women during pregnancy, although this problem is difficult to detect on a routine prenatal visit.

C. Associated Perinatal Effects

Several associations and complications have been reported in opiate-using mothers and their infants.[26]
1. Concurrent use of other substances
Opiate-using mothers have greater consumption levels of alcohol, cigarettes, and other street drugs.
2. Increased incidence of preterm deliveries and IUGR

3. Increased incidence of intrauterine hypoxia and fetal distress[27]

D. Long-Term Sequelae

Infants and children of opiate-addicted mothers are at increased risk for growth and developmental disorders. However, the degree to which these disorders can be ascribed to intrauterine exposure to opiates versus multiple associated environmental risks remains difficult to measure.[16]

E. Diagnostic Options

Screening options for opiates are virtually the same as those discussed in the previous section dealing with cocaine abuse (see Crack and Cocaine use during Pregnancy section).

F. Treatment

Similar to programs geared toward the cocaine-using pregnant woman, treatment for opiate users must be comprehensive in scope and must address many of the areas listed in the treatment summary section.[28]

III. ABUSE OF ALCOHOL DURING PREGNANCY

A. Perinatal Associations

Alcohol use during pregnancy has been strongly associated with birth defects in the offspring of drinking mothers. One third of pregnant women who ingest six or more drinks per day during pregnancy have offspring with signs of fetal alcohol syndrome (FAS), the leading cause of preventable mental retardation.[29] Although maternal alcohol consumption of less than two drinks (1 ounce of alcohol) per day has not been associated with an increase in birth defects, it is possible that unmeasured deleterious effects do occur.[30] As such, abstinence should be recommended for all pregnant women. Patients who refuse or are unable to comply with this recommendation should be considered at risk for alcohol-related maternal and infant complications.

Even if regular, daily use is not discovered in alcohol use screening during pregnancy, clinicians should specifically ask about the presence of binge drinking, defined as intake of five or more alcoholic drinks on any one occasion. Data from the National Survey on Drug Use and Health (NSDUH) estimated the prevalence of binge drinking among pregnant women to be 4.1% in 2002 and 2003.[1] Risk factors for binge drinking during pregnancy include being unmarried, being employed, and currently smoking.[31] Half of all pregnancies in the United States are unintended, and many women are not aware of their pregnancy status until 6 to 8 weeks of gestation. Therefore, women may unknowingly expose their fetuses to large amounts of alcohol concentration if they have a drinking binge during this critical time. Clinicians need to inquire about binge drinking in both pregnant and nonpregnant patients, and inform patients of the risks associated with binge drinking.

Physician advice to avoid alcohol during pregnancy has been shown to be influential in a patient's decision-making process. Women receiving advice not to drink during routine health maintenance care self-report a lower risk for alcohol use during pregnancy.[32]

B. Prevalence of Alcohol Abuse (Risk Drinking)

The prevalence of alcohol abuse in prenatal populations ranges from 4% to 14% (depending on the characteristics of the practice population), as compared with 7% in the general female population. Although this problem may be more prevalent in certain low socioeconomic settings, all patient groups have a substantial percentage of women with alcohol abuse issues.

C. Adverse Perinatal Outcomes

1. Prenatal
   Alcoholism during pregnancy may serve as a proximate marker for other risk factors, such as smoking, domestic abuse, depression, and poor social support. When some or all of these conditions contribute to the pregnant woman receiving sporadic or nonexistent prenatal care, the risk for adverse perinatal outcomes, such as prematurity and IUGR, is even greater.
2. Neonatal
   Alcohol risk-taking (>1 ounce of alcohol or 2 drinks/day) during pregnancy has well-defined teratogenic effects that may result in central nervous system dysfunction, growth deficiencies, a cluster of facial abnormalities, and other major and minor malformations. An infant has FAS when all of these categories of effects are present (Table 5-5).[33] When a subset of these effects is present, they are termed fetal alcohol effects. Clinicians should be adept at recognizing this syndrome (Figure 5-1).[26]

TABLE 5-5 Principal Features of the Fetal Alcohol Syndrome Observed in 245 Affected Patients

Feature	Manifestation
Central Nervous System Dysfunction	
Intellectual	Mild-to-moderate mental retardation*
Neurologic	Microcephaly*
	Poor coordination, hypotonia
Behavioral	Irritability in infancy*
	Hyperactivity in childhood
Growth Deficiency	
Prenatal	<2 SD for length and weight*
Postnatal	<2 SD for length and weight*
	Disproportionately diminished adiposity
Facial Characteristics	
Eyes	Short palpebral fissures*
Nose	Short, upturned
	Hypoplastic philtrum*
Maxilla	Hypoplastic
Mouth	Thinned upper vermilion*
Retrognathia in infancy*	
Micrognathia or relative prognathia in adolescence	

*Feature seen in more than 80% of patients.
SD, Standard deviation.
From Clarren S, Smith D: The fetal alcohol syndrome, *N Engl J Med* 298:1063-1067, 1978.

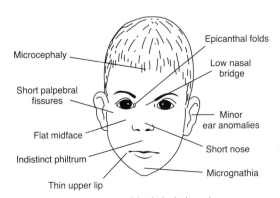

Microcephaly
Short palpebral fissures
Flat midface
Indistinct philtrum
Thin upper lip
Epicanthal folds
Low nasal bridge
Minor ear anomalies
Short nose
Micrognathia

FIGURE 5-1. Appearance of fetal alcohol syndrome.

D. Long-Term Sequelae

Infants born with FAS have long-term sequelae, most notably mild to moderate mental retardation. Even infants born of alcoholic mothers with no apparent stigmata of FAS are at increased risk of delayed-onset fetal alcohol effects, including hyperactivity and mental retardation.[20] Long-term studies into adolescence indicate that intellectual and behavioral deficits in these children often widen, in part mediated by unstable family environments.[34]

E. Diagnostic Options

1. Self-reporting
   This method of screening often carries the risk for underreporting referred to previously.
2. Application of systematic screening tools
   a. CAGE questionnaire (Table 5-6): The CAGE questionnaire was developed in 1970 and remains one of the most reliable and easy screening instruments for the detection of alcoholism.[35] A single affirmative answer on this screening should alert the provider to the possibility of alcohol abuse, although most studies using the CAGE survey have used two positive answers as the threshold for further evaluation.[30] The validity of this instrument has not been determined within a prenatal population.
   b. T-ACE questionnaire (Table 5-7)[36]: This modified version of the CAGE questionnaire has proved to be a sensitive, reliable screening instrument for excessive alcohol intake in a study involving women initiating prenatal care at Brigham and Women's Hospital in Boston.[37] The questionnaire requires only 1 minute to administer and the tolerance question is considered the strongest predictor of excessive alcohol consumption. As a screening tool, the T-ACE has a sensitivity of 69%, specificity of 89%, and

TABLE 5-6 The CAGE Questionnaire

C	Ever felt need to **C**ut down drinking?
A	Ever felt **A**nnoyed by criticism of drinking?
G	Had **G**uilty feelings about drinking?
E	Ever take morning **E**ye-opener?

From Ewing J: Detecting alcoholism: the CAGE questionnaire, *JAMA* 252:1905-1907, 1984.

TABLE 5-7 T-ACE Questionnaire

T	How many drinks does it take to make you feel high (**T**olerance)?
A	Have people **A**nnoyed you by criticizing your drinking?
C	Have you felt you ought to **C**ut down on your drinking?
E	Have you ever had a drink first thing in the morning to steady your nerves or get rid of a hangover (**E**ye-opener)?

Found to be significant identifiers of risk drinking, that is, alcohol intake sufficient to potentially damage the embryo/fetus.
From Sokol R, Martier S, Ager J: The T-ACE questions, *Am J Obstet Gynecol* 160:863–870, 1989.

positive predictive value of 23% in a population that has a 4.3% incidence rate of consuming 2 or more drinks per day. The T-ACE is scored by assigning two points to an affirmative response on the tolerance (T) question and one point each to the others. A score of 2 or greater qualifies as a positive screening test.

F. Treatment

1. Preconception diagnosis and intervention
   The primary prevention of FAS can be accomplished with proper identification and treatment of women with alcohol abuse before conception. Family planning counseling and encouragement of contraceptive use should be included in early treatment efforts until the woman is sober and regularly participating in an outpatient recovery program.
2. Treatment options
   a. Provision of referral to freestanding alcohol treatment programs
   b. Establishment of on-site treatment capabilities in high-risk settings that have direct tie-ins to other social support services
   c. Participation with community-based coalitions that provide additional outreach, education, and intensive case management; these programs have been developed to address special populations in which the incidence of FAS is markedly increased[38]
   d. Recognition that for some patients, especially adolescents, pregnancy may provide an opportunity to intervene to decrease current or future substance abuse use[39]

IV. METHAMPHETAMINE ABUSE DURING PREGNANCY

The use of methamphetamine (slang names: ice, meth, speed, crystal, glass, and crank) has increased dramatically in recent years. Methamphetamine can be smoked, injected, swallowed, inhaled, or snorted. A few studies are beginning to examine the effects of methamphetamine use on the fetus. Methamphetamine use causes increased maternal blood pressure and heart rate, which may lead to premature delivery or spontaneous abortion. Methamphetamine use constricts blood vessels in the placenta, reducing blood flow to the fetus with the possible result of IUGR.[40] Problems seen in the newborn include jitteriness, trouble sleeping, and poor feeding. No known increase in specific birth defects has been found in infants exposed to methamphetamine in utero. It is unknown whether prenatal exposure to methamphetamine can cause behavioral or intellectual problems later in life.[41] The full effect of methamphetamine use during pregnancy on the newborn is currently unknown, but studies are under way to determine this necessary information.

V. SUMMARY RECOMMENDATIONS

Intervention strategies dealing with substance abuse and pregnancy have not been studied in a randomized, prospective fashion. The following recommendations are based on successful demonstration projects.[28]

A. Screening

Assess for past or current use of potentially harmful drugs in a systematic fashion, both in the preconceptual and prenatal periods. Screening instruments, such as the T-ACE, can be incorporated into a larger questionnaire that asks for detailed information on past or current use of substances when the initial screen is indicative of a problem. Intermittent use of toxicology screening during pregnancy should be considered.

B. Treatment

Develop a treatment plan that incorporates office staff and community resources to assist with both substance abuse counseling and unmet social service needs, such as housing, nutrition, and education. Optimal prenatal care for the substance-abusing patient can be provided when a mechanism exists to track progress and compliance with recommended care. Lay or professional staff can be used for this purpose.

C. Outcomes

Recognize that a patient with substance abuse issues has, in general, a higher behavioral risks profile, which may contribute to adverse perinatal outcomes. Ongoing risk assessment of the pregnancy is necessary, and appropriate interventions should be offered when available.

D. Postpartum and Early Childhood Care

All of the supportive services provided for substance-abusing pregnant women during the prenatal period should be continued and strengthened during the year after childbirth. With the stress of a new baby, a new mother may revert to previous "coping patterns" (i.e., drug use) unless new coping skills are presented and developed in the prenatal visits. Close follow-up with continued counseling and support may prevent relapse.

E. Prevention

Physicians can and should play a role in the primary, secondary, and tertiary prevention of this major public health epidemic, both in the office and in community settings.

REFERENCES

1. Substance use during pregnancy: 2002-2003, *The NSDUH Report*, June 2, 2005. Available at: http://www.oas.samhsa.gov/2k5/pregnancy/pregnancy.htm.
2. Francis H, Smith D: Substance abuse, pregnancy and HIV. Available at: http://www.cdc.gov/hiv/projects/perinatal/materials/ps2_Francis.pdf. Accessed November 11, 2006.
3. At-risk drinking and illicit drug use: ethical issues in obstetric and gynecologic practice. ACOG Committee Opinion No. 294. American College of Obstetricians and Gynecologists, *Obstet Gynecol* 103:1021-1031, 2004.
4. Volpe J: Effect of cocaine use on the fetus, *N Engl J Med* 327:399-405, 1992.
5. Singer L, Garber R, Kliegman R: Neurobehavioral sequelae of fetal cocaine exposure, *J Pediatr* 119:667-672, 1991.
6. Schutzman D, Frankenfield-Chernicoff M, Clatterbaugh HE et al: Incidence of intrauterine cocaine exposure in a suburban setting, *Pediatrics* 88:825-827, 1991.
7. George S, Price J, Hauth JC et al: Drug abuse screening of childbearing-age women in Alabama public health clinics, *Am J Obstet Gynecol* 165:924-927, 1991.
8. Brantley M, Rochat R, Floyd V et al: Population-based prevalence of perinatal exposure to cocaine—Georgia, 1994, *MMWR* 45(41):887-891, 1996.
9. Robins L, Mills J: Effects of in utero exposure to street drugs, *Am J Public Health* 83(suppl):3-32, 1993.
10. Slutsker L: Risks associated with cocaine use during pregnancy, *Obstet Gynecol* 79:778-789, 1992.
11. Gillogley KM, Evans AT, Hansen RL et al: The perinatal impact of cocaine, amphetamine and opiate use detected by universal intrapartum screening, *Am J Obstet Gynecol* 163:1535-1542, 1990.
12. Ness RB: Cocaine and tobacco use and the risk of spontaneous abortion, *N Engl J Med* 340:333-339, 1999.
13. Amaro H, Fried L, Cabral H et al: Violence during pregnancy and substance use, *Am J Public Health* 80:575-579, 1990.
14. Hans SL: Demographic and psychosocial characteristics of substance-abusing pregnant women, *Clin Perinatol* 26(1):55-74, 1999.
15. Bass M, Kravath R, Glass L: Death-scene investigation in sudden infant death, *N Engl J Med* 315:100-105, 1986.
16. Zuckerman B, Bresnahan K: Developmental and behavioral consequences of prenatal drug and alcohol exposure, *Pediatr Clin North Am* 38:1387-1405, 1991.
17. Frank D, Augustyn M, Knight W et al: Growth, development, and behavior in early childhood following prenatal cocaine exposure: a systematic review, *JAMA* 285:1613-1625, 2001.
18. Christmas J, Knisely J, Dawson K et al: Comparison of questionnaire screening and urine toxicology for detection of pregnancy complicated by substance use, *Obstet Gynecol* 80:750-754, 1992.
19. Ostrea E, Brady M, Gause S et al: Drug screening of newborns by meconium analysis: a large-scale, prospective epidemiologic study, *Pediatrics* 89:107-113, 1992.
20. Graham K, Koren G, Klein J et al: Determination of gestational cocaine exposure by hair analysis, *JAMA* 262:3328-3330, 1989.
21. Beasley VL: Personal communication, November 11, 2006.
22. Lester BM: Substance use during pregnancy: time for policy to catch up with research [on-line], *Harm Reduction J* 1:5, 2004. Available at: http://www.Harmreductionjournal.com/content/1/1/05.
22a. *Whitner v. State*, 328 S.C. 1, 492 S.E. 2d 777 (1997).
23. Chasnoff I, Landress H, Barrett M: The prevalence of illicit-drug or alcohol use during pregnancy and discrepancies in mandatory reporting in Pinellas County, Florida, *N Engl J Med* 322:1202-1206, 1990.
24. Howell EM, Chasnoff IJ: Perinatal substance abuse treatment: findings from focus groups with clients and providers, *J Subst Abuse Treat* 17:139-148, 1999.
25. Feldman J, Minkoff H, McCalla S et al: A cohort study of the impact of perinatal drug use on prematurity in an inner-city population, *Am J Public Health* 82:726-728, 1992.
26. Little B, Snell L, Klein V et al: Maternal and fetal effects of heroin addiction during pregnancy, *J Reprod Med* 35:159-162, 1990.
27. Wolman I, Niv D, Yovel I et al: Opioid-addicted parturient, labor, and outcome: a reappraisal, *Obstet Gynecol Surv* 44:592-596, 1989.
28. Suffet F, Brotman R: A comprehensive care program for pregnant addicts: obstetrical, neonatal and child development outcomes, *Int J Addict* 19:199-219, 1984.
29. Cyr M, Moulton A: Substance abuse in women, *Obstet Gynecol Clin North Am* 17:905-922, 1990.
30. Mills J, Graubard B: Is moderate drinking during pregnancy associated with an increased risk for malformations? *Pediatrics* 80:309-314, 1987.
31. Ebrahim SH, Diekman ST, Floyd RL et al: Comparison of binge drinking among pregnant and non-pregnant women, United States, 1991–1995, *Am J Obstet Gynecol* 180:1-7, 1999.

32. Jones-Webb R, McKiver M, Pirie P et al: Relationships between advice and tobacco and alcohol use during pregnancy, *Am J Prev Med* 16(3):244-247, 1999.

33. Clarren S, Smith D: The fetal alcohol syndrome, *N Engl J Med* 298:1063-1067, 1978.

34. Streissguth A, Aase J, Clarren S et al: Fetal alcohol syndrome in adolescents and adults, *JAMA* 265:1961-1967, 1991.

35. Ewing J: Detecting alcoholism. The CAGE questionnaire, *JAMA* 252:1905-1907, 1984.

36. Sokol R, Martier S, Ager J: The T-ACE questions: practical prenatal detection of risk-drinking, *Am J Obstet Gynecol* 160:863-870, 1989.

37. Chang G, Goetz MA, Wilkins-Haug L et al: Identifying prenatal alcohol use: screening instruments versus clinical predictors, *Am J Addict* 8:87-93, 1999.

38. Masis K, May P: A comprehensive local program for the prevention of fetal alcohol syndrome, *Public Health Rep* 106:484-489, 1991.

39. Flanagan P, Kokotailo P: Adolescent pregnancy and substance abuse, *Clin Perinatol* 26:55-74, 1999.

40. Smith L, Yonekura M, Wallace T et al: Effects of prenatal methamphetamine exposure on fetal growth and drug withdrawal symptoms in infants born at term, *J Dev Behav Pediatr* 24:17-23, 2003.

41. Organization of Teratology Information Services (OTIS): *Dextroamphetmine/methamphetamine and pregnancy.* Available at: http://www.otispregnancy.org/pdf/methamphetamines.pdf. Accessed November 11, 2006.

S E C T I O N D Smoking in Pregnancy

Elizabeth G. Baxley, MD

Smoking continues to be one of the most important preventable risk factors for pregnancy complications.

I. MAGNITUDE OF THE PROBLEM

A. Epidemiology

Despite extensive publicity regarding its dangers, tobacco use in pregnancy continues to be high.[1] In the period between 1990 and 2003, a decline in the overall rate of smoking reported by pregnant women declined from 18.4% to 11%.[2,3] However, some of the decline may relate to reluctance women have toward disclosing their smoking status because of societal pressures. Between 14% and 25% of women have been shown to conceal their smoking from health-care providers.[4,5]

Smoking rates among pregnant women vary by demographic characteristics.

1. Age

   Pregnant adolescents have the greatest smoking rates of all age groups, with 18% of women younger than 19 years reporting tobacco use while pregnant.[6,7]

   a. Mothers older than 35 years smoke significantly less than younger women.[6]

2. Race/Ethnicity

   a. Among race and ethnic groups, Native American, Puerto Rican, white, non-Hispanic, and Hawaiian women have the greatest rates of smoking during pregnancy; Chinese women have the lowest rates.[8,9]

3. Socioeconomic status

   a. Women with low incomes and those from low education groups have greater smoking rates.[8]

4. Parity/Marital status

   a. Multiparous women are more frequent, "heavier" smokers than primiparous women.[6,8]

   b. Single women have greater smoking rates than married women.[6]

Mothers who smoke also tend to seek prenatal care less often, as evidenced by this group having greater rates of four or fewer prenatal visits as compared with nonsmokers.[6]

B. Smoking-Related Problems in Pregnancy

The adverse effects of maternal smoking are well documented. Physiologically, increased rates of carboxyhemoglobin predispose to fetal hypoxia. Maternal smoking also results in reduced blood flow through the placenta, and nicotine and other compounds in smoke are suspected of having direct effects on the placenta, as well as having been demonstrated to be neuroteratogenic to the fetus.[10]

Complications that have been associated with smoking in pregnancy include:

1. Low birth weight (LBW)

   LBW newborns, those weighing less than 2500 g at birth, occur as a result of prematurity, IUGR, or both. Mothers of small-for-gestational-age infants smoke more often and in greater amounts than mothers of infants of average gestational age, with neonatal weight correlating negatively with the number of cigarettes smoked daily.[6,11] In a prospective study of 160 women, maternal smoking in the third trimester was shown to be a strong and independent predictor of birth weight percentages. For each additional cigarette per day that a woman smoked in the third trimester, an estimated 27-g reduction in birth weight occurred that appeared to be a reduction in fetal growth velocity rather than an increase in preterm birth frequency.[12] Efforts at reducing cigarette consumption during the third trimester can lead to improvements in birth weight,[10] whereas cessation before the third trimester would eliminate much of the reduced birth weight caused by maternal smoking.[13] Analyses of birth certificate data estimate that elimination of smoking during pregnancy would reduce the incidence of singleton LBW by 10.4%.[14] Passive exposure to smoke is also associated with LBW infants, particularly if the exposure is longer than 2 hours per day.[11]

2. Intrauterine growth restriction (IUGR)

A large, population-based study demonstrated that IUGR increased from 5.7% in nonsmokers to 15.8% in women who smoked more than 10 cigarettes/day.[6] Cigarette smoking in the second trimester has been significantly associated with fetal growth restriction in both white and African American women, in a dose–response relation.[15]

3. Placental abruption[6,12]

A metaanalysis of seven case–control and six cohort studies on a total of more than one million pregnancies demonstrated a strong relation between cigarette smoking and placental abruption.[16] Maternal smoking was associated with a 90% increase in the risk for placental abruption (odds ratio, 1.9; 95% CI, 1.8-2.0). A dose–response effect was demonstrated with increasing number of cigarettes smoked. The population attributable risk percentage of this effect suggests that 15% to 25% of placental abruption is due to cigarette smoking. The risk for abruption is greater when pregnant smokers also have chronic hypertension, mild or severe preeclampsia, or chronic hypertension with superimposed preeclampsia.

4. Preterm delivery and preterm premature rupture of the membranes

Smoking increases the risk for both preterm delivery and preterm premature rupture of membranes, directly in proportion to the number of cigarettes smoked each day. The odds ratio for preterm delivery was 1.2 (95% CI, 1.13-1.28) and for preterm premature rupture of the membranes was 1.3 (95% CI, 1.12-1.40).[6]

5. Perinatal mortality, including SIDS

Population estimates suggest that elimination of smoking during pregnancy would reduce infant deaths by 5%.[12,17]

6. Asthma

Rates of childhood asthma are increased in women who smoke during pregnancy. The impact on asthma prevalence appears to be as a direct effect, and also through indirect relation related to greater rates of preterm births and LBW.[18] Overall, these children have a 25% greater risk for development of asthma in first 7 years of life if their mothers smoked less than 10 cigarettes/day and a 36% greater risk if their mothers smoked more than 10 cigarettes/day.[19]

Additional pregnancy-related complications associated with maternal smoking include greater rates of ectopic pregnancy, placenta previa, meconium stained amniotic fluid, decreased Apgar scores, and clinical asphyxia and need for neonatal intubation.[6,12,20,21]

Paradoxically, maternal smoking is associated with a lower incidence in hypertensive disorders of pregnancy.[22,23] In a population-based retrospective analysis of 170,254 pregnancies in Germany, a dose-related reduction in the incidence of preeclampsia was seen among pregnant smokers, with the rate of preeclampsia being inversely proportional to the number of cigarettes smoked per day.[6] However, this inverse association between cigarette smoking during pregnancy and preeclampsia must be balanced with the other harmful effects that have strong associations with tobacco use.

Smoking during pregnancy has also been associated with adverse effects that continue into the newborn period, childhood, and young adulthood.

1. Impact on nutrition

Maternal smoking is a significant predictor of infant nutrition. Greater rates of childhood obesity have been reported among children of mothers who smoked during pregnancy.[24] Mothers who smoke during all or part of their pregnancy are less likely than nonsmokers to initiate breast-feeding or to continue breastfeeding beyond 12 weeks.[25] Smokers are also more likely than nonsmokers to introduce solid food by 12 weeks.

2. Impact on childhood illness

a. Infant colic has been reported at greater rates among newborns of mothers who smoked during pregnancy.[26]

b. A study of nearly 2000 Danish children reported that children born to mothers who smoked 15 or more cigarettes/day during pregnancy had hospitalization rates before 8 months of age that were twice that of children whose mothers did not smoke or smoked less than 15 cigarettes/day. This effect of in utero exposure was shown to be independent of postpartum smoking habits of either the mother or father.[27]

c. In children up to 5 years of age, a population attributable risk of 39.4% for acute middle ear infections is related to in utero exposure to cigarette smoke at the first prenatal visit.[28,29]

II. SMOKING CESSATION PROGRAMS IN PREGNANCY

A. Effectiveness

Between 15% and 42% of women smokers stop before their first prenatal visit,[29,30] and approximately 46% of prepregnancy smokers quit during pregnancy.[31,32] Successful smoking cessation is largely dependent on the patient's ability to make difficult changes in her life; quitting use of an addictive substance rarely occurs suddenly and without preparation. Motivation for cessation is greatest early in the pregnancy.[33] Effective counseling for pregnant smokers can be enhanced by understanding each woman's readiness for change (Figure 5-2). Because the effects of tobacco use in pregnancy have been shown to be dose related, even these efforts at cutting down should be strongly encouraged.

Smoking cessation programs have been attempted in numerous prenatal programs with varying effectiveness and limited long-term success, ranging from 4% to 20% in low-income groups and from 16% to 26% in higher income groups.[8] Approximately 25%

of women relapse before delivery.[34,35] Smoking relapse rates are particularly high when there are other smokers in the immediate environment.

Cochrane reviewed 51 randomized controlled trials involving 20,931 women and 6 cluster-randomized trials with more than 7500 women to provide information on the effectiveness of smoking cessation interventions and perinatal outcomes.[36] In 48 trials on effectiveness, there was a significant reduction in smoking in the intervention groups (RR, 0.94; 95% CI, 0.93-0.95), an absolute difference of 6 in 100 women continuing to smoke. The 36 trials with validated smoking cessation had a similar reduction (RR, 0.94; 95% CI, 0.92-0.95). Smoking cessation interventions reduced LBW (RR, 0.81; 95% CI, 0.70-0.94) and preterm birth (RR, 0.84; 95% CI, 0.72-0.98). There was a 33-g (95% CI, 11-55) increase in mean birth weight. In two trials, the intervention strategy of rewards plus social support resulted in a significantly greater smoking reduction than other strategies (RR, 0.77; 95% CI, 0.72-0.82). Five trials of smoking relapse prevention (N = 800 women) showed no statistically significant reduction in relapse.

B. Techniques

Nonpharmacologic smoking cessation techniques that have been studied in pregnancy include counseling, cognitive behavioral therapy, hypnosis, and acupuncture. Interventions that appear to be effective in reducing smoking include advice by physician, group

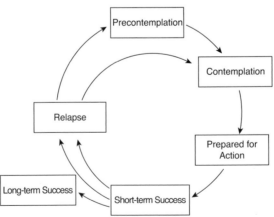

FIGURE 5-2. Stages of change model. Adapted from National Cancer Institute: Strategies to control tobacco use in the United States: a blueprint for public health action in the 1990's, Publication No. 92-3316, Bethesda, MD, 1991, National Institutes of Health, 1991.

sessions, and behavioral therapy based on self-help manuals.[37]

Metaanalyses indicate that brief counseling of 5 to 10 minutes increases validated smoking cessation by 70% in pregnant women.[8] This brief intervention was most effective among women who smoked fewer than 20 cigarettes/day and when conducted by trained health-care providers using the 5 As technique[38]:

1. **Ask** about smoking status.
   A multiple-choice question has been shown to improve disclosure of smoking by 40% over the usual question "Do you smoke?"[3]
2. **Advise** to stop smoking by providing individualized, strong, clear messages about the benefits of stopping and risks of continued smoking on pregnancy.
3. **Assess** willingness to quit in next 30 days. If yes, go to next step; if no, repeat these steps at subsequent prenatal visits.
4. **Assist** by providing pregnancy-specific, self-help smoking cessation materials.
   Table 5-8 lists a variety of resources available to the pregnant woman and her prenatal care provider to help her quit smoking.[30] Great Start (1-866-66-START) is a national pregnancy-specific smokers'

quit-line operated by the American Legacy Foundation.

5. **Arrange** follow-up visits to track the progress of patient's efforts.

Pregnant women should be informed about the specific risks of smoking during pregnancy, such as the risk for delivering a baby with LBW and preterm. Women who smoke or who have recently stopped should be offered smoking cessation interventions.[36] Although quitting in early pregnancy yields the greatest benefits for the pregnant woman and fetus, quitting at any point can be beneficial.[37]

III. PHARMACOLOGIC APPROACH TO SMOKING CESSATION IN PREGNANCY

A. Use of Nicotine Delivery Systems in Pregnancy

Use of nicotine replacement products or other pharmaceuticals have not been sufficiently evaluated to determine their efficacy or safety, and they are not U.S. Food and Drug Administration approved for use in pregnancy.[30] Only one randomized controlled trial has been done on trial of

TABLE 5-8 Resources for Smoking Cessation

Organization	Materials Available	Phone Number or URL	Cost
American Academy of Family Medicine	"Patient Stop Smoking Guide"	http://www.aafp.org/online/etc/ medialib/aafp_org/documents/ clinical/pub_health/askact/ guide.Par.0001.File.tmp/ StopSmokeGd07.pdf	Free
			$80 nonmembers
American Cancer Society	"The Most Often Asked Questions about Smoking, Tobacco, and Health…and the Answers"	http://www.cancer.org/docroot/ PED/content/PED_10_2x_ Questions_About_Smoking_ Tobacco_and_Health.asp	Free
American Lung Association	"Smoking & Pregnancy"	http://www.lungusa.org/site/pp. asp?c=dvLUK9O0E&b=33573 or 1-800-LUNG-USA (1-800-586-4872)	Free
National Institutes of Health, National Cancer Institute	"Clearing the Air"	http://www.smokefree.gov/pubs/ clearing_the_air.pdf	Free

nicotine replacement, using transdermal patch, and it showed no difference from placebo; however, the numbers were small and the trial was underpowered to whether nicotine replacement was effective.[39] Infants born to women in the nicotine group did have significantly higher birth weights than those in the placebo group, suggesting that the growth restriction caused by smoking is probably not attributable to nicotine.

In a small study conducted at the Mayo Clinic, serial measurements of maternal urinary nicotine and cotinine levels and indicators of fetal well-being, such as fetal heart rate and reactivity, systolic/diastolic ratio of blood flow in the umbilical artery, and biophysical profile scores, were made at baseline while the mother was smoking, abstaining from smoking, and using a nicotine patch for 4 days in an inpatient special care unit. Nicotine patch therapy was not found to be associated with indications of fetal compromise during the in-hospital phase of nicotine patch therapy in pregnant smokers who were abstaining.[40] The small sample size and short study period warrant further follow-up studies. Nicotine gum and patches cause dose-related increases in maternal blood pressure and heart rate and lesser effects on fetal heart rate, but each of these changes is less pronounced than those caused by smoking.[41] An argument can been made that the potential risks of this therapeutic use in pregnancy are outweighed by the benefits of smoking cessation.

If nicotine replacement is to be recommended, products with intermittent dosages, such as gum or inhaler, should be tried first.[42] If a patch used, it should be removed at night to reduce fetal nicotine exposure.[43]

B. Use of Bupropion

1. Bupropion use during pregnancy

   Although pharmacotherapy with bupropion may improve smoking cessation rates in pregnancy, few studies have examined the safety and efficacy of this medication to treat pregnant smokers. In one prospective matched, controlled observational study of 22 pregnant smokers, bupropion appears to be effective for smoking cessation, with 10 (45%) of 22 women taking the drug stopping smoking, as compared with 3 (14%) of 22 control subjects ($p = 0.047$).[44] As for safety of the drug, in a study with completed follow-up on 136 women exposed to bupropion during the first trimester of pregnancy, there were 105 live births and no major malformations.[45] The mean birth weight was 3450 g, the mean gestational age at delivery was 40 weeks, and the number of spontaneous abortions was 20. There was one stillbirth and one neonatal death. The only statistically significant difference between the exposed and comparison groups was an increase in the rate of spontaneous abortions in the bupropion group ($p = 0.009$). However, the greater rates of spontaneous abortions were similar to other studies examining the safety of antidepressants during pregnancy. A registry has been established by Glaxo Wellcome to assess the safety of bupropion use in pregnancy.[46] Health-care providers are encouraged to register patients by calling 1-800-336-2176 (toll-free) or (910) 256-0549 or http://www.pregnancyregistry.gsk.com/bupropion.html.

2. Bupropion use during breastfeeding

   Bupropion is excreted in breast milk; however, no accumulation of the parent drug or its metabolites has been detected in infant plasma, and no adverse effects have been noted.[47,48] As with all medications in pregnancy, the decision to use bupropion should be a risk–benefit decision that is made after careful discussion with the patient.

IV. POSTPARTUM SMOKING CESSATION EFFORTS

Even if smoking cessation efforts are sustained throughout the pregnancy, 60% to 70% of women who quit during pregnancy relapse in the first postpartum year, and half do so in the first 6 weeks.[31,49-53] Risk factors for postpartum relapse include[48,49,54,55]:

1. Having a partner who smokes
2. Having friends who smoke
3. Lacking confidence in ability to remain smoke free
4. Concern about losing the weight gained during pregnancy
5. Younger maternal age
6. Prior heavy smoking before pregnancy
7. Quitting in the third trimester

   Successful programs at reducing postpartum relapse rates have some of the following characteristics[49,53,56]:

1. Target smoking habits of the partner, others living in the home, and close friends

2. Support women with positive encouragement rather than negative nagging
3. Encourage women's social networks to support her in her efforts
4. Initiate and continue throughout pregnancy and through early childhood care
5. Distinguish between women with concrete plans for not relapsing and those who have not thought out possible challenges

V. SUMMARY

Numerous medical complications of pregnancy have been associated with smoking during pregnancy. Although quitting smoking before conception or early in pregnancy is most beneficial, there are health benefits from cessation at any time. A woman who still smokes should continue to be encouraged to quit. Maternity care providers should ensure that smoking cessation programs are available and accessible to all women in their care. High-risk groups should receive enhanced targeted education and incentives for quitting.

VI. SOR A RECOMMENDATIONS

RECOMMENDATIONS	REFERENCES
Smoking cessation programs in pregnancy reduce the proportion of women who continue to smoke, and reduce LBW and preterm birth.	*35*
Pregnant women should be informed about the specific risks of smoking during pregnancy, such as the risk for delivering a baby with LBW and preterm. The benefits of quitting at any stage should be emphasized.	*36*
Women who smoke or who have recently stopped smoking should be offered smoking cessation interventions. Interventions that appear to be effective in reducing smoking include advice by physician, group sessions, and behavioral therapy based on self-help manuals.	*36*
Women who are unable to quit smoking during pregnancy should be encouraged to reduce smoking quantity.	*36*

REFERENCES

1. Hellerstein S, Sachs G: Smoking and reproductive health, *ACOG Tech Bull* 180, 1993.
2. Smoking during pregnancy—United States 1990-2002. Centers for Disease Control and Prevention, *MMWR Morb Mortal Wkly Rep* 53:911-915, 2004.
3. Hamilton BE, Martin JA, Sutton PD: Births: preliminary data for 2003. Centers for Disease Control and Prevention, National Center for Health Statistics, *Natl Vital Stat Rep* 53(a):1-17, 2004.
4. Mullen PD, Carbonari JP, Tabak ER et al: Improving disclosure of smoking by pregnant women, *Am J Obstet Gynecol* 165:409-413, 1991.
5. Windsor RA, Barker D: Health care service delivery issues and systems. Paper presented at consensus workshop on smoking cessation in pregnancy, US Department of Health and Human Services, Health Resources and Services Administration, Rockville, MD, April 9-10, 1998.
6. National Center for Health Statistics (NCHS): *Health, United States, 2004: with chartbook on trends in the health of Americans,* Hyattsville, MD, 2004, NCHS. Available at: http://www.ncbi.nlm.nih.gov/books/bv.fcgi?call=bv.View..ShowTOC&rid=healthus04. Accessed August 26, 2007.
7. Hammoud AO, Bujold E, Sorokin Y et al: Smoking in pregnancy revisited: findings from a large population-based study, *Am J Obstet Gynecol* 192:1856-1863, 2005.
8. Mathews TJ: Smoking during pregnancy, 1990–96, *Natl Vital Stat Rep* 47:1-12, 1998.
9. Mullen PD: Maternal smoking during pregnancy and evidence-based intervention to promote cessation, *Prim Care Clin Office Pract* 26(3):577-589, 1999.
10. U.S. Department of Health and Human Services (DHHS): *The health consequences of smoking: a report of the Surgeon General,* Washington, DC, 2004, DHHS. Available at: www.cdc.gov/tobacco/sgr/sgr_2004/chapters.htm
11. Martin T, Bracken M: Association of low birth weight with passive smoke exposure in pregnancy, *Am J Epidemiol* 124:633-642, 1986.
12. Bernstein IM, Mongeon JA, Badger GJ et al: Maternal smoking and its association with birth weight, *Obstet Gynecol* 106(5 pt 1):986-991, 2005.
13. U.S. Department of Health and Human Services (DHHS): *The health consequences of smoking: a report of the Surgeon General,* Washington, DC, 2004, DHHS. Available at: http://www.cdc.gov/tobacco/data_statistics/sgr/sgr_2004/index.htm. Accessed August 26, 2007.
14. Ventura SJ, Hamilton BE, Mathews TJ et al: Trends and variations in smoking during pregnancy and low birth weight: evidence from the birth certificate 1990-2000, *Pediatrics* 111:1176-1180, 2003.
15. Sprauve ME, Lindsay MK, Drews-Botsch CD et al: Racial patterns in the effects of tobacco use on fetal growth, *Am J Obstet Gynecol* 181:822-827, 1999.
16. Ananth CV, Smulian JC, Vintzileos AM: Incidence of placental abruption in relation to cigarette smoking and hypertensive disorders during pregnancy: a meta-analysis of observational studies, *Obstet Gynecol* 93:622-628, 1999.
17. Salihu HM, Aliyu MH, Pierre-Louis BJ et al: Levels of excess infant deaths attributable to maternal smoking during pregnancy in the United States, *Matern Child Health J* 7:219-227, 2003.
18. Li YF, Langholz B, Salam MT et al: Maternal and grandmaternal smoking patterns are associated with early childhood asthma, *Chest* 127:1232-1241, 2005.

19. Jouni JK, Jaakkola MD, Gissler M: Maternal smoking in pregnancy, fetal development, and childhood asthma, *Am J Public Health* 94(1):136-140, 2004.

20. Castles A, Adams EK, Melvin CL et al: Effects of smoking during pregnancy: five meta-analyses, *Am J Prev Med* 16:208-215, 1999.

21. Salafia C, Shiverick K: Cigarette smoking and pregnancy II: vascular effects, *Placenta* 20:273-279, 1999.

22. Conde-Agudelo A, Althabe F, Belizan JM et al: Cigarette smoking during pregnancy and risk of pre-eclampsia: a systematic review, *Am J Obstet Gynecol* 181:1026-1035, 1999.

23. McCormick M, Brooks-Gun J: Factors associated with smoking in low income pregnant women: relationship to birth weight, stressful life events, social support, health behaviors, and mental distress, *J Clin Epidemiol* 43:441-448, 1990.

24. von Kries R, Toschke AM, Koletzko B et al: Maternal smoking during pregnancy and childhood obesity, *Am J Epidemiol* 156:954-961, 2002.

25. Edwards N, Sims-Jones N, Breithaupt K: Smoking in pregnancy and postpartum: relationship to mothers' choices concerning infant nutrition, *Can J Nurs Res* 30:83-98, 1998.

26. Sondergaard C, Henriksen TB, Obel C et al: Smoking during pregnancy and infantile colic, *Pediatrics* 108:342-346, 2001.

27. Wisborg K, Henriksen TB, Obel C et al: Smoking during pregnancy and hospitalization of the child, *Pediatrics* 104:e46, 1999.

28. Stathis SL, O'Callaghan DM, Williams GM et al: Maternal smoking during pregnancy is an independent predictor for symptoms of middle ear disease at five years' postdelivery, *Pediatrics* 104:e16, 1999.

29. Quinn VP, Mullen PD, Ershoff DH: Women who stop smoking spontaneously prior to prenatal care and predictors of relapse before delivery, *Addict Behav* 16(1-2):29-40, 1991.

30. Windsor RA, Lowe JB, Perkins LL et al: Health education for pregnant smokers: its behavioral impact and cost benefit, *Am J Public Health* 83(1):201-206, 1993.

31. ACOG Committee Opinion #316. Smoking cessation during pregnancy, *Obstet Gynecol* 106(4):883-888, October 2005.

32. Coleman GJ, Joyce T: Trends in smoking before, during and after pregnancy in ten states, *Am J Prev Med* 24:29-35, 2003.

33. McBride CM, Curry SJ, Lando HA et al: Prevention of relapse in women who quit smoking during pregnancy, *Am J Public Health* 89:706-711, 1999.

34. Ershoff DH, Quinn VP, Mullen PD: Relapse prevention among women who stop smoking early in pregnancy: a randomized clinical trial of a self-help intervention, *Am J Prev Med* 11(3):178-184, 1995.

35. Floyd RL, Rimer BK, Giovino GA et al: A review of smoking in pregnancy: effects on pregnancy outcomes and cessation efforts, *Annu Rev Public Health* 14:379-411, 1995.

36. Lumley J, Oliver SS, Chamberlain C et al: Interventions for promoting smoking cessation during pregnancy, *Cochrane Database Syst Rev* (4):CD001055, 2004.

37. Smoking Cessation Clinical Practice Guideline Panel and Staff: The Agency for Health Care Policy and Research smoking cessation clinical practice guideline, *JAMA* 275(16):1270-1280, 1996.

38. Fiore MC, Bailey WC, Cohen SJ et al: *Treating tobacco use and dependence. Clinical practice guideline,* Rockville, MD, 2000, US Department of Health and Human Services, Public Health Service.

39. Wisborg K, Henriksen TB, Jespersen LB et al: Nicotine patches for pregnant smokers: a randomized controlled trial, *Obstet Gynecol* 96:967-971, 2000.

40. Ogburn PL Jr, Hurt RD, Croghan IT et al: Nicotine patch use in pregnant smokers: nicotine and cotinine levels and fetal effects, *Am J Obstet Gynecol* 181:736-743, 1999.

41. Dempsey DA, Benowitz NL: Risks and benefits of nicotine to aid smoking cessation in pregnancy, *Drug Saf* 24:277-322, 2001.

42. Benowitz N, Dempsey D: Pharmacotherapy for smoking cessation during pregnancy, *Nicotine Tob Res* 6(suppl 2):S189-S202, 2004.

43. Windsor R, Oncken C, Henningfield J et al. Behavioral and pharmacological treatment methods for pregnant smokers: issues for clinical practice, *J Am Med Womens Assoc* 55:304-310, 2000.

44. Chan B, Einarson A, Koren G: Effectiveness of bupropion for smoking cessation during pregnancy, *J Addict Dis* 24(2):19-23, 2005.

45. Chun-Fai-Chan B, Koren G, Fayez I et al: Pregnancy outcome of women exposed to bupropion during pregnancy: a prospective comparative study, *Am J Obstet Gynecol* 192(3):932-936, 2005.

46. Eldridge RR, Ephross SA, Heffner CR et al: Monitoring pregnancy outcomes following prenatal drug exposure through prospective pregnancy registries and passive surveillance: a pharmaceutical company commitment, *Prim Care Update Ob Gyns* 5(4):190-191, 1998.

47. Briggs GG, Samson JH, Ambrose PJ et al: Excretion of bupropion in breast milk, *Ann Pharmacother* 27:431-433, 1993.

48. Baab SW, Peindl KS, Piontek CM et al: Serum bupropion levels in 2 breastfeeding mother-infant pairs, *J Clin Psychiatry* 63(10):910-911, 2002.

49. McBride C, Pirie P: Postpartum smoking relapse, *Addict Behav* 15:165-168, 1990.

50. Fang WL, Goldstein AO, Butzan AY et al: Smoking cessation in pregnancy: a review of postpartum relapse prevention strategies, *J Am Board Fam Pract* 17:264-275, 2004.

51. Fingerhut LA, Kleinman JC, Kendrick JS: Smoking before, during and after pregnancy, *Am J Public Health* 80:541-544, 1990.

52. McBride CM, Pirie PL, Curry SJ: Postpartum relapse to smoking: a prospective study, *Health Educ Res* 7:381-390, 1992.

53. Mullen PD, Quinn VP, Ershoff DH: Maintenance of non-smoking postpartum by women who stopped during pregnancy, *Am J Public Health* 80:992-994, 1990.

54. Ratner PA, Johnson JL, Botoroff JL et al: Twelve-month follow-up of a smoking relapse prevention program for postpartum women, *Addict Behav* 25:81-92, 2000.

55. Mullen PD, Richardson MA, Quin VP et al: Postpartum return to smoking: who is at risk and when, *Am J Health Promot* 11:323-330, 1997.

56. Gielen AC, Windsor R, Faden R et al: Evaluation of a smoking cessation intervention for pregnant women in an urban prenatal clinic, *Health Educ Res* 12:247-254, 1997.

SECTION E Group Prenatal Care: CenteringPregnancy®

Kathryn J. Trotter, RN, MSN, CNM, FNP

I. DESCRIPTION OF METHOD

A. Group Prenatal Care

A growing family-centered maternity care option now being offered by some midwives and physicians is an innovative model of group prenatal care called CenteringPregnancy®. After the initial one or two traditional examination room visits, women receive their care in small groups of 8 to 12 women with similar due dates where individual risk assessment, education, and support are all encompassed in the group space. The program has 10 defined 90-minute sessions implemented from weeks 16 through 40 of pregnancy. Education components are developed through a 10-session curriculum that includes topics such as early pregnancy concerns including adjustment to pregnancy, fetal development, nutrition for pregnancy and lactation, birthing options, postpartum issues, newborn feeding choices and care, sexuality, birth-control options, and parenting styles. All prenatal care occurs within the group setting except for the initial intake done before group assignment, medical concerns involving need for privacy, and cervical assessments late in the pregnancy.

B. Group Participants

In this group setting, women receive basic prenatal risk assessments, can share support from other women, and obtain knowledge and skills related to pregnancy, childbirth, and early parenting. Groups are facilitated by an obstetric provider and an assistant trained in the CenteringPregnancy® program. Consistency in leadership is paramount to providing continuity to the group and ensuring comprehensive content presentation. Furthermore, the model is interdisciplinary in design and encourages women to take responsibility for themselves; leading to a shift in the patient provider power base and empowering these women.[1] Other professionals who can assist as group leaders include social workers, nutritionists, physical therapists, birthing unit nurses, and parent educators.

C. Role of Partners and Children

Partners are encouraged to attend sessions, as are other important support persons such as friends and grandparents. However, women are highly encouraged to find childcare for these group visits so they can concentrate on their own needs.

D. Components of the Session

Each session is divided into two more formal discussion and education periods, with the prenatal assessment occurring for the first 20 minutes and finishing during the midsession break, at which time refreshments are available. Handouts and self-assessment worksheets facilitate the discussion and are completed during the initial minutes.

E. Role of Patients

Within the group space, women participate actively in their risk assessment by weighing themselves, taking their blood pressure, determining the gestational age, and charting these entries. As they access their charts, women become familiar with the entries and ask questions about recorded findings. This demystifies the experience and contributes to the women's control over their pregnancies and care.

F. Individual Prenatal Care Component

Each woman has individual time with the practitioner to share particular concerns, review her progress, measure the fundus, and listen to fetal heart tones. This assessment is conducted on the edge of the group either on a mat on the floor, on a table (low-lying massage table works well), or in a reclining chair. A contract for follow-up is made at this time (immediately at the end of group or separate date) for any issue that involves more privacy for assessment or is too involved for a quick resolution.

G. Adapting the Model to the Practice

Practices will inherently adapt this model to their site and their patients' needs, but the essential elements of this model are shown in Table 5-9.

TABLE 5-9 **Essential Elements of CenteringPregnancy®**

Entire session occurs within the group space

Women are involved in self-care activities

A facilitative leadership style used

Stability of group leadership

Group is conducted in a circle

Composition of the group is stable but not rigid

Group size is optimal to promote the process, usually 8-12 members

Group honors contribution of each member

Attention to general content outline

Involvement of family support people is optional

Opportunity for socialization within the group is provided

Emphasis varies depending on needs of group

Ongoing evaluation of outcomes

II. PRINCIPLES THAT SUPPORT THIS METHOD

A. Educational

Adult learning is important to understand life's experiences, and pregnancy, as a motivational time for most women, can be an excellent time to offer self-care education. The need for prenatal education has become especially acute with early discharge after delivery and no assurance of home follow-up. The format for patient education is interactive, guided by the needs and experience of the women and the knowledge and wisdom of the practitioner.

B. Social Support

The support component of the program may be most important because women with good support systems may be more able to be more effective problem-solvers. As the same group of women and couples meet together over the span of 10 sessions, support develops naturally.[2] This "networking" is facilitated by name tags, interviewing, formal sharing during discussions, and informal conversation during refreshment break and during risk-assessment times. As women bond, they may assist each other outside of the group, such as with transportation or childcare. Near the end of the program, an opportunity to exchange names, addresses, and phone numbers is suggested.

C. Effectiveness of Care

The design of the program is consistent with the Institute of Medicine's recommendations for redesign of health-care processes to provide services based on the following: scientific knowledge to all those likely to benefit, a patient-centered orientation, timely delivery of care, efficiency, and equity in the care process regardless of sex, ethnicity, geography, and socioeconomic status.[3] A patient-centered team approach has been recommended in the *Future of Family Medicine Report*, together with innovative methods of care that address financial issues of reimbursement.[4]

III. CONCERNS OF IMPLEMENTATION

A. Health Insurance Portability and Accountability Act Regulations

Health Insurance Portability and Accountability Act (HIPAA) regulations are addressed in the general orientation of the group participants at the first session. The women and any partners are asked to sign a patient confidentiality agreement. The initial intake done in the traditional examination room will have addressed most of these sensitive areas.

B. Minimizing Disruption

Disruptive elements to group are decreased by the general rule that pagers and phones are to be on vibrate mode or turned off and children should be present only on rare occasions. The facilitator should be skilled in handling inappropriate talking or lack of respectful listening by members. Clinic staff should be made aware that when the CenteringPregnancy® group is in closed-door session, no interruptions should occur unless they are emergent.

C. Billing/Reimbursement

Billing is currently paid by insurance carriers as prenatal care at standard rates. An effort is being made to negotiate additional payment for preparation for childbirth services at standard rates reimbursed for childbirth education classes.

D. Incorporating the New Model

Although groups actually offer patients more contact time with clinicians and more customization of care, many people assume that a system of one-on-one visits enhances intimacy and individualization. More than likely, many women and providers are comfortable with the familiar model and may be hesitant to consider a new approach. Moreover, learning to facilitate groups can be a challenge, and even skilled practitioners require training. Institution investment in both clinician education and system innovation is important for this model to succeed.[3]

IV. OUTCOMES

Little or no evidence exists to support effectiveness of traditional one-on-one prenatal care.[5] Nonetheless, as an alternative to established methodology, the effectiveness of group prenatal care has been questioned and requires demonstration to change models of care delivery.[6]

A Cochrane systematic review of trials for increased social support during pregnancy found no reduction in LBW but some reduced risk for cesarean birth with increased support measures.[7] To date, four published reports exist that suggest this group care model contributes to improved perinatal outcomes. Both pilot and cohort studies comparing this group care model versus traditional care have demonstrated decreases in LBW and prematurity as compared with control subjects,[6,8] as well as greater breastfeeding rates among adolescents enrolled in the CenteringPregnancy® method of care.[9] Results of a 5-year randomized controlled trial documented a 33% reduction in the odds of preterm birth. Women in group prenatal care were more likely to receive adequate prenatal care, had more prenatal care knowledge, and were more likely to initiate breastfeeding.[10] (For further information about the model or training workshops, including tips for starting the model in your location, go to the Centering Pregnancy and Parenting Association website: www.centeringpregnancy.org.)

REFERENCES

1. Rising SS: Centering pregnancy. An interdisciplinary model of empowerment, *J Nurse Midwifery* 43(1):46-54, 1998.
2. Trotter K, Sterling L, Strickland C et al: Put eight pregnant women in the same room, *Fam Pract Manag* 34:14, 2004.
3. Institute of Medicine: *Crossing the quality chasm: a new health system for the 21st century*, Washington, DC, 2001, National Academy Press.
4. The future of family medicine: a collaborative project of the family medicine community, *Ann Fam Med* 2:S3-S32, 2004.
5. Berwick DM: Disseminating innovations in health care, *JAMA* 289:1969-1975, 2003.
6. Novick G: CenteringPregnancy® and the current state of prenatal care, *J Midwifery Womens Health* 49:405-411, 2004.
7. Hodnett ED, Fredericks S: Support during pregnancy for women at increased risk of low birth weight babies, *Cochrane Database Syst Rev* (3):CD000198, 2003.
8. Ickovics JR, Kershaw TS, Westdahl C et al: Group prenatal care and preterm birth weight: results from a matched cohort study at public clinics, *Obstet Gynecol* 102:1061-1067, 2003.
9. Grady MA, Bloom KC: Pregnancy outcomes of adolescents enrolled in a CenteringPregnancy Program, *J Midwifery Womens Health* 49:412-420, 2004.
10. Ickovics JR, Kershaw TS, Westdahl C et al: Group prenatal care and perinatal outcomes: a randomized control trial, *Obstet Gynecol* 110:330-339, 2007.

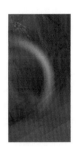

Diagnosis and Management of First-Trimester Complications

SECTION A Diagnosis

Mark Deutchman, MD

Early pregnancy loss is a common event. The incidence rate of miscarriage in recognized pregnancies is between 10 and 20%, but loss of pregnancy before clinical recognition is much greater, bringing the overall miscarriage rate to about 30%.[1,2] The risk for miscarriage of clinically recognized pregnancy increases with age, reaching 40% at age 40 and 80% at age 45.[3] Ectopic pregnancy is potentially life-threatening and occurs in from 1 in 40 to 1 in 100 pregnancies, the rate having increased fourfold between 1970 and 1992.[4]

I. EPIDEMIOLOGY AND RISK FACTORS

About 20% of clinically diagnosed pregnancies are complicated by bleeding, and the odds ratio of miscarriage is about 2.6 in such cases compared with pregnancies without bleeding.[5]

Risk factors or causes for first-trimester pregnancy loss and other first-trimester complications are listed in Table 6-1. Those risk factors of particular importance in the development of ectopic pregnancy or recurrent pregnancy loss are identified in the "Comments" column of Table 6-1.

II. PATHOGENESIS

As illustrated in Table 6-1, many potential causes and conditions are associated with the first-trimester complications of miscarriage and ectopic pregnancy.

The pathogenesis of these complications can be framed to include one or more of these categories:

1. Chromosomally abnormal conceptus
2. Implantation
   The implantation of the pregnancy is in the wrong location, such as the fallopian tube in the case of ectopic pregnancy.
3. Environmental factors
   The death of the conceptus occurs because of toxins, teratogens, infection, or an abnormal intrauterine environment. Regardless of the cause, the physician's task is to determine that the conceptus is nonviable and help the patient choose her treatment options.

III. CLINICAL FEATURES

Pregnancy and its complications should be considered in any woman of childbearing age who presents with abdominal pain, vaginal bleeding, or both. Qualitative urine and blood pregnancy testing is widely available and inexpensive, and should be initiated early in the process of patient evaluation to establish whether pregnancy is in the differential diagnosis. The following features characterize the patient who should be suspected of having a complication of pregnancy during the first trimester:

1. Abdominal pain
2. Vaginal bleeding
3. Uterus smaller than expected for gestational age
4. Uterus larger than expected for gestational age
5. Fetal heartbeat not audible after 10 to 12 weeks of gestational age

TABLE 6-1 **Risk Factors or Causes for First-Trimester Pregnancy Loss and Other First-Trimester Complications**

Risk Factor or Cause	Comment
Chromosomal abnormalities	Cause up to 70% of first-trimester miscarriages[6] Parental chromosomal abnormalities are 20 times more common in parents experiencing recurrent miscarriages than in the normal population[7]
Infections	Toxoplasmosis, rubella, cytomegalovirus
Environmental and workplace toxins	For example, PCP (pentachlorophenol)
Hormonal irregularities—progesterone defect	Particular risk for recurrent miscarriage[7]
Uterine abnormalities	Fibroids and congenital anomalies of the uterus are a particular risk for recurrent miscarriage[7]
Incompetent cervix	Particular risk for recurrent miscarriage[7]
Smoking	
Alcohol	
Illicit drugs	
High coffee intake	≥ 4 cups/day = miscarriage odds ratio of 4.0[7]
Immune disorders, including lupus	Particular risk for recurrent miscarriage[7]
Hematologic disorders—thrombophilias	Particular risk for recurrent miscarriage[7]
Polycystic ovarian syndrome	Particular risk for recurrent miscarriage[7]
Severe maternal kidney disease	
Maternal congenital heart disease	
Maternal diabetes, uncontrolled	
Maternal thyroid disease	
Radiation exposure	
Toxic or teratogenic medication	Accutane
Severe malnutrition	
Bacterial vaginosis—probably with some degree of endometritis	Odds ratio of miscarriage up to 9.0[8]
Group B beta strep	
Use of nonsteroidal antiinflammatory drugs (e.g., ibuprofen and aspirin) at the time of conception[9]	
Advancing maternal age and/or advancing paternal age	Miscarriage risk is particularly increased if mother is older than 35 AND father is older than 40[10]
Previous tubal infection or pelvic inflammatory disease	Up to 50% of patients with ectopic pregnancy have this risk factor[4]
Previous tubal surgery including tubal ligation	Particular ectopic pregnancy risk[4]
Endometriosis	Particular ectopic pregnancy risk[4]
Progesterone-only contraception	Fivefold increase in ectopic pregnancy[4]
Intrauterine contraceptive device (IUD) use	When pregnancy occurs with IUD in place, 5% are ectopic with a nonmedicated IUD and 15% are ectopic with a progesterone-medicated IUD[4]
"Morning-after pill" contraception	10-fold increase in ectopic pregnancy if contraception fails[4]
Assisted reproductive technology	Particular ectopic pregnancy risk, possibly because of preexisting fallopian tube abnormalities
Prior ectopic pregnancy	Particular ectopic pregnancy risk[4]

See comments about factors of particular importance in the development of ectopic pregnancy or recurrent pregnancy loss.

IV. DIAGNOSIS

Making a prompt and correct diagnosis is facilitated by awareness of the differential diagnosis suggested by the patient's clinical features. In the pregnant woman with pain and/or bleeding during the first trimester, the differential diagnosis includes both pregnancy- and nonpregnancy-related conditions.

A. Pregnancy-Related Conditions

Pregnancy-related conditions to consider when making a diagnosis in the first semester include:
1. Normal intrauterine pregnancy
2. Threatened miscarriage (abortion)
3. Complete, spontaneous miscarriage (abortion)
4. Incomplete miscarriage (abortion) with retained products of conception
5. Subchorionic hemorrhage
6. Missed abortion, embryonic demise, embryonic resorption, blighted ovum
7. Ectopic pregnancy
8. Hydatidiform mole

B. Nonpregnancy-Related Conditions

Nonpregnancy-related conditions to consider when making a diagnosis in the first semester include:
1. Appendicitis
2. Adnexal torsion
3. Tuboovarian abscess or other manifestation of pelvic infection
4. Ureteral stone with colic
5. Cystitis or pyelonephritis
6. Ruptured ovarian cyst
7. Corpus luteum cyst

C. Making the Diagnosis

A prompt diagnosis usually can be made by combining history, physical examination, laboratory test results, and diagnostic ultrasonography. It is extremely important to consider and search for ectopic pregnancy because it is a potentially life-threatening condition.
1. History
   Pregnancies are dated from the first day of the last normal menstrual period before conception (menstrual dating), not from the conception date itself. To estimate the age of the pregnancy and

obtain other information needed to assess the patient's risk for abnormal pregnancy, the following information should be sought at a minimum:
   a. Last menstrual period
      It is important to date the last menstrual period and whether it was normal. A light, late period suggests that the patient conceived the month prior to the month in which she had the light, late period.
   b. Previous pregnancy history
   c. Recent use of contraception
   d. Recent medications taken
   e. Recent febrile illnesses
   f. Recent attempts at abortion
   g. Risk factors for ectopic pregnancy (see Table 6-1)
   h. Onset, duration, and severity of pain and bleeding: if generalized abdominal pain is present or if pain is referred to the shoulder area, the possibility of ruptured ectopic pregnancy with hemoperitoneum is great.
   i. History of any tissue being passed and whether tissue was saved for pathologic examination
   j. History of rubella immunization
   k. Blood type and Rh if known
   l. General health status
2. Physical examination
   a. Vital signs, including supine and standing blood pressure: Syncopal symptoms or a decline in systolic blood pressure of 20 mmHg suggest hypovolemia caused by excessive vaginal bleeding from miscarriage or intraperitoneal bleeding from ruptured ectopic pregnancy.
   b. General physical examination: This should assess for cardiopulmonary health and signs of acute surgical abdomen.
   c. Vaginal speculum examination: Note presence and severity of bleeding.
   d. Condition and appearance of the cervix: Is the os open? Is any tissue being passed?
   e. Appearance of the posterior fornix: Is there bulging caused by fluid or blood in the cul-de-sac (pouch of Douglas)?
   f. Consider obtaining cervical cultures for gonorrhea and chlamydia.
   g. Consider obtaining urine sample by urethral catheterization, if needed.
   h. Bimanual pelvic examination: This examination should focus on findings that will help diagnose ectopic pregnancy.[11]

i. Size, position, and texture of the uterus: Ectopic pregnancy is unlikely if the uterus is greater than 8 weeks' size.

j. Presence of tenderness: Unilateral or bilateral tenderness and pain with cervical motion is suspicious for ectopic pregnancy. Pain associated with spontaneous miscarriage is more likely to be midline.

k. Presence of pelvic masses: Any pelvic mass should suggest ectopic pregnancy until proved otherwise.

3. Use of handheld Doppler to listen for a fetal heartbeat

This is often best done during the bimanual pelvic examination when the fundus can be identified with the vaginal hand and the transducer aimed at the fundus with the abdominal hand. Using this technique, the physician can detect a fetal heartbeat almost always by 10 to 12 weeks, even in obese patients. If a fetal heartbeat is heard, miscarriage is ruled out for the present, and the likelihood of ectopic pregnancy is extremely low because most ectopic pregnancies become clinically apparent before 9 to 10 weeks (Figure 6-1).

4. Choice of additional tests

Findings of history and physical examination determine the necessity and urgency of additional testing. All patients must have initial urine or blood pregnancy testing performed. Complete blood count, blood type, and Rh analysis should be obtained routinely.

If a fetal heartbeat is heard by Doppler, the likelihood of ectopic pregnancy is extremely low and no additional tests are needed beyond those ordered for routine prenatal care and scheduling of a follow-up visit. Even when a fetal heartbeat is heard, the woman should be counseled that spontaneous miscarriage is still possible.

If no fetal heartbeat is heard, the choice of additional testing depends on the severity of the patient's symptoms and the availability of serum hormone testing and ultrasonography. Although serum hormone testing, in the form of human chorionic gonadotropin (hCG) and progesterone levels, can help establish a diagnosis, ultrasonography promptly yields a definitive diagnosis in a high percentage of patients and should be the first-line test if readily available.[12]

5. Ultrasonography

Diagnostic ultrasonography is the key to prompt, efficient diagnosis of first-trimester pregnancy problems once the history has been taken and the physical examination has been performed. Scanning may be performed by the transabdominal route, the transvaginal route, or both. The transabdominal route provides a wider field of view, whereas the transvaginal route yields more detailed spatial resolution and greater diagnostic power because higher frequency transvaginal transducers produce more detailed spatial resolution. The transvaginal approach avoids intervening bowel and subcutaneous tissue[12] (Figure 6-2).

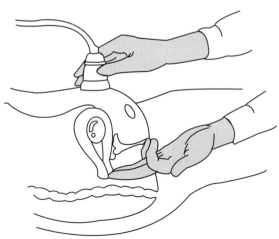

FIGURE 6-1. Use of handheld Doppler to detect fetal heartbeat early. The uterine fundus is identified with the vaginal hand, and the Doppler transducer is aimed at the uterine fundus with the abdominal hand.

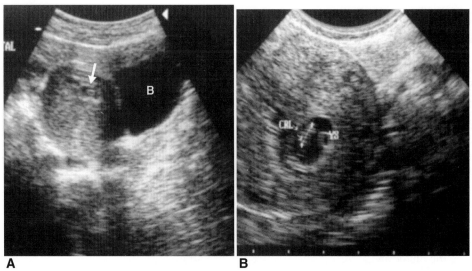

FIGURE 6-2. A, Transabdominal sagittal scan showing vague intrauterine findings *(arrow)*. B, Bladder. **B,** Transvaginal scan of the same patient on the same day demonstrating an embryo with crown rump length *(CRL)* measured and yolk sac *(YS)* visible. Cardiac activity was visible in this 7-mm embryo, corresponding to ≥7 weeks.

a. Normal sonographic landmarks by menstrual age

   i. Gestational sac (also called *chorionic sac*): The earliest sonographic sign of intrauterine pregnancy is the chorionic sac or gestational sac (Figure 6-3). This is a small, lucent area within the uterus surrounded by a brighter, more echogenic

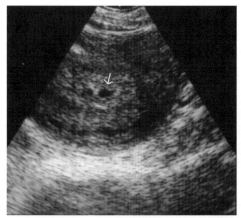

FIGURE 6-3. The chorionic sac, or gestational sac *(arrow)*; in this case, only a few millimeters in diameter. No yolk sac or embryo is yet visible.

ring composed of chorionic villi. The chorionic sac is seen as early as 35 to 40 menstrual days.[13] The chorionic sac is empty when first seen. It should be rounded in shape and located in the uterine fundus. The chorionic sac grows at 1.1 mm/day up to 80 days.[14]

   ii. The menstrual age of the pregnancy in days: This can be calculated by measuring the mean diameter of the chorionic sac in millimeters and adding 30.[14] The mean diameter of the chorionic sac is calculated by adding length plus width plus height and dividing by 3: menstrual age in days (±4 days) = mean sac diameter in millimeters + 30.

   iii. Yolk sac: The earliest structure of embryonic origin to be seen within the chorionic sac is the yolk sac (Figure 6-4). This structure is spherical and appears attached to the chorionic sac wall at one point and should not be larger than 4.5 mm when the mean sac diameter is between 12 and 30 mm (42-60 menstrual days).[15]

   iv. Embryo: The embryo is first seen as a fetal pole between the yolk sac and chorionic sac wall (Figure 6-5A). Embryonic

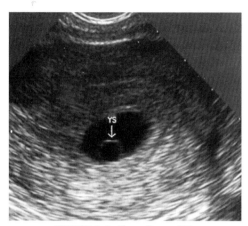

FIGURE 6-4. The yolk sac *(YS).*

cardiac activity often can be seen at the fetal pole before an embryo can be measured easily (see Figure, 6-5*B*). Embryonic cardiac motion can be documented with an M-mode tracing (see Figure, 6-4*B*).

v. Calculating the gestational age: The crown-rump length of the embryo provides the most accurate assessment of gestational age and is calculated as follows. Menstrual age in weeks = crown rump length in centimeters + 6.5 (Figure 6-6).[16] The yolk sac must *not* be included in the crown-rump measurement.

vi. Embryonic cardiac activity: Embryonic cardiac activity is usually seen by the time the crown-rump length is 5 to 8 mm (7 weeks) but should always be seen by the time the crown-rump length is 14 mm (8 weeks).[16-18] When first seen, the embryonic heart rate is about 100 beats/min.[18] If the heart rate is less than 85 beats/minute, subsequent embryonic demise is highly likely, particularly if the heart rate is less than 85 beats/min after 8 weeks.[15]

b. Subchorionic hemorrhage appearance and significance[19]: Subchorionic hemorrhage is seen as a wedge- or crescent-shaped lucent area adjacent to the chorionic sac (Figure 6-7). The location is more significant than the size, with hemorrhages that undermine the placental implantation site more often associated with pregnancy loss. Patients with a subchorionic hemorrhage should be counseled to expect additional bleeding. A subchorionic hemorrhage should not be mistaken for a second (twin) chorionic sac. In some studies, this finding is associated with a 30% miscarriage rate.

c. Complete, spontaneous miscarriage: An empty uterus with a bright endometrial echo is seen in cases of spontaneous complete miscarriage (Figure 6-8).

d. Incomplete miscarriage: Bright echogenic material greater than 5 mm in diameter is characteristic of incomplete miscarriage (Figure 6-9).[20] Mixed sonolucent and bright echogenic material also may be seen.

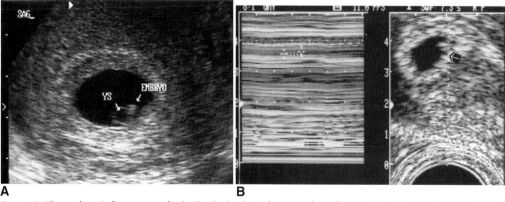

A   **B**

FIGURE 6-5. **A,** The embryo is first seen as the fetal pole (embryo) between the yolk sac *(YS)* and chorionic sac wall. **B,** Left: Early embryonic cardiac activity documented by M-mode. Right: The M-mode beam passes through the fetal pole *(arrow)* at the edge of the chorionic sac.

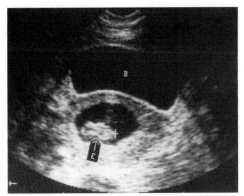

FIGURE 6-6. Transabdominal transverse image of 9½-week intrauterine pregnancy illustrating the fluid-filled urinary bladder *(B)* overlying the pregnant uterus. The embryo *(E)*, with a crown-rump length of 27 mm, is seen between the calipers.

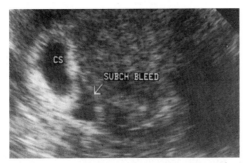

FIGURE 6-7. Transvaginal scan of uterus containing a chorionic sac *(CS)* with an adjacent subchorionic hemorrhage *(SUBCH BLEED)*.

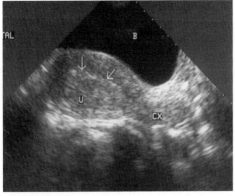

FIGURE 6-8. Midline sagittal transabdominal scan of the uterus *(U)* and cervix *(CX)*, with overlying bladder *(B)* illustrating the endometrial echo *(arrows)*.

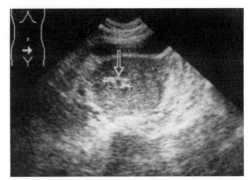

FIGURE 6-9. Transabdominal transverse scan of a uterus containing a 23-mm echogenic area *(arrow)* indicating retained tissue.

e. Missed abortion: When the embryo dies but is entirely retained with the uterus, a variety of findings is possible.

   i. Embryo demise: An embryo is seen with no cardiac motion. In general, embryos that are 5 to 8 mm in crown-rump length must exhibit a heartbeat during real-time scanning (Figure 6-10).[21]

   ii. Embryonic resorption or blighted ovum: A sonolucent sac is seen in the uterus with either no embryo or only some echogenic debris (Figure 6-11). In general, a chorionic sac of mean diameter 16 to 20 mm must have an embryo within it to be normal.[14,19]

f. Ectopic pregnancy: An extrauterine embryo with a heartbeat is positive proof of ectopic pregnancy but is seen in only 10% to 24% of cases (Figure 6-12).[22,23] The use of transvaginal scanning dramatically improves the likelihood of identifying extrauterine pregnancy.[24]

   i. Adnexal masses and/or free fluid: The presence of adnexal masses, free fluid, or both is strongly predictive of ectopic pregnancy (Table 6-2).[22] The sonographic appearance of free pelvic fluid is shown in Figure 6-13.

   ii. Pseudogestational sac: A pseudogestational sac may be seen in some cases of ectopic pregnancy.[25,26] It is a small sonolucent area within the uterus (Figure 6-14) that can be confused with a chorionic (gestational) sac. Distinguishing features are the lack of a surrounding echogenic

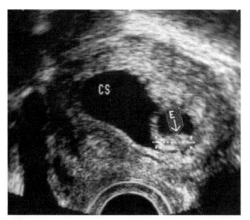

FIGURE 6-10. Coronal transvaginal scan of a uterus containing a dead embryo *(E)* between the electronic calipers. No cardiac motion was seen despite the crown-rump length of 1.6 cm corresponding to ≥8 weeks. *CS,* Chorionic sac.

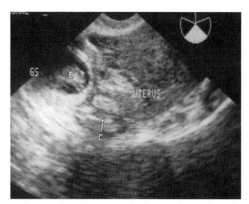

FIGURE 6-12. Coronal transvaginal scan of a confirmed ectopic pregnancy *(GS)* to the right of the uterus, behind which are blood clots *(C)*. The extrauterine embryo *(E)* showed cardiac motion.

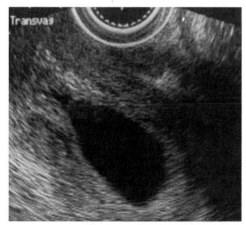

FIGURE 6-11. Transvaginal scan of an "empty" chorionic sac in a case of embryonic resorption; also called *blighted ovum*.

TABLE 6-2 Ancillary Findings Predictive of Risk for Ectopic Pregnancy

Finding	Risk for Ectopic Pregnancy (%)
No mass or free fluid	20
Any free fluid	71
Echogenic mass	85
Moderate-to-large amount of fluid	95
Echogenic mass with fluid	100

Adapted from Brown DJ, Emerson DS, Felker RE et al: Diagnosis of early embryonic demise by endovaginal sonography, *J Ultrasound Med* 9:631-636, 1990.

ring of chorionic villi and the lack of a yolk sac or fetal pole within.

iii. Simultaneous intrauterine and extrauterine pregnancy: This condition is rare, occurring in 1 in 30,000 pregnancies in the general population or as many as 1 in 6000 patients undergoing ovulation induction.[27] A ruptured corpus luteum cyst, which produces free fluid in the cul-de-sac together with an intrauterine pregnancy, can be confused with simultaneous intrauterine and extrauterine pregnancy.

g. Hydatidiform mole: This condition is characterized by typical complex echoes filling the uterus (Figure 6-15).

h. Twin intrauterine pregnancy: A subchorionic hemorrhage should not be mistaken for a second chorionic sac. Avoid making the diagnosis of twin intrauterine pregnancy until two embryos and two heartbeats are seen. The spontaneous loss rate of twin gestation is greater than that of singletons, with combined miscarriage and reduction from twins to singleton reaching 30% to 40% after initial diagnosis. Even after twins are diagnosed sonographically, the

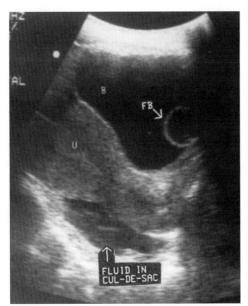

FIGURE 6-13. Sagittal transabdominal scan showing a large amount of free fluid behind the uterus in a ruptured ectopic pregnancy. The urinary bladder *(B)* and the Foley catheter balloon *(FB)* are seen above the uterus *(U)*.

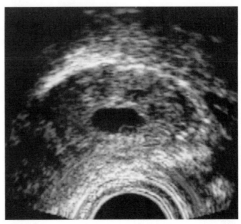

FIGURE 6-14. Coronal transvaginal scan of a uterus containing a "pseudosac" in an ectopic pregnancy. The pseudosac is not surrounded by an echogenic chorionic ring.

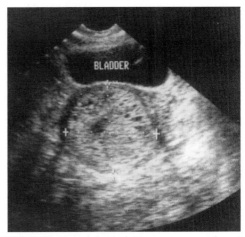

FIGURE 6-15. Transabdominal transverse scan of a uterus containing typical echoes of hydatidiform mole.

rate of spontaneous reduction to singleton is 20% to 33%.[28]

6. Examination of passed tissue

If the patient brings in tissue she has passed vaginally, it should be examined for an embryo or chorionic villi. If either is seen, ectopic pregnancy is virtually ruled out (except in the case of simultaneous intrauterine and extrauterine pregnancy). To look for chorionic villi, suspend the tissue in saline and view it either with the naked eye or under low-power magnification using a colposcope. Chorionic villi appear as tiny, frondlike structures. Some patients with an ectopic pregnancy pass a decidual cast (Arias–Stella reaction), which may resemble products of conception grossly but contains no chorionic villi.[29]

7. Culdocentesis

Culdocentesis provides a way to sample free fluid seen in the cul-de-sac on ultrasonography. Although ultrasonography can visualize free fluid, culdocentesis is still a useful test in many settings.[30] If nonclotting blood with a hematocrit of 15% or greater is determined, an ectopic pregnancy is the diagnosis until proved otherwise.[31]

Analysis of pelvic fluid obtained by culdocentesis also can differentiate hemorrhage from the fluid from a ruptured corpus luteum cyst. Culdocentesis is performed as follows:

a. Counsel the patient.

b. Insert a sterile vaginal speculum.

c. Prepare the cervix and posterior fornix with povidone-iodine or other antiseptic solution.

d. Inject a few milliliters of 1% lidocaine (Xylocaine) with epinephrine into the posterior lip of the cervix.

e. Grasp the anesthetized cervix with a tenaculum.

f. Anesthetize the tissue of the posterior fornix with less than 1 ml of 1% Xylocaine with epinephrine.

g. Puncture the posterior fornix with a 20- or 21-gauge needle and aspirate. If ultrasonography is immediately available, the target fluid pocket and needle can be simultaneously imaged, making the procedure faster and less painful for the patient.

8. Serum hCG testing

a. Quantitative hCG levels: Quantitative hCG levels increase predictably during early pregnancy, doubling every 2 to 3 days during the 4th to 8th weeks of pregnancy.[32] Various reporting standards exist, but most current tests follow the International Reference Preparation (IRP),[33] or third international standard, which are equivalent.[24]

b. The "discriminatory zone": This is the level of hCG by which a gestational sac can be seen sonographically. The diagnostic value of this concept is that if an intrauterine gestational sac is not visible by the time the hCG is at or above this threshold, the pregnancy has a high likelihood of being ectopic or otherwise abnormal. This value is reported differently in various studies. A prudent approach is to use a cutoff of 1500 IU/L if ancillary findings such as an adnexal mass or cul-de-sac fluid are seen, but to use a greater cutoff of 2000 IU/L if no ancillary sonographic signs are present.[34] The yolk sac should be visible by the time the hCG reaches about 5000 IU/L IRP and an embryo with cardiac motion by about 17,000 IU/L IRP.

c. Clinical utility of hCG testing: Single or serial quantitative hCG tests can be particularly helpful when transvaginal sonography fails to show an intrauterine pregnancy or definitive signs of ectopic pregnancy. Ectopic pregnancy is virtually ensured in such cases if the hCG level is greater than 2000 mIU/ml, particularly if serial testing shows it to be either increasing or not decreasing.[35]

9. Quantitative serum progesterone testing

This has been used to help identify patients with abnormal pregnancies. Living intrauterine pregnancies are associated with quantitative progesterone levels of 25 ng/ml or greater. Values less than that level are strongly associated with various forms of pregnancy loss and ectopic pregnancy.[36,37] Progesterone levels less than 5 ng/ml are invariably associated with pregnancy loss including, but not limited to, ectopic pregnancy.[38]

10. Cost of testing

Results of serum hormone tests are generally not as immediately available as ultrasonography. The cost of multiple serum hormone tests is likely to exceed the cost of a single diagnostic ultrasound examination.[39]

V. PITFALLS AND CONTROVERSIES

A. Ultrasound of the Endometrium

The utility of sonographic measurement of the thickness of the endometrium when no gestational sac is seen has been investigated. In one study, pregnancy was abnormal in 97% of cases in which the thickness was 8 mm or less.[40] However, another study found endometrial thickness measurements *not* to be helpful in differentiating intrauterine from ectopic pregnancy.[41]

VI. EVIDENCE-BASED SUMMARY RECOMMENDATIONS USING SOR

No SOR A level recommendations are available in this area. There are a number of recommendations that receive a SOR B level:

1. Patients with a serum hCG level greater than 2000 mIU/mL and a nondiagnostic transvaginal ultrasound are at increased risk for ectopic pregnancy.[42]

2. Obtain a repeat serum hCG determination at least 2 days after the initial presentation because it is useful in characterizing the risk for ectopic pregnancy and the probability of a viable intrauterine pregnancy.[42]

REFERENCES

1. Wilcox AJ, Weinberg CR, O'Connor JF et al: Incidence of early loss of pregnancy, *N Engl J Med* 319:189, 1988.
2. Wang X, Chen C, Wang L et al: Conception, early pregnancy loss, and time to clinical pregnancy: a population-based prospective study, *Fertil Steril* 79:577-584, 2003.
3. Nybo Andersen AM, Wohlfahrt J, Christens P et al: Maternal age and fetal loss: population based register linkage study, *BMJ* 320:1708, 2000.
4. Smith MN: Ectopic pregnancy. Available at: http://www.nlm.nih.gov/medlineplus/ency/article/000895.htm#Causes,%20incidence,%20and%20risk%20factors. Accessed July 3, 2005.
5. Sotiriadis A, Papatheodorou S, Makrydimas G: Threatened miscarriage: evaluation and management, *BMJ* 329(7458): 152-155, 2004.

6. Hogge WA: The clinical use of karyotyping spontaneous abortions, *Am J Obstet Gynecol* 189:397-402, 2003.

7. Li TC, Makris M, Tomsu M et al: Recurrent miscarriage: aetiology, management and prognosis, *Hum Reprod Update* 8:463-481, 2002.

8. Leitich H, Bodner-Adler B, Brunbauer M: Bacterial vaginosis as a risk factor for preterm delivery: a meta-analysis, *Am J Obstet Gynecol* 189:139-147, 2003.

9. Li DK, Liu L, Odouli R: Exposure to non-steroidal anti-inflammatory drugs during pregnancy and risk of miscarriage: population based cohort study, *BMJ* 327:368, 2003.

10. de La Rochebrochard E, Thonneau P: Paternal age and maternal age are risk factors for miscarriage; results of a multicentre European study, *Hum Reprod* 17:1649-1656, 2002.

11. Glass RH, Golbus MS: Pregnancy wastage. In Creasy RK, Resnick R, editors: *Maternal fetal medicine,* Philadelphia, 1989, WB Saunders.

12. Laing FC, Frates MC: Ultrasound evaluation during the first trimester of pregnancy. In Callen PW, editor: *Ultrasonography in obstetrics and gynecology,* ed 4, Philadelphia, 2000, WB Saunders.

13. Fossum GT, Davajan V, Kletzky OA: Early detection of pregnancy with transvaginal ultrasound, *Fertil Steril* 49:788-791, 1988.

14. Nyberg DA, Mack LA, Laing FC et al: Distinguishing normal from abnormal gestational sac growth in early pregnancy, *J Ultrasound Med* 6:23-27, 1987.

15. Howe RS, Isaacson KJ, Alber JL et al: Embryonic heart rate in human pregnancy, *J Ultrasound Med* 10:367-371, 1991.

16. Timor-Trisch EL, Rottem S: Pathology of the early intrauterine pregnancy. In Timor-Trisch IE, Rottem S, editors: *Transvaginal sonography,* New York, 1991, Elsevier.

17. Brown DJ, Emerson DS, Felker RE et al: Diagnosis of early embryonic demise by endovaginal sonography, *J Ultrasound Med* 9:631-636, 1990.

18. Pennell RG, Baltarowich OH, Kurtz AB et al: Complicated first-trimester pregnancies: evaluation with endovaginal ultrasound versus transabdominal technique, *Radiology* 165:79-83, 1987.

19. Rempen A: Diagnosis of viability in early pregnancy with vaginal sonography, *J Ultrasound Med* 9:711-716, 1990.

20. Timor-Trisch EL, Rottem S: Pathology of the early intrauterine pregnancy. In Timor-Trisch IE, Rottem S, editors: *Transvaginal sonography,* New York, 1991, Elsevier.

21. Kurtz AB, Shlansky-Goldberg RD, Choi HY et al: Detection of retained products of conception following spontaneous abortion in the first trimester, *J Ultrasound Med* 10:387-395, 1991.

22. Brown DJ, Emerson DS, Felker RE et al: Diagnosis of early embryonic demise by endovaginal sonography, *J Ultrasound Med* 9:631-636, 1990.

23. Mahony BS, Filly RA, Nyberg DA et al: Sonographic evaluation of ectopic pregnancy, *J Ultrasound Med* 4:221-228, 1985.

24. Rempen A: Vaginal sonography in ectopic pregnancy. A prospective evaluation, *J Ultrasound Med* 7:381-387, 1988.

25. Graczykowski JW, Seifer DB: Diagnosis of acute and persistent ectopic pregnancy, *Clin Obstet Gynecol* 42(1):9-22, 1999.

26. Nelson P, Bowie JD, Rosenberg ER: Early pregnancy or decidual cast: an anatomic-sonographic approach, *J Ultrasound Med* 2:543-547, 1983.

27. Nyberg DA, Laing FC, Filly RA et al: Ultrasonographic differentiation of the gestational sac of early intrauterine pregnancy from the pseudogestational sac of ectopic pregnancy, *Radiology* 146:755-759, 1983.

28. Yaghoobian J, Pinck RL, Ramanthan K et al: Sonographic demonstration of simultaneous intrauterine and extrauterine gestation, *J Ultrasound Med* 5:309-312, 1986.

29. Grobman WA, Peaceman AM: What are the rates and mechanisms of first and second triimester pregnancy loss in twins? *Clin Obstet Gynecol* 41(1):36-45, 1998.

30. Goldstein SR: *Endovaginal ultrasound,* New York, 1988, A.R. Liss.

31. Vande Krol L, Abbott JT: The current role of culdocentesis, *Am J Emerg Med* 10(4):354-358, 1992.

32. Droegemueller W: Ectopic pregnancy. In Danforth DN, editor: *Obstetrics and gynecology,* Philadelphia, 1986, JB Lippincott.

33. Pittaway DE, Reish RL, Wentz AC: Doubling times of human chorionic gonadotropic increase in early viable intrauterine pregnancies, *Am J Obstet Gynecol* 152:299-302, 1985.

34. Painter PC: Discordant hCG results in pregnancy. A method in crisis, *Diagn Clin Test* 27:20-24, 1989.

35. Tay JI, Moore J, Walker JJ: Ectopic pregnancy (regular review), *BMJ* 320:916-919, 2000.

36. Mol BW, Hajenius PJ, Engelsbel S et al: Serum human chorionic gonadotropin measurement in the diagnosis of ectopic pregnancy when transvaginal ultrasonography is inconclusive, *Fertil Steril* 70(5):972-981, 1998.

37. Hahlin M, Wallin JA, Sjoblom P et al: Single progesterone assay for early recognition of abnormal pregnancy, *Hum Reprod* 5:622-626, 1990.

38. Yeko TR, Gorrill MJ, Hughes LH et al: Timely diagnosis of early ectopic pregnancy using a single blood progesterone measurement, *Fertil Steril* 48:1084-1050, 1987.

39. Mol BW, Lijmer JG, Ankum WM et al: The accuracy of single serum progesterone measurement in the diagnosis of ectopic pregnancy: a meta-analysis, *Hum Reprod* 13(11):3220-3227, 1998.

40. Deutchman ME: Advances in the diagnosis of first-trimester pregnancy problems, *Am Fam Phys* 44:15S-30S, 1991.

41. Spandorfer SD, Barnhart KT: Endometrial stripe thickness as a predictor of ectopic pregnancy, *Fertil Steril* 66(3):474-477, 1996.

42. Mol BWJ, Hajenius PJ, Engelsbel S et al: Are gestational age and endometrial thickness alternatives for serum human chorionic gonadotropin as criteria for the diagnosis of ectopic pregnancy? *Fertil Steril* 72:643-635, 1999.

SECTION B Management of Ectopic Pregnancy

Mark Deutchman, MD

Ectopic pregnancy is a potentially life-threatening condition. Patients with abnormal bleeding or pelvic pain, or both, who are found to have ectopic pregnancy or who are strongly suspected of having ectopic pregnancy require establishment of a diagnostic and management plan and close follow-up to avoid the potentially catastrophic complication of tubal rupture with massive hemorrhage and shock. The use of assisted reproductive techniques in women with preexisting tubal abnormalities has not only increased the overall incidence of ectopic pregnancy, but has increased the incidence of unusual forms of the condition such as cornual, interstitial, and heterotopic (simultaneous intrauterine and ectopic) pregnancy. Many choices in treatment are possible depending on clinical factors and available resources.[1] Two major considerations must be balanced when choosing the type of treatment for ectopic pregnancy.

A. Short-Term Consideration

Short-term consideration addresses the likelihood of success in eliminating the ectopic pregnancy and not leaving any persistent trophoblastic tissue behind.

B. Long-Term Consideration

Long-term consideration addresses the effect of the treatment on future fertility.

I. MANAGEMENT

Table 6-3 lists management options and clinical factors that affect their utility.

A. Open Surgical Treatment with Salpingectomy

When a woman presents with hemoperitoneum and shock after tubal rupture, little or no chance exists for conservative therapy, and open surgical treatment with salpingectomy is usually indicated. A population-based study[4] identified four risk factors for tubal rupture:
1. Never having used contraception
2. A history of tubal damage and infertility
3. Induction of ovulation
4. hCG level greater than 10,000 mIU/ml

B. Conservative Surgical Treatment

When an *unruptured* ectopic pregnancy is identified with the use of ultrasonography and hCG testing, a range of conservative treatments becomes possible. Conservative surgical treatment options include techniques for removing the ectopic pregnancy while preserving the fallopian tube. These options include removing the ectopic pregnancy from the fallopian tube and closing the incision in

TABLE 6-3 Management Options for Ectopic Pregnancy

Management Option	Factors to Consider
Open surgical treatment with salpingectomy	Large ectopic mass with or without rupture and hemoperitoneum
Conservative surgical treatment, open or laparoscopic[2]: Salpingostomy Salpingotomy Segmental resection Fimbrial expression	Unruptured fallopian tube Desire for future fertility Hemodynamically stable
Medical treatment with methotrexate alone[3] or with methotrexate plus mifepristone	Unruptured ectopic; mass <4 cm; low human chorionic gonadotropin level
Expectant waiting for spontaneous resolution	Mainly patients with "occult" ectopic pregnancy

the tube or leaving the incision open, removing a segment of the tube and repairing the tube, or squeezing the ectopic pregnancy out of the fimbriated end of the fallopian tube. All of these techniques can be performed through an open laparotomy or by the laparoscopic approach. The laparoscopic approach is less successful than open treatment because of greater rates of persistent trophoblastic tissue, but it is overall superior because of the following outcomes[5]:
1. Lower cost
2. Less blood loss
3. Less analgesic requirement
4. Shorter operating time and hospital stay
5. Shorter convalescent time

C. Medical Management

Methotrexate, a folic acid antagonist, is being used extensively to treat ectopic pregnancy in properly selected women.[3] Various regimens administer methotrexate orally (PO), intramuscularly (IM), or by direct injection into the ectopic pregnancy by the laparoscopic route or under sonographic guidance. Considerations in the use of methotrexate include:
1. Patient selection
2. Route of administration
3. Initial dosage
4. Repeat dosage (if necessary)

5. Side effects
6. Combination therapy with mifepristone (progesterone receptor inhibitor)
7. Efficacy compared with surgical therapy
8. Cost compared with surgical therapy
9. Long-term fertility compared with surgical therapy

Reasonable clinical selection criteria for use of methotrexate in women with ectopic pregnancy are[3,5,7]:

1. Stable vital signs
2. No medical contraindication to methotrexate therapy (normal liver enzymes, normal blood count, normal platelet count)
3. Patient reliable for follow-up
4. Unruptured ectopic pregnancy
5. Absence of embryonic cardiac motion
6. Ectopic mass 3 to 4 cm or less
7. Starting hCG levels less than 5000 mIU/ml; greater levels increase the risk for treatment failure and need for additional doses

A variety of methotrexate regimens has been published, including single or multiple doses given IM or by direct injection into the ectopic mass by laparoscopic approach. Single-dose intramuscular regimens are commonly calculated at 1 mg/kg or 50 mg/m^2. Serum hCG testing is performed on the 4th and 7th posttreatment days and followed until the level reaches 5 mIU/ml, which may take 3 to 4 weeks. The hCG initially increases slightly but should decline 15% between days 4 and 7; if not, the dose should be repeated or surgical therapy performed. Serum progesterone levels may be followed instead of hCG; a decline to 1.5 ng/ml is considered a successful end point and usually occurs by about 2 to 3 weeks.[8]

D. Expectant Management

Waiting for spontaneous resolution without either medical or surgical treatment is another option. It is based on the fact that some tubal pregnancies undergo spontaneous abortion or resorption. One randomized trial from 1955 showed that about half of expectantly managed patients escaped the need for surgery.[9] Modern reports have focused on identifying patients appropriate for expectant management, including those whose hCG is less than 1000 mIU/ml and declining.[7,10-13] These women tend to be those in whom the ectopic pregnancy is "occult" with no sonographically identifiable adnexal mass. Patients must be managed with serial hCG, hematocrits,

physical examinations, and ultrasound as needed until clinical resolution and hCG level is less than 5 mIU/ml.

II. CLINICAL COURSE: EFFICACY OF TREATMENT AND EFFECT ON SUBSEQUENT FERTILITY

A. Efficacy

These statements summarize information about the efficacy of various forms of treatment for ectopic pregnancy based on Cochrane reviews and metaanalyses[5]:

1. The open surgical approach

   This is the most effective treatment for ectopic pregnancy. The laparoscopic approach is more likely to leave persistent trophoblastic tissue behind.[5]

2. Laparoscopic salpingostomy

   The success rate of laparoscopic salpingostomy for removal of ectopic pregnancy is reported to be 91% (range, 72-100%)[7] compared with the expected 100% for open surgery.

3. Multiple-dose methotrexate therapy

   Laparoscopic salpingostomy and multiple-dose methotrexate therapy are similarly successful.[5,7] The primary treatment success rate statistics of multiple-dose methotrexate versus laparoscopic salpingostomy are: relative risk (RR), 1.2; 95% confidence interval (CI), 0.93-1.4.[5] However, methotrexate treatment is associated with more quality-of-life impairment. This impairment is due to those cases in which the method fails, tubal rupture occurs, and surgical intervention is required, resulting in increased costs, hospital stays, and lost productivity.[5]

   Laparoscopic salpingostomy is more effective in treating ectopic pregnancy than local injection of methotrexate by either laparoscopic or sonographic guidance.[5] Single-dose intramuscular methotrexate is less effective than multiple-dose intramuscular methotrexate.[5] The patients in whom intramuscular methotrexate therapy saves costs are those with the lowest initial hCG levels.[5]

4. Expectant management

   The effectiveness of expectant management (simple observation without medication or surgery) is reported to be 69.2%.[7] Most studies include patients in whom transvaginal ultrasound fails to identify a pregnancy and in whom hCG levels are very low and decreasing.

B. Fertility after Treatment for Ectopic Pregnancy

Laparoscopic conservative surgery versus open conservative surgery appears to produce similar tubal patency and fertility rates[5]:
1. Tubal patency (RR, 0.89; 95% CI, 0.74-1.1)
2. Fertility (RR, 1.2; 95% CI, 0.88-1.5)
   Systemic methotrexate (multiple-dose intramuscular regimen) versus laparoscopic salpingostomy appears to produce similar tubal preservation and fertility rates[5]:
3. Tubal preservation (RR, 0.98; 95% CI, 0.87-1.1)
4. Fertility (74 patients trying to conceive 18 months after treatment for ectopic pregnancy)
   a. Methotrexate group (34 women)
      i. 12 spontaneous intrauterine pregnancies
      ii. 3 spontaneous ectopic pregnancies
   b. Laparoscopic salpingectomy group (40 women)
      i. 16 spontaneous intrauterine pregnancies
      ii. 4 spontaneous ectopic pregnancies

III. CONTROVERSIES

The following questions remain controversial in the treatment of ectopic pregnancies:
1. Does the addition of mifepristone to methotrexate improve the effectiveness of medical treatment of ectopic pregnancy? Resolution of this question requires further studies.[5,6]
2. Which treatment for tubal ectopic pregnancy is most cost-effective: medical or laparoscopic? The answer to this question depends on the likelihood of failure of medical therapy necessitating follow-up surgical therapy. The most powerful predictor of medical therapy failure appears to be hCG level. In women with initial hCG levels less than 1500 mIU/ml, methotrexate appears to be more cost-effective, but when the initial hCG level exceeds 3000 mIU/ml, methotrexate is more expensive.[14]
3. Women being treated with methotrexate for tubal pregnancy commonly experience pain. Whether this pain indicates the need for surgery can be a difficult clinical decision. In one study, only 20% of women with pain severe enough to require evaluation or hospitalization required surgery.[15]

IV. SOR A RECOMMENDATIONS

RECOMMENDATIONS	REFERENCES
Laparoscopic surgery is the cornerstone of treatment in the majority of women with tubal pregnancy.	*5*
Compared with laparoscopic conservative surgery (salpingostomy), local methotrexate is not a treatment option.	*5*
If the diagnosis of tubal pregnancy can be made noninvasively, medical treatment with systemic methotrexate in a multiple-dose intramuscular regimen is an alternative treatment option, but only in hemodynamically stable women with an unruptured tubal pregnancy and no signs of active bleeding presenting with low initial serum hCG concentrations, and after properly informing these patients about the risks and benefits of the available treatment options.	*5*

REFERENCES

1. Leach RE, Ory SJ: Modern management of ectopic pregnancy, *J Reprod Med* 34:324-338, 1989.
2. Stangel JJ, Reyniak JV, Stone ML: Conservative surgical management of tubal pregnancy, *Obstet Gynecol* 48:241-244, 1976.
3. American College of Obstetricians and Gynecologists: Medical management of tubal pregnancy, *ACOG Pract Bull* (3), 1998.
4. Job-Spira N, Fernandez H, Bouyer J et al: Ruptured tubal ectopic pregnancy: risk factors and reproductive outcome: results of a population-based study in France, *Am J Obstet Gynecol* 180:938-944, 1999.
5. Hajenius PJ, Mol F, Mol BW et al: Interventions for tubal ectopic pregnancy, *Cochrane Database Syst Rev* (1):CD000324, 2007.
6. Garbin O, de Tayrac R, de Poncheville L et al: Medical treatment of ectopic pregnancy: a randomized clinical trial comparing methotrexate-mifepristone and methotrexate-placebo, *Cochrane Central Register of Controlled Trials The Cochrane Collaboration*, (2), 2005. (Review of: Traitement medical des grossesses extra-uterines: un essai clinique randomise comparant methotrexate-mifepristone et placebo-methotrexate, *J Gynecol Obstet Biol Reprod (Paris)* 5:391-400, 2004.)
7. Tulandi T, Sammour AP: Evidence-based management of ectopic pregnancy, *Curr Opin Obstet Gynecol* 12:289-292, 2000.
8. Saraj AJ, Wilcox JG, Najmabadi S: Resolution of hormonal markers of ectopic gestation: a randomized trial comparing single-dose intramuscular methotrexate with salpingostomy, *Obstet Gynecol* 92:989-994, 1998.
9. Lund J: Early ectopic pregnancy: comments on conservative treatment, *J Obstet Gynaecol Br Emp* 62:70-76, 1955.

10. Adoni A, Milwidsky A, Hurwitz A et al: Declining β-hCG levels: an indicator for expectant approach in ectopic pregnancy, *Int J Fertil* 31:40-42, 1986.
11. Cohen MA, Sauer MV: Expectant management of ectopic pregnancy, *Clin Obstet Gynecol* 42:48-54, 1999.
12. Garcia AJ, Aubert JM, Sama J et al: Expectant management of presumed ectopic pregnancies, *Fertil Steril* 48:395-400, 1987.
13. Mashiach S, Carp JH, Serr DM: Nonoperative management of ectopic pregnancy, *J Reprod Med* 27:127-132, 1982.
14. Mol BW, Hajenius PJ, Engelsbel S, et al: Treatment of tubal pregnancy in the Netherlands: an economic comparison of systemic methotrexate administration and laparoscopic salpingostomy, *Am J Obstet Gynecol* 181:945-951, 1999.
15. Lipscomb GH, Puckett KJ, Bran D et al: Management of separation pain after single-dose methotrexate therapy for ectopic pregnancy, *Obstet Gynecol* 93:590-593, 1999.

SECTION C Management of Miscarriage

David Turok, MD, MPH

The most common complication in the first 12 weeks of pregnancy is early pregnancy failure, a condition that rarely presents serious health risks to women.[1] Early pregnancy failure is either the result of incomplete abortion, anembryonic pregnancy, or embryonic demise. Because these conditions occur in approximately 15% of clinically detected pregnancies, practitioners delivering obstetric care are certain to encounter them regularly and must be familiar with their management.

The paradigm of management for miscarriage has changed radically since the late 1980s. It was previously recommended that all patients with early pregnancy failure undergo dilation and curettage (D&C). However, this practice has been challenged, and now mounting evidence exists to support expectant management and medical treatment of this condition.[2-4] This chapter focuses on the three acceptable management options for early pregnancy failure: expectant management, medical management with misoprostol, and D&C. Miscarriage is frequently a traumatic experience for patients that can be eased with anticipatory guidance. Management of a first-trimester pregnancy loss is not complete until a plan has been developed for contraception and/or future attempts at pregnancy.

I. DIAGNOSIS

Any woman with first-trimester bleeding needs to be evaluated to rule out ectopic pregnancy and early pregnancy failure. This frequently requires multiple examinations and laboratory testing to be certain of the diagnosis. Ultrasound is the single most effective tool in this situation and needs to be combined with quantitative hCG levels if a gestational sac is not visualized by ultrasound. If ectopic pregnancy has been eliminated as a diagnostic possibility, the bleeding patient may have threatened abortion or early pregnancy failure.

A. Threatened Abortion

Threatened abortion occurs with bleeding that takes place with a viable early pregnancy that requires observation.

B. Early Pregnancy Failure

Early pregnancy failure is a pregnancy less than 13 weeks that will not develop any further.

1. Complete abortion
   The patient has passed the gestational tissue, the uterus has returned to normal nonpregnant size, and bleeding has slowed or resolved. If a gestational sac (membranes) with attached chorionic villi can be identified in the passed tissue, you can be certain of the diagnosis and the patient needs no further treatment for this condition. Identifying the components of passed tissue is made easier by rinsing the tissue through a strainer with cold water and placing it in a clear tray with backlighting or placing it in a plastic bag and holding it up to the light.

2. Incomplete abortion
   This occurs when a patient has bleeding with a nonviable early pregnancy and has passed some but not all of the tissue.

3. Anembryonic pregnancy
   This describes the situation when a gestational sac is visible by ultrasound with a mean sac diameter of more than 20 mm without an embryo or yolk sac or if the diameter is 20 mm or less with no change in 1 week.[5] A mean sac diameter of 16 mm has been reported in some texts as diagnostic of an anembryonic pregnancy, but gestational sacs of this size have been shown to later develop viable embryos.[6] In the past, this has been referred to as a *blighted ovum*. The term *anembryonic pregnancy* is preferred because it clearly describes the situation.

4. Embryonic demise
   This term describes an embryo larger than 5 mm (6 weeks) without cardiac activity.[7] An embryonic demise without bleeding or cervical dilation was

previously referred to as a missed abortion. This is not a clear or descriptive term and its use should be abandoned.

II. TREATMENT

A. Patients with Heavy Bleeding

Patients with heavy bleeding and/or signs of hypovolemia need immediate resuscitation and uterine curettage. These patients should have blood drawn for a hematocrit, blood type and Rh, and quantitative hCG.

Before attempting uterine evacuation, an ultrasonographic assessment of the pregnancy is extremely helpful and may clarify clinical suspicions. This assures the presence of an intrauterine pregnancy and prevents you from attempting to begin removing the gestational tissue when there is a pregnancy of longer than 13 weeks where fetal parts may not pass through the cervix or there could be significant hemorrhage that could not be controlled in an office or emergency department setting. In the emergent setting, if a bimanual examination demonstrates that the uterus is more than 12 weeks, there is heavy bleeding, and gestational tissue is visible in or beyond the cervical os, it is certainly advisable to remove the tissue as long as backup vacuum curettage is available.

Most patients with early pregnancy failure will not present with heavy vaginal bleeding. These patients require a thorough explanation of the cause of the condition and available treatment options. An early study of spontaneous abortions showed that half are due to anembryonic pregnancies.[8] When gestational tissue contains an embryo, 50% to 60% demonstrate a chromosomal abnormality.[9]

The next step in management is to counsel patients regarding their treatment options, which include D&C, medical management with misoprostol, and expectant management.

1. Dilatation and curettage

   Since the invention of the uterine curette, D&C has been the recommended method of treatment for early pregnancy failure.[10] This may have been a reasonable approach in an era where ultrasound and highly sensitive hCG tests were not available and obtaining gestational tissue by D&C ruled out the potentially lethal diagnosis of ectopic pregnancy. In addition, before the legalization of abortion in the United States, many incomplete abortions were the result of poorly performed illegal and unsafe attempts at termination of pregnancy,

which carried a high rate of infection.[11] Evidence-based medicine has brought a thorough critique of the practice of D&C, a surgical procedure that was widely used without any controlled studies supporting the practice.[12]

D&C is a reasonable approach for some patients but is by no means necessary in all cases of early pregnancy failure. It is certainly the method of choice where there is heavy vaginal bleeding associated with current or impending hypovolemia, and in the patient who desires the most rapid resolution of the pregnancy. It is also useful as a backup method when a patient who has pursued expectant or medical management has not completed the process.

Although D&C traditionally has been performed in the operating room, this dramatically increases cost and waiting time for patients. Outpatient D&C is safe and effective, and is the method that is used for almost all the 1.3 million elective abortions performed yearly in the United States.[13] Patients should be offered one or more of the following: local anesthesia with a lower uterine field block (a superior modification of a paracervical block [Figure 6-16]), oral narcotics taken 15 to 30 minutes before the procedure, or conscious sedation with intravenous narcotics and midazolam. A Cochrane review evaluating the instruments of choice for evacuating the uterus in this situation showed a clear preference for vacuum aspiration over sharp curettage.[14] Vacuum aspiration was associated with less blood loss, less pain, and shorter procedure times. The lower uterine field block improved pain scores 25% in women undergoing first-trimester therapeutic abortions[15] using 20 ml of 1% lidocaine.

2. Manual vacuum aspiration (MVA)

   Outpatient first-trimester D&C can be easily accomplished with MVA. MVA is performed with a reusable 60-ml syringe that can provide vacuum pressure equivalent to electric vacuum aspirators (Figure 6-17). MVA has been studied extensively, and a literature review of the use of MVA for early pregnancy failure showed a 98% success rate in more than 5000 cases.[16] MVA is a cheaper and acceptable alternative to electric vacuum aspiration. In a study comparing patients presenting to the emergency department with incomplete abortion at less than 12 weeks, those treated with MVA with conscious sedation had fewer charges ($827 vs. $1404; $p < 0.01$) and shorter hospital times

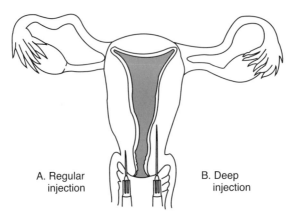

A. Regular injection

B. Deep injection

FIGURE 6-16. A 1.5-inch 22- to 25-gauge needle is used to inject 20 ml of 1% lidocaine. Using 10-ml syringes facilitates visualization. One milliliter is injected superficially at 6 sites (12, 2, 4, 6, 8, and 10 o'clock), then 3 to 4 ml is injected 1.5 inches deep at 4, 6, 8, and 10 o'clock positions. (From Wiebe ER: Comparison of the efficacy of different local anesthetics and techniques of local anesthesia in therapeutic abortions, *Am J Obstet Gynecol* 167:131-134, 1992.)

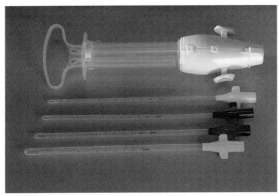

FIGURE 6-17. Manual vacuum aspirator (MVA) with suction cannulae (see Color Plates). (Courtesy IPAS, Carrboro, NC.)

(5.66 vs. 19.26 hours; $p < 0.01$) compared with those who had a D&C in the operating room.[17] These savings are not as striking as a recent retrospective comparison of costs for 715 patients presenting with first-trimester bleeding. The total cost for patients who were managed with office D&C was $1,773 versus $4,948 for patients treated with a D&C in the operating room.[18] In a trial evaluating patient acceptance of MVA versus electric vacuum aspiration in first-trimester abortion, there was equal acceptability of the two methods.[19] A full discussion of the method of D&C for early pregnancy failure is beyond the scope of this text but is available elsewhere in the literature.[20]

B. Use of Antibiotic Prophylaxis

Antibiotic prophylaxis for early pregnancy failure has been evaluated in a Cochrane review. Results were based on a single trial with low compliance to the treatment regimen and limited follow-up. The review concluded that "there is not enough evidence to evaluate a policy of routine antibiotic prophylaxis to women with incomplete abortion."[21]

C. Medical Management

Misoprostol is a prostaglandin E_1 analog known to cause increased uterine tone. Although misoprostol is not FDA approved for the management of early pregnancy failure, it has been increasingly administered for this indication since the first report of its use in 1992.[22] The studies that followed were a heterogenous group with small sample sizes, a variety of control groups, gestational ages treated, description of type of abortion, definition of success, route of misoprostol administration (vaginal vs. oral), and tremendous variation in misoprostol dose (400-800 μg) and dosing frequency (once every 4 hours vs. several days apart).[23-38]

Some of these studies were included in a Cochrane review on the subject that concluded that misoprostol is the prostaglandin of choice in this setting, a greater dose is more effective (800 μg), and the vaginal route is more effective than oral administration.[39]

One study looked specifically at patient satisfaction among 218 women randomized to surgical versus medical therapy. The study showed statistically significant greater patient satisfaction among patients who received medical therapy and completed the process. However, for medical patients who did not complete the process, they were less satisfied than the surgical group.[40]

Recently, a large, adequately powered, multicentered, National Institutes of Health sponsored, randomized control trial of medical versus surgical treatment for early pregnancy failure was published.[41] The trial included patients with anembryonic pregnancy, embryonic death, and incomplete abortion at 5 to 12 weeks of gestation by ultrasound. They were randomized to misoprostol 800 μg vaginally or vacuum aspiration in a 3:1 ratio. This dose and route of misoprostol administration are the standard of care for medical abortion when misoprostol is used in conjunction with mifepristone for early medical abortion.[42] Patients in the misoprostol group received their first dose on day 1 in conjunction with ibuprofen and codeine. This was repeated on day 3 if a gestational sac was still seen by transvaginal ultrasound. Vacuum aspiration was performed on day 8 for patients in the misoprostol group if expulsion was still not complete. By day 3, 71% of the 491 women assigned to the misoprostol group had a complete abortion, and that number increased to 84% by day 8. There was no difference in rare outcomes of hemorrhage or infection, both occurring in less than 1% of patients. Eighty-three percent of patients in both groups would recommend this treatment to others. This study firmly establishes the safety and acceptability of 800 μg misoprostol placed vaginally for the treatment of early pregnancy failure. Until another regimen is shown to be superior, this

TABLE 6-4 **Sample Medications and Instructions for Patients Using Misoprostol for Treatment of Early Pregnancy Failure**

1. Misoprostol 200 μg 4 tablets placed vaginally, may repeat in 72 hours if no tissue passed. Disp #8.

2. Ibuprofen 800 mg po q8 hours prn cramping. Disp #30.

3. Hydrocodone/acetaminophen 7.5/500 mg 1-2 po q4 hours prn pain. Disp #15. May take first within 15 minutes of placing misoprostol tablets to prevent pain of cramping.

4. Phenergan 25 mg po q6 hours prn nausea. Disp #10. May take first within 15 minutes of placing misoprostol tablets to prevent nausea side effects of misoprostol.

dosing should be the standard of care for medical treatment of early pregnancy failure.

Although serious side effects are rare, patients undergoing this treatment need to be advised that they will have intense bleeding and cramping that will likely begin within 24 hours of the first dose of misoprostol. If this lasts longer than 2 hours, they should be seen immediately. Nausea and fever are common adverse effects of misoprostol. These side effects can be managed with nonsteroidal antiinflammatory drugs, oral narcotics, and antiemetics. Prescriptions for these should accompany the prescription for misoprostol (Table 6-4). Contraindications to misoprostol use for early pregnancy failure include history of allergy to misoprostol or other prostaglandins, suspicion of ectopic pregnancy, signs of pelvic infection and/or sepsis, or hemodynamic instability. Precaution should be used in patients with anemia or a history of a bleeding disorder. Patients who have an intrauterine device (IUD) should have the IUD removed before misoprostol administration. Patients who are breastfeeding should be advised that small quantities of misoprostol or its metabolite may be present in their breast milk without any known adverse consequences.[43]

D. Expectant Management

Expectant management is a safe and effective method of treatment for stable patients with early pregnancy failure. A large review and a comprehensive observational study support success rates from 81% to 92.5%.[44,45] In the later study, success rates were reported by diagnosis, with 91% of patients with incomplete abortion completing their miscarriage spontaneously, 76% for embryonic demises, and 66% for anembryonic pregnancies. These patients had a complication rate of 1%.

Patients electing expectant management should be informed that there will be a period of heavy cramping and bleeding that usually lasts 1 to 2 hours. This is likely to occur sometime within the next 2 weeks. It is perfectly reasonable to wait beyond 4 weeks if it is the patient's desire. It is also reasonable to offer patients a combination of the three treatment options where they can pursue expectant management for a certain time period and then use medical therapy if unsuccessful and, finally, D&C if that is unsuccessful. Family physicians offering their patients expectant management and medical treatment need to be able to perform a D&C or have a backup in place who can assist in the rare event that this is necessary.

E. Follow-up Care

For patients who have completed the miscarriage process by one of the above treatment methods, there are several issues to address. The first issue is plans for future pregnancy. Because almost half of pregnancies in the United States are unplanned, it is extremely important to address contraception. Patients may begin any method of contraception immediately. A Cochrane review of immediate postabortal IUD insertion supports this as a safe and practical method, though cautions that expulsion rates may be greater.[46]

For patients who desire another pregnancy, it has been recommended to wait 3 months for further attempts at conception to reduce the risk for miscarriage in the subsequent pregnancy. This has been refuted in a study of 187 women where a group with an interpregnancy interval of less than 3 months had an abortion rate of 16%, which was not statistically significant from the group with longer interpregnancy interval (18%).[47] Patients should be counseled to begin folic acid supplementation to reduce the risk for neural tube defects 3 months before attempting any conception.

Rh status must be known, and all Rh-negative patients who are not sensitized with first-trimester abortion should receive 50 μg of anti-D immunoglobulin.[48] This "mini-dose" is used because of the small red cell mass. This can be done before or after the miscarriage is complete. If this is a patient's

second or third early pregnancy loss, the workup for recurrent pregnancy loss should be discussed.

Miscarriage represents a loss to the pregnant woman and her partner. A wide variety of reactions manifests to this loss largely based on patient expectations of the pregnancy. It is important to dispel feelings of guilt and to convey to patients that this is not their fault and did not result from anything they did or did not do. In addition, offer comfort and support, and assure patients that they have an excellent chance of a normal pregnancy in the future if they desire this.

Many strategies to reduce rates of miscarriage have been evaluated. Cochrane reviews of studies evaluating miscarriage rates have shown no benefit to bed rest,[49] vitamin supplements,[50] or progestins.[51] Neither is there benefit in the use of β agonist for threatened miscarriage.[52]

III. SOR A RECOMMENDATIONS

RECOMMENDATIONS	REFERENCES
Expectant management, D&C, and medical management are acceptable treatment options for women with early pregnancy failure.	38, 40, 41, 43, 44
Vacuum aspiration is safe and less painful than sharp curettage for the management of incomplete abortion.	13
All women with early pregnancy loss should receive 50 μg anti-D immunoglobulin.	41
IUD placement immediately after spontaneous or induced first-trimester abortion is safe and effective.	45
No evidence exists to support the routine use of progestins to prevent miscarriage in early pregnancy.	50
Vitamin supplementation does not decrease the risk for miscarriage.	48

REFERENCES

1. Saraiya M, Green CA, Berg CJ et al: Spontaneous abortion-related deaths among women in the United States—1981-1991, *Obstet Gynecol* 94:172-176, 1999.
2. Ballagh SA, Harris HA, Demasio K: Is curettage needed for uncomplicated incomplete spontaneous abortion? *Am J Obstet Gynecol* 179:1279-1282, 1998.
3. Creinin MD, Schwartz JL, Guido RS et al: Early pregnancy failure—current management concepts, *Obstet Gynecol Surv* 56:105-113, 2001.

4. Ankum WM, Waard MW, Bindels PJE: Regular review: management of spontaneous miscarriage in the first trimester: an example of putting informed shared decision making into practice, *BMJ* 322:1343-1346, 2001.

5. RCR/RCOG Working Party: *Early pregnancy assessment,* London, 1996, RCOG Press.

6. Rowling SE, Coleman BG, Langer JE et al: First-trimester US parameters of failed pregnancy, *Radiology* 203:211-217, 1997.

7. Goldstein SR: Significance of cardiac activity on endovaginal ultrasound in very early embryos, *Obstet Gynecol* 80:670-672, 1992.

8. Hertig AT, Sheldon WH: Minimal criteria required to prove prima facie case of traumatic abortion or miscarriage: an analysis of 1,000 spontaneous abortions, *Ann Surg* 117:596, 1943.

9. Abortion. In Cunningham FG, Leveno KJ, Bloom SL et al, editors: *Williams obstetrics,* ed 22, New York, 2005, McGraw-Hill.

10. Alloway TJ: The immediate use of the uterine scoop or curette in the treatment of abortions, versus waiting or the expectant plan, *Am J Obstet Gynecol* 16:133-141, 1883.

11. Dunn RD: A five-year study of incomplete abortions at San Francisco Hospital, *Am J Obstet Gynecol* 33:149-153, 1937.

12. Hemminki E: Treatment of miscarriage: current practice and rationale, *Obstet Gynecol* 91:247-253, 1998.

13 Finer LB, Henshaw SK: Abortion incidence and services in the United States in 2000, *Perspect Sexual Reproduct Health* 35:6-15, 2003. Available at: www.guttmacher.org/pubs/journals/3500603. html. Accessed September 10, 2007.

14. Forna F, Gulmezoglu AM: Surgical procedures to evacuate incomplete abortion , *Cochrane DatabaseSyst Rev* (1): CD001993, 2001.

15. Wiebe ER: Comparison of the efficacy of different local anesthetics and techniques of local anesthesia in therapeutic abortions, *Am J Obstet Gynecol* 167:131, 1992.

16. Greenslade FC, Leonard AH, Benson J et al: *Manual vacuum aspiration: a summary of clinical and programmatic experience worldwide,* Carrboro, NC, 1993, IPAS.

17. Blumenthal PD, Remsburg RE: A time and cost analysis of the management of incomplete abortion with manual vacuum aspiration, *Int J Gynecol Obstet* 45:261-267, 1994.

18. Schauberger CW, Mathiason MA, Rooney BL: Ultrasound assessment of first-trimester bleeding, *Obstet Gynecol* 105(2): 333-338, 2005.

19. Bird ST, Harvey SM, Beckman LJ et al: Similarities in women's perceptions and acceptability of manual vacuum aspiration and electric vacuum aspiration for first trimester abortion, *Contraception* 67:207-212, 2003.

20. Grimes DA: Management of abortion. In Rock JA, Jones HW III, editors: *TeLinde's operative gynecology,* ed 9, Philadelphia, 2003, Lippincott Williams & Wilkins.

21. May W, Gulmezoglu AM, Ba-ThikeK: Antibiotics for incomplete abortion, *Cochrane Database Syst Rev* (4):CD001779, 1999.

22. El-Refaey H, Hinshaw K, Henshaw R et al: Medical management of missed abortion and anembryonic pregnancy, *BMJ* 305:1399, 1992.

23. Autry A, Jacobson G, Sandhu R et al: Medical management of non-viable early first trimester pregnancy, *Int J Gynaecol Obstet* 67:9-13, 1999.

24. Bagratee JS, Khullar V, Regan L et al: A randomized controlled trial comparing medical and expectant management of first trimester miscarriage, *Hum Reprod* 19:266-271, 2004.

25. Blanchard K, Taneepanichskul S, Kiriwat O et al: Two regimens of misoprostol for treatment of incomplete abortion, *Obstet Gynecol* 103:860-865, 2004.

26. Chung TK, Lee DT, Cheung LP et al: Spontaneous abortion: a randomized, controlled trial comparing surgical evacuation with conservative management using misoprostol, *Fertil Steril* 71(6):1054-1059, 1999.

27. Coughlin LB, Roberts D, Haddad NG et al: Medical management of first trimester incomplete miscarriage using misoprostol, *J Obstet Gynaecol* 24:67-68, 2004.

28. Creinin MD, Moyer R, Guido R: Misoprostol for medical evacuation for early pregnancy failure, *Obstet Gynecol* 89:768-772, 1997.

29. Demetroulis C, Saridogan E, Kunde D et al: A prospective randomized control trial comparing medical and surgical treatment for early pregnancy failure, *Hum Reprod* 16:365-369, 2001.

30. Henshaw RC, Cooper K, El-Rafaey H et al: Medical management of miscarriage: non-surgical uterine evacuation of incomplete and inevitable abortion, *BMJ* 306:894-895, 1993.

31. Hughes J, Ryan M, Hinshaw K et al: The costs of treating miscarriage: a comparison of medical and surgical management, *Br J Obstet Gynaecol* 103:1217-1221, 1996.

32. Johnson N, Priestnall M, Marsay T et al: A randomised trial evaluating pain and bleeding after a first trimester miscarriage treated surgically or medically, *Eur J Obstet Gynecol Reprod Biol* 72:213-215, 1997.

33. Muffley PE, Stitely ML, Gherman RB: Early intrauterine pregnancy failure: a randomized trial of medical versus surgical treatment, *Am J Obstet Gynecol* 187:321-325, 2002.

34. Ngai SW, Chan YM, Tang OS et al: Vaginal misoprostol as medical treatment for first trimester spontaneous miscarriage, *Hum Reprod* 16:1493-1496, 2001.

35. Nielsen S, Hahlin M, Platz-Christensen J: Randomised trial comparing expectant with medical management for first trimester miscarriages, *Br J Obstet Gynaecol* 106:804-807, 1999.

36. Sahin HG, Sahin HA, Kocer M: Randomized outpatient clinical trial of medical evacuation and surgical curettage in incomplete miscarriage [published erratum in Eur J Contracept Reprod Health Care 2002;7:iv], *Eur J Contracept Reprod Health Care* 6:141–144, 2001.

37. Tang OS, Lau WN, Ng EH et al: A prospective randomized study to compare the use of repeated doses of vaginal with sublingual misoprostol in the management of first trimester silent miscarriages, *Hum Reprod* 18:176, 2003.

38. Wood SL, Brain PH: Medical management of missed abortion: a randomized clinical trial, *Obstet Gynecol* 99:563-566, 2002.

39. Neilson JP, Hickey M, Vazquez J: Medical treatment for early fetal death (less than 24 weeks). *Cochrane Database of Systematic Reviews* (3):CD002253, 2006.

40. Lee DT, Cheung LP, Haines CJ et al: A comparison of the psychologic impact and client satisfaction of surgical treatment with medical treatment of spontaneous abortion: a randomized clinical trial, *Am J Obstet Gynecol* 185:953-958, 2001.

41. Zhang J, Gilles JM, Barnhart K et al: A comparison of medical management with misoprostol and surgical management for early pregnancy failure, *N Engl J Med* 353:761-769, 2005.

42. ACOG: ACOG practice bulletin. Clinical management guidelines of obstetrician-gynecologists. Number 67, October 2005. Medical management of abortion, *Obstet Gynecol* 106:871-882, 2005.

43. Consensus statement: instructions for use—misoprostol for treatment of incomplete abortion and miscarriage. Presented at expert meeting on misoprostol sponsored by Reproductive Health Technologies Project and Gynuity Health Projects, New York, NY, June 4, 2004.

44. Geyman JP, Oliver LM, Sullivan SD: Expectant, medical, surgical treatment of spontaneous abortion in first trimester of pregnancy? A pooled quantitative literature evaluation, *J Am Board Fam Pract* 12:55-64, 1999.

45. Luise C, Jermy K, May C et al: Outcome of expectant management of spontaneous first trimester miscarriage: observational study, *BMJ* 324:873-875, 2002.

46. Grimes D, Schulz K, Stanwood N: Immediate postabortal insertion of intrauterine devices, *Cochrane Database Syst Rev* (4):CD001777, 2004.

47. Vlaanderen W, Fabriek LM, van Tuyll van Serooskerken C: Abortion risk and pregnancy interval, *Acta Obstet Gynecol Scand* 67(2):139-140, 1988.

48. ACOG practice bulletin: Prevention of Rh D Alloimmunization. Number 4, May 1999. Clinical management guidelines for obstetrician-gynecologists. American College of Obstetrics and Gynecology, *Int J Gynaecol Obstet* 66(1):63-70, 1999.

49. Aleman A, Althabe F, Belizán J et al: Bed rest during pregnancy for preventing miscarriage, *Cochrane Database Syst Rev* (2): CD003576, 2005.

50. Rumbold A, Middleton P, Crowther CA: Vitamin supplementation for preventing miscarriage, *Cochrane Database Syst Rev* (2):CD004073, 2005.

51. Oates-Whitehead RM, Haas DM, Carrier JAK: Progestogen for preventing miscarriage, *Cochrane Database Syst Rev* (4): CD003511, 2003.

52. Lede R, Duley L: Uterine muscle relaxant drugs for threatened miscarriage, *Cochrane Database Syst Rev* (3):CD002857, 2005.

CHAPTER 7

Complications of Pregnancy

S E C T I O N   A   Gestational
Diabetes Mellitus

Richard Beukema, MD, Miranda Raiche,
MD, and David Turok, MD, MPH

Gestational diabetes mellitus (GDM) is defined as glucose intolerance acquired or first detected during pregnancy.[1,2] Women with GDM represent nearly 90% of all pregnancies complicated by diabetes. GDM has been associated with future progression to type 2 diabetes, hypertension in pregnancy, fetal macrosomia, shoulder dystocia, increased rate of cesarean section (CS), fetal hypoglycemia, and hyperbilirubinemia. This chapter focuses on the pathophysiology, epidemiology, diagnosis, and treatment of GDM.

I. PATHOPHYSIOLOGY

Glucose physiology changes during pregnancy, allowing for efficient nutrient storage for mother and fetus during feeding. In the latter months of normal pregnancies, increased insulin resistance and hyperinsulinemia occur.[3,4] Human placental lactogen, progesterone, prolactin, and cortisol levels are all increased in this period and have been implicated in insulin resistance. Their levels parallel the size of the fetus and placenta. Insulin resistance leads to a blunting of the action insulin takes on skeletal muscles that results in postprandial hyperglycemia. GDM has been described as a failure of the pancreas to respond to the increased demands of pregnancy, thus acting as a pancreatic stress test. The mechanism of this limited insulin secretion is not well understood, but pancreatic beta-cell dysfunction is likely linked to body composition and genetic factors, explaining the racial and familial prevalence of GDM in certain populations. The beta-cell dysfunction of GDM is a marker for future type 2 DM because up to 50% of women with GDM will later experience development of type 2 DM,[5] with most cases developing within 10 years. The fetal effects of GDM may be explained by the hyperglycemia-hyperinsulinemia hypothesis[6] based on the fact that glucose crosses the placenta whereas insulin does not. Maternal hyperglycemia results in fetal hyperglycemia and increased fetal insulin secretion, thus enhancing fetal anabolism.[7] Fetal tissues have varying degrees of insulin sensitivity with adipose, muscle, and large organs such as heart and liver being most responsive, whereas the brain is least affected. GDM may result in an infant with a large shoulder-to-head ratio, with a high birth weight with relatively normal head size and body length.[8] Fetal hyperglycemia is also associated with an increased metabolic rate, particularly in the third trimester. Animal models have estimated a 30% increase in oxygen consumption secondary to hyperglycemia and subsequent hypoxemia. In response to the increasing metabolic rate, the fetus increases its red cell mass. This can be associated with polycythemia and increased blood viscosity, leading to underperfusion of vital organs.[6] The increased red blood cell mass likely explains the increased risk for neonatal hyperbilirubinemia.

II. EPIDEMIOLOGY

A. Incidence

The incidence of gestational diabetes varies among populations and is most commonly estimated to be between 3% and 6%.[9,10] Ethnic groups with a greater rate of GDM include Hispanic, African, Native American, South Asian, East Asian, and Pacific Islander populations.[9] Recent trends show an increasing rate among all ethnic groups. A study of

36,403 singleton pregnancies in the Kaiser Permanente of Colorado system, which universally screens for GDM, showed an increase from 2% to 4% between January 1994 and December 2002 across all ethnic groups.[11] Currently, there are approximately 135,000 cases of GDM per year in the United States. A societal increase in body mass index (BMI) and glucose intolerance will likely drive this number upward in the future.

B. Classification

Diabetes is generally classified using the White classification:
1. A1—gestational diabetes not requiring insulin
2. A2—gestational diabetes requiring insulin

C. Risk Factors for Gestational Diabetes

Risk factors for gestational diabetes include[9]:
1. Previous history of GDM
2. Previous history of macrosomia, polyhydramnios, shoulder dystocia, and infant birth trauma
3. Age older than 25 years
4. Obesity or a BMI of greater than 25
5. Ethnicity: Native American, South Asian, East Asian, Latino, Pacific Islander, or indigenous Australian
6. Family history of diabetes in first-degree relative
7. Multifetal pregnancy[12]

D. Complications

Interpretation of data regarding maternal and fetal risk is problematic because of the lack of differentiation of gestational diabetes from preexisting diabetes and the frequent comorbidities of maternal obesity and hypertension.
1. Maternal
   The most remarkable outcome of gestational diabetes is the future risk for development of type 2 diabetes mellitus (DM). A 2002 metareview estimated a range of incidence rates between 2.6% and more than 70%.[5] The wide range was due to the different populations being studied and the length of follow-up, though most studies in the review showed an incidence between 15 and 45% with the highest rates in the first 5 years after delivery and lower rates after 10 years. The most common risk factor associated with subsequent type 2 DM is an increased fasting glucose.[5] Recurrence rates of GDM have been estimated at approximately one third.[13] Women with gestational

diabetes are more likely to have gestational hypertension, preeclampsia, operative delivery and earlier interventions to cause delivery.[9,14]
2. Fetal/Neonatal
   Women with GDM have an increased relative risk (RR) of having large-for-gestational age (LGA) infants of 1.54 (95% confidence interval [CI], 1.35-1.74) not explained by maternal obesity.[9,15] There is also an increased risk of shoulder dystocia, brachial plexus injuries, birth trauma, hyperbilirubinemia and neonatal hypoglycemia.[9,16,17] The association of fetal death and GDM has been debated for decades, and the data are confounded by the risks associated with overweight mothers.[9] Women who are overweight (BMI 25-29.9) or obese (BMI $\geq$ 30) before pregnancy have an increased risk for demise with an odds ratio (OR) of 1.9 to 2.7 and 2.1 to 2.8, respectively.[18]

III. DIAGNOSIS

A. Screening

A range of recommendations for screening for GDM has been published from various professional organizations. These guidelines range from recommendations for universal screening to risk-factor–based screening to recommendations for not screening because of insufficient evidence. Whether to screen for GDM has been a long-term issue of controversy. The U.S. Preventative Services Task Force (USPSTF) concluded that evidence was insufficient to recommend for or against screening for gestational diabetes,[19] as did the most recent Cochrane review.[10] The USPSTF did, however, find fair to good evidence that screening combined with diet and insulin therapy can reduce the rate of fetal macrosomia in GDM. The USPSTF cited the potential harm of false-positive results and a negative perception of health that may be associated with universal screening.

The American Diabetes Association (ADA) recommends risk assessment for clinical characteristics associated with a high risk for GDM (marked obesity, history of GDM, glycosuria, or a strong family history of diabetes) at the first prenatal visit.[20] Those women at high risk for GDM should be screened early as described later. The ADA states that women at low risk for GDM may forego screening. However, they must meet all the following characteristics: age younger than 25 years, normal weight, not in a high-risk ethnic group, no history of GDM or poor obstetric outcome, no first-degree relative with diabetes. Women who do not fall in the above categories are classified as "average risk" and are recommended to be tested between 24 and 28 weeks.

In 2001, an American College of Obstetricians and Gynecologists (ACOG) Practice Bulletin states: "All pregnant patients should be screened for GDM, whether by patient's history, clinical risk factors, or a laboratory screening test to determine blood glucose levels. The optimal method of screening is controversial, and there are insufficient data from which to draw firm conclusions."[9] The article notes that even in a population of mostly white patients, the above criteria of low-risk patients would exclude only 10% from screening[21] and universal screening may be more practical. During the next few years, additional publications will address screening for and treating GDM as two large-scale prospective studies are under way.[22,23]

1. Timing of screening
   a. Early screening based on risk factors: A first-trimester 50-g glucola test is recommended for patients with a history of prior gestational diabetes, a strong family history of diabetes, marked maternal obesity, maternal glycosuria, delivery of a previous macrosomic infant, or history of birth trauma.[20] It must be emphasized that testing should be repeated at 24 to 28 weeks if a first-trimester screen is negative. This screening is conducted to identify women at increased risk for development of pregestational diabetes.
   b. Universal screening between 24 and 28 weeks (Table 7-1)[20]
   c. Late screening based on complications: Additional screening may be considered later in pregnancy for those patients who experience

development of complications known to be associated with diabetes, such as macrosomia, polyhydramnios, or unexplained fetal death in utero.

2. Method of screening
   a. One-step testing: Patients at high risk for GDM may forego the 1-hour glucose challenge test (GCT) and proceed to the 3-hour glucose tolerance test (GTT) using the below values for the diagnosis of GDM.
   b. Two-step testing
      i. Fifty-gram 1-hour screening GCT: The most common screening test is the 50-g 1-hour GCT. For this test, a 50-g oral glucose load is administered to a pregnant woman without regard to fasting state, and a blood sugar measurement is made 1 hour later. Venous blood samples are necessary, as handheld capillary glucose monitors carry too much variation and have a 3% to 5% higher reading. Some patients cannot tolerate the 50-g glucola test because of gastric irritation. A possible alternative is to have the patient eat 28 jelly bellies in a 5-minute period.[24]

There are various cutoff values for the 1-hour GCT. The lower values will offer increased sensitivity but decreased specificity, whereas greater values will offer higher specificity but lower sensitivity. The most widely used cutoff value for the GCT, ≥140 mg/dl (7.8 mmol/L), is approximately 80% to 93% sensitive for GDM; an estimated 14% to 18% of women will screen positive with a positive predictive value between 17% and 18% with an estimated specificity of 86%

TABLE 7-1 Comparison of Differing Cutoff Values for Glucose Challenge Test

Cutoff Values	Sensitivity	Specificity	Percentage Screening Positive	Positive Predictive Value
140 mg/dl (7.8 mmol/L)	80-93%	86-89%	14-18%	17-18%
130 mg/dl (7.2 mmol/L)	90-99%	80-82%	20-25%	13-16%

The calculation of the positive and negative predictive values is based on an estimated prevalence of gestational diabetes mellitus of 3%. Adapted from Modanlou HD, Komatsu G, Dorchester W et al: Large-for-gestational-age neonates: anthropometric reasons for shoulder dystocia, *Obstet Gynecol* 60:417-422, 1982; and Lamar ME, Kuehl TJ, Cooney AT: Jelly beans as an alternative to a fifty-gram glucose beverage for gestational diabetes screening, *Am J Obstet Gynecol* 181:1154-1157, 1999.

to 89%. If one uses the more strict cutoff value of ≥130 mg/dl (7.2 mmol/L), the sensitivity is estimated to be between 90% and 99%, 20% to 25% of women will screen positive, and the positive predictive value is estimated to be between 13% and 15%[17,25] with an estimated specificity of 80% to 82%.

A random glucose value of ≥200 mg/dl (11.1 mmol/L) or a fasting serum glucose value greater than 126 mg/dl (7.0 mmol/L) meets the diagnostic criteria of diabetes if repeated.[20] Women with either of these values do not need to have a GTT, and if the results are confirmed, should initiate monitoring.

ii. The 100-g GTT (Table 7-2): When screening suggests a need for further diagnostic testing or the patient is at high risk, a 3-hour GTT is administered after an overnight fast for at least 8 but not more than 14 hours. Three days of unrestricted diet and physical activity precede the test; however, one must not smoke before the test. One must avoid carbohydrate depletion (<150 g carbohydrates/day) before the GTT because it may cause artificially high glucose values.[9] A fasting blood sugar is obtained and a 100-g glucose load is administered. Venous blood sugar samples are then obtained at 1, 2, and 3 hours after the glucose load. Two or more positive values are diagnostic of gestational diabetes.

GDM was historically diagnosed by whole-blood glucose greater than two standard deviations above the mean for each of the respective values.[26] The two sets of criteria are due to different methods of converting whole-blood glucose to venous plasma or serum glucose values; Carpenter and Coustan[27] also accounted for the change to an enzymatic method. Historically, the National Diabetes Data Group criteria have most often been used. Some centers have adopted a more strict approach to cutoff values with the Carpenter and Coustan criteria, which leads to a diagnosis of gestational diabetes in 54% more pregnant women than with current standards.[28] A previously mentioned clinical trial that showed improved outcome with the treatment of gestational diabetes used the lower Carpenter and Coustan values,[29] which are also endorsed by the ADA and other expert groups.[17] The ACOG endorses either criteria.

IV. PREVENTION

Women known to be at risk for gestational diabetes can be counseled preconceptually with regard to weight loss, diet, and activity. Fasting and 2-hour postprandial glucose levels and hemoglobin A1c values can be checked before pregnancy to identify women with previously unrecognized type 2 diabetes. Without this counseling and careful planning of pregnancy, many women with

TABLE 7-2 Criteria for Abnormal Result on 100-g, 3-Hour Oral Glucose Tolerance Tests in Pregnant Women

Blood Sample	Carpenter and Coustan*	National Diabetes Data Group†
Fasting	95 mg/dl (5.3 mmol/L)	105 mg/dl (5.8 mmol/L)
1 hour	180 mg/dl (10.0 mmol/L)	190 mg/dl (10.5 mmol/L)
2 hour	155 mg/dl (8.6 mmol/L)	165 mg/dl (9.2 mmol per L)
3 hour	140 mg/dl (7.8 mmol/L)	145 mg/dl (8.0 mmol/L)

Gestational diabetes mellitus is diagnosed if two or more of the values (venous serum or plasma glucose levels) are met or exceeded

Adapted from *Carpenter MW, Coustan DR: Criteria for screening tests for gestational diabetes, *Am J Obstet Gynecol* 144:768-773, 1982; and †National Diabetes Data Group: Classification and diagnosis of diabetes mellitus and other categories of glucose intolerance, *Diabetes* 28:1039-1057, 1979.

asymptomatic non–insulin-dependent DM present at 10 to 12 weeks of gestation with poor glucose control. Treatment at this time is much less effective at reducing malformations because early organogenesis has already taken place.

V. TREATMENT

In 2005, the publication of the Australian Carbohydrate Intolerance in Pregnancy Trial Group[30] showed significant decreases in "serious perinatal outcomes" in aggressively managed women with gestational diabetes. The prospective, randomized controlled trial (RCT) randomized 1000 pregnant women with abnormal glucose tolerance at 24 to 34 weeks of gestation to routine care or aggressive diabetic management. The study excluded women with preexisting diabetes by always screening with a fasting glucose and a 75-g 2-hour GTT. Women with a fasting glucose of $\geq$140 mg/dl (7.8 mmol/L) or with 2-hour GTT values greater than 198 mg/dl (11 mmol/L) were excluded because of meeting criteria for type 2 diabetes. Women in the intervention group participated in nutrition and activity counseling, and monitored blood glucose four times daily. Insulin therapy was instituted if fasting glucose was more than 99 mg/dl (5.5 mmol/L) or 2-hour postprandial values were greater than 126 mg/dl (7.0 mmol/L). The main outcome was a difference in serious perinatal outcome, a composite outcome that included fetal and neonatal death, shoulder dystocia, bone fracture at delivery, and nerve palsy. Serious perinatal outcome occurred in 7 of the 506 women in the intervention group and in 23 of the 524 women who received routine care ($p<0.01$). There were no perinatal deaths in the treatment group, but five in the control group (not significant). The number needed to treat to prevent one serious perinatal outcome was 34 (95% CI, 20-103). Of note, quality-of-life measures were evaluated thoroughly in this study and were similar in the two groups, but the treated group had fewer cases of depression (8% vs. 17%).The main objective of GDM treatment is to reduce adverse neonatal and maternal outcomes, such as macrosomia, shoulder dystocia, large for gestational age, neonatal intensive care unit (NICU) admissions, neonatal hypoglycemia, and cesarean delivery to the levels of pregnant women without diabetes.

Treatment of GDM requires active participation and understanding by the patient, because she needs to comply with diet, home self–blood glucose monitoring, and possibly medications. Treatment of GDM focuses on maintaining strict glucose control through diet, exercise, oral diabetic medication, or insulin injections.

A. Blood Glucose Monitoring

The ideal frequency of self-monitoring of blood glucose has not been established for patients with GDM. Commonly, blood glucose is checked four times per day: morning fasting to rule out fasting hyperglycemia, and 2 hours postprandial after the three main meals. For women who have demonstrated control with diet alone, there is neither objective evidence nor guidelines available to direct frequency of glucose monitoring. For these patients, it is possible to decrease the frequency of blood glucose monitoring to four times per day, 2 days a week. One should begin more frequent monitoring if two values per week exceed set limits. Postprandial testing is preferable to preprandial testing. In one randomized study of GDM patients who require insulin therapy, a comparison of postprandial and preprandial blood glucose showed those who measured their glucose levels after meals had statistically significant larger declines in hemoglobin A1c (-3.0 vs. -0.6%), lower birth weight infants (3649 vs. 3848 g), fewer infants with hypoglycemia (3% vs. 21%) and fewer cesarean deliveries (12% vs. 42%).[31]

The blood glucose levels recommended by the ADA are morning fasting blood glucose $\leq$105 mg/dl and 2-hour postprandial levels $\leq$130 mg/dl.[32] However, tighter glycemic control has been associated with fewer LGA (birth weight >90th percentile for gestational age) and macrosomic (birth weight $\geq$4000 g) neonates.[33,34] For this reason, many organizations and experts have recommend tighter glycemic control, with goal fasting blood glucose levels less than 90 to 105 mg/dl and 2-hour postprandial glucose levels less than 120 mg/dl.[9,35,36]

Hemoglobin A1c concentration is used to retrospectively monitor nongestational diabetes, but its role in monitoring gestational diabetes is unknown. Hemoglobin A1c concentration is not useful in the diagnosis of GDM.[37] Preliminary data reveal that the reference range of hemoglobin A1c in normal glucose-tolerant pregnant women is 4.0% to 5.5%.[38] Given the retrospective nature of hemoglobin A1c and the quickly evolving nature of GDM, it is not a timely enough indicator for management of GDM.

B. Diet

Registered dietitians and certified diabetes educators are tremendous resources for patients with any type of diabetes. The education they provide is particularly helpful when tight glycemic control is needed. However, a recent Cochrane review found that there was insufficient evidence to recommend dietary therapy in patients with altered glucose metabolism.[39] The review found no difference in the prevalence of macrosomia or cesarean deliveries in women with impaired glucose tolerance randomly assigned to receive dietary therapy or no dietary therapy. No trials evaluating dietary therapy met criteria to be included in the Cochrane review of efficacy of treatments.

Current recommendations for the ideal diet for women with gestational diabetes are based on expert opinion.[15,32,40] The ADA recommends nutrition counseling with a registered dietitian if possible. The diet must adequately meet the needs of pregnancy and be consistent with maternal blood glucose goals, but caloric restriction should be approached with caution. Recommended daily caloric intake is based on pre-pregnancy BMI. Obese women (BMI, ≥30) with GDM generally can restrict calories by 30% to 33%, to about 25 kcal/kg/day. Normal to overweight women (BMI, 20-29.9) with GDM should be prescribed 30 to 35 kcal/kg/day. Restricting carbohydrates has been shown to decrease maternal glucose levels and improve both maternal and fetal outcomes.[32] Restricting carbohydrates to 35% to 40% of total calories per day or reducing the glycemic index to 60% of daily intake is recommended. Though caloric restriction is recommended, ketonemia should be avoided because of a demonstrated relation between maternal ketones and intelligence quotient at 3 and 9 years of age in the offspring of mothers with GDM.[41,42]

C. Exercise

Women without medical or obstetric contraindications may start or continue an exercise program of moderate intensity.[15,20] It is thought that exercise improves glycemic control; however, one study suggests that neonatal outcomes are unchanged.[43]

D. Oral Hypoglycemic Medications

For women who do not respond favorably to dietary treatment alone, insulin therapy has been the mainstay of treatment for gestational diabetes. An oral medication that is safe and effective for the treatment of gestational diabetes has long been anticipated for added ease and patient acceptability. First-generation sulfonylureas cross the placenta and are not recommended because of concern for teratogenicity and neonatal hypoglycemia.[20] However, glyburide, a second-generation sulfonylurea, does not cross the placenta in measurable quantities, and studies have evaluated its safety and efficacy in the treatment of gestational diabetes.[44,45] In the largest study, 404 women with GDM were randomized to receive either glyburide or insulin, with the primary end point being achievement of glycemic control. Four percent of the glyburide group did not achieve good glycemic control and were switched to insulin therapy. Maternal outcomes such as cesarean delivery and preeclampsia were similar in both groups. Neonatal outcomes were similar for glyburide versus insulin, with no statistical significance in LGA (12% vs. 13%, respectively), birth weight, macrosomia (7% vs. 4%), hypoglycemia (9% vs. 6%), hyperbilirubinemia (6% vs. 4%), admission to NICU (6% vs. 7%), congenital anomalies (2% vs. 2%), stillbirth (0.5% vs. 0.5%), and neonatal deaths (0.5% vs. 0.5%).[46]

Although not endorsed by the ADA or ACOG, it has become common practice to use glyburide for the treatment of GDM because several other studies have reinforced its effectiveness and safety.[44,45,47] A usual starting dosage is 2.5 mg daily, increased at 2.5-mg intervals to a maximum daily dosage of 20 mg/day split twice daily. The failure rate is approximately 20%. Glyburide success is predicted if dietary failure occurred after 30 weeks of gestation, or if fasting blood sugar levels are less than 110 mg/dl and 1-hour postprandial levels are less than 140 mg/dl (sensitivity 98%, specificity 65%).[44] Predictors of glyburide treatment failure are women diagnosed before 25 weeks of gestational age, older maternal age, multiparity, higher fasting glucose levels, obesity, and a history of GDM.[48] Another benefit to patients is that glyburide is cost-effective compared with insulin.[49]

Metformin is used in patients with polycystic ovarian syndrome and continued through the first trimester of pregnancy; it is currently pregnancy category B.[50] However, before this medication is recommended for use in the treatment of GDM, further studies are needed to document its safety and efficacy.

E. Insulin

When the therapies described earlier fail to control hyperglycemia, women with gestational diabetes are started on insulin therapy. Traditionally, the starting daily dosage of insulin is 0.7 unit/kg/day, but overweight and obese women usually need 0.9 or 1 units/kg/day.[35] Using regular and NPH insulin, two thirds the total daily dose is given in the morning, two thirds of that being NPH and one third regular insulin, and the remaining one third of the total dose is given in the evening, split half NPH and half regular insulin. Insulin requirements typically increase throughout pregnancy as insulin resistance increases, requiring weekly evaluation of blood glucose levels and insulin regimens.

In the literature, only human insulin has been recommended because of the lack of data regarding insulin analogs, such as insulin lispro (Humalog) and glargine (Lantus).[35] Insulin lispro crosses the placenta at high doses or when bound to anti-insulin antibodies. Studies have demonstrated that insulin lispro does not cross the placenta at the doses commonly used for GDM.[51] In addition, anti-insulin antibodies are typically seen in individuals with type 1 diabetes, not in women with gestational diabetes. Several small studies suggest that insulin lispro (Humalog) and insulin aspart (Novolog) are safe and more effective at controlling postprandial glucose excursions than regular human insulin.[51,52] Also, insulin lispro was not detected in the cord blood of any of four neonates whose mothers received continuous intravenous (IV) therapy during labor.[51] ACOG cites the above-mentioned studies that insulin lispro does not cross the placenta and may be useful in improving postprandial glucose concentrations.[9] At this time, despite their widespread use, insulin analogs in GDM are not endorsed by all organizations because of lack of data demonstrating safety, and further research needs to be done.[20,35]

F. Antepartum Fetal Assessment

No evidence is available to support the effectiveness or the optimal regimen of antepartum fetal surveillance in women with GDM. A 2001 ACOG Practice Bulletin declared that there was insufficient evidence to recommend routine antenatal testing for women who are well-controlled with diet therapy and have no other complicating factors.[9] Expert opinion recommends that women who require oral hypoglycemic agents or insulin undergo biweekly antenatal testing starting at approximately 32 weeks of gestation. Acceptable forms of surveillance are nonstress test (NST), modified biophysical profile (NST and amniotic fluid index [AFI]), or full biophysical profile.[9]

G. Timing and Route of Delivery

The most dreaded complication of GDM is shoulder dystocia and associated permanent brachial plexus injury, bone fracture, or death. As described previously, shoulder dystocia and birth trauma are associated with an increased shoulder-to-head ratio and an increased fetal weight. Fortunately, these outcomes are rare. The overall occurrence of shoulder dystocia is approximately 1% of vaginal deliveries, 4% to 40% of which experience brachial plexus injury. Of those infants experiencing a brachial plexus injury, 75% to 81% resolve within the first months of life.[53] However, maternal diabetes is one of the most significant risk factors for shoulder dystocia, with an increased RR of six times that of nondiabetic pregnancies. The incidence of a shoulder dystocia of an infant weighing ≥4.5 kg is 4% to 22% in a mother without diabetes versus 20% to 50% in a mother with diabetes.[53] Clinicians face difficult decisions regarding delivery when fetal macrosomia is suspected. A recent Cochrane review on the subject included only 1 trial of 200 women, the majority of whom had GDM, comparing elective induction at 38 weeks versus expectant management. No increased risk for CS with elective induction existed, and there was a significantly decreased risk for macrosomia (RR, 0.56). There were no shoulder dystocia cases in the induction group, but three mild dystocia cases in the expectant management group.[54]

Debate continues regarding cesarean delivery when fetal macrosomia is suspected. Of particular concern is the error rate of approximately 13% (± 2 standard deviations) in estimating fetal weight by ultrasonography.[55] However, an estimated weight of ≥4000 g has a positive likelihood ratio of 5.7 (95% CI, 4.3-7.6).[56] An analysis of elective CS in mothers with diabetes with estimated fetal weights (EFWs) of greater than 4000 g or greater than 4500 g estimates that 489 and 443 CSs, respectively, would be needed to prevent 1 permanent brachial plexus injury.[57] However, the ACOG states that it would appear reasonable to recommend that patients with GDM be counseled regarding possible cesarean delivery without labor when the EFW is ≥4500 g. When the estimated weight is 4000 to 4500 g, additional factors such as the patient's age, delivery history, clinical pelvimetry, and the progress of labor may be helpful to consider in determining the mode of delivery.[9] In another study of 75,979 vaginal births, 84% of women with diabetes showed evidence of shoulder dystocia when the birth weight was ≥4000 g.[57] The author concluded that "elective cesarean delivery is strongly recommended for diabetics with fetal weights ≥4250 grams."[58] When the second stage of labor in a patient with GDM is prolonged, one should proceed to operative vaginal delivery with caution because this is also significantly associated with shoulder dystocia.[53]

H. Intrapartum Management

It is important to maintain euglycemia during labor to prevent neonatal hypoglycemia. Studies have shown that good glycemic control, antepartum and peripartum, results in less neonatal hypoglycemia, though this has usually been a secondary end point and has not been studied independently.[33,35] Women who use insulin for treatment of GDM usually discontinue scheduled insulin either at the onset of spontaneous labor or the night before a scheduled induction. Women with GDM controlled with diet alone should have blood glucose concentration checked on arrival at labor and delivery. This needs to be repeated only if the first value is greater than 120 mg/dl or if the patient eats. Those treated with glyburide or insulin need hourly blood glucose checks, though many do not require insulin during labor if fasting. Blood glucose is usually checked with a bedside monitor, with a target range of 80 to 110 mg/dl. If insulin is needed, either subcutaneous or continuous infusion is used.[59] An insulin drip is set up with a continuous IV infusion of normal saline (NS) at a rate of 125 ml/hr and varying drip rates of regular insulin based on blood glucose measurements (Table 7-3). The insulin drip usually can be stopped immediately after delivery.

I. Postpartum Management

1. Maternal

   After delivery, insulin resistance quickly decreases. Women with diet-controlled GDM generally will have normal glucose levels after delivery and do not require further monitoring until a 2-hour GTT at 6 weeks after delivery. Patients who were taking oral hypoglycemic medication or insulin should have fasting and 2-hour postprandial blood sugars monitored to determine any ongoing need

TABLE 7-3 Sample Intrapartum Insulin and Intravenous Fluid Drip

Blood Glucose (mg/dl)	Intravenous Insulin	Intravenous Fluid at 125 ml/hr
<120	0	D5LR
120-140	1 unit/hr	D5LR
141-180	1.5 units/hr	Normal saline
181-220	2.0 units/hr	Normal saline
>220	2.5 units/hr	Normal saline

for medication. Women should be encouraged to breastfeed because this improves lipid and blood glucose metabolism.[60]

2. Neonatal

   Neonates need to have serum measures of blood glucose to check for hypoglycemia. The first measurement should be within 30 minutes of birth. If the blood sugar is less than 40 mg/dl, the infant may be given oral dextrose, IV dextrose, or fed formula or breast milk. Neonates of mothers with diabetes should have fasting glucose checks before the first three feedings. If the neonate has hypoglycemia, then postprandial blood glucose should be evaluated as well. Sometimes a continuous IV infusion of dextrose is needed, which can then be slowly weaned as hypoglycemia resolves. Hyperbilirubinemia, polycythemia, and hyperviscosity are other potential neonatal problems. Finally, all infants should have a careful physical examination for cardiac, renal, gastrointestinal, or musculoskeletal anomalies. The risk for respiratory distress syndrome is not increased in infants of mothers with well-controlled diabetes at term.

VI. CONSULTATION AND REFERRAL

Many family physicians and midwives obtain an obstetric or perinatology consultation if the patient with gestational diabetes cannot maintain adequate glucose control with diet alone. Consultation may be helpful in any case in which the patient, family, or physician is uncomfortable or concerned. If insulin is required and consultant facilities are readily available, some clinicians prefer to transfer care of the patient for the duration of the pregnancy. If referral is less available, comanagement can often be conducted by the family physician with consultation as needed by the obstetrician or perinatologist. Clinicians should monitor for complications such as hypertension, proteinuria, polyhydramnios, suspected fetal macrosomia, intrauterine growth restriction (IUGR), or other signs of fetal compromise and should use the consultants in an appropriate manner to manage these conditions.

VII. LONG-TERM CONSEQUENCES AND PATIENT EDUCATION

A. Maternal

1. Risk for diabetes
   Woman with gestational diabetes have a high risk for development of type 2 diabetes and should be screened for type 2 diabetes 6 weeks after delivery. Screening is recommended with a 2-hour 75-g GTT, but two random blood sugar tests greater than 200 mg/dl or a fasting sugar level greater than 126 mg/dl also make the diagnosis. For those women who have a negative screen, annual screening should be initiated. A systemic literature review found that the incidence of type 2 diabetes increases rapidly in the first 5 years after the pregnancy with GDM, and then seems to plateau at around 10 years.[5] The review found the cumulative incidence of type 2 diabetes after the index pregnancy to be between 2.6% and 70%. Many practitioners accept a lifetime risk for development of type 2 diabetes after GDM of about 30% to 50%. Women with increased fasting blood sugar concentrations during pregnancy develop type 2 diabetes at a faster rate than those with only increased postprandial sugar concentrations. It is known that people with glucose intolerance can avoid development of diabetes with diet and exercise. This has yet to be studied in women with a history of gestational diabetes, but it stands to reason that a woman with a history of GDM could reduce her chance of development of type 2 diabetes with these steps as well. Counseling of the patient and her family regarding diet, exercise, weight control, and signs and symptoms of DM should continue at the postpartum visit and at yearly examinations.

2. Thyroiditis
   This common postpartum problem may be overlooked by the provider, and it is seen more often in women with other endocrinopathies, such as DM. Further discussion of this diagnosis appears in Chapter 20.

3. Birth control options and birth planning
   It is important to discuss contraception with all women during pregnancy so they have a clear plan when the postpartum period arrives. Women who have had GDM are at increased risk for development of GDM or type 2 DM that may affect future pregnancies. If a patient experiences development of type 2 diabetes, it is important to achieve euglycemia during the preconception period to minimize the risk for birth defects and other neonatal complications. No limitation exists on the type of contraception that a woman with a history of GDM may use; however, because medroxyprogesterone causes weight gain, this may not be a prudent choice.

B. Pediatric

Offspring of mothers with diabetes are at increased risk for being overweight throughout childhood and into adulthood. This is associated with both intrauterine growth and parental obesity.[61] Offspring of GDM mothers have increased risk for impaired glucose tolerance, DM, and metabolic syndrome, and in one study, this was not correlated with LGA versus appropriate-for-gestational-age birth weight.[62] Healthy eating habits and lifestyle should be encouraged throughout childhood to all children, especially to those with risk factors for being overweight and DM, in the hopes of preventing future adverse outcomes.

VIII. SUMMARY

Family physicians have an excellent opportunity to identify women with asymptomatic type 2 DM during routine screening or preconceptional counseling. Gestational diabetes is a common obstetric condition associated with increased perinatal morbidity and possibly also with fetal mortality. Screening pregnant patients at risk for GDM may reduce adverse perinatal outcomes associated with this condition. There are several acceptable screening methods.

Family physicians are familiar with testing, monitoring, and treatment of type 1 and type 2 DM in nonpregnant patients. With knowledge of modified values in the pregnant patient, family physicians are able to manage most pregnancies complicated by GDM. Consultation and referral are appropriate in selected settings and situations. There is insufficient evidence to support the need for elective induction for suspected macrosomia. Expectant management at term (using some form of antenatal fetal surveillance, usually NSTs) for women with GDM requiring insulin or oral diabetes medications is appropriate. The family physician should provide comprehensive postpartum care with a particular emphasis on encouraging breastfeeding and effective contraception for women at increased risk for development of type 2 diabetes.

REFERENCES

1. American Diabetes Association: Gestational diabetes mellitus, *Diabetes Care* 21:S60-S62, 1998.
2. Reinauer H, Home PD, Kanagasabapathy AS et al: *Laboratory diagnosis and monitoring of diabetes mellitus,* Geneva, 2002, World Health Organization.
3. Moore TR: Diabetes in pregnancy. In Creasy R, Resnik R, editors: *Maternal-fetal medicine,* ed 4, Philadelphia, 1999, WB Saunders.
4. Buchanan TA: Metabolic changes during normal and diabetic pregnancies. In Reece EA, Coustan DR, editors: *Diabetes mellitus in pregnancy,* ed 2, London, 1995, Churchill Livingstone.
5. Kim K, Newton K, Knopp R: Gestational diabetes and the incidence of type 2 diabetes: a systematic review, *Diabetes Care* 25:1862-1868, 2002.
6. Pedersen J: Weight and length at birth of infants of diabetic mothers, *Acta Endocrinol* 16:330-342, 1954.
7. Eidelman A, Samueloff A: The pathophysiology of the fetus of the diabetic mother, *Semin Perinatol* 26:232-236, 2002.
8. Naeye R: Infants of diabetic mother: a quantitative, morphologic study, *Pediatrics* 35:980-987, 1965.
9. American College of Obstetricians and Gynecologists (ACOG): Gestational diabetes, *ACOG Pract Bull* 1-14, September 30, 2001.
10. Tuffnell DJ, West J, Walkinshaw SA: Treatments for gestational diabetes and impaired glucose tolerance in pregnancy, *Cochrane Database Syst Rev* (1):CD003395, 2006.
11. Dabelea D, Snell-Bergeon JK, Harstfield CL et al: Increasing prevalence of gestational diabetes mellitus (GDM) over time and by birth cohort: Kaiser Permanente of Colorado GDM Screening Program, *Diabetes Care* 28:579-584, 2005.
12. Norwitz ER, Edusa V, Park JS: Maternal physiology and complications of multiple pregnancy, *Semin Perinatol* 29:338-348, 2005.
13. MacNeil S, Dodds L, Hamilton DC et al: Rates and risk factors for recurrence of gestational diabetes, *Diabetes Care* 24:659-662, 2001.
14. Tallarigo L, Giampietro O, Penno G et al: Relation of glucose tolerance to complications of pregnancy in non-diabetic women, *N Engl J Med* 315:989-992, 1986.
15. Casey BM, Lucas MJ, McIntire DD et al: Pregnancy outcomes in women with gestational diabetes compared with the general obstetric population, *Obstet Gynecol* 90:869-873, 1997.
16. Modanlou HD, Komatsu G, Dorchester W et al: Large-for-gestational-age neonates: anthropometric reasons for shoulder dystocia, *Obstet Gynecol* 60:417-422, 1982.
17. Kjos SL, Buchanan TA: Gestational diabetes mellitus, *N Engl J Med* 341:1749-1756, 1999.
18. Fretts RC: Etiology and prevention of stillbirths, *Am J Obstet Gynecol* 193:1923-1935, 2005.
19. Preventive Services Task Force (USPSTF): Screening for gestational diabetes mellitus: recommendation and rationale, *Am Fam Physician* 68:331-335, 2003.
20. American Diabetes Association, Position statement: gestational diabetes mellitus, *Diabetes Care* 27:S88-S90, 2004.
21. Danielenko-Dixon DR, Van Winter JT, Nelson RL: Universal versus selective gestational diabetes screening: application of the 1997 American Diabetes Association recommendations, *Am J Obstet Gynecol* 181:798-802, 1999.
22. HAPO Study Cooperative Research Group. The Hyperglycemia and Adverse Pregnancy Outcome (HAPO) Study, *Int J Gynaecol Obstet* 78:69-77, 2002.
23. Landon MB, Thom E, Spong CY et al: A planned randomized controlled trial of strict glycemic control and tertiary level obstetric care versus routine obstetric care in the management of gestational diabetes: a pilot study, *Am J Obstet Gynecol* 177:190-195, 1997.
24. Lamar ME, Kuehl TJ, Cooney AT: Jelly beans as an alternative to a fifty-gram glucose beverage for gestational diabetes screening, *Am J Obstet Gynecol* 181:1154-1157, 1999.
25. Esakoff TF, Cheng YW, Caughey AB: Screening for gestational diabetes: different cut-offs for different ethnicities? *Am J Obstet Gynecol* 193:1040-1044, 2005.
26. O'Sullivan JB, Mahan CM: Criteria for the oral glucose tolerance test in pregnancy, *Diabetes* 13:278-285, 1964.
27. Carpenter MW, Coustan DR: Criteria for screening tests for gestational diabetes, *Am J Obstet Gynecol* 144:768-773, 1982.
28. Schwartz ML, Ray WN, Lubarsky SL: The diagnosis and classification of gestational diabetes mellitus: is it time to change our tune? *Am J Obstet Gynecol* 180:1560-1571, 1999.
29. Langer O, Yogev Y, Orli M et al: Gestational diabetes: the consequences of not treating, *Am J Obstet Gynecol* 192:989-897, 2005.
30. Crowther CA, Hiller JE, Moss JR et al: Effect of treatment of gestational diabetes mellitus on pregnancy outcomes, *N Engl J Med* 352:2477-2486, 2005.
31. De Veciana M, Major CA, Morgan MA et al: Postprandial versus preprandial blood glucose monitoring in women with gestational diabetes mellitus requiring insulin therapy, *N Engl J Med* 333:1237-1241, 1995.
32. American Diabetes Association: Gestational diabetes mellitus, *Diabetes Care* 27:S88-S90, 2004.
33. Langer O, Rodriguez DA, Xenakis EMJ et al: Intensified versus conventional management of gestational diabetes, *Am J Obstet Gynecol* 170:1036-1046, 1994.
34. Langer O, Mazze R: The relationship between large-for-gestational-age infants and glycemic control in women with gestational diabetes, *Am J Obstet Gynecol* 159:1478-1483, 1988.
35. Langer O: Management of gestational diabetes: pharmacologic treatment options and glycemic control, *Endocrinol Metab Clin N Am* 35:53-78, 2006.
36. Metzger BE, Coustan DR, and the Organizing Committee: Summary and recommendations of the fourth international workshop-conference on gestational diabetes mellitus, *Diabetes Care* 21(S2):B161-B168, 1998.
37. Agarwal MM, Dhatt GS, Punnose J et al: Gestational diabetes: a reappraisal of HgbA1c as a screening test, *Acta Obstet Gynecol Scand* 84(12):1159-1163, 2005.
38. Lapolla A, Paleari R, Dalfrà MG et al: A study on reference range for HbA1C in pregnancy (Abstract 26). Presented at 5th International Workshop-Conference on Gestational Diabetes, Chicago, IL, November 11-13, 2005.
39. Walkinshaw SA: Dietary regulation for "gestational diabetes," *Cochrane Database Syst Rev* (2):CD000070, 2003.
40. Turok DK, Ratcliffe SD, Baxley EG: Management of gestational diabetes mellitus, *Am Fam Physician* 68:1767-1772, 2003.

41. Rizzo T, Metzger BE, Burns WJ et al: Correlations between antepartum maternal metabolism and child intelligence, *N Engl J Med* 325:911-916, 1991.
42. Rizzo TA, Dooley SL, Metzger BE et al: Prenatal and perinatal influences on long-term psychomotor development in offspring of diabetic mothers, *Am J Obstet Gynecol* 173:1753-1758, 1995.
43. Avery MD, Leon AS, Kopher RA: Effects of a partially home-based exercise program for women with gestational diabetes, *Obstet Gynecol* 89:10-15, 1997.
44. Chmait R, Dinise T, Moore T: Prospective observational study to establish predictors of glyburide success in women with gestational diabetes mellitus, *J Perinatol* 24:617-622, 2004.
45. Kremer CJ, Duff P: Glyburide for the treatment of gestational diabetes, *Am J Obstet Gynecol* 190:1438-1439, 2004.
46. Langer O, Conway DL, Berkus MD et al: A comparison of glyburide and insulin in women with gestational diabetes mellitus, *N Engl J Med* 343:1134-1138, 2000.
47. Jacobson GF, Ramos GA, Ching JY et al: Comparison of glyburide and insulin for the management of gestational diabetes in a large managed care organization, *Am J Obstet Gynecol* 193:118-124, 2005.
48. Barbour L, Kahn B, Davies J et al: Predictors of glyburide failure in the treatment of gestational diabetes (Abstract 4). Presented at the 5th International Workshop-Conference on Gestational Diabetes, Chicago, IL, November 11-13, 2005.
49. Goetzl L, Wilkins I: Glyburide compared to insulin for the treatment of gestational diabetes mellitus: a cost analysis, *J Perinatol* 22:403-406, 2002.
50. American College of Obstetricians and Gynecologists: ACOG Practice Bulletin. Clinical management guidelines for obstetrician-gynecologists: number 41, December 2002, *Obstet Gynecol* 100:1389-1402, 2002.
51. Jovanovic L, Ilic S, Pettitt DJ et al: Metabolic and immunologic effects of insulin lispro in gestational diabetes, *Diabetes Care* 22:1422-1427, 1999.
52. Pettitt, DJ, Ospina P, Kolaczynski JW et al: Comparison of an insulin analog, insulin aspart, and regular human insulin with no insulin in gestational diabetes mellitus, *Diabetes Care* 26:183-186, 2003.
53. Dildy G, Clark S: Shoulder dystocia: risk identification, *Clin Obstet Gynecol* 43:265-281, 2000.
54. Boulvain M, Stan C, Irion O: Elective delivery in diabetic pregnant women (review), *Cochrane Database Syst Rev* (2): CD001997, 2001.
55. Nahum GG, Stanislaw H: Ultrasonographic prediction of term birth weight: how accurate is it? *Am J Obstet Gynecol* 188:566-574, 2003.
56. Coomarasamy A, Connock M, Thornton J: Accuracy of ultrasound biometry in the prediction of macrosomia: a systematic quantitative review, *BJOG* 112:1461-1466, 2005.
57. Rouse DJ, Owen J, Goldenberg RL et al: The effectiveness and costs of elective cesarean delivery for fetal macrosomia diagnosed by ultrasound, *JAMA* 276:1480-1486, 1996.
58. Langer O, Berkus MD, Juff RW: Shoulder dystocia: should the fetus weighing ≥4000 grams be delivered by cesarean section? *Am J Obstet Gynecol* 165:831-837, 1991.
59. Caplan RH, Pagliara AS, Beguin EA et al: Constant intravenous insulin infusion during labor and delivery in diabetes mellitus, *Diabetes Care* 5:6-10, 1982.
60. Kjos SL, Henry O, Lee RM et al: The effect of lactation on glucose and lipid metabolism in women with recent gestational diabetes, *Obstet Gynecol* 82:451-455, 1993.
61. Schaefer-Graf UM, Pawliczak J, Passow D et al: Birth weight and parental BMI predict overweight in children from mothers with gestational diabetes, *Diabetes Care* 28:1745-1750, 2005.
62. Boney CM, Verma A, Tucker R et al: Metabolic syndrome in childhood: association with birth weight, maternal obesity, and gestational diabetes mellitus, *Pediatrics* 115:e290-e296, 2005.

SECTION B Multiple Gestation

Ellen L. Sakornbut, MD

Multiple-gestation pregnancies are associated with increased risks for mothers and infants. Risk stratification includes consideration of the exact type of multiple gestation and the other medical, social, and obstetric risk factors in the pregnancy. The detection of multiple gestation as early as possible in the pregnancy is essential in monitoring for growth problems and prevention of preterm birth. Early diagnosis is also helpful in prognosis, especially for determination of chorionicity and amnionicity.

I. MULTIPLE GESTATION AND ADVERSE OUTCOMES

A. Associations
Increasing numbers of multiple-gestation pregnancies correlate with older maternal ages and treatment of infertility. A large, population-based, cohort study in Canada demonstrated an increased rate of maternal complications such as gestational-onset DM, preeclampsia, cardiac complications of pregnancy, hematologic complications, operative interventions (including hysterectomy), postpartum hemorrhage, transfusion, and amniotic fluid embolism.[1]

B. Adverse Neonatal Outcomes
Adverse neonatal outcomes are increased in multiple gestation, and disparity exists in outcomes based on ethnicity in U.S. populations, with disproportionately poorer outcomes in blacks than whites.[2] Multiple gestation is a major risk factor for cerebral palsy.[3] Preterm labor, preterm spontaneous rupture of membranes, preterm birth, and low birth weight occur in up to 50% of multiple gestations. Multiple gestations account for 20% of the mortality in very-low-birth-weight (VLBW)

infants and 30% of the mortality in VLBW not attributable to congenital anomalies.[4] Increased rates of preterm births in monozygous multiple gestations may occur secondary to acute polyhydramnios, which has a weak association with preterm premature rupture of membranes.[5]

Discordant growth in multiple gestation is an independent predictor for adverse outcome. The average discordance in birth weight in twins with poor outcomes is 19% compared with 12% in a cohort of twins with normal outcomes.[6] In the absence of abnormal growth or IUGR, neonatal outcomes are similar for multiple gestation and singleton births at the same gestational age.[7] Abnormal or discordant growth may occur as a result of abnormal placental implantation, velamentous cord insertion or unequal sharing of a single placenta, and twin-twin transfusion syndrome.

II. CLINICAL FINDINGS

A. Common Presentations
Common presentations of multiple gestation include size/dates discrepancy, increased maternal serum α-fetoprotein (MSAFP) level, hyperemesis gravidarum, auscultation of two distinctly different fetal heart rates, or palpation of greater than two fetal poles on Leopold maneuvers.

B. Missed Diagnosis
Missed diagnosis occurs more often when the patient presents with the late onset of prenatal care. Poor attention to dating criteria and historical data increase the risk that a patient will be assigned an inaccurate and overly advanced gestational age. If preterm labor occurs, it may be assumed that the patient is at term. Diagnosis of twin presentation is unusual at the time of delivery but can occur even after delivery of the first infant.

C. Incidental Diagnosis
The finding of a twin pregnancy is commonly made since the advent of ultrasound in a first trimester ultrasound. It is not uncommon for one pregnancy to fail, resulting in "the disappearing twin."[8] In this instance, the existence of a twin would otherwise be unsuspected because fetal resorption in early pregnancy does not result in fetus papyraceus. Occasionally, fetal death of a twin in the second trimester may go undetected until delivery of a live fetus, as well as a small macerated twin (fetus papyraceus).

D. Risk Factors
Risk factors for multiple gestation include infertility therapy and use of gonadotrophic medication (dizygotic twins), positive family history (maternal) of dizygotic twins, increasing parity, and increasing maternal age.

III. VARIATIONS OF MULTIPLE GESTATION

A. Zygosity
Monozygous twins occur as a result of splitting of the embryo after fertilization of a single egg. The incidence of monozygotic twins does not vary worldwide (1/200-250). The incidence of dizygotic twins varies with ethnic groups.

B. Chorionicity and Amnionicity
Monochorionic placentation may result in a monoamnionic, monochorionic (MoMo) pregnancy or diamnionic, monochorionic (DiMo) pregnancy. Both of these represent monozygotic origin. Dichorionic, diamnionic (DiDi) twin gestation may be monozygotic (with early splitting of zygote) or dizygotic.[9]

IV. COMPLICATIONS RESULTING FROM MONOCHORIONIC PREGNANCY

Although premature birth is increased in dichorionic pregnancy, monochorionic pregnancy results in 3 to 10 times the mortality rate of dichorionic because of increased rates of IUGR, discordant growth, twin-twin transfusion syndrome, congenital anomalies, and single intrauterine fetal demise (IUFD).[10] Discordant growth can also occur with monochorionic pregnancy because of asymmetric cord insertion with unequal sharing of the placenta.

A. Twin-Twin Transfusion Syndrome
1. Pathophysiology
   Some degree of arterial and venous communication is found in the placental circulations of most monochorionic pregnancies. The degree of arteriovenous and arterioarterial communication determines whether a transfusion syndrome has occurred. Characteristics of a transfusion syndrome include[11]:

a. High-to-low pressure shunting (arterial to venous) creates a donor and a recipient twin. The degree of shunting in any given situation depends on the number of connections between the fetal circulations; the proportion of arterio-arterial, arteriovenous, and venovenous connections; and other anatomic factors.

b. The donor twin experiences hypovolemia, oliguria, or anuria, and is usually polycythemic. The recipient twin is subject to hypervolemia, polyuria, hypertension, and finally, fetal hydrops or heart failure. Anemia is dilutional.

c. Chronic disseminated intravascular coagulation (DIC) and damage to multiple fetal tissues may occur in twin-twin transfusion, regardless of whether IUFD has occurred.

2. Sonographic findings
Sonographic findings include oligohydramnios and small or absent bladder filling in the donor twin, and polyhydramnios and increased bladder filling in the recipient.

3. Growth discordance
Growth discordance is also diagnosed during ultrasound examination. Although serial examinations are most useful in observing twins to evaluation normality of growth, even a single examination may reveal substantial differences in biometric measurements and EFW.
Mortality rates vary for twin A and B with degree of growth discordance. If birth weight differences are less than 10%, perinatal mortality rates are the same. As growth discordance increases to a 25% difference in birth weight, the OR in perinatal death rate increases to 1.7.[12]

4. Treatment
Treatment of the twin-twin transfusion syndrome may be necessary to prevent fetal loss. Severe twin-twin transfusion syndrome occurs in approximately 15% of monochorionic twin pregnancies with high mortality rates if untreated. Patients referred with early diagnosis to perinatal centers may benefit from fetoscopic laser occlusion of anastomosing vessels or amniodrainage with severe polyhydramnios.[13]

5. Summary
Monoamnionic, monochorionic pregnancies are rare but have high risk for complications. Fetal loss is common as a result of cord accidents and anomalies. Route of delivery is generally operative because of risk for cord entanglement with delivery. Fetal survival is only about 60% in the older

literature but appears to be improving in more recent studies.

V. DIAGNOSIS OF MULTIPLE GESTATION

Establishment of diagnosis at the time of ultrasound examination should not occur without clear visualization of two heads, two heartbeats, and so forth. The diagnosis of twins then should not be made until triplets are excluded. This may be more difficult in late pregnancy. Chorionicity and amnionicity should be determined as soon as possible in gestation.

A. Chorionicity and Amnionicity
Early in pregnancy, the so-called gestational sac is actually a chorionic sac. Dichorionic twins in early pregnancy will present with two (thick) gestational sacs on transabdominal or transvaginal ultrasound. In early pregnancy, the amnion has not yet fused to chorion and is seen as a wispy structure on transvaginal ultrasound surrounding the fetal pole with the yolk sac adjacent to the embryo but external to its boundaries. Dual amnionic sacs are usually visualized only in this instance with transvaginal ultrasound.

B. Ultrasound Features
Ultrasound features of a dichorionic pregnancy in the second and third trimester include the following:
1. A "thick" membrane that is easily visualized: This feature may not be reliable.
2. Clear visualization of two distinctly separate placental masses: They may appear to be fused secondary to crowding.
3. The "twin peak" sign: This is represented by a small triangle of chorionic tissue at the juncture of the membranes and the placenta (dichorionic).

If a separating membrane cannot be found in late gestation, a gentle tap to the maternal abdomen may elicit a "fluid wave" across the membrane, causing sufficient displacement for visualization during the ultrasound examination.

VI. MANAGEMENT

A. Early Diagnosis
Early diagnosis assists the practitioner in defining subsequent management strategies. Early assessment of all risk factors will aid in determining an

appropriate site for care. The monoamnionic, mono-chorionic twin pregnancy should be referred to a high-risk center. Multiple gestations greater than twins should be referred. Obstetric referral or consultation should be considered for all twins, especially monochorionic. The risk associated with a first-trimester "vanishing twin" is probably not significantly increased.

B. Preterm Birth Prevention

Prophylactic hospitalization for bed rest in the third trimester has not been found to be protective against preterm labor and has been shown to be associated with poorer outcomes than outpatient management.[13] A recent Cochrane review found insufficient evidence to support or refute prevention of preterm birth with oral betamimetics.[14] Cerclage under ultrasound guidance has not been successful in preventing premature birth.[15]

C. Nutrition

The prevention of anemia requires the use of iron and folate supplementation (see Chapter 8, Section E). Optimal weight gain is about 44 lb (20 kg).[16,17]

D. Other Prenatal Surveillance and Interventions

Clinicians should monitor for urinary tract infections, asymptomatic bacteriuria, and pregnancy-induced hypertension. A prospective RCT of low-dose aspirin did not demonstrate reduction in preeclampsia in this high-risk group.[5]

E. Antenatal Surveillance of Fetal Growth

Each fetus is assigned a designation on the first ultrasound, and biometry is performed. Discordance of crown-rump length in the first trimester signifies a severe problem with the pregnancy, triggering immediate investigation. Greater than 10% discordance in crown-rump length between 11 and 14 weeks of gestation is associated with a 10-fold risk for chromosomal abnormality, major structural anomaly, or both.[18]

Serial ultrasound scans are indicated to assess for concordant fetal growth. Fetal growth velocity appears to be diminished in twin pregnancies during the third trimester using serial measurements of fetal biparietal diameter and abdominal circumference.[19] Growth discordance of 15% to 20% or greater should alert the clinician to a potentially serious problem.[20-22] "Pseudo" twin-to-twin transfusion syndrome has been

described; growth discordance appeared to have been the result of velamentous cord insertion in half the cases seen.[23] Conventional antenatal fetal surveillance should be used if any maternal/fetal complications arise or are suspected (see Chapter 11).

F. Management of a Second- or Third-Trimester Intrauterine Fetal Demise

Demise of one twin carries up to a 38% risk for death to the surviving twin and a 46% risk for neurologic injury to the co-twin. Antenatal necrosis of cerebral white matter has been noted more frequently in association with twin-twin transfusion syndrome and death of a co-twin.[24] Causes of IUFD in the second and third trimester include twin-twin transfusion syndrome, chronic DIC, severe IUGR, placental insufficiency, and abruption.[25] Maternal coagulopathy, although described with IUFD, does not appear to be common in any series of surviving twin pregnancy.

REFERENCES

1. Walker MC, Murphy KE, Pan S et al: Adverse maternal outcomes in multifetal pregnancies, *BJOG* 111(11):1294-1296, 2004.
2. Tan H, Wen SW, Walker M et al: The effect of parental race on fetal and infant mortality in twin gestations, *J Natl Med Assoc* 96(10):1337-1343, 2004.
3. Gabriel R, Grolier F, Graesslin O: Can obstetric care provide further improvement in the outcome of preterm infants? *Eur J Obstet Gynecol Reprod Biol* 117(suppl):S25-S28, 2004.
4. Magee BD: Role of multiple births in very low birth weight and infant mortality, *J Reprod Med* 49(10):812-816, 2004.
5. Caritis S, Sibai B, Hauth J et al: Low-dose aspirin to prevent preeclampsia in women at high risk, *N Engl J Med* 338(11):701-705, 1998.
6. Vergani P, Locatelli A, Ratti M et al: Preterm twins: what threshold of birth weight discordance heralds major adverse neonatal outcome? *Am J Obstet Gynecol* 191(4):1441-1445, 2004.
7. Garite TJ, Clark RH, Elliott JP et al: Twins and triplets: the effect of plurality and growth on neonatal outcome compared with singleton infants, *Am J Obstet Gynecol* 191(3):700-707, 2004.
8. Landy HJ, Weiner S, Corson SL et al: The "vanishing twin": ultrasonographic assessment of fetal disappearance in the first trimester, *Am J Obstet Gynecol* 155:14-19, 1986.
9. Benirschke K: The placenta in twin gestation, *Clin Obstet Gynecol* 33:18-31, 1990.
10. Pasquini L, Wimalasundera RC, Fisk NM: Management of other complications specific to monochorionic twin pregnancies, *Best Pract Res Clin Obstet Gynaecol* 18(4):577-599, 2004.
11. Crowther CA: Hospitalisation and bed rest for multiple pregnancy, *Cochrane Database Syst Rev* (1):CD000110, 2001.
12. Snijder MJ, Wladimiroff JW: Fetal biometry and outcome in monochorionic vs. dichorionic twin pregnancies: a retrospective

cross-sectional matched-control study, *Ultrasound Med Biol* 24:197-201, 1998.

13. Huber A, Hecher K: How can we diagnose and manage twin-twin transfusion syndrome? *Best Pract Res Clin Obstet Gynaecol* 18(4):543-556, 2004.

14. Yamasmit W, Chaithongwongwatthana S, Tolosa JE et al: Prophylactic oral betamimetics for reducing preterm birth in women with a twin pregnancy, *Cochrane Database Syst Rev* (3):CD004733, 2005.

15. Roman AS, Rebarber A, Pereira L et al: The efficacy of sonographically indicated cerclage in multiple gestations, *J Ultrasound Med* 24(6):763-768, 2005.

16. Spellacy WN, Handler A, Ferre CD: A case-control study of 1253 twin pregnancies from a 1982–1987 perinatal data base, *Obstet Gynecol* 75:168-171, 1990.

17. Worthington-Roberts B: Weight gain patterns in twin pregnancies with desirable outcomes, *Clin Nutr* 7:191-196, 1988.

18. Kalish RB, Gupta M, Perni SC et al: Clinical significance of first trimester crown-rump length disparity in dichorionic twin gestations, *Am J Obstet Gynecol* 191(4):1437-1440, 2004.

19. Taylor GM, Own P, Mires GJ: Foetal growth velocity in twin pregnancies, *Twin Res* 1:9-14, 1998.

20. Deter RL, Stefos T, Harrist RB et al: Detection of intrauterine growth retardation in twins using individualized growth assessment: I. Evaluation of growth outcome at birth, *J Clin Ultrasound* 20:573-577, 1992.

21. Deter RL, Stefos T, Harrist RB et al: Detection of intrauterine growth retardation in twins using individualized growth assessment: II. Evaluation of third-trimester growth and prediction of growth outcome at birth, *J Clin Ultrasound* 20:579-585, 1992.

22. Rode ME, Jackson M: Sonographic considerations with multiple gestation, *Semin Roentgenol* 34:29-34, 1999.

23. Mari G, Detti L, LeviD' Ancona R et al: "Pseudo" twin-to-twin transfusion syndrome and fetal outcome, *J Perinatol* 18:399-403, 1998.

24. Bejar R, Vigliocco G, Gramajo H et al: Antenatal origin of neurologic damage in newborn infants. II. Multiple gestations, *Am J Obstet Gynecol* 162:1230-1236, 1990.

25. Peterson IR, Nyholm HC: Multiple pregnancies with single intrauterine demise: description of twenty-eight pregnancies, *Acta Obstet Gynaecol Scand* 78:202-206, 1999.

S E C T I O N C Vaginal Bleeding in the Second and Third Trimesters

John C. Houchins, MD

Vaginal bleeding may represent a minor problem, such as a cervical polyp, or it may be the presenting feature of a catastrophic occurrence, such as a severe placental abruption. This section delineates the causes of vaginal bleeding, a diagnostic approach, and management strategies, especially those pertinent to the preterm gestation.

I. CAUSES OF VAGINAL BLEEDING IN THE SECOND AND THIRD TRIMESTER

Causes of vaginal bleeding in the second and third trimester include:

1. Second-trimester miscarriage
2. Cervical dilatation of preterm labor
3. Cervical and vaginal causes of bleeding
   a. Cervicitis and vaginitis—causative agents include chlamydia, group B streptococcus, gonorrhea, *Trichomonas,* bacterial vaginosis, and *Candida*
   b. Cervical polyp
   c. Cervical and vaginal lacerations (traumatic)
   d. Cervical carcinoma
4. Intrauterine causes
   a. Molar pregnancy
   b. Placenta previa
   c. Abruptio placentae
   d. Vasa previa
   e. Marginal sinus rupture
   f. Uterine leiomyomata
5. Coagulopathy—either pregnancy related or preexisting

II. DIAGNOSTIC APPROACH

A. Patients with Minimal Bleeding

Patients with spotting or minimal postcoital bleeding (less than a pad) can be evaluated in an expeditious manner in the office, assuming there are no other complicating factors, such as preterm labor or abdominal pain. They may be evaluated by ultrasound examination in a timely manner as outpatients. They should abstain from intercourse until the cause of bleeding is ascertained and report immediately more serious bleeding, decreased fetal movement, abdominal pain, or symptoms of labor.

B. Speculum Examination

No contraindication exists to a gentle speculum examination, regardless of whether the location of the placenta is known. This examination often provides key diagnostic information and can be performed in the office or labor room. The cervical cultures for pathogens and a wet preparation and potassium hydroxide (KOH) should be performed if signs or symptoms indicate possible infection. If mucopurulent cervical discharge or obvious cervical inflammation is present, empiric therapy may be indicated before culture results are available.

C. Heavy Vaginal Bleeding

Patients experiencing significant vaginal bleeding ("as much as a period") present an obstetric emergency and should be evaluated in labor and delivery (see Chapter 16, Section D). It is imperative to determine placental location in all patients with heavy vaginal bleeding.

III. MAJOR CAUSES OF VAGINAL BLEEDING: CLINICAL FEATURES AND MANAGEMENT STRATEGIES

A. Placenta Previa

Placenta previa occurs when the placenta partially or completely covers the cervical os.

1. Incidence

   Placenta previa is a common incidental finding on early ultrasound scans, occurring in 1 of 20 pregnancies. Only 1 in 200 pregnancies, or 1 in 10 of patients with this early diagnosis, has a placenta previa after 30 weeks of gestation. This has been described as placental migration; other theories have attributed this to the development of the lower uterine segment as pregnancy progresses. One study estimates that if the placenta overlaps the internal cervical os by 23 mm or less at 11 to 14 weeks, there is a 92% chance that there will be no placenta previa at term.[1] The concept of trophotropism has been introduced whereby the placenta is thought actually to grow toward a site in the uterus with improved vascularity.[2]

2. Clinical presentation

   Placenta previa occasionally presents in a previously undiagnosed patient with bleeding in labor. This condition presents commonly between 27 and 32 weeks of gestation with painless bleeding, sometimes after coitus. Patients with large, central placenta previas tend to present earlier, and bleeding tends to recur. Abruptio placentae can also be seen in conjunction with placenta previa. One series documented the largest blood loss in patients with combined previa and abruption.[3] The risk for placenta previa increases in patients with a persistent transverse or breech presentation.

3. Risk factors
   a. Previous uterine scar (risk increasing with increased number of CSs and decreased interval between births[4])
   b. Multiple gestation
   c. Previous abnormal placental implantation
   d. Advanced maternal age
   e. Increasing parity

4. Diagnosis

   The diagnosis of placenta previa versus a marginal or low-lying placenta often poses a diagnostic challenge. A marginal placenta previa can be partially circumferential around the cervical os without covering it. A Stallworthy placenta is low-lying and perceived to be a placenta previa because the chorionic surface is "rolled" over the cervical os.[2] It is important also to keep in mind that a full bladder can distort the cervix and lower uterine segment to give the appearance of a placenta previa where none exists. For this reason, among others, transvaginal ultrasound, during which a full bladder is not required, has been shown to be safe[5] and superior to transabdominal ultrasound in diagnosing placenta previa, especially when the placenta is posterior.[6] This approach should be used whenever the transabdominal scan leaves the diagnosis in doubt.

5. Complications

   Complications of placenta previa include the following:
   a. IUGR
   b. Postpartum hemorrhage
   c. Placenta accreta (especially in multiparas with previous CS)

6. Management strategies
   a. Incidental finding of placenta previa on an early ultrasound scan has no implications as to patient management except to obtain a repeat scan after 30 weeks of gestation.
   b. Prematurity is the major cause of perinatal mortality and morbidity. Therefore, management is directed toward prolongation of pregnancy if possible. In a symptomatic patient with a large central previa or a viable but severely preterm gestation, this may necessitate transfer to a perinatal center in case of recurrent bleeding.
   c. Although there has been some controversy about the use of tocolysis, it does not appear to be contraindicated to prolong the very preterm pregnancy, as long as the fetus is

not compromised and hemorrhage is not massive. Medium-sized retrospective studies have shown tocolysis does not add any risk to the fetus,[7] and possibly adds benefit such as increased birth weight.[8] However, no prospective randomized trials have shown a clear benefit to tocolysis. Magnesium sulfate is preferred to terbutaline, indomethacin, and nifedipine, and it has been the most widely used agent for tocolysis.[3,9]

d. One series demonstrated a perinatal mortality of 7.6% in pregnancies with second-trimester bleeding caused by placenta previa alone, even if the pregnancy was prolonged until the third trimester.[9]

e. When determining a route of delivery, the exact relation of the placenta to the cervical os should be determined, if necessary, by transvaginal or transperineal scan. Chances for a vaginal delivery increase dramatically (60% vs. 10%) when the placenta is 2.0 cm from the internal os.[10]

f. In the presence of known placenta previa in the third trimester, it is useful to look for placenta accreta using ultrasound with bladder filling, using transvaginal scanning if necessary.[3] Color Doppler imaging using the transvaginal approach has been shown to be an effective means of diagnosing placenta accreta.[11]

g. Fatal or exsanguinating hemorrhage is extremely uncommon in the absence of instrumentation or digital examination.

h. Cervical cerclage may reduce the risk for delivery before 34 weeks, birth weight less than 2000 g, and 5-minute Apgar less than 6. However, the studies providing the basis for this are small and have other methodological problems.[12,13]

i. In cases when the mother and the fetus are stable, and bleeding has stopped, two retrospective studies[14,15] and one RCT[16] suggest that outpatient management can be as safe as inpatient management for first and second bleeding episodes.

j. No RCTs provide guidance as to how many days of quiescence should be achieved before discharge is safe. Two to 3 days of no bleeding before discharge appears prudent. Hospitalization for the duration of the pregnancy usually follows the third bleeding episode.

k. In a stable situation, delivery should be planned once fetal lung maturity can be safely assumed using ACOG dating criteria or using fetal lung maturity studies.

B. Abruptio Placenta

Abruptio placenta occurs when there has been a premature separation, either partial or complete, of the placenta from the uterine wall.

1. Incidence
   Uterine abruptio occurs in 0.5% to 1.1% of all pregnancies,[17] with approximately 0.2% severe enough to result in fetal death.

2. Clinical presentation
   The presentation of this disorder is extremely variable, with hemorrhage, bloody amniotic fluid, or concealed hemorrhage being possible. A placental abruption often presents with pain in the abdomen or back. Abruptions are commonly graded on a scale of 1 to 3 based on amount of bleeding (often diagnosable only after delivery), degree of uterine irritability, and fetal well-being. Grade 1 abruptions have little bleeding, slight irritability, and reassuring fetal heart tracings. Grade 2 abruptions have moderate bleeding, have irritable to tetanic uterine activity, and show evidence of fetal compromise. Grade 3 abruptions are characterized by severe bleeding, painful and tetanic uterine activity, and fetal death. The relative percentage of each of these is 40%, 45%, and 15%, respectively.[17] The clinical presentation is discussed further in Chapter 16, Section D.

3. Risk factors
   Risk factors are additive. Hypertensive disorders are the most common risk factor, being present in 36% to 59% of all patients with severe abruptio.[18] Uterine anomalies and leiomyomata were uncommon causes of abruptio in one large series,[18] implying less risk than previously suggested with leiomyomata.[2,19]
   Many forms of substance abuse, especially tobacco (RR, 2.46), alcohol, and cocaine, are associated with an increased risk for abruptio placentae. Other conditions associated with abruptio include[20]:
   a. Sudden decompression of an overdistended uterus (ruptured membranes in polyhydramnios)
   b. Chronic hypertension and preeclampsia (RR, 4.39)
   c. Blunt abdominal trauma (see Chapter 9, Section C)
   d. Grand multiparity (RR, 3.60)

e. History of previous abruptio placenta (RR, 4.50)[21]

f. Velamentous cord insertion (RR, 2.53)

g. Advanced maternal age (RR, 1.62)

h. Previous CS (RR, 1.7)[21]

It is important to keep in mind, however, that most cases of abruption occur in low-risk pregnancies and are not predictable.[20]

4. Diagnosis

The diagnosis of abruptio may be made on ultrasound, but diagnostic priority should be given to clinical features. A negative ultrasound scan does not eliminate the diagnosis of abruptio.

5. Complications

Complication rates of abruption are common and increase if the fetus is stillborn at admission. The following complications are most frequent. Complication rates are listed as those for viable versus stillborn fetus at admission.[22]

a. Bleeding severe enough to require transfusion: 30.1% versus 63.3%

b. DIC: 7.2% versus 28.3%

c. Acute renal failure: 2.0% versus 5.0%

d. Acute respiratory distress syndrome: 2.0% versus 5.0%

e. Composite: 11.3% versus 68.3%

6. Strategies for antepartum management

a. Second-trimester abruptions have been thought to carry a poor prognosis for the pregnancy. Studies suggest that partial abruption in a severely preterm fetus may be managed conservatively if maternal and fetal parameters are stable.[3,9,23] Preterm patients who are stable should be considered for transfer to a tertiary facility.

b. The value of Doppler testing in the management of abruptio has not been demonstrated,[20,21,24] except in the case of accompanying IUGR. Antepartum assessment otherwise consists of NST and serial sonographic examination for fetal growth.[23,25]

c. Although previously considered controversial, tocolysis appears to be safe and helpful in delaying preterm birth and its associated morbidity in patients with partial abruptio and significantly preterm fetuses.[3,7,9,23] Magnesium sulfate appears to be preferable to β-sympathomimetics and nifedipine because of their hemodynamic effects. Indomethacin is contraindicated because of its effect on clotting.

d. It should be remembered that all Rh-negative patients with significant antenatal bleeding should receive 300 mg Rh-immunoglobulin (RhoGAM). If a larger fetomaternal bleed is suspected, a Kleihauer–Betke test may be performed to determine the number of units of RhoGAM indicated.

C. Bleeding of Unknown Origin

No cause will be found in approximately 30% of cases of second- and third-trimester bleeding.[26,27] These patients remain at greater risk for premature labor and delivery, and the associated morbidity and mortality. The infants of these pregnancies may also be at greater risk for minor neurodevelopmental abnormalities compared with gestational- and birth-weight–matched control infants.[27]

REFERENCES

1. Mustafá SA, Brizot ML, Carvalho MHB et al: Transvaginal ultrasonography in predicting placenta previa at delivery: a longitudinal study, *Ultrasound Obstet Gynecol* 20(4):356-359, 2002.

2. Finberg HJ, Benirschke K: Recent observations on the ultrasound diagnosis of placenta previa and placenta accreta with correlation to the principles of placental pathophysiology. Presented at the Proceedings of the American Institute of Ultrasound in Medicine, Annual Meeting, 1992.

3. Nielson EC, Varner MW, Scott JR: The outcome of pregnancies complicated by bleeding in the second trimester, *Surg Gynecol Obstet* 173:371-374, 1991.

4. Getahun D, Oyelese Y, Salihu H et al: Previous cesarean delivery and risks of placenta previa and placental abruption, *Obstet Gynecol* 107(4):771-778, 2006.

5. Timor-Tritsch IE, Yunis R: Confirming the safety of transvaginal sonography in patients suspected of placenta previa, *Obstet Gynecol* 81:742-744, 1993.

6. Sherman SJ, Carlson DE, Platt ID et al: Transvaginal ultrasound: does it help in the diagnosis of placenta previa? *Ultrasound Obstet Gynecol* 2:256-260, 1992.

7. Towers CV, Pircon RA, Heppard M: Is tocolysis safe in the management of third-trimester bleeding? *Am J Obstet Gynecol* 180:1572-1578, 1999.

8. Besinger RE, Moniak CW, Paskiewicz LS et al: The effect of tocolytic use in the management of symptomatic placenta previa, *Am J Obstet Gynecol* 172:1770-1775, 1995.

9. Saller DN, Nagey DA, Pupkin MJ et al: Tocolysis in the management of third trimester bleeding, *J Perinatol* 10:125-128, 1990.

10. Bhide A, Prefumo F, Moore J et al: Placental edge to internal os distance in the late third trimester and mode of delivery in placenta praevia, *BJOG* 110(9):860-864, 2003.

11. Lerner JP, Deane S, Timor-Tretsch IE: Characterization of placenta accreta using transvaginal sonography and color Doppler imaging, *Ultrasound Obstet Gynecol* 5:198-201, 1995.

12. Cobo E, Conde-Agudelo A, Delgado J et al: Cervical cerclage: an alternative for the management of placenta previa? *Am J Obstet Gynecol* 179:122-125, 1998.

13. Arias F: Cervical cerclage for the temporary treatment of patients with placenta previa, *Obstet Gynecol* 71:545-548, 1988.
14. Droste S, Keil K: Expectant management of placenta previa: cost-benefit analysis of outpatient treatment, *Am J Obstet Gynecol* 170:1254-1257, 1994.
15. Mouer JR: Placenta previa: antepartum conservative management, inpatient versus outpatient, *Am J Obstet Gynecol* 170:1683-1685, 1994.
16. Wing DA, Paul RH, Millar LK: Management of the symptomatic placenta previa: a randomized, controlled trial of inpatient versus outpatient expectant management, *Am J Obstet Gynecol* 175:806-811, 1996.
17. Gabbe S: *Obstetrics—normal and problem pregnancies,* ed 4, London, 2002, Churchill Livingstone.
18. Pritchard JA, Cunningham G, Pritchard SA et al: On reducing the frequency of severe abruptio placentae, *Am J Obstet Gynecol* 165:1345-1351, 1991.
19. Rice, KHH, Mahony BS: The clinical significance of uterine leiomyomas in pregnancy, *Am J Obstet Gynecol* 160:1212-1216, 1989.
20. Toivonen S, Heinonen S, Anttila M et al: Reproductive risk factors, Doppler findings, and outcome of affected births in placental abruption: a population-based analysis, *Am J Perinatol* 19:451-460, 2002.
21. Tikkanen M, Nuutila M, Hiilesmaa V et al: Prepregnancy risk factors for placental abruption, *Acta Obstet Gynecol Scand* 85(1):40-44, 2006.
22. Witlin AG, Sibai BM: Perinatal and maternal outcome following abruptio placentae, *Hypertens Pregnancy* 20(2):195-203, 2001.
23. Combs CA, Nyberg DA, Mack LA et al: Expectant management after sonographic diagnosis of placental abruptio, *Am J Perinatol* 9:170-174, 1992.
24. Rafla NM: The use of Doppler umbilical artery waveforms in placental abruptio: a report of two cases, *Eur J Obstet Gynaecol* 38:167-168, 1990.
25. Ajayi RA, Soothill PW, Campbell S et al: Antenatal testing to predict outcome in pregnancies with unexplained antepartum hemorrhage, *Br J Obstet Gynaecol* 99:122-125, 1992.
26. Chan CCW, To WWK: Antepartum hemorrhage of unknown origin—what is its clinical significance? *Acta Obstet Gynecol Scand* 78:186-190, 1999.
27. Spinillo A, Fazzi E, Stronati M et al: Early morbidity and neurodevelopmental outcome in low-birthweight infants born after third trimester bleeding, *Am J Perinatol* 11:85-90, 1994.

S E C T I O N D **Vaginal Birth after Cesarean**

Valerie J. King MD, MPH

I. EPIDEMIOLOGY

The influence of fad and fashion on the practice of childbirth is perhaps nowhere more evident than in the pendulum swings around vaginal birth after cesarean (VBAC). Cesarean delivery was uncommon in the United States before the twentieth century, but it became more common as improvements in anesthesia, blood banking, surgical technique, and antibiotic therapy were developed. The dictum of "once a cesarean, always a cesarean," attributed to Cragin, influenced U.S. practice for most of the twentieth century. Between 1970 and 1980, the rate of cesarean delivery more than tripled from about 5% to more than 16%. This rapid increase together with consumer demands for the option of VBAC prompted the 1980 National Institutes of Health (NIH) Consensus Development Conference on Cesarean Childbirth. The conference's expert panel recommended that for carefully selected women with a previous low-transverse cesarean, a safe trial of labor could be undertaken in facilities with appropriate services available.[1]

TOLAC became more common between 1980 and the mid 1990s. The VBAC rate peaked at 28.3% in 1996.[2] Beginning in 1984 and continuing through 1998, the ACOG encouraged a TOLAC in women with one prior transverse lower segment uterine incision. The initial NIH criteria began to be relaxed with increasing experience with VBAC and pressures to control both costs and the burgeoning cesarean rate. Some insurers and managed care providers went so far as to require TOLAC and refuse payment for elective repeat cesarean delivery (ERCD).[1]

In 1996, McMahon and colleagues' landmark population-based study of more than 6000 Nova Scotian women found that the symptomatic uterine rupture rate for women who elected a TOLAC was 0.27% greater than for women who had an ERCD.[3] This rate was greater than previously thought and, together with other emerging data about the risks of TOLAC, led to narrowed parameters for the practice of TOLAC and more restrictive practice guidelines.[1,4]

The total cesarean rate in the United States increased 6% in 2004 to an all-time high of 29.1%. Contributing to this increase is the nationwide decline in VBAC. The VBAC rate has declined 67% since 1996 and stood at 9.2% in 2004.[5]

II. RISKS AND BENEFITS OF TRIAL OF LABOR AFTER PRIOR CESAREAN BIRTH

No RCTs have compared the maternal and fetal outcomes of TOLAC versus ERCD. The best data on the RRs and benefits of TOLAC and ERCD come from prospective cohort studies, but only lower quality evidence is available for some outcomes.

Overall, poor outcomes as a result of TOLAC are rare. However, some outcomes such as uterine rupture are true obstetric emergencies that must be dealt with promptly to avoid maternal and fetal morbidity and mortality. The risks of TOLAC must be balanced against the risks for experiencing multiple cesarean deliveries. It is increasingly recognized that prior cesarean delivery is a risk factor for such outcomes as abnormal placentation and fetal loss in subsequent pregnancies. The risks and benefits of TOLAC must not only be weighed against risks in the current pregnancy, but also evaluated in the context the woman's plans for future childbearing.

The lowest risk to the woman and her fetus is probably achieved by an uncomplicated TOLAC leading to a successful VBAC. The greatest risks are found in TOLAC labors that result in complications and ultimate emergency repeat cesarean delivery. An ERCD confers intermediate risk. Thus, the best and worst outcomes are both associated with the choice of TOLAC. This feature, together with our inability to precisely predict successful, uncomplicated VBAC, make decisions about TOLAC and ERCD complex for both women and their caregivers.

A. Harms and Benefits of Trial of Labor

1. Uterine rupture

   The evidence base is fair to poor for this outcome because of inconsistencies in definitions used across studies. A high-quality systematic review was commissioned by the Agency for Healthcare Research and Quality (AHRQ).[6] The review reports on outcomes from two large population-based retrospective cohort studies, 15 prospective cohort studies, 2 case–control studies, and 2 case series. Data on symptomatic uterine rupture came from 11 observational studies with more than 20,000 deliveries among them. The additional risk for uterine rupture with TOLAC compared with ERCD is 2.7 events per 1000 TOLAC attempts (95% CI, 0.73-4.7/1000).[7] Based on data from the studies included in this systematic review, 370 ERCD deliveries (95% CI, 213-1370) would have to be performed to prevent 1 symptomatic uterine rupture.[8] In 2005, the American Academy of Family Physicians (AAFP) published an update of this systematic review that did not find additional studies that would contribute to the question of uterine rupture with TOLAC.[1]

Landon and colleagues[9,10] recently reported the results of the multicenter National Institute of Child Health and Human Development (NICHD) Maternal and Fetal Medicine Units (MFMU) network study of more than 33,000 women undergoing TOLAC or ERCD in U.S. academic medical centers. Nearly 18,000 women underwent a TOLAC, and 95% of them had a single prior cesarean delivery. There were 124 cases of uterine rupture among these women. Nine uterine ruptures occurred among 975 women with a history of multiple cesarean deliveries. The remaining 115 cases of uterine rupture occurred in the 16,915 women who had a history of a single prior cesarean.[10] No cases of uterine rupture were reported among 15,801 women who had ERCD.[9] The investigators determined risk factors for uterine rupture by constructing multiple logistic regression models to control for covariates and confounders. The ORs for risk factors in the final model are presented in Table 7-4.

2. Maternal mortality

   No maternal deaths were reported across the studies in Guise and colleagues' systematic reviews.[6,7] The MFMU study recorded 3 maternal deaths among 17,898 TOLAC patients (0.02%) and 7 maternal deaths among 15,801 women who had ERCD (0.04%). This difference was not statistically significant (OR, 0.38; 95% CI, 0.10-1.46).[9]

3. Perinatal mortality

   Estimation of perinatal mortality is imprecise because of the rarity of the outcome and inconsistencies in reporting and outcome assessment

---

TABLE 7-4 Factors Associated with Uterine Rupture

Factors	Odds Ratio (95% Confidence Interval)
Multiple prior cesarean deliveries	1.69 (0.75-3.29)
Oxytocin augmentation	2.31 (1.35-4.05)
Induction of labor	2.81 (1.56-5.22)
Epidural use	1.23 (0.76-2.10)
Prior vaginal delivery	0.82 (0.53-1.25)
Years since last cesarean (per year)	0.92 (0.86-0.98)
Dilation at admission ≥4 cm	0.96 (0.85-1.08)

across studies. Among the 11 observational studies in this systematic review, 6 had no perinatal deaths reported. Rates in the other five studies varied widely. Overall, there were 6 perinatal deaths associated with 74 symptomatic ruptures, corresponding to an increase of 1.4 perinatal deaths (95% CI, 0-9.8) per 10,000 TOLAC attempts.[8]

The MFMU study reported 18 cases of antepartum stillbirth among 15,338 TOLAC attempts and 8 among the 15,014 ERCDs at 37 to 38 weeks of gestation (OR, 2.93; 95% CI, 1.27-6.75). At 39 weeks of gestation or greater, there were 16 cases of antepartum stillbirth in the TOLAC group and 5 in the ERCD group (OR, 2.70; 95% CI, 0.99-7.38). There were two cases of intrapartum stillbirth, one in each gestational age period and both in the TOLAC group. There were 13 neonatal deaths and 12 cases of hypoxic-ischemic encephalopathy (HIE) in the TOLAC group versus no deaths and 7 cases of HIE in the ERCD group. Two of the neonatal deaths and seven cases of HIE in the TOLAC group were related to uterine rupture.[9] Concerns exist about potential selection bias in this study, as well as speculation about whether differences among the women included in the TOLAC and ERCD groups, such as gestational age, might account for at least some of the outcomes observed. For example, it was unclear whether women with an antepartum stillbirth may have chosen a TOLAC after the stillbirth had been diagnosed.[11]

4. Hysterectomy
The AHRQ systematic review found five cohort studies that reported hysterectomy related to uterine rupture. A total of 7 hysterectomies occurred in 60 incidents of symptomatic rupture. Given these data, 3.4 women having a TOLAC would experience a hysterectomy because of a uterine rupture per 10,000 TOLAC attempts.[6,8] The MFMU study did not find a statistically significant difference in hysterectomy rates with 41 among 17,898 in the TOLAC group and 47 among 15,801 in the ERCD group (OR, 0.77; 95% CI, 0.51-1.17).[9]

5. Need for transfusion
Two good-quality studies in the AAFP update of the AHRQ systematic review found conflicting results regarding the need for maternal transfusion with TOLAC versus ERCD. The first study found rates of 1.1% for TOLAC versus 1.3% for ERCD. The second study found a statistically significant difference with 0.72% for TOLAC and 1.72% for ERCD.[1] The MFMU study found a statistically greater incidence of transfusion in the TOLAC group compared with the ERCD group; 1.7% versus 1.0% (OR, 1.71; 95% CI, 1.41-2.08).[9]

6. Infection
Assessment of the magnitude of this outcome is also hampered by poor-quality evidence and inconsistent definitions across studies. The ranges of infectious complications, including both wound infections and puerperal infections, are 5.3% to 6.7% for TOLAC and 6.4% to 9.7% for ERCD.[7] The MFMU study evaluated rates of endometritis among women undertaking a TOLAC compared with those having ERCD. They found that rates of endometritis were greater in the TOLAC group: 2.9% versus 1.8% (OR, 1.62; 95% CI, 1.40-1.87).[9]

B. Risks of Prior Cesarean Delivery on Subsequent Pregnancies

The literature on the RRs of TOLAC and ERCD has concentrated on those that occur in the "index" or current pregnancy in which a TOLAC may or may not be considered. However, newer data about the risks of multiple repeat cesarean deliveries are beginning to emerge. It is clear that as the number of cesarean deliveries a woman has had increase, so do her risks for placenta previa, placenta accreta, placental abruption, cesarean hysterectomy, and unexplained stillbirth.

1. Maternal outcomes: abnormal placentation and hysterectomy
Faiz and Ananth[12] published a review of abnormal placentation after prior cesarean delivery using literature published between 1966 and 2000. They found 58 observational studies, including 32 retrospective hospital-based cohort studies, 15 hospital-based case–control studies, 6 population-based case–control studies, and 5 population-based retrospective cohort studies. The study populations ranged from 6576 to more than 1.8 million pregnancies. The authors found 21 studies that investigated the relation between previous cesarean and placenta previa. Their pooled OR estimates ranged from 1.9 (95% CI, 1.7-2.2) to 3.5 (95% CI, 2.7-4.6), with the lower estimates based on the four studies they considered to be well-designed.

An update of Faiz and Ananth's systematic review[12] was conducted for the NIH State-of-the-Science Conference on Cesarean Delivery on Maternal

Request.[13] This update searched for literature published from 2000 to 2005, using the original search strategy that Faiz and Ananth used. The authors located 131 articles and included 13 in their analysis. Adjusted ORs for placenta previa with one or more cesarean deliveries ranged from 1.32 (95% CI, 1.04-1.68) to 4.7 (95% CI, 1.9-11.4), comparable with the ranges found in the original study. One study published after Viswanathan and colleagues' review[13] is large, population based, and relevant to this issue. Data from the Missouri longitudinally linked birth certificate and fetal morality files from 1989 to 1997 were used by Getahun and colleagues[14] to examine the association among cesarean delivery, placenta previa, and abruption in subsequent pregnancies. The study looked at second and third births for each mother and included more than 156,000 women with their first 2 pregnancies. Among women with a history of a prior cesarean delivery, there were 116,814 subsequent vaginal deliveries and 39,661 subsequent cesarean births. The pregnancy after a cesarean delivery was more likely to be complicated by placenta previa (RR, 1.5; 95% CI, 1.3-1.8) compared with vaginal delivery. Women who had a cesarean delivery in both the first and second pregnancies had a two-fold increased risk for placenta previa in the subsequent pregnancy (RR, 2.0; 95% CI, 1.3-3.0). Women who had a cesarean delivery for their first birth were more likely to experience a placental abruption compared with women who had a vaginal first birth (RR, 1.3; 95% CI, 1.2-1.5). As with placenta previa, the risk for placental abruption in the third pregnancy increased markedly with a history of two prior cesarean deliveries (RR, 1.3; 95% CI, 1.0-1.8). Pregnancy occurring within a year from the time from the first cesarean delivery was associated with grater risks for both placenta previa (RR, 1.7; 95% CI, 0.9-3.1) and placental abruption (RR, 1.5; 95% CI, 1.1-2.3) compared with pregnancy spacing of more than a year.[14]

Pare and colleagues[15] conducted a decision analysis comparing the rates of hysterectomy for placenta accreta or other indications among women with one prior cesarean delivery who had a TOLAC versus those who had an ERCD. They found that for women planning no additional pregnancies, a policy of TOLAC in the second pregnancy led to 80 additional hysterectomies per 100,000 deliveries than did ERCD (267/100,000 vs. 187/100,000). However, for women planning at least one more pregnancy, a policy of ERCD led to an excess of 558 hysterectomies per 100,000 deliveries. The authors conclude that the downstream risks of multiple CSs outweigh the immediate risks of TOLAC for women who plan to have at least two children after a first pregnancy in which a cesarean is required.[14]

The NIH State-of-the Science Conference held in March 2006 examined the question of cesarean delivery on maternal request. Although this conference was dealing with issues of elective cesarean delivery, some of the data reviewed are applicable to the question of VBAC. The conference statement recommends that because of the increasing risks for placenta accreta and placenta previa with each subsequent cesarean procedure, cesarean on maternal request not be recommended for women desiring "several" children, but it did not specify a particular number.[13,16]

2. Fetal and neonatal outcomes

Smith and colleagues[17] conducted a linked longitudinal vital statistics study using Scottish registry data from 1980 to 1998. They included 120,633 singleton second pregnancies and compared the rate of unexplained antepartum stillbirth among women who had cesarean versus vaginal first deliveries. A significant increase was noted in the incidence of unexplained antepartum stillbirth among women with a prior cesarean delivery (2.39 vs. 1.44 per 10,000 women per week). The excess risk was apparent from 34 weeks onward (hazard ratio [HR], 2.23; 95% CI, 1.48-3.36). The HR estimate increased when controlling for maternal and obstetric characteristics (HR, 2.74; 95% CI, 1.74-4.30). The absolute risk of unexplained antepartum stillbirth at or after 39 weeks doubled for women with a history of a previous cesarean birth (0.5/1000 vs. 1.1/1000).

III. FACTORS ASSOCIATED WITH SUCCESSFUL TRIAL OF LABOR OR NEED FOR REPEAT CESAREAN BIRTH

A. Overall Rates of Vaginal Delivery in Women with a Prior Cesarean Birth

Based on a comprehensive systematic review, 80% of women with spontaneous onset of labor and a history of a prior cesarean delivered vaginally (range, 65-89%).[7] An average of 68% of women who received oxytocin in these studies delivered vaginally (range, 56-82%), although the difference compared with women who labored spontaneously was not statistically significant. A total of eight prospective cohort studies contributed to these findings. A large, population-based, cohort study of 6138 women from Nova Scotia, Canada, found that 52.9% of women with 1 prior nonvertical cesarean elected a trial of labor. Of these, 1962 (60.4%) women delivered vaginally.[3] More recently, the large multicenter MFMU study, which included more than 14,000 women undertaking TOLAC, found that 73.6% had a successful TOLAC.[9]

Many studies are reviewing factors that influence the ultimate mode of delivery for women who have had a prior cesarean birth. Most of these studies are of poor quality because of their lack of attention to confounding factors. The MFMU study by Landon and colleagues is large, recent, and had good data quality control. Although it was conducted in multiple university settings across the United States, it probably represents the most accurate picture for current obstetric practice in this country. No such large studies have been conducted exclusively in family medicine or midwifery settings. The MFMU study is also important because it helps to elucidate the relative importance of factors that are associated with vaginal delivery after cesarean birth.[9,10,18]

B. Demographic Factors Associated with Vaginal Birth after Cesarean

The MFMU study examined single demographic and historical factors that were associated with VBAC.[9] Univariate analysis demonstrated the following factors as statistically significant as individual predictors of TOLAC success. African American and Hispanic women were less likely to deliver vaginally (OR, 0.69; 95% CI, 0.63-0.65; and OR, 0.65; 95% CI, 0.59-0.72, respectively). Unmarried women and those who smoked were slightly less likely to have successful TOLAC (OR, 0.88; 95% CI, 0.82-0.95; and OR, 0.87; 95% CI, 0.78-0.96, respectively). Insurance status was associated with VBAC, with women having private insurance being more likely to deliver vaginally. Women with nonprivate insurance and those who were uninsured had lower rates of successful TOLAC (OR, 0.88; 95% CI, 0.81-0.95; and OR, 0.74; 95% CI, 0.66-0.83). Obese women with a BMI of greater than or equal to 30 were less likely to have a vaginal birth than those with a BMI less than 30 (OR, 0.55; 95% CI, 0.51-0.60).

C. Obstetric and Historical Factors Associated with Successful Trial of Labor after Cesarean

Landon and colleagues[9,10,18] also evaluated individual obstetric factors that were associated with successful TOLAC. The indication for the prior cesarean operation was associated with vaginal delivery in this population. Compared with malpresentation as a reason for the prior cesarean, dystocia, nonreassuring fetal well-being, and other reasons were associated with lower rates of vaginal delivery (OR, 0.34; 95% CI, 0.30-0.37; OR, 0.51; 95% CI, 0.45-0.58; and OR, 0.67; 95% CI, 0.58-0.67, respectively). Women who were less than 2 years from their prior cesarean birth were less likely to deliver vaginally (OR, 0.70; 95% CI, 0.64-0.76). The authors found that induction or augmentation of labor was associated with decreased rates of vaginal delivery (OR, 0.50; 95% CI, 0.45-0.55; and OR, 0.68; 95% CI, 0.62-0.75, respectively). Admission cervical dilation of greater than 4 cm was, not surprisingly, associated with greater rates of TOLAC success. Women who had cervical dilation of 4 cm or less at admission had more than 60% fewer vaginal deliveries (OR, 0.39; 95% CI, 0.36-0.42). Use of epidural anesthesia was positively related to vaginal delivery. Women who did not have an epidural were less likely to deliver vaginally (OR, 0.37; 95% CI, 0.33-0.41). However, the authors believed that this finding may have been related to women who intended to have a cesarean delivery but arrived in labor and ultimately had spinal anesthesia for their operation. Compared with women who were at 41 weeks of gestation or more, women who were 37 to 41 weeks of gestation also had greater rates of vaginal delivery (OR, 0.61; 95% CI, 0.55-0.68).

D. Summary of Factors Associated with Successful Trial of Labor after Cesarean

Although these individual demographic and obstetric factors were all related to TOLAC success, few factors remained statistically significant when multiple logistic regression was used to control for multiple factors simultaneously. The MFMU study found six factors that were associated with successful TOLAC: having had a previous vaginal delivery, infant birth weight less than 4000 g, spontaneous labor, white race, no maternal comorbid diseases (diabetes,

TABLE 7-5 Factors Associated with Successful Vaginal Birth after Cesarean Section

Factors	Odds Ratio (95% Confidence Interval)
Prior vaginal delivery	3.9 (3.6-4.3)
Birth weight <4 kg	2.0 (1.8-2.3)
White race	1.8 (1.6-1.9)
Prior indication not dystocia	1.7 (1.5-1.8)
Spontaneous labor	1.6 (1.5-1.8)
No maternal disease	1.2 (1.1-1.4)

asthma, thyroid diseases, seizure disorder, chronic hypertension requiring medications, renal disease, and connective tissue disease), and the previous cesarean not because of dystocia.[9,10,18] Overwhelmingly, the most predictive factor in favor of a vaginal delivery was a history of a prior vaginal delivery. The predictive factors in the multivariate analysis are listed in Table 7-5.

Landon and colleagues[9,10,18] also examined combinations of predictive factors that were associated with vaginal delivery. For example, women with a history of previous dystocia who were induced, had no prior vaginal deliveries, and were obese had the lowest vaginal delivery rate at 39.8%. Women with malpresentation as the reason for their prior cesarean birth, but who had had a vaginal birth previously, were nonobese, and labored spontaneously had high rates of vaginal delivery (94.8%). Regardless of the indication for the prior cesarean, nonobese women with spontaneous onset of labor and a prior vaginal birth had vaginal delivery rates in excess of 90%.

E. Influence of Maternal Preferences on Trial of Labor after Cesarean

A woman's choice of TOLAC or ERCD obviously influences her route of delivery. Eden and colleagues'[19] systematic review was part of the overall AHRQ-sponsored comprehensive systematic review[6] that examined childbirth preferences after cesarean birth and how these preferences influenced subsequent choice of TOLAC or ERCD. The review located 1758 potential studies, but found only 1 good-quality study and 10 fair-quality studies that met their inclusion

criteria. Five poor-quality studies were excluded. Methodologic limitations included generally small sample sizes, missing information on TOLAC and VBAC rates, heterogeneity of included populations, use of measures for which validity and reliability were not reported, variation in assessment time, and ambiguity about who interviewed patients. However, looking across these studies, the authors found that the following factors appeared to have some influence on choice of TOLAC or ERCD: race, individual patient preferences, family obligations, safety, patient knowledge of VBAC, and physical support.

Nonwhite women were less likely to choose TOLAC; although in one prospective cohort study that reported on these factors, there also appeared to be underlying differences in medical knowledge between African American and white women, as well apparent differences in the cultural value placed on vaginal birth.

All 11 included studies reported on some aspect of patient preference, although no single factor was examined in the same manner by all studies. Factors reported in these studies included desire for a vaginal delivery, prior history of vaginal delivery, avoidance of labor, and perceptions of the prior cesarean birth. In five studies of six mentioning it, women reported that they chose TOLAC to experience vaginal birth. Two of the 11 studies found that women who had previously had a vaginal delivery were more likely to elect a TOLAC. Four of 11 studies reported that fear of labor or fear of having a difficult labor and ultimately needing a cesarean operation were cited as strong reasons for choosing ERCD.

Women's family situations were mentioned more often than safety factors as determinants of preferred delivery mode. Five of six studies reporting it found that women chose TOLAC because of perceived easier recovery. Women choosing ERCD in 2 of 11 studies cited convenience as the primary reason. In 3 of 11 studies, women who did not desire more children or who wanted to have tubal ligation elected to have ERCD.

Four of 11 studies reported safety factors as important considerations in the choice for preferred delivery mode. However, women choosing ERCD and TOLAC both cited safety factors as the reason for their choice. In another study, women were not aware of the actual probabilities of adverse events for themselves or their infants with ERCD or TOLAC. None of the four studies where safety was cited as a determining factor reported on whether women had been given information about actual complication rates or whether they remembered or used these rates if they had been provided to them.

Knowledge about VBAC may also be related to choice of TOLAC or ERCD. Three of the 11 studies described an educational intervention. The one RCT did not find an overall difference in choice of TOLAC in the group exposed to an educational intervention beginning at 21 weeks of gestation. This RCT may not have been able to demonstrate a difference because up to half of women decide on their preferred mode of delivery before pregnancy and another third will have decided by the middle of pregnancy. Any educational intervention will likely need to begin early, even at the time of the initial cesarean delivery and certainly before the next pregnancy.

It also appears that local hospital and clinician practices may influence the selection of TOLAC. Melnikow and colleagues[20] reviewed medical records of 369 randomly selected women with a history of previous cesarean delivery who had a subsequent birth between 1992 and 1993 in a California acute-care hospital. The records were examined for evidence of counseling about VBAC. The hospitals were stratified for low-, moderate-, or high-risk adjusted rates of cesarean delivery. Women who delivered in hospitals with low overall rates of cesarean delivery were significantly more likely to have VBAC compared with women who delivered in hospitals with moderate or high rates of cesarean delivery (71% vs. 39% vs. 31%; $p < 0.05$). Records of women who delivered in low cesarean facilities were more likely to have documentation of counseling about TOLAC (99% vs. 85% vs. 79%; $p < 0.001$).[20]

IV. MANAGEMENT OF TRIAL OF LABOR AFTER CESAREAN

A. Management of Trial of Labor after Cesarean

The recommendations for selection of patients and management of labor for TOLAC from major professional organizations in the United States, Canada, and the United Kingdom are summarized later in Section VI. No RCTs of TOLAC versus ERCD exist, so the strength of evidence for these recommendations is generally fair to poor, based on observational data and expert opinion. There are no level A recommendations regarding TOLAC.[1,21-25] Evidence about the more controversial aspects of labor management is detailed in the following section.

B. Induction and Augmentation of Labor

Several studies have evaluated the risk for uterine rupture with induction of labor using oxytocin, prostaglandins, or both versus spontaneous labor and ERCD. A recent ACOG committee opinion on induction for VBAC summarizes this recent literature and finds that the potential increase in uterine rupture should be discussed with the mother and fully documented before induction is undertaken.[22] ACOG recommends that selecting women with a greater likelihood of vaginal delivery and avoiding the sequential use of prostaglandins and oxytocin may offer the lowest risk for uterine rupture. Induction may be needed for maternal or fetal indications and remains a reasonable option. The use of misoprostol is not recommended in women who have had prior cesarean deliveries or major uterine surgery because of the high rate of rupture (2 of 17 women) in a RCT using a 25-μg dose of misoprostol.[26] This RCT was stopped early because of the excess risk for uterine rupture with misoprostol.

A recent systematic review of 14 fair-quality studies examined the benefits and risks of inducing labor in women with prior cesarean delivery.[27] The review found that induction of labor was more likely to result in cesarean delivery. For women with spontaneous onset of labor, 20% had a cesarean delivery with a range among the studies from 11% to 35%. For women who received oxytocin, an average of 32% had cesarean births with a range between 18% and 44% in these studies. Some studies compared spontaneous onset of labor and the use of prostaglandins (PGE_2 agents), and found that use of prostaglandins was associated with a higher cesarean delivery rate than was spontaneous labor (48% [range, 28-51%] vs. 24% [range, 18-51%]). Among five population-based studies, there was a nonsignificant increase in uterine ruptures among women who received oxytocin compared with those who had spontaneous labor. The pooled OR was 2.10 (95% CI, 0.76-5.78). However, it is not clear from these studies which induced women received only oxytocin. In at least one of these studies, some women also received misoprostol. Furthermore, it is not possible to tell which women in these studies received oxytocin for induction only or also for augmentation of labor. The MFMU study[10] found an increase in rates of uterine rupture with both induction (OR, 2.81; 95% CI, 1.56-5.22) and oxytocin augmentation (OR, 2.31;

95% CI, 1.35-4.05) of labor. In this study, the use of augmentation was associated with a one-third lower rate of vaginal delivery. The AHRQ systematic review and the AAFP update of that review found that the need for augmentation of labor was associated with an approximately 10% decreased likelihood of vaginal delivery.[1,6]

C. Continuous Electronic Fetal Monitoring

Continuous electronic fetal monitoring is recommended by most professional organizations because a nonreassuring fetal heart rate pattern can be the first sign of uterine rupture. However, this recommendation is not held universally and is based largely on expert opinion. For example, The Institute for Clinical Systems Improvement in the U.S. recommends that either intermittent auscultation or continuous electronic fetal heart monitoring should be done during active labor.[28] The American College of Nurse-Midwives recommends that women be monitored either with continuous electronic fetal monitoring or with intermittent monitoring using a structured protocol.[23] The National Institute for Health and Clinical Excellence guideline from the United Kingdom advocates that women should be offered electronic fetal monitoring in labor and that during induction of labor women should be monitored closely, "with access to electronic fetal monitoring..."[25]

D. Use of Epidural Anesthesia

Because searing or continuous pain at the site of the prior uterine incision can be a sign of uterine rupture, there was concern that the use of epidural anesthesia could mask this symptom and lead to delayed recognition of uterine rupture. However, the majority of evidence indicates that the use of epidural anesthesia appears to be safe for women who have had a prior cesarean delivery. In the MFMU study, epidural anesthesia was not statistically significantly associated with uterine rupture.[9,10] There was a slightly greater rate of vaginal delivery for women who had used epidural anesthesia in this study, but this may have been due to women who planned cesarean deliveries arriving at the hospital in labor and receiving spinal anesthesia.

E. Controversies Regarding Hospital Staffing

The ACOG 1999 practice guideline on vaginal birth after prior cesarean recommended that TOLAC be attempted only in institutions capable of performing immediate cesarean delivery.[4] A revised 2004 ACOG guideline reaffirmed this recommendation.[21] Many hospitals, unable to afford adequate staffing or simply with this staffing level unavailable, stopped providing TOLAC services. Rural hospitals have been more often affected by the guideline than urban hospitals. The 2005 AAFP evidence review and guidelines recommended that TOLAC not be restricted to hospitals with full-time operative coverage. The AAFP recommended that an individual plan to accommodate each woman desiring a VBAC be developed with a rigorous informed consent process.

Zweifler and colleagues[29] conducted a study of more than 380,000 attempted and failed VBACs and repeat cesarean deliveries in California over a 7-year period before and after the 1999 ACOG recommendation. More than 138,000 of the deliveries took place in rural hospitals. The authors found no significant overall association between delivery method and neonatal death among rural hospitals, but that the neonatal death rate increased slightly (OR, 1.21; 95% CI, 0.76-1.95) in rural California hospitals after the ACOG guideline was promulgated.

V. RECOMMENDATIONS FROM U.S. PROFESSIONAL ORGANIZATIONS

A. American College of Obstetricians and Gynecologists Recommendations

ACOG recommendations are as follows[21]:

1. Most women with one prior low transverse CS are candidates for VBAC and should be counseled about VBAC and offered a TOL.
2. Women with a prior lower segment vertical incision that does not extend into the fundus may be offered a TOL.
3. VBAC is contraindicated in women with a previous classical uterine incision or extensive transfundal uterine surgery.
4. After weighing the individual risks and benefits of VBAC, the ultimate decision to attempt the procedure or undergo a repeat cesarean delivery should be made by the patient and her physician with the discussion thoroughly documented in the medical record.
5. Epidural anesthesia may be used.
6. The use of prostaglandins for cervical ripening or induction of labor should be discouraged.

7. VBAC should be attempted in institutions equipped to respond to emergencies with physicians immediately available to provide emergency care.
8. Contraindications for VBAC:
   a. Previous classical or T-shaped uterine incision
   b. Previous uterine rupture
   c. Medical or obstetric complications that preclude vaginal delivery
   d. Inability to perform an emergency cesarean delivery because of unavailable surgeon, anesthesia, staff, or facility
   e. Two prior uterine scars and no vaginal deliveries

B. American Academy of Family Physicians Recommendations

AAFP recommendations are as follows[1]:
1. Women with one prior CS with a low transverse incision are candidates for and should be offered a TOL.
2. Patients desiring TOL should be counseled about positive and negative factors influencing likelihood of a successful VBAC.
3. Positive factors include:
   a. Maternal age younger than 40 years
   b. Prior vaginal delivery, particularly prior successful VBAC
   c. Favorable cervical factors
   d. Spontaneous labor
   e. Nonrecurrent indication for prior CS
4. Negative factors include:
   a. Increased number of prior CSs
   b. Gestational age greater than 40 weeks
   c. Birth weight greater than 4000 grams
   d. Induction or augmentation of labor
5. Prostaglandins should not be used for cervical ripening or induction because of their association with greater rates of uterine rupture and decreased rates of successful vaginal delivery.
6. TOL should not be restricted only to facilities with available surgical teams present throughout labor because there is no evidence that these additional resources result in improved outcomes. It is also appropriate that a management plan for uterine rupture or other potential emergencies requiring rapid CS should be documented for each woman undergoing TOL.
7. No evidence-based recommendation regarding the best way to present the risks and benefits of TOL to patients currently can be made. However,

maternity care professionals need to explore all the issues that may affect a woman's decision, including issues such as recovery time and safety.

C. American College of Nurse-Midwives Recommendations

American College of Nurse-Midwives Recommendations are as follows[23]:
1. TOL contraindicated for women with a prior classical or T-shaped incision, other transfundal surgery, contracted pelvis, or medical/obstetric complications that would preclude vaginal delivery.
2. Midwifery practices should work with hospitals, emergency response systems, and physicians to develop patient education and informed consent materials, practice guidelines, and standards for referral.
3. Women who desire TOLAC should be formally counseled during the prenatal period.
4. Informed consent should include the probability of VBAC success, risks associated with TOLAC (including uterine rupture), and risks for emergency cesarean delivery. Women should also be informed that the best outcomes are associated with performance of an indicated cesarean delivery within 15 minutes.
5. The use of specific consent forms for VBAC should be used to aid in patient education and documentation.
6. During labor, fetal heart rate monitoring should be accomplished by either continuous monitoring or intermittent monitoring using a high-risk protocol (e.g., every 15 minutes in active labor and every 5 minutes in second stage).
7. The highest VBAC success rates are obtained when labor begins spontaneously and progresses normally. Abnormal labor progress can be a marker for dystocia, which is associated with greater rates of uterine rupture.
8. Induction of labor should be done only when the benefits outweigh the risks and only in a hospital after consultation with a physician available to perform a cesarean delivery.
9. Prostaglandins for cervical ripening are discouraged and use of misoprostol is contraindicated in women with scarred uteri.
10. The use of herbal or homeopathic uterotonics is not well supported by scientific evidence, and no data regarding safety of these products in women with a uterine scar are available. Given that other uterotonics appear to increase the risk for uterine

rupture, the use of herbal and homeopathic agents should be discouraged, and if they are used, require full informed consent by the patient.

VI. RECOMMENDATIONS FROM INTERNATIONAL PROFESSIONAL ORGANIZATIONS

A. Canada: Society of Obstetricians and Gynaecologists of Canada

Society of Obstetricians and Gynaecologists of Canada issued a new evidence-based guideline containing 19 recommendations for management of vaginal birth after a previous CS in February 2005.[24]

Key recommendations include:

1. Women with one prior CS should be offered TOL with appropriate discussion of risks and benefits.
2. TOL for women with more than one prior CS is associated with a greater rate of uterine rupture but is likely to be successful.
3. Women delivering within 18 to 24 months of a CS should be counseled that they are at a greater risk for uterine rupture during labor.
4. Multiple gestation, DM, postdatism, and suspected fetal macrosomia do not contraindicate TOLAC.
5. Women should deliver in facilities with access to timely cesarean delivery with an approximate time frame of 30 minutes for urgent surgery.
6. Continuous electronic fetal monitoring is recommended.
7. Suspected uterine rupture requires urgent attention and expedited delivery.
8. Induction of labor with oxytocin may be associated with an increased risk for uterine rupture and should be used carefully and with appropriate counseling.
9. Induction with prostaglandins is contraindicated because of the risk for uterine rupture.
10. Foley catheters may be used for cervical ripening.
11. Augmentation of spontaneous labor is not contraindicated.
12. Every effort should be made to obtain the previous operative report(s) to determine the type of uterine incision used and the circumstances of the delivery. In cases where the scar type is unknown but the likelihood of a lower transverse incision is high, TOLAC can be offered.

B. United Kingdom: Royal College of Obstetricians and Gynaecologists and the National Institute of Health and Clinical Excellence

Key recommendations of the Royal College of Obstetricians and Gynaecologists and the National Institute of Health and Clinical Excellence include[25]:

1. Given that the risks and benefits of vaginal birth after CS compared with repeat CS are uncertain, decisions about mode of delivery should take into consideration maternal preferences and priorities, a general discussion of the overall risks and benefits of CS, the risk for uterine rupture, and the risk for perinatal morbidity and mortality.
2. Women who have had a previous CS and who want to have a vaginal birth should be supported in this decision. They should also be informed that uterine rupture is a rare complication, but that it is increased among women who are having a planned vaginal birth compared with a planned repeat CS (35/10,000 vs. 12/10,000). They should also be informed that the risk for infant death, although small, is greater for a planned vaginal birth compared with a planned CS (10/10,000 vs. 1/10,000). The effect of planned vaginal birth on cerebral palsy is uncertain.
3. Women who have had a prior CS should be offered electronic fetal monitoring during labor and care in a unit with immediate access to CS and on-site blood transfusion services.
4. Women who have had a prior CS can be offered induction of labor, but both they and the professionals caring for them should be aware that there is an increased risk for uterine rupture when labor is induced with nonprostaglandin agents (80/10,000) or prostaglandins (240/10,000).
5. Pregnant women with both previous CS and a previous vaginal birth should be informed that they have an increased likelihood of vaginal birth compared with women who have never before had a vaginal birth.

REFERENCES

1. American Academy of Family Physicians (AAFP): Trial of labor after cesarean (TOLAC), formerly trial of labor versus elective repeat cesarean section for the woman with a previous cesarean section, AAFP Policy Action, Leawood, KS, March 2005, AAFP.
2. Menacker F: Trends in cesarean rates for first births and repeat cesarean rates for low-risk women: United States, 1990-2003.

National vital statistics reports; vol 54, no 4, Hyattsville, MD, 2005, National Center for Health Statistics.

3. McMahon MJ, Luther ER, Bowes WA et al: Comparison of a trial of labor with an elective second cesarean section, *N Engl J Med* 335:689-695, 1996.

4. American College of Obstetricians and Gynecologists (ACOG): Clinical management guidelines for obstetrician-gynecologists: vaginal delivery after previous Cesarean delivery, *ACOG Practice Bulletin 5,* Washington, DC, 1999, ACOG.

5. Hamilton BE, Martin JA, Ventura SJ et al: Births: preliminary data for 2004. National vital statistics reports, vol 54, no 8, Hyattsville, MD, 2005, National Center for Health Statistics.

6. Guise J, McDonagh M, Hashima J et al: Vaginal birth after cesarean (VBAC). Evidence report/technology assessment (Prepared by the Oregon Health & Science University Evidence-based Practice Center under Contract No. 290-97-0018), Rockville, MD, 2003, Agency for Healthcare Research and Quality Publication.

7. Guise J, Berlin M, McDonagh M et al: Safety of vaginal birth after cesarean: a systematic review, *Obstet Gynecol* 103:420-429, 2004.

8. Guise J, McDonagh M, Osterweil P et al: Systematic review of the incidence and consequences of uterine rupture in women with previous caesarean section, *BMJ* 329:1-7, 2004.

9. Landon MB, Hauth JC, Leveno KJ et al: Maternal and perinatal outcomes associated with a trial of labor after prior cesarean delivery, *N Engl J Med* 351:2581-2589, 2004.

10. Landon MB, Spong CY, Thom E et al: Risk of uterine rupture with a trial of labor in women with multiple and single prior cesarean delivery, *Obstet Gynecol* 108(1):12-20, 2006.

11. Bujold E, Gauthier RJ, Hamilton E: Commentary: maternal and perinatal outcomes associated with a trial of labor after prior cesarean delivery, *J Midwifery Womens Health* 50(5): 363-364, 2005.

12. Faiz AS, Ananth CV: Etiology and risk factors for placenta previa: an overview and meta-analysis of observational studies, *J Matern Fetal Neonatal Med* 13:175-190, 2003.

13. Viswanathan M, Visco AG, Hartmann K et al: Cesarean delivery on maternal request. Evidence report/technology assessment No. 133 (Prepared by the RTI International-University of North Carolina Evidence-based Practice Center under Contract No. 290-02-0016.), Agency for Healthcare Research and Quality (AHRQ) Publication No. 06-E009, Rockville, MD, 2006, AHRQ.

14. Getahun D, Oyelese Y, Salihu H et al: Previous cesarean delivery and risks of placenta previa and placental abruption, *Obstet Gynecol* 107:771-778, 2006.

15. Pare E, Quinones JN, Macones GA: Vaginal birth after caesarean section versus elective repeat caesarean section: assessment of maternal downstream health outcomes, *BJOG* 113:75-85, 2006.

16. National Institutes of Health (NIH) State-of-the-Science Panel: NIH State-of-the-Science panel conference statement. Cesarean delivery on maternal request. March 27-29, 2006, *Obstet Gynecol* 107(6):1386-1397, 2006.

17. Smith GC, Pell JP, Dobbie R: Caesarean section and the risk of unexplained stillbirth in subsequent pregnancy, *Lancet* 362:1779-1784, 2003.

18. Landon MB, Leindecker S, Spong CY et al: The MFMU Cesarean Registry: factors affecting the success of trial of labor after previous cesarean delivery, *Am J Obstet Gynecol* 193:1016-1023, 2005.

19. Eden KB, Hashima JN, Osterweil P et al: Childbirth preferences after cesarean birth: a review of the evidence, *Birth* 31(1):49-60, 2004.

20. Melnikow J, Romano P, Gilbert WM et al: Vaginal birth after cesarean in California, *Obstet Gynecol* 98:421-426, 2001.

21. American College of Obstetricians and Gynecologists (ACOG): Vaginal birth after previous cesarean delivery, *ACOG Practice Bulletin 54,* Washington, DC, 2004, ACOG.

22. American College of Obstetricians and Gynecologists (ACOG): Induction of labor for vaginal birth after cesarean delivery, *ACOG Committee Opinion 342,* Washington, DC, 2006, ACOG.

23. American College of Nurse-Midwives: Vaginal birth after previous cesarean section. Position statement, Silver Spring, MD, December 2000.

24. Society of Obstetricians and Gynaecologists of Canada: Guidelines for vaginal birth after previous caesarean birth. No. 155, February 2005, *J Obstet Gynaecol Can* 27(2):164-174, 2005.

25. National Institute for Health and Clinical Excellence (NICE): *Clinical guideline 13: caesarean section,* April 2004. Available at: www.nice.org.uk/CG013NICEguideline. Accessed September 4, 2007.

26. Wing DA, Lovett K, Paul RH: Disruption of prior uterine incision following misoprostol for labor induction in women with previous caesarean delivery, *Obstet Gynecol* 91:828-830, 1998.

27. McDonagh MS, Osterweil P, Guise JM: The benefits and risks of inducing labour in patients with prior caesarean delivery: a systematic review, *BJOG* 112:1007-1015, 2005.

28. Institute for Clinical Systems Improvement (ICSI): *Health care guideline: vaginal birth after cesarean,* ed 10, Bloomington, MN, October 2004, ICSI.

29. Zweifler J, Garza A, Huges S et al: Vaginal birth after Cesarean in California before and after a change in guidelines, *Ann Fam Med* 4:228-234, 2006.

SECTION E Small-for-Dates Pregnancy

Ellen L. Sakornbut, MD

The clinical issue of a small-for-dates pregnancy revolves around whether a pregnancy is developing normally. Fetal growth continues as one of the only ways that clinicians can assess the normality of fetal physiology and the uteroplacental unit. Assessment of growth may not be accurate, and consistent evaluation over a series of prenatal visits is probably of more value than any single examination. In addition, population growth curves provide evidence of normal but smaller individuals in any population. This is compounded by the ever-changing face of our communities where ethnic diversity may result in a mismatch between the population reference standards and the individual growth potential of a given fetus. In other words, small is often perfectly normal, and intervention unnecessary or harmful.

I. CAUSATIVE FACTORS OF A SMALL-FOR-DATES PRESENTATION

A. Inaccurate Pregnancy Dating

Fetuses that are discovered to be small for dates are typically first suspected during prenatal visits when the uterine size is routinely measured and compared with established pregnancy dating parameters. With ample clinical experience, first-trimester uterine size as determined by bimanual examination can be accurately correlated with dates; however, size-date discrepancy in early pregnancy usually represents abnormal pregnancy (missed abortion, molar pregnancy, etc.), uterine abnormality (such as fibroids), or wrong dates. Size-date correlation by physical examination may become more difficult between 13 and 20 weeks of gestation, particularly in the presence of clinical factors such as maternal obesity. By 20 weeks, accurate dating by examination, early ultrasound, or both should be established. If clinical dates are not confirmed by 20 weeks, growth assessment can be performed only by serial examinations.

B. Importance of Accurate Assessment of Fetal Growth

Improper measurement of fundal height may lead to a concern for small-for-gestational age (SGA). The measurement should extend from the symphysis to the most superior aspect of the fundus. Generally speaking, the fundus should be at the umbilicus at 20 weeks of gestation, and rise by 1 cm/week. Reliability of the size-date correlation should remain consistent until 32 weeks of gestation. Small discrepancies between gestational age and fundal height measurements are usually not significant, but measurements that lag 3 to 4 cm behind expected may be significant. After 32 weeks, fundal height may less well predict fetal size depending on descent into the pelvis, fetal lie, and abdominal laxity. At this time, it is more helpful to estimate fetal weight by Leopold maneuvers rather than reliance on fundal height measurements. The acquisition of physical examination skills in assessment of uterine and fetal size requires experience and repeated correlation with outcome. Accuracy in detection of deviation from normal is dependent on both patient and clinician factors.

C. Abnormal Fetal Growth

Normal biologic variation will account for some size-date discrepancies. The constitutionally small fetus usually has at least one parent of limited stature. Ethnic background should be considered in judging fetal growth. However, the constitutionally small fetus still displays interval change, and a leveling off of growth should be investigated. Size-date discrepancies of the pregnancy may include abnormal growth of the fetus, oligohydramnios, or both.

II. INTRAUTERINE GROWTH RESTRICTION

The fetus that is SGA may be constitutionally small and normal or may have restricted growth through a pathologic mechanism. The incidence of IUGR is about 5% in the general pregnant population, but it can increase to as much as 10% in high-risk populations. The majority (70%) of growth restriction in fetuses is asymmetric (AIUGR), in which growth of the head and long bones is spared relative to that of abdomen and viscera. This pattern reflects compromised fetal nutrition, with decreased subcutaneous fat, brown fat, and liver glycogen stores. As the process continues, fetal measurements may become more symmetric when long bone and, finally, central nervous system growth falls off. About 30% of growth-restricted fetuses display symmetric growth abnormalities throughout the pregnancy (SIUGR). The majority of these fetuses suffer from chromosomal abnormalities, intrauterine infections (such as TORCH [toxoplasmosis, other, rubella, cytomegalovirus and herpes] infections), or other major anomalies.

A. Risk Factors for Intrauterine Growth Restriction

Risk factors for IUGR are listed in Table 7-6, together with possible pathophysiology of these conditions.

B. Fetal Complications

Fetal complications of AIUGR include a greater likelihood of encountering fetal intolerance of labor, greater rates of meconium aspiration syndrome, and increased incidence of stillbirth related to chronic uteroplacental insufficiency.

C. Maternal Complications

Maternal complications associated with IUGR include preeclampsia and complications seen in thrombophilic disorders, such as abruption. Some thrombophilic disorders are more strongly associated with growth restriction.[1] The most commonly identified inherited thrombophilias consist of factor V Leiden and the prothrombin gene mutation G20210A. Factor

TABLE 7-6 Conditions Associated with Intrauterine Growth Restriction

Chronic Medical Conditions	Obstetric Complications
Chronic hypertension and chronic renal disease (preeclampsia)	Pregnancy-induced hypertension
Diabetes mellitus, classes C, D, or R	Multiple gestation
Systemic lupus erythematosus	Placental abnormalities—partial abruption, placenta previa, circumvallate placenta, and velamentous cord insertion
Sickle cell anemia and other severe anemias	Intrauterine infection (TORCH infections, listeria)
Cyanotic congenital heart disease	Previous history of intrauterine growth restriction
Other maternal cardiac diseases with poor cardiac output	Fetal abnormalities
Therapeutic medications, including phenytoin (Dilantin), trimethadione, warfarin (Coumadin)	Chromosomal abnormalities—trisomies, Turner syndrome, cri-du-chat
Tobacco use	Congenital malformations
Alcohol and other substance abuse (opiates, cocaine)	
Thrombophilias (antiphospholipid antibody [APA], factor V Leiden, protein C and S)	
Malnutrition	
Chronic lead poisoning	
Low socioeconomic status, especially with poor	
Social support	

V Leiden is associated with a 2.9-fold (95% CI, 2.0-4.3) increased risk for severe preeclampsia, and a 4.8-fold (95% CI, 2.4-9.4) increased risk for fetal growth retardation.[2] Currently, clinical trials using heparin or low-molecular-weight heparin and low-dose aspirin have not demonstrated prevention of either preeclampsia or IUGR in women with thrombophilic disorders.[3-5]

D. Neonatal Complications

Neonatal complications include hypoglycemia, hypothermia, polycythemia-hyperviscosity, hyperbilirubinemia, asphyxia, meconium aspiration syndrome, respiratory distress syndrome, and hypocalcemia. Infants are often initially poor feeders. Infants with SIUGR sustain additional risks related to their congenital abnormalities or systemic illness.

E. Long-Term Sequelae of Intrauterine Growth Restriction

The long-term sequelae of IUGR depend, to some extent, on the cause. The prognosis of infants diagnosed with intrauterine infections, genetic syndromes, or congenital anomalies is variable. Discussion of these issues is beyond the scope of this textbook.

When the diagnosis of IUGR is not accompanied by another inherent pathology, the long-term consequences appear to be those of continued impairment in growth, neurodevelopmental abnormalities, and increased risk for metabolic syndrome and ischemic heart disease.

1. Short stature
   Catch-up growth may occur in growth-restricted infants, but growth abnormalities and short stature are common. Growth hormone levels are usually within references ranges, but insulin-like growth factor binding proteins levels are low. Growth hormone treatment is effective, albeit sometimes at higher doses, indicating relative insensitivity to growth hormone.[6]

2. Linkage to long-term neurologic impairment
   Multiple studies have linked growth restriction to long-term minor neurologic impairment, such as learning disabilities, but study designs and findings display considerable heterogeneity.[7,8] Confounding factors, such as maternal smoking, make it difficult to substantiate these concerns. Other authors suggest a stronger influence of parental factors, such as child-rearing style and maternal smoking, on childhood cognitive development as compared with IUGR.[9]

3. Metabolic syndrome and insulin resistance

A growing body of information links IUGR to development of the metabolic syndrome and insulin resistance with its attendant consequences. The development of insulin resistance has been demonstrated in early childhood[10,11] and young adulthood.[12] In one large prospective study, insulin levels, glucose tolerance, and BMI were followed sequentially with an increased risk for impaired glucose tolerance or diabetes by early adulthood among those who were SGA at birth but typically demonstrated an increase in BMI after 2 years of age.[13]

III. DIAGNOSIS OF INTRAUTERINE GROWTH RESTRICTION

A. Clinical Diagnosis

A diagnosis of growth restriction can be suspected on the basis of lagging fundal height, palpation of a fetus that appears small for dates, or abnormal measurements on ultrasound. The diagnosis of growth restriction almost always relies on previous accurate establishment of the gestational age or with sequential examinations that show abnormal growth rates.

B. Biometric Evaluation

Growth charts for all biometric measurements of the fetus exist with established percentiles for each gestational age. If a fetus is assigned an average uterine age of 18 weeks, this merely implies that the fetal measurements, on average, are at the 50th percentile for 18 weeks. Growth charts should be used that are compatible with the ethnic composition of the population measured. Once a fetus has been assigned a gestational age by thorough and accurate means of clinical or ultrasound dating, or both, growth percentiles for a given gestational age can be assigned on later ultrasound examinations.

Growth restriction has been defined as less than the 10th percentile for gestational age (some authors use less than the 5th percentile). A more specific definition of AIUGR is a fetal ponderal index (the weight of the fetus divided by the length) that is less than the 10th percentile.[14] This defines the "thin" fetus, as described previously, but may be difficult to prove by clinical or ultrasound means because the length and weight of the fetus can only be estimated in utero. Multiple body ratios have been developed to define normal proportions of fetal measurements; the most pertinent in growth assessment are the femur length/abdominal circumference ratio[15,16] and

the head circumference/abdominal circumference ratio.[17] Others advocate the use of the abdominal circumference alone as most reflective of fetal nutritional status.[18,19] Single ultrasound examinations rarely are helpful because the most meaningful information is obtained by plotting serial fetal measurements with an abnormal growth velocity.

C. Diagnosis of Symmetric Intrauterine Growth Restriction

SIUGR is diagnosed using serial ultrasound scans that demonstrate abnormal progression of all fetal growth parameters. Rarely, it may be diagnosed by a single ultrasound scan that can be compared with unequivocal information about the gestational age of the fetus.

IV. SCREENING FOR INTRAUTERINE GROWTH RESTRICTION

A. Screening in Women at Low Risk

Large prospective clinical trials do not demonstrate clinical benefit from routine screening of low-risk women in the third trimester with ultrasound biometric examination. In one study, the sensitivity of ultrasound detection was only 32%.[20] A randomized trial of ultrasound at 34 weeks in 1500 women at low risk demonstrated no differences in perinatal outcome.[21] Another randomized trial found the intervention rate to be almost doubled (31.3% vs. 16.9%; $p < 0.0001$) with no difference in the rate of admission to the NICU.[22] Jahn and co-workers[20] found an increased risk for premature delivery and NICU admissions because of iatrogenic prematurity, whereas the largest trial, a Swedish population-based trial comparing 50,000 screened women and 150,000 women not screened, did not find an increase in operative delivery, perinatal mortality, or neonatal admission to intensive care.[23] The difference in findings between studies may be accounted for by the clinical setting and clinical protocols initiated when a diagnosis of growth restriction was suspected. However, all studies are consistent that screening did not produce clinical benefits.

B. Screening in Women at High Risk

Screening for IUGR in women at high risk has generally been suggested in women with hypertension, whether pregnancy-induced or preexisting, vascular disease, known thrombophilic disorders, and chronic renal disease. In addition, women whose fundal height lags 3 cm or more behind on measurements between 20 and 32 weeks are candidates for further investigation. If a patient is to be screened, ultrasound should be performed between 32 and 34 weeks of gestation or as part of an overall assessment of a significant pregnancy complication, such as preeclampsia. Ultrasound examinations for growth must include a measurement of the abdomen, head, and femur, with attention to normal body ratios and using previously recorded measurements for comparison. A careful anatomic survey should be performed, as well as an assessment for fluid volume.

1. Biometric ultrasound examination
   Ability to predict IUGR by biometric examinations has been an area of investigation and some controversy since early use of obstetric ultrasound. A discussion of these issues is beyond the scope of this textbook. Overall, positive predictive values for ultrasound biometry are increased in women at high risk. Approaches include an emphasis on either EFW or measurement of the fetal abdominal circumference. Growth percentiles may be customized to more accurately reflect the maternal height, prepregnancy weight, fetal sex, ethnic group, and parity.[24] In the setting of high-risk pregnancies, a diagnosis of IUGR using either EFW less than the 10th percentile in weight or an abdominal circumference less than the 10th percentile is predictive of operative delivery for fetal distress and admission to the NICU.[25-27]

2. Second-trimester Doppler uterine artery studies
   Preliminary studies show an association between notching of the uterine artery waveform during the second trimester and an increased risk for preeclampsia and IUGR.[28,29] On the basis of this finding, one RCT found a difference in outcome in women at high risk when treated with low-dose aspirin after demonstration of uterine artery waveform notching between 14 and 16 weeks. The study group showed a significant decrease in rates of preeclampsia and IUGR as compared with control subjects not treated with aspirin.[30]

V. PREVENTION OF INTRAUTERINE GROWTH RESTRICTION

A. Hypertensive Disorders of Pregnancy

Treatment of hypertension does not prevent IUGR and may exacerbate the risk. A metaregression analysis of 34 trials with a total of 2640 women evaluated the outcome of reducing mean arterial pressure (MAP) with antihypertensive agents in hypertensive pregnancies. Treatment of hypertension with antihypertensives has been associated with a decrease in birth weight. Over the range of reported mean differences in MAP, a 10-mmHg decline in MAP was associated with a 176-g decrease in birth weight.[31]

B. Nutrient Supplementation

A Cochrane systemic review found that balanced energy/protein supplementation was associated with modest increases in maternal weight gain and mean birth weight, and a substantial reduction in risk for SGA birth. Supplementation of calories with high protein content or isocaloric high-protein diets resulted in a slight increase in SGA birth.[32] This review examines studies from developing countries and may not be clinically relevant in U.S. populations.

VI. MANAGEMENT OF INTRAUTERINE GROWTH RESTRICTION

A. Further Diagnostic Testing

Genetic amniocentesis and/or TORCH titers may be performed if an anatomic survey indicates major anomalies, a large (hydropic) placenta, and/or other findings indicative of intrauterine infections, although no data exist regarding the change in outcome. Routine screening of IUGR infants with postnatal workups for TORCH infections produces minimal yields.[33]

B. Limited Treatment Options for Suspected Intrauterine Growth Restriction

In the presence of otherwise reassuring fetal assessment or in cases in which the diagnosis is not well established, conservative management is justified with modification of risk factors where possible. A series of Cochrane reviews found insufficient evidence to support modalities such as bed rest[34] and calcium channel blockers[35] for suspected impaired fetal growth.

C. Broaden Physician Management

Although intervention may not be needed at the time of delivery, the clinician must consider the resources available and consider consultation or referral for management of this high-risk condition.

D. Fetal Surveillance and the Timing of Delivery

Because IUGR may occur in conjunction with significant maternal complications, the timing of maternal delivery may be determined by deterioration of maternal condition. Oligohydramnios is considered to be a serious finding, signifying uteroplacental insufficiency in the absence of severe urinary obstruction or bilateral renal agenesis (see Section H).

1. Risks versus benefits

   Risks for preterm delivery should be weighed against the risks of continuing the pregnancy. A large RCT evaluated pediatric outcomes at or beyond 2 years of age. A total of 588 pregnancies between 24 and 36 weeks of gestation referred because of IUGR and concern for fetal compromise were randomly assigned to immediate delivery (n = 296) or delayed delivery (n = 292) until the obstetrician was no longer uncertain of the necessity for delivery.[36] No difference was found in outcomes comparing the two groups. The majority of newborns with poor outcomes were those less than 31 weeks of gestation.

2. Antepartum monitoring

   RCTs using Doppler velocimetry (DV) as a screening test for fetal well-being in patients with IUGR demonstrated reduced incidence of cesarean delivery for fetal distress compared with the NST, with no increase in neonatal morbidity.[37,38] Using DV, an abnormal systolic/diastolic ratio is predictive of increased fetal distress, admission to the NICU, and neonatal respiratory distress in fetuses evaluated because of an EFW less than the 10th percentile or abdominal circumference less than the 2.5th percentile.[39]

   A metaanalysis of trials using DV in hypertensive conditions and IUGR found clinical significance compared with trials with more generalized risk populations. Doppler assessment of pregnancies resulted in significant reduction in antenatal admissions, inductions of labor, elective deliveries (inductions of labor and elective CSs), and CSs. By perinatal audit it was determined that DV prevented potentially avoidable perinatal deaths as compared with controls.[40]

   The frequency of monitoring has not been fully determined. In a pilot study, SGA fetuses with normal DV on entry were randomized to twice weekly or every 14 days. Pregnancy intervention (induction) was more common in the twice-weekly group. No differences in neonatal outcomes were detected. A much larger trial is required to determine the safety and potential benefits of less frequent surveillance of SGA fetuses with normal results of umbilical artery DV studies.[41]

VII. SUMMARY

Fetal growth is monitored during pregnancy as a means of assessing the normality of the process. Growth is best assessed by establishment of accurate dates by 20 weeks. Although the SGA fetus may be normal, the diagnosis of abnormal growth restriction should prompt additional evaluation and surveillance in an effort to prevent poor perinatal outcome.

VIII. SOR A RECOMMENDATIONS

RECOMMENDATIONS	REFERENCES
Biometric ultrasound screening in women at low risk does not lead to an improvement in perinatal outcomes.	21-23
Reducing the MAP with antihypertensive medication is associated with a reduction in birth weight.	32
Doppler assessment of the pregnancy complicated by a SGA fetus allows differentiation between those pregnancies needing intervention (delivery) and pregnancies that can be allowed to continue with expectant management	41
Doppler assessment of the fetus with IUGR as compared with NST decreases the frequency of CS without increasing the risk for admission to an NICU.	38, 39

REFERENCES

1. Paidas MJ, Ku DH, Langhoff-Roos J et al: Inherited thrombophilias and adverse pregnancy outcome: screening and management, *Semin Perinatol* 29(3):150-163, 2005.
2. Dudding TE, Attia J: The association between adverse pregnancy outcomes and maternal factor V Leiden genotype: a meta-analysis, *Thromb Haemost* 91(4):700-711, 2004.
3. Spaanderman ME, Aardenburg R, Ekhart TH et al: Prepregnant prediction of recurrent preeclampsia in normotensive thrombophilic formerly preeclamptic women receiving prophylactic antithrombotic medication, *J Soc Gynecol Investig* 12(2):112-117, 2005.
4. Kalk JJ, Huisjes AJ, de Groot CJ et al: Recurrence rate of pre-eclampsia in women with thrombophilia influenced by low-molecular-weight heparin treatment? *Neth J Med* 62(3):83-87, 2004.
5. Yu VY, Upadhyay A: Neonatal management of the growth-restricted infant, *Semin Fetal Neonatal Med* 9(5):403-409, 2004.

6. Ali O, Cohen P: Insulin-like growth factors and their binding proteins in children born small for gestational age: implication for growth hormone therapy, *Horm Res* 60(suppl 3):115-123, 2003.

7. Veelken N, Stollhoff K, Claussen M: Development and perinatal risk factors of very low-birth-weight infants. Small versus appropriate for gestational age, *Neuropediatrics* 23(2):102-107, 1992.

8. Roth S, Chang TC, Robson S et al: The neurodevelopmental outcome of term infants with different intrauterine growth characteristics, *Early Hum Dev* 55(1):39-50, 1999.

9. Sommerfelt K, Andersson HW, Sonnander K et al: Cognitive development of term small for gestational age children at five years of age, *Arch Dis Child* 83:25-30, 2000.

10. Chiarelli F, diRicco L, Mohn A et al: Insulin resistance in short children with intrauterine growth retardation, *Acta Paediatr* 88:62-65, 1999.

11. Ong KK, Ahmed ML, Emmett PM et al: Association between catch-up growth and obesity in childhood: prospective cohort study, *BMJ* 320:967-971, 2000.

12. Jaquet D, Gaborian A, Czernichow P et al: Insulin resistance early in adulthood in subjects born with intrauterine growth retardation, *J Clin Endocrinol Metab* 85:1401-1406, 2000.

13. Bhargava SK, Sachdev HS, Fall CH et al: Relation of serial changes in childhood body-mass index to impaired glucose tolerance in young adulthood, *N Engl J Med* 350(9):865-875, 2004.

14. Vintzileos AM, Lodeiro JG, Feinstein SJ et al: Value of fetal ponderal index in predicting intrauterine growth retardation, *Obstet Gynecol* 67:585-588, 1986.

15. Hadlock FP, Deter RL, Harrist RB et al: A date-independent predictor of intrauterine growth retardation: femur-length/abdominal circumference ratio, *Am J Roentgenol* 141:979-984, 1983.

16. Hadlock FP, Deter RL, Harrist RB: Sonographic detection of abnormal fetal growth patterns, *Clin Obstet Gynecol* 27:342-351, 1984.

17. Campbell S, Thomas A: Ultrasound measurement of the fetal head to abdomen circumference ratio in the assessment of growth retardation, *Br J Obstet Gynaecol* 84:165-174, 1977.

18. Seeds JW: Impaired fetal growth: ultrasonic evaluation and clinical management, *Obstet Gynecol* 64:577-584, 1984.

19. Warsof, SL, Cooper DJ, Little D et al: Routine ultrasound screening for antenatal detection of intrauterine growth retardation, *Obstet Gynecol* 67:33-39, 1986.

20. Jahn A, Razum O, Berle P: Routine screening for intrauterine growth retardation in Germany: low sensitivity and questionable benefit for diagnosed cases, *Acta Obstet Gynaecol Scand* 77:643-648, 1998.

21. Duff GB: A randomized controlled trial in a hospital population of ultrasound measurement screening for the small for dates baby, *Aust N Z J Obstet Gynaecol* 33(4):374-378, 1993.

22. McKenna D, Tharmaratnam S, Mahsud S et al: A randomized trial using ultrasound to identify the high-risk fetus in a low-risk population, *Obstet Gynecol* 101(4):626-632, 2003.

23. Sylvan K, Ryding EL, Rydhstroem H: Routine ultrasound screening in the third trimester: a population-based study, *Acta Obstet Gynecol Scand* 84(12):1154-1158, 2005.

24. De Jong CL, Francis A, Van Geijn HP et al: Customized fetal weight limits for antenatal detection of fetal growth restriction, *Ultrasound Obstet Gynecol* 15(1):36-40, 2000.

25. Yoshida S, Unno N, Kagawa H et al: Prenatal detection of a high-risk group for intrauterine growth restriction based on sonographic fetal biometry, *Int J Gynaecol Obstet* 68(3):225-232, 2000.

26. Smith-Bindman R, Chu PW, Ecker JL et al: US evaluation of fetal growth: prediction of neonatal outcomes, *Radiology* 223(1):153-161, 2002.

27. Williams KP, Nwebube N: Abdominal circumference: a single measurement versus growth rate in the prediction of intrapartum Cesarean section for fetal distress, *Ultrasound Obstet Gynecol* 17(6):493-495, 2001.

28. Vainio M, Kujansuu E, Koivisto AM et al: Bilateral notching of uterine arteries at 12-14 weeks of gestation for prediction of hypertensive disorders of pregnancy, *Acta Obstet Gynecol Scand* 84(11):1062-1067, 2005.

29. El-Hamedi A, Shillito J, Simpson NA et al: A prospective analysis of the role of uterine artery Doppler waveform notching in the assessment of at-risk pregnancies, *Hypertens Pregnancy* 24(2):137-145, 2005.

30. Ebrashy A, Ibrahim M, Marzook A et al: Usefulness of aspirin therapy in high-risk pregnant women with abnormal uterine artery Doppler ultrasound at 14-16 weeks pregnancy: randomized controlled clinical trial, *Croat Med J* 46(5):826-831, 2005.

31. von Dadelszen P, Magee LA: Fall in mean arterial pressure and fetal growth restriction in pregnancy hypertension: an updated metaregression analysis, *J Obstet Gynaecol Can* 24(12):941-945, 2002.

32. Kramer MS, Kakuma R: Energy and protein intake in pregnancy, *Cochrane Database Syst Rev* (1):CD000148, 2003.

33. Khan NA, Kazzi SN: Yield and costs of screening growth-retarded infants for TORCH infections, *Am J Perinatol* 17:131-135, 2000.

34. Gulmezoglu AM, Hofmeyr GJ: Bed rest in hospital for suspected impaired fetal growth, *Cochrane Database Syst Rev* (2):CD000034, 2000.

35. Gulmezoglu AM, Hofmeyr GJ: Calcium channel blockers for potential impaired growth, *Cochrane Database Syst Rev* (2):CD000079, 2000.

36. Thornton JG, Hornbuckle J, Vail A et al: GRIT study group. Infant wellbeing at 2 years of age in the Growth Restriction Intervention Trial (GRIT): multicentred randomised controlled trial, *Lancet* 364(9433):513-520, 2004.

37. Williams KP, Farquharson DF, Bebbington M et al: Screening for fetal well-being in a high-risk pregnant population comparing the nonstress test with umbilical artery Doppler velocimetry: a randomized controlled clinical trial, *Am J Obstet Gynecol* 188(5):1366-1371, 2003.

38. Almstrom H, Axelsson O, Cnattingius S et al: Comparison of umbilical-artery velocimetry and cardiotocography for surveillance of small-for-gestational-age fetuses, *Lancet* 340(8825):936-940, 1992.

39. Baschat AA, Weiner CP: Umbilical artery Doppler screening for detection of the small fetus in need of antepartum surveillance, *Am J Obstet Gynecol* 182(1 pt 1):154-158, 2000.

40. Westergaard HB, Langhoff-Roos J, Lingman G et al: A critical appraisal of the use of umbilical artery Doppler ultrasound in high-risk pregnancies: use of meta-analyses in evidence-based obstetrics, *Ultrasound Obstet Gynecol* 17(6):466-476, 2001.

41. McCowan LM, Harding JE, Roberts AB et al: A pilot randomized controlled trial of two regimens of fetal surveillance for small-for-gestational-age fetuses with normal results of umbilical artery Doppler velocimetry, *Am J Obstet Gynecol* 182(1 pt 1):81-86, 2000.

SECTION F Large-for-Dates Pregnancy Including Macrosomia

Thomas J. Gates, MD

Between 20 and 35 weeks of gestation, the fundal height in centimeters roughly corresponds to the weeks of gestation. *Large-for-dates* refers to a pregnancy where the fundal height exceeds the number of weeks of gestation by 3 or more centimeters. The differential diagnosis of large-for dates pregnancy is wide, but includes *macrosomia,* which is an EFW beyond a specific weight cutoff, usually either 4500 (9 lb 15 ounces) or 4000 g (8 lb 13 ounces). *Large-for-gestational age* refers to newborns whose actual birth weight exceeds the 90th percentile for gestational age (4060 g at 40 weeks).

I. CAUSATIVE FACTORS OF LARGE-FOR-DATES PREGNANCY

A. Obesity
In obese women who are pregnant, the measured fundal height may appear to be increased in all trimesters of pregnancy. Macrosomia, however, is also more common in the obese patient.

B. Short Stature
Women whose height is short also may appear to be larger than their dates suggest, although the fundal height measurements typically correlate properly at between 20 and 32 weeks.

C. Inaccurate Measurement
Fundal height measurements carry a degree of subjectivity, such that variation of several centimeters may be recorded by different examiners on the same patient at the same gestational age. This variation is enhanced in the patient with obesity or excessive maternal weight gain.

D. Inaccurate Dates
The most common cause of fundal height measurements exceeding menstrual dates is improper dating of the pregnancy. In these cases, the designated last menstrual period may actually represent bleeding that took place after the onset of pregnancy, such as implantation bleeding of the placenta. The patient who presents late for prenatal care poses a significant diagnostic problem when fundal height exceeds that expected with menstrual dating because reliability of ultrasound dating declines with advancing gestational age.

E. Polyhydramnios
The increase in uterine size may represent an increase in amniotic fluid rather than fetal size. This commonly presents in the late second and third trimester.

F. Multiple Gestation
Two (or more) fetuses will cause the fundal height to measure large for dates. Multiple gestation is often discovered by ultrasound obtained because of concern over a large fundal height measurement.

G. Uterine Leiomyomata
Women with preexisting leiomyomata may experience growth of these benign tumors during pregnancy. Even when fibroid growth does not occur, their mere presence may cause the uterus to measure larger than would be expected by the fetus, amniotic fluid, and placenta alone.

H. Molar Pregnancy
In the first trimester, an enlarged uterus may signify a molar pregnancy, particularly if fetal heart tones are not heard by Doppler when anticipated.

II. WORKUP OF LARGE-FOR-DATES PREGNANCY

Women who consistently measure 3 or more centimeters greater than their gestational age in weeks should have an ultrasound examination to determine the cause. Ultrasound should reliably differentiate among inaccurate dating, multiple gestation, polyhydramnios, and fetal macrosomia, but most women who clinically measure large for dates will have no specific cause found on ultrasound.

III. MACROSOMIA

A. Natural History
Although most women who measure large-for-dates will not have large babies, macrosomia is important to diagnose because it can lead to significant maternal and neonatal complications. Women with macrosomic fetuses have a 2-fold increased risk for cesarean delivery, a 1.9-fold risk for postpartum hemorrhage, and a 5-fold risk for shoulder dystocia. Complications in the neonate include fractures of the clavicle

and humerus, and brachial plexus injuries. The risk for brachial plexus injury to a macrosomic infant born vaginally is between 4% and 8%.[1] Although 90% of these injuries resolve spontaneously by 1 year of age, providers of obstetric care should be aware that permanent brachial plexus injury is a major cause of malpractice litigation.

B. Epidemiology and Risk Factors

Ten percent of all newborns in the United States weigh more than 4000 g, whereas 1.5% weigh more than 4500 g.[1] A number of risk factors have been described, but as many as 34% of macrosomic infants are born to mothers with no risk factors.[2] Some evidence exists that the incidence of macrosomia has increased since 1990, and that most of the increase can be accounted for by an increase in maternal obesity and a decrease in maternal smoking.[3] A large case–control study identified the following risk factors, in order of decreasing importance[4]:

1. Maternal diabetes, both gestational and pregestational
   This has traditionally been considered the strongest risk factor, with cohort studies showing up to a threefold increased risk for macrosomia in women with diabetes.[3] If gestational diabetes is unrecognized and untreated, the risk for macrosomia may be as great as 44%.[1,5] A recent randomized prospective trial of mild gestational diabetes showed that those in the more intensively treated group had a 0.47 RR for macrosomia.[6] Some controversy exists about the relative importance of maternal diabetes compared with maternal obesity; many argue that obesity is the more important predictor.[1,4,7]

2. Prior history of macrosomia
   Women who have had a previous infant weighing more than 4000 g are 5 to 10 times more likely to deliver an infant exceeding 4500 g, compared with women without this history.[1] Risk factors for macrosomia include the following:
   a. Maternal prepregnancy weight: A large, retrospective study showed 2-fold increased risk for macrosomia for prepregnancy BMI of 25 to 29.9 and a 3-fold risk for BMI of 30 or greater.[3] The risk from maternal obesity appears to be independent of the risk conferred by gestational diabetes.[7]
   b. Weight gain during pregnancy: In nondiabetic nulliparas, women exceeding the Institute of Medicine recommendations for weight gain during pregnancy (25-35 lb for BMI 19.8-26.0; 15-25 lb for BMI >26.0) had an adjusted OR of 2.2 for birth weight of both 4000 and 4500 g.[8] Another retrospective study found that BMI greater than 29 and gestational weight gain of more than 35 pounds were the two factors most strongly predictive of macrosomia; when both were present, there was a fourfold greater incidence of macrosomia.[9]
   c. Multiparity: For parity of more than 4, the adjusted OR of an LGA baby was 3.28.[3]
   d. Male fetus: Adjusted OR of LGA baby was 1.6 to 2.0.[4,7]
   e. Gestational age more than 40 weeks: The OR was 2.0.[4]
   f. Ethnicity: Hispanic and Native American women appear to be at greater risk.[1,4]

C. Diagnosis

An accurate diagnosis of macrosomia can be made only by weighing the newborn after delivery; the prenatal diagnosis of macrosomia remains imprecise.[1] Several studies of varying methodology have suggested that ultrasound prediction of fetal weight is no more accurate than prediction based on clinical examination alone.[1,10] Ultrasound diagnosis of macrosomia has a positive predictive value of only 30% to 44%, but a negative predictive value of 97% to 99%; thus, it may be most useful in ruling out the diagnosis.[1]

D. Management of Suspected Fetal Macrosomia

There is a dearth of high-quality evidence on which to make recommendations, and current approaches are in flux. In the absence of definitive studies, three alternative management strategies are possible: early induction of labor, elective CS, and allowing pregnancy to continue without intervention.

1. Induction of labor
   Retrospective studies have suggested no benefit and a possible increase in CS rates when labor is induced because of suspected fetal macrosomia.[1] A 1998 Cochrane review located just two randomized prospective studies, involving a total of 313 women. No significant difference was found in the rate of cesarean delivery, instrumental delivery, or neonatal injury.[11] Larger trials addressing this question are currently in progress.

2. Elective CS
   No prospective RCTs have measured the benefit of elective CS in preventing the complications of

macrosomia. An observational study in women with diabetes, with CS recommended when ultrasound EFW exceeded 4250 g, resulted in a lower rate of shoulder dystocia but a higher cesarean rate, compared with historical control subjects.[12] A cost–benefit analysis suggested that screening for macrosomia with ultrasound and performing elective CS for EFW greater than 4500 g would require 3695 CSs to prevent 1 case of permanent brachial plexus injury. However, in women with diabetes, the number would be 443.[13] ACOG states that the evidence "does not support a policy of prophylactic cesarean delivery for suspected fetal macrosomia with estimated weights less than 5000 grams," but that women should be presented with accurate statistics concerning the fetal and maternal risks of both vaginal and cesarean delivery. Without citing any studies, ACOG also states that "most, but not all, authors agree that consideration should be given to cesarean delivery" when the EFW exceeds 5000 g.[1]

3. Synthesis of literature

In the absence of high-quality evidence that either induction of labor or prophylactic cesarean delivery improve outcomes, the default position would seem to be nonintervention and a trial of labor. Numerous cohort and case–control studies have demonstrated the relative safety of vaginal delivery of macrosomic infants.[1] For example, in a review of 227 infants with an actual birth weight of more than 4500 g, 15% of women were delivered by elective CS. Of the 192 who had a trial of labor, 82% delivered vaginally. The incidence of shoulder dystocia was 18.5%, with half of those infants having either an Erb's palsy or a clavicular fracture, but with no permanent sequelae detected in any infant at 2 months of age.[14]

E. Clinical Recommendations

1. Macrosomia is difficult to diagnose. Clinical diagnosis is probably as accurate as ultrasound; ultrasound has a high negative predictive value, and thus may be most helpful in ruling out macrosomia. Studies are lacking that address how best to learn (or teach) the clinical estimation of fetal weight.

2. At this time, limited evidence suggests that early induction of labor is not an effective strategy for management of suspected macrosomia.

3. Limited evidence exists to suggest that elective CS in women with diabetes with an EFW greater than 4250 g may decrease the incidence of shoulder

dystocia. In women without diabetes, it seems intuitive that there is some weight beyond which CS is indicated, but there is no good evidence for what that cutoff should be.

4. Aggressive treatment of gestational diabetes decreases the incidence of macrosomia and decreases the composite outcome of serious neonatal complication (neonatal death, shoulder dystocia, fracture, or nerve palsy).

5. Because preexisting obesity and gestational weight gain are important and additive risk factors for macrosomia, it would seem prudent to counsel women accordingly. However, currently, no convincing evidence is available that any proposed dietary or lifestyle interventions are effective in preventing macrosomia.

F. SOR A RECOMMENDATION

RECOMMENDATION	REFERENCE
Aggressive treatment of gestational diabetes decreases the incidence of macrosomia and decreases the composite outcome of serious neonatal complication (neonatal death, shoulder dystocia, fracture, or nerve palsy).	6

REFERENCES

1. ACOG Committee on Practice Bulletins: *ACOG Practice Bulletin,* No. 22:1-11, November 2000.
2. Boyd ME, Usher RH, McLean FH: Fetal macrosomia: prediction, risks, proposed management, *Obstet Gynecol* 61:715-722, 1983.
3. Surkan PJ, Hsieh CC, Johansson A et al: Reasons for increasing trends in large for gestational age births, *Obstet Gynecol* 104:720-726, 2004.
4. Okun N, Verma A, Mitchell BF et al: Relative importance of maternal constitutional factors and glucose intolerance of pregnancy in the development of newborn macrosomia, *J Matern Fetal Med* 6:285-290, 1997.
5. Adams KM, Hongzhe L, Nelson RL et al: Sequelae of unrecognized gestational diabetes, *Am J Obstet Gynecol* 178:1321-1332, 1998.
6. Crowther CA, Hiller JE, Moss JR et al: Effect of treatment of gestational diabetes mellitus on pregnancy outcomes, *N Engl J Med* 352:2477-2486, 2005.
7. Ehrenberg HM, Mercer BM, Catalano PM: The influence of obesity and diabetes on the prevalence of macrosomia, *Am J Obstet Gynecol* 191:964-968, 2004.
8. Stotland NE, Hopkins LM, Caughey AB: Gestational weight gain, macrosomia, and risk of cesarean birth in nondiabetic nulliparas, *Obstet Gynecol* 104:671-677, 2004.

9. Johnson JWC, Longmate JA, Frentzen B: Excessive maternal weight and pregnancy outcome, *Am J Obstet Gynecol* 167:353-372, 1992.
10. Sherman DJ, Arieli S, Tovbin J et al: A comparison of clinical and ultrasonic estimation of fetal weight, *Obstet Gynecol* 91:212-217, 1998.
11. Irion O, Boulvain M: Induction of labour for suspected fetal macrosomia, *Cochrane Database Syst Rev* (2):CD000938, 2000.
12. Conway DL, Langer O: Elective delivery of infants with macrosomia in diabetic women: reduced shoulder dystocia versus increased cesarean deliveries, *Am J Obstet Gynecol* 178:922-925, 1998.
13. Rouse DJ, Owen J, Goldenberg RL, Cliver SP: The effectiveness and costs of elective cesarean delivery for fetal macrosomia diagnosed by ultrasound, *JAMA* 276:1480-1486, 1996.
14. Lipscomb KR, Gregory K, Shaw K: The outcome of macrosomic infants weighing at least 4500 grams, *Obstet Gynecol* 85:558-564, 1995.

SECTION G Disorders of Amniotic Fluid Including Oligohydramnios and Polyhydramnios

Mark L. Rast, MD

I. AMNIOTIC FLUID PHYSIOLOGY

Amniotic fluid is a "complex and dynamic milieu that changes as pregnancy progresses."[1] Amniotic fluid contains nutrients and growth factors that facilitate fetal growth and produce mechanical cushioning and antimicrobial effectors that protect the fetus and allow assessment of fetal maturity and disease. Amniotic fluid initially originates from maternal plasma, but by the second half of pregnancy, fetal urination and swallowing contribute significantly to the volume of amniotic fluid. By 28 weeks, amniotic fluid reaches a volume of about 800 ml, where it plateaus until near term and then begins to decrease. By 42 weeks, it has declined to about 400 ml.[2]

Four pathways have been identified that comprise amniotic fluid circulation: production by excretion of fetal urine; secretion of oral, nasal, tracheal, and pulmonary fluids; removal of amniotic fluid by fetal swallowing; and an intermembranous pathway that transfers fluids and solutes from the amniotic to the fetal circulation across the amniotic membranes.[3]

Based on this physiology, fetal anomalies of the gastrointestinal or genitourinary systems are associated with disorders of amniotic fluid that can have adverse effects on the outcome of a pregnancy.

II. OLIGOHYDRAMNIOS

Oligohydramnios is defined as less than 5th percentile of amniotic fluid volume expected for gestational age.[4] Amniotic fluid index (AFI), which is measured by summing the depth of amniotic fluid in the four quadrants of the uterine cavity using ultrasound, has been shown to be the most acceptable method for assessing the fluid status in a singleton gestation.[5] Oligohydramnios complicates 0.5% to 8% of all pregnancies. The prognosis of oligohydramnios is highly dependent on gestational age and the presence of at-risk maternal or fetal conditions.[6]

A. Oligohydramnios in the First and Second Trimesters

In fetuses with severe oligohydramnios between 13 and 24 weeks, 51% have fetal abnormalities (1% are aneuploidy), 34% have preterm premature rupture of membranes, 7% abruption, and 5% growth restriction.[6] The finding of oligohydramnios during this period of pregnancy should elicit a careful search for these and other causes often in conjunction with obstetric or maternal fetal medicine consultation.

1. Prognosis and survival rates
   Prognosis and survival rates are significantly diminished (10%) when severe oligohydramnios is present in conjunction with fetal anomalies.
2. Genetics consultation
   Most authorities recommend genetic amniocentesis when severe oligohydramnios is noted in the second trimester or if fetal anomalies are noted on the ultrasound. Patients can then be counseled accordingly. Specific therapies are possible for some conditions, for example, bladder amniotic fluid shunt for posterior urethral valves.[7]

B. Oligohydramnios at Term

Oligohydramnios occurs in 1% to 5% of pregnancies at term. Because adverse outcomes occur in high-risk pregnancies complicated by low amniotic fluid volume, oligohydramnios commonly prompts labor induction. However, isolated (not associated with any other problem) oligohydramnios at term (AFI < 5) has not been clearly shown to be associated with poor maternal or fetal outcomes. Management may be individualized based on factors such as parity, cervical ripeness, and patient preference.[8] Ek and colleagues[9] randomly assigned 54 patients beyond 40 weeks to either induction of labor or expectant management. No differences were found for any important maternal or neonatal outcome. Driggers and co-workers showed that an AFI less than or equal to 5 cm within 7 days of delivery in the third trimester was not associated with decreasing umbilical artery pH and base excess.[10] Another study suggests that DV may help predict those pregnancies with oligohydramnios that are at greater risk for adverse outcomes. In a retrospective study of 76 patients with oligohydramnios not secondary to PROM or congenital anomalies, those with normal Doppler studies had no incidence of adverse outcome. Carroll and colleagues' recommendation is to avoid intervention in cases of oligohydramnios with normal Doppler studies.[11]

1. Isolated oligohydramnios at term

   Sherer states that "intuitively, decreased amniotic fluid volume in a structurally normal fetus is considered to reflect impaired uteroplacental blood flow.[12] Redistribution of oxygenated blood toward essential organs (brain, heart, adrenals) resulting in decreased peripheral and renal perfusion would explain decreased urine output and associated oligohydramnios." However, the evidence has not borne this out.

   Sherer goes on to note that "although induction of labor in postterm patients with oligohydramnios (AFI < 5) is considered the standard of care, adherence to this practice clearly results in subsequent increases in labor complications and the incidence of operative delivery without significantly improving outcomes." He then suggests that "evidence is accumulating that in the presence of an appropriate for gestational age fetus, with reassuring fetal well-being and the absence of maternal disease oligohydramnios is not associated with an increased incidence of adverse perinatal outcome."[12] Ross and colleagues also note that "evidence is mounting that isolated oligohydramnios at term is not a marker for fetal compromise."[13]

2. Management of isolated oligohydramnios at term

   A number of recent studies have questioned the practice of immediate induction for isolated oligohydramnios noted at term (>37 weeks).

Leeman and Almond[14] note the following:

a. Isolated term oligohydramnios, defined by an AFI less than 5 cm, has not been shown to be associated with poor maternal or fetal outcomes. Management may be individualized based on factors such as parity, cervical ripeness, and patient preference.

b. Maternal hydration with oral water has been shown to increase AFI in a few hours, likely because of improved uteroplacental perfusion. This is a reasonable alternative to immediate labor induction in women with isolated term oligohydramnios.

c. An isolated finding of so-called "borderline AFI" (5-8 cm) is not an indication for labor induction. Labor induction has been shown to increase the use of cesarean delivery, particularly for the primiparous woman with an unripe cervix. No studies to date have addressed whether labor induction improves outcomes for this indication.

III. POLYHYDRAMNIOS

Polyhydramnios is defined as a volume of amniotic fluid greater than 95th percentile for gestational age or a maximum vertical pocket of more than 8 cm. Approximately 1% of all pregnancies are complicated by polyhydramnios. Severity is often classified by ultrasound criteria: mild—8- to 11-cm pocket; moderate—12- to 16-cm pocket; severe—>16-cm pocket.[15]

Congenital anomalies in many organ systems are associated with polyhydramnios. The most common are those that interfere with fetal swallowing and fetal absorption of fluid. Abnormalities such as esophageal or duodenal atresia are often associated with increased fluid volume. Obstruction of the gastrointestinal tract can also occur with entities such as large dysplastic kidneys. Neuromuscular disorders can cause the fetus to have disordered and decreased swallowing, with anencephaly being the most extreme example.[16] Other causes of polyhydramnios include maternal diabetes, fetal infection, aneuploidy, and multiple gestations. Two studies[15,17] reviewing the causes of polyhydramnios in 90 and 120 cases revealed the following:

1. Idiopathic: 60% in both studies[15,17]
2. Fetal anomalies: 19%[15] and 12%[17]
3. Multiple gestation: 7.5%[15] and 9%[17]
4. Maternal diabetes: 5%[15] and 19%[17]

IV. EVALUATION

A. Ultrasound

Evaluation begins with a comprehensive ultrasound to assess whether fetal anomalies or hydrops is present. Amniocentesis with karyotype should be strongly considered, especially in cases of early-onset polyhydramnios and severe polyhydramnios. In Dashe and co-workers' study[18] of polyhydramnios, 80% of infants with anomaly as the cause of the polyhydramnios were detected before birth. The most common missed anomalies were tracheoesophageal fistula, cleft palate, and cardiac septal defects.

B. Laboratory Evaluation

If ultrasound does not identify a possible cause, then laboratory evaluation to assess for maternal diabetes, congenital infection, and fetal-maternal hemorrhage (Kleihauer–Betke test) can be considered.

C. Maternal Effects

The maternal effect of polyhydramnios is related to its severity. Uterine overdistension can occur with subsequent problems including preterm labor, premature preterm rupture of membranes, prolapsed cord, maternal respiratory compromise, and postpartum atony and secondary hemorrhage.[19]

D. Treatment

Several treatments for polyhydramnios have been suggested; however, the level of evidence is weak—no RCTs exist. Amniocentesis has been used to reduce amniotic fluid volume, and some have tried PG synthetase inhibitors (primarily indomethacin [Indocin]) to decrease amniotic fluid production. Indocin must be used with caution, particularly later in pregnancy, because of the potential risk for ductus constriction.[19]

In cases of severe polyhydramnios at term, one can consider abdominal or transcervical amnioreduction before or early in labor to help prevent rapid, severe uterine decompression with spontaneous rupture of membranes, which increases the risk for cord prolapse and abruption.[20]

REFERENCES

1. Underwood MA, Gilbert WM, Sherman MP: State of the Art: amniotic fluid: not just fetal urine anymore, *J Perinatol* 25: 341-348, 2005.
2. Brace RA, Wolf EJ: Normal amniotic fluid changes throughout pregnancy, *Am J Obstet Gynecol* 161:382-388, 1989.
3. Sherer DM: A review of amniotic fluid dynamics and the enigma of isolated oligohydramnios, *Am J Perinatol* 19: 253-266, 2002.
4. Brace RA: Physiology of amniotic fluid regulation, *Clin Obstet Gynecol* 40(2):280-289, 1997.
5. Moore TR, Cayle JE: The amniotic fluid index in normal human pregnancy, *Am J Obstet Gynecol* 162:1168-1172, 1990.
6. Magann EF, Sanderson M, Martin RW et al: The amniotic fluid index, single deepest pocket, and 2-diameter pocket in human pregnancy, *Am J Obstet Gynecol* 182:1581-1588, 2000.
7. Marino T: Ultrasound abnormalities of amniotic fluid, membranes, umbilical cord, and placenta, *Obstet Gynecol Clin N Am* 31:177-200, 2004.
8. Kilpatrick SJ: Therapeutic interventions for oligohydramnios: amnioinfusion and maternal hydration, *Clin Obstet Gynecol* 40:303-313, 1997.
9. Ek S, Andersson A, Johansson A et al: Oligohydramnios in uncomplicated pregnancies beyond 40 completed weeks. A prospective, randomized, pilot study on maternal and neonatal outcomes, *Fetal Diagnostic Ther* 20:182-185, 2005.
10. Driggers RW, Holcroft CJ, Blakemore KJ et al: An amniotic fluid index of less than or equal to 5 cm within 7 days of delivery in the third trimester is not associated with decreasing umbilical artery pH and base excess, *J Perinatol* 24:72-76, 2004.
11. Carroll BC, Bruner JP: Umbilical artery Doppler velocimetry in pregnancies complicated by oligohydramnios, *J Reprod Med* 45:462-466, 2000.
12. Sherer DM: A review of amniotic fluid dynamics and the enigma of isolated oligohydramnios, *Am J Perinatol* 19: 253-266, 2002.
13. Ross MG, Brace RA, NIH Workshop: NICHD conference summary: amniotic fluid biology—basic and clinical aspects, *J Matern Fetal Med* 10:2-19, 2001.
14. Leeman L, Almond D: Isolated oligohydramnios at term: is induction indicated? *J Fam Pract* 54(1):25-32, 2005.
15. Hill LM, Breckle R, Thomas ML et al: Polyhydramnios: ultrasono-graphically detected presence and neonatal outcome, *Obstet Gynecol* 69:21-25, 1987.
16. Stoll CG, Alembik Y, Dott B: Study of 156 cases of polyhydramnios and congenital malformations in a series of 118,265 consecutive births, *Am J Obstet Gynecol* 165:586-590, 1991.
17. Ben-Chetrit A, Hochner-Celnikier D, Ron M et al: Hydramnios in the third trimester of pregnancy: a change in the distribution of accompanying fetal anomalies as a result of early ultrasonographic prenatal diagnosis, *Am J Obstet Gynecol* 162:1344-1345, 1990.
18. Dashe JS, McIntire DD, Ramus RM et al: Hydramnios: anomaly presence and sonographic detection, *Obstet Gynecol* 100:134-139, 2002.
19. Moise KJ: Polyhydramnios, *Clin Obstet Gynecol* 40(2): 266-279, 1997.
20. Leung WC, Jouannic JM, Hyatt J et al: Procedure related complications of rapid amniodrainage in the treatment of polyhydramnios, *Ultrasound Obstet Gynecol* 23:154-158, 2004.

Section H Possible Indicators of Fetal Abnormalities

Barbara F. Kelly, MD

In 2007, new guidelines for screening all pregnancies for fetal chromosomal abnormalities were published by the ACOG.[1] These guidelines include counseling all parents, not just those at increased risk, such as advanced maternal age, on noninvasive and invasive screening and diagnostic options currently available clinically to detect the fetus with chromosomal abnormalities. Now screening options for trisomy 21, as well as trisomies 18 and 13, are available in the first trimester. These include both maternal serum screening and ultrasound screening for nuchal translucency (NT), and allow for earlier detection and diagnosis of the chromosomally abnormal fetus.[1] The strategies for screening are increasingly complex, and clinicians are faced with a challenging array of testing options, varying cost considerations, and the fact that some options such as NT screening will be available only in selected centers rather than in every practice setting. These screening options do result in phenomenal detection rates up to 96%, which is approaching the gold standard of amniocentesis. Clinicians need to understand that among similar options, small changes in detection rates may not be that clinically relevant given that the risk for having an abnormal fetus is small. Then again, we are all aware that the impact on an affected pregnancy is enormous. Clinicians should carefully weigh the various options presented, their patient population, and their practice setting to decide which screening strategy is accessible and meets the needs of their patients. Even with the best screening available to date, the risk cannot be reduced to zero. Counseling should include a review of screening and diagnostic options, detection rates, false-positive rates, risks, benefits, and alternatives allowing patients to make informed choices for their family.[1]

Clinicians are faced with the task of monitoring many pregnancies to find the few that are abnormal. Many fetal abnormalities can be detected with current screening strategies. Ideal management includes preconception counseling with genetic screening to impact pregnancy decisions and family planning.

This section covers both first- and second-trimester screening options, ultrasound testing, and diagnostic options such as chorionic villus sampling (CVS; first trimester) and amniocentesis (second trimester).

I. EPIDEMIOLOGY

A. Chromosomal Abnormalities
Chromosomal abnormalities are relatively common. About 1 in 13 conceptions is chromosomally abnormal, and chromosomal anomalies are associated with 50% of first-trimester spontaneous losses. Chromosomal defects with a significant clinical impact occur in 0.65% of all births and are associated with up to 11.5% of stillbirths and neonatal deaths.[2] The most common autosomal trisomy in live births is trisomy 21 (Down syndrome), which has the most clinically applicable antepartum screening and diagnosis strategies available. Current screening may also detect other significant chromosomal aneuploidies such as trisomies 18 and 13.[3]

B. Major Anatomic Defects
Major anatomic defects occur in about 2% of all births. Major congenital defects, mental retardation, or genetic abnormality are evident at birth in 3% to 4% of newborns. The prevalence of these abnormalities doubles by the age of 7 to 8 years.[2]

C. Maternal Age Risk
The risk for a chromosomal aneuploidy increases with increasing maternal age, but most pregnancies occur in younger women. Currently, about half of trisomy 21 births are to mothers younger than 35.[4,5] Amniocentesis traditionally has been offered to woman age 35 years or older at the time of delivery because of the much greater risk for aneuploidy of about 1 in 200, which balances the rate of fetal loss with amniocentesis of about 1 in 200.[3] Recent changes in fetal chromosomal screening options have been developed, and now screening options and invasive testing should be offered to all pregnant women regardless of age.[1]

D. Offering Screening in All Pregnancies
1. Screening in the first trimester
   First-trimester screening with serum markers including pregnancy-associated plasma protein A (PAPP-A) and the free beta subunit of human chorionic gonadotropin (β-hCG) and/or ultrasound

for NT recently has been introduced. Several protocols combining both first- and second-trimester screening have been suggested using serum markers and ultrasonographic findings alone and in combination.[1]

NT should be performed only in centers that meet strict criteria including specific training, standardization of images, use of appropriate ultrasound equipment, and ongoing quality assessment.[1] Many areas of the United States do not have access to this level of expertise locally. These technologies add expense to routine pregnancy care, and the cost impacts of such screening will need further study. It will take some time to develop centers accessible to all maternity patients across the United States. In addition, these screening procedures have been studied in tightly regulated research protocols, and it remains to be seen how well these screening procedures will perform when translated into the routine care of pregnant women. Current NT screening centers may find that the increase in demand for services overwhelms screening availability, particularly given the narrow window for screening between 10 4/7 and 13 6/7 weeks for each pregnancy. These systems issues, as well as cost-effectiveness issues, will need to be addressed as medical systems, patients, and clinicians adjust to these new screening modalities.

2. α-Fetoprotein (AFP)
   a. High AFP level: Maternal serum AFP (MSAFP) level is increased in neural tube defects (NTDs) and other fetal structural defects. Since the advent of AFP screening, the NTD birth rate declined from 1.3 to 0.6 per 1000 births.[6]
   b. Low AFP level: A low MSAFP level is associated with an increased risk for aneuploidy, particularly trisomy 21.[7]
3. Maternal serum triple screen (MSTS)
   Three second-trimester maternal serum markers (AFP, hCG, and unconjugated estriol [uE3]) used in combination (MSTS) combine for a 70% detection rate for trisomy 21 fetuses.[1,8]
4. Maternal serum quadruple screen (QUAD screen)
   The addition of inhibin-A (INH-A) as a fourth serum marker improves the detection rate for trisomy 21 to about 80%.[1,9,10]
5. Fetal cells and DNA/RNA
   Fetal cells in maternal circulation have been identified and studied, and may have about the same sensitivity as the serum markers with increased specificity.[6] There are ongoing research efforts to identify fetal DNA and RNA in maternal serum that may become clinically applicable in the future.[11,12]

E. Use of Ultrasound as a Screening Tool for Fetal Abnormalities

Ultrasound is used for screening (NT), diagnosis (fetal anatomy), and gestational age determination.

F. Preconception Counseling

1. General recommendations
   All women of childbearing age should be taking at least 400 μg (0.4 mg) folic acid daily before conception and continuing through pregnancy. This intervention has been proved to decrease NTDs and may improve other birth defects as well. Folic acid supplementation before pregnancy may prevent more than 50% of serious NTDs such as spina bifida and anencephaly.[13]
2. Women with previous pregnancy with NTD
   Women who have had a prior affected pregnancy with a NTD should consume 4 mg folic acid before and during the pregnancy. This is associated with a 71% decrease in the risk for a NTD reoccurrence.[13]

G. Risk Assessment

Risk assessment begins with preconception care and continues throughout the pregnancy. Genetic screening should include those autosomal recessive disorders that are more common in specific ethnic groups such as hemoglobinopathies, thalassemias, cystic fibrosis (CF), among others.[14] These disorders have prenatal testing options as follows:

1. Sickle cell and hemoglobinopathies
   Sickle cell and other hemoglobinopathies are best diagnosed in pregnancy by hemoglobin electrophoresis. This determines trait or disease and other hemoglobin variants such as hemoglobin C and β-thalassemia.[14,15]
2. Thalassemia
   A reasonable screen for thalassemia is the mean cell volume (MCV) value in a CBC. If the MCV is low (<80 μ^3), the clinician can proceed with a hemoglobin electrophoresis. This will identify most hemoglobinopathies such as sickle cell, hemoglobin C, and β-thalassemia, but unfortunately, α-thalassemia is diagnosed only with DNA

testing. If a diagnosis is made, the partner should also be offered testing to assess fetal risk.[15]

3. CF screening

Screening should be offered to all pregnant women with a special emphasis on those with a family history of CF, couples with one partner with the disease, and couples in which one is white.[16]

a. Standard screening test for CF: This should include the 25 disease-causing mutations in the cystic fibrosis transmembrane regulator (CTFR) gene that have a frequency of more than 0.1% in North American CF patients.[16]

b. Risk for disease: Risk can be reduced but not canceled with the screening. For European whites, the risk for having a child with CF is 1 in 3300, and that risk decreases to 1 in 16,240 with one negative partner.[16]

c. Two screening strategies
   i. Concurrent: screen both partners at the same time
   ii. Sequential: screen the available or the high-risk partner first and screen the other partner only if one is positive

The screening strategy choice depends on the other diseases being screened for and the time constraints of testing.[16]

d. Results reporting: Couple screening reports the results to the couple as a unit as positive only if both parents are screen positive and as negative if only one or neither parent is a carrier. The goal of screening is that the at-risk pregnancy can be identified and not the healthy carrier of the recessive gene. Sequential screening reports results to each partner as well as the couple, and allows for those screened to know their individual status.[16]

H. Medical and Social History

Lifestyle issues including tobacco and alcohol and other substance use and abuse should be evaluated. Health issues including immunizations, medications, and disease management (hypertension, DM, depression) should be addressed as well. Multiple spontaneous abortions, stillbirth, or positive family history suggest a potential chromosomal disorder. Family members with multiple malformations or mental retardation may provide clues for chromosomal abnormalities. Those with autosomal recessive disorders may have no family history of affected offspring and yet still carry the recessive gene.[14]

II. PATHOGENESIS

Trisomy 21 and other autosomal trisomies are usually the result of meiotic nondisjunction, which increases as maternal age increases. NT, the ultrasonographic finding of an increased amount of clear fluid behind the fetal neck, may be related to an increase in lymph fluid caused by the delayed development of lymph ducts.[3] Multiple other causative factors may be involved including cardiac failure, venous congestion, fetal anemia, and congenital infection.[17] This finding translates later in gestation to a thickened nuchal fold that is a marker for trisomy 21 during the second trimester.

III. CLINICAL SCREENING OPTIONS

A. Preconception Counseling

Patients with preexisting diseases such as diabetes, genetic disorders, prior unfavorable pregnancy outcomes, and those with increased risks conferred by age, ethnic group, or occupation may benefit from prepregnancy consultations to plan for and manage a pregnancy.[18]

B. Screening

1. Informed consent counseling

This should occur before screening, be nondirective, and include the type of screening offered, interpretation of results, and management of an abnormal screen.

2. Genetic counseling should be offered to those with the following characteristics:

a. Family history of a genetic disorder

b. Personal history of recurrent early pregnancy loss (defined as 2 or more consecutive <15-week pregnancy losses),[19] fetal deaths, or an abnormal offspring

c. Advanced maternal age (35 or older at the time of delivery for singletons; 33 or older with multifetal pregnancies)

d. Abnormal screening results[14]

The underlying rate of 2% to 3% for major anomalies at birth needs to be emphasized with parents. Despite screening for particular disorders, others may occur that were not anticipated, and there is no guarantee of a perfectly healthy infant. Anticipatory guidance and planning for the birth of an affected infant into a family improves parental adjustment and allows for advance medical decisions to be made. Couples who face a genetic disorder or birth defect can be empowered to help with decision making around a variety of pregnancy and delivery issues and neonatal care issues. This sense of control over such decisions improves emotional adjustment after the diagnosis of an abnormal fetus.[20]

3. First-trimester screening

   Prenatal screening and diagnosis during the first trimester has the advantage of timely reassurance or early diagnosis for parents in a window of time where privacy can be maintained and clinical options are increased.

   a. First-trimester maternal serum analytes: PAPP-A and β-hCG are measured between 9.0 weeks and 13 6/7 weeks of gestation. Combining both serum marker levels with maternal age increases the detection rate for trisomy 21 to 65% to 70%. This is comparable with current second-trimester screening detection rates.[10,21,22]

   b. First-trimester ultrasound findings: NT measures an area of clear subcutaneous fluid in the posterior fetal neck between 11 and 13 6/7 weeks of gestation. NT is increased in trisomy 21 and other chromosomal aneuploidies such as trisomy 13, trisomy 18, Turner syndrome, genetic syndromes, and fetal anatomic anomalies, particularly cardiac anomalies. Combined with maternal age, NT can detect up to 87% of fetuses with trisomy 21.[10] Those with enlarged NT should be offered follow-up ultrasound and fetal echocardiography in the second trimester.[22] In multifetal gestations, serum screening is less sensitive and NT may be attempted to screen these fetuses.[1] NT should be offered only at centers with ongoing quality assessment, specific training, and appropriate equipment.[1]

   c. Combination first-trimester screening: Maternal serum analytes (PAPP-A and β-hCG) combined with NT measurement can detect all aneuploidies up to 96% of the time, including trisomy 21 at up to a 97% detection rate and trisomies 13 and 18 up to 100% of the time.[23,24]

   d. Integrated testing: This is a screening strategy integrating both first- and second-trimester screening results into a single risk assessment[1] (see second-trimester screening in Table 7-7)

TABLE 7-7 Sensitivity and Specificity for Screening Tests for Down Syndrome

Screening Test	Sensitivity	Specificity	Positive Predictive Value*	Negative Predictive Value*
First Trimester				
NT measurement	64-70%[10]	95%	2.6%	99.93%
NT, PAPP-A, β-hCG	82-87%[10]	95%	3.3%	99.97%
Second Trimester				
MSTS (AFP, hCG, uE3)	69%[10]	95%	2.7%	99.93%
Quad (AFP, hCG, uE3, INH-A)	81%[10]	95%	3.1%	99.96%
First plus Second Trimester				
Integrated (NT, PAPP-A, quad)	94-96%[10]	95%	3.7%	99.99%
Serum integrated (PAPP-A, quad)	85-88%[10]	95%	3.3%	99.97%
Stepwise sequential	95%[10]	95%	3.7%	99.99%
Contingent sequential	88-94%[48]	95%	3.5%	99.98%

False-positive rate at 5% for all tests.
*Positive and negative predictive values are calculated using a prior probability of 1 in 504 or the current prevalence of Down syndrome at 16 weeks in the United States.[48]
NT, Nuchal translucency; PAPP-A, pregnancy-associated plasma protein A; β-hCG, beta subunit of human chorionic gonadotropin; MSTS, maternal serum triple screen; AFP, α-fetoprotein; uE3, unconjugated estriol; quad, serum quadruple screen; INH-A, inhibin-A.
Adapted from American College of Obstetricians and Gynecologists: ACOG Committee on Practice Bulletins #77. Screening for fetal chromosomal abnormalities, *Obstet Gynecol* 109(1):217-227, 2007, using data generated from FASTER Trial[10] and predicted detection rates.[49]

e. Women with abnormal first-trimester screening should be offered genetic counseling and diagnostic testing such as CVS or amniocentesis.[1]

f. Pregnancies with abnormal first-trimester serum markers or an increased NT (>3.5 mm) may be at risk for adverse pregnancy outcomes (fetal loss $<$ 24 weeks, fetal demise, low birth weight, or preterm birth), but it remains unclear whether outcomes improve with third-trimester fetal surveillance.[1]

4. Second-trimester maternal serum screening

a. MSTS or quad screen: Testing is offered to pregnant women to screen for anatomic and chromosomal abnormalities, and is routinely done between 15 and 22 weeks of gestation with the ideal window at 16 to 18 weeks.[3] This test may be offered to those presenting for care after 13 6/7 weeks or in combination with first-trimester screening.[1]

b. Increased AFP level: The AFP level is increased in pregnancies that involve fetuses with NTDs.[6] NTDs occur in 1 to 2 per 1000 pregnancies, but 90% to 95% occur in those without a prior family history.[13] Congenital anomalies including ventral defects such as gastroschisis or omphalocele also are associated with increased AFP levels. Other associated defects include Finnish nephrosis, Turner syndrome with cystic hygroma, fetal bowel obstruction, and teratoma. Increased levels may be because of inaccurate pregnancy dating, multiple gestation, or fetal demise.[25] NTD screening with AFP or ultrasound evaluation, or both, should be offered to women undergoing only first-trimester aneuploidy screening.[1]

c. Evaluating an increased MSAFP level: Ultrasound evaluation should be offered as the first step in the evaluation of an abnormal AFP level.

    i. Anencephaly may be detected as early as the first trimester by ultrasound and should be detected on routine standard second-trimester ultrasound examinations.

    ii. Open spina bifida, meningocele, and myelomeningocele usually can be detected 90% to 95% of the time in second-trimester scanning.[25]

    iii. Ventral defects such as gastroschisis, omphalocele, and exstrophy of the bladder usually are detected by standard ultrasound scanning.

    iv. Genetic amniocentesis should be offered to those with omphalocele because of the high rate of chromosomal abnormalities associated with this malformation.[26]

    v. Amniocentesis for karyotyping, AFP level, and acetylcholinesterase levels may be offered for diagnosis of an increased AFP level.[25]

    vi. Pregnancies with increased MSAFP levels, despite normal ultrasound and normal karyotype, remain at risk for poor pregnancy outcomes including preterm delivery, growth restriction, placental abruption, stillbirth, and preeclampsia. Further screening protocols for these pregnancies have been suggested.[27]

d. A low MSAFP level is associated with chromosomal defects. Combining maternal age and MSAFP level defines risk and provides an individual risk ratio. This ratio is screen positive when it meets or exceeds that of a 35-year-old woman usually about 1:270.[25]

e. The triple combination of AFP with hCG and uE3 (MSTS) increases the detection rate for chromosomal aneuploidies and other chromosomal abnormalities (see Table 7-7).

    i. For trisomy 21, the triple test has a 60% to 75% detection rate and a specificity of 95% (false-positive rate of 5%).[3,28]

    ii. Trisomy 21 is associated with low AFP, increased hCG, and low uE3 levels.[28]

    iii. Trisomy 18 is associated with decreased levels of all three analytes, and the MSTS can detect up to 90% of these affected fetuses.[29]

f. The quad screen adds Inhibin-A (INH-A) to MSTS to increase the detection rate for trisomy 21 from 70% to 81% with a specificity of 95%.

5. Abnormal maternal serum screening

These analyte values are highly dependent on accurate gestational dating. The first response to an abnormal serum screen should be to get a standard ultrasound examination to confirm pregnancy dating. If the pregnancy dating is in error by a week or more, the results should be recalculated. If the pregnancy is found to be less than 15 weeks, a specimen can be redrawn at the appropriate gestational age. If the pregnancy is found to be further than 22 weeks, the testing cannot be done.

a. Role of ultrasound: Confirmation of gestational age and number of fetuses by standard ultrasound is the usual first response to abnormal serum screening results. A genetic ultrasound can also be done to look for anatomic abnormalities or more subtle findings called *markers*. Normal ultrasound findings can further refine the risk assessment, making it less likely to actually have an abnormal fetus.

b. Amniocentesis: Assuming confirmation of dates and normal anatomy by a standard ultrasound examination, patients with an abnormal maternal serum screening result should be offered both genetic counseling and amniocentesis. Amniocentesis can provide chromosome analysis and also measurement of amniotic fluid levels of AFP, as well as acetylcholinesterase levels if indicated by increased MSAFP levels.[25]

C. Screening Strategies

Given that most pregnancies are normal and that the abnormalities discussed in this section are relatively rare, most of these strategies are comparable, and a given patient population, local expertise, and time of entry into care will impact screening strategy decisions. Counseling should reflect gestational age, obstetric history, family history, NT availability, test sensitivity and specificity, risk of invasive procedures, result timing, and subsequent options for pregnancy interventions. Test results should be communicated as a numeric risk that can then be contrasted with individual pretest probability and invasive testing risk profiles to assist patient understanding and decision making.

Although the average pretest probability of trisomy 21 is 1 in 500, there is a spectrum of prevalence between 1 in 80 and 1 in 900 depending on a woman's age. Thus, the negative predictive value of testing is much greater in a woman at low risk than at average risk, which is demonstrated in Table 7-7. This, in essence, an average risk of 1 in 500 results in a difference of missing 1 diagnosis in 10,000 women for the most aggressive screening strategy listed versus 7 in 10,000 for current second-trimester MSTS. If the pretest probability is even less than average at 1 in 900, then the NPV is 99.96 or missing 4 trisomy 21 fetuses in 10,000 patients screened. These numbers may aid in both clinician and patient understanding of the impact of screening (see Table 7-7).

Screening options for those entering care in the second trimester remain maternal serum screening (MSTS or quad), standard ultrasound evaluation, or both. Women entering care in the first trimester should be offered a strategy that includes both first- and second-trimester screening. Not all communities will have access to NT screening locally because this testing can be done only by qualified sonographers using appropriate equipment. Clinicians will need to review screening options and decide which strategy best meets their patients' needs.[1]

First- and second-trimester results should be interpreted together because interpreting each individually increases the false-positive rate.

1. Integrated screening
   Integrated screening reports risk in the second trimester only after both first- and second-trimester markers are evaluated. Integrating serum markers without NT results in an 85% to 88% detection rate, or if combined with NT, results in a 94% to 96% detection rate.[10] The advantage is higher sensitivity with a lower false-positive rate, but the disadvantage is a 3- to 4-week delay in screening completion, and thus the loss of CVS as a diagnostic option.

2. Sequential screening
   a. Stepwise strategy: Women at high risk are offered genetic counseling and invasive testing, and women at low risk are offered second-trimester screening.
   b. Contingent: First-trimester results are classified as high (offered CVS), intermediate (offered second-trimester screening), or low risk (no further screening).[1]

D. Summary Maternal Serum Screening Recommendations

1. Screening and invasive testing for aneuploidy should be available and offered to all women who present for care before 20 weeks of gestation. Clinicians should be aware of these screening strategies and consider their patient population and community resources in choosing a strategy for their practice.

2. First-trimester screening using both NT and serum markers is comparable with quad screening in the second trimester for use in general population screening.

3. NTD screening should continue to be offered in the second trimester.

4. Multiple-gestation pregnancies present special challenges in screening, and available screening is less sensitive than in singleton pregnancies.

5. After first-trimester screening, second-trimester screening for trisomy 21 is not indicated unless it is performed and analyzed as part of integrated, stepwise sequential, or contingent sequential testing.

6. NT should be limited to centers with specific training, appropriate equipment, and ongoing quality assessment in performing a standardized NT examination.[1]

E. Second-Trimester Ultrasound Summary

Those with abnormal serum screens with dating confirmation by routine ultrasound should be offered diagnostic evaluation. Increased AFP level is associated with NTD and other structural defects, many of which can be identified by a standard ultrasound examination evaluating the spine and fetal anatomy. Chromosomal aneuploidies such as trisomies 21, 18, and 13 all are associated with anatomic structural abnormalities or ultrasound findings known as markers.[30,31] A normal ultrasound without any evidence of trisomy 21 by markers decreases the risk for aneuploidy. Studies vary and suggest that a normal ultrasound may decrease the risk for trisomy 21 by anywhere from 45% to 80%.[3,32,33] Thus, a normal ultrasound may be sufficiently reassuring with this decrease in risk to impact the decision to proceed with invasive diagnostic evaluation.

F. Genetic Ultrasound

Fetal aneuploidy is associated with major structural defects and various ultrasonographic markers. Trisomy 21 markers include increased nuchal fold, short femur, short humerus, pyelectasis, and hyperechoic bowel. These markers may be transient during gestation and may not indicate an underlying structural abnormality.[31] Some of these findings are highly associated with an abnormal fetal karyotype, and the more markers a fetus has the more likely it is to be abnormal.[4,31] The finding of a major organ or structural abnormality or the finding of two or more minor anatomic abnormalities indicates a high risk for fetal aneuploidy. These women should be offered invasive diagnostic testing and genetic counseling.[3] A genetic sonogram performed specifically for these ultrasonographic markers improves the odds of detecting the truly abnormal fetus to about 50% and may provide the information needed to clarify the individual risk and allow for only the very high-risk fetuses to undergo invasive diagnostic testing such as amniocentesis.[31]

IV. DIAGNOSIS

Screening can provide a risk profile, but this should be followed up with informed patient counseling including genetic counseling and offering diagnostic options such as CVS in the first trimester or amniocentesis in the second trimester. Patients undergoing these procedures have concluded that the indications for invasive testing warrant the fetal risk.

A. Amniocentesis (15-20 weeks)

Amniocentesis, or removing amniotic fluid that contains fetal cells with a transabdominal approach and ultrasound guidance, has been demonstrated to have a fetal loss rate of less than 0.5%.[3] Amniotic fluid is analyzed for chromosomes, AFP level, or acetylcholinesterase level for open NTDs. The diagnostic accuracy of cytogenetic testing by amniocentesis is more than 99%.[34] Risks include spontaneous abortion, infection, needle injuries, and preterm labor. Early amniocentesis (11-13 weeks) has been studied but carries an unacceptably high risk for fetal injury or fetal loss of about 2.5% and a greater rate of fetal cell culture failures.[35]

B. Chorionic Villus Sampling (10-12 weeks)

CVS is the current first-trimester diagnostic test of choice and is usually done between 10 and 12 weeks of gestation. CVS samples the chorionic villi either transcervically or transabdominally under ultrasound guidance.[3] Earlier diagnosis provides opportunity for more private pregnancy decisions, a more rapid turnaround for results (a few days), and safer termination options for the pregnancy. The risk for spontaneous pregnancy loss is 1% to 2%.[36] The CVS loss rate is 0.6% to 0.8% greater than that of traditional amniocentesis. This may reflect the timing earlier in gestation and the expected additional spontaneous loss rate between 9 and 16 weeks of gestation.[3] There have been reports of limb reduction and oromandibular defects associated with CVS. The rate for limb reduction is 6 per 10,000, which mirrors that of the general population. These defects seem to be more common in CVS performed before 9 weeks of gestation. CVS performed after 9 menstrual weeks has a low risk for these facial and limb defects that matches that of the general population.[3,37] Contraindications include active cervical infections (for the transcervical approach), and uterine position, maternal body habitus, or difficulty with ultrasonographic images may make the procedure difficult.[3] CVS cannot be used for detection of NTDs. Culture success rates, such as amniocentesis, are more than 99%. Because of the nature of the testing, approximately 2% have ambiguous results because of chromosomal mosaicism.[38]

C. Additional Diagnostic Options

1. Cordocentesis or percutaneous umbilical blood sampling
   This involves obtaining blood from the umbilical vein under direct ultrasound guidance. The fetal blood can then be karyotyped in 24 to 48 hours. The loss rate is reported to be less than 2%.[3,39]

2. Preimplantation genetic diagnosis
   Newer technologies have continued to evolve and provide the ability to test early embryos before implantation with in vitro fertilization techniques. These have been used to identify some chromosomal abnormalities and genetic disorders such as CF and Tay–Sachs disease. The list of detectable disorders continues to expand such that consultation with reproductive specialists or geneticists may be indicated.[40]

3. Fetal cell sorting
   Fetal cells can be found in maternal circulation. Free fetal DNA and fetal RNA have been isolated in maternal serum. Although currently research tools, these technologies in the future may create opportunities for noninvasive diagnosis of fetal chromosomal defects or other disorders.[12,41]

4. Fluorescence in situ hybridization (FISH)
   FISH technology involves the binding of specific DNA probes to partial or entire chromosomes and is used to diagnose aneuploidies or chromosomal deletions. This technology provides a diagnosis in 24 to 48 hours for some abnormalities (chromosomes 13, 18, 21, X, and Y) compared with 1 to 2 weeks for culturing amniotic cells or chorionic villi and subsequent karyotype analysis. To date, this testing needs confirmation with routine chromosome analysis because FISH does not detect translocations, inversions, deletions, or chromosomal abnormalities of all chromosomes.[42]

5. Three-dimensional (3D) ultrasound
   3D ultrasound offers even more options in the area of fetal screening and diagnosis of abnormal pregnancies. 3D ultrasound can improve the diagnosis detected on routine 2D scanning and may impact patient management decisions. 3D ultrasound is most helpful in facial anomalies, hand and foot abnormalities, axial spine defects, and NTDs. These images are particularly helpful in the accurate localization of spinal defects and may help in demonstrating anomalies not apparent in 2D scanning or with patients who are difficult to scan because of fetal positioning or maternal obesity. 3D images may be helpful in complex anomalies, providing additional information not only to the sonographer/clinician but also allowing patients to see and understand an anomaly better.[43] 3D imaging has improved our estimation of fetal weight impacting the diagnosis of IUGR.[44] 3D ultrasound has been shown to diagnose fetal sex earlier, which may impact those at risk for X-linked chromosomal disorders.[45] In one study, 3D imaging impacted the clinical management of 5% of clinical anomalies identified by 2D scanning.[43]

V. TREATMENT

A. Folic Acid

All women of childbearing age should be taking 400 μg (0.4 mg) folic acid daily to decrease their risk for NTDs and possibly other birth defects. For those with a prior history of NTD affected pregnancy, the recommendation is to take 4 mg folic acid daily. This dose has been shown in these high-risk patients to decrease the risk for NTD recurrence by 71%.[13] Recently, the United States has fortified foods with folic acid, but the recommendation of a supplemental folic acid dose remains and can be accomplished simply with a daily women's formula multivitamin.

B. Treatment Options

The choice to terminate a pregnancy based on karyotype findings or fetal structural abnormalities is a difficult one. Decisions should be based on individual risk profiles and findings from screening and diagnostic testing. A couple who would not consider termination as an option should still be offered screening and diagnostic testing if appropriate so that this information is available to manage the pregnancy, delivery, and immediate and subsequent care of the newborn. This knowledge may impact decisions around delivery including the use of and interpretation of fetal monitoring and the indications for an assisted or cesarean delivery. Preparation for the management and care of the newborn can be made in advance, including the decision of where to deliver and how much resuscitation is appropriate, as well as management plans for the medical care of an abnormal newborn.[46] Treatment options vary and include both intrauterine surgical management and immediate postdelivery care. Consultation with perinatal and neonatal specialists and preparation for both the care of the mother and the newborn can improve outcomes. Information gained about genetic, structural, or metabolic disorders may impact future pregnancy and family planning.

VI. SOR A RECOMMENDATIONS

RECOMMENDATION	REFERENCE
Folic acid supplementation before pregnancy and during the first 2 months of pregnancy protects against NTDs. Folate may increase the risk for multiple gestation. A multivitamin taken alone does not provide this protection.	47

REFERENCES

1. American College of Obstetricians and Gynecologists (ACOG): ACOG Committee on Practice Bulletins #77. Screening for fetal chromosomal abnormalities, *Obstet Gynecol* 109(1): 217-227, 2007.
2. Milunsky A, Milunsky J: Genetic counseling: preconception, prenatal, and perinatal. In Milunsky A, editor: *Genetic disorders and the fetus,* Baltimore: 1998, The Johns Hopkins University Press.
3. American College of Obstetricians and Gynecologists: ACOG Committee on Practice Bulletins #27: prenatal diagnosis of fetal chromosomal abnormalities, *Obstet Gynecol* 97(5 pt 1, suppl):1-12, 2001.
4. Nicolaides KH: Screening for chromosomal defects, *Ultrasound Obstet Gynecol* 21(4):313-321, 2003.
5. Benn PA: Advances in prenatal screening for Down syndrome: I. General principles and second trimester testing, *Clin Chim Acta* 323:1-16, 2002.
6. Evans MI, O'Brien JE, Harrison H: Second trimester screening. In Ransom SB, Dombrowski MP, Evans MI et al, editors: *Contemporary therapy in obstetrics and gynecology,* Philadelphia, 2002, WB Saunders.
7. Merkatz IR, Nitowsky HM, Macri JN et al: An association between low maternal serum alpha-fetoprotein and fetal chromosomal abnormalities, *Am J Obstet Gynecol* 148(7):886-894, 1984.
8. Wald NJ, Cuckle HS, Densem JW et al: Maternal serum screening for Down's syndrome in early pregnancy, *BMJ* 297:883-887, 1988.
9. Wald NJ, Densem JW, George L et al: Prenatal screening for Down's syndrome using inhibin-A as a serum marker, *Prenat Diagn* 16:143-153, 1996.
10. Malone FD, Canick JA, Ball RH et al: First-trimester or second-trimester screening, or both, for Down's syndrome, *N Engl J Med* 353(19):2001-2011, 2005.
11. Holzgreve W, Hahn S: Prenatal diagnosis using fetal cells and free fetal DNA in maternal blood, *Clin Perinatol* 28:353-365, 2001.
12. Qinyu G, Liu Q, Bai Y et al: A semi-quantitative microarray method to detect fetal RNA's in maternal plasma, *Prenat Diagn* 25(10):912-918, 2005.
13. American Academy of Pediatrics Committee on Genetics: Folic acid for the prevention of neural tube defects, *Pediatrics* 104(2):325-327, 1999.
14. Bubb JA, Mathews AL: What's new in prenatal screening and diagnosis? *Prim Care* 31:561-582, 2004.
15. American College of Obstetricians and Gynecologists Committee on Genetics: Committee Opinion Number 238. Genetic screening for hemoglobinopathies, *Obstet Gynecol* 96(1):C1-C2, 2000.
16. American College of Obstetricians and Gynecologists and the American College of Medical Genetics: *Preconception and prenatal carrier screening for cystic fibrosis: clinical and laboratory guidelines,* Washington, DC, 2001, American College of Obstetricians and Gynecologists.
17. Pathophysiology of increased nuchal transluceny. In: Nicolaides KH, Sebire NJ, Snijders RJM, editors: *The 11-14 week scan: the diagnosis of fetal abnormalities,* London, 1999, The Parthenon Publishing Group.
18. Donnai D: Genetic counseling and the pre-pregnancy clinic. In Brock DJH, Rodeck CH, Ferguson-Smith MA, editors: *Prenatal diagnosis and screening,* London, 1992, Churchill Livingstone.
19. American College of Obstetricians and Gynecologists: ACOG Committee on Practice Bulletins #24: management of recurrent early pregnancy loss, *Obstet Gynecol* 97(2): 1-12, 2001.
20. Matthews AL: Known fetal malformations during pregnancy: a human experience of loss, *Birth Defects Orig Artic Ser* 26(3):168-175, 1990.
21. Cuckle HS, van Lith JMM: Appropriate biochemical parameters in first-trimester screening for Down syndrome, *Prenat Diagn* 19:505-512, 1999.
22. Benn PA: Advances in prenatal screening for Down syndrome: II. First trimester testing, integrated testing, and future directions, *Clin Chim Acta* 324(1-2):1-11, 2002.
23. Nicolaides KH: Nuchal translucency and other first-trimester sonographic markers of chromosomal abnormalities, *Am J Obstet Gynecol* 191:45-67, 2004.
24. Spencer K, Spencer CE, Power M et al: Screening for chromosomal abnormalities in the first trimester using ultrasound and maternal serum biochemistry in a one-stop clinic: a review of three years prospective experience, *BJOG* 110(3): 281-286, 2003.
25. Ross HL, Elias S: Maternal serum screening for fetal genetic disorders, *Fetal Diagn Ther* 24(1):33-47, 1997.
26. Hsu LY: Prenatal diagnosis of chromosomal abnormalities through amniocentesis. In Milunsky A, editor: *Genetic disorders of the fetus,* Baltimore, 1998, The Johns Hopkins University Press.
27. Katz VL, Chescher NC, Cefalo RC: Unexplained elevations of maternal serum alpha-fetoprotein, *Obstet Gynecol Surv* 45(11):719-726, 1990.

28. Wald NJ, Watt HC, Hackshaw AK: Integrated screening for Down's syndrome based on tests performed during the first and second trimesters, *N Engl J Med* 341(7):461-467, 1999.

29. Palomaki GE, Neveux LM, Knight GJ et al: Maternal serum-integrated screening for trisomy 18 using both first- and second-trimester markers, *Prenat Diagn* 23(3):243-247, 2003.

30. Sanders RC, Blackmon LR, Hogge WA et al: Structural fetal abnormalities, the total picture. St. Louis, 1996, Mosby.

31. Nyberg DA, Souter VL, El-Bastawissi A et al: Isolated sonographic markers for detection of fetal Down syndrome in the second trimester of pregnancy, *J Ultrasound Med* 20(10): 1053-1063, 2001.

32. Nyberg DA, Luthy DA, Cheng EY et al: Role of prenatal ultrasonography in women with positive screen for Down syndrome on the basis of maternal serum markers, *Am J Obstet Gynecol* 173:1030-1035, 1995.

33. Vintzileos AM, Guzman ER, Smulian JC et al: Indication-specific accuracy of second-trimester genetic ultrasonography for the detection of trisomy 21, *Am J Obstet Gynecol* 181(5, pt 1):1045-1048, 1999.

34. Jackson LG, Zachary JM, Fowler SE et al: A randomized comparison of transcervical and transabdominal chorionic-villus sampling, *N Engl J Med* 327(9):594-598, 1992.

35. The Canadian Early and Mid-trimester Amniocentesis Trial (CEMAT) Group: Randomized trial to assess the safety and fetal outcome of early and mid-trimester amniocentesis, *Lancet* 351:242-247, 1998.

36. Gardner RJM, Sutherland GR: Prenatal diagnostic procedures. *Chromosome abnormalities and genetic counseling,* ed 3, Oxford, 2004, Oxford University Press.

37. Kuliev A, Jackson LG, Froster U et al: Chorionic villus sampling safety. Report of World Health Organization/EURO meeting in association with the Seventh International Conference on Early Prenatal Diagnosis of Genetic Diseases, Tel Aviv, Israel, *Am J Obstet Gynecol* 174:807-811, 1996.

38. Gardner RJM, Sutherland GR: Chromosome abnormalities detected at prenatal diagnosis. *Chromosome abnormalities and genetic counseling,* ed 3, Oxford, 2004, Oxford University Press.

39. Ghidini A, Sepulveda W, Lockwood CJ et al: Complications of fetal blood sampling, *Am J Obstet Gynecol* 168(5):1339-1344, 1993.

40. Zhuang GL, Zhang D: Preimplantation genetic diagnosis, *Int J Gynaecol Obstet* 82:419-423, 2003.

41. Jackson LG: Fetal cells and DNA in maternal blood, *Prenat Diagn* 23:837-846, 2003.

42. American College of Medical Genetics: Technical and clinical assessment of fluorescence in situ hybridization: an ACMG/ASHG position statement. I. Technical considerations, *Genet Med* 2(6):356-361, 2000.

43. Dyson RL, Pretorius DH, Budorick NE et al: Three-dimensional ultrasound in the evaluation of fetal anomalies, *Ultrasound Obstet Gynecol* 16(4):321-328, 2000.

44. Platt LD: Three-dimensional ultrasound, *Ultrasound Obstet Gynecol* 16:295-298, 2000.

45. Lev-Toaff AS, Ozhan S, Pretorius DH et al: Three-dimensional multiplanar ultrasound for fetal gender assignment: value of the mid-sagittal plane, *Ultrasound Obstet Gynecol* 16:345-350, 2000.

46. Clark SL, DeVore GR: Prenatal diagnosis for couples who would not consider abortion, *Obstet Gynecol* 73:1035-1037, 1989.

47. Lumley J, Watson L, Watson M et al: Periconceptual supplementation with folate and/or multivitamins for preventing neural tube defects, *Cochrane Database Syst Rev* (3):CD001056, 2001.

48. Egan JFX, Benn PA, Borgida AF et al: Efficacy of screening for fetal Down syndrome in the United States from 1974 to 1997, *Obstet Gynecol* 96:979-985, 2000.

49. Cuckle HS, Benn PA, Wright D: Down syndrome screening in the first and/or second trimester: model predicted performance using meta-analysis parameters, *Semin Perinatol* 29:252-257, 2005.

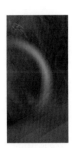

CHAPTER 8

Chronic Medical Conditions in Pregnancy

SECTION A Pulmonary Problems in Pregnancy

Matthew K. Cline, MD

I. ASTHMA

Asthma is the most common chronic respiratory disease that coexists with pregnancy, with a prevalence rate of 3.7% to 8.4% in pregnant women from 1997 to 2001.[1] This rate is similar to the 8.4% incidence rate of asthma in women 18 to 44 years of age who are not pregnant in the 2001-2003 National Health Interview Survey.[2] It is a chronic inflammatory disorder characterized by recurrent episodes of wheezing, breathlessness, chest tightness, and cough, and it is associated with widespread, but variable, airflow limitation that is at least partially reversible, either spontaneously or with treatment.

A. Epidemiology, Pathogenesis, and Interaction with Pregnancy

The traditional view of asthma as an illness that is primarily bronchospastic in nature is no longer valid. The pathophysiology of asthma is more clearly defined in terms of *chronic airway inflammation* and *bronchial hyperactivity*, with reversible episodes of airway obstruction.

1. Effect of pregnancy on asthma[3]

   Pregnancy can have a varying effect on asthma. Studies that assess pulmonary function before and during pregnancy for patients with asthma have reported the following results:
   a. 69% of women will have improvement in symptoms
   b. 31% of women will experience worsening of symptoms

   The course of asthma is typically consistent for a given woman during successive pregnancies, emphasizing the importance of taking a careful pregnancy and medical history. Women with more severe, uncontrolled asthma before pregnancy are more likely to experience worsening during pregnancy, precipitated most often by upper respiratory tract infections, followed by noncompliance with medical therapy. General concordance exists between rhinitis symptoms during pregnancy and the status of asthma; treatment of rhinitis is a reasonable secondary goal for pregnant women with asthma.[4]

   The peak incidence of exacerbations is between the 24th and 36th weeks of pregnancy, whereas the fewest symptoms are experienced during weeks 37 to 40. Asthma generally remains quiescent during labor and delivery. Changes in asthma severity during pregnancy are more than just random fluctuations, as symptoms generally revert toward the prepregnancy state within 3 months from delivery. The course of asthma has been associated with sex of the fetus. Women pregnant with boys tend to have improved symptoms during pregnancy compared with women pregnant with girls, possibly because of greater androgen production by male fetuses (Table 8-1).[5]

2. Complications

   Asthma has been associated with several pregnancy complications, based on retrospective studies done

TABLE 8-1 Changes in Respiratory System during Pregnancy

Increased minute ventilation

Caused by increased circulating progesterone in the first trimester, increases 40% by term, also known as *pregnancy-induced hyperventilation,* or the dyspnea of early pregnancy

Increased oxygen consumption and basal metabolic rate

Normal blood gases in pregnancy have a greater Po_2 (102-106 mm Hg) and a lower Pco_2 (28-30 mm Hg)

A $Pco_2 > 35$ mm Hg or a $Po_2 < 70$ mm Hg represents a more severe compromise during an asthma exacerbation during pregnancy

Increased tidal volume

Tidal volume increases by 20-40%, thought to be due to increase in progesterone from placenta

Decreased residual volume and functional residual capacity

Caused by mechanical effects on the gravid uterus on the diaphragm

Pregnant women experiencing acute asthma do better in a seated position

Increased vital capacity and total lung capacity

These increase by 100-200 ml and 300 ml, respectively, at term, once fetus engages in the pelvis

Before fetal descent there is no significant change in either

No change in FEV_1 and PEF

Can be used for assessment of response to therapy

Arterial Po_2 in the fetus is one third to one fourth the arterial Po_2 in the adult

Fetal umbilical vein blood has greatest fetal Po_2 (average, 31.9 mm Hg) and can never exceed maternal venous Po_2

A maternal $Po_2 < 60$ mm Hg directly reduces oxygen supply to the fetus

Reduction in uterine blood flow caused by endogenous sympathetic discharge or exogenous vasoconstrictors may further compromise fetal oxygenation

FEV_1, Forced expiratory volume in 1 second; PEF, peak expiratory flow.
From Gardner MO, Doyle NM: Asthma in pregnancy, *Obstet Gynecol Clin North Am* 31:385-413, 2004.

after initiation of antiinflammatory therapy.[6]

a. Preeclampsia (odds ratio [OR], 1.77)
b. Cesarean delivery (OR, 1.58)
c. Placental abruption (OR, 1.41)
d. Preterm delivery (OR, 1.40)
e. Low-birth-weight (LBW)/small-for-gestational-age (SGA) infants (OR, 1.16)

In women who have asthma exacerbations during pregnancy, there have also been associations with longer infant and maternal hospital length of stay; a fivefold increase in rates of maternal pneumonia; transient tachypnea of the term newborn, especially with male infants; and neonatal hyperbilirubinemia if mothers received oral steroids during pregnancy.

Although the risks for these complications are increased in pregnancies complicated by asthma, the risks can be minimized with good asthma control.[7]

B. Clinical Features and Diagnosis

The presentation of asthma in the pregnant woman is similar to that in nonpregnant women, with intermittent wheezing, cough, and shortness of breath. Exacerbations are episodic and can be precipitated by presence of viral upper respiratory infection; exposure to certain allergens such as dust mites, animal dander, or cigarette smoke; and exercise. Other associated symptoms and possible triggers include gastroesophageal reflux, psychosocial stress, and reactions to medications or other chemicals.

The cardinal feature of asthma is the reversibility of airway obstruction by medications that act on the bronchial smooth muscle, such as β-adrenergic agents, together with antiinflammatory agents. Recurrence of symptoms is also a requirement for the diagnosis of asthma because most clinicians would consider the single episode of wheezing associated with infection or allergic exposure to represent acute bronchospasm rather than the chronic and recurrent condition that asthma represents.

In addition to findings on physical examination, such as wheezes, prolonged expiratory phase, dyspnea at rest and with talking, and use of accessory respiratory muscles, pulmonary function tests during an acute attack will show significant decreases in forced expiratory volume in 1 second (FEV_1) and peak expiratory flow (PEF). These should both return to normal, or near normal, during asymptomatic periods. In most cases, a chest radiograph is not necessary. However, if radiographs are needed, they should be done with abdominal shielding.

C. Surveillance during Pregnancy

1. Treatment goals
   The three main goals of asthma management during pregnancy are as follows:
   a. Reduction in the number of asthma exacerbations
   b. Prevention of severe, acute bronchospasm
   c. Assurance of adequate maternal and fetal oxygenation
2. Pulmonary surveillance[8]
   a. Initial objective evaluation of pulmonary function by spirometry, including vital capacity, forced vital capacity, and FEV_1, will aid in early recognition of an exacerbation.
   b. Measuring peak expiratory flow rate (PFR) provides a good approximation of the FEV_1, and can be done easily and inexpensively using a portable peak flow meter. The normal PFR ranges between 350 and 500 L/min in the pregnant patient.
   c. PFR should be obtained at every office visit and can be used at home by patients to monitor the course of their disease before the onset of symptoms. A "personal best" PFR should be should be determined for each patient during a time when their asthma is well controlled.
3. Pregnancy surveillance
   Women with well-controlled asthma require no specific changes in management of their pregnancy. However, in women with severe or poorly controlled asthma, the National Asthma Education and Prevention Program (NAEPP) Expert Panel Report[8] recommends consideration of serial sonography for evaluation of fetal growth

and to rule out growth restriction beginning at 32 weeks. Other monitoring, though not specifically recommended by the Expert Panel, can be considered as well. For example, in patients with FEV_1 or PFR less than 80% predicted throughout the pregnancy, the rate of preterm labor is increased (number needed to harm = 17), which may lead to evaluation with fetal fibronectin or other tests.[9]

D. Management

1. Nonpharmacologic management
   a. Attempts should be made to identify and remove potentially avoidable triggering factors, including dust mites, molds, animal dander, tobacco smoke, pollen, exercise, emotional stress, aspirin, or nonsteroidal antiinflammatory drugs.
   b. Airtight covers should be used for mattresses and pillows. Contact with household cleaning products should be avoided.
   c. Smoking cessation should be emphasized during prenatal visits. Smoking rates are greater among pregnant women with asthma than pregnant women without lung disease.[10]
   d. Reduce patient anxiety by giving her an opportunity to express her concerns. Educate them regarding their illness and its relation to pregnancy.
2. Allergy immunotherapy
   a. Diagnostic skin testing should be deferred during pregnancy because of potentially serious systemic reactions.
   b. Allergy immunotherapy appears safe for patients to continue during pregnancy if they were already receiving it, though dose reduction is recommended to further decrease the risk for systemic reaction, and immunotherapy should be discontinued if increases in doses would be required to achieve therapeutic doses.[1]
   c. Immunotherapy should not be initially started during pregnancy because the propensity for systemic reactions is unpredictable, the likelihood of systemic reactions is greatest during initiation, there is a natural latency of immunotherapy effect, and it is difficult to tell in advance who will actually benefit from immunotherapy.
   d. Influenza vaccine should be administered in any trimester during the influenza season (October to mid-May), as it is a killed virus vaccine with an established safety profile.[11]

3. Pharmacologic management
   a. The potential risks of untreated exacerbations, and their associated hypoxia, make pharmacologic intervention for gestational asthma often necessary. Risks of pharmacologic therapy are generally few.
   b. In general, inhalation therapy is preferable over use of systemic medications. Use of a spacer device maximizes delivery of medication.
   c. Asthma medications that are used during pregnancy are appropriate for use during lactation.
   d. In 1993, the U.S. National Asthma Education Program Working Group on Asthma issued consensus guidelines on preferred medicine for asthma during pregnancy. Although there have been updates to the general recommendations made by the NAEPP in 1997 and 2002, the next update for management strategies in pregnancy was published in 2004. The medication recommendations below are taken from this guideline, which is based on a systematic review of the evidence on the safety of asthma medications from more than 220 articles published from 1990 to 2003.[8]
      i. Inhaled β_2-agonist bronchodilators are the cornerstone for immediate relief of asthma exacerbations; albuterol has the best safety data and has the advantages of relative beta selectivity, long duration of action, and lack of teratogenicity in animals.[3]
      ii. Regular prophylactic inhaled glucocorticoid therapy is the cornerstone of chronic management; budesonide is the preferred inhaled corticosteroid in pregnancy because more information is available on its safety in this setting than for any other steroid. However, there are also data to support the use of beclomethasone, with outcome data and a safety profile that shows 25% fewer asthma exacerbations and a 55% reduction in need for repeat hospitalization during pregnancy when compared with women not receiving inhaled steroids.[12,13] Large case series of patients receiving inhaled corticosteroid therapy have shown no evidence of increased risk for intrauterine growth restriction (IUGR) or SGA babies.[14]

4. Categories of asthma severity and relation to treatment options
   a. Mild intermittent
      i. Symptoms 1 to 2 times/week and pulmonary function maintained at 80% of baseline
      ii. Inhaled β agonists alone usually sufficient
      iii. Not associated with fetal or maternal complications
   b. Mild persistent
      i. Symptoms are greater than two times a week but not more than once a day.
      ii. Inhaled β agonists are used for acute symptoms.
      iii. Daily inhaled antiinflammatory medication, such as budesonide or beclomethasone, is used to reduce symptoms.
      iv. Inhaled cromolyn sodium and leukotriene receptor antagonists are alternatives to this, but not preferred therapies for mild and moderate persistent asthma. Although cromolyn has a solid record of safety, its efficacy is not as good as inhaled corticosteroids. Leukotriene receptor antagonists have little direct human data for safety in pregnancy, but animal studies are reassuring; their best role might be as an adjunct agent for asthma control in patients for whom they have already been proved effective.
      v. Evaluate and treat for sinusitis if signs and symptoms suggest this as a trigger.
      vi. Evaluate and treat for gastroesophageal reflux if nocturnal symptoms present. Ranitidine and metoclopramide are both U.S. Food and Drug Administration (FDA) category B agents.
   c. Moderate persistent
      i. Symptoms occur daily, not controlled with episodic use of inhaled β_2 agonists; nocturnal symptoms present at least once a week.
      ii. Pulmonary function is generally at 60% to 80% of baseline.
      iii. Add inhaled antiinflammatory agents if not already started, and consider using a moderate dose.
      iv. Symptom control may be improved with addition of long-acting β agonist. Salmeterol has the longest track record in the United States.

v. A short course of oral corticosteroid therapy is indicated, if symptoms are not controlled with inhalation management.

vi. Theophylline therapy with sustained release oral preparation, aiming for serum steady-state level of 5 to 12 µg/ml, is generally considered an alternative therapy because of its side effect profile. A randomized controlled trial (RCT) comparing theophylline with inhaled beclomethasone showed similar incidence of asthma exacerbations in pregnant patients taking each medicine, but a greater incidence of discontinuation of theophylline because of negative side effects.[15]

d. Severe persistent

i. This occurs in less than 0.1% of pregnancies and refers to continuous symptoms despite adequate trial of inhaled bronchodilators and antiinflammatory agents, or less than 10 days of relief after oral steroid therapy.

ii. Pulmonary function is typically less than 60% of baseline.

iii. This is associated with increased preterm labor, gestational hypertension, and LBW when spirometry consistently abnormal throughout pregnancy (FEV_1 or PFR persistently <80% predicted).[9]

iv. Treatment in this stage may require continuous oral corticosteroids. Surveillance should include observing for increased risk for maternal gestational diabetes, maternal adrenal insufficiency, and fetal IUGR (Table 8-2).

5. Management of acute asthma exacerbation

a. An acute asthma exacerbation is the most common respiratory crisis during pregnancy. If treated immediately, these have been shown to have no deleterious effect on the length of gestation, third stage of labor, birth weight, or risk for fetal malformations.

b. Treatment of acute asthma exacerbation involves:

i. Supplemental oxygen (3-4 L/min by nasal cannula) to achieve Po_2 ≥70 mmHg and/or o_2 saturation by pulse oximetry ≥95%. Because of the dissociative properties of fetal hemoglobin, decreases in maternal Po_2, especially to less than 60 mmHg, can quickly result in profound fetal hypoxia. Even small increases in maternal oxygen saturation in the hypoxic pregnant woman may produce significantly increased fetal oxygen saturation.

ii. Intravenous (IV) fluids should be administrated at a rate of at least 100 ml/hr, depending on patient's current oral intake and hydration status.

iii. Nebulized albuterol (2 mg in 2 ml saline) should be administered every 15 to 30 minutes, up to three doses, until respiratory distress is corrected (Po_2 ≥70, Pco_2 ≤35 mmHg). This can be tapered to maintenance dosing every 4 hours once the patient is stable.

iv. In patients on chronic steroids, or those who do not improve during first hour of treatment with β agonists,

---

TABLE 8-2 Doses of Inhaled Corticosteroids

Drug	Delivered Dose per Puff	Low Daily Dose	Medium Daily Dose	High Daily Dose
Beclomethasone MDI	40 or 80 µg	80-240 µg	240-480 µg	>480 µg
Budesonide DPI	200 µg	200-600 µg	600-1200 µg	>1200 µg
Flunisolide MDI	250 µg	500-1000 µg	1000-2000 µg	>2000 µg
Fluticasone MDI	44, 110, 220 µg	88-264 µg	264-660 µg	>660 µg
Triamcinolone MDI	100 µg	400-1000 µg	1000-2000 µg	>2000 µg

DPI, Dry powder inhaler; MDI, metered-dose inhaler.
Adapted from Asthma and pregnancy—update 2004. NAEPP Working Group Report on Managing Asthma during Pregnancy: recommendations for pharmacologic treatment—update 2004, NIH Publication No. 05-3279, Bethesda, MD, 2004, U.S. Department of Health and Human Services; National Institutes of Health; National Heart, Lung, and Blood Institute.

IV methylprednisolone should be given at a dosage of 60 mg every 8 hours for up to 48 hours. Taper as the patient improves to a daily oral dose of 60 mg prednisone or equivalent.[8]

v. Metered dose or nebulized ipratropium should be considered for patients who respond poorly to the previous treatments.

6. Labor and delivery management
   a. A significant exacerbation of asthma is unusual during labor.
   b. Maintenance asthma medications should be continued during labor.
   c. Symptoms that persist despite use of maintenance medications should be treated with nebulized albuterol.
   d. If no response to inhaled β agonists, IV methylprednisolone should be given (60 mg IV every 8 hours).
   e. Women who have been on maintenance or frequent periodic doses of oral steroids during pregnancy should be given supplemental parenteral corticosteroids to deal with the stresses of labor and delivery. An example of a regimen for this would be 100 mg hydrocortisone intravenously on admission, followed by 100 mg every 8 hours for 24 hours.
   f. Labor management is essentially the same as for women without asthma, *with a few specific caveats:*
      i. Prostaglandin $F_2\alpha$ (Prepidil, Cervidil, or Dinoprost) has been reported to cause increased airway resistance and clinical bronchospasm, and should be avoided. However, intravaginal prostaglandin E_2 (misoprostol) for cervical ripening before labor induction has not been reported to cause bronchospasm, even in women with asthma.[16]
      ii. Methylergonovine, ergonovine, and 15-methyprostaglandin $F_2\alpha$ (carboprost tromethamine [Hemabate]) should be avoided in treating postpartum hemorrhage because they may exacerbate asthma.[1] Oxytocin is a safe alternative.
      iii. β-Blockers should be avoided for intrapartum management of hypertension. Magnesium sulfate and calcium channel blockers are preferred in this setting.
      iv. Epidural anesthesia is the preferred method of analgesia during labor

because it has minimal impact on the respiratory system and its mechanics.

E. Pitfalls and Controversies

Pregnant woman are less likely to receive appropriate treatment for their asthma than nonpregnant women. In the Multicenter Asthma Research Collaboration, conducted across 36 emergency departments in 18 states, pregnant women did not differ from nonpregnant women by duration of asthma symptoms or initial peak flow rate. However, only 44% of pregnant women were treated with corticosteroids as compared with 66% of nonpregnant women. At a 2-week follow-up visit, pregnant women were 2.9 times more likely to report an ongoing exacerbation.[17]

Those who care for asthmatic women during pregnancy often have a challenging time of balancing the possible side effects of medications, especially in the first trimester, with the pitfalls of poorly controlled asthma. The NAEPP Expert Panel statement is appropriate to help guide therapy in this setting: "It is safer for pregnant women with asthma to be treated with asthma medication than for them to have asthma symptoms and exacerbations."[8]

II. PNEUMONIA

Pneumonia is an inflammation of the bronchioles and alveoli. Although it can be caused by noninfectious causative agents, such as inhalation of smoke or irritant substances, most cases are the result of infection with viruses, bacteria, or fungal organisms. In one series, pneumonia was the primary diagnosis in 4.2% of the antepartum admissions for nonobstetric causes during pregnancy.[18] Much of the information discussed in this section is based on guidelines or information for nonpregnant adults; the specific considerations unique to the pregnant patient are presented in greater detail.

A. Epidemiology and Risk Factors

Epidemiologic features and risk factors of pneumonia include:

1. During pregnancy, the incidence of pneumonia is between 1.5 and 2.7 per 1000, which is similar to the nonpregnant population of the same age range.[19]
2. Risk factors that have been associated with an increased risk for pneumonia during pregnancy include smoking, asthma, other lung disorders such

as cystic fibrosis, significant anemia, human immunodeficiency virus (HIV) positivity, and cocaine use.[20]

3. Complications of pneumonia in pregnancy include increased rates of miscarriage, preterm labor, and decreased birth weight. Before the widespread availability of antibiotics, pneumonia was associated with a maternal mortality rate of 20% or more; the rate in the most recent case series is less than 3%.[21]

B. Microbiology and Clinical Features

Microbiologic aspects and clinical features of pneumonia include:

1. Overall, the causative organisms of pneumonia in pregnancy are similar to that in the general population, with *Streptococcus pneumoniae* being most common. It typically presents with abrupt onset of fever, chills, productive cough, and blood-tinged sputum. The associated chest radiograph may show a lobar infiltrate, and effusions are common. Blood cultures in adults are positive about 11% of the time. A Gram stain of the sputum may show characteristic diplococci; although not recommended in the outpatient setting, the Infectious Diseases Society of America (IDSA) practice guideline update for community-acquired pneumonia (CAP) in adults recommends an expectorated sputum for Gram stain and culture in patients admitted to the hospital.[22] However, as the yield from Gram stain of the sputum is often less than 10%, the American Thoracic Society practice guideline for the management of adults with CAP does not recommend that they be obtained.[23]

2. Additional common bacterial agents are *Haemophilus influenzae* and *Moraxella catarrhalis*. These may present with a slower onset of fever, productive cough, and chills, and often produce a patchy infiltrate on chest radiograph.

3. Atypical agents, such as *Mycoplasma pneumoniae* and *Chlamydia pneumoniae,* present with a gradual onset of malaise, low-grade fever, and nonproductive cough; headache and earache are also common. In 1 case series, 2 of 19 cases in which a pathogen was identified in pregnant women with pneumonia were caused by *M. pneumonia*.[21]

4. *Legionella pneumophila,* in contrast with the other atypical organisms, presents with high fever, nausea and vomiting, dyspnea, pleuritic pain, and a patchy infiltrate that can involve multiple lobes within the lung. The same case series found this organism in 1 of 19 pneumonias diagnosed during pregnancy.

5. Viral pneumonia can be caused by multiple organisms, but influenza is the most important agent in pregnancy. Although most cases of influenza in pregnancy are uncomplicated, maternal mortality rates of more than 50% were seen in the pandemics of 1918 and 1957. Mortality today is thought to be caused by secondary infection with *H. influenzae* and *Staphylococcus aureus.* Influenza virus does not appear to be teratogenic, but maternal infection can lead to pregnancy complications.[24] Currently, American College of Obstetrics and Gynecology (ACOG) and the Advisory Committee for Immunization Practices recommend the influenza vaccine for all pregnant women, in all trimesters, who are pregnant during the months of October to mid-May each year.

C. Diagnosis

1. Use of chest radiographs

   In patients with a history suggestive of pneumonia, the IDSA guideline recommends a chest radiograph to substantiate the diagnosis of pneumonia and to assist in assessing severity.[25] The acceptable cumulative radiation dose during pregnancy is up to 5 rad, and a posteroanterior and lateral chest radiograph exposes the fetus to only 0.00007 rad. The most sensitive time period for the developing central nervous system (CNS) is between 10 and 17 weeks; therefore, nonurgent radiologic procedures should be delayed during this time. However, in the evaluation of a patient with possible pneumonia, this potential low exposure to radiation is acceptable.[26]

2. Laboratory investigation

   In patients who present with significant dyspnea or multilobar disease, additional studies are warranted because they can assist in the determination of appropriateness of outpatient versus inpatient management. These include a complete blood cell count (CBC) with differential; a chemistry panel including glucose, renal function, and electrolytes; a pulse oximetry (with arterial blood gas recommended in the setting of known underlying pulmonary disease, to help assess carbon dioxide retention); blood cultures at two sites; sputum Gram stain and culture; and consideration of an HIV test for those between 15 and 55 years old. The American Thoracic Society guideline for CAP reviews risk stratification of patients using age (>65, thus not useful in pregnancy), medical history, and results of the above tests to help decide location of treatment.[23] Factors that support hospitalization are as follows:

a. Coexisting illness (lung disease such as asthma, diabetes, renal failure, congestive heart failure, liver disease, or postsplenectomy state such as sickle cell disease)
b. Altered mental status
c. Respirations > 30/min, or temperature <35 or >40°C
d. White blood cell count less than 4000 or >30,000 per microliter
e. Arterial blood gas on room air with Pao_2 < 60 mmHg or $Paco_2$ > 50 mmHg
f. Creatinine level > 1.2 mg/dl
g. Pleural effusion or multilobe involvement by chest radiograph

In a case series of pregnant patients with diagnosis of pneumonia, use of these factors for risk stratification of women with CAP was found to be accurate in predicting those who would have a complicated hospital course.[27] In other words, absence of the previous criteria in a pregnant patient presenting with CAP can help identify those who can be managed with outpatient therapy and close follow-up.

3. During influenza season, in patients with a suggestive clinical history, the possibility of influenza pneumonia should be considered. Diagnosis of acute influenza can be assisted by use of a rapid immunoassay from a nasopharyngeal or throat swab for influenza A and B, helping to clarify options for treatment.

D. Treatment

1. Bacterial pneumonia

Among the antimicrobial agents recommended for adults with CAP, the following are appropriate choices for pregnancy[22]:

a. For an immunocompetent pregnant woman who can be managed as an outpatient, the first-line agent is a macrolide (azithromycin or erythromycin). If aspiration is suspected or the patient is allergic to macrolides, amoxicillin/clavulanate can be used.
b. For otherwise healthy women who require hospitalization, a β-lactam, such as ceftriaxone, should be used with a macrolide.

c. If aspiration is suspected, a penicillin with β-lactamase inhibitor such as ampicillin/sulbactam is appropriate. In situations in which underlying pulmonary disease is present, an antipseudomonal penicillin with a macrolide is recommended.
d. The recommended duration of therapy ranges from 72 hours after the patient becomes afebrile to a total of 14 days.
e. Supportive therapy such as IV hydration, supplemental oxygen, and management of any associated bronchospasm is an important part of care.

2. Influenza

a. Four medications available for treatment of acute influenza include amantadine, rimantadine, oseltamivir, and zanamivir. The latter two inhibit the viral neuraminidase enzyme and are effective against both influenza A and B, whereas amantadine and rimantadine are effective against influenza A only.
b. Each of the four medications to treat influenza is categorized as FDA category C agents because there are no human trials to assess safety in pregnancy. However, amantadine and rimantadine are teratogenic in rats at a high dose. No significant toxic effects have been noted in rats or rabbits with oseltamivir or zanamivir, so these appear to be the preferred agents.[28] Zanamivir is administered in inhaled form, whereas all other antiviral agents are given orally. ACOG recommends use of antiviral agents in pregnancy only if the potential benefits justify the potential risks.[11] Benefits from these agents occur only if started within 72 hours of the onset of symptoms.
c. Specific agents may be indicated based on recent patterns of resistance (the most updated guideline each year is available at the Centers for Disease Control and Prevention [CDC] website: www.cdc.gov/flu). For the 2005-2006 influenza season, the Centers for Disease Control and Prevention (CDC) issued an advisory to avoid use of amantadine and rimantadine because of significant increases in resistance of the prevalent strain of influenza A to these drugs.[29]

E. Prevention

A study of the effect of influenza during 17 interpandemic influenza seasons demonstrated that the relative risk for hospitalization for selected cardiorespiratory conditions among pregnant women enrolled in Medicaid increased 4.7-fold during the last month of gestation when compared with women in their first 6 months postpartum.[30] Women in their third trimester of pregnancy with influenza were hospitalized at a rate of 2.5 per 1000 pregnant women, comparable with that of nonpregnant women who had high-risk medical conditions. Researchers estimate that an average of 1 to 2 hospitalizations can be prevented for every 1000 pregnant women vaccinated. Because of the increased risk for influenza-related complications, women who will be pregnant during the influenza season should be vaccinated; this can occur in any trimester. No adverse fetal effects have been noted with inactivated influenza vaccine.[31] Although pneumococcal vaccine has not been shown to be harmful in pregnancy, it is not currently recommended for use in pregnancy.

F. Pitfalls and Controversies

1. Yost and colleagues' study[27] of 133 patients with pneumonia yielded an important pitfall: 14 patients were initially hospitalized with an alternative diagnosis, including 2 who received exploratory laparotomies for presumed appendicitis. Other admission diagnoses that were subsequently found to be patients with pneumonia included pyelonephritis (two patients), viral syndrome (four patients), and asthma exacerbation (three patients).
2. Guidelines for CAP in adults often recommend a fluoroquinolone as the first-line agent for presumptive treatment. These are not appropriate for use in pregnancy based on safety concerns.

III. TUBERCULOSIS

Though rates of tuberculosis (TB) in the United States have been declining since 1992, this follows an increase in reported cases from 1985 to the early 1990s thought to be associated with increased prevalence in HIV-positive patients.[32] The majority of cases of active TB infection occur as activation of latent infection. Because of this, identification and treatment of latent TB in pregnancy remains an important part of prenatal care.

A. Epidemiology and Risk Factors

Epidemiologic features and risk factors of pneumonia include:
1. In 2003, 14,874 cases of TB were reported in the United States, for a rate of 5.1 cases per 100,000 people. Rates were greatest in Asians (29.3/100,000), followed by non-Hispanic blacks (11.6/100,000), Hispanics (10.3/100,000), and Native Americans (8.3/100,000). The lowest rates are among non-Hispanic whites (1.4/100,000), though declines in the previous 10 years have been noted in all ethnic and age groups.
2. Risk factors for latent tuberculosis infection (LTBI) parallel the criteria used in patient selection for a targeted approach to purified protein derivative (PPD) skin testing in pregnancy. These are based on risk factors for recent TB infection or progression from LTBI to active disease.[33]
   a. Risk factors for recent TB infection
      i. Contact with persons with active TB
      ii. Immigration from areas with endemic TB
      iii. Homelessness
      iv. Illicit IV drug use
      v. Working in institutional settings with patients at risk for TB
   b. Risk factors for progression to active TB disease
      i. HIV infection
      ii. Diabetes, including type I, type II, and gestational
      iii. Transplant recipients
      iv. Immunosuppressed states, including chronic steroid use
      v. Chronic renal failure
      vi. History of gastrectomy, because of risk for disseminated disease, as stomach acid is inhibitor of the tubercle bacillus
      vii. Presence of pulmonary fibrosis
3. Screening is performed by use of an intradermal injection of 0.1 ml of 5 tuberculin units of PPD into the forearm, and is read in 48 to 72 hours. In patients without any risk factors, 15 mm of induration is considered positive. In those with diabetes, institutional risk for exposure, underlying lung or renal disease, or who have emigrated from areas with high TB rates, 10 mm of induration is positive. In immunosuppressed populations and those with recent exposure to persons with active TB infection, 5 mm of induration is considered a positive result. A positive screening PPD should be followed by a chest radiograph to assess for evidence of active disease, with abdominal shielding during pregnancy.

B. Pathogenesis

Infection with *Mycobacterium tuberculosis* is transmitted through respiratory droplets expectorated by those with active disease. Congenital transmission through the placenta is uncommon. Newborns are usually infected through the respiratory tract from close contacts.[34] Once the pathogen has infected the lung, the host immune response usually contains it via a local inflammatory response, and the patient remains asymptomatic. However, the organism can remain dormant within the lung for decades and then reactivate to cause active pulmonary disease in settings of decreased cellular immunity.

Although pregnancy has not been shown to affect the course or likelihood of reactivation of pulmonary TB, a case series of patients with TB during pregnancy reveals an increase in the incidence of pregnancy-induced hypertension, bleeding during pregnancy, and miscarriage.[35]

C. Clinical Features

LTBI is asymptomatic and can only be discovered in pregnancy through PPD testing. Active pulmonary TB or reactivation of LTBI presents as cough with bloody sputum, fever, night sweats, weight loss, and weakness. In this setting, a chest radiograph may reveal patchy lung infiltrates or scarring and cavitation in the upper lobes of the lungs. Reliance on the PPD test to suggest active TB is not recommended because these patients often have negative skin tests.

D. Diagnosis

In patients suspected of having active pulmonary TB, treatment should be started immediately while diagnostic evaluation continues. Three first-morning sputa should be collected for AFB smear and culture. Family members should be screened for LTBI or active disease if the index patient is confirmed to have active TB. Should hospital admission be necessary, respiratory isolation should be used pending definitive culture results.

E. Treatment

Treatment of LTBI and active pulmonary TB during pregnancy is derived from guidelines for treatment of adults, with special attention to the safety of the medications used in pregnancy. Local patterns of drug resistance, as well as sensitivities from cultured organisms, need to taken into account in devising an appropriate regimen.

For LTBI, the preferred agent in pregnancy is isoniazid (INH), given either daily or twice weekly, together with daily pyridoxine, for 9 months. INH has not been shown to have any teratogenic effects even if given during the first trimester. In addition,

because of low levels found in breast milk, breastfeeding can be continued during INH treatment. However, some concern exists that the incidence of hepatotoxicity of INH is increased during pregnancy and immediately postpartum, such that monthly monitoring for symptoms of liver damage, together with serum liver function tests, is recommended for the duration of treatment.[36]

For patients suspected of having active pulmonary TB during pregnancy, it is appropriate to begin three-drug therapy during the evaluation. The recommended drugs for use during pregnancy are INH, rifampin, and ethambutol, each daily for a period of 2 months. This is followed by INH and rifampin daily for 7 months.[37] This regimen has the best safety profile of those available during pregnancy.[28] In addition to hepatic irritation from INH, hepatitis has also been reported with rifampin use, stressing the importance of monthly liver function testing while taking these drugs. Concerns of a relation between rifampin use and limb defects in the fetus appear to be equivalent to the incidence in the general population. The most common side effect of ethambutol is optic neuritis. Patients who take this medication should have eye examinations at the onset and completion of therapy and at any time that any changes in vision are noted. Breastfeeding is not contraindicated on this regimen.

F. Clinical Course and Prevention

Treatment response to LTBI and active pulmonary TB during pregnancy is generally equivalent to that in the nonpregnant adult. Prevention of TB, both latent and active, depends on the ability to identify those with latent disease and decrease their risk for reactivation in the future, as well as identification and treatment of active cases and their contacts with effective antituberculous medications.

G. Pitfalls and Controversies

Treatment of asymptomatic LTBI during pregnancy is controversial because of concerns of increased hepatotoxicity of INH in pregnancy, as well as the fact that pregnancy does not increase the likelihood of progression to active disease. Decisions in this setting require discussion with the patient and individualization of the treatment plan. The CDC guideline on treatment of TB recommends treatment of LTBI during pregnancy with INH, supplemented with 25 mg/day pyridoxine, for 9 months.[38] Laboratory monitoring for hepatotoxicity is essential. One argument against a delay of chemoprophylaxis until after delivery is the experience from prenatal clinics in Los Angeles County, where approximately 90% of patients failed to return to receive their preventive therapy after the birth of their child.[39]

IV. SOR A RECOMMENDATION

RECOMMENDATION	REFERENCES
Inhaled corticosteroid should be used for all persistent asthma. It is safe and associated with decrease in acute asthma episodes and hospital admissions (number needed to treat [NNT] = 5.8 to prevent 1 admission)	12, 13

REFERENCES

1. Kwon HL, Triche EW, Belanger K et al: The epidemiology of asthma during pregnancy: prevalence, diagnosis, and symptoms, *Immunol Allergy Clin N Am* 26:29-62, 2006.
2. Schiller JS, Adams PF, Nelson ZC: Summary health statistics for the U.S. population: National Health Interview Survey, 2003, *Vital Health Stat* 10(224):1-104, 2005.
3. Kwon HL, Belanger K, Bracken MB: Effect of pregnancy and stage of pregnancy on asthma severity: a systematic review, *Am J Obstet Gynecol* 190:1201-1210, 2004.
4. Kircher S, Schatz M, Long L: Variables affecting asthma course during pregnancy, *Ann Allergy Asthma Immunol* 89(5): 463-466, 2002.
5. Beecroft N, Cochrane GM, Milburn HJ: Effect of sex of fetus on asthma during pregnancy: blind prospective study, *BMJ* 317(7162):856-857, 1998.
6. Demissie K, Breckenridge MB, Rhoads GG: Infant and maternal outcomes in the pregnancies of asthmatic women, *Am J Respir Crit Care Med* 158(4):1091-1095, 1998.
7. Schatz M, Zeiger R, Hoffman C et al: Perinatal outcomes in pregnancies of asthmatic women: a prospective controlled analysis, *Am J Respir Crit Care Med* 151:1170-1174, 1995.
8. Asthma and pregnancy—update 2004. NAEPP Working Group Report on Managing Asthma during Pregnancy: recommendations for pharmacologic treatment—update 2004, NIH Publication No. 05-3279, Bethesda, MD, 2004, U.S. Department of Health and Human Services; National Institutes of Health; National Heart, Lung, and Blood Institute.
9. Schatz M, Dombrowski MP, Wise R et al: Spirometry is related to perinatal outcomes in pregnancy women with asthma, *Am J Obstet Gynecol* 194:120-126, 2006.
10. Kurinczuk JJ, Parsons DE, Dawes V et al: The relationship between asthma and smoking during pregnancy, *Women Health* 29(3):31-47, 1999.
11. ACOG Committee on Obstetric Practice: ACOG committee opinion number 305, November 2004. Influenza vaccination and treatment during pregnancy, *Obstet Gynecol* 104: 1125-1126, 2004.
12. Wendel PJ, Ramin SM, Barnett-Hamm C et al: Asthma treatment in pregnancy: a randomized controlled study, *Am J Obstet Gynecol* 175:150-154, 1996.
13. Dombrowski M, Thom E, McNellis D: Maternal-Fetal Medicine Units (MFMU) studies of inhaled corticosteroids during pregnancy, *J Allergy Clin Immunol* 103:S356-S359, 1999.
14. Namazy J, Schatz M, Long L et al: Use of inhaled steroids by pregnant asthmatic women does not reduce intrauterine growth, *J Allergy Clin Immunol* 113:427-432, 2004.
15. Dombrowski MP, Schatz M, Wise R et al: Randomized trial of inhaled beclomethasone dipropionate versus theophylline for moderate asthma during pregnancy, *Am J Obstet Gynecol* 190:737-744, 2004.
16. Wendel PJ, Ramin SM, Barnett-Hamm C et al: Asthma treatment in pregnancy: a randomized controlled study, *Am J Obstet Gynecol* 175:150-154, 1996.
17. Cydulka RK, Emerman CL, Schreiber D et al: Acute asthma among pregnancy women presenting to the emergency department, *Am J Respir Crit Care Med* 160:887-892, 1999.
18. Grazmararian KD, Peterson R, Jamieson DJ et al. Hospitalizations during pregnancy among managed care enrollees, *Obstet Gynecol* 100:94-100, 2002.
19. Berkowitz K, LaWala A: Risk factors associated with the increasing prevalence of pneumonia during pregnancy, *Am J Obstet Gynecol* 163:981-985, 1990.
20. Goodnight WH, Soper DE: Pneumonia in pregnancy, *Crit Care Med* 33:S390-S397, 2005.
21. Richey SD, Roberts SW, Ramin KD et al: Pneumonia complicating pregnancy, *Obstet Gynecol* 84:525-528, 1994.
22. Mandell LA, Bartlett JG, Dowell SF et al: Update of practice guidelines for the management of community-acquired pneumonia in immunocompetent adults, *Clin Infect Dis* 37:1405-1433, 2003.
23. American Thoracic Society: Guidelines for the management of adults with community-acquired pneumonia, *Am J Respir Crit Care Med* 163:1730-1754, 2001.
24. Irving WL, James DK. Stephenson T et al: Influenza virus infection in the second and third trimesters of pregnancy: a clinical and seroepidemiological study, *BJOG* 107:1282-1289, 2000.
25. Bernstein JM: Treatment of community-acquired pneumonia: IDSA guidelines, *Chest* 115:9S-13S, 1999.
26. Toppenberg KS, Hill DA, Miller DP: Safety of radiographic imaging during pregnancy, *Am Fam Physician* 59:1813-1818, 1999.
27. Yost NP, Bloom SL, Richey SD et al: An appraisal of treatment guidelines for antepartum community-acquired pneumonia, *Am J Obstet Gynecol* 183:131-135, 2000.
28. Briggs GG, Freeman RK, Yaffe SJ: *Drugs in pregnancy and lactation,* ed 7, Philadelphia, 2005, Lippincott Williams & Wilkins.
29. *Guidelines & recommendations: Influenza antiviral medications: 2005-2006 interim chemoprophylaxis and treatment guidelines.* Available at: http://www.cdc.gov/flu/professionals/treatment/0506antiviralguide.htm. Accessed January 14, 2006.
30. Neuzil KM, Reed GW, Mitchel EF et al: Impact of influenza on acute cardiopulmonary hospitalizations in pregnant women, *Am J Epidemiol* 148:1094-1102, 1998.
31. Harper SA, Fukuda K, Uyeki TM et al: Prevention and control of influenza: recommendations of the Advisory Committee on Immunization Practices (ACIP), *MMWR Recomm Rep* 53(RR-6):1-40, 2004.
32. Centers for Disease Control and Prevention (CDC): *Reported tuberculosis in the United States, 2003,* Atlanta, September 2004, U.S. Department of Health and Human Services, CDC.

33. Munsiff S, Nilsen D, Dworkin F: *Guidelines for testing and treatment of latent tuberculosis infection,* New York, April 2005, NYC Dept of Health & Mental Hygiene, Bureau of TB Control.

34. Cantwell MF, Shehab ZM, Costello AM et al: Congenital tuberculosis, *N Engl J Med* 330:1051-1054, 1994.

35. Bjeredal T, Bahna SL, Lehmann EH: Course and outcome of pregnancy in women with pulmonary tuberculosis, *Scand J Respir Dis* 56:245-250, 1975.

36. Targeted tuberculin testing and treatment of latent tuberculosis infection. American Thoracic Society, *MMWR Recomm Rep* 49(RR-6):1-51, 2000.

37. Center for Disease Control and Prevention (CDC): *Tuberculosis and pregnancy update,* June 2005, Atlanta, June 2005, CDC, Division of Tuberculosis Elimination.

38. American Thoracic Society, CDC, and Infectious Diseases Society of America: Treatment of tuberculosis, *MMWR Recomm Rep* 52(RR-11):1-77, 2003.

39. Davidson PT: Managing tuberculosis during pregnancy, *Lancet* 346:199, 1995.

S E C T I O N   B   Cardiovascular Conditions

Ellen L. Sakornbut, MD

I. STRUCTURAL HEART DISEASE

A. General Approach

Some women with heart conditions can be safely managed in pregnancy by the family physician, whereas others should receive consultation or referral for pregnancy management. Nonetheless, the family physician may encounter these referred patients in emergency situations, particularly in rural areas. In addition, women with heart disease should receive preconception counseling, and much of the information included in this section is included for this purpose. Delay in age of childbearing and increasing numbers of survivors with congenital heart disease increases the likelihood of encountering pregnant women with cardiac conditions.

Although rheumatic heart disease is less common now in U.S. and European populations, it is still common in non-Western populations. In general, women with stenotic lesions, such as mitral stenosis and aortic stenosis, are at greater risk for deterioration of their condition during pregnancy than women with predominately regurgitant valvular disease. The risk for congestive heart failure during pregnancy in women who have structural heart disease is as high as 38%, and prematurity and LBW are increased.[1] Women who have undergone valve replacement, have adequate left ventricular function, and are anticoagulated appropriately experience relatively good pregnancy outcomes.

Women with repaired congenital shunt lesions (ventricular septal defect, atrial septal defect [ASD], and tetralogy of Fallot) experience generally good outcomes, with some tendency to smaller fetal weights as long as they had good cardiac function before pregnancy. For all types of heart disease, women with New York Heart Association classification I or II (no symptoms or symptoms only with heavy activity) have perinatal mortality rates that are only slightly greater than women without heart disease. In contrast, the perinatal mortality rates with class III or IV heart disease are 12% and 31%, respectively. Approximately one sixth of all maternal deaths are due to cardiac disease, the majority from peripartum cardiomyopathy, myocardial infarction, and aortic dissection.[2] Table 8-3 summarizes cardiac conditions associated with high maternal and fetal mortality rates.

B. Cardiovascular Changes in Pregnancy

Peripartum changes in cardiovascular physiology (Table 8-4) that affect women with structural heart disease include the following:

1. Increased intravascular volume
   As much as a 50% increase by the early to middle third trimester may lead to congestive heart failure or increased ischemia in patients with valvular heart disease or myocardial dysfunction. It may also result in formation or dissection of an aneurysm in patients at risk, such as those with Marfan syndrome.

2. Decreased systemic vascular resistance
   This may worsen a right-to-left shunt.

3. Pregnancy-associated hypercoagulability
   The risk for arterial thromboembolic disease is increased, especially in patients with atrial fibrillation and artificial valves.

4. Marked shifts in cardiac output and intravascular volume during labor
   Cardiac output increases during the first stage of labor. Preload may be increased by the release of pressure on the inferior vena cava and a physiologic transfusion from the contracted uterus after delivery. In cases of postpartum hemorrhage, preload may be decreased, which adversely affects

TABLE 8-3 Cardiac Conditions Associated with High Maternal/Fetal Mortality

Condition	Maternal Effects	Fetal Effects
Mitral stenosis, severe, valve < 1.0 cm	Up to 25% maternal mortality if pulmonary hypertension present	
Aortic stenosis, severe	Cardiac, cerebral ischemia	Decreased uterine blood flow; 30% fetal loss
Eisenmenger syndrome	30-40% maternal mortality	30% fetal loss if mother survives
Marfan syndrome, with dilated aortic root > 4 cm or valvular lesions	30-40% maternal mortality; 30-50% maternal mortality secondary to aortic dissection	
Primary pulmonary hypertension	Up to 50% maternal mortality	40% perinatal mortality if mother survives

TABLE 8-4 Cardiovascular Changes in Pregnancy

Blood volume	40-50% increase
Heart rate	10-20% (15 beats/min) increase
Cardiac output	30-50% increase (4.5-6.8 L/min)
Systemic vascular resistance	Decreased
Mean arterial blood pressure	Decreased

TABLE 8-5 Cardiac Conditions That Require Subacute Bacterial Endocarditis Prophylaxis

Prosthetic heart valves, mechanical or porcine

Valvular heart lesions such as mitral stenosis and aortic stenosis

Ventricular septal defect (not atrial septal defect)

Idiopathic hypertrophic subaortic stenosis

Patent ductus arteriosus

Mitral valve prolapse with significant regurgitation

Marfan syndrome

Coarctation of the aorta

Data compiled from Hameed and colleagues,[1] Yentis and colleagues,[7] and Vongpatanasin and colleagues.[8]

patients with pulmonary hypertension or fixed cardiac output. Tachycardia may be poorly tolerated in patients with valvular obstructive lesions.

C. Intrapartum Management in Patients with Significant Structural Heart Disease

1. Subacute bacterial endocarditis (SBE)
   SBE prophylaxis is required in many cardiac conditions for delivery. Table 8-5 summarizes conditions needing this intervention. Table 8-6 summarizes antibiotic regimens used for SBE prophylaxis.
2. Labor management
   Labor management for patients with significant structural heart disease includes careful monitoring of fluid status, often with the use of central catheter monitoring to assess right and left heart pressures. Epidural anesthesia is used in most patients to control fluctuations in cardiac output. Valsalva maneuver should be minimized by allowing the mother to "labor down" in the second trimester. Lateral recumbent positioning and oxygen

TABLE 8-6 Protocol for Subacute Bacterial Endocarditis Prophylaxis

Ampicillin 1 g, intravenously or intramuscularly, 30 minutes to 1 hour before procedure; repeat every 8-12 hours for 2 doses *or*

Vancomycin 1 g intravenously for patient who is allergic to penicillin

Plus

Gentamicin 1.5 mg/kg, intramuscularly or intravenously (not to exceed 120 mg); repeat every 8 hours for 2 doses *or*

Streptomycin 1 g intramuscularly; repeat every 12 hours for 2 doses administration are used if there are any concerns about fetal well-being. Clinical setting and resources for management should be appropriate to the risk status of these patients.

3. Preterm labor

    If treatment is required, this should be managed with magnesium sulfate. β-Sympathomimetic agents should be avoided.

4. Ergot alkaloids, such as methylergonovine maleate (Methergine), should be avoided for patients at risk for pulmonary congestion.[3]

5. Oxytocin as a bolus injection may cause transient, but significant, hypotension.[4]

D. Specific Diagnoses

Specific diagnoses of structural heart disease include:

1. Mitral stenosis

    Mitral stenosis may be relatively asymptomatic until pregnancy-associated hemodynamic changes, such as increased cardiac output and heart rate, cause an increase in the diastolic pressure gradient across the mitral valve. This results in increased left atrial and pulmonary capillary wedge pressure, leading to pulmonary edema. Critical mitral stenosis, with a valve cross section of less than 1.0 cm^2, carries a high risk for life-threatening complications.[5]

    Tachycardia or atrial fibrillation results in decreased filling of the left ventricle with resultant pulmonary edema, although left ventricular function may be normal. Atrial fibrillation also increases the risk for embolic phenomena and cerebrovascular accident. Digoxin should be used in atrial fibrillation to prevent a rapid ventricular rate and is safe for use in pregnancy. β-Blockers may also be used to control tachycardia. High doses of β-blockers may be necessary because of high circulating levels of catecholamines. When using β-blockers, metoprolol and pindolol are preferred, with atenolol being classified as FDA category D.

    Balloon valvotomy or valvuloplasty has a good safety record in pregnancy.[6] It reduces adverse events such as congestive heart failure and arrhythmias, but it has not been demonstrated to significantly improve maternal and fetal outcomes.[3]

    Antibiotic prophylaxis includes rheumatic fever prophylaxis with daily oral penicillin V or monthly benzathine penicillin, as well as SBE prophylaxis in labor. Epidural anesthesia and assisted delivery are often used, and Valsalva in second stage should be avoided. There is increased risk for postpartum pulmonary edema with mobilization of extravascular fluid.

2. Aortic stenosis

    Aortic stenosis carries high maternal mortality rates if the stenosis is severe. Fetal loss rates of up to 30% have been reported, especially if surgical correction is necessary during pregnancy. Angina and syncope are worrisome symptoms associated with transient inadequacy of cardiac output.

    Intrapartum management includes avoidance of acute increase in afterload or decrease in preload. Regional anesthesia may cause hypotension and a decrease in cardiac output.

3. Atrial septal defect (ASD)

    ASD (specifically secundum ASD) is the most common congenital lesion that may escape diagnosis in childhood. Most patients with ASD tolerate pregnancy well, but a few experience development of congestive heart failure. A potentially devastating complication is a right-to-left arterial embolus with Valsalva maneuver. If Eisenmenger syndrome (pulmonary hypertension with a right-to-left intracardiac shunt) is present, the maternal mortality rate is as great as 40%.[7,8]

4. Ventricular septal defect

    Ventricular septal defects are usually detected in early childhood. Surgical correction should take place before pregnancy. Patients with a small ventricular septal defect or previous surgery to repair a ventricular septal defect tolerate pregnancy well. SBE prophylaxis is indicated. A large left-to-right shunt puts the patient at risk for development of pulmonary hypertension and Eisenmenger syndrome with the high maternal mortality rates reported previously. An increased risk for congestive heart failure exists in patients with uncorrected lesions.

5. Marfan syndrome

    Marfan syndrome carries a risk for aortic dissection, with greater risk in symptomatic patients with mitral prolapse, aortic insufficiency, or aortic root dilatation. The risk for dissection is as high as 60% in patients with an aortic root larger than 4 cm. Pregnancy should be avoided in these women. Patients at high risk who choose to undertake or continue pregnancy are treated with bed rest and β-blockade. A prospective study demonstrated that patients without aortic root dilatation typically remain unchanged during pregnancy and have good outcomes.[9]

Transesophageal echocardiography and magnetic resonance imaging may be used to diagnose aortic dissection. Patients with progressive aortic root dilation during pregnancy should have surgical correction at or before the aortic root reaches 5.5 cm.[10]

The offspring of a patient with Marfan syndrome carries a 50% risk for inheriting the autosomal dominant gene for this syndrome.

6. Mitral valve prolapse

   Mitral valve prolapse is common in young women, most of whom are asymptomatic. No antenatal treatment is indicated if symptoms are minor. Symptomatic arrhythmias are treated with activity restriction and β-blockers.

   SBE prophylaxis is indicated for delivery when patients have demonstrated significant regurgitation or valve thickening on echocardiogram.[11] However, clinicians should be aware that modern color-flow Doppler techniques demonstrate clinically insignificant regurgitant flow across normal heart valves in many patients who have no disease state and are not at risk for endocarditis. Many women have flow murmurs in pregnancy, but mitral regurgitant murmurs are soft in quality, blowing, and generally heard throughout systole, best in the mitral area and radiating to the apex or axilla.

7. Idiopathic hypertrophic subaortic stenosis (IHSS)

   IHSS carries a good prognosis for most pregnant women because of the increased blood volume. Syncope may occur with vasovagal attacks or blood loss. β-Blockade is indicated for symptoms of dyspnea and angina. Epidural anesthesia, because of its systemic vasodilatation, should be avoided. Postpartum hemorrhage may exacerbate this cardiac condition and should be managed aggressively. SBE prophylaxis is indicated.

8. Pregnancy-related cardiomyopathy

   Peripartum cardiomyopathy is defined as occurring from 1 month before delivery to 5 months after delivery in a woman without a history of heart disease. The highest risk period occurs during the first 3 months after delivery. In actuality, peripartum and early pregnancy-associated cardiomyopathy appear to present as a spectrum of disease. Studies comparing women with early pregnancy cardiomyopathy do not demonstrate significant differences in characteristics or prognosis with those presenting in the peripartum period.[12]

The incidence of peripartum cardiomyopathy is from 1 in 1300 to 4000 pregnancies; occurrence is more common in older patients, multiparas, African Americans, and patients with multiple gestation. The cause is unclear, but possible linkages include pregnancy-induced hypertension, viral myocarditis, autoimmune disorders such as lupus and anti-phospholipid antibody syndrome (APS), and beriberi.

Approximately 50% of patients will normalize their ejection fraction by 6 months after delivery, with a greater prognosis if the initial ejection fraction is more than 30%. Inotropic contractile reserve demonstrated on dobutamine stress echocardiography correlates with ejection fraction in follow-up and can be used to assess prognosis for long-term recovery of cardiac function.[13]

A small series of reports demonstrated that subsequent pregnancy after a diagnosis of peripartum cardiomyopathy results in a greater than 10% reduction in ejection fraction in the majority of patients. Mortality rates are high despite optimal medical management.[12] Prognosis is better if cardiac function normalizes within 6 months.

9. Preexisting dilated cardiomyopathy

   Less information is available for this condition than for pregnancy-associated cardiomyopathy. Comparisons of women who carry a diagnosis of peripartum cardiomyopathy and preexisting dilated cardiomyopathy appear to demonstrate better prognosis in subsequent pregnancy for women with nonpregnancy-associated cardiomyopathy who are stable.[14]

10. Coarctation of the aorta

    Coarctation of the aorta may go undiagnosed until pregnancy and may be associated with bicuspid aortic valve, ASD, or congenital cerebral aneurysm. Increased risk exists for aortic dissection, stroke, congestive heart failure, or endocarditis. Fetal growth is normal. Activity should be limited with increased bed rest. SBE prophylaxis is indicated. Labor management includes avoidance of bearing down and increase of systolic blood pressure (BP).

11. Cyanotic congenital heart disease

    Cyanotic congenital heart disease carries an increased risk for congenital heart disease in the fetus, as do other congenital heart lesions. A large series of tetralogy of Fallot patients found the incidence of congenital anomalies in their pregnancies to be 6%.[15]

Poor prognostic indicators include polycythemia, with a hematocrit greater than 60% and oxygen saturation less than 80%. The risk for IUGR is increased. SBE prophylaxis is indicated. Patients with surgical correction tend to do better, but some have residual valvular defects or postoperative effects that may affect overall health status.

12. Other valvular heart disease

    Other valvular defects, such as aortic insufficiency and mitral insufficiency, are generally tolerated better in pregnancy than stenotic lesions. Those with acquired valvular disease may include women with valvular insufficiency who have used appetite-suppressant medication. These patients need SBE prophylaxis.

13. Prosthetic valves

    Anticoagulation of women with mechanical heart valves remains an area of controversy. Although general principles regarding management of thromboembolic disorders in pregnancy may be useful, patients with mechanical heart valves remain at the greatest risks for thromboembolic disease during the hypercoagulable state of pregnancy. Prosthetic valve thrombosis has occurred with women on all anticoagulation regimens but is more common with heparin than with warfarin. In addition to considerations of teratogenesis, other pregnancy-related concerns include the incidence of bleeding complications, such as abruption, and the management of anticoagulants close to term and during labor. Therapeutic options include the following:

    a. Warfarin: This is inexpensive, easy to administer, and must be monitored to achieve an INR of 2.5 to 3.5. Yet, it is classified by the FDA as category D because of an associated embryopathy that includes IUGR, eye, nasal, CNS, and cardiac anomalies. The reported risk is between 5% and 25% of infants exposed in the first trimester,[16] though a large Asian study[17] did not find an increased rate of embryopathy. It is currently unclear whether warfarin embryopathy is dose dependent; the majority of affected fetuses in one study occurred in pregnancies where mothers received more than 5 mg Coumadin daily to effect anticoagulation.[18] Second- and third-trimester exposure to warfarin is associated with possible complications of fetal hemorrhage, abruption, and stillbirth. The largest review of women with prosthetic heart valves included studies with 976 women over 3 decades.

Warfarin embryopathy was eliminated as a concern when heparin was substituted in the first trimester, but maternal deaths from valve thromboses increased from 1.8% to 4.2%.[19]

b. Heparin: Heparin has a long track record of use in pregnancy, is safe for the fetus, and can be used either subcutaneously in the antepartum period or intravenously in the peripartum period. The subcutaneous dosage of heparin for anticoagulation is greater than with venous thrombosis prophylaxis, and patients generally need more than 30,000 units daily. Unfractionated heparin (UFH) should be dosed to achieve the activated partial thromboplastin time (aPTT) at two to three times normal in patients with valvular prostheses. In the third trimester, women have increased heparin-carrying proteins and may require a dose increase. Other considerations with heparin include the risk for thrombocytopenia and osteoporosis with long-term administration. In the intrapartum setting, heparin infusion should be stopped 12 hours before delivery is anticipated and can be restarted, in the absence of hemorrhagic problems, 4 to 6 hours after delivery.

c. Low-molecular-weight heparin (LMWH): LMWH is more expensive than heparin or warfarin and is injected subcutaneously. Recent clinical trials demonstrate safety and efficacy in pregnancy, but this LMWH is not approved by the FDA for use with prosthetic heart valves.[20,21] LMWH should be monitored and dose-adjusted to achieve an anti–factor Xa level of a minimum of 0.6 to 1.0 unit/ml 4 to 6 hours after injection to reduce the possibility of valve thromboses.[22] It can be stopped 12 hours before delivery without an increase in hemorrhagic complications.[23]

d. Patients with heterograft prostheses (e.g., porcine): These patients have a much lower risk for embolic phenomena and need not be anticoagulated if asymptomatic. All patients with prosthetic valves require SBE prophylaxis.

    All methods of anticoagulation have been associated with the life-threatening consequence of valvular thrombosis. Recent consensus guidelines for anticoagulation are presented in Table 8-7.[24] Warfarin has the greatest efficacy in preventing valvular thromboses. Its use throughout pregnancy may be most important in women with older prosthetic mitral valves, despite the risk for teratogenicity.

TABLE 8-7 Consensus Guidelines for Anticoagulation

Low-molecular-weight heparin (LMWH) adjusted dose throughout pregnancy to achieve anti–factor Xa level of 0.6-1.0 unit/ml

or

Adjusted-dose unfractionated heparin throughout pregnancy to maintain partial thromboplastin time two to three times normal

or

Unfractionated heparin (UFH) or LMWH in the first trimester, warfarin in the second and third trimester, and resumption of UFH or LMWH 2 weeks before delivery and scheduled induction at 40 weeks

---

From Bates SM, Greer IA, Hirsh J et al: Use of antithrombotic agents during pregnancy: the Seventh ACCP Conference on Antithrombotic and Thrombolytic Therapy, *Chest* 126(3 suppl):627S-644S, 2004.

14. Pulmonary hypertension

A systematic review of pulmonary hypertension treatment over two decades documents a poor prognosis with maternal mortality rates of 30% and 56% in primary and secondary pulmonary hypertension, respectively.[25] However, neonatal survival rates are as high as 87% to 89% in pregnancies with maternal survival.[26] New pharmacologic treatments for pulmonary hypertension that have been used successfully in pregnancy include sildanefil/L-arginine[27] and epoprostenol.[28] These studies represent isolated case reports of women with medical emergencies in late pregnancy and not prolonged treatment; therefore, currently, it is unclear how helpful they will be in improving overall outcomes.

II. ARRHYTHMIAS

A. Prevention

Elimination of stimulants and avoidance of fatigue may be helpful in preventing arrhythmias.

B. Medications and Other Therapies

Decisions about the use of medications to treat arrhythmias depend on assessing both the indication and risk/benefit ratio.[29,30]

1. Adenosine

Adenosine (FDA category C) has not been shown to be harmful in pregnancy and is the drug of choice for acute termination of maternal supraventricular tachycardia.

2. Verapamil

Verapamil (FDA category C) may also be used to treat maternal supraventricular tachycardia and is not teratogenic. Cases of fetal bradycardia and heart block have been reported.

3. Digoxin

Digoxin (FDA category C) is not teratogenic and appears to be without fetal toxicity. An increased dose may be needed in pregnancy.

4. Lidocaine

Lidocaine (FDA category B) is generally safe in pregnancy; fetal levels are typically half those of maternal levels. Uterine artery constriction has been noted at high levels but not at therapeutic levels. Fetal accumulation may be greater in the presence of fetal acidosis.

5. Amiodarone

Amiodarone (FDA category D) has been associated with congenital anomalies; it should be used only for arrhythmias refractory to other medications. Approximately 38% iodine by weight, amiodarone has been associated with fetal and neonatal hypothyroidism, fetal bradycardia, and goiter.[31,32] It is excreted substantially in breast milk, and safety in breastfeeding mothers is thus of concern.

6. Cardioversion

This is safe in pregnancy, when indicated.

REFERENCES

1. Hameed A, Karaalp IS, Tummala PP et al: The effect of valvular heart disease on maternal and fetal outcome of pregnancy, *J Am Coll Cardiol* 37(3):893-899, 2001.
2. Ray P, Murphy GJ, Shutt LE: Recognition and management of maternal cardiac disease in pregnancy, *Br J Anaesth* 93(3): 428-439, 2004.
3. Malhotra M, Sharma JB, Arora P et al: Mitral valve surgery and maternal and fetal outcome in valvular heart disease, *Int J Gynaecol Obstet* 81(2):151-156, 2003.
4. Hendricks CH, Brenner WE: Cardiovascular effects of oxytocic drugs used postpartum, *Am J Obstet Gynecol* 108:751-760, 1970.
5. Lesniak-Sobelga A, Trasc W, KostKiewicz M et al: Clinical and echocardiographic assessment of pregnant women with valvular heart diseases—maternal and fetal outcome, *Int J Cardiol* 94(1):15-23, 2004.
6. Nercolini DC, da Rocha Loures Bueno R, Eduardo Guerios E et al: Percutaneous mitral balloon valvuloplasty in pregnant women with mitral stenosis, *Catheter Cardiovasc Interv* 57(3):318-322, 2002.
7. Yentis SM, Steer PJ, Plaat F: Eisenmenger's syndrome in pregnancy: maternal and fetal mortality in the 1990s, *Br J Obstet Gynaecol* 105(8):921-922, 1998.
8. Vongpatanasin W, Brickner ME, Hillis LD et al: The Eisenmenger syndrome in adults, *Ann Intern Med* 128:745-755, 1998.

9. Meijboom LJ, Vos FE, Timmermans J et al: Pregnancy and aortic root growth in the Marfan syndrome: a prospective study, *Eur Heart J* 26(9):914-920, 2005.

10. Elkayam U, Ostrzega E, Shotan A et al: Cardiovascular problems in pregnant women with the Marfan's syndrome, *Ann Intern Med* 123:117-122, 1995.

11. Treizenberg D, Helmen J, Pearson M et al: Clinical inquires: which patients with mitral valve prolapse should get endocarditis prophylaxis? *J Fam Pract* 53(3):223-228, 2004.

12. Elkayam U, Akhter MW, Singh H et al: Pregnancy-associated cardiomyopathy: clinical characteristics and a comparison between early and late presentation, *Circulation* 111(16):2050-2055, 2005.

13. Dorbala S, Brozena S, Zeb S et al: Risk stratification of women with peripartum cardiomyopathy at initial presentation: a dobutamine stress echocardiography study, *J Am Soc Echocardiogr* 18(1):45-48, 2005.

14. Bernstein PS, Magriples U: Cardiomyopathy in pregnancy: a retrospective study, *Am J Perinatol* 18(3):163-168, 2001.

15. Veldtman GR, Connolly HM, Grogan M et al: Outcomes of pregnancy in women with tetralogy of Fallot, *J Am Coll Cardiol* 44(1):174-180, 2004.

16. Danik S: Anticoagulation in pregnant women with prosthetic heart valves, *Mt Sinai J Med* 71(5):322-329, 2004.

17. Geelani MA, Singh S, Verma A et al: Anticoagulation in patients with mechanical valves during pregnancy, *Asian Cardiovasc Thorac Ann* 13(1):30-33, 2005.

18. Vitale N, Feo M, De Santo LS et al: Dose-dependent fetal complications of warfarin in pregnant women with mechanical heart valves, *J Am Coll Cardiol* 33:1637-1641, 1999.

19. Chan WE, Anand S, Ginsberg JS: Anticoagulation in pregnant women with mechanical heart valves, *Arch Intern Med* 160:191-196, 2000.

20. Rowan JA, McLintock C, Taylor RS et al: Prophylactic and therapeutic enoxaparin during pregnancy: indications, outcomes and monitoring, *Aust N Z J Obstet Gynaecol* 43(2):123-128, 2003.

21. Huxtable LM, Tafreshi MJ, Ondreyco SM: A protocol for the use of enoxaparin during pregnancy: results from 85 pregnancies including 13 multiple gestation pregnancies, *Clin Appl Thromb Hemost* 11(2):171-181, 2005.

22. Oran B, Lee-Parritz A, Ansell J: Low molecular weight heparin for the prophylaxis of thromboembolism in women with prosthetic mechanical heart valves during pregnancy, *Thromb Haemost* 92(4):747-751, 2004.

23. Maslovitz S, Many A, Landsberg JA et al: The safety of low molecular weight heparin therapy during labor, *Matern Fetal Neonatal Med* 17(1):39-43, 2005.

24. Bates SM, Greer IA, Hirsh J et al: Use of antithrombotic agents during pregnancy: the Seventh ACCP Conference on Antithrombotic and Thrombolytic Therapy, *Chest* 126(3 suppl):627S-644S, 2004.

25. Weiss BM, Zemp L, Seifert B et al: Outcome of pulmonary vascular disease in pregnancy: a systematic overview from 1978 through 1996, *J Am Coll Cardiol* 31:1650-1657, 1998.

26. Bonnin M, Mercier FJ, Sitbon O et al: Severe pulmonary hypertension during pregnancy: mode of delivery and anesthetic management of 15 consecutive cases, *Anesthesiology* 102(6):1133-1137, 5A-6A, 2005.

27. Lacassie HJ, Germain AM, Valdes G et al: Management of Eisenmenger syndrome in pregnancy with sildenafil and L-arginine, *Obstet Gynecol* 103(5 pt 2):1118-1120, 2004.

28. Geohas C, McLaughlin VV: Successful management of pregnancy in a patient with eisenmenger syndrome with epoprostenol, *Chest* 124(3):1170-1173, 2003.

29. Gowda RM, Khan IA, Mehta NJ et al: Cardiac arrhythmias in pregnancy: clinical and therapeutic considerations, *Int J Cardiol* 88(2-3):129-133, 2003.

30. Joglar JA, Page RL: Treatment of cardiac arrhythmias during pregnancy: safety considerations, *Drug Saf* 20:85-94, 1999.

31. Bartalena L, Bogazzi F, Braverman LE et al: Effects of amiodarone administration during pregnancy on neonatal thyroid function and subsequent neurodevelopment, *J Endocrinol Invest* 24(2):116-130, 2001.

32. Lomenick JP, Jackson WA, Backeljauw PF: Amiodarone-induced neonatal hypothyroidism: a unique form of transient early-onset hypothyroidism, *J Perinatol* 24(6):397-399, 2004.

S e c t i o n   C   Chronic Hypertension

Lawrence Leeman, MD, MPH

Chronic hypertension is one of the most common medical conditions complicating pregnancy, affecting about 3% of pregnant women.[1,2] Adverse maternal and perinatal outcomes occur primarily because of superimposed preeclampsia, IUGR, or placental abruption. Women with severe untreated chronic hypertension are at risk for adverse maternal outcomes secondary to end-organ damage. This section covers the diagnosis and management of pregnant women with chronic hypertension.

I. EPIDEMIOLOGY AND PATHOGENESIS

Chronic hypertension is more common in pregnant women who are older than 40 years, African American, or obese. Primary idiopathic hypertension is the most common cause of chronic hypertension in pregnancy. Women whose hypertension is severe, resistant to medicines, of sudden onset, or with specific abnormal physical examination or laboratory findings are more likely to have a cause of secondary hypertension.[3] Renal disease (intrinsic medical renal disease and renal artery stenosis) is the most common cause of secondary hypertension. Pheochromocytoma, hyperaldosteronism, Cushing disease, and coarctation of the aorta are quite uncommon causes of secondary hypertension.

II. DIAGNOSIS

A. Chronic Hypertension

Pregnant women may have a diagnosis of chronic hypertension before conception, or a presumptive diagnosis may be made in the presence of sustained hypertension before 20 weeks of gestation. A systolic BP of ≥140 mmHg or a diastolic BP of ≥90 mmHg on 2 occasions at least 4 hours apart is necessary for diagnosis.[4] Diastolic BP is measured by Korotkoff stage V (disappearance of sounds). Severe chronic hypertension (stage 3) is diagnosed when the systolic BP is ≥180 mmHg or diastolic BP ≥110 mmHg.[4] Table 8-8 reviews the steps recommended to obtain accurate BP measurements.

B. Preeclampsia

The presence of more than 300 mg protein in a 24-hour urine collection is diagnostic for preeclampsia in the setting of new-onset hypertension unless it was present before conception.

C. Gestational Hypertension

Women who present in pregnancy beyond 20 weeks with increased BP without proteinuria or a known history of chronic hypertension are classified as having gestational hypertension. This is a heterogeneous group, including women who will eventually experience development of proteinuria and be diagnosed with preeclampsia, women who will have persistent hypertension after 12 weeks postpartum and be diagnosed with chronic hypertension, and women who do not experience development of preeclampsia and whose BP normalizes after delivery consistent with a diagnosis of transient hypertension of pregnancy. Women presenting for their initial prenatal care visit after 20 weeks may present a diagnostic dilemma in distinguishing gestational from chronic hypertension. They require close surveillance for the development of preeclampsia. Preeclampsia ultimately develops in approximately 50% of women diagnosed with gestational hypertension at between 24 and 35 weeks.[5] Women with severe gestational hypertension have worse perinatal outcomes than women with mild preeclampsia, including preterm delivery, SGA, and placental abruption.[6]

III. TREATMENT

A. Evaluation of Renal Function

All women with chronic hypertension need an evaluation of their baseline renal function with serum blood urea nitrogen (BUN) and creatinine level and a 24-hour urine collection for creatinine clearance and proteinuria. Women with serum creatinine levels less than 1.4 mg/dl have an increased risk for development of preeclampsia and IUGR; however, they generally have good pregnancy outcomes with preservation of baseline renal function.[4] Women with chronic hypertension with increased baseline proteinuria have an increased risk for preterm delivery (OR, 3.1; 95% confidence interval [CI], 1.8-5.3) and IUGR (OR, 2.8; 95% CI, 1.6-5.0).[7] Women with a creatinine level ≥1.5 mg/dl are at greater risk for adverse pregnancy outcomes and deterioration of renal function during pregnancy.[8]

B. Treatment with Antihypertensive Medicines

Treatment with antihypertensive medicine during pregnancy to achieve "tight" control (aiming for a diastolic BP < 90 mmHg) has no proven benefit to the fetus, nor has it been shown to prevent the development of preeclampsia.[2,9,10] Excessively lowering the BP in a woman with chronic hypertension may result in decreased placental perfusion and adverse perinatal outcomes. A metaanalysis demonstrated an association between reduction in maternal BP secondary to treatment with hypertensive medicines and an increase in SGA infants, as well as a decrease in mean birth weight.[11] Treatment with antihypertensive medicines is required for severe chronic hypertension to prevent maternal end-organ damage (cerebrovascular accident, myocardial ischemia, and

---

TABLE 8-8 Accurate Blood Pressure Measurement

Seated quietly in a chair with feet on the floor for at least 5 minutes

No caffeine, tobacco, or exercise for 30 minutes

Arm supported at level of the heart

Appropriate cuff size (bladder encircles at least 80% of arm)

At least two measurements

From Chobanian AV, Bakris GL, Black HR et al: The Seventh Report of the Joint National Committee on Prevention, Detection, Evaluation, and Treatment of High Blood Pressure: the JNC 7 report, *JAMA* 289:2560-2572, 2003.

renal injury) when the BP is persistently greater than 160/100 mmHg.[2,4]

C. Choice of Oral Antihypertensive Medicines during Pregnancy

Following is a list of oral antihypertensive medicines used during pregnancy to manage chronic hypertension:

1. Methyldopa
   Methyldopa is the medicine that has traditionally been used for treatment of chronic hypertension in pregnancy and the only medicine with reassuring long-term follow-up studies.[12] Although it remains a first-line medicine, some women will not tolerate the side effects of fatigue and dry mouth or will require the addition of a second medicine.
2. Labetalol
   Labetalol may be used as a first-line antihypertensive medicine in pregnancy and is usually well tolerated.
3. Nifedipine and hydralazine
   These are alternative medicines that are commonly used in pregnancy.[13]
4. Angiotensin-converting enzyme (ACE) inhibitors and angiotensin II receptor antagonists
   These medications should not be used during pregnancy because of association with IUGR, oligohydramnios, neonatal renal failure, and death.[2]
5. β-Blockers and thiazide diuretics
   These medications remain controversial. β-Blockers, specifically atenolol, have been associated with IUGR,[10,14] and thiazide diuretics can exacerbate the intravascular fluid depletion of preeclampsia if chronic hypertension becomes complicated by superimposed preeclampsia.[10]

D. Monitoring for Superimposed Preeclampsia

Preeclampsia will develop in approximately 25% of women with chronic hypertension.[4] The incidence rate is greater in women who have had hypertension for more than 4 years, preeclampsia in a prior pregnancy, or a baseline diastolic BP greater than 100 mmHg.[7] The development of superimposed preeclampsia may be diagnosed based on new-onset proteinuria, an increase in systolic BP to 180 mmHg or diastolic BP to 110 mmHg or more in a woman whose hypertension has previously been well controlled, or development of increased liver enzymes or thrombocytopenia (<100,000/mm).[4]

E. Surveillance for Intrauterine Growth Restriction

Women with chronic hypertension are at risk for IUGR. Serial ultrasound examinations every 4 weeks starting at 30 to 32 weeks have been recommended to detect IUGR, although National High Blood Pressure Education Program (NHBPEP) guidelines suggest that serial fundal height measurements by the same examiner may be adequate screening.[4,15]

F. Antenatal Assessment of Fetal Well-Being

The NHBPEP guidelines do not recommend the use of routine antenatal testing for women with chronic hypertension unless IUGR or superimposed preeclampsia develops.[4] Antenatal testing with nonstress tests or biophysical profiles (BPPs) has been recommended for women with severe chronic hypertension and/or those who require antihypertensive medicines.[16] Use of umbilical artery Doppler velocimetry for women with IUGR or hypertension was demonstrated in a 2000 Cochrane analysis[17] to decrease the need for induction of labor and in a 2003 RCT to decrease the incidence of cesarean delivery for fetal distress compared with nonstress tests as the primary antepartum surveillance method.[18] The timing of initiation of the antenatal testing will be dependent on severity of disease.

G. Timing of Delivery

Women with chronic hypertension should be delivered by their due date even if superimposed preeclampsia or IUGR has not developed.[16] Induction can prevent perinatal morbidity and mortality caused by placental abruption or uteroplacental insufficiency. Placental abruption occurs in 0.7% to 1.5% of women with mild chronic hypertension, which is close to the baseline rate. The incidence of placental abruption in women with chronic hypertension and superimposed preeclampsia is 3%.[7]

H. Intrapartum Management

Continuous fetal monitoring is recommended for the patient with suspected IUGR, preeclampsia, or severe chronic hypertension because of the increased incidence of placental abruption and potential for uteroplacental insufficiency.[19] Women in active labor with severe chronic hypertension may be treated with IV labetalol or hydralazine in a similar fashion to women with severe preeclampsia.[20]

I. Postpartum Care and Lactation

After delivery, the decision to continue antihypertensive medicines is based on the guidelines for nonpregnant women, which support use of medicines in patients with systolic BP greater than 140 mmHg or diastolic BP greater than 90 mmHg.[3] Methyldopa and labetalol have low levels in breast milk and are generally considered safe, as is nifedipine.[21] Avoid use of ACE inhibitors and angiotensin II receptor antagonists because of potential effects on neonatal renal function.

IV. CLINICAL COURSE AND PREVENTION

Preconception counseling for women with chronic hypertension involves the recommendation of dietary changes and weight loss, discussion of the effect of chronic hypertension on pregnancy, and detection of end-organ damage. A serum creatinine and urinalysis to detect hypertensive nephropathy are important because women with an increased serum creatinine level, particularly greater than 1.5 mg/dl, should be counseled regarding potential irreversible progression of their renal disease because of pregnancy.[8] Early prenatal care to ensure accurate dating and adjustment of antihypertensive medicines should be encouraged. Women who smoke tobacco should be strongly urged to stop because of the association of tobacco with placental abruption and IUGR.

Physicians must carefully observe all pregnant women with chronic hypertension for signs of superimposed preeclampsia or IUGR. Women with chronic hypertension should be given aspirin starting at 12 weeks to decrease the likelihood of development of preeclampsia (number needed to treat [NNT] = 69) and the associated adverse outcomes of preterm delivery (NNT = 83) and fetal death (NNT = 227).[22] Calcium supplementation should also be offered to women with chronic hypertension because it has been shown to decrease the risk for development of preeclampsia in women with low baseline calcium supplementation or those at high risk for development of hypertension.[23] Women with mild chronic hypertension without these secondary complications usually have excellent maternal and neonatal outcomes, and care must be taken to avoid iatrogenic outcomes caused by inappropriate use of antihypertensive medicines or unneeded labor induction.

V. SOR A RECOMMENDATIONS

RECOMMENDATIONS	REFERENCES
Low-dose aspirin has small-to-moderate benefits for prevention of preeclampsia (NNT = 69), preterm delivery (NNT = 83), and fetal death (NNT = 227) in women at greater risk for development of preeclampsia.	22
Calcium supplementation decreases the risk for development of hypertension and preeclampsia, particularly among women with low baseline calcium supplementation or those at high risk for development of hypertension. The risk for preterm delivery is decreased in women at high risk of development of hypertension in pregnancy.	23
Insufficient evidence is available to recommend using antihypertensive medicines to achieve "tight" control (aiming for a diastolic BP < 90 mmHg) versus "less tight" control (aiming for a diastolic BP of 100-110 mmHg).	9
Use of umbilical artery Doppler velocimetry for women with severe hypertension or IUGR is associated with a decreased need for labor induction or cesarean delivery compared with nonstress testing.	17, 18

REFERENCES

1. Agency for Healthcare Research and Quality: Management of chronic hypertension during pregnancy. Summary evidence report/technology assessment: Number 14, AHRQ Publication No. 00-E010, August 2000. Available at: http://www.ahrq.gov/clinic/epcsums/pregsum.htm. Accessed August 28, 2005.
2. American College of Obstetricians and Gynecologists: ACOG practice bulletin No. 29: chronic hypertension in pregnancy, *Obstet Gynecol* 98(suppl):177-185, 2001.
3. Chobanian AV, Bakris GL, Black HR et al: The Seventh Report of the Joint National Committee on Prevention, Detection, Evaluation, and Treatment of High Blood Pressure: the JNC 7 report, *JAMA* 289:2560-2572, 2003.
4. National High Blood Pressure Education Program Working Group on High Blood Pressure in Pregnancy: Report of the National High Blood Pressure Education Program Working Group on High Blood Pressure in Pregnancy, *Am J Obstet Gynecol* 183:S1-S22, 2000.
5. Barton JR, O'Brien JM, Bergauer NK et al: Mild gestational hypertension remote from term: progression and outcome, *Am J Obstet Gynecol* 184:979-983, 2001.

6. Buchbinder A, Sibai BM, Caritis S et al: Adverse perinatal outcomes are significantly higher in severe gestational hypertension than in mild preeclampsia, *Am J Obstet Gynecol* 186:66-71, 2002.

7. Sibai B, Lindheimer MD, Hauth J et al: Risk factors for preeclampsia, abruptio placentae, and adverse neonatal outcomes among women with chronic hypertension. National Institute of Child Health and Human Development Network of Maternal-Fetal Medicine Units, *N Engl J Med* 339:667-671, 1998.

8. Jones DC, Hayslett JP: Outcome of pregnancy in women with moderate or severe renal insufficiency, *N Engl J Med* 335:226-232, 1996.

9. Abalos E, Duley L, Steyn DW et al: Antihypertensive drug therapy for mild to moderate hypertension during pregnancy, *Cochrane Database Syst Rev* (1):CD002252, 2007.

10. Magee LA, Duley L: Oral beta blockers for mild to moderate hypertension during pregnancy, *Cochrane Database Syst Rev* (3):CD002863, 2003.

11. Von Dadelszen P, Ornstein MP, Bull SB et al: Fall in mean arterial pressure and fetal growth restriction in pregnancy hypertension: a meta-analysis, *Lancet* 355:87-92, 2000.

12. Cockburn J, Moar VA, Ounsted M et al: Final report of study on hypertension during pregnancy: the effects of specific treatment on the growth and development of the children, *Lancet* 1982;1:647-649.

13. James PR, Nelson-Piercy C: Management of hypertension before, during, and after pregnancy, *Heart* 90:1499-1504, 2004.

14. Butters L, Kennedy S, Rubin PC: Atenolol in essential hypertension during pregnancy, *BMJ* 301:587-589, 1990.

15. Sibai BM: Diagnosis and management of gestational hypertension and preeclampsia, *Obstet Gynecol* 102:181-192, 2003.

16. Sibai B: Chronic hypertension in pregnancy, *Obstet Gynecol* 100:369-377, 2002.

17. Neilson JP, Alfirevic Z: Doppler ultrasound for fetal assessment in high risk pregnancies, *Cochrane Database Syst Rev* (2):CD000073, 2000.

18. Williams KP, Farquharson DF, Bebbington M et al: Screening for fetal well-being in a high-risk pregnant population comparing the nonstress test with umbilical artery Doppler velocimetry: a randomized controlled clinical trial, *Am J Obstet Gynecol* 188:1366-1371, 2003.

19. American College of Obstetricians and Gynecologists: ACOG practice bulletin No. 62: intrapartum fetal heart rate monitoring, *Obstet Gynecol* 105:1161-1169, 2005.

20. Duley L, Henderson-Smart DJ: Drugs for treatment of very high blood pressure during pregnancy, *Cochrane Database Syst Rev* (3):CD001449, 2006.

21. American Academy of Pediatrics Committee on Drugs: Transfer of drugs and other chemicals into human milk, *Pediatrics* 108:776-789, 2001.

22. Duley L, Henderson-Smart DJ, Knight M et al: Antiplatelet agents for preventing pre-eclampsia and its complications, *Cochrane Database Syst Rev* (2):CD004659, 2007.

23. Atallah AN, Hofmeyr GJ, Duley L: Calcium supplementation during pregnancy for preventing hypertensive disorders and related problems, *Cochrane Database Syst Rev* (1):CD001059, 2002.

SECTION D

Thromboembolic Disease and Chronic Anticoagulation

Jeffrey T. Kirchner, DO, FAAFP

I. PRECONCEPTION EXPOSURE TO ANTICOAGULANTS

Women receiving chronic anticoagulation with vitamin K antagonists such as warfarin should ideally discontinue this drug before conception because of its multiple teratogenic effects (pregnancy category X). Some data suggest that warfarin is safe if given before week 6 of pregnancy. Thus, one preconception option is to continue this anticoagulant with frequent monitoring of pregnancy tests and substitute heparin when pregnancy is achieved. The following sections discuss risks associated with warfarin include embryopathy, CNS abnormalities, and coagulopathy.[1,2]

A. Embryopathy
First-trimester exposure to warfarin may result in nasal hypoplasia and skeletal abnormalities, including stippled epiphyses.

B. Central Nervous System Abnormalities
Multiple CNS abnormalities including optic atrophy may result from exposure during any trimester. Neurodevelopmental problems in children exposed during the second and third trimesters have also been reported.

C. Coagulopathy
Warfarin can cause an anticoagulant effect in the fetus, which could be problematic, especially at the time of delivery.

II. HISTORY OF THROMBOPHILIC DISEASE

About 50% of gestational venous thrombotic events (VTEs) are associated with heritable thrombophilia. A thorough evaluation of a woman's personal and family history for inheritable thromboembolic disease should be obtained. Screening for inherited coagulation disorders, including antithrombin deficiency, homozygosity for the C667T methylene tetrahydrofolate reductase mutation, and factor V Leiden, should be considered.[2,3]

Although there are conflicting outcome data, current guidelines recommend that women with recurrent pregnancy loss, second-trimester miscarriage, history of intrauterine death, or severe or recurrent preeclampsia be screened for congenital thrombophilias. Screening women for anti-phospholipid antibodies (APLAs), which have been associated with VTEs and recurrent miscarriage, is recommended. Specific treatment with heparin and aspirin has proved effective in reducing miscarriage rates.[2] Although women with thrombophilia are at risk for development of VTEs and complications, the absolute risk remain low. Current evidence does not support universal screening for thrombophilia.[4,5]

III. ANTICOAGULANT OPTIONS DURING PREGNANCY

UFH historically has been the drug of choice for anticoagulation in preconception and pregnancy. It should be administered subcutaneously every 12 hours in a dose-adjusted fashion, typically 150 to 200 units/kg, with a goal to maintain a midinterval aPTT of 1.5 to 2 times normal.

LMWH including enoxaparin and dalteparin can be used as an alternative to UFH (pregnancy category B). Metabolism of these agents can be altered in pregnancy, and a recommended target goal is an anti–factor Xa level of 0.5 to 1.2 IU/ml. These agents have been shown have a lower risk for bleeding complications, heparin-induced thrombocytopenia, and osteoporosis.[7] They are becoming the therapy of choice in this setting. Neither UFH nor LMWH cross the placenta. However, data are still limited to suggest one form of heparin is safer or more effective than the other.[2,4,5]

IV. ANTENATAL PROPHYLAXIS

Pregnancy is associated with a twofold increase in the risk for a first deep venous thrombosis (DVT). The frequency is similar during all three trimesters. Ninety percent of cases occur in the left leg. The risk is greater in women with a previous VTE or thrombophilia.

Based on prior history of thromboembolic disease, prophylaxis against future VTE may be appropriate.

Recommendations vary depending on whether the previous VTE was associated with pregnancy.[2,6]

A. History of One Prior Venous Thrombotic Event Associated with Risk Factor

Women with one prior VTE associated with a transient risk factor that is no longer present (e.g., surgery) can be managed with routine clinical surveillance but should receive postpartum anticoagulation for 4 to 6 weeks.

B. History of One Prior Idiopathic Venous Thrombotic Event

Women with a single idiopathic VTE who are not receiving long-term anticoagulation therapy can be managed clinically or may receive minidose or moderate-dose UFH or LMWH, followed by postpartum anticoagulation for 4 to 6 weeks.

C. History of Venous Thrombotic Event in Pregnancy or in Women with Known Risk Factors

Women with a previous VTE during pregnancy, or related to estrogen use (e.g., related oral contraceptives), or who have additional risk factors (e.g., obesity), should receive antenatal prophylaxis with minidose UFH or LMWH.

D. History of Venous Thrombotic Event and Thrombophilia

Women with a single episode of VTE and thrombophilia (i.e., have antithrombin deficiency or are homozygotes or compound heterozygotes for prothrombin G20210A or factor V Leiden) or with a strong family history of thrombosis should receive minidose or moderate-dose UFH, prophylactic or intermediate-dose LMWH, followed by postpartum anticoagulation for 4 to 6 weeks.

E. History of Two or More Venous Thrombotic Events and/or Receiving Long-Term Anticoagulation

Women who have had two or more VTEs or are receiving long-term anticoagulation, or both, should receive adjusted-dose UHF or adjusted-dose LMWH, followed by long-term resumption of an anticoagulant in the postpartum period.

F. Women with Prosthetic Heart Valves

Women with prosthetic heart valves should receive adjusted-dose LMWH throughout the pregnancy to keep anti–factor Xa level at 1 to 1.2 units/ml. Alternatively, they can receive adjusted-dose UFH to keep the aPTT at twice control or the anti–factor Xa level of 0.35 to 0.70 unit/ml. Addition of low-dose aspirin (75-162 mg/day) can be considered for women at high risk. Long-term anticoagulation with warfarin should be resumed after delivery.

G. Women with History of Deep Venous Thrombosis

All women with a previous DVT should use graduated elastic compression stockings antenatally and postpartum.

V. DIAGNOSIS OF VENOUS THROMBOTIC EVENT DURING PREGNANCY

The diagnostic approach during pregnancy is essentially the same as for the nonpregnant patient, but most of the commonly performed diagnostic tests have not been validated in pregnancy.[9,10] The clinical picture is often confounded by the compressive effect of the gravid uterus on the iliac vein, which may produce unilateral or bilateral leg swelling and mimic DVT. The role of D-dimer is also limited because its concentrations increase during pregnancy and it has not been validated in prospective studies.[11] If DVT is suspected based on clinical findings of leg swelling and pain, the following modalities can help confirm the diagnosis.

A. Venous Doppler

Venous Doppler or ultrasonography is the method of choice for diagnosis of DVT.[9,12] It can visualize blood flow, augmentation, and effects of compression. It has greater sensitivity for detecting proximal DVT as opposed to distal thrombi. The sensitivity and specificity are 96% and 99%, respectively, before 20 weeks of gestation.[12] False-positive results may occur from uterine compression.

B. Venography

Venography should be done if ultrasonography is not available or equivocal in the case of high clinical probability. The venogram can visualize the deep calf veins, popliteal veins, and distal three fourths of the superficial femoral veins. Full visualization of the entire pelvic system with this technique requires injection of both feet. Risks associated with venography include systemic reactions, contrast extravasation and tissue necrosis, induction of venous thrombosis, and radiation exposure.[9]

C. Magnetic Resonance Imaging

Magnetic resonance imaging can diagnose pelvic extension of thrombus and isolated pelvic thrombosis. It can also better distinguish true thrombus from pelvic vein compression. An advantage of is the lack of ionizing radiation to the fetus. There are limited data with this modality in pregnancy, and drawbacks include high costs and availability.[9,13]

D. Spiral Computed Tomography

Spiral computed tomography (CT) is a rapid and noninvasive method for diagnosing pulmonary embolism associated with DVT. Sensitivity and specificity are quite good at 90% and 95%, respectively.[10] It does expose the mother and fetus to low levels of ionizing radiation.

E. Radioisotope Studies

Because of radiation exposure, radioisotopes should generally be avoided during pregnancy. Ventilation-perfusion scintigraphy scanning may be necessary to establish the diagnosis of PE but, where available, is being replaced by spiral CT scanning.

VI. TREATMENT OF ACUTE VENOUS THROMBOTIC EVENT DURING PREGNANCY

If a VTE occurs during pregnancy, two treatment options include[2,6,8]:
1. IV UFH for 5 days, followed by at least 3 months of adjusted-dose subcutaneous UFH, *or*
2. LMWH or adjusted-dose subcutaneous UFH or LMWH for both initial and long-term treatment

Therapy with either medication should continue throughout the course of the pregnancy and continue for at least 6 weeks after delivery. Better bioavailability, safety profile in terms of osteoporosis and thrombocytopenia, and the lack of need to monitor aPTT make LMWH the preferred regimen for most patients. In women with a very high risk for recurrence, a temporary inferior vena cava filter can be used.

VII. INTRAPARTUM AND EMERGENCY MANAGEMENT OF VENOUS THROMBOTIC EVENT

See discussion of this topic in Chapter 16, Section H.

A. Use of Heparin during Labor

It is recommended the adjusted-dose heparin be discontinued 24 hours before elective induction of labor or planned cesarean delivery to prevent an unwanted anticoagulant effect during pregnancy. If spontaneous labor occurs and the aPTT is markedly prolonged, protamine sulfate may be given.[2] The recommended dose is 1 mg to neutralize 100 units heparin, based on the amount of heparin given over the previous 2 hours. It should be given in doses of 50 mg or less intravenously over 10 minutes to limit adverse events. Bleeding complications are uncommon with LMWH, but the same 24-hour time period is recommended for discontinuation. For very-high-risk patients (e.g., proximal DVT within 2 weeks of labor), therapeutic IV UHF can be discontinued 4 to 6 hours before delivery to limit the duration of time without anticoagulation (Table 8-9).

VIII. POSTPARTUM VENOUS THROMBOTIC EVENT AND ANTICOAGULANT USE IN BREASTFEEDING

The puerperium is associated with a 14-fold increased risk for a first DVT. The risk is greatest after cesarean delivery. Evaluation of VTE in the postpartum period is the same as during pregnancy. Heparin and LMWHs are not secreted into breast milk and can be given safely to nursing mothers. The use of warfarin is also safe for breastfeeding women.

REFERENCES

1. Jilma B, Kamath S, Hip KY: Antithrombotic therapy in special circumstances. I. pregnancy and cancer, *BMJ* 326:37-40, 2003.
2. Bates SM, Greer IA, Hirsh J et al: Use of antithrombotic agents during pregnancy: the Seventh ACCP Conference on Antithrombotic and Thrombolytic Therapy, *Chest* 126(3 suppl): S627-S644, 2004.
3. Samama CM, Albaladejo P, Benhamou D et al: Venous thromboembolism prevention in surgery: clinical practice guidelines, *Eur J Anaesthesiol* 23(2):95-116, 2006.
4. Robertson L, Wu O, Langhorne P et al. Thrombophilia in pregnancy: a systematic review, *Br J Haematol* 132(2):171-196, 2006.
5. Lee RV: Thromboembolism in pregnancy: a continuing conundrum, *Ann Intern Med* 143:749-750, 2005.
6. Debelak D, Neher JO, St Anna L: How can we best treat and monitor VTE during pregnancy? *J Fam Pract* 54:998-999, 2005.
7. Greer IA, Nelson-Piercy C: Low-molecular-weight heparins for thromboprophylaxis and treatment of venous thromboembolism in pregnancy: a systematic review of safety and efficacy, *Blood* 106:401-407, 2005.
8. Greer IA: Venous thromboembolism and anticoagulant therapy in pregnancy, *Gend Med* 2(suppl A):S10-S17, 2005.
9. Nijkeuter M, Ginsberg JS, Huisman MV: Diagnosis of deep vein thrombosis and pulmonary embolism in pregnancy: a systematic review, *J Thromb Haemost* 4(3):496-500, 2006.
10. Righini M, Bounameaux H: Diagnosis of suspected deep venous thrombosis and pulmonary embolism during pregnancy, *Rev Med Suisse* 1(4):286-289, 2005.

TABLE 8-9 **Dosing of Heparin Types**

Type of Heparin	Minidose	Moderate Dose	Adjusted Dose	Prophylactic Dose	Intermediate Dose
Unfractionated	5000 units SC every 12 hours	Adjusted SC every 12 for target anti–factor Xa of 0.1-0.3 unit/ml	Adjusted SC every 12 hours for midinterval therapeutic aPTT	NA	NA
Low-molecular-weight	NA	NA	Dalteparin 100 units/kg every 12 hours	Dalteparin 5000 units SC every 24 hours	Dalteparin 5,000 units SC every 12 hours
Low-molecular weight	NA	NA	Enoxaparin 1 mg/kg every 12 hours	Enoxaparin 40 mg SC every 24 hours	Enoxaparin 40 mg SC every 24 hours

SC, Subcutaneously; NA, not applicable; aPPT, activated partial thromboplastin time.

11. Kyrle PA, Eichinger S: Deep vein thrombosis, *Lancet* 365:1163-1174, 2005.
12. Sharma S: *Venous thromboembolism in pregnancy. Pulmonary medicine and pregnancy,* Available at: www.emedicine.com/med/topic1958.htm. Accessed December 21, 2005.
13. Sampson FC, Goodacre SW, Thomas SM, van Beek EJ: The accuracy of MRI in diagnosis of suspected deep vein thrombosis: systematic review and meta-analysis, *Eur Radiol* 17:175-181, 2007.

SECTION E Hematologic Conditions in Pregnancy

Jacqueline E. Julius, MD, and Jeffrey T. Kirchner, DO, FAAFP

I. ANEMIA

During pregnancy, anemia is defined as a hemoglobin level less than 10.5 g/dl in the second trimester and less than 11.0 g/dl in the first and third trimesters. The most common causes of anemia in pregnancy are iron and folate deficiency. Less common causes are vitamin B_{12} deficiency, parasitic infections, hemoglobinopathies, malignancy, and chronic blood loss.

A. Iron Deficiency Anemia

Iron deficiency anemia can cause increased risk for maternal infection. It is also associated with infant and child morbidity and mortality from prematurity, LBW, lower infant iron reserve, and heavier placentas. In addition, these infants can have developmental, cognitive, and growth delay. According to the World Health Organization (WHO), iron deficiency from inadequate dietary intake is the most common nutritional deficiency in pregnancy. The WHO recommends using hemoglobin for monitoring iron deficiency; however, serum ferritin is the most accurate measure of iron stores.[1]

1. Severe anemia (hemoglobin level < 7 g/dl)
   This condition causes an increased risk for maternal heart failure, decreased hemoglobin reserve, and fatigue. Malhotra and colleagues[2] demonstrated that the increased risk for prolonged labor, longer mean duration of spontaneous labor, LBW, transfusion requirement, and operative deliveries were statistically significant in these women. However, a few of these operative deliveries were prophylactic to prevent maternal heart failure.[2]

2. Treatment
   Iron supplementation during pregnancy should increase pregnancy and postpartum hemoglobin to greater than 10.0 g/dl. Recommendations are 60 mg of elemental iron per day for nonanemic pregnant women if used for greater than 6 months, and 120 mg per day if less than 6 months or anemia is present. In a recent Cochrane review, iron supplementation was demonstrated to increase the hemoglobin concentration, but the evidence is limited on whether this improves outcomes.[1]
   a. Side effects: Potential side effects of iron supplementation are hemoconcentration, causing LBW and prematurity, and increased production of reactive oxygen species. Gastrointestinal side effects of iron are constipation, diarrhea, nausea, vomiting, and dyspepsia.
   b. Weekly iron prophylaxis: Weekly iron prophylaxis appears to be as effective as daily administration in maintaining the hemoglobin level without anemia[3] and prevents hemoglobin levels associated with prenatal complications, especially hemoconcentration.[4] Mukhopadhyay and co-workers[3] used 200 mg of elemental iron weekly versus 100 mg daily. Weekly supplementation can decrease adverse effects of treatment.[4]
   c. Parenteral iron supplementation: IV iron sucrose in pregnancy has fewer adverse effects and more rapid increase in hemoglobin than oral supplementation.[5] Both IV and intramuscular iron cause anaphylaxis, allergic reactions, skin discoloration, venous thrombosis, myocardial infarctions, and death. Therefore, in severe anemia, the benefits of parenteral iron may outweigh the risks. Transfusion therapy is indicated if the degree of anemia is severe.
   d. Postpartum treatment: Limited studies are available on postpartum treatment of clinically significant anemia, the severity of the anemia, and oral iron supplementation. Other treatment options that improve postpartum hemoglobin are blood transfusions, subcutaneous erythropoietin, and IV iron sucrose.[6,7] Iron sucrose is not recommended in mothers who are breastfeeding.[7]

II. MEGALOBLASTIC ANEMIA

A. Folate Deficiency

All pregnant women require folate supplementation because of depletion by the rapidly growing fetus. Without additional folate, greater than 30% have low folate levels and more than 3% develop megaloblastic anemia. Routine folate during pregnancy decreases the incidence of developing a hemoglobin concentration less than 10 to 10.5 g/dl.[8]

1. Folate supplementation

   All pregnant women should ingest 0.4 to 1 mg/day folic acid. Women with a personal or family history of neural tube defects, type I diabetes, use of folate antagonist (e.g., methotrexate and aminopterin), or use of valproic acid or carbamazepine should ingest 4 to 5 mg/day folic acid.

2. Beneficial effects

   There is insufficient evidence to show a benefit or risk in terms of maternal and fetal outcomes if the anemia is treated with folate.[8] However, Wilson and colleagues suggest preconceptual supplementation decreases the incidence of congenital heart defects, urinary tract abnormalities, pyloric stenosis, limb defects, and oral facial clefts.[9]

3. Adverse effects

   Adverse effects of high-dose folic acid are masking of vitamin B_{12} deficiency, pruritus, rash, bronchospasm, and malaise.[9]

B. Vitamin B_{12} Deficiency

This is a rare cause of anemia during pregnancy. A small study by Milman and colleagues[10] demonstrated that P-cobalamin levels decreased from 18 to 39 weeks with the lowest levels in the third trimester. These low levels did not correlate with low hemoglobin levels.

III. HEMOGLOBINOPATHIES

More than 270 million people are heterozygous for hemoglobin disorders. The most common types are sickle cell and thalassemia. Carrier screening should be offered to populations at risk, including African Americans, Greeks, Italians, Turks, Arabs, Southern Iranians, and Asian Indians. The recommended screening tests are a CBC and hemoglobin electrophoresis. Solubility testing is not recommended because it fails to detect some hemoglobin abnormalities. Sampling of DNA from chorionic villus sampling or amniocentesis is the best test for determining the presence of a fetal hemoglobinopathy. Genetic counseling and screening is recommended for parents with other children diagnosed with disease.

A. Sickle Hemoglobin

There are numerous sickle cell disorders, and all involve persons with at least one hemoglobin S consisting of the β-chain with an amino acid substitution.

A person can be heterogeneous or homogeneous for hemoglobin S, or even have a combination of hemoglobinopathies (including hemoglobin S with hemoglobin C or hemoglobin S with α or β-thalassemia mutations).[11]

1. Sickle cell trait

   Sickle cell trait affects 1 in 12 African Americans. These individuals are typically asymptomatic; however, they should have genetic counseling when contemplating pregnancy because their offspring can have sickle cell disease if the other parent has either sickle cell trait or disease.

2. Sickle cell disease (hemoglobin SS)

   Sickle cell disease causes increased maternal and fetal morbidity and mortality. Maternal complications include preterm labor, premature rupture of membranes, hospitalization for pain crises, and postpartum infection. Risks to the fetus are IUGR, LBW, and preterm delivery.[11] Emphasis on preterm labor symptoms is important because 30% to 50% these women deliver before 36 weeks of gestation. In addition, they are at risk for pyelonephritis and should be treated for asymptomatic bacteriuria if it occurs during pregnancy. Exposure to parvovirus B19 infection is best avoided because of the risk for maternal aplastic anemia and fetal bone marrow suppression.[12] Therapeutic recommendations are ensuring the mother receives 4 mg folic acid per day for the excessive cell turnover and adequate treatment of painful crisis with IV fluids, supplemental oxygen, opiates, and transfusions. Fetal monitoring must be interpreted with caution because these individuals are often receiving narcotics. Prophylactic exchange transfusions 4 to 6 weeks before delivery are controversial. Only one RCT showed benefit by reduction in pain crises and severe anemia, but no change in pregnancy outcome.[11]

B. Thalassemia

Thalassemia is a reduction in synthesis of the globin chains. Therefore, in screening, the mean cell volume is low (<80 fentoliters).

1. α-Thalassemia

   α-Thalassemia occurs when two or more α-globins have a gene deletion. If only one α-globin is affected, the person is not clinically affected and laboratory results are normal. If α-thalassemia occurs with an individual with sickle cell disease, the disease is less severe. No additional folate supplementation is recommended.[11] α-Thalassemia trait occurs with a mutation in two of the α-globins.

The individuals are carriers having an asymptomatic microcytic anemia and the gene they can pass on to their children. Management of pregnancy is unchanged.

a. Hemoglobin H disease: In this case, there is a deletion of three α-globins causing a mild to moderate hemolytic anemia. Good pregnancy outcomes are reported, but the number of documented cases is limited. There is risk for worsening anemia, preeclampsia, preterm birth, or new-onset heart failure. Transfusion with iron chelation may be required.[12]

b. α-Thalassemia major (hemoglobin Bart's disease): This occurs if no α-globins are present, and it leads to hydrops fetalis and intrauterine death. Treatment with fetal exchange transfusion is usually required.[12] Women carrying a fetus with hemoglobin Bart's disease are also at risk for preeclampsia.

2. β-Thalassemia

Individuals with β-thalassemia have a mutation in one or both of the β-globin genes, causing a decrease in β-globins present.[11] Recommendations are 4 mg/day folic acid in women with β-thalassemia.[12]

a. β-Thalassemia minor: This is caused by a heterozygous mutation on the β-globin gene, producing a mild asymptomatic anemia. In pregnancy, a greater risk for IUGR and oligohydramnios has been documented, but no change in perinatal outcomes has been noted. Women should receive supplementation only as required for iron deficiency in pregnancy.[11]

b. β-Thalassemia major (Cooley's anemia): This occurs with a homozygous mutation of the β-globin gene. These patients with β-thalassemia major have poor growth and delayed sexual development from hemosiderin deposition. Without treatment, including exchange transfusions and chelation, death occurs by 10 years of age. Pregnancy can be safe if the woman is receiving intense therapy and has a normal baseline cardiac status. Serial antenatal ultrasounds should be preformed to monitor fetal growth.[11]

IV. BLEEDING DISORDERS

A. Thrombocytopenia

Thrombocytopenia is defined as a platelet count less than 150,000/μl. The overall incidence in pregnancy is 5% to 8%. Women diagnosed with a platelet count less than 75,000/μl, history of idiopathic thrombocytopenia purpura (ITP), or ITP would benefit from a hematology consult because of the potential for maternal and fetal morbidity and mortality.[13]

1. Gestational thrombocytopenia

This is the most common cause of thrombocytopenia (75%) and is a diagnosis of exclusion. Characteristics are an asymptomatic mild-to-moderate thrombocytopenia in the second to third trimester with no previous history and normal platelets preconception and in the early prenatal period. Platelets return to normal at 2 to 12 weeks after delivery, and fetal platelets are not affected. The cause is unknown. This condition possesses no risks to maternal or fetal outcomes. Recommendations are routine measuring of platelets per trimester but no other specific treatment. The platelet level usually is greater than 75,000/μl for women with gestational thrombocytopenia. If the level becomes less than 75,000/μl, then further investigation needs to occur and a hematology consult should be considered.[13]

2. Pregnancy-induced hypertensive disorders

Twenty-one percent of all thrombocytopenias in pregnancy are related to pregnancy-induced hypertension, with 4% to 12% of women with severe preeclampsia having thrombocytopenia as part of the HELLP (hemolysis, elevated liver enzymes, and low platelets) syndrome. Thrombocytopenia can occur before onset of hypertension. Risks to the fetus are IUGR in the full-term neonate, but a bleeding risk has not been demonstrated. However, there is an increased bleeding risk in the preterm neonate with maternal pregnancy-induced hypertension. Treatment of HELLP syndrome is delivery. Platelet transfusions are indicated only in the presence of active bleeding with a platelet count less than 20,000 or to increase the platelet count to greater than 50,000 for a cesarean section. After delivery, the platelet count usually normalizes within 72 hours.[13]

3. Immune-mediated thrombocytopenia

This accounts for about 4% of all thrombocytopenias.[13]

a. ITP: Women with ITP usually have prepregnancy thrombocytopenia caused by (IgG) immune-mediated platelet destruction. Platelet levels are usually less than 100,000/μl, and patients often present with spontaneous mucocutaneous bleeding. Affected persons have normal red and white cell counts, do not have splenomegaly, and exhibit normal to increased megakaryocytes in the bone marrow. Potential risks are fetal thrombocytopenia from maternal IgG crossing the placenta, IUGR, and prematurity. Spontaneous intracranial hemorrhage in the mother may occur if platelet counts are less than 20,000/μl. Treatment with prednisone (1 mg/kg/day for 2-3 weeks, then slow taper to maintain platelet level) is recommended if platelet counts are less than 50,000/μl. Generally, two thirds of patients see improvement in their platelet counts within 1 week and one fourth usually go into remission with treatment. Intravenous immunoglobulin (IVIG) is indicated if prednisone is unsuccessful, if the platelet count is less than 10,000/μl in the third trimester, if bleeding occurs with a platelet count of less than 30,000/μl, or if an operative delivery is required. Other treatment options are platelet transfusion or splenectomy. Mode of delivery should be determined based on obstetric indications. Maternal treatment does not correlate with fetal outcome. Recommendations include getting serial platelet counts on the neonate because of the risk for thrombocytopenia.[13]

b. Neonatal alloimmune thrombocytopenia: Maternal IgG antiplatelet antibodies to fetal platelet antigens, especially PA1 (paternal in origin), cross the placenta and destroy fetal platelets. This occurs in 1 in 1000 to 2000 live births, with 50% in the first pregnancy. Diagnosis usually occurs after birth, with the neonate presenting with ecchymosis, petechiae, or bleeding after circumcision. A fetal ultrasound may show intracranial hemorrhage, hydrocephalus, porencephalic cysts, or fetal hydrops. The mother does not usually present with thrombocytopenia. Diagnosis is by percutaneous umbilical artery sampling for PLA1 antibodies in fetal circulation and fetal platelet count if there is a maternal history or concerning ultrasound findings. Treatment is IVIG together with steroids given maternally in combination with fetal platelet transfusions. Caesarian delivery is recommended if the fetus is found to have a platelet count of less than 50,000/μl; however, this has not been demonstrated to prevent intracranial hemorrhage.

4. Medication-induced thrombocytopenia
Medications used during pregnancy that may cause thrombocytopenia include heparin, penicillin, rifampin, aspirin, acetaminophen, methyldopa, ranitidine, cimetidine, and some anticonvulsants.[13]

5. Other causes
Other causes of thrombocytopenia include systemic lupus erythematosus (SLE), APS, disseminated intravascular coagulation, HIV infection, thrombotic thrombocytopenia purpura, hemolytic uremic syndrome, and fatty liver.[13]

B. Common Coagulopathies

Factor levels fluctuate during pregnancy to a more hypercoagulable state, but return to normal by day 7 to 10 after delivery. Therefore, in women with hereditary coagulopathies, there is a 16% to 22% postpartum risk for early hemorrhage and 11% to 24% of a late hemorrhage. These women must be warned of the signs of hemorrhage and have a 2-week postpartum visit.[14]

1. Von Willebrand disease
Von Willebrand disease is the most common inherited bleeding disorder. Von Willebrand factor (vWF) antigen levels and activity increase during pregnancy. Epidural anesthesia can be used if third-trimester factor levels are normal, but it presents a slightly increased risk for neuraxial hematoma. The safety of desmopressin (which causes a release of vWF from endothelial cells) in pregnancy is unknown, but a few studies show no adverse effects. It also is safe in women who breastfeed.

2. Hemophilia A and B
These are X-linked deficiencies of factors VIII and IX, respectively. Therefore, women affected are usually carriers and will need genetic counseling in regard to risk for inheritance, especially in male offspring. Factor VIII increases during pregnancy, and factor IX usually does not change with pregnancy. Factor levels are measured during the third trimester because unpredictable fluctuations occur. In addition, the levels should be determined before performing any maternal procedures.

a. Treatment during pregnancy: It is important that delivery occur in a hospital with the ability to transfuse the needed factor. Caesarean delivery is reserved for obstetric indications.

b. Neonate: The maternal factor level that is low should be measured in the neonate cord blood. If a bleeding disorder is present, an ultrasound should be performed to rule intracranial hemorrhage.

V. THROMBOEMBOLIC DISEASE

A. Thrombophilic Disorders

During pregnancy, physiologic changes occur that increase coagulation factors and decrease anticoagulation activity. Pregnancy induces a hypercoagulable state with five to six times greater risk for venous thrombosis than in nonpregnant women.[15] Women with thrombophilic disorders are at increased risk for IUGR, recurrent spontaneous abortion, late stillbirth, and abruption, possibly from thrombosis of the placenta. If a history of one prior complication is present, there is a greater than 20% risk for another complication occurring in subsequent pregnancies.[16] These thrombophilic disorders are factor V Leiden, prothrombin gene mutation G20210, antithrombin III deficiency, protein S deficiency, protein C deficiency, hyperhomocystinemia, anti-cardiolipin (aCL) antibodies, lupus anticoagulant, APLAs, and recently, protein Z deficiency.[17,18] Women can be affected by more than one of the thrombophilic disorders, significantly increasing their risk for complications.

1. Screening
   Screening should occur for the above thrombophilic disorders in the presence of a late pregnancy loss, recurrent spontaneous abortion(s), previous unexplained thrombus, or significant family history of thrombus.[17] Limited evidence exists for screening for thrombophilic disorders if IUGR, severe preeclampsia, or placental abruption occurs.[16]

2. Treatment
   Heparin use has helped infants attain increased gestational age, greater birth weight, and umbilical artery flow. LMWH has decreased pregnancy complications by 80%. LMWH is more beneficial at reducing pregnancy complications than aspirin alone. However, more randomized trials are needed in this area (see Section D for further information on treatment).

B. Essential Thrombocythemia

Essential thrombocythemia (ET) is a condition with a platelet level greater than 600×10^9/L, hyperplastic megakaryocytes, and giant platelets with abnormal function.[19] ET is more common in women than men, and about one fifth of patients are younger than 40 years. Approximately one third of patients are asymptomatic at presentation, with others experiencing both venous and arterial thromboembolic

events. Minor hemorrhages occur in 20% of patients, especially with platelet counts greater than 1000×10^9/L, which reduces vWF.[20]

1. ET in pregnancy
   About 50% of pregnancies in women with ET experience complications. Spontaneous abortion is the most common pregnancy complication (41%). Also seen are IUGR, preeclampsia, placental abruption, and fetal death from placental thrombosis. Maternal problems are less common, with an overall incidence rate of about 8%, compared with the effects on the fetus, possibly because of the maternal physiologic decrease in platelet count.

2. Treatment
   Women with ET who become pregnant should have perinatal and hematologic consultations, with serial platelet counts and fetal monitoring. In addition, these individuals should be screened for other coagulation disorders. Potential treatments during pregnancy are aspirin, heparin, interferon-α, and plateletpheresis. Epidural anesthesia is usually contraindicated because of the risk for epidural hematoma.

VI. SOR A RECOMMENDATIONS

RECOMMENDATIONS	REFERENCES
Use folic acid to prevent neural tube defects in the preconception and conception periods. Use 400 μg/day to 1 mg/day for individuals at low risk and 4-5 mg/day for individuals at high risk.	9
Screen ethnicities at risk for hemoglobinopathies by CBC and hemoglobin electrophoresis.	11
Give genetic counseling to those families at risk for having a child with hemoglobinopathy.	11

REFERENCES

1. Pena-Rosas JP, Viteri FE: Effects of routine oral iron supplementation with or without folic acid for women during pregnancy, *Cochrane Database Syst Rev* (3):CD004736, 2006.
2. Malhotra M, Sharma JB, Batra S et al: Maternal and perinatal outcome in varying degrees of anemia, *Int J Gynaecol Obstet* 79(2):93-100, 2002.

3. Mukhopadhyay A, Bhatla N, Kriplani A et al: Daily versus intermittent iron supplementation in pregnant women: hematological and pregnancy outcome, *J Obstet Gynaecol Res* 30(6):409-417, 2004.

4. Casanueva E, Viteri FE, Mares-Galindo M et al: Weekly iron as a safe alternative to daily supplementation for nonanemic pregnant women, *Arch Med Res* 37(5):674-682, 2006.

5. Al RA, Unlubilgin E, Kandemir O et al: Intravenous versus oral iron for treatment of anemia in pregnancy: a randomized trial, *Obstet Gynecol* 106(6):1335-1340, 2005.

6. Dodd J, Dare MR, Middleton P: Treatment for women with postpartum iron deficiency anemia, *Cochrane Database Syst Rev* (4):CD004222, 2004.

7. Broche DE, Gay C, Armand-Branger S et al: Severe anemia in the immediate postpartum period. Clinical practice and value of intravenous iron, *Gynecol Obstet Fertil* 32:613-619, 2004.

8. Mahomed K: Folate supplementation in pregnancy, *Cochrane Database Syst Rev* (2):CD000183, 2000.

9. Wilson RD, Davies G, Desilets V et al: Genetics Committee and Executive and Council of the Society of Obstetricians and Gynecologists of Canada: The use of folic acid for the prevention of neural tube defects and other congenital anomalies, *J Obstet Gynaecol Can* 25(11):959-973, 2003.

10. Milman N, Byg KE, Bergholt T et al: Cobalamin status during normal pregnancy and postpartum: a longitudinal study comprising 406 Danish women, *Eur J Haematol* 76(6):521-525, 2006.

11. ACOG Committee: ACOG practice bulletin. Clinical management guidelines for obstetrician-gynecologists number 64, July 2005 (replaces committee opinion number 238, July 2000): hemoglobinopathies in pregnancy, *Obstet Gynecol* 106(1):203-210, 2005.

12. Rappaport VJ, Velazquez M, Williams K: Hemoglobinopathies in pregnancy, *Obstet Gynecol Clin North Am* 31(2):287-317, 2004.

13. Levy JA, Murphy LD: Thrombocytopenia in pregnancy, *J Am Board Fam Pract* 15(4):290-297, 2002.

14. Demers C, Derzko C, David M et al: Society of Obstetricians and Gynecologists of Canada: gynecological and obstetric management of women with inherited bleeding disorders, *J Obstet Gynaecol Can* 27(7):707-732, 2005.

15. Kujovich JL: Thrombophilia and pregnancy complications, *Am J Obstet Gynecol* 191(2):412-424, 2004.

16. Paidas MJ, Ku DH, Langhoff-Roos J et al: Inherited thrombophilias and adverse pregnancy outcome: screening and management, *Semin Perinatol* 29(3):150-163, 2005.

17. Lin J, August P: Genetic thrombophilias and preeclampsia: a meta-analysis, *Obstet Gynecol* 105(1):182-192, 2005.

18. Kutteh WH, Triplett DA: Thrombophilias and recurrent pregnancy loss, *Semin Reprod Med* 24(1):54-66, 2006.

19. Vantroyen B, Vanstraelen D: Management of essential thrombocythemia during pregnancy with aspirin, intraferon, alpha-2a, and no treatment, *Acta Haematol* 107:158-169, 2002.

20. Griesshammer M, Grunewald M, Michiels JJ: Acquired thrombophilia in pregnancy: essential thrombocythemia, *Semin Thromb Hemost* 29(2):205-212, 2003.

S E C T I O N   F

Gastrointestinal Conditions

Ellen L. Sakornbut, MD

I. INFLAMMATORY BOWEL DISEASE

Ulcerative colitis and Crohn's disease are relatively common conditions in women of childbearing age.

A. Ulcerative Colitis

1. Fertility

   Fertility is normal in patients with ulcerative colitis, except in patients who have had some surgical procedures (see later).

2. Adverse perinatal outcomes

   There are no increases in miscarriage or stillbirth in quiescent disease, but stillbirth is increased in women with poor disease control.[1] Several large, population-based studies suggest an increase in limb deficiencies, obstructive urinary congenital abnormalities, and infants with multiple congenital abnormalities.[2,3] Pregnancy outcomes in women with ulcerative colitis include an increase in frequency of LBW infants, especially if a flare occurs during the pregnancy.[4] The risk for exacerbation during pregnancy is cited as between 20% and 50% the yearly risk in nonpregnant patients, and relapse rates decrease in both ulcerative colitis and Crohn's disease during the postpartum period.[5] The risk for exacerbation is decreased if the disease is quiescent at conception.

3. Genetic links

   Genetic links have been found, with an increased risk for familial transmission.

B. Crohn's Disease

1. Fertility

   Reduced fertility is noted, but no increases in first-trimester pregnancy loss, fetal abnormality, or stillbirths are seen when the disease is quiescent. If Crohn's disease is active at conception, the spontaneous abortion rate is increased.[6]

2. Adverse perinatal outcomes

   The onset of Crohn's disease during pregnancy is associated with increased fetal risk. Compared with healthy women, patients with Crohn's disease have an increased risk for preterm birth and

LBW, but the risk is greatest with exacerbations during pregnancy.[2]

Most patients experience improvement in their disease during pregnancy. The reasons behind this are unclear, but a study of maternal and newborn human leukocyte antigens (HLAs) showed improvement of symptoms when there was disparity in HLA class II between mother and fetus, suggesting that the maternal immune response to paternal HLAs plays a role in pregnancy-induced remission.[7]

A history of previous surgery for Crohn's disease is associated with a greater spontaneous abortion rate.[8] Patients who have an ileostomy may deliver vaginally.

3. Genetic links

Genetic links are present with an increased risk for familial transmission.

C. Pharmacologic Treatment

Women on chronic medications for inflammatory bowel disorders can safely conceive and continue most medication during pregnancy and with breastfeeding.

1. 5-Aminosalicylic acid medications

These medications, such as sulfasalazine and mesalazine, have been used extensively and are safe during pregnancy.[9] Discontinuing these medications briefly when the patient is close to delivery may be advisable because binding to fetal albumin may result in neonatal hyperbilirubinemia. It should be started immediately after delivery to avoid relapse and is safe if breastfeeding. The dosage of mesalazine should be limited to 2 g/day.

2. Prednisone

This drug is discussed earlier in other sections of this chapter. Prednisone is relatively safe for use in pregnancy, but high dosages (1-2 mg/kg/day) are associated with an increased risk for oral clefts if used in the first trimester.

3. Immunomodulators

Azathioprine and 6-mercaptopurine have been used extensively in pregnancy and do not increase rates of congenital malformations, abortions, or stillbirths.[10-12] There appears to be some increase in IUGR with these two agents, and concerns exist about impaired fetal immunity. Cyclosporine, usually prescribed in severe, steroid-resistant ulcerative colitis and for extraintestinal manifestations, is not teratogenic. Despite concerns about alteration of immune function in newborns exposed to immunomodulator medication, no changes are detected in infant CBCs, immunoglobulin subclasses, lymphocyte subpopulations, serum levels of antibodies, or response to hepatitis B vaccination when compared with nonexposed infants.[13]

No adverse events have been reported with exposure to infliximab during pregnancy. Medications that should be discontinued before conception or as early as possible in pregnancy include cyclophosphamide (teratogenicity) and methotrexate (abortifacient).

4. Antibiotics

Antibiotics that may be used for short courses, such as metronidazole and ciprofloxacin, have not been associated with pregnancy complications in women with inflammatory bowel disease. Metronidazole has a much greater track record of safety in pregnancy than ciprofloxacin, because quinolones have been associated with cartilage problems in animal studies.

D. Surgical Treatment

Fertility is decreased in women who have undergone an ileal pouch-anal anastomosis for ulcerative colitis,[14] but women who do get pregnant can be managed in labor expectantly with route of delivery determined by usual criteria.[15,16] Pouch function may be altered transiently because of pressure from the gravid uterus, with return of usual pouch function normally occurring after delivery. In women with permanent change in pouch function, route of delivery does not appear to be a significant factor.

E. Breastfeeding

Breastfeeding is not associated with an increased relapse rate of inflammatory bowel disease. Instead, it appears that relapses may be related to reluctance to take medication while breastfeeding.[17]

II. PEPTIC ULCER DISEASE

The frequency of peptic ulcer disease is not increased in pregnancy. Most patients with dyspepsia have gastroesophageal reflux (see Chapter 4, Section E). Medications with extensive safety profiles include sucralfate (not systemically absorbed) and antacids. Prospective controlled trials from multicenter teratology information networks[18,19] and a metaanalysis of cohort studies[20] support no increased risk for malformations with H2 blockers and proton-pump inhibitors, with the majority of cases involving ranitidine and omeprazole.

III. SOR A RECOMMENDATIONS

RECOMMENDATIONS	REFERENCES
Vaginal delivery is not contraindicated in patients who have had surgery for inflammatory bowel disease such as ileal-anal pouch anastomosis.	15, 16
H2 blockers and proton-pump inhibitors are safe for use during pregnancy.	18-20

REFERENCES

1. Alstead EM, Nelson-Piercy C: Inflammatory bowel disease in pregnancy, *Gut* 52(2):159-161, 2003.
2. Norgard B, Puho E, Pedersen L et al: Risk of congenital abnormalities in children born to women with ulcerative colitis: a population-based, case-control study, *Am J Gastroenterol* 98(9):2006-2010, 2003.
3. Dominitz JA, Young JC, Boyko EJ: Outcomes of infants born to mothers with inflammatory bowel disease: a population-based cohort study, *Am J Gastroenterol* 97(3):641-648, 2002.
4. Bush MC, Patel S, Lapinski RH et al: Perinatal outcomes in inflammatory bowel disease, *J Matern Fetal Neonatal Med* 15(4):237-241, 2004.
5. Castiglione F, Pignata S, Morace F et al: Effect of pregnancy on the clinical course of a cohort of women with inflammatory bowel disease, *Ital J Gastroenterol* 28:199-204, 1996.
6. Nielsen OH, Andreasson B, Bondesen S et al: Pregnancy in Crohn's disease, *Scand J Gastroenterol* 19:724-732, 1984.
7. Kane S, Kisiel J, Shih L et al: HLA disparity determines disease activity through pregnancy in women with inflammatory bowel disease, *Am J Gastroenterol* 99(8):1523-1526, 2004.
8. Hudson M, Flett G, Sinclair TS et al: Fertility and pregnancy in inflammatory bowel disease, *Int J Obstet Gynecol* 58:229-237, 1997.
9. Norgard B, Fonager K, Pedersen L et al: Birth outcome in women exposed to 5-aminosalicylic acid during pregnancy: a Danish cohort study, *Gut* 52(2):243-247, 2003.
10. Moskowitz DN, Bodian C, Chapman ML et al: The effect on the fetus of medications used to treat pregnant inflammatory bowel-disease patients, *Am J Gastroenterol* 99(4):656-661, 2004.
11. Katz JA: Pregnancy and inflammatory bowel disease, *Curr Opin Gastroenterol* 20(4):328-332, 2004.
12. Francella A, Dyan A, Bodian C et al: The safety of 6-mercaptopurine for childbearing patients with inflammatory bowel disease: a retrospective cohort study, *Gastroenterology* 124(1):9-17, 2003.
13. Cimaz R, Meregalli E, Biggiogerro M et al: Alterations in the immune system of children from mothers treated with immunosuppressive agents during pregnancy, *Toxicol Lett* 149(1-3):155-162, 2004.
14. Johnson P, Richard C, Ravid A et al: Female infertility after ileal pouch-anal anastomosis for ulcerative colitis, *Dis Colon Rectum* 47(7):1119-1126, 2004.
15. Kitayama T, Funayama Y, Fukushima K et al: Anal function during pregnancy and postpartum after ileal pouch anal anastomosis for ulcerative colitis, *Surg Today* 35(3):211-215, 2005.
16. Hahnloser D, Pemberton JH, Wolff BG et al: Pregnancy and delivery before and after ileal pouch-anal anastomosis for inflammatory bowel disease: immediate and long-term consequences and outcomes, *Dis Colon Rectum* 47(7):1127-1135, 2004.
17. Kane S, Lemieux N: The role of breastfeeding in postpartum disease activity in women with inflammatory bowel disease, *Am J Gastroenterol* 100(1):102-105, 2005.
18. Garbis H, Elefant E, Diav-Citrin O et al: Pregnancy outcome after exposure to ranitidine and other H2-blockers. A collaborative study of the European Network of Teratology Information Services, *Reprod Toxicol* 19(4):453-458, 2005.
19. Diav-Citrin O, Arnon J, Shechtman S et al: The safety of proton-pump inhibitors in pregnancy: a multicentre prospective controlled study, *Aliment Pharmacol Ther* 21(3):269-275, 2005.
20. Nikfar S, Abdollahi M, Moretti ME et al: Use of proton pump inhibitors during pregnancy and rates of major malformations: a meta-analysis, *Dig Dis Sci* 47(7):1526-1529, 2002.

S E C T I O N G Neurologic Conditions

Ellen L. Sakornbut, MD

I. SEIZURE DISORDERS

A. Clinical Background

The prevalence rate of existing seizure disorders in pregnancy is between 0.3% and 0.6%. Approximately 1 million women of childbearing age in the United States have idiopathic epilepsy. Other causes of seizures include arteriovenous malformations, posttraumatic seizures, and tuberous sclerosis. An increased risk for arteriovenous malformation hemorrhage or enlargement exists during pregnancy. Epilepsy also demonstrates some genetic linkage. Women with tuberous sclerosis should receive genetic counseling. It has been thought that the risk for congenital defects is increased in women with epilepsy, independent of the use of antiepileptic drugs (AEDs); this is not supported by large retrospective epidemiologic studies,[1] prospective cohort design studies,[2-4] or metaanalyses using the Cochrane and other large databases.[5]

B. Preconception Assessment and Planning

AEDs may decrease ovulatory function and fertility through its effects on sex hormone binding globulin. Polycystic ovarian changes and increased androgen levels have been seen with use of valproate.[6] However, enzyme-inducing AEDs may decrease the effectiveness of oral contraceptives by increasing their metabolism. If postponement of pregnancy is desired, a higher-dose oral contraceptive or alternative contraceptive method may be indicated. Newer AEDs such as felbamate, gabapentin, lamotrigine, tiagabine, and vigabatrin do not interfere with hormonal contraception.[7] Women desiring pregnancy should be supplemented with folic acid and treated with monotherapy, if possible, to reduce the risk for major congenital anomalies.

Preconception assessment includes consideration of the frequency of seizures and number of medications required for control. A reduction in number of medications, change of medication, or trial "off" medications should be considered in selected patients. For example, patients with petit mal (absence) seizures will often experience clinical remission before adulthood and may be able to stop their medical therapy. A Cochrane review found evidence for waiting 2 or more seizure-free years before discontinuing medications in children, particularly in individuals with abnormal electroencephalograms or partial seizures. Insufficient evidence exists to recommend timing of withdrawal of AEDs in children with generalized seizures or in adults who are seizure free.[8] Thus, the decision about whether to stop medication in a seizure-free woman remains one of individual risk assessment. If continued medication is necessary, trimethadione poses a significant risk, with high rates of major congenital anomalies and spontaneous abortion,[9] and should be discontinued with a change to another medication, such as ethosuximide. Discontinuance of medication is not recommended in patients who continue to have seizures because uncontrolled seizures pose an immediate risk to both mother and fetus.

C. Effects of Pregnancy on Seizures

Approximately one in five women with epilepsy has worsening of seizures during pregnancy.[10,11] Patients with rare seizures are less likely to deteriorate, whereas those with seizures occurring at least monthly almost always experience increased seizures. These effects are usually temporary and revert after delivery.

Physiologic changes of pregnancy, such as increased minute ventilation, hyponatremia, hypocalcemia, and expanded extracellular volume (increased volume of distribution), reduce the seizure threshold. Fatigue and emotional stress may make patients more prone to seizures.

Anticonvulsant levels may fluctuate as a result of changes in extravascular fluid, renal clearance, decline in plasma proteins, hepatic enzyme activity, missed doses because of nausea and vomiting, or with medication noncompliance attributable to patient anxiety about medication risks.[12] Metabolism of many AEDs is altered during pregnancy, and most patients will need serial monitoring throughout pregnancy (Table 8-10).

D. New-Onset Seizures

Patients who have new-onset seizures during pregnancy (and who are determined not to be eclamptic) or who have seizures that occur only in pregnancy, should be evaluated for vascular malformations, such as a cavernous angioma.[13] Diagnostic testing should include CT scanning for intracranial hemorrhage, possibly followed by magnetic resonance imaging.

E. Effects of Seizures on Pregnancy

Effects of seizures on pregnancy include:
1. Spontaneous abortion
   The incidence of early pregnancy loss appears to be increased.[14,15]
2. Congenital anomalies
   Pregnancies in women treated for epilepsy have an incidence of congenital abnormalities that is approximately two to three times that of the general population. Perinatal mortality is increased because of this increase in congenital malformations.
3. Folic acid absorption
   Maternal folate absorption is decreased in patients treated with anticonvulsants.
4. Perinatal morbidity
   Fetal acidosis, hypoxia, and fetal heart rate abnormalities may accompany seizures. Seizures, especially status epilepticus, may result in fetal death, presumably as a result of altered uteroplacental circulation and hypoxia. In addition, uncontrolled seizures pose a significant risk to the mother, and maternal injuries during seizures may affect fetal well-being.

TABLE 8-10 Use of Antiepileptic Drugs in Pregnancy

Medication	Clearance in Pregnancy	Effects on Fetus	Effects on Newborn	Breastfeeding
Phenytoin	Increased	7-10% incidence of fetal anticonvulsant syndrome; cognitive function may be altered; folate absorption is decreased	No depression/withdrawal; neonatal hypocalcemia and tetany are possible	Levels 25-35% of maternal; not contraindicated
Phenobarbital	Increased	Increased risk for oral clefts, cardiac defects[41]	Neonatal depression/withdrawal in 10-20%	Levels 10-30% of maternal; may cause neonatal depression
Primidone		Increased risk of major congenital anomalies	Neonatal depression possible	May cause sedation in neonates
Carbamazepine	Increased	Fetal anticonvulsant syndrome, craniofacial defects	No depression/withdrawal	Levels 40% of maternal, no depression
Ethosuximide		6% of exposed fetuses with malformations	No depression/withdrawal	Levels approximately same as maternal; no ill effects known
Valproate		Dose-dependent (>1 g/day or 70 μg/ml) increase in fetal malformations (neural tube defects, cardiac, limb)[42,43]	No depression/withdrawal	Breast milk levels are 2% of maternal serum levels; no contraindication to breastfeeding
Lamotrigine	Increased (up to 330%) 32 weeks, then decreased[44]	No increased risk with monotherapy[45]	Slow metabolism in neonate	Ineffective metabolism in newborn and may accumulate to therapeutic levels,[46] probably contraindicated
Gabapentin		No additional risk known but little data	No adverse effects observed[47]	No data
Topiramate		Extensive transfer across placenta	No adverse effects observed[22]	Excreted extensively in milk, but no adverse effects noted[48]
Oxcarbazepine		No additional risk known but little data	No adverse effects observed[49]	No data
Diazepam—use only intravenously for status epilepticus		Fetal levels exceed maternal (first-trimester chronic use associated with cleft lip/palate)	Slow metabolism in neonate with intrapartum use associated with poor suck, hypotonia, apnea, and hypothermia	May cause poor feeding, sedation; avoid if possible

F. Medications

AED registries have resulted in increased availability of information regarding anticonvulsant use in pregnancy. Most study designs are cohort, and RCTs are rare (see Table 8-10). The quality of information from clinical trials may be diminished because of the heterogeneity of causes manifesting as seizure disorders.

1. Vitamin K deficiency coagulopathy

   Deficient clotting has been proposed as a risk to newborns when mothers are treated with enzyme-inducing AEDs. The proposed mechanism for coagulopathy is a reduction in clotting factors II, VII, IX, and X caused by altered absorption and metabolism of vitamin K. Proposed preventive measures included antenatal maternal vitamin K administration during the last months of pregnancy[16] or 2.5 to 5 mg intravenously or subcutaneously while in labor, but there is no evidence that such therapy changes outcomes or is actually needed. It is common practice in Western countries to administer 1 mg vitamin K intramuscularly to neonates at birth. A large, prospective, clinical trial comparing newborns exposed to enzyme-inducing AEDs with those not exposed found no increase in bleeding complications in the exposed group (all newborns received intramuscular vitamin K at birth).[17] Those few newborns with prolonged prothrombin times measured in cord blood corrected within 2 hours when intramuscular vitamin K was administered at birth.[18]

2. Long-term effects of AEDs on cognitive function

   Blinded neuropsychological evaluations of school-age children found decreased verbal intelligence quotient (IQ) and/or impaired memory function in children with in utero valproate exposure when compared with children exposed to other AEDs or not exposed to AEDs.[19-21] A recent Cochrane review noted the limited quality of most studies, as well as limited information on valproate, but some trend toward poorer neurodevelopmental outcomes in children exposed to polytherapy.[22]

3. Fetal anticonvulsant syndrome

   Fetal anticonvulsant syndrome includes combinations of the following: IUGR and postnatal growth problems, cognitive dysfunction, mild motor and development delays, facial dysmorphism (midface hypoplasia), hypertelorism, frontal bossing, a long upper lip, digit hypoplasia, and microcephaly. Other congenital anomalies may also be present, such as congenital heart disease, diaphragmatic hernias, cleft lip/palate, or abnormal genitalia. Physical findings of fetal anticonvulsant syndrome are approximately two to three times more likely in newborns exposed to anticonvulsant monotherapy than in nonexposed newborns, and are approximately four times more likely when polytherapy is used.[23] The incidence of fetal anticonvulsant syndrome is increased with polytherapy because of competition for metabolism.[24] Whenever possible, monotherapy is recommended to decrease this risk. A possible mechanism associated with fetal anticonvulsant syndrome is carnitine deficiency, and multiple AEDs have been demonstrated to interfere with placental carnitine transport, including phenytoin, valproate, and gabapentin.[25] Cognitive dysfunction is correlated with microcephaly in AED-exposed children, but other findings of fetal anticonvulsant syndrome, either midface or digit hypoplasia, are also correlated with decreased performance and verbal IQ scores.[15] Major malformations, such as cardiac disease, do not display this correlation.

4. Folic acid supplementation

   Folic acid supplementation is hypothesized to decrease the risk for related congenital defects (cardiovascular, oral clefts, neural tube defects, and urinary tract defects) in AEDs (carbamazepine, phenytoin, phenobarbital) and dihydrofolate reductase inhibitors (trimethoprim, triamterene). Current evidence suggests that folic acid supplementation decreases the risk for folic acid–related defects in dihydrofolate reductase inhibitors, but not in AEDs.[26]

5. Intrapartum care

   Parenteral anticonvulsants may be administered during labor if there are concerns about the patient oral receiving medication, because of vomiting or delayed gastric emptying. This is probably not necessary in early labor, when oral medication is suitable. Valium should be used only for noneclamptic status epilepticus because its metabolism and clearance in the newborn will be prolonged. Vitamin K should be administered to the newborn to prevent associated clotting defects.

6. Postnatal care

   Decisions about breastfeeding will depend on infant status, type of medication, and maternal factors, and they should be individualized. Infants should be monitored for lethargy, poor feeding, and signs of withdrawal.

II. MIGRAINE HEADACHE

Patients with catamenial migraines generally improve with pregnancy. The frequency of migraine headache, regardless of type, is decreased in 80% of women[27]; therefore, use of migraine prophylaxis is usually not a concern during pregnancy. Because many patients experience reduction in headaches during pregnancy, increase in headache frequency or intensity should provoke consideration of other entities such as preeclampsia, benign intracranial hypertension, (pseudotumor cerebri), or intracranial lesions.

A. Treatment

Nonpharmacologic measures (rest, stress-reduction, etc.) should always be utilized to prevent or relieve headaches. Prophylaxis with β-blockers should be considered only in patients with frequent, severe migraine, using metoprolol and pindolol. Magnesium sulfate, 1 g IV given over 15 minutes,[28] narcotic pain medication, or antiemetic medication could be considered for treatment of acute headaches.

B. Medications to Avoid

Ergot alkaloids can cause vascular constriction and uterine contraction, and they have been associated with birth defects. They should not be used during pregnancy. A controlled clinical trial of sumatriptan exposure in the first trimester showed no teratogenic effect compared with disease-matched and nonteratogen control subjects.[29] No studies exist about triptan use in later pregnancy or effects on uterine blood flow. Currently, there seems to be no reason to use these medications for therapy in pregnant women.

III. MULTIPLE SCLEROSIS

A. Relapse Rates

Relapse rates are not increased during pregnancy but may be increased after delivery. Women treated with IV steroids monthly in the first 6 months after delivery may experience lower relapse rates.[30] In addition, pregnancy does not appear to contribute to the overall progression of multiple sclerosis.[31-33] A retrospective study of patients with relapsing-remitting multiple sclerosis found reduction in the number of relapses in patients treated with IVIG when compared with patients who did not receive immunoglobulin.[34] No RCTs currently confirm this finding.

B. Urinary Tract Infection

Patients with urinary retention caused by a neurogenic bladder are at increased risk for urinary tract infection and may need to practice intermittent self-catheterization. More frequent urine cultures should be obtained in these patients.

C. Postpartum

Half of perinatal relapses occur in the first 3 months after delivery. No contraindication to breastfeeding exists. Patients should be careful to get adequate rest because fatigue influences symptoms.

IV. MYASTHENIA GRAVIS

Myasthenia gravis is more common in women than men, with onset usually in the second or third decade of life. The disease may complicate the course of pregnancy in multiple ways. One third of patients experience exacerbation during pregnancy, and two thirds remain unchanged. Because of the complexity of management and risks to the neonate, these patients should be delivered in a tertiary setting. The following information is provided for assistance in emergency management and patient counseling.[35,36]

A. Intrapartum Issues

The risk for premature labor is increased as a result of anticholinesterase medication. β-Sympathomimetic drugs and betamethasone have been associated with maternal respiratory crisis.

B. Myasthenic Crisis

Myasthenic crisis presents as severe weakness and respiratory insufficiency, and may be precipitated by labor. It must be distinguished from cholinergic crisis, which is usually associated with nausea, tearing, cramping, and diarrhea. Edrophonium improves myasthenic crisis but not a cholinergic crisis.

C. Medications

The mainstay of treatment continues to be anticholinesterase medications. In addition, corticosteroids, azathioprine, and cyclosporine may be useful. Their use in pregnancy is discussed elsewhere in this chapter. Methotrexate should not be used in pregnancy or by women trying to become pregnant. No safety information is available for mycophenolate mofetil. In the intrapartum setting, magnesium sulfate should not be used because high levels inhibit the release of acetylcholine, causing collapse and apnea. Numerous anesthetics can also cause untoward effects.

D. Neonatal Myasthenia

Neonatal myasthenia occurs in 4% to 20% of neonates due to transplacental passage of acetylcholine receptor antibodies. This syndrome is more severe in the premature infant.

E. Postpartum Exacerbations

Exacerbations are common in the first 6 weeks after delivery. Patients may breastfeed while taking anticholinesterase medications.

V. PARAPLEGIA AND QUADRIPLEGIA

A. Urinary Tract Infections

Urinary tract infections are common complications. Women should be trained to avoid urinary retention, using bladder evacuation by the Credé maneuver (involving the exertion of pressure over the bladder to express urine from the bladder), self-catheterization, or double voiding. Urine cultures should be done on an intermittent basis dependent on patient history. Acidification of the urine may be accomplished with vitamin C, 500 mg four times a day, and may be helpful to prevent recurrent infection.

B. Preterm Labor

The risk for preterm birth is increased, and patients should be observed closely in the third trimester for signs and symptoms of preterm labor.

C. Labor Management

All patients have sacral anesthesia. If the lesion is above T11, labor is painless. Lesions above T5-T6 are above the level of splanchnic outflow. Autonomic hyperreflexia may occur during labor, because of bladder distension before labor occurs, or with cesarean delivery. Signs and symptoms of this massive sympathetic outflow include hypertension, severe vasoconstriction, secondary bradycardia, sweating, pounding headache, and flushing. Normal BPs in Westgren and colleagues' series of spinal cord injury patients were low.[36] Epidural anesthesia is administered early in labor to prevent or treat autonomic hyperreflexia.[37] In cases of autonomic hyperreflexia caused by a distended bladder, it should be emptied. Patients may give birth vaginally, but if cesarean delivery is indicated, regional anesthesia should be used.[38]

VI. BENIGN INTRACRANIAL HYPERTENSION

Benign intracranial hypertension, sometimes referred to as *pseudotumor cerebri*, can occur at any trimester in pregnancy. The syndrome generally presents as unremitting headaches with funduscopic findings of increased intracranial pressure. The diagnosis is established as in nonpregnant women. Treatment is directed at relief of symptoms and preservation of vision, with outcomes similar to the nonpregnant state. Medical therapy includes nonketotic diet, serial lumbar punctures, diuretics, steroids, and analgesics.[39] Acetazolamide is associated with birth defects in animal studies, but it has been used in small series of women without apparent adverse pregnancy outcomes.[40] In addition, surgical management options include optic nerve fenestration and lumboperitoneal shunt, but risks of anesthesia and surgery during pregnancy must be weighed against ophthalmologic concerns.

REFERENCES

1. Artama M, Auvinen A, Raudaskoski T et al: Antiepileptic drug use of women with epilepsy and congenital malformations in offspring, *Neurology* 64(11):1874-1878, 2005.
2. Holmes LB, Harvey EA, Coull BA et al: The teratogenicity of anticonvulsant drugs, *N Engl J Med* 344(15):1132-1138, 2001.
3. Wyzinski DF, Nambisan M, Surve T et al: Increased rate of major malformations in offspring exposed to valproate during pregnancy, *Neurology* 64:961-965, 2005.
4. Kaneko S, Battino D, Andermann E et al: Congenital malformations due to antiepileptic drugs, *Epilepsy Res* 33(2-3): 145-158, 1999.
5. Fried S, Kozer E, Nulman I et al: Malformation rates in children of women with treated epilepsy: a meta-analysis, *Drug Saf* 27(3):197-202, 2004.
6. Isojarvi JI, Tauboll E, Herzog AG: Effects of antiepileptic drugs on reproductive endocrine function in individuals with epilepsy, *CNS Drugs* 19(3):207-223, 2005.
7. Morrell MJ: The new antiepileptic drugs and women: efficacy, reproductive health, pregnancy, and fetal outcome, *Epilepsia* 37(suppl 6):S34-S44, 1996.
8. Sirven JI, Sperling M, Winterchuk DM: Early versus late antiepileptic drug withdrawal for people with epilepsy in remission, *Cochrane Database Syst Rev* (3):CD001902, 2001.
9. Jick SS, Terris BZ: Anticonvulsants and congenital malformations, *Pharmacotherapy* 17:561-564, 1997.
10. Taganelli P, Regesta G: Epilepsy, pregnancy, and major birth anomalies: an Italian prospective, controlled study, *Neurology* 42(suppl 5):89-93, 1992.
11. Sabers A, Rogvi-Hansen B, Dam M et al: Pregnancy and epilepsy: a retrospective study of 151 pregnancies, *Acta Neurol Scand* 97:164-170, 1998.

12. Pennell PB: Antiepileptic drug pharmacokinetics during pregnancy and lactation, *Neurology* 61(6 suppl 2):S35-S42, 2003.
13. Awada A, Watson T, Obeid T: Cavernous angioma presenting as pregnancy-related seizures, *Epilepsia* 38:844-846, 1997.
14. Schupf N, Ottman R: Reproduction among individuals with idiopathic/cryptogenic epilepsy: risk factors for spontaneous abortion, *Epilepsia* 38:824-829, 1997.
15. Mountain KR, Hirsch J, Gallus AS: Neonatal coagulation defect due to anticonvulsant drug treatment in pregnancy, *Lancet* 1:265-268, 1970.
16. Kaaja E, Kaaja R, Matila R et al: Enzyme-inducing antiepileptic drugs in pregnancy and the risk of bleeding in the neonate, *Neurology* 58(4):549-553, 2002.
17. Hey E: Effect of maternal anticonvulsant treatment on neonatal blood coagulation, *Arch Dis Child Fetal Neonatal Ed* 81(3):F208-F210, 1999.
18. Vinten J, Adab N, Kini U et al: Neuropsychological effects of exposure to anticonvulsant medication in utero, *Neurology* 64(6):949-954, 2005.
19. Adab N, Kini U, Vinten J et al: The longer term outcome of children born to mothers with epilepsy, *J Neurol Neurosurg Psychiatry* 75(11):1575-1583, 2004.
20. Gaily E, Kantola-Sorsa E, Hiilesmaa V et al: Normal intelligence in children with prenatal exposure to carbamazepine, *Neurology* 62(1):28-32, 2004.
21. Adab N, Tudur SC, Vinten J et al: Common antiepileptic drugs in pregnancy in women with epilepsy, *Cochrane Database Syst Rev* (3):CD004848, 2004.
22. Holmes LB, Harvey EA, Coull BA et al: The teratogenicity of anticonvulsant drugs, *N Engl J Med* 344(15):1132-1138, 2001.
23. Pennell PB: The importance of monotherapy in pregnancy, *Neurology* 60(11 suppl 4):S31-S38, 2003.
24. Wu SP, Shyu MK, Liou HH et al: Interaction between anticonvulsants and human placental carnitine transporter, *Epilepsia* 45(3):204-210, 2004.
25. Holmes LB, Coull BA, Dorfman J et al: The correlation of deficits in IQ with midface and digit hypoplasia in children exposed in utero to anticonvulsant drugs, *J Pediatr* 146(1):118-122, 2005.
26. Hernandez-Diaz S, Werler MM, Walker AM et al: Folic acid antagonists during pregnancy and the risk of birth defects, *N Engl J Med* 343(22):1608-1614, 2000.
27. Maggioni F, Alessi C, Maggino T et al: Headache during pregnancy, *Cephalgia* 17(7):765-769, 1997.
28. Demirkaya S, Vural O, Doar B et al: Efficacy of intravenous magnesium sulfate in the treatment of acute migraine attacks, *Headache* 41(2):171-177, 2001.
29. Shuhaiber S, Pastiszak A, Schick B et al: Pregnancy outcome following first trimester exposure to sumatriptan, *Neurology* 51:581-583, 1998.
30. De Seze J, Chapelotte M, Delalande S et al: Intravenous corticosteroids in the postpartum period for reduction in multiple sclerosis, *Mult Scler* 10(5):596-597, 2004.
31. Dwosh E, Guimond C, Duquette P et al: The interaction of MS and pregnancy: a critical review, *Int MS J* 10:38-42, 2003.
32. Flachenecker P, Hartung P: Multiple sclerosis and pregnancy: overview and status of the European multicenter PRIMS study, *Nervenarzt* 66:97-104, 1995.
33. Sadovnick AD, Eisen K, Hashimoto SA et al: Pregnancy and multiple sclerosis: a prospective study, *Arch Neurol* 51:1120-1124, 1994.
34. Achiron A, Kishner I, Dolev M et al: Effect of intravenous immunoglobulin treatment on pregnancy and postpartum-related relapses in multiple sclerosis, *J Neurol* 251(9):1133-1137, 2004.
35. Ferrero S, Pretta S, Nicoletti A et al: Myasthenia gravis: management issues during pregnancy, *Eur J Obstet Gynecol Reprod Biol* 121(2):129-138, 2005.
36. Westgren N, Hultling C, Levi R et al: Pregnancy and delivery in women with a traumatic spinal cord injury in Sweden, 1980-91, *Obstet Gynecol* 81:926-930, 1993.
37. Pereira L: Obstetric management of the patient with spinal cord injury, *Obstet Gynecol Surv* 58(10):678-687, 2003.
38. American College of Obstetrics and Gynecology: ACOG committee opinion. Obstetric management of patients with spinal cord injuries. Number 275, September 2002. Committee on Obstetric Practice. American College of Obstetrics and Gynecology, *Int J Gynaecol Obstet* 79(2):189-191, 2002.
39. Tang RA, Dorotheo EU, Schiffman JS et al: Medical and surgical management of idiopathic intracranial hypertension in pregnancy, *Curr Neurol Neurosci Rep* 4(5):398-409, 2004.
40. Lee AG, Pless M, Falardeau J et al: The use of acetazolamide in idiopathic intracranial hypertension during pregnancy, *Am J Opthalmol* 139(5):855-859, 2005.
41. Arpino C, Brescianini S, Robert E et al: Teratogenic effects of antiepileptic drugs: use of an International Database on Malformations and Drug Exposure (MADRE), *Epilepsia* 41(11):1436-1443, 2000.
42. Mawer G, Clayton-Smith J, Coyle H et al: Outcome of pregnancy in women attending an outpatient epilepsy clinic; adverse features associated with higher doses of sodium valproate, *Seizure* 11(8):512-518, 2002.
43. Samren EB, van Duijin CM, Koch S et al: Maternal use of antiepileptic drugs and the risk of major congenital malformations: a joint European prospective study of human teratogenesis associated with maternal epilepsy, *Epilepsia* 38:981-990, 1997.
44. Pennell PB, Newport DJ, Stowe ZN et al: The impact of pregnancy and childbirth on the metabolism of lamotrigine, *Neurology* 62(2):292-295, 2004.
45. Cunnington M, Tennis P: International Lamotrigine Pregnancy Registry Scientific Committee. Lamotrigine and the risk of malformations in pregnancy, *Neurology* 64(6):955-960, 2005.
46. Liporace J, Kao A, D'Abreu A: Concerns about lamotrigine and breastfeeding, *Epilepsy Behav* 5(1):102-105, 2004.
47. Montouris G: Gabapentin exposure in human pregnancy: results from the Gabapentin Pregnancy Registry, *Epilepsy Behav* 4(3):310-317, 2003.
48. Ohman I, Vitols S, Luef G et al: Topiramate kinetsics during delivery, lactation, and in the neonate: preliminary observations, *Epilepsia* 43(10):1157-1160, 2002.
49. Montouris G: Safety of the newer antiepileptic drug oxcarbazepine during pregnancy, *Curr Med Res Opin* 21(5):693-701, 2005.

SECTION H Renal Disease

Ellen L. Sakornbut, MD

I. EFFECTS OF CHRONIC RENAL FAILURE ON PREGNANCY OUTCOME

First-trimester serum creatinine values up to 0.8 mg/dl are accepted as normal in pregnancy. Values between 0.8 and 1.4 mg/dl are considered as mildly impaired, with a serum creatinine greater than or equal to 1.4 mg/dl classified as moderately impaired. Renal function should be monitored serially in all women with renal disease in pregnancy.

Patients with chronic renal disease but normal or mildly decreased function usually have good pregnancy outcomes. Most experts agree that pregnancy should be avoided in patients with a baseline creatinine level greater than 2.0 mg/dl. The incidence of maternal and fetal complications, including preeclampsia, IUGR, and abruption, is significantly increased in patients with a creatinine level of 3.0 mg/dl or more. Most patients with severe untreated renal insufficiency are infertile.

II. END-STAGE RENAL DISEASE

A. Dialysis

Fertility is markedly reduced in women with end-stage renal disease. However, the majority of women undergoing long-term dialysis are able to become pregnant. In these women, and in women started on dialysis after becoming pregnant, 50% to 70% are able to complete their pregnancy.[1,2] Greater rates of pregnancy complications, including prematurity, IUGR, hypertension, disorders of amniotic fluid volume, and second- and third-trimester losses, occur in these pregnancies.[3] Treatment protocols include increasing erythropoietin doses to maintain a hemoglobin level of 10 to 11 g, as well as an increase in dialysis frequency and volumes.

B. Transplant Recipients

Several large series of pregnancies in female transplant recipients have demonstrated live birth rates of greater than 70%. The incidence of hypertension, both preexisting and new onset, is between 19% to 50% in these women, with increased complications that include urinary tract infections in 13% to 17%, graft dysfunction in up to 30%, and reversible or permanent graft rejection in approximately 10%. The cesarean delivery rate is high, as much as 60% to 70% in some series, but this may reflect management that is predicated on very high risk. Preterm labor and preterm birth are also common, between 40% and 60%, and IUGR occurs in about 20% of births.[4-8]

There does not appear to be a significant risk for congenital anomalies in women treated with prednisone, azathioprine, cyclosporine, or tacrolimus.[9] Little evidence is available about newer immunosuppressant medications used in transplantation. Recommendations from available studies include delay of pregnancy until patients are stable at approximately 2 years after transplant. Transplant recipients are also at risk for intrauterine infections with cytomegalovirus, toxoplasmosis, and herpes simplex.[10]

III. CHRONIC RENAL CONDITIONS

Because women of childbearing age with chronic renal disease may be taking ACE inhibitors, the clinician should be mindful of potential pregnancy in these women and discontinue use before conception, or as soon as pregnancy is diagnosed.

A. Chronic Pyelonephritis

More than one in four women with a history of vesicoureteric reflux and surgical correction have recurrent infection in pregnancy and should be monitored closely.[11] Patients may benefit from antibiotic suppressive therapy. Outcomes are better if renal function is well preserved and BP remains within normal range. Two large case series of younger adults followed for reflux nephropathy examined outcomes in nearly 300 pregnancies.[12,13] The incidence of preeclampsia was 14% in normotensive women but increased to 42% in women with preexisting hypertension, together with an increase in preterm birth. Women with mild-to-moderate renal impairment were also at increased risk for deterioration of renal function.

B. Nephrotic Syndrome

Albumin levels are normally 1 g lower in pregnancy; therefore, a diagnosis of nephrotic syndrome cannot be made using this as a criterion. Pregnancy prognosis depends on the cause of nephrotic syndrome and the presence or absence of hypertension and renal function compromise. If renal function is normal, and the patient is not hypertensive, outcomes are generally good. The patient may become significantly edematous; diuretics should not be used because intravascular volume is decreased.

C. Glomerulonephritis

Some types of glomerular disease are associated with a benign prognosis. Maternal and fetal outcomes are generally good in women with primary membranous glomerulonephritis, and repeated pregnancies do not cause deterioration of renal function.[14] Maternal and fetal outcomes also do not appear to be significantly different from the general population in women with thin basement membrane nephropathy (nonimmunoglobulin A mesangial proliferative nephropathy).[15] Outcomes are generally poorer if renal function is decreased or if hypertension is present. The incidence of preeclampsia is increased.

D. Diabetic Nephropathy

The effect of pregnancy on long-term renal function in women with diabetic nephropathy is debatable, with some studies finding no impact of pregnancy on creatinine clearance[16] and other series finding decreasing creatinine clearance after pregnancy among some women. This is possibly attributable to poor control of hypertension.[17] The incidence of preeclampsia is high. Prognosis is worse with concomitant hypertension (see Section I for a more detailed discussion of diabetes mellitus [DM]).

E. Lupus-Related Renal Disease

Although initially thought to be associated with increasing rates of renal dysfunction, a prospective study comparing pregnant and nonpregnant women with lupus nephritis did not demonstrate increased renal deterioration during pregnancy.[18] Class III to IV disease is associated with high rates of hypertensive complications, seen in more than one third of pregnancies.[19]

F. Permanent Urinary Diversion

Patients with permanent urinary diversion should be monitored for acute pyelonephritis or outflow obstruction in late pregnancy.

G. Polycystic Kidney Disease

There is a slight increase in preeclampsia in women with polycystic kidney disease. Genetic counseling is always indicated because adult polycystic kidney disease is an autosomal dominant disorder.

H. Single Kidney

Pyelonephritis was common in one series of women with a single kidney, but outcomes overall were good, with 78% of newborns born at term.[20]

I. Pelvic Kidney

Women with pelvic kidney may be more prone to infection. Some types of urinary tract anomalies such as pelvic kidney may interfere with fetal descent.

REFERENCES

1. Moranne O, Samouelian V, Lapeyre F et al: Pregnancy and hemodialysis, *Nephrologie* 25(7):287-292, 2004.
2. Chao AS, Huang JY, Lien R et al: Pregnancy in women who undergo long-term hemodialysis, *Am J Obstet Gynecol* 187(1): 152-156, 2002.
3. Romaoo JE Jr, Luders C, Kahhale S et al: Pregnancy in women on chronic dialysis: a single center experience with 17 cases, *Nephron* 78:416-422, 1998.
4. Sivaraman P: Management of pregnancy in transplant recipients, *Transplant Proc* 36(7):1999-2000, 2004.
5. Ghanem ME, El-Baghdadi LA, Badawy AM et al: Pregnancy outcome after renal allograft transplantation: 15 years experience, *Eur J Obstet Gynecol Reprod Biol* 121(2):178-181.
6. Byrd L, Donnai P, Gokal R: Outcome of pregnancy following renal transplantation, *J Obstet Gynaecol* 20(1):15-18, 2000.
7. Al-Khader AA, Al-Ghamdi, Basri N et al: Pregnancies in renal transplant recipients—with a focus on the maternal issues, *Ann Transplant* 9(3):62-64, 2004.
8. Al-Khader AA, Basri N, Al-Ghamdi et al: Pregnancies in renal transplant recipients—with a focus on babies, *Ann Transplant* 9(3):65-67, 2004.
9. Kainz A, Harabacz I, Cowlrick IS et al: Review of the course and outcome of 100 pregnancies in 84 women treated with tacrolimus, *Transplantation* 70(12):1718-1721, 2000.
10. Hou S: Pregnancy in chronic renal insufficiency and end-stage renal disease, *Am J Kidney Dis* 33:235-245, 1999.
11. Mor Y, Leibovitch I, Zalts R et al: Analysis of the long-term outcome of surgically corrected vesico-ureteric reflux, *BJU Int* 92(1):97-100, 2003.
12. Kohler JR, Tencer J, Forsberg L et al: Long-term effects of reflux nephropathy on blood pressure and renal function in adults, *Nephron Clin Pract* 93(1):C35-C46, 2003.
13. North RA, Taylor RS, Gunn TR: Pregnancy outcome in women with reflux nephropathy and the inheritance of vesico-ureteric reflux, *Aust N Z J Obstet Gynaecol* 40(3):280-285, 2000.
14. Malik GH, Al-Harbi AS, Al-Mohaya S et al: Repeated pregnancies in patients with primary membranous glomerulonephritis, *Nephron* 91(1):21-24, 2002.
15. Packham D: Thin basement membrane nephropathy in pregnancy, *Semin Nephrol* 25(3):180-183, 2005.
16. Rossing K, Jacobsen P, Hommel E et al: Pregnancy and progression of diabetic nephropathy, *Diabetologia* 45(1):36-41, 2002.
17. Biesenbach G, Grafinger P, Stoger H et al: How pregnancy influences renal function in nephropathic type 1 diabetic women depends on their pre-conceptional creatinine clearance, *J Nephrol* 12(1):41-46, 1999.

18. Tandon A, Ibanez D, Gladman DD et al: The effect of pregnancy on lupus nephritis, *Arthritis Rheum* 50(12):3941-3946, 2004.
19. Carmona F, Font J, Moga I et al: Class III-IV proliferative lupus nephritis and pregnancy: a study of 42 cases, *Am J Reprod Immunol* 53(4):182-188, 2005.
20. Shektman MM, Petrova SB: Pregnancy and labor in females with solitary kidney, *Ter Arkh* 72(6):39-42, 2000.

SECTION I **Endocrine Conditions**

David Turok, MD, MPH, and Ted R. Schultz, MD

I. THYROID DISEASE IN PREGNANCY: INTRODUCTION

Although thyroid disease is prevalent among women of childbearing age and is the second most common endocrine disorder seen in pregnancy, the combined incidence of perinatal hypothyroidism and hyperthyroidism is less than 1%. Although markedly abnormal thyroid function is associated with infertility, less severe disease may affect pregnancy duration, course, and fetal/neonatal health. This section describes normal changes in thyroid function during pregnancy and the diagnosis and treatment of common thyroid disorders.

II. EPIDEMIOLOGY

The majority of abnormal serum thyroid function in pregnancy is subclinical and does not require treatment. In the largest study to date on thyroid dysfunction in pregnancy, overt hyperthyroidism was found in 3.6 of 1000 pregnant women screened before 20 weeks of gestation,[1] with Graves' disease accounting for 90% to 95% of all cases. The rate for subclinical hyperthyroidism was 17 in 1000. The rates were 1.8 in 1000 for overt hypothyroidism and 23 in 1000 for subclinical disease.[2]

III. MATERNAL AND FETAL THYROID PHYSIOLOGY

Pregnancy is associated with a mild, sometimes palpable enlargement of the thyroid gland. Some thyroid function tests are predictably altered by physiologic changes associated with pregnancy (Table 8-11). Thyroxine-binding globulin (TBG) increases are driven by an increase in estrogen levels. Total T_4 and triiodothyronine (T_3) values are also increased, but free L-thyroxine (FT_4) and T_3 values remain in the normal range because of increased TBG. Serum levels of thyroid-releasing hormone (TRH) and TSH remain normal during pregnancy. TSH and FT_4 are the preferred markers of disease and treatment. Subclinical hyperthyroidism is characterized by a depressed thyroid-stimulating hormone (TSH) level and a normal FT_4 value, whereas in subclinical hypothyroidism there is an increased TSH and a normal FT_4 value.

Because human chorionic gonadotrophin (hCG) and TSH share a common α subunit, the first-trimester hCG peak causes an increase in thyroid hormone activity and a resultant increase in FT_4 values, though this increase remains within the normal nonpregnant range.[3] Increased FT_4 causes a compensatory depression of TSH levels, which are also within laboratory norms.[4-6] Iodide levels in the maternal circulation decrease throughout pregnancy because of fetal use of iodide and increased maternal GFR, which increases iodide excretion.[7]

Normal fetal development is dependent on maternal euthyroidism. Fetal thyroid hormone production does not start until the end of the first trimester, and then increases steadily through the second and

TABLE 8-11 Changes in Thyroid Function with Pregnancy and Thyroid Disease

Maternal Status	Thyroid-Stimulating Hormone	L-Thyroxine (FT₄)	Thyroxine-Binding Globulin	Total T₄
Normal pregnancy	No change	No change	Increased	Increased
Hyperthyroidism	Decreased	Increased	No change	Increased
Hypothyroidism	Increased	Decreased	No change	Decreased

third trimesters, reaching normal adult levels by term.[8] TSH does not cross the placenta, whereas small quantities of T_4 and T_3 do. The presence of some T_4 and T_3 in the fetal circulation at birth can prevent signs and symptoms of overt neonatal hypothyroidism. Over time, however, the maternal hormone disappears; this is the basis for repeat testing of neonatal thyroid function in state screening programs in the United States.

IV. DIAGNOSIS AND TREATMENT

A. Preconception Care and Risk Assessment

Women usually require a euthyroid state to conceive. Infertility is common in clinically hypothyroid patients with anovulatory cycles. Treatment of hypothyroidism reverses this problem, and it is important to ensure patients have clear reproductive or contraceptive plans when initiating treatment for hypothyroidism. Preconception or early prenatal patients should have a TSH checked if they have a personal history of thyroid disorders, prior treatment for thyroid disease, medications that may affect thyroid function, prior or current use of iodine- or lithium-containing products, or head and neck radiation.

B. General Screening for Maternal Subclinical Hypothyroidism

Universal screening for hypothyroidism was advocated by two studies in 1999 that associated hypothyroidism during pregnancy with lower IQ scores in children up to 9 years old.[9,10] These studies were observational, and although they support an association of subclinical maternal hypothyroidism with lower performance in childhood neuropsychologic testing, they did not test any intervention. Thus, universal screening with thyroid function tests during pregnancy is not recommended, but rather should be based on history of thyroid disease, symptoms, and physical findings.[11,12]

C. Hyperthyroidism in Pregnancy

1. Clinical features and laboratory evaluation
   Many of the signs and symptoms of hyperthyroidism can also be found in normal pregnancy. Anxiety, increased appetite, fatigue, heat intolerance, tremor, emotional lability, tachycardia, and thyroid enlargement are common to both conditions.

However, unanticipated weight loss, as well as the exophthalmos and pretibial myxedema of hyperthyroidism, are uncommon in normal pregnancy. Hyperthyroidism is diagnosed by a decrease in serum TSH and an increase in free T_4 values. Although Graves' disease is caused by hyperstimulation of the TSH receptor by thyroid-stimulating immunoglobulin and TSH binding inhibitory immunoglobulin, these do not need to be routinely checked.[12] Other causes of hyperthyroidism in pregnancy include central excess production of TSH, gestational trophoblastic disease (i.e., hydatidiform mole and choriocarcinoma), toxic multinodular goiter, and subacute thyroiditis. Hyperemesis gravidarum can create a biochemical hyperthyroidism in 66% of patients, but these resolve without treatment by 18 weeks of gestation.[13]

2. Treatment
   Hyperthyroidism in pregnancy is associated with increased risk for preterm delivery, severe preeclampsia, LBW, maternal heart failure, and fetal death.[14,15] Improved outcomes have been documented with preconceptive treatment, as compared with initiating therapy during pregnancy.[16] As such, every effort should be made to provide definitive treatment before pregnancy and to ensure effective contraception for the patient until her medical condition is stabilized.[17,18]
   The most common treatment for Graves' disease in the United States is radioiodine ablation. It is recommended that women avoid pregnancy for 4 months after treatment to avoid ablation of the fetal thyroid.[19] Fetuses that are inadvertently exposed to I^{131} beyond 10 to 12 weeks of gestation are at high risk for induced congenital hypothyroidism. Because of the poor outcome associated with this, termination of pregnancy is recommended.
   The thioamides propylthiouracil (PTU) and methimazole are the treatment of choice for sustained hyperthyroidism during pregnancy. Both of these drugs block organification of iodide, but PTU has been preferred for use in pregnancy because it also blocks peripheral conversion of T_4 to T_3. In addition, there were early associations between methimazole use in pregnancy and fetal aplasia cutis (a reversible scalp defect), as well as a belief that methimazole crosses the placenta more readily than PTU. Recent studies have refuted both of these claims,[20-22] and it may be time to consider the advantages of once daily dosing with methimazole.

Both of these drugs are safe for breastfeeding, although PTU is present in lower quantities in breast milk. Side effects of these medications include agranulocytosis, hepatitis, thrombocytopenia, rash, nausea, fever, and arthritis.

The goal of thioamide therapy is to maintain FT_4 in the high normal range at the lowest possible dose to minimize fetal exposure to medication, thus reducing fetal risk for hypothyroidism. PTU can be initiated at 300 to 450 mg/day in divided doses and tapered to 100 to 200 mg/day as the patient's symptoms improve and her FT_4 level comes into the high normal range. The corresponding doses for methimazole are 30 to 40 mg/day at initiation and 5 to 15 mg at maintenance. One third of patients improve sufficiently so that the medications may be discontinued in the third trimester.[18] FT_4 should be monitored every 2 to 4 weeks after initiation of therapy.

β-Blockers may be used on a short-term basis for control of symptoms. A goal of therapy is maternal heart rate less than 90 beats/min. Long-term administration of β-blockers in pregnancy has been associated with growth restriction and poor fetal outcome, but most of these studies are difficult to interpret because of methodologic problems and the confounding influence of the disease state treated.[23] In cases of thyrotoxicosis when medical management has failed, a total or subtotal thyroidectomy should be considered.

One percent of pregnancies affected by hyperthyroidism are complicated by thyroid storm.[14] The diagnosis is made in a hyperthyroid patient with fever, tachycardia, mental status changes, vomiting, diarrhea, and cardiac arrhythmia. This condition is frequently triggered by labor, delivery, surgery, or infection. This is a medical emergency that requires a precise coordinated plan of several medications, each of which has a specific role in suppressing thyroid function. These include PTU to block thyroid hormone synthesis and inhibit peripheral conversion of T_4 to T_3, potassium iodide and dexamethasone to prevent expulsion of hormone from the thyroid gland, propranolol to prevent the adrenergic effects of excess thyroid hormone, and phenobarbital to reduce agitation.[24]

3. Fetal and neonatal concerns
   When a pregnancy is complicated by thyrotoxicosis and requires administration of the accompanying medications, the fetus is at risk for hyperthyroidism or hypothyroidism. Fetal hyperthyroidism may be characterized by fetal tachycardia (>160 beats/min), IUGR, and craniosynostosis.[25] A pregnant woman with active Graves' disease, or one who has been treated previously with radioablative or surgical therapy, will have active thyroid-stimulating immunoglobulin (TSI) and thyroid-stimulating hormone-binding inhibitory immunoglobulin (TBII) that cross the placenta. These antibodies can stimulate or inhibit the fetal thyroid.[26] Clinically significant fetal or neonatal disease is rare because of a balance between the stimulatory effects of the antibodies and inhibitory effects of the medication. Ironically, neonates of mothers previously treated with ablative thyroid therapy and not currently taking antithyroid medication are at greater risk for neonatal Graves' disease because of the lack of suppression from maternal medication.[27] Careful surveillance of fetal growth is helpful in pregnancies with current or previously treated hyperthyroidism. Fetal growth anomalies in the setting of hyperthyroidism will likely benefit from tertiary medical care.

When maternal hyperthyroidism is controlled by thioamides, neonatal hyperthyroidism may not be present at birth. Falling maternal immunoglobulins and decreasing thioamide levels can lead to symptoms such as mild irritability, tachycardia, poor feeding, goiter, heart failure, jaundice, exophthalmos, and thrombocytopenia.[16] Cord blood and neonatal serum for free T_4 and TSH should be used for diagnostic thyroid evaluation on the first or second day of life.

D. Hypothyroidism in Pregnancy

1. Clinical features and laboratory evaluation
   Hypothyroidism is caused by inadequate production of thyroid hormone. Classic symptoms include modest weight gain, fatigue, cold intolerance, hair loss, dry skin, and constipation. The size of the thyroid gland ranges from enlarged to undetectable. Making the diagnosis is imperative because of its complications. Preeclampsia, anemia, placental abruption, spontaneous abortion, and preterm delivery (mostly for induction caused by hypertensive disease in pregnancy) are all seen at an increased frequency.[28-30] The most dramatic and concerning adverse effect of uncontrolled maternal hypothyroidism is congenital hypothyroidism in neonates, which can result in neurologic and cognitive impairments.

Iodine replacement in iodine-deficient women before the third trimester reduces the incidence of moderate-to-severe neurologic abnormalities in their offspring from 9% to 2% ($p < 0.008$).[31] The diagnosis of hypothyroidism is made in symptomatic women when the serum TSH level is increased and free T_4 value is decreased. In subclinical hypothyroidism, TSH level is increased with a normal free T_4 value. The most common cause of hypothyroidism in pregnancy is chronic autoimmune thyroiditis, or Hashimoto disease. Autoantibodies to thyroglobulin and antimicrosomal antibodies can be measured. These autoantibodies can cross the placenta and cause hypothyroidism in the neonate.[18] Chronic autoimmune thyroiditis is common in women with insulin-dependent diabetes, occurring in 20% of patients with class D and F disease.[32]

Other causes of hypothyroidism in pregnancy include postthyroid ablation or surgical excision, primary atrophic hypothyroidism, central hypothyroidism (TRH or TSH deficiency), and infiltrative disease. Drugs associated with hypothyroidism include carbamazepine, phenytoin, lithium, iodides, and thioamides. A causal association exists between lithium and iodides with hypothyroidism. An unusual cause of maternal and fetal hypothyroidism in the United States is iodine deficiency with subsequent goiter. However, globally, this is the most common cause of maternal and neonatal hypothyroidism.

2. Treatment
Women with preexisting hypothyroidism may require up to a 50% increase in dosage of levothyroxine during pregnancy.[33] A recent prospective study examined levothyroxine dosing to maintain normal levels of TSH in 20 hypothyroid women.[34] The study found that levothyroxine dose increased by 29% by 10 weeks of gestation and 48% by 20 weeks. This led the authors to recommended close monitoring and a 30% increase in levothyroxine dose when pregnancy is confirmed. No studies have found improved clinical outcomes. Initiation of therapy in a newly diagnosed patient may be started at an average dosage of 0.10 to 0.15 mg/day levothyroxine. TSH levels need to be monitored every 4 to 6 weeks, and dosages adjusted accordingly. If a previous diagnosis of hypothyroidism is in doubt and the patient is receiving replacement therapy, medication should be continued. A therapeutic trial off thyroid replacement medication should not be attempted during pregnancy.

3. Fetal and neonatal concerns
Fetal hypothyroidism is associated with craniosynostosis, cardiomegaly, and prematurity. It may occur as a result of inadvertent I^{131} administration before the diagnosis of pregnancy or due to maternal PTU therapy because PTU crosses the placenta. Fetal hypothyroidism has been established in utero with percutaneous umbilical vein sampling and treated with intraamniotic instillation of L-thyroxine.

Neonatal hypothyroidism may present as a prolonged gestation, fetal macrosomia, feeding and respiratory difficulties, constipation, abdominal distension, vomiting, and prolonged jaundice. Other features are a large posterior fontanelle caused by delayed bony maturation; coarse, dry skin; hypothermia; and umbilical hernia. Although routine neonatal screening occurs in most states, in an infant with suspicious findings or in situations of known increased risk, the initial diagnosis should not await the results of routine screening. T_4 values less than 4 μg/100 ml and TSH values greater than 80 μU/100 ml are diagnostic. T_4 values of 4 to 7 μg/100 ml and TSH values of 20 to 80 μU/100 ml are borderline and require further evaluation.

E. Thyroid Masses

Slight enlargement of the thyroid is common in pregnancy. The enlarged gland should be soft and homogeneous in texture and nontender to palpation. Unless symptoms of thyroid disease are present, this clinical finding does not require thyroid hormone testing. Women with a thyroid mass, in contrast, should have thyroid function testing, an ultrasound scan of the thyroid, and fine-needle aspiration biopsy. Radionucleotide scanning is contraindicated in pregnancy. Pregnancy does not appear to affect the course of papillary thyroid cancer. Patients can have surgical management in either the second trimester or after delivery with no difference in outcome.[35]

V. DIABETES: INTRODUCTION

The epidemiology of diabetes in pregnancy has changed. Previously, type 1 diabetes mellitus (DM) was more recognized in pregnancy. However, with the national epidemic of obesity, type 2 DM is more prevalent. This is particularly true in immigrant and low-income communities commonly cared for by family physicians. DM is one of the most important and prevalent chronic diseases in women of childbearing age, and it can be associated with significant morbidity if not managed carefully. Although new insulin preparations, the insulin pump, and self-monitoring of blood glucose have revolutionized the care of pregnant women with diabetes, these pregnancies are still associated with significant risks. Thus, it is critical that every office visit with diabetic women of childbearing age should include a clear plan for contraception or preconceptional planning. This chapter focuses on guidelines for management of pregnancies in women with preexisting type 1 and type 2 DM. Few well-designed clinical trials exist on the subject; thus, many of the recommendations are based on expert opinion and observational studies.

VI. EPIDEMIOLOGY

Millions of American women younger than 45 years have diabetes, and more than 100,000 of these women have pregnancies affected by diabetes annually, accounting for 2% to 3% of all live births.[36] Ninety percent of these are due to gestational DM (see Chapter 7, Section A). Yet, approximately 10,000 pregnant women each year have preexisting type 1 or type 2 DM.

VII. PATHOGENESIS

Maternal glucose metabolism changes dramatically during pregnancy to aid nutrient storage. These changes are marked by increasing insulin resistance, driven in large part by placental hormones human placental lactogen, progesterone, prolactin, and cortisol. The pathophysiology of diabetes in pregnancy was understood 50 years ago.[37] Whereas glucose crosses the placenta, insulin does not. During pregnancy, increased maternal serum glucose concentrations cause resultant increases in fetal glucose. Greater fetal glucose concentrations cause fetal hyperinsulinemia. Insulin is a critical growth hormone, and the most insulin-sensitive tissues are fat and muscle. Fetuses of mothers with poorly controlled DM are large, and the increased mass is concentrated around the shoulders and chest, creating a large shoulder-to-head ratio.[38] This focal increased mass drives the increased rate of shoulder dystocia, the most feared intrapartum complication for mothers with diabetes.

Fetuses whose mothers have type 1 or type 2 DM are also at increased risk for fetal death late in the third trimester.[39,40] One potential explanation of this is based on the association of fetal hyperglycemia and increased metabolic rate. To compensate for this increased demand, the fetus increases its red cell mass. This may lead to polycythemia and increased blood viscosity, which can result in underperfusion of vital organs, and possibly fetal death.[41] Women with preexisting type 1 and 2 DM also commonly have hypertension and microvascular disease, which can lead to poor placental function and increase the risk for fetal growth restriction.

VIII. CLINICAL FEATURES

Because pregnancy risks are great for patients with DM, contraceptive status should be reviewed at every office visit with diabetic women of childbearing age. There should be documentation of a clear plan for contraception or preconceptional planning.

A. Type 1 Diabetes

Before the discovery of insulin in 1922, the maternal mortality rate in diabetic pregnancies was more than 50%. These patients have increased risk for miscarriage, fetal malformations, preeclampsia, birth trauma, and progression of maternal retinopathy. Tight glycemic control from the preconception period through delivery has normalized the majority of these risks in women with type 1 DM. Preconception care is crucial for the well-being of these patients and their potential offspring, and it has been shown to be cost-effective.[42] It is best to develop a plan of care for women with type 1 DM before conception that involves all available resources, including nutrition/diabetes counselors, endocrinology, ophthalmology, and perinatology/obstetric backup or referral if available. Unfortunately, the majority of women with type 1 DM do not seek preconception counseling.[43] Approximately 60% have unplanned pregnancies.[44]

B. Type 2 Diabetes

Women with non–insulin-dependent, or type 2, DM are commonly encountered in practice. This condition is increasingly common for patients older than 30, especially in women whose family histories or ethnic backgrounds put them at increased risk. Screening for diabetes early in pregnancy for patients at high risk enhances the likelihood of diagnosing previously undetected type 2 DM. Data on the pregnancy outcomes of patients with preexisting type 2 DM have shown statistically significant increases in perinatal morality

(4.1-6.6%) and congenital malformations (3.4-6.7%) over the general population.[45-47] Management for this group has been based on studies conducted on patients with type 1 DM and a mixture of patients with type 1, type 2, and gestational diabetes.

IX. DIAGNOSIS

The American Diabetes Association (ADA) and the WHO revised diagnostic criteria for DM in 1997 to include the presence of a random venous plasma glucose concentration greater than 200 mg/dl in a symptomatic patient (polyuria, polydipsia, ketoacidosis), or a fasting plasma glucose concentration greater than 126 mg/dl on two different days. The older WHO definition of a 2-hour oral glucose tolerance test of more than 200 mg/dl after a 75-g glucose load is no longer recommended for routine clinical use.[48]

Pregnant women with diabetes historically have been categorized by the White classification system (Table 8-12).[49] First published in 1932, this system correlates pregnancy risk with the duration of diabetes and complications present at the onset of pregnancy, acknowledging the higher pregnancy risk associated with increasing vasculopathy. Our understanding of diabetes has evolved into a more simplified classification scheme that reflects current understanding (Table 8-13).[50]

X. ANTENATAL TREATMENT

A. Preconception Risk Assessment

The chances of successful pregnancy outcome are influenced by effective patient self-management and compliance, careful family planning, the presence or absence of vascular complications, and involvement from several members of the health-care team. Women should be counseled on the importance of achieving tight control of their diabetes before they become pregnant to reduce the risk for congenital anomalies related to hyperglycemia during the period of organogenesis.[51,52] Tight control is defined as maintaining euglycemia as measured by normal glycohemoglobin levels. Preconception and early pregnancy control of diabetes has been shown to reduce the incidence of anomalies to the same rate seen in the general population.[53]

Patients with type 1 and type 2 DM without vascular complications require intensive supervision, education, and good control to maximize their chances for successful pregnancies. Patients with vascular disease are at significant risk for both maternal and fetal complications and should have specialty consultation before becoming pregnant. Women with diabetes with coexisting coronary artery disease are at high maternal risk and should not become pregnant or strongly consider pregnancy termination if they do become pregnant.

TABLE 8-13 Classification of Pregestational Diabetes

1. Type 1 diabetes
   a. Uncomplicated
   b. Complicated (presence of hypertension, retinopathy, nephropathy, or cardiovascular disease)
2. Type 2 diabetes
   a. Uncomplicated
   b. Complicated

TABLE 8-12 White Classification for Diabetes in Pregnancy

Class A1, A2	Gestational diabetes
Class B	Onset of disease after age 20, no vascular complications
Class C	Onset between ages 10 and 19 or duration 10 to 19 years, no vascular complications
Class D	Onset of disease before age 10 or greater than 20 years' duration, and those with benign retinopathy including microaneurysms, exudates, or venous dilatation
Class F	Patients with renal disease who have impaired creatinine clearance or proteinuria of at least 400 mg/24 hours, measured in the first trimester
Class R	Patients with proliferative retinopathy
Class T	Patients who have undergone renal transplant
Class H	Patients with diabetes and coronary artery disease

B. Fetal Considerations

Congenital anomalies are the leading cause of perinatal mortality in diabetes. The relative risk of congenital anomalies ranges from 2.0 to 7.9 compared with the rate in the nondiabetic population.[17,54-56] The most common anomalies are cardiac defects, neural tube defects (especially anencephaly), hemivertebrae, caudal regression, and renal anomalies.[57,58] MSAFP levels may be up to 60% less in diabetics than in nondiabetic women with pregnancies of the same gestational age. Therefore, thresholds for detection of neural tube defects must be set lower for patients with diabetes.

In the third trimester, fetal complications revolve around the risk for abnormal fetal growth. Macrosomia is found in all classes of diabetics where hyperglycemia exists. The relative risk for shoulder dystocia for babies born to mothers with diabetes is 5.2, an effect that is compounded by increasing neonatal weight. Despite the increased risk for shoulder dystocia, the rate of birth trauma in these infants is not significantly different than normal control infants (3.4% vs. 2.5%).[59] Conversely, the incidence of LBW infants is also increased in pregnancies of women with diabetes because of greater rates of growth restriction, preterm delivery, and preeclampsia.

C. Maternal Considerations

In addition to its relation to fetal outcomes, of concern in pregnant women with diabetes is how pregnancy impacts the disease progression. Among the most common diabetic complications, nephropathy, retinopathy, and hypertension are of greatest concern in pregnancy.

1. Nephropathy

   In normotensive mothers with nephropathy but normal creatinine clearance, generally good fetal outcomes are expected. Irreversible worsening of renal function is rare in pregnancy. The exception to this is in women with serum creatinine levels greater than 1.5 mg/dl or baseline 24-hour urine protein totals of more than 3 g.[60] In a study of 11 women with moderate-to-severe renal disease, 5 patients were believed to have an accelerated course to dialysis caused by worsening renal function during pregnancy.[61] In this same study, women with existing diabetic nephropathy had a significantly greater risk for preeclampsia, placental insufficiency, and preterm delivery. Renal function should be assessed early in pregnancy with a BUN, serum creatinine, and a 24-hour urine collection for protein with creatinine clearance. This should be repeated in each trimester. This information can also be helpful in distinguishing preeclampsia from chronic hypertension in the third trimester.

   Because of the increased risk for preeclampsia, women with diabetes with hypertension, renal compromise, or other risk factors for pregnancy-induced hypertension should have serum uric acid, serum creatinine, urine protein levels, and creatinine clearance monitored. Low-dose daily aspirin therapy and calcium supplementation, which showed promise in early clinical trials, have not been shown to prevent preeclampsia for patients at high risk in large, multicenter, randomized trials.[62,63]

2. Retinopathy

   Women with diabetes should have a retinal examination early in pregnancy. Controversy exists regarding the impact of pregnancy on diabetic retinopathy. Because of reports of worsening retinopathy in pregnancy,[64] the examination should be repeated in pregnancy only if retinopathy is detected on the initial examination. Laser photocoagulation is the treatment of choice for diabetic retinopathy and could be safely performed, if needed, in pregnancy.

3. Hypertension

   Five to 10% of pregnant women with diabetes have concomitant chronic hypertension, and all are at increased risk for preeclampsia. Those with preexisting hypertension and nephropathy represent a group with particularly high risk for preeclampsia, uteroplacental insufficiency, and stillbirth. Patients may continue antihypertensive medications throughout pregnancy, with the exception that ACE inhibitors or angiotensin II receptor blockers are to be avoided.

D. Antepartum Care Guidelines

1. Disease monitoring

   Early in pregnancy, patients should undergo a dilated retinal examination and studies of renal function, including BUN, creatinine, and 24-hour urine collection for creatinine clearance and protein. Evaluation of glycemic control during periconception and organogenesis can be made with home glucose monitoring and following glycohemoglobin levels. If an early hemoglobin A1c is more than 8.5%, the patient should undergo fetal echocardiography at 18 to 20 weeks because of the increased risk for cardiac defects.[65] Septal defects, either ventricular or atrial, may be missed with this procedure, but this should not significantly affect management.

2. Pregnancy dating

Accurate dating of the pregnancy should be accomplished by clinical measures and ultrasonography. Follow-up ultrasound should be performed in the second trimester to screen for anomalies and in the early third trimester for evaluation of fetal growth. Although macrosomia may be an indicator of poor diabetic control, it can be found even in patients who have good control.[66] Polyhydramnios may be an indicator of poor control or the presence of a fetal anomaly.

E. Dietary Management

No single "diabetic" or "ADA" diet exists. A regular diet is crucial to maintain good glycemic control and should be based on formal nutritional assessment. A successful diet should be culturally appropriate and account for preexisting obesity, desired weight gain during pregnancy (13-18 kg for BMI < 20; 12-16 kg for BMI = 20-29; approximately 7 kg for BMI > 29), gestational age, physical activity level, coexisting renal disease, and lipid goals. A starting point is a diet consisting of 30 to 35 kcal/kg of ideal body weight divided into three meals and three snacks per day. If maternal weight is more than 120% of ideal, the caloric target should be 24 kcal/kg/day.[67] The diet composition should be high in fiber but limited in high glycemic carbohydrates (e.g., simple sugars). Caloric distribution should be 40% to 50% complex, high-fiber carbohydrates; 20% protein; and 30% to 40% fat, primarily from unsaturated sources.

F. Insulin Therapy: Goals and Management

A baseline hemoglobin A1c level is helpful in differentiating patients with good diabetes control (hemoglobin A1c level < 7.0 g/dl) and those who need tighter control. Home glucose monitoring is an essential step in assessing the adequacy of current treatment and modifying it to normalize blood glucose with the following targets: fasting <95 mg/dl (5.4 mmol/L), 1-hour postprandial values <140 mg/dl, 2-hour postprandial values <120 mg/dl (6.6 mmol/L), or preprandial values <100 mg/dl (5.6 mmol/L).[68] Blood sugar values in this range are associated with the fewest neonatal complications

and episodes of maternal hypoglycemia.[5,69] Tight control is advocated, as opposed to very tight control (all blood glucose levels < 5.6 mmol/L = 100 mg/dl), because very tight control has not been shown to result in improved outcomes but is associated with greater incidence of hypoglycemia, especially in the first trimester. The increased attention to 2-hour postprandial blood sugars is based on the Diabetes in Early Pregnancy Study, which showed that the incidence rate of macrosomia was 20% when these values were less than 120 mg/dl and 30% when they were greater.[70]

Blood sugars should be checked often enough to provide the patient and provider with adequate information to maintain euglycemia. The exact frequency necessary to do this is unclear from the literature. A common practice is to check five times daily: fasting, 2-hour postprandial after each main meal, and at bedtime. In women with type 2 diabetes, the bedtime check can be omitted because it is unlikely to provide additional useful information. A large prospective study of more than 1000 women with gestational diabetes (both diet only and insulin controlled) in each arm showed that the group that monitored blood sugar seven times daily (the above schedule plus two preprandial checks) had fewer cesarean deliveries and neonatal intensive care unit admissions than a group that monitored four times daily.[71] No similar data are available for management of women with preexisting type 1 and 2 DM during pregnancy.

Human insulin remains the standard for treatment of pregnant patients with both type 1 and 2 DM. However, as newer insulin analogs such as insulin lispro (Humalog) and glargine (Lantus) offer increased convenience and enhanced compliance, providers have begun using them despite limited data documenting their safety.[72] Several small studies suggest that insulin lispro (Humalog) and insulin aspart (Novolog) are safe and more effective at controlling postprandial glucose variations than regular human insulin.[73,74] However, insulin lispro was not detected in the cord blood of any of four neonates whose mothers received continuous IV therapy during labor.[42]

Just as with glucose monitoring, there is no one best method for insulin administration in pregnancy. The standard approach is to divide total daily insulin use into Regular and NPH. Two thirds of the daily dose is given in the morning, 30 minutes before breakfast. Of this, two thirds is NPH and one third is standard Regular. Half of the remaining one third is given as Regular insulin before dinner and the other half as NPH insulin given at bedtime. One study composed of women with both type 1 and type 2 DM showed improved glycemic control with insulin administered four times daily as opposed to two times daily during pregnancy.[75] Because of the shorter half-life of insulin during pregnancy, it is convention to change the evening NPH dose to bedtime. This is done to avoid nocturnal hypoglycemia when the NPH effect would be peaking at 2:00 to 3:00 AM.

Using a nighttime dose of Ultralente and very-short-acting lispro (Humalog) before meals is becoming increasingly popular in the management of type 1 diabetes in pregnancy. Use of lispro (Humalog) allows patients to administer their insulin immediately before meals and avoid the postprandial hypoglycemia that occurs when Regular insulin is still working but the meal has already been absorbed. Humalog is pregnancy category B and is considered safe for use.[76] Another excellent option is the insulin pump. This continuous subcutaneous insulin infusion uses Humalog insulin at an adjustable basal rate and gives boluses at mealtimes. There are several reports of successful use of the pump in pregnancy, dating back to 1981.[77]

Insulin requirements change throughout pregnancy. Early in pregnancy, most patients require less insulin, and hypoglycemic reactions may be encountered more frequently. Insulin requirements increase with increasing levels of placental hormones at 14 to 16 weeks. Patients with type 1 DM are at risk for life-threatening ketoacidosis, which may be precipitated by infection or other stressors and represents a major hazard to both mother and fetus. It requires intensive inpatient treatment. Because of the increased infection risk associated with DM, a urine culture should be performed at least every trimester, and patients should immediately report any signs of viral or bacterial infection to their provider.

G. Oral Hypoglycemics and Pregnancy

The use of oral medications is extremely attractive and there is mounting evidence that the sulfonylurea glyburide may be used safely and effectively in pregnancies affected by gestational DM.[78-80] However, no studies have documented the use of glyburide in pregnant patients with preexisting type 2 DM. Although metformin has been used in the first trimester in patients with polycystic ovarian syndrome, no studies have evaluated its use in pregnant patients with type 2 DM or in the second or third trimesters of pregnancy. For now, insulin will remain the drug of choice for maintaining euglycemia in pregnancies complicated by preexisting diabetes.

H. Assessment of Fetal Well-Being

Third-trimester ultrasound is frequently performed to assess fetal growth and rule out IUGR. Antepartum testing should begin at 32 to 34 weeks for women with type 1 and 2 diabetes, and may consist of weekly or twice weekly nonstress tests, biophysical profiles (BPPs), or modified BPPs.[81,82] Patients with diabetes-related vascular disease have the greatest risk for abnormal antenatal testing necessitating early delivery.[83] Doppler flow studies have been demonstrated to improve perinatal outcomes in the presence of IUGR (see Chapter 11, Section B).

XI. INTRAPARTUM MANAGEMENT

The timing of delivery involves a balancing of the risks for fetal compromise and prematurity. In the patient with uncomplicated, well-controlled diabetes with reassuring antenatal testing, the pregnancy can continue until 39 to 40 weeks of gestation. If complications such as preeclampsia or IUGR are present, management should follow guidelines for those conditions. If delivery must occur so early that antenatal steroids are required, close glucose monitoring and increased insulin doses will be necessary for several days. Alternatively, an insulin drip may be used for managing these situations. In women with poorly controlled diabetes, an amniocentesis for fetal lung maturity is advised before considering delivery before 39 weeks.[68] This is based on a delay in the presence of markers of pulmonary maturity from amniotic fluid testing in women with diabetes.[84]

Induction of labor for suspected fetal macrosomia increases cesarean delivery rates without decreasing the risk for shoulder dystocia and resultant birth trauma.[85] Based on clinical factors and birth history, consideration should be given to cesarean delivery to prevent birth trauma only if estimated fetal weight exceeds 4500 g.[86]

Maintenance of euglycemia during labor is important to prevent neonatal hypoglycemia. Blood glucose should be checked hourly during active labor with a bedside monitor, and insulin drip titrated to

TABLE 8-14 Sample Intrapartum Insulin and Intravenous Fluid Drip

Blood Glucose	IV Insulin	IVF (125 ml/hr)
<120 mg/dl	0	D_5LR
120-140 mg/dl	1 unit/hr	D_5LR
141-180 mg/dl	1.5 units/hr	Normal saline
181-220 mg/dl	2.0 units/hr	Normal saline
>220 mg/dl	2.5 units/hr	Normal saline

IV, Intravenous; IVF, intravenous fluid; D_5LR, dextrose in 5% lactated Ringer solution.

achieve goal blood glucose values (Table 8-14).[87] The target range is 80 to 110 mg/dl. Patients with type 2 DM will likely require greater doses of insulin. However, in women who are fasting, little or no insulin may be required. The insulin drip can be stopped immediately after delivery.

XII. POSTPARTUM ISSUES

Insulin requirements decline sharply after delivery, and a standard approach is to cut insulin doses by half. Breastfeeding should be strongly encouraged for all of the usual benefits. In addition, it has also been shown to significantly decrease the future likelihood of type 2 diabetes in infants who were exclusively breastfed versus those exclusively bottle-fed (OR, 0.41).[88] For patients with type 2 DM who require continued treatment for optimal blood sugar control, insulin is the safest drug to use while breastfeeding.

Infants of mothers with diabetes need to be observed for hypoglycemia and are at increased risk for other neonatal complications, including hypocalcemia, hypomagnesemia, polycythemia, hyperbilirubinemia, renal vein thrombosis, and hypertrophic cardiomyopathy.

Family planning is a critical issue and should have been discussed during prenatal care. Options should focus on long-term contraceptive methods with high efficacy. For patients with vasculopathy or completed families, vasectomy or female sterilization are ideal choices. The intrauterine device is an excellent option for women who desire a long-term reversible contraceptive method and is safe for use in women with diabetes. Progestin-only methods (progestin-only pills and depo-medroxyprogesterone acetate [Depo-Provera]) are also acceptable for use in women with diabetes, whereas low-dose combined oral contraceptive pills may be considered in patients without vasculopathy.

XIII. SUMMARY

Diabetes presents many preconception and perinatal management challenges to the maternity care provider. With the current increase in rates of obesity and more aggressive screening for type 2 DM, more women will be identified preconceptually with DM. Family planning, preconceptual risk assessment/education, timing of pregnancy, tight blood sugar control, and antenatal assessment of potential pregnancy complications and fetal well-being are essential to achieving successful outcomes.

REFERENCES

1. Casey BM, Dashe JS, Wells CE et al: Subclinical hyperthyroidism and pregnancy outcomes, *Obstet Gynecol* 107:337-341, 2006.
2. Casey BM, Dashe JS, Wells CE et al: Subclinical hypothyroidism and pregnancy outcomes, *Obstet Gynecol* 105:239-245, 2005.
3. Ecker JL, Musci TJ: Treatment of thyroid disease in pregnancy, *Obstet Gynecol Clin North Am* 24:575-589, 1997.
4. Amir SM, Osanthonondh R, Berkowitz RW et al: Human chorionic gonadotropin and thyroid function in patients with hydatiform mole, *Am J Obstet Gynecol* 150:723-728, 1984.
5. Fantz CR, Fantz CR, Dagogo-Jack S et al: Thyroid function during pregnancy, *Clin Chem* 45:2250-2258, 1999.
6. Kimura M, Amino N, Tamaki H et al: Physiologic thyroid activation in normal early pregnancy is induced by circulating hCG, *Obstet Gynecol* 75:775-778, 1990.
7. Burrow GN, Fisher DA, Larsen PR: Maternal and fetal thyroid function, *N Engl J Med* 331:1072-1078, 1994.
8. Thorpe-Beeston JG, Nicolaides KH, Felton CV et al: Maturation of the secretion of thyroid hormone and thyroid-stimulating hormone in the fetus, *N Engl J Med* 324:532-536, 1991.
9. Haddow JE, Palomaki GE, Allan WC et al: Maternal thyroid deficiency during pregnancy and subsequent neuropsychological development of the child, *N Engl J Med* 341:549-555, 1999.
10. Pop VJ, Kuijpens JL, van Baar AL et al: Low maternal free thyroxine concentrations during early pregnancy are associated with impaired psychomotor development in infancy, *Clin Endocrinol (Oxf)* 50:149-155, 1999.
11. U.S. Preventive Task Force Guidelines: Screening for thyroid disease: recommendation statement, *Ann Intern Med* 140:125-127, 2004.
12. American College of Obstetricians and Gynecologists: ACOG practice bulletin. Clinical management guidelines for obstetrician-gynecologists. Number 37, August 2002. (Replaces Practice Bulletin Number 32, November 2001). Thyroid disease in pregnancy. *Obstet Gynecol* 100:387-396, 2002.

13. Goodwin TM, Montoro M, Mestman JH: Transient hyperthyroidism and hyperemesis gravidarum: clinical aspects, *Am J Obstet Gynecol* 167:648-652, 1992.

14. Davis LE, Lucas MJ, Hankins GD et al: Thyrotoxicosis complicating pregnancy, *Am J Obstet Gynecol* 160:63-70, 1989.

15. Millar LK, Wing DA, Leung AS et al: Low birth weight and preeclampsia in pregnancies complicated by hyperthyroidism, *Obstet Gynecol* 84:946-949, 1994.

16. Creasy RK, Resnik R, Iams J, editors: *Maternal-fetal medicine,* ed 5, Philadelphia, 2004, W.B. Saunders.

17. Cefalo RC: Thyroid disorders. In Cefalo RC, Moos MK, editors: *Preconceptional health promotion: a practical guide,* Rockville, MD, 1988, Aspen Publishers.

18. Hamburger JL: Diagnosis and management of grave's disease in pregnancy, *Thyroid* 2:219-225, 1992.

19. Gittoes NJ, Franklyn JA: Hyperthyroidism. Current treatment guidelines, *Drugs* 55:543-553, 1998.

20. Momotani N, Noh JY, Ishikawa N et al: Effects of propylthiouracil and methimazole on fetal thyroid status in mothers with Graves' hyperthyroidism, *J Clin Endocrinol Metab* 82:3633-3636, 1997.

21. Van Dijke CP, Heydendail RJ, De Kleine MJ: Methimazole, carbimazole and congenital skin defects, *Ann Intern Med* 106:60-61, 1987.

22. Wing DA, Millar LK, Koonings PP et al: A comparison of propylthiouracil versus methimazole in the treatment of hyperthyroidism in pregnancy, *Am J Obstet Gynecol* 170:90-95, 1994.

23. Rubin PC: Beta-blockers in pregnancy, *N Engl J Med* 305:1323-1326, 1981.

24. Burch HB, Wartofsky L: Life-threatening thyrotoxicosis. Thyroid storm, *Endocrinol Metab Clin North Am* 22(2):263-277, 1993.

25. Becks GP, Burrow G: Thyroid disease and pregnancy, *Med Clin North Am* 75:121-150, 1991.

26. McKenzie JM, Zakarija M: Fetal and neonatal hyperthyroidism and hypothyroidism due to maternal TSH receptor antibodies, *Thyroid* 2:155-163, 1992.

27. Laurber P, Nygaard B, Glinoer D et al: Guidelines for TSH-receptor antibody measurements in pregnancy: results of an evidence-based symposium organized by the European Thyroid Association, *Eur J Endocrinol* 139:584-586, 1998.

28. Davis LF, Leveno KJ, Cunningham FG: Hypothyroidism complicating pregnancy, *Obstet Gynecol* 72:108-112, 1988.

29. Leung AS, Millar LK, Koonings PP et al: Perinatal outcome in hypothyroid pregnancies, *Obstet Gynecol* 81:349-353, 1993.

30. Abalovich M, Gutierrez S, Alcaraz G et al: Overt and subclinical hypothyroidism complicating pregnancy, *Thyroid* 12:63-68, 2002.

31. Cao XY, Jiang XM, Dou ZH et al: Timing of vulnerability of the brain to iodine deficiency in endemic cretinism, *N Engl J Med* 331:1739-1744, 1994.

32. Soler NG, Nicholson H: Diabetes and thyroid disease during pregnancy, *Obstet Gynecol* 54:318-321, 1979.

33. Mandel SJ, Larsen PR, Seely EW et al: Increased need for thyroxine during pregnancy in women with primary hypothyroidism, *N Engl J Med* 323:91-96, 1990.

34. Alexander EK, Marqusee E, Lawrence J et al: Timing and magnitude of increases in levothyroxine requirements during pregnancy in women with hypothyroidism, *N Engl J Med* 351:241-249, 2004.

35. Nam KH, Yoon JH, Chang HS et al: Optimal timing of surgery in well-differentiated thyroid carcinoma detected during pregnancy, *J Surg Oncol* 91:199-203, 2005.

36. Ventura SJ, Martin JA, Curtin SC et al: Births: final data for 1998, *Natl Vital Stat Rep* 48(3):1-100, 2000.

37. Pedersen J: Weight and length at birth of infants of diabetic mothers, *Acta Endocrinol* 16:330-342, 1954.

38. Naeye R: Infants of diabetic mother: a quantitative, morphologic study, *Pediatrics* 35:980-988, 1965.

39. Lauenborg J, Mathiesen E, Ovesen P et al: Audit on stillbirths in women with pregestational type 1 diabetes, *Diabetes Care* 26:1385-1389, 2003.

40. Macintosh MC, Fleming KM, Bailey JA et al: Perinatal mortality and congenital anomalies in babies of women with type 1 or type 2 diabetes in England, Wales, and Northern Ireland: population based study, *BMJ* 333:177-180, 2006.

41. Eidelman A, Samueloff A: The pathophysiology of the fetus of the diabetic mother, *Semin Perinatol* 26:232-236, 2002.

42. Rosenn B, Miodovnik M, Combs CA et al: Preconception management of insulin-dependent diabetes: improvement of pregnancy outcome, *Obstet Gynecol* 77:846-849, 1991.

43. Janz NK, Herman WH, Becker MP et al: Diabetes and pregnancy. Factors associated with seeking pre-conception care, *Diabetes Care* 18:157-165, 1995.

44. Holing EV, Brown ZA, Beyer CS et al: Why don't women with diabetes plan their pregnancies? *Diabetes Care* 21:889-893, 1998.

45. Cundy T, Gamble G, Townend K et al: Perinatal mortality in type 2 diabetes mellitus, *Diabet Med* 17(1):33-39, 2000.

46. Clausen TD, Mathiesen E, Ekbom P et al: Poor pregnancy outcome in women with type 2 diabetes, *Diabetes Care* 28(2):323-328, 2005.

47. Boulot P, Chabbert-Buffet N, d'Ercole C et al: French multicentric survey of outcome of pregnancy in women with pregestational diabetes, *Diabetes Care* 26(11):2990-2993, 2003.

48. Expert Committee on the Diagnosis and Classification of Diabetes Mellitus, *Diabetes Care* 20:1183-1197, 1997.

49. White P: *Diabetes in childhood and adolescence,* Philadelphia, 1932, Lea & Febiger.

50. Metzger BE, Phelps RL, Dooley SL: The mother in pregnancies complicated by diabetes mellitus. In Porte D, Sherwin RS, Baron A, editors: *Ellenberg and Rifkin's diabetes mellitus,* New York, 2002, McGraw-Hill.

51. Miller E, Hare JW, Cloherty JP et al: Elevated maternal hemoglobin A1c in early pregnancy and major congenital anomalies in infants of diabetic mothers, *N Engl J Med* 304:1331-1334, 1981.

52. Molsted-Peterson L, Tygstrup I, Pedersen J: Congenital malformations in newborn infants of diabetic women, *Lancet* 1:1124-1126, 1964.

53. Fuhrman K, Reiher H, Semmler K et al: The effect of intensified conventional insulin therapy before and during pregnancy on malformation rate in offspring of diabetic mothers, *Exp Clin Endocrinol* 83:173-177, 1984.

54. Chung CS, Myrianthopoulos NC: Factors affecting risks of congenital malformations. II. Effect of maternal diabetes, *Birth Defects* 11:1-38, 1975.

55. Cousins L: Congenital anomalies among infants of diabetic mothers, *Am J Obstet Gynecol* 147:333-338, 1983.

56. Grix A: Malformations in infants of diabetic mothers, *Am J Med Genet* 13:131-137, 1982.

57. Milunsky A, Alpert A, Kitzmiller JL et al: Prenatal diagnosis of neural tube defects. VIII. The importance of serum alpha-fetoprotein screening in diabetic pregnant women, *Am J Obstet Gynecol* 142:1030-1032, 1982.

58. Mills JL, Baker L, Goldman AS: Malformations in infants of diabetic mothers occur before the seventh gestational week. Implications for treatment, *Diabetes* 28:292-293, 1979.

59. Mimouni F, Miodovnik M, Rosenn B et al: Birth trauma in insulin-dependent diabetic pregnancies, *Am J Perinatol* 9:205-208, 1992.

60. Purdy LP, Hantsch CE, Molitch ME et al: Effect of pregnancy on renal function in patients with moderate-to-severe diabetic renal insufficiency, *Diabetes Care* 19:1067-1074, 1996.

61. Khoury JC, Miodovnik M, LeMasters G, Sibai B: Pregnancy outcome and progression of diabetic nephropathy. What's next? *J Matern Fetal Neonatal Med* 11:238-244, 2002.

62. Caritis S, Sidai B, Hauth J et al: Low-dose aspirin to prevent pre-eclampsia in women at high risk, *N Engl J Med* 338:701, 1998.

63. Levine RJ, Hauth JC, Curet LB et al: Trial of calcium to prevent preeclampsia, *N Engl J Med* 337:69-76, 1997.

64. Rosenn B, Miodovnik M, Kranias G et al: Progression of diabetic retinopathy in pregnancy: association with hypertension in pregnancy, *Am J Obstet Gynecol* 166:1214-1218, 1992.

65. Shields LE, Gan EA, Murphy HF et al: The prognostic value of hemoglobin A1c in predicting fetal heart disease in diabetic pregnancies, *Obstet Gynecol* 81:954-957, 1993.

66. Miller E, Hare JW, Cloherty JP et al: Elevated maternal hemoglobin A1c in early pregnancy and major congenital anomalies in infants of diabetic mothers, *N Engl J Med* 304:1331-1334, 1981.

67. American Diabetes Association: Prepregnancy counseling and management of women with preexisting diabetes or previous gestational diabetes. *Medical management of pregnancy complicated by diabetes*, ed 3, Alexandria, VA, 2000, ADA.

68. ACOG Committee on Practice Bulletins: ACOG Practice Bulletin. Clinical management guidelines for obstetricians-gynecologists. Number 60, March 2005. Pregestational diabetes mellitus, *Obstet Gynecol* 105:675-685, 2005.

69. Farrag OM: Prospective study of 3 metabolic regimens in pregnant diabetics, *Aust N Z J Obstet Gynaecol* 27:6-9, 1987.

70. Jovanovic-Peterson L, Peterson CM, Red DG et al: Maternal postprandial glucose levels and infant birth weight: the diabetes in early pregnancy study, *Am J Obstet Gynecol* 164:103-111, 1991.

71. Langer O, Rodriguez DA, Xenakis EMJ et al: Intensified versus conventional management of gestational diabetes, *Am J Obstet Gynecol* 170:1036-1047, 1994.

72. Langer O: Management of gestational diabetes: pharmacologic treatment options and glycemic control, *Endocrinol Metab Clin North Am* 35:53-78, 2006.

73. Pettitt DJ, Ospina P, Kolaczynski JW et al: Comparison of an insulin analog, insulin aspart, and regular human insulin with no insulin in gestational diabetes mellitus, *Diabetes Care* 26:183-186, 2003.

74. Jovanovic L, Ilic S, Pettitt DJ et al: Metabolic and immunologic effects of insulin lispro in gestational diabetes, *Diabetes Care* 22:1422-1427, 1999.

75. Nachum Z, Ber-Shlono I, Weives E et al: Twice daily versus four times daily insulin dose regimens in pregnancy: randomized control trial, *Br Med J* 319:1223-1227, 1999.

76. Jovanovic L, Ilic S, Pettitt DJ et al: Metabolic immunologic effects of insulin lispro in gestational diabetes, *Diabetes Care* 22:1422-1427, 1999.

77. Potter JM, Reckless JPD, Cullen DR: The effect of continuous subcutaneous insulin infusion and conventional insulin regimens on 24-hour variations of blood glucose and intermediary metabolism in the third trimester of diabetic pregnancy, *Diabetologia* 21:534-539, 1981.

78. Langer O, Conway D, Berkus M et al: A comparison of glyburide and insulin in women with gestational diabetes mellitus, *N Engl J Med* 343:1134-1138, 2000.

79. Chmait R, Dinise T, Moore T: Prospective observational study to establish predictors of glyburide success in women with gestational diabetes mellitus, *J Perinatol* 24:617-622, 2004.

80. Kremer CJ, Duff P: Glyburide for the treatment of gestational diabetes, *Am J Obstet Gynecol* 190:1438-1439, 2004.

81. Golde SH, Montoro M, Good-Anderson B et al: The role of nonstress tests, fetal biophysical profile, and contraction stress tests in the outpatient management of insulin-requiring diabetic pregnancies, *Am J Obstet Gynecol* 148:269-273, 1984.

82. Diamond MP, Vaughn WK, Salyer SL et al: Antepartum fetal monitoring in insulin-dependent diabetic pregnancies, *Am J Obstet Gynecol* 153:528-533, 1985.

83. Landon MB, Langer O, Gabbe SG et al: Fetal surveillance in pregnancies complicated by insulin-dependent diabetes mellitus, *Am J Obstet Gynecol* 167:617-621, 1992.

84. Piper JM: Lung maturation in diabetes in pregnancy: if and when to test, *Semin Perinatol* 26:206-209, 2002.

85. Sanchez-Ramos L, Bernstein S, Kaunitz AM: Expectant management versus labor induction for suspected fetal macrosomia: a systematic review, *Obstet Gynecol* 100:997-1002, 2002.

86. Rouse DJ, Owen J, Goldenber RL et al: The effectiveness and costs of elective cesarean delivery for fetal macrosomia diagnosed by ultrasound, *JAMA* 276:1480-1486, 1996.

87. Caplan RH, Pagliara AS, Beguin EA et al. Constant intravenous insulin infusion during labor and delivery in diabetes mellitus, *Diabetes Care* 5:6-10, 1982.

88. Perez-Bravo F, Carrasco E, Gutierrez-Lopez MD et al: Genetic predisposition and environmental factors leading to the development of insulin-dependent diabetes mellitus in Chilean children, *J Mol Med* 74:105-109, 1996.

S E C T I O N   J   Autoimmune Conditions

Ellen L. Sakornbut, MD

Multiple conditions exist in which autoantibodies affect pregnancy outcome through transplacental passage, effects on the placenta, or changes in maternal physiology.

I. RHEUMATOID ARTHRITIS

A. Natural History in Pregnancy

The clinical course of rheumatoid arthritis is generally improved during pregnancy, with more than 70% experiencing improvement.[1] The reduction in disease activity is reflected in patient scoring on quality-of-life measurements[2] and by clinical scoring.[3] This may be due to changes in cytokines and cytokine inhibitors.[4] Other than rare cases of vasculitis, there do not appear to be any increased risks to the fetus for patients with rheumatoid arthritis.

B. Use of Medications

Although methotrexate is considered cytotoxic, inadvertent first-trimester exposure has not been associated with significant teratogenic risk.[5] It should be discontinued in the preconception period, or as soon as pregnancy is diagnosed. A case series of pregnancies with exposure to infliximab showed no increase in congenital abnormalities.[6] Plaquenil, cyclosporine, and sulfasalazine are discussed later in reference to lupus. Corticosteroids may be used for symptomatic reduction during flares. Nonsteroidal antiinflammatory agents should be used only with caution for symptom relief and should be stopped at least 8 weeks before anticipated delivery to prevent persistent fetal circulation, premature constriction of the ductus, impaired renal function in the fetus, or bleeding risks in the mother.[7]

C. Intrapartum Management

Patients with hip contractures may experience some need for modification of delivery practices. A lateral Sims' position may be more comfortable.

II. SYSTEMIC LUPUS ERYTHEMATOSUS

A. Natural History in Pregnancy

The natural history of lupus in pregnancy is variable. Patients with quiescent disease at the time of conception often do well. Conflicting information exists about the tendency for lupus to flare during pregnancy.[7,8] Although concern exists that pregnancy was associated with progression of renal disease, prospective, case–control studies do not support this conclusion.[9]

Patients who score high on disease activity are more likely to experience pregnancy loss and poor outcome. A case series of patients found that only 25% of patients with high disease activity scores experience term birth compared with approximately 60% when disease activity is low. The rate of miscarriage and perinatal loss is significantly increased in patients with high disease activity.[10]

Preeclampsia is extremely common in women with nephropathy as compared with those without nephropathy. Patients with active nephritis remain at greater risk for poor pregnancy outcome than those with quiescent nephritis.[11] Risk factors associated with greater risk for premature birth include a flare during pregnancy and preexisting hypertension. Thrombocytopenia is also a risk factor for the development of preeclampsia.[12]

B. Use of Medications

1. Steroids

   In general, autoimmune conditions that necessitate corticosteroid therapy are best treated with prednisone or hydrocortisone because they are oxidized to relatively inactive forms by the placenta. Consideration of steroid therapy should be based on maternal indications and may be influenced by the desirable effect on the fetus of stabilizing the maternal condition. High-dose steroids should be avoided in the first trimester because of the risk for oral clefts but can be used in the second and third trimester if necessary. Patients who are receiving long-term steroid therapy require stress doses of corticosteroids for infection, labor and birth, and surgical procedures. Fetal adrenal suppression is extremely rare in women treated with steroids.

2. Other medications

   Because lupus flares during pregnancy increase the risk for premature birth, women who are controlled on medication should be considered for continuance of medication during pregnancy to prevent an acute flare. Like many other medications, no RCTs have established the safety of hydroxychloroquine in pregnancy. A large database following cases treated during pregnancy has not found an increase in adverse effects such as teratogenicity or other adverse outcomes.[13] Audiologic evaluation of newborns exposed to hydroxychloroquine does not demonstrate ototoxicity.[14] Sulfasalazine, cyclosporine, and azathioprine may also be used if required for disease control. Little information is available about mycophenolate, mofetil, and tumor necrosis factor inhibitors such as etanercept, infliximab, and adalimumab. Cytotoxic drugs, such as methotrexate and cyclophosphamide, should not be used.[15]

C. Neonatal Lupus

Neonatal lupus may occur as a complication in patients who produce anti-SSA (Ro) and anti-SSB/La antibodies. The neonate may demonstrate typical skin lesions, hemolytic anemia, and thrombocytopenia.

The most serious manifestation of neonatal lupus is congenital complete heart block (CHB), caused by fibrosis and inflammation of the cardiac conduction system. Although the anti-SSA or anti-SSB antibodies, or both, are present in more than 85% of women whose infants experience development of CHB, only 2% of women with these antibodies will deliver an affected child, making it likely that specific fetal factors must also be present for the condition to develop. The pathway probably involves apoptosis of cardiocytes, surface translocation of Ro and La antigens, binding of maternal autoantibodies, secretion of tumor growth factor-β from the scavenging macrophages, and modulation of cardiac fibroblasts to a type that causes scarring of the conduction pathways.[16,17]

The dermatologic and hematologic manifestations of neonatal lupus resolve within 6 months, suggesting mediation by maternal antibodies. Most cases of CHB are diagnosed soon after birth, but late-onset cardiac manifestations are possible. Many infants affected by CHB require permanent cardiac pacing. If CHB affects the fetus sufficiently, fetal hydrops and intrauterine demise may result. Maternal steroid therapy has not been demonstrated to prevent or reverse congenital CHB.[18] Although steroid use is relatively low risk in pregnancy, risks associated with systemic steroids do not appear justified on the basis of anti-SSA and SSB antibodies alone. Currently, no clinical trials have demonstrated any benefit to other types of immunoregulation.

III. ANTI-PHOSPHOLIPID ANTIBODY SYNDROME

APS refers to a group of patients who experience arterial and/or venous thromboses and recurrent pregnancy loss due to producing IgG antibodies toward phospholipids. Complications seen during pregnancy include placental infarction, IUGR, miscarriage, thrombocytopenia, preeclampsia-eclampsia, and hemolytic anemia. Multiple antibodies appear to be of relevance, including anticardiolipin (aCL) antibodies, and those directed against phospholipid-binding proteins such as β_2-glycoprotein I (anti–β_2-GBI), antiprothrombin (aPT), and annexin V (anti-Anx V).[19] Antibodies toward annexin V are found more frequently in women who experienced recurrent pregnancy loss, whereas the greatest risk for thrombosis is found in patients with antiprothrombin.[19,20] In addition, lupus anticoagulant appears to be a clear-cut marker for increased risk for thrombosis.[21]

Approximately 85% of women with APS have primary APS and do not experience development of systemic lupus. In a longitudinal study of women with APS, the presence of Coombs positivity had statistical significance (OR, 66.4; 95% CI, 1.6-2714; $p = 0.027$) for the development of systemic lupus erythematosus (SLE).[22] Conversely, 10% to 30% of patients with SLE are at increased risk for fetal loss, preeclampsia, and IUGR as a result of APS.

1. Screening for APS

   Given that the prevalence of APLAs in pregnant women appears to be approximately 5%, the utility of screening for APS in a general population has been debated.[23] aCL antibodies are found in 10% to 20% of women with recurrent pregnancy loss, 37% of women with lupus, and 24% of women requiring in vitro fertilization.[11] Screening does not appear to be beneficial in the general population, but testing for APS in these higher risk groups is probably advantageous.[24]

2. Management of APS

   Use of either LMWH or UFH in combination with low-dose aspirin has been effective in improving pregnancy outcomes in patients with APS. In addition, high-dose immunoglobulin has also been efficacious in selected patients.[25]

IV. OTHER CONNECTIVE TISSUE DISORDERS

A. Sjögren Syndrome

Sjögren syndrome has been studied in a relatively small series demonstrating increased fetal loss with a relative risk of 2.7 (95% CI, 1.1-6.5; $p = 0.023$). This risk is similar to that with SLE, but fetal growth restriction and prematurity were seen less frequently than in pregnancies with lupus.[26] Some patients with Sjögren syndrome are at risk to deliver infants with neonatal lupus and/or congenital CHB due to anti-Ro and anti-LA antibodies.

B. Scleroderma and Systemic Sclerosis

Most information is available from small case series and anecdotal reports of pregnancies complicated by renal crisis or esophageal tears in patients with esophageal disease.[27] The largest series of pregnancies in women with systemic sclerosis[28,29] demonstrate rates of preterm birth at almost 30%, with some increase in SGA infants as compared with women with rheumatoid arthritis and healthy women. Placental pathology is noted frequently in scleroderma pregnancies with a decidual vasculopathy.[30] It does not appear that pregnancy accelerates the rate of complications in patients with these connective tissue disorders, including renal crisis.

REFERENCES

1. Buyon JP: The effects of pregnancy on autoimmune diseases, *J Leukoc Biol* 63:281-287, 1998.
2. Forger F, Oestensen M, Schumacher A et al: Impact of pregnancy on health related quality of life evaluated prospectively in pregnant women with rheumatic diseases by the Short Form-36 Health Survey, *Ann Rheum Dis* 2005;64:1494-1499.
3. Ostensen M, Fuhrer L, Mathieu R et al: A prospective study of pregnant patients with rheumatoid arthritis and ankylosing spondylitis using validated clinical instruments, *Ann Rheum Dis* 63(10):1212-1217, 2004.
4. Ostensen M, Forger F, Nelson JL et al: Pregnancy in patients with rheumatic disease: anti-inflammatory cytokines increase in pregnancy and decrease post partum, *Ann Rheum Dis* 64(6):839-844, 2005.
5. Lewden B, Vial T, Elefant E et al: Low dose methotrexate in the first trimester of pregnancy: results of a French collaborative study, *J Rheumatol* 31(12):2360-2365, 2004.
6. Katz JA, Antoni C, Keenan GF et al: Outcome of pregnancy in women receiving infliximab for the treatment of Crohn's disease and rheumatoid arthritis, *Am J Gastroenterol* 99(12): 2385-2392, 2004.
7. Mintz R, Niz J, Gutierrez G et al: Prospective study of pregnancy in systemic lupus erythematosus: results of a multidisciplinary approach, *J Rheumatol* 13:732-739, 1986.
8. Ruiz-Irastorza G, Lima F, Alves J et al: Increased rate of lupus flares during pregnancy and the puerperium: a prospective study of 78 pregnancies, *Br J Rheumatol* 35:133-138, 1996.
9. Tandon A, Ibanez D, Gladman DD et al: The effect of pregnancy on lupus nephritis, *Arthritis Rheum* 50(12):3941-3946, 2004.
10. Clowse ME, Magder LS, Witter F et al: The impact of increased lupus activity on obstetric outcomes, *Arthritis Rheum* 52(2):514-521, 2005.
11. Rahman FZ, Rahman J, Al-Suleiman SA et al: Pregnancy outcome in lupus nephropathy, *Arch Gynecol Obstet* 271(3): 222-226, 2005.
12. Molad Y, Borkowski T, Monselise A et al: Maternal and fetal outcome of lupus pregnancy: a prospective study of 29 pregnancies, *Lupus* 14(2):145-151, 2005.
13. Costedoat-Chalumeau N, Amoura Z, Huong du LT et al: Safety of hydroxychloroquine in pregnant patients with connective tissue diseases. Review of the literature, *Autoimmun Rev* 4(2):111-115, 2005.
14. Borba EF, Turrini-Filho JR, Kuruma KA et al: Chloroquine gestational use in systemic lupus erythematosus: assessing the risk of child ototoxicity by pure tone audiometry, *Lupus* 13(4):223-227, 2004.
15. Ostensen M: Disease specific problems related to drug therapy in pregnancy, *Lupus* 13(9):746-750, 2004.
16. Buyon JP, Clancy RM: Neonatal lupus: basic research and clinical perspectives, *Rheum Dis Clin North Am* 31(2):299-313, 2005.
17. Buyon JP, Clancy RM: Autoantibody-associated congenital heart block: TGFbeta and the road to scar, *Autoimmun Rev* 4(1):1-7, 2005.
18. Breur JM, Visser GH, Kruize AA et al: Treatment of fetal heart block with maternal steroid therapy: case report and review of the literature, *Ultrasound Obstet Gynecol* 24(4):467-472, 2004.
19. Bizzaro N, Tonutti E, Villalta D et al: Prevalence and clinical correlation of anti-phospholipid-binding protein antibodies in anticardiolipin-negative patients with systemic lupus erythematosus and women with unexplained recurrent miscarriages, *Arch Pathol Lab Med* 129(1):61-68, 2005.
20. Bertolaccini ML, Atsumi K, Khamashta MA et al: Autoantibodies to human prothrombin and clinical manifestations in 207 patients with systemic lupus erythematosus, *J Rheumatol* 25:1104-1108, 1998.
21. Galli M, Barbui T: Antiphospholipid syndrome: clinical and diagnostic utility of laboratory tests, *Semin Thromb Hemost* 31(1):17-24, 2005.
22. Gomez-Puerta JA, Martin H, Amigo MC et al: Long-term follow-up in 128 patients with primary antiphospholipid syndrome: do they develop lupus? *Medicine (Baltimore)* 84(4):225-230, 2005.
23. Harris EN, Spinnato JA: Should anticardiolipin tests be performed in otherwise healthy pregnant women? *Am J Obstet Gynecol* 165:1272-1277, 1991.
24. Stuart RA, Kornman LH, McHugh NJ: A prospective study of pregnancy outcome in women screened at a routine antenatal clinic for anticardiolipin antibodies, *Br J Obstet Gynaecol* 100:599-600, 1993.
25. Nishiguchi T, Kobayashi T: Antiphospholipid syndrome: characteristics and obstetrical management, *Curr Drug Targets* 6(5):593-605, 2005.
26. Julkunen H, Kaaja R, Kurki P et al: Fetal outcome in women with primary Sjögren's syndrome. A retrospective case-control study, *Clin Exp Rheumatol* 13:65-71, 1995.
27. Chin KA, Kaseba CM, Weaver JB: Scleroderma in pregnancy, *Obstet Gynaecol* 18(3):238-242, 1998.
28. Steen VD, Medsger TA Jr: Fertility and pregnancy outcome in women with systemic sclerosis, *Arthritis Rheum* 42(4): 763-768, 1999.
29. Steen VD: Pregnancy in women with systemic sclerosis, *Obstet Gynecol* 94(1):15-20, 1999.
30. Doss BJ, Jacques SM, Mayes MD et al: Maternal scleroderma: placental findings and perinatal outcome, *Hum Pathol* 29(12):1524-1530, 1998.

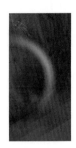

Commonly Encountered Medical Problems in Pregnancy

Infectious illnesses are commonly encountered in pregnancy. Many are self-limited and can be addressed solely from the perspective of patient comfort and safe use of medication in pregnancy. Some have substantial impact on the course and outcome of pregnancy. Others pose a significant danger to the neonate. Several conditions are associated with increased complications in pregnancy.

I. GENERAL GUIDELINES FOR THE USE OF ANTIBIOTICS IN PREGNANCY
Stephen D. Ratcliffe, MD, MSPH

A. Safe Use in Pregnancy
Antibiotics that are classified as category A or B in pregnancy include penicillins, cephalosporins, clindamycin, erythromycin (except estolate because of increased hepatotoxicity in pregnancy), nitrofurantoin, nystatin, azithromycin, and spectinomycin.

B. Use with Caution in Pregnancy
Antibiotics that are classified as category C include acyclovir, vancomycin, and miconazole. Class C antibiotics that should be used only with specific precautions include chloramphenicol, sulfonamides, aminoglycosides, trimethoprim, and metronidazole.

1. Chloramphenicol
   Chloramphenicol is classified as category C, but its use may result in "gray baby syndrome" if used close to term; therefore, it should be avoided except in situations of specific need.
2. Sulfonamides
   Sulfonamides theoretically increase the risk for kernicterus in the neonate because of competitive binding of albumin sites. Their use should be avoided in late pregnancy, if possible.
3. Gentamicin
   Gentamicin and other aminoglycosides may cause ototoxicity in the fetus. Their use should include the monitoring of levels.
4. Trimethoprim
   Trimethoprim is a folate antagonist. Concerns exist about its teratogenicity; it should not be used in the first trimester. In the second and third trimesters, concern for its antagonistic effects on folate should be balanced with other clinical considerations.
5. Metronidazole
   Metronidazole should not be used in the first trimester, although a recent metaanalysis did not find an association between its use in this period and an increased risk for birth defects.[1] It has a class B designation.

C. Unsafe for Use in Pregnancy
Antibiotics classified as category C that should be completely avoided during pregnancy except in severe circumstances in which other medications are not efficacious include quinolones, tetracycline and derivatives, and newer macrolides.

1. Quinolones
   Quinolones are classified as category C and have been found to cause cartilage degeneration in

animal studies; no information is available about human fetal effects. Quinolones should not be used if class A or B antibiotics can be used as an effective treatment.
2. Tetracycline and derivatives
   Tetracycline and derivatives are associated with staining of the teeth in the fetus and in young children. Their use should be avoided in pregnancy, but inadvertent first-trimester use is not known to be teratogenic. Severe hepatic toxicity has been reported with use during pregnancy.
3. Newer macrolides
   Azithromycin is a category B drug and can be used safely. Clarithromycin has been associated with increased embryonic loss and malformations in animal studies. It is classified as category C and should not be used if at all possible.

REFERENCE

1. Cano-Paton T, Carvajal A, Martin de Diego I et al: Is metronidazole teratogenic? A meta-analysis, *Br J Clin Pharmacol* 44:179-182, 1997.

II. CHLAMYDIA
Rachel Elizabeth Hall, MD, FAAFP

A. Epidemiology

1. Incidence/Prevalence
   Chlamydia trachomatis is the most common bacterial sexually transmitted disease (STD), with an estimated 3 million cases occurring each year in the United States.[1] Depending on the population, clinicians can expect to find chlamydial infection in 2% to 50% of their obstetric patients.[2-4]
2. At-risk groups
   Chlamydial infections are encountered in all age and socioeconomic groups. Age is the most important risk factor, with younger women (age < 25 years) more at risk. Other risk factors are single status, black race, history of STDs, new or multiple sex partners, cervical ectopy, and inconsistent use of barrier contraception.[1]

B. Natural History

1. Signs and symptoms
   Chlamydia infections may demonstrate no specific signs or symptoms. They also may present with mucopurulent cervicitis, excessive friability of the cervix at the time of pelvic examination, or spotting, especially after sexual intercourse.
2. Pelvic inflammatory disease (PID)
   Approximately 25% of untreated chlamydial infections develop into PID, with a number of life-long sequelae including pelvic pain, ectopic pregnancy, and infertility.
3. PID and pregnancy
   Upper genital tract infection (PID) is an unusual complication during pregnancy. This may pose a confusing and concerning clinical picture because of consideration of ectopic pregnancy. Demonstration of an intrauterine gestation is essential in a first-trimester patient with pelvic pain (see Chapter 6, Section B).
4. Differential diagnosis
   The differential diagnosis of chlamydia cervicitis includes trichomonal, gonorrhea, ureaplasma, and mycoplasma infections.

C. Effects on Perinatal Outcome

1. Prenatal
   Chlamydia infections are associated with increased rates of preterm labor (PTL), premature rupture of membranes, low birth weight (LBW), and preterm contractions. It is estimated 12% to 20% of women with chlamydia will miscarry.[5]
2. Neonatal
   Chlamydia conjunctivitis occurs in about 15% to 44% of neonates whose mothers are infected with chlamydia, and late-onset pneumonia occurs in 1% to 22% of these infants,[3] usually developing between 2 and 19 weeks after birth.
3. Late-onset endometritis
   More than 50% of patients presenting with late-onset endometritis, occurring between 2 days and 6 weeks after birth, have positive cultures for chlamydia.[6] Chlamydia does not have an association with endometritis occurring in the first 2 days after delivery.[7]
4. Treatment of chlamydia in pregnancy
   Successful treatment of chlamydial infection reduces the risk for preterm delivery (PTD) by 84%, premature rupture of membranes by 69%, preterm contractions by 87%, and LBW by 55%.[3] In addition, antepartum treatment of infected pregnant women has been shown to decrease rates of infection in offspring from 50% to 7%.[3]

D. Diagnosis

1. Symptomatic infection
   Identification of cervicitis occurs via mucopurulent discharge, excessive friability, or complaints

of spotting (including postcoital spotting). Wet preparation demonstrates increased leukocytes but no evident cause.

2. Routine screening
   Routine screening in populations at increased risk is recommended. The Centers for Disease Control and Prevention (CDC) defines this group to include women younger than 25 years, with other STDs, with a new partner or more than one in the preceding 3 months, and women who do not use a barrier method of contraception. The CDC also recommends repeat screening for these at-risk groups early in the third trimester.[8] Early screening improves overall pregnancy outcome, whereas third-trimester screening is most effective at preventing fetal transmission.[1]

3. Preterm labor
   Chlamydia testing of any patient who presents with PTL or preterm premature rupture of membranes (PPROM) should be considered because of the high rates of transmitted infection to the fetus, although there are no randomized controlled trial (RCT) data to support this intervention.

4. Testing techniques
   Acceptable testing techniques include rapid monoclonal fluorescent-antibody staining (DFA), enzyme-linked immunoassay (EIA), culture, direct gene probe, and DNA amplification assays (polymerase chain reaction [PCR], ligase chain reaction).[9] DFA and EIA carry a sensitivity of 70% to 80% and specificity of 96% to 100%,[1] whereas cervical culture has a sensitivity of 70% to 90%, but a specificity that approaches 100%.[8,10] The direct gene probe technology has a sensitivity of 76% to 96% and specificity of 98%.[11] The ligase chain reaction technology can be performed on urine specimens and achieves a sensitivity of 96% and a specificity of 99%.[10] The superior sensitivity and specificity of the DNA amplification tests result in a higher positive and negative predictive value for at-risk populations, defined by the CDC as having a prevalence of chlamydia greater than 5%. Practitioners should check the availability and costs of the newer technologies to determine what is most cost-effective in their practices.

E. Treatment

1. Erythromycin
   The CDC recommends erythromycin base 500 mg four times a day for 7 days with alternative regimens of 250 mg base four times a day for 14 days, erythromycin ethylsuccinate 800 mg four times a day for 7 days, or 400 mg four times a day for 14 days.[8] The lower dose regimens have fewer reports of side effects, but there are not enough data to support lower dose regimens at this time unless the patient cannot tolerate the higher dose regimens.[3] No evidence has been reported of an increased risk for pyloric stenosis among infants born to mothers exposed to erythromycin during pregnancy.[12] Erythromycin estolate should not be used in pregnancy.

2. Amoxicillin
   An additional recommended first-choice treatment option is amoxicillin 500 mg three times a day for 7 days.[8] Metaanalyses confirm equivalent or better test of cure rates and compliance with this regimen when compared with erythromycin.[3]

3. Clindamycin
   Clindamycin (450 mg four times a day for 2 weeks) is also an acceptable regimen but is much more costly than those listed above.

4. Azithromycin
   Azithromycin (1 g as a single dose) is the other alternative to erythromycin recommended by the CDC.[8] Azithromycin is derived from erythromycin, and a recent metaanalysis calculated the microbiological cure rate for azithromycin to be 92% compared with 81% for erythromycin. This may be because of increased compliance, especially if the treatment is given at the site of medical care. There are limited data on the safety of azithromycin in pregnancy; however, it has been widely used in obstetric practice since the late 1990s with no reports of serious adverse outcomes.[3]

5. Other regimens
   Tetracycline derivatives, quinolones, and clarithromycin are not indicated in pregnancy.

6. Test-of-cure (TOC)/treatment of partners
   TOC culture or other testing technique should be performed 3 weeks after completion of therapy.[3,8] This is recommended because compliance with longer regimens, or those with frequent reports of side effects (such as erythromycin), may not achieve eradication. Treatment of the patient's sexual partner is essential.

7. Repeat screening for high-risk patients
   Patients judged to be at high risk for contracting chlamydia, such as adolescents, should undergo repeat chlamydial testing in the third trimester because recurrent infection is common.[11]

F. Prevention

Strong evidence exists that population-based screening for asymptomatic chlamydial infections results in a decreased prevalence of this infection and its complications.[13] The CDC recommends screening women who are 25 or younger. Women older than 25 who have recently begun a new sexual relationship are also candidates for screening in the asymptomatic state.

G. SOR A Recommendations

RECOMMENDATIONS	REFERENCES
Amoxicillin is an acceptable alternative therapy for the treatment of chlamydia in pregnancy when compared with erythromycin. Clindamycin and azithromycin may be considered if erythromycin and amoxicillin are contraindicated or not tolerated.	14
Clinicians should routinely screen all sexually active women aged 25 and younger, and other asymptomatic women at increased risk for infection for chlamydial infection.	1

REFERENCES

1. United States Preventive Services Task Force: Screening for chlamydial infection recommendations and rationale, *Am J Prev Med* 20:90-94, 2001.
2. Cram LF, Zapata MI, Toy EC et al: Genitourinary infections and their association with preterm labor, *Am Fam Physician* 65:241-248, 2002.
3. Genc MR: Treatment of genital *Chlamydia trachomatis* infection in pregnancy, *Best Pract Res Clin Obstet Gynaecol* 16:913-922, 2002.
4. Rastogi S, Das B, Salhan S et al: Effect of treatment for *Chlamydia trachomatis* during pregnancy, *Int J Gynaecol Obstet* 80:129-137, 2003.
5. Logan S, Browne J, McKenzie H et al: Evaluation of endocervical, first-void urine and self-administered vulval swabs for the detection of *Chlamydia trachomatis* in a miscarriage population, *BJOG* 112:103-106, 2005.
6. Hoyme UB, Kiviat N, Eschenbach DA: The microbiology and treatment of late post-partum endometritis, *Obstet Gynecol* 68:226-230, 1986.
7. Watts DH, Eschenbach DA, Kenny GE: Early post-partum endometritis: the role of bacteria, genital mycoplasmas, and *Chlamydia trachomatis*, *Obstet Gynecol* 73:52-57, 1989.
8. Sexually transmitted diseases treatment guidelines 2002. Centers for Disease Control and Prevention, *MMWR Recomm Rep* 51(RR-6):1-78, 2002.
9. Wendel PJ, Wendel GD: Sexually transmitted diseases in pregnancy, *Semin Perinatol* 17:443-451, 1993.
10. Gaydos CA, Howell MR, Quinn TC et al: Use of ligase chain reaction with urine versus cervical culture for detection of *Chlamydia trachomatis* in an asymptomatic military population of pregnant and non-pregnant females attending papanicolaou smear clinics, *J Clin Microbiol* 36:1300-1304, 1998.
11. Miller JM: Recurrent chlamydial colonization during pregnancy, *Am J Perinatol* 15:307-309, 1998.
12. Louik C, Werler MM, Mitchell AA: Erythromycin use during pregnancy in relation to pyloric stenosis, *Am J Obstet Gynecol* 186:288-290, 2002.
13. Scholes D, Stergachis A, Heidrich FE et al: Prevention of pelvic inflammatory disease by screening for cervical chlamydial infection, *N Engl J Med* 334:1842-1846, 1994.
14. Brockelhurst P, Rooney G: Interventions for treating genital Chlamydia trachomatis infection in pregnancy, *Cochrane Database Syst Rev* (2):CD000054, 2000.

III. GONORRHEA
Rachel Elizabeth Hall, MD, FAAFP

A. Epidemiology

The CDC estimates that there are 600,000 new cases of *Neisseria gonorrhea* infection each year,[1] with an estimated 40,000 cases in pregnant women.[2] It is the second most common reportable disease in the United States, second only to *C. trachomatis*.[3] Reported cases are increasing among whites and Hispanics and decreasing among blacks, but the rate for blacks still remains 20 times greater than that for whites.[3] Overall, rates are greatest among women aged 15 to 24 and men aged 20 to 24.[3] Risk factors for gonorrhea are the same for pregnant and nonpregnant women, and include age younger than 25, history of gonorrhea infection or other sexually transmitted infections, new or multiple sexual partners, inconsistent condom use, sex work, and drug use.[3]

B. Natural History

The endocervical canal and urethra are usually infected with *N. gonorrhea* bacteria. Symptoms include dysuria, vaginal discharge, and abnormal vaginal bleeding. Signs include mucopurulent endocervical discharge and/or cervical friability and erythema.[4,5]

C. Diagnosis

Recovery rate of cultures is greater if appropriate technique is observed (endocervical canal thoroughly swabbed, careful use of transport media or direct plating on Thayer–Martin culture media, increased pickup with urethral and anal culture). The sensitivity of culture is between 80% and 90%.[5] Gram stain of cervical discharge is unacceptable for diagnosis because of normal vaginal commensal organisms (sensitivity 50–70%, specificity 97%). Insufficient evidence is available to support the use of wet mount to predict which patients are at increased risk for gonorrhea.[6,7] DNA probe technology and PCR techniques are now readily available in many practice settings. These tests are rapidly replacing culture techniques.

D. Effects on Perinatal Outcome

The effects of gonorrhea infection on perinatal outcome include[4,5]:

1. Effects on the mother and fetus
   a. PID (rare, in first trimester)
   b. Septic abortion
   c. PPROM
   d. PTL
   e. Chorioamnionitis
   f. Puerperal sepsis
2. Effects on the neonate
   Infection develops in about one third of exposed neonates (including infants born by cesarean section after rupture of membranes).[5,8]
   a. Gonococcal ophthalmia neonatorum[8]
      This results in acute purulent conjunctivitis in the first week of life; untreated infants may develop corneal ulceration, panophthalmitis, and loss of the eye. Before topical silver nitrate or erythromycin prophylaxis, this was a major cause of blindness.
   b. Other neonatal infections include:
      i. Gonococcemia
      ii. Septic arthritis
      iii. Pharyngitis
      iv. Proctitis
      v. Vaginitis
      vi. Scalp abscesses
      vii. Meningitis

E. Management Guidelines

Management guidelines for gonorrheal infection include[5]:

1. β-Lactamase resistance
   Currently, this is common in the United States. Recommended first-line therapy is ceftriaxone 125 mg intramuscularly once. A recent study showed both this regimen, as well as 400 mg oral cefixime, to be efficacious for all forms of gonorrhea infection in pregnancy.[2]
2. Cephalosporin allergy
   Previously, spectinomycin 2 g intramuscularly was given; however, the manufacturer has recently

discontinued this medicine. An alternative may be single-dose oral azithromycin 2 g, but its efficacy and safety in pregnancy is yet to be proven. Emerging resistance also is a concern. The CDC currently recommends consideration of desensitization to cephalosporins.[9]

3. Other precautions
   Quinolones should not be used in pregnancy. The patient's partner should be treated. A TOC and third-trimester testing should be performed because of risk for treatment failures and recurrent infection. If using the culture method, TOC can be done as early as 3 to 7 days after treatment[4]; other forms such as the DNA probe should be performed 3 weeks after treatment. There is also a high coinfection rate with chlamydia; therefore, consideration of dual treatment regimens is recommended.[1,2]

F. SOR A Recommendation

RECOMMENDATION	REFERENCE
Use prophylactic ocular topical medication for all newborns against gonococcal ophthalmia neonatorum.	3

REFERENCES

1. Sexually transmitted diseases treatment guidelines 2002. Centers for Disease Control and Prevention, *MMWR Recomm Rep* 51(RR-6):1-78, 2002.
2. Ramus R, Sheffield J, Mayfield J et al: A randomized trial that compared oral cefixime and intramuscular ceftriaxone for the treatment of gonorrhea in pregnancy, *Am J Obstet Gynecol* 185:629-632, 2001.
3. U.S. Preventive Services Task Force: Screening for gonorrhea: recommendation statement; publication no. 05-0579-A, Rockville, MD, May 2005, Agency for Healthcare Research and Quality (AHRQ).
4. Ament LA, Whalen E: Sexually transmitted diseases in pregnancy: diagnosis, impact, and intervention, *J Obstet Gynecol Neonatal Nurs* 25:657-666, 1996.
5. Gonorrhea and chlamydial infections. ACOG Technical Bulletin Number 190-March 1994 (replaces No. 89, November 1985), *Int J Gynaecol Obstet* 45:169-174, 1994.
6. Bohmer JT, Schemmer G, Harrison F et al: Cervical wet mount as a negative predictor for gonococci- and *Chlamydia trachomatis*-induced cervicitis in a gravid population, *Am J Obstet Gynecol* 181:283-287, 1999.
7. Majeroni BA, Schank JN, Horwitz M et al: Use of wet mount to predict *Chlamydia trachomatis* and *Neisseria gonorrhoeae* cervicitis in primary care, *Fam Med* 28:580-583, 1996.
8. Fletcher JL, Gordon RC: Perinatal transmission of bacterial sexually transmitted diseases. Part I: syphilis and gonorrhea, *J Fam Pract* 30:448-456, 1990.

9. Centers for Disease Control: Notice to readers: discontinuation of spectinomycin, *MMWR* 55:370, 2006.

IV. SYPHILIS
Rachel Elizabeth Hall, MD, FAAFP

A. Epidemiology
1. Incidence/Prevalence

   Syphilis is a life-threatening, chronic infection caused by the *Treponema pallidum* spirochete. It is acquired via sexual or congenital transmission. An increase in congenital syphilis occurred in the late 1980s, especially in populations in which drug abuse is common and among patients with late entry into prenatal care.[1] The latter occurred, in part, because of a revised case definition by the CDC that considers infants of mothers who have not received any or appropriate treatment during pregnancy to have presumed congenital infection.[2] Prevalence in pregnancy is estimated between 0.02% and 4.5% for northern Europe and the United States, affecting an average of 30 cases per 10,000 live births in the United States in 1996.[3]

B. Natural History
1. Primary syphilis

   This is the initial phase of infection and is usually accompanied by the presence of a painless chancre and regional lymphadenopathy. The chancre can persist up to 8 weeks if the infection is untreated. The lymphadenopathy persists well after this.

2. Secondary syphilis

   This phase of the infection begins about 6 weeks after the appearance of the chancre and is marked by the following signs and symptoms.[4]
   a. Macular papular rash (90%)
   b. Silver-gray mucosal patches (30%)
   c. White-gray intertriginous patches (condylomata lata) (20%)
   d. Constitutional symptoms, such as fever, headache, malaise, arthralgia, myalgia (70%)

3. Latent syphilis

   The signs and symptoms of secondary syphilis resolve in 3 to 12 weeks without treatment. About 25% of patients will have relapsing symptoms during the first 12-month period, called *early latent syphilis*. During this initial asymptomatic period, patients are still highly infectious. Late latent syphilis begins after a period of 12 months. Relapses are uncommon and overall infectivity is less than with early latent syphilis.

4. Late/Tertiary syphilis

   About 25% of patients who do not receive treatment acquire late or tertiary syphilis. Manifestations include:
   a. Gummata: These are locally destructive granulomatous lesions that occur in body tissues including muscle, bone, and skin.
   b. Cardiovascular disease: This results in a vasculitis of the aorta that leads to the formation of an aneurysm, most commonly in the ascending portion.
   c. Neurosyphilis: Meningovascular disease results in strokelike syndromes or in seizure disorders. Parenchymal involvement also can result in strokelike symptoms or in tabes dorsalis.

C. Effects on Perinatal Outcome
Pregnancy does not appear to affect the natural history of syphilis. Syphilis, however, exerts many deleterious effects on pregnancy.[2,4] The level of risk to the fetus is directly related to the maternal state of infection, with earlier infection resulting in worse outcomes for the pregnancy.[3]

1. Increased perinatal morbidity/mortality

   About 40% to 50% of women who do not receive treatment for syphilis during pregnancy experience the following complications:
   a. Spontaneous abortion: can occur throughout pregnancy
   b. Stillbirth
   c. Prematurity

2. Congenital syphilis[4]

   Vertical transmission is more common in primary syphilis (70-100%), secondary syphilis (40-50%), and early latent syphilis with bacteremic relapse (30%).[5] In addition, it was previously thought that transmission could not occur before 18 weeks of gestation, but more recent research proves the spirochete can infect the fetus as early as 9 to 10 weeks.[3] The revised CDC definitions of confirmed and presumed congenital syphilis are found in Table 9-1. There are two phases of congenital syphilis:
   a. Early congenital syphilis: In neonates with early congenital syphilis, clinical presentation includes hepatosplenomegaly, abdominal distention, nephrotic syndrome, petechiae, hemolytic anemia, thrombocytopenia, osteochondritis, periostitis, central nervous system involvement,

TABLE 9-1 Congenital Syphilis Case Definition

Case Type	Description
Confirmed	Infant in whom *Treponema pallidum* is identified by dark-field microscopy, fluorescent antibody, or other specific stains in specimens from lesions, placenta, umbilical cord, or autopsy material
Presumed	An infant whose mother had untreated or inadequately treated syphilis at delivery, regardless of findings for the infant
	Any infant or child with a reactssive treponemal test for syphilis and one of the following:
	Evidence of CS on physical examination
	Evidence of CS on long-bone radiograph
	Reactive CSF on a VDRL test
	Increased CSF cell count or protein (without other cause)
	Nontreponemal serologic titers fourfold greater than the mother's (drawn at birth)
	Reactive test for FTA-ABS antibody

From Centers for Disease Control and Prevention (CDC): Guidelines for the prevention and control of congenital syphilis, *MMWR Morb Mortal Wkly Rep* 37(suppl 1):1-13, 1988.
CS, Congenital syphilis; VDRL, Venereal Disease Research Laboratory; CSF, cerebrospinal fluid; FTA-ABS, fluorescent treponemal antibody absorption.
Inadequate treatment consists of any nonpenicillin therapy or penicillin given less than 30 days before delivery.

and mucocutaneous manifestations. Full discussion of congenital infection and its management is beyond the scope of this chapter.

    b. Late congenital syphilis: This is a clinical syndrome that presents after 2 years of age and is a result of an inflammatory response to the initial or persistence of infection. Malformations/abnormalities include abnormal teeth (Hutchinson's teeth), healed chorioretinitis, eighth nerve deafness, cranial nerve palsies, mental retardation, and bony abnormalities such as frontal bossing and saddle-nose deformities.

D. Diagnosis

1. Maternal infection[6]
   a. Direct detection: Fluid can be expressed from cutaneous lesions or aspirated from lymph nodes and examined using a dark-field microscope to directly visualize spirochetes. High spirochete loads and an experienced examiner are required. When these conditions are met, the sensitivity is about 80%.
   b. Nontreponemal tests: The Venereal Disease Research Laboratory (VDRL) or rapid plasma reagin (RPR) are the screening tests of choice. The sensitivity is only 78% to 86% for primary infections, increases to 100% for secondary, remains high at 95% to 98% for latent infections,

and decreases to 72% to 73% for tertiary syphilis. The specificity remains at 97% to 99% for all stages of the infection, yielding a false-positive rate of 1% to 3%. False-positive tests may occur in the setting of other infections, malignancies, autoimmune disorders, aging, and illicit parenteral drug use.[4]

    c. Treponemal tests: The two available tests are the fluorescent treponemal antibody absorption (FTA-ABS) and the microhemagglutination (MHA). These tests have sensitivities and specificities comparable with the nontreponemal methods and are used to confirm the diagnoses of a positive VDRL or RPR. If the nontreponemal test is positive and the treponemal test is nonreactive without clinical evidence of disease, both tests should be repeated within 4 weeks. If the FTA or MHA remains negative, it can be assumed that the nontreponemal test was a false-positive result.

2. Prenatal diagnosis of fetal syphilis[2]
   The diagnosis of fetal syphilis can be made when the mother is seropositive for infection and the ultrasound identifies hydrops fetalis characterized by skin thickening, intraabdominal and pleural effusions, hepatomegaly, and polyhydramnios. Cordocentesis and amniocentesis may be used to confirm the diagnosis.

3. Diagnosis of congenital syphilis (see Table 9-1)
   Lack of prenatal care is most associated with failure to prevent congenital syphilis, with only 52% of mothers of infants with congenital syphilis having at least one prenatal visit. Those with prenatal care typically presented for their first visit at a mean of 22 weeks.[3]

E. Treatment

If clinical or serologic evidence of infection is present, the patient should be treated per CDC guidelines. The CDC recommends all seropositive women be treated unless history of adequate treatment and documentation of appropriate decline in titers can be obtained. In addition, they solely recommend penicillin for the treatment of syphilis during pregnancy, as no alternatives have been proved effective for its treatment during pregnancy.[7] A Cochrane review confirmed the efficacy of penicillin in pregnancy; however, more research is needed to determine optimal treatment regimens.[8]

1. Primary, secondary, and early latent disease[4]
   Administer benzathine penicillin 2.4 million units intramuscularly once. Some authors recommend two injections spaced by 1 week. For latent disease with unknown duration or greater than 1 year, treatment should be weekly for 3 weeks. RPR or VDRL titers should be monitored on a monthly basis to document response to therapy. A fourfold decline in the titer should occur after 3 to 6 months, and an eightfold decline by 6 to 12 months.[2] The treponemal antibody level (FTA or MHA) will remain positive despite treatment. Treatment failures are rare among women with primary or tertiary syphilis.[9] Failure rates of 5% to 6% in secondary and 2% in early latent syphilis have been reported.

2. Penicillin-allergic patients
   The approximate 5% to 10% of women who are allergic to penicillin can be identified with skin testing and safely undergo oral penicillin desensitization.[10] Preliminary data suggest ceftriaxone may be an effective therapeutic alternative in these patients,[11] but further research with greater numbers of patients (study referenced included only 11 women) will be necessary for the CDC to change its recommendations.

3. Jarisch–Herxheimer reaction[12]
   The Jarisch–Herxheimer reaction is common in the earlier stages of syphilis (60-100%); up to 45% of women allergic to penicillin treated during early syphilis will experience the reaction.[3]

It is characterized by maternal fever, tachycardia, hypotension, myalgias, and headache. Pregnant patients may experience, in addition, uterine contractions, decreased fetal movement, fetal tachycardia, and decreased variability noted by fetal monitoring. Transient late decelerations have also been noted with monitoring of contractions. This reaction should be treated with hydration, rest, and acetaminophen for fever. Patients with reduced fetal movement and contractions should receive fetal heart rate monitoring until signs and symptoms resolve. Klein and colleagues[12] recommend obtaining a baseline fetal ultrasound before initiating syphilitic therapy, and providing more intensive monitoring and follow-up for women with abnormal studies.

4. Congenital syphilis
   Treatment regimens are available through the CDC and are beyond the scope of this textbook.[7]

F. Prevention

Clinicians can largely prevent congenital syphilis by screening all pregnancies for the maternal syphilis and tracking all confirmed cases with serial serologies to confirm successful treatment. Clinicians working with at-risk populations (inner-city populations with suspected use or access to illicit drugs, especially cocaine) should screen for maternal syphilis at the onset of care, at 28 weeks of gestation, and again at birth.[7,13] Good evidence exists that models of clinician-community partnerships with Women, Infants and Children, Medicaid, Aid to Families with Dependent Children, and family-planning clinics improve the detection and treatment of maternal syphilis.[14]

G. SOR A Recommendations

RECOMMENDATIONS	REFERENCES
Screen all pregnant women for syphilis infection and consider rescreening high-risk populations at the beginning of the third trimester and/or at delivery.	15
Penicillin is the agent of choice for treatment of syphilis during pregnancy.	7, 8

REFERENCES

1. Rolfs RT, Nakashima AK: Epidemiology of primary and secondary syphilis in the United States, 1981 through 1989, *JAMA* 264:1432-1437, 1990.

2. Sanchez PJ, Wendel GD: Syphilis in pregnancy, *Clin Perinatol* 24:71-90, 1997.
3. Genc M, Ledger WJ: Syphilis in pregnancy, *Sex Transm Infect* 76:73-79, 2000.
4. Sheffield JS, Wendel GD: Syphilis in pregnancy, *Clin Obstet Gynecol* 42:97-106, 1999.
5. Fletcher JL, Gordon RC: Perinatal transmission of bacterial sexually transmitted diseases. Part I: syphilis and gonorrhea, *J Fam Pract* 30:448-456, 1990.
6. Larsen SA, Steiner BM, Rudolph AH: Laboratory diagnosis and interpretation of tests for syphilis, *Clin Microbiol Rev* 8:1-21, 1995.
7. Sexually transmitted diseases treatment guidelines 2002. Centers for Disease Control and Prevention, *MMWR Recomm Rep* 51(RR-6):1-78, 2002.
8. Walker GJA: Antibiotics for syphilis diagnosed during pregnancy, *Cochrane Database Syst Rev* (3):CD001143, 2001.
9. Alexander JM, Sheffield JS, Sanchez PJ et al: Efficacy of treatment for syphilis in pregnancy, *Obstet Gynecol* 93:5-8, 1999.
10. Wendel GD, Stark BJ, Jamison RB et al: Penicillin allergy and desensitization in serious infections during pregnancy, *N Engl J Med* 322:270-271, 1985.
11. Zhou P, Gu Z, Xu J et al: A study evaluating ceftriaxone as a treatment agent for primary and secondary syphilis in pregnancy, *Sex Transm Dis* 32:495-498, 2005.
12. Klein VR, Cox SM, Mitchell MD et al: The Jarisch-Herxheimer reaction complicating syphilotherapy in pregnancy, *Obstet Gynecol* 75:375-380, 1990.
13. Hollier LM, Hill J, Sheffield JS et al: State laws regarding prenatal syphilis in the United States, *Am J Obstet Gynecol* 4:1178-1183, 2003.
14. Swain GR, Kowalewski SJ, Schubot DB: Reducing the incidence of congenital syphilis in Milwaukee: a public private partnership, *Am J Public Health* 88:1101-1102, 1998.
15. U.S. Preventive Services Task Force: Screening for syphilis infection, *Ann Fam Med* 4:362-365, 2004.

V. GROUP B STREPTOCOCCUS
Stephen D. Ratcliffe, MD, MSPH

A. Epidemiology

1. Prevalence
   About 30% of women are colonized with group B streptococcus (GBS) at some time during pregnancy, with two thirds of them being colonized at the time of delivery.[1] Of the women who are culture-positive at the time of labor, neonatal colonization of the mucous membranes occurs in 50% to 70%. Of these colonized infants, 1% to 3% will experience development of symptomatic infection.[2,3] Without the use of intrapartum antibiotic prophylactic treatment of GBS carriers, the overall number of infants who experience development of early-onset group B streptococcus (EOGBS) infection is about 1.8 per 1000.[3] With the widespread use of prenatal GBS screening, this rate has decreased to 0.37 of 1000 live births.[4] The GBS "attack" rate varies greatly depending on the presence or absence of concurrent risk factors. In the early 1990s, there were approximately 8,000 neonatal GBS infections in the United States each year. About 80% to 85% of these infections occur in the first 7 days of life, are thought to occur from vertical transmission at or before birth, and are termed *EOGBS*. The remaining infections are called *late-onset GBS* and occur from 7 days to 3 months of age.

2. Risk factors for colonization with GBS include:
   a. Age younger than 21
   b. Low socioeconomic status
   c. Sexual activity
   d. Low parity
   e. Hispanic and black ethnicity[5]

B. Natural History

1. Timing of colonization[1]
   Women who are GBS-positive during pregnancy have the following natural history: one third remains culture positive throughout the pregnancy; one third are intermittently positive; and one third are positive only once.

2. Risk factors that affect vertical transmission of GBS include:
   a. Women who are chronically colonized with heavy GBS growth
   b. Women with GBS bacteriuria[3]
   c. Prematurity (<37 weeks of gestation)
   d. Rupture of membranes greater than 18 hours
   e. Intrapartum fever
   f. Having a sibling with previous invasive GBS

3. EOGBS
   The case fatality rate for EOGBS infections has decreased from about 50% in the 1970s to 10% in the 1990s.[6] Nevertheless, these are otherwise healthy infants who continue to experience significant morbidity and mortality from vertical transmission of GBS at or before birth.

4. Late-onset GBS
   These infections can also be devastating to the older infant and may be acquired by vertical or horizontal spread. Intrapartum interventions described in this section are not effective in preventing the late-onset type.

C. Effects on Perinatal Outcome

1. Association with PTL and PPROM
   Heavy, persistent growth of GBS and GBS bacteriuria are associated with an increased risk for PTL

and PPROM.[3] RCTs have not been able to demonstrate a reduction in PTL or PPROM with the treatment of this infection in pregnancy.[7,8]

2. Asymptomatic bacteriuria (ASB)
   Fifteen percent of ASB in pregnancy is caused by GBS. This condition is associated with increased risk for PTL, PPROM, chorioamnionitis, and increased EOGBS.

3. Increased risk for chorioamnionitis and endometritis
   Women who are chronic carriers of GBS are at increased risk for having these intrapartum and postpartum complications.[9]

4. Other puerperal infections
   Women colonized with GBS are at increased risk for pelvic cellulitis and septic thrombophlebitis.[10]

D. Diagnosis

1. Culture
   Culture remains the gold standard. However, clinicians should use selective broth medium and obtain cultures from the anterior vagina, perineum, and anorectal area to ensure accurate detection of the GBS. Failure to use this culture medium and the multiple culture sites results in a false-negative rate or sensitivity of about 50%.[1]

2. Rapid streptococcal tests
   It is desirable to have a rapid turnaround test that a clinician could use in the intrapartum setting. The sensitivity of the currently available tests is insufficient to detect GBS in patients who are not heavily colonized. In 1997, the U.S. Food and Drug Administration issued a warning not to use these rapid strep tests but to rely instead on cultures using the selective broth medium.[11] Evidence has been reported that the rapid detection of GBS in the intrapartum setting can be done using PCR testing with a sensitivity of 97% and specificity of 98.8%.[12] This test currently is not available commercially.

E. Management: Prevention of Early-Onset Group B Streptococcus Infection

The focus on management has shifted over the past decade to the intrapartum setting. Four RCTs show that the vertical transmission of GBS from an infected mother to her newborn can be effectively prevented with the use of intrapartum antibiotics.[13,14] Infant colonization is decreased (number needed to treat [NNT] = 2.3), and neonatal GBS infection is decreased (NNT = 20). On the basis of the studies, neonatal mortality is not improved (odds ratio [OR], 0.12; 95% confidence interval [CI], 0.10-2.00). This is likely due to insufficient numbers in the studies. However, further RCTs in this area will most likely not occur because of the risk posed to infants in the control group.

Current management practices include:

1. Antibiotic selection
   a. Aqueous penicillin G (5 million units IV, then 2.5 million units every 4 hours until delivery) is the treatment of choice because of its narrow antimicrobial spectrum, thus having less of a chance of inducing antibiotic-resistant bacteria.[6]
   b. Ampicillin (2 g bolus IV followed by 1 g every 4 hours until delivery)
   c. Cefazolin (2 g bolus IV followed by 1 g every 8 hours until delivery) is the drug of choice for patients allergic to penicillin who are not at high risk for anaphylactic reactions (i.e., patients who have a history of immediate hypersensitivity to the penicillin by having immediate hives or angioedema).[15]
   d. Clindamycin can given to the mother who is allergic to penicillin (900 mg IV every 8 hours until delivery) and is at high risk for anaphylaxis. No prospective trials have measured the effectiveness of clindamycin in the treatment of GBS. Fifteen percent of genitourinary GBS isolates are resistant to clindamycin.[16] Therefore, patients allergic to penicillin should undergo susceptibility testing of clindamycin and erythromycin.
   e. Erythromycin (500 mg IV every 6 hours) is a less desirable alternative because of unpredictable levels of antibiotic crossing the placenta. The incidence rate of GBS strains resistant to erythromycin has ranged from 7% to 25%.
   f. Vancomycin (1 g IV every 12 hours until delivery) is the treatment of choice for patients who are allergic to penicillin, have GBS resistant to clindamycin and erythromycin, and are at increased risk for anaphylactic reactions if cephalosporins are used.
   g. Broad-spectrum coverage: Regimens such as ampicillin and gentamicin should be used if chorioamnionitis is present.

2. Timing of antibiotic use in labor
   Two or more doses of intravenous antibiotics or having an interval of 4 or more hours between

antibiotic dosing and delivery are effective in reducing infant colonization rates to less than 3%.[17]

3. Recent history of GBS treatment strategies

Until 1996 there was considerable controversy as to the best approach to prevent EOGBS. The American Academy of Pediatrics (AAP) recommended screening cultures at 26 to 28 weeks of gestation and the intrapartum treatment of positive cultures when one of the following obstetrical risk factors was present: fever, rupture of membranes longer than 18 hours, history of sibling with invasive GBS, gestational age less than 37 weeks, and GBS bacteriuria in current pregnancy.[18,19] The American College of Obstetricians and Gynecologists (ACOG) recommended that no prenatal cultures be performed, but that a risk factor–guided intrapartum treatment regimen should be followed.[20]

In 1996, the CDC issued consensus guidelines that were endorsed by the AAP and ACOG.[20,21] They provided clinicians with two treatment strategies:

a. Culture- and risk factor–based approach: Clinicians obtain GBS cultures from the lower genital tract of all of their patients between 35 and 37 weeks of gestation and offer chemoprophylaxis for culture-positive women when they are in labor. If culture results were not available, patients received intrapartum chemoprophylaxis if one or more of the following risk factors were present: gestation less than 37 weeks, duration of membrane rupture greater than 18 hours, maternal temperature greater than 100.4°F, and a previous infant with GBS infection. It was estimated that this approach resulted in intrapartum antibiotic use for about 27% of women and prevented 90% of EOGBS cases.[22]

b. Risk factor–alone approach: This approach offered antibiotic chemoprophylaxis to those women who have one or more of the previously mentioned risk factors. It estimated that this approach resulted in intrapartum antibiotic use for about 18% of women and prevented 69% of EOGBS cases.[22]

4. Current CDC recommendations

In August 2002, the CDC issued revised guidelines recommending universal screening for vaginal and rectal GBS colonization of women between 35 and 37 weeks of gestation.[23] This was based on a growing body of evidence showing that this treatment strategy reached more of the targeted population than the risk factor–alone approach. A large, multistate study conducted by the CDC demonstrated that 18% of all women who were GBS culture positive would not have received intrapartum antibiotic coverage by the risk factor–alone approach.[24] The relative risk of EOGBS among infants of screened mothers versus those who were treated based on risk factors was 0.46 (95% CI, 0.36-0.60). The Society of Obstetricians and Gynecologist of Canada subsequently endorsed this approach.[25]

a. Intrapartum prophylaxis with intravenous penicillin indicated

i. Previous infant with invasive GBS disease

ii. GBS bacteriuria (regardless of the level of colony-forming units) during current pregnancy

iii. Positive GBS screening culture during current pregnancy

iv. Unknown GBS status and delivery at less than 37 weeks of gestation, duration of amniotic membrane rupture more than 18 hours, and intrapartum temperature greater than 101.4°F

b. Intrapartum prophylaxis not indicated

i. Previous pregnancy with a positive GBS screening culture

ii. Planned cesarean delivery performed in the absence of labor or membrane rupture regardless of maternal GBS culture

iii. Negative vaginal and rectal GBS screening culture in late gestation during the current pregnancy, regardless of intrapartum risk factors

c. Threatened PTD

The CDC recommends managing the PTL patient whose GBS status is unknown with the use of intrapartum antibiotic prophylaxis.

d. Neonatal care[24,26]

i. Healthy-appearing infant at 37 or more weeks of gestation who received intrapartum antibiotics more than 4 hours before delivery: no diagnostic workup, could be sent home in 24 hours in reliable home environment

ii. Healthy-appearing infant at 37 or more weeks of gestation who did not receive intrapartum antibiotics more than 4 hours before delivery: no diagnostic workup, observe 48 hours

iii. Healthy-appearing infant at less than 35 weeks of gestation with unknown GBS status: limited diagnostic workup (complete blood cell count with differential and blood culture) and observe 48 hours

iv. Maternal antibiotics for suspected chorioamnionitis or signs of suspected neonatal sepsis: full diagnostic evaluation including chest radiograph, lumbar puncture, and empiric therapy.

F. Impact of Centers for Disease Control and Prevention Screening Recommendations

1. Decreasing incidence of EOGBS
   In tracking the incidence of EOGBS from the period of no surveillance or no treatment for GBS (1990-1992) to risk factor–based protocols (1993-1996) to screening-based protocols (1997-2002), the incidence of EOGBS decreased from 2.0 to 1.1 to 0.4 per 1000 births.[27]

2. Cases of EOGBS despite screening
   Screening for GBS within 5 weeks of delivery and the use of intrapartum antibiotic prophylaxis have decreased the incidence of EOGBS, but cases of this dangerous infection still occur despite negative cultures. Retrospective reviews indicate that clinical evidence of chorioamnionitis and neonatal sepsis must be recognized and treated to help prevent fatal complications of this infection.[4]

3. Association between prenatal screening and decrease in maternal morbidity
   Locksmith and colleagues[9] analyzed the impact of using one of three GBS treatment strategies over a 7-year period involving more than 20,000 deliveries. Two of the three strategies were the ones recommended by the CDC in 1996. They were unable to detect an improvement in neonatal outcome under the universal screening protocol. The group that underwent universal screening had a 30% decrease in chorioamnionitis (NNT = culture 23 patients and treat 4 patients in labor) and endometritis (NNT = culture 31 patients and treat 5.3 patients in labor).

4. Association between prenatal screening/intrapartum treatment and subsequent neonatal infection
   a. No increase in non-GBS neonatal infections: Concerns exist that the widespread use of intrapartum antibiotics to prevent EOGBS would be linked to an increase in the incidence of non-GBS invasive infections in neonates. Two case–control studies have demonstrated no increase in the incidence of non-GBS invasive neonatal infections in the era of screening and treating women who are carriers of GBS or meet either criteria for treatment.[28,29]

   b. No increase in ampicillin-resistant infection: This screening has not been associated with an increase in ampicillin-resistant early-onset infection.[27] Two factors that are associated with an increase in the ampicillin resistant infections are a history of chorioamnionitis or use of intrapartum antibiotics longer than 24 hours.[29]

G. Primary Prevention: Development of a Group B Streptococcus Vaccine

Extensive research has been undertaken to develop conjugated vaccines against the major serotypes of GBS. One of these vaccines produced a fourfold or greater increase in antibody production in more than 90% of women of childbearing age.[30] The primary prevention of EOGBS is a promising strategy for the future.

H. SOR A Recommendation

RECOMMENDATION	REFERENCE
Vertical transmission of GBS from an infected mother to the newborn can be effectively prevented with the use of intrapartum antibiotics. Infant colonization is decreased (NNT = 2.3), and neonatal GBS infection is decreased (NNT. = 20).	14

REFERENCES

1. McKenna D, Iams J: Group B streptococcal infections, *Semin Perinatol* 22:267-276, 1998.
2. Ferrieri P, Cleary P, Seeds A: Epidemiology of group B streptoccocal carriage in pregnant women and newborn infants, *J Med Microbiol* 10:103-114, 1976.
3. Regan JA, Klebanoff MA, Nugent RP: The epidemiology of group B streptococcal colonization in pregnancy, *Obstet Gynecol* 77:604-610, 1991.
4. Puopolo K, Madoff LC, Eichenwald EC: Early-onset group B streptococcal disease in the era of maternal screening, *Pediatrics* 115:1240-1246, 2005.
5. Goldenberg R, Klebanoff M, Nugent R et al: Bacterial colonization of the vagina during pregnancy in four ethnic groups, *Am J Obstet Gynecol* 174:1618-1621, 1996.
6. Schuchat A: Group B streptococcus, *Lancet* 353:51-56, 1999.

7. Regan J, Klebanoff M, Nugent R et al: Colonization with group B streptococci in pregnancy and adverse outcome. VIP Study Group, *Am J Obstet Gynecol* 174:1354-1360, 1996.

8. Klebanoff M, Regan J, Rau A et al: Outcome of the Vaginal Infections and Prematurity Study: results of a clinical trial of erythromycin among pregnant women colonized with group B streptococci, *Am J Obstet Gynecol* 172:1540-1545, 1995.

9. Locksmith G, Clark P, Duff P: Maternal and neonatal infection rates with three different protocols for prevention of group B streptococcal disease, *Am J Obstet Gynecol* 180:416-422, 1999.

10. Yancey M, Duff P, Clark P et al: Peripartum infection associated with vaginal group B streptococcal colonization, *Obstet Gynecol* 84:816-819, 1994.

11. United States Food and Drug Administration. *FDA safety alert: risks of devices for direct detection of group B streptococcal antigen,* Rockville, MD, 1997, Department of Health and Human Services.

12. Bergeron MG, Danbing K, Menard C et al: Rapid detection of group B streptococci in pregnant women at delivery, *N Engl J Med* 343:175-179, 2000.

13. Boyer KM, Gotoff SP: Prevention of early onset neonatal group B streptococcal disease with selective intrapartum chemoprophylaxis, *N Engl J Med* 314:1665-1669, 1986.

14. Smaill F: Intrapartum antibiotics for group B streptococcal colonisation, *Cochrane Database Syst Rev* (2):CD000115, 2000.

15. Schrag S, Gorwitz R, Fultz-Butts K et al: Prevention of perinatal group B streptococcal disease. Revised guidelines from CDC, *MMWR Recomm Rep* 51(RR-11):1-22, 2002.

16. Pearlman M, Pierson C, Faix R: Frequent resistance of clinical group B streptococci isolates to clindamycin and erythromycin, *Obstet Gynecol* 92:258-261, 1998.

17. Pylipow M, Gaddis M, Kinney J: Selective intrapartum prophylaxis for group B streptococcus colonization: management and outcome of newborns, *Pediatrics* 93:631-635, 1994.

18. American Academy of Pediatrics, Committee on Infectious Diseases 1991–1992: Recommendations for prevention of early-onset neonatal GBS infection, 1992, American Academy of Pediatrics.

19. American Academy of Pediatrics: Revised guidelines for prevention of early-onset group B streptococcal (GBS) infection. American Academy of Pediatrics Committee on Infectious Disease and Committee on Fetus and Newborn, *Pediatrics* 99:489-496, 1997.

20. ACOG committee opinion: Prevention of early-onset group B streptococcal disease in newborns. Number 173–June 1996. Committee on Obstetric Practice. American College of Obstetrics and Gynecologists, *Int J Gynaecol Obstet* 54:197-205, 1996.

21. Prevention of perinatal group B streptococcal disease: a public health perspective. Centers for Disease Control and Prevention, *MMWR Recomm Rep* 45(RR-7):1-24, 1996.

22. Rouse D, Goldenberg R, Cliver S et al: Strategies for the prevention of early-onset neonatal group B streptococcal sepsis: a decision analysis, *Obstet Gynecol* 83:483-494, 1994.

23. Schrag S, Gorwitz R, Fultz-Butts K, Schuchat A: Prevention of perinatal group B streptococcal disease. Revised guidelines from CDC, *MMWR Recomm Rep* 51(RR-11):1-22, 2002.

24. Schrag SJ, Zell ER, Lynfield R et al: A population-based comparison of strategies to prevent early-onset group B streptococcal disease in neonates, *N Engl J Med* 347:233-239, 2002.

25. Money DM, Dobson S: The prevention of early onset neonatal group B streptococcal disease, *J Obstet Gynaecol Can* 26:826-840, 2004.

26. Apgar BS, Greenberg G, Yen G: Prevention of group B streptococcal disease in the newborn, *Am Fam Physician* 71:903-910, 2005.

27. Chen KT, Puopolo KM, Eichenwald EC et al: No increase in rates of early-onset neonatal sepsis by antibiotic-resistant group B Streptococcus in the era of intrapartum antibiotic prophylaxis, *Am J Obstet Gynecol* 192:1167-1171, 2005.

28. Sinha A, Yokoe D, Platt R: Intrapartum antibiotics and neonatal invasive infections caused by organisms other than group B streptococcus, *J Pediatr* 142:492-497, 2003.

29. Rentz AC, Samore MH, Stoddard GJ et al: Risk factors associated with ampicillin-resistant infection in newborns in the era of group B streptococcal prophylaxis, *Arch Pediatr Adolesc Med* 158:556-560, 2004.

30. Kasper D, Paoletti L, Wessels M et al: Immune response to type III group B streptococcal polysaccharide-tetanus toxoid conjugate vaccine, *J Clin Invest* 98:2308-2314, 1996.

VI. BACTERIAL VAGINOSIS
Stephen D. Ratcliffe, MD, MSPH

A. Epidemiology

Bacterial vaginosis (BV) is the most common vaginal infection. It affects between 15% and 20% of women in the general population. It is a clinical syndrome where the vaginal flora has changed from one of being 95% lactobacilli to a mixed one where there are increased concentrations of *Gardnerella vaginalis, Mobiluncus, Bacteroides,* and *Mycoplasma* species.[1]

B. Natural History

Women who are symptomatic with BV present with a malodorous, homogeneous vaginal discharge. Vulvar pain, irritation, and itching are usually not present with BV infections. About 50% of BV infections are asymptomatic.[1]

C. Association of Bacterial Vaginosis with Adverse Perinatal Outcome

Prospective studies show an independent association between BV and increased rates of spontaneous abortion, PPROM, PTL, chorioamnionitis, and postcesarean endometritis.[2-5]

D. Diagnosis

1. Amsel criteria

   The Amsel criteria, developed in 1983, is the method most commonly used in clinical practice[6] (Table 9-2). The presence of three or more of these factors supports a diagnosis of BV. Primary care clinicians can develop the laboratory skills to make this diagnosis.

TABLE 9-2 Amsel Criteria

1. Thin, homogeneous discharge
2. pH greater than 4.5
3. Positive whiff test (fishy odor after placing a few drops of potassium hydroxide with the vaginal specimen)
4. Presence of 25% or greater of clue cells (epithelial cells heavily coated with bacilli that cause a stippled appearance)

  a. Presence of clue cells: Using this finding as the sole criterion for diagnosing BV has a sensitivity of 92%, a specificity of 97%,[7] and a number needed to diagnose (NND) of 1.12 (for a discussion of number needed to diagnose, see Chapter 3, Section F, Part II)

  b. Using pH: Using pH as the sole criterion results in a sensitivity of 87%, a specificity of 45%,[7] and a NND of 3.13.

  c. Whiff test: Using the whiff test alone to diagnose BV results in a sensitivity of 81%, a specificity of 99%,[7] and a NND of 1.25.

2. Nugent method
   The Nugent method uses a Gram stain to identify coccobacilli that are present with BV. A score greater than or equal to 7 diagnoses BV. Using Amsel's criteria as a gold standard, the Nugent method showed a sensitivity of 97%, a specificity of 98%,[7] and a NND of 1.05. This method requires trained microbiologists. This method has been used extensively in the research setting to diagnose BV.

3. Diamine swab test
   This is a commercially available test that has a sensitivity of 97%, a specificity of 83%,[8] and a NND of 1.25.

4. Papanicolaou (Pap) smear
   Using the Nugent method as the comparison gold standard, the sensitivity and specificity of the Pap smear was 43% and 94%, respectively,[9] giving this test a NND for BV of 2.7.

5. Vaginal culture
   Using the Nugent method as the comparison gold standard, the sensitivity and specificity of vaginal culture was 78% and 98%,[9] respectively, with an NND of 1.32.

6. Method of obtaining vaginal specimen
   Strauss and colleagues[10] demonstrated that patients who submitted self-obtained specimens had substantial agreement (weighted κ = 0.82) with physician-obtained specimens that used Gram stain and pH determinations of BV status.

E. Evidence Regarding Treatment of Bacterial Vaginosis in Pregnancy

1. Symptomatic patients
   The CDC Guideline for STD Treatment for 2006 recommends treatment of all symptomatic patients with BV during pregnancy with one of the methods outlined in Table 9-3.[10a]

2. Asymptomatic patients
   Extensive literature is available about the effect of diagnosing and treating asymptomatic BV in pregnancy.

  a. Screening/treatment of asymptomatic BV in the patient at low risk: One of the first multicenter RCTs of screening and treating asymptomatic BV in women at low risk identified women with BV between 16 and 24 weeks of gestation.[11] Those randomized into the treatment arm received two 2-g doses of metronidazole. Women who remained positive for BV were treated again in the 24- to 30-week period. Treatment of these women positive for BV did not reduce PTD or any other relevant perinatal complications.

    An RCT using 7 days of an intravaginal treatment with 2% clindamycin at the first prenatal visit between 10 and 17 weeks of gestation did not decrease the rate of preterm deliveries.[12] A similar RCT using intravaginal clindamycin (home treatment for a week) did not decrease the rate of preterm deliveries but was associated with a decrease in deliveries before 32 weeks of gestation.[13]

    In contrast with the above studies, Ugwumadu and co-workers conducted an RCT of 6120 women who were screened for BV using the

TABLE 9-3 Recommended Regimens for Bacterial Vaginosis for Pregnant Women

Metronidazole 500 mg orally twice a day for 7 days
or
Metronidazole 250 mg orally three times a day for 7 days
or
Clindamycin 300 mg orally twice a day for 7 days

Sexually transmitted diseases treatment guidelines, 2006, *MMWR* 55(RR-11):51-52, 2006.

Nugent method who underwent second-trimester treatment with oral clindamycin (300 mg twice daily for 5 days) versus placebo.[14] The treatment group had a statistically significant decrease in PTD (<24 weeks) and late miscarriage (>13 weeks).

b. Screening/treatment of asymptomatic BV in the patient at high risk: Evidence that supports the effectiveness of screening and treatment of asymptomatic BV in patients with a history of PTD to reduce the risk for subsequent PTD is lacking in a 2005 Cochrane review[15] and two recent metaanalyses.[16,17] However, this screening and treatment may decrease the risk for PPROM and LBW infants.[15] This evidence is based on only 2 trials of 114 women.

F. Antibiotic Treatment of Women in Fetal Fibronectin–Positive Women

The detection of fetal fibronectin (FFN) in vaginal secretions after 22 weeks of gestation is associated with an increased risk for PTD.[18] A preliminary RCT suggested that the treatment of women who tested positive for FFN with two courses of metronidazole decreased the incidence of PTD.[19] A large cohort of women (16,317) were screened at 21 to 26 weeks of gestation for the presence of vaginal FFN and 6.6% (715) were positive.[20] These women were randomized to treatment with metronidazole and erythromycin versus placebo. This treatment did not result in a decrease in deliveries before 32, 35, or 37 weeks of gestation. Therefore, based on the best data available, in the setting of a patient who tested positive for FFN before 26 weeks of gestation, treatment with metronidazole and erythromycin does not seem to affect the incidence of PTD.

G. SOR A Recommendations

RECOMMENDATIONS	REFERENCES
Screening and treatment of asymptomatic BV in pregnancy in the general population does not result in a decrease of PTD.	15-17
Screening and treatment of asymptomatic BV in pregnancy for women with a previous history of PTD may decrease the risk for PPROM (NNT = 4.0) and LBW infants (NNT = 4.8) but does not decrease the incidence of PTD.	15

REFERENCES

1. Eschenbach D: Bacterial vaginosis and anaerobes in obstetric-gynecologic infection, *Clin Infect Dis* 16:S282-S287, 1993.
2. Gibbs R: Chorioamnionitis and bacterial vaginosis, *Am J Obstet Gynecol* 169:460-462, 1993.
3. Hillier S, Nugent R, Eschenbach D et al: Association between bacterial vaginosis and preterm delivery of a low-birth-weight infant, *N Engl J Med* 333:1737-1742, 1995.
4. Kimberlin D, Andrews W: Bacterial vaginosis: association with adverse pregnancy outcome, *Semin Perinatol* 22:242-250, 1998.
5. Leitich H, Bodner-Adler B, Brunbauer M et al: Bacterial vaginosis as a risk factor for preterm delivery: a meta-analysis, *Am J Obstet Gynecol* 189:139-147, 2003.
6. Amsel R, Totten P, Spiegel C et al: Nonspecific vaginitis: diagnostic and microbial and epidemiological associations, *Am J Med* 74:14-22, 1983.
7. Coppolillo EF, Perazzi BE, Famiglietti AM et al: Diagnosis of bacterial vaginosis during pregnancy, *J Low Genit Tract Dis* 7:117-121, 2003.
8. O'Dowd T, West R, Winterburn P et al: Evaluation of a rapid diagnostic test for bacterial vaginosis, *Br J Obstet Gynaecol* 103:366-370, 1996.
9. Tokyol C, Aktepe OC, Cevrioglu AS et al: Bacterial vaginosis: comparison of Pap smear and microbiological test results, *Mod Pathol* 17:857-860, 2004.
10. Strauss RA, Eucker B, Savitz DA et al: Diagnosis of bacterial vaginosis from self-obtained vaginal swabs, *Infect Dis Obstet Gynecol* 13:31-35, 2005.
10a. Centers for Disease Control and Prevention: Sexually transmitted diseases treatment guidelines, 2006, *MMWR* 55:51-52, 2006. Available at: www.cdc.gov/std/treatment. Accessed September 19, 2007.
11. Carey JC, Klebanoff MA, Hauth JC et al: Metronidazole to prevent preterm delivery in pregnant women with asymptomatic bacterial vaginosis. National Institute of Child Health and Human Development Network of Maternal-Fetal Medicine Units, *N Engl J Med* 342:534-540, 2000.
12. Kekki M, Kurki T, Pelkonen J et al: Vaginal clindamycin in preventing preterm birth and peripartal infections in asymptomatic women with bacterial vaginosis: a randomized, controlled trial, *Obstet Gynecol* 97:643-648, 2001.
13. Larsson PG, Fahraeus L, Carlsson B et al: Late miscarriage and preterm birth after treatment with clindamycin: a randomized consent design study according to Zelen, *BJOG* 113:629-637, 2006.
14. Ugwumadu A, Manyonda I, Reid F et al: Effect of early oral clindamycin on late miscarriage and preterm delivery in asymptomatic women with abnormal vaginal flora and bacterial vaginosis: a randomized controlled trial, *Lancet* 361:983-988, 2003.
15. McDonald H, Brocklehurst P, Parsons J: Antibiotics for treating bacterial vaginosis in pregnancy, *Cochrane Database Syst Rev* (1):CD000262, 2005.
16. Riggs M, Klebanoff JA: Treatment of vaginal infections to prevent preterm birth: a meta-analysis, *Clin Obstet* 47:796-807, 2004.
17. Okun N, Gronau KA, Hannah ME: Antibiotics for bacterial vaginosis or *Trichomonas vaginalis* in pregnancy: a systematic review, *Obstet Gynecol* 105:857-868, 2005.
18. Andrews WW, Goldenberg RL: What we have learned from an antibiotic trial in fetal fibronectin positive women, *Semin Perinatol* 27:231-238, 2003.
19. Goldenberg RL, Klebanoff M, Carey JC et al: Metronidazole treatment of women with a positive fetal fibronectin test result, *Am J Obstet Gynecol* 185:485-486, 2001.

20. Andrews WW, Sibai BM, Thom EA et al: Randomized clinical trial of metronidazole plus erythromycin to prevent spontaneous preterm delivery in fetal fibronectin-positive women, *Obstet Gynecol* 101:847-855, 2003.

VII. CANDIDA VULVOVAGINITIS
Rachel Elizabeth Hall, MD, FAAFP

A. Epidemiology
Candida vulvovaginitis is one of the most common vaginal infections. It is estimated that three of four women will have at least one candidal vulvovaginitis in their childbearing years. The incidence of this condition is increasing, with approximately 13 millions cases reported in the United States per year.[1] Candida vulvovaginitis is also more common during pregnancy because of multiple factors.[2,3]

1. Microbiology
   Most infections are caused by *Candida albicans.* Non-albicans species such as *Candida tropicalis* and *Candida glabrata* are becoming increasingly common and can be a source of antifungal resistance.
2. Conditions associated with candidal infections
   a. Diabetes mellitus
   b. Cushings or Addison's disease
   c. Hypothyroidism or hyperthyroidism
   d. Malignancies
   e. Human immunodeficiency virus (HIV)
   f. Pregnancy
   g. Vaginal trauma
3. Other predisposing risk factors
   a. Antibiotic therapy
   b. Hormone therapy
   c. Corticosteroids
   d. Radiotherapy or chemotherapy
   e. Immunosuppressive therapy
   f. Multiple sexual partners
   g. Tight-fitting/synthetic-fiber clothing

B. Natural History
Candida vaginitis may be asymptomatic or symptomatic; it is characterized by heavy, white, curdlike vaginal discharge, often with severe vaginal or vulvar pruritus and inflammation. No signs or symptoms of candida infection are specific for the diagnosis.[4]

C. Effect on Perinatal Outcome
Infection in pregnancy may be more difficult to eradicate; recurrence is common. Otherwise, there are no other effects on perinatal outcome.[3,5]

D. Diagnosis
1. Physical examination
   Marked vulvar erythema and swelling may be seen in women with symptomatic infections. A thick, white, curdlike discharge is often present.
2. Microscopic diagnosis
   This infection can be detected as budding yeast or hyphae on potassium hydroxide (KOH) preparation. It may be seen on Pap smear or on urinalysis if there is a contaminated specimen.

E. Management
Multiple regimens exist for the treatment of vulvovaginal candidiasis in pregnancy, with generally longer course of any medication used to effect remission of symptoms. One study found that 4 days of topical therapy cured about half of the infections in pregnant women, whereas there was a 90% cure rate when a 7-day course was used.[5] A TOC is not necessary[4]; patients need follow-up only if symptoms persist or recur within 2 months.[6] The CDC recommends only topical therapy,[1,4,6] but treatment with low-dose fluconazole (150-mg single dose) is generally considered safe. It is well documented that a regimen of daily doses exceeding 400 mg in the first trimester is teratogenic.[7] Treatment of sexual partners is not recommended but may be considered in light of recurrent infections.[6] Note that oral therapy is contraindicated during pregnancy.[1,4]

1. Clotrimazole (over the counter, class B).
   Several studies have demonstrated the safety of clotrimazole in pregnancy.[3]
   1% cream, 5 g for 7 to 14 days or vaginal tablets 100 mg for 7 days, 200 mg for 3 days, or 500 mg for a single dose
2. Miconazole (over the counter, class C)
   2% cream, 5 g for 7 to 14 days or 100-mg vaginal tablet, 200-mg vaginal tablet for 3 days or 500-mg vaginal tablet for 1 day
3. Nystatin (prescription, class B)
   100,000-unit vaginal tablet for 14 days
4. Butoconazole (prescription, class C)
   2% cream, 5 g for 3 days
5. Terconazole (prescription, class C)
   0.4% cream, 5 g for 7 days or 0.8% cream 5 g for 3 days
6. Tioconazole (prescription, class C)
   6.5% ointment, 5-g single dose
7. Nystatin cream (prescription, class B)
   14-day treatment, not as effective

8. Boric acid capsules
   600-mg gelatin capsules per dose for two doses
9. Gentian violet
   One application a week for 2 weeks (effective but messy)

F. SOR A Recommendation

RECOMMENDATION	REFERENCES
Topical azole therapies, applied for 7 days, are recommended for treatment of vulvovaginal candidiasis in pregnancy.	5, 6

REFERENCES

1. Tobin MJ: Vulvovaginal candidiasis: topical vs. oral therapy, *Am Fam Physician* 51:1715-1720, 1995.
2. Fonck K, Kidula N, Jaoko W et al: Validity of the vaginal discharge algorithm among pregnant and non-pregnant women in Nairobi, Kenya, *Sex Transm Infect* 76:33-38, 2000.
3. Moudgal VV, Sobel JD: Antifungal drugs in pregnancy: a review, *Exp Opin Drug Saf* 2:475-483, 2003.
4. Association for Genitourinary Medicine, Medical Society for the Study of Venereal Disease: *2002 national guideline on the management of vulvovaginal candidiasis*, London, 2002, Association for Genitourinary Medicine, Medical Society for the Study of Venereal Disease.
5. Young GL, Jewell D: Topical treatment for vaginal candidiasis (thrush) in pregnancy, *Cochrane Database Syst Rev* (4): CD000225, 2001.
6. Sexually transmitted diseases treatment guidelines 2002. Centers for Disease Control and Prevention, *MMWR Recomm Rep* 51(RR-6):1-78, 2002.
7. Briggs GG, Freeman RK, Yaffe SJ: *Drugs in pregnancy and lactation,* ed 7, Philadelphia, 2005, Lippincott Williams & Wilkins.

VIII. TRICHOMONAS VAGINALIS
Stephen D. Ratcliffe, MD, MSPH

A. Epidemiology
The prevalence of *Trichomonas vaginalis*, a unicellular flagellated protozoan, in the prospective Vaginitis in Pregnancy (VIP) study was 12.6% (n = 13,816).[1] In that study, the prevalence among black women was 22.8% compared with 6.6% among Hispanic and 6.1% among white women. Other factors that were associated with an increased risk for *Trichomonas* infection include being unmarried, lower income, lower educational attainment, and smoking. *Trichomonas* infection is also associated with an increased risk for concurrent gonorrhea, chlamydia, GBS, and BV.[2]

B. Natural History
Infection often presents with copious frothy, greenish to clear, watery vaginal discharge; vaginal pruritus; dyspareunia; or dysuria. Spotting may be a common presentation because of cervical inflammation. Physical examination may reveal vaginal erythema, often accompanied by cervicitis, sometimes described as a strawberry cervix.[3]

C. Effect on Perinatal Outcome
T. vaginalis infection in pregnancy is associated with a 40% increase in premature, LBW infants.[2,4] Women with this infection are also more likely to have PPROM, postpartum endometritis, stillborn fetuses, and neonatal deaths than are women without *Trichomonas* infection.

Despite the association of *Trichomonas* infection with adverse perinatal outcomes, the treatment of *Trichomonas* infection in pregnancy is associated with an increase in the incidence of preterm birth.[5,6] The available evidence does not support the routine screening and treatment of this common vaginal infection.

D. Diagnosis
Most office settings use a microscopic vaginal wet prep to diagnose symptomatic infections. Motile flagellated organisms are diagnostic of infection. However, the VIP study demonstrated that *Trichomonas* infections are common in the absence of the classical symptoms, and thus are often underdiagnosed.[1] The sensitivity of the wet prep was 55.8%, specificity 98.5%, positive predictive value 78.4%, and negative predictive value 95.7% using culture as the standard diagnostic test.

E. Management
Although there is no evidence to routinely screen and treat this vaginal infection, many women are often symptomatic and will require treatment. A Cochrane review demonstrated a 90% cure rate with a single 2-g dose of oral metronidazole.[6] Sexual partners should be treated as well. Evidence supports that metronidazole is not teratogenic in humans, although some clinicians delay the use of metronidazole past the period of organogenesis.[7]

F. SOR A Recommendation

RECOMMENDATION	REFERENCE
Treatment of T. vaginalis in pregnancy with metronidazole reduces the risk for persistent infection but increases the incidence of preterm birth.	5

REFERENCES

1. Cotch M, Pastorek J, Nugent R et al: *Trichomonas vaginalis* associated with low birth weight and preterm delivery, *Sex Transm Dis* 24:353-560, 1997.
2. Pastorek J, Cotch M, Martin D et al: Clinical and microbiological correlates of vaginal trichomoniasis during pregnancy, *Clin Infect Dis* 23:1075-1080, 1996.
3. Ament L, Whalen E: Sexually transmitted diseases in pregnancy: diagnosis, impact, and intervention, *J Obstet Gynecol Neonatal Nurs* 25:657-666, 1996.
4. Sutton M, Sternberg M, Nsuami M et al: Trichomoniasis in pregnant human immunodeficiency virus-uninfected Congolese women: prevalence risk factors, and association with low birth weight, *Am J Obstet Gynecol* 181:656-662, 1999.
5. Okun N, Gronau KA, Hannah ME: Antibiotics for bacterial vaginosis or *Trichomonas vaginalis* in pregnancy: a systematic review, *Obstet Gynecol* 105:857-868, 2005.
6. Gulmezoglu AM: Interventions for trichomoniasis in pregnancy, *Cochrane Database Syst Rev* (3):CD000220, 2002.
7. Burtin P, Taddio A, Ariburnu O et al: Safety of metronidazole in pregnancy: a meta-analysis, *Am J Obstet Gynecol* 172:525-529, 1995.

IX. HERPES SIMPLEX, TYPE II (GENITAL)

Stephen D. Ratcliffe, MD, MSPH

A. Epidemiology

The third National Health and Nutrition Examination Surveys (NHANES III) showed that the age-adjusted prevalence of herpes simplex virus type 2 (HSV-2) among female individuals 12 years and older was 21%, a 30% increase compared with the survey done in 1980.[1] The groups identified as having the highest seroprevalence include black women, Mexican American women, and women living in poverty, having numerous sexual partners, and using illicit drugs. Between NHANES II and III there was a fivefold increase in the seroprevalence of HSV-2 among white adolescents and a twofold increase among white women in their twenties. Most people (90%) with positive serology in this study reported no history of previous herpes infections.

The most recent NHANES IV that measured the health status in the United States between 1999 and 2004 demonstrated some remarkable improvements in the seroprevalence of HSV-2 among US women.[2] The age-adjusted prevalence decreased to 17%, a 19% decrease from a decade earlier. Patients' knowledge of their HSV-2 status increased from 10% to 14%.

B. Natural History

1. Primary genital HSV infection and pregnancy
   A large, prospective study of HSV-seronegative women demonstrated that approximately 2% of these women acquire this infection during pregnancy.[3] Thirty percent are acquired in the first and second trimesters and 40% in the third trimester. It is this latter group that is at increased risk for vertical transmission of the virus to the newborn because of insufficient time to mount a maternal IgG response.
   The primary genital HSV infection is characterized by multiple vesicular lesions and may have systemic symptoms of fever and regional lymphadenopathy. Antibodies to HSV-1 and HSV-2 are absent. This initial infection is often asymptomatic. This is supported by Hensleigh and colleagues' study[4] that demonstrated in a prospective cohort that only 1 of 23 women presenting with symptoms consistent with primary genital herpes simplex infection had negative serologic testing to support this diagnosis.[4]

2. Nonprimary first-episode genital HSV
   This occurs with a first-time genital infection to HSV-1 when antibodies to HSV-2 are already present or with a first-time genital infection with HSV-2 when antibodies to HSV-1 are already present. Nonprimary first episode infections have fewer systemic symptoms and a briefer duration of viral shedding.[5]

3. Recurrent infection
   Recurrent infections are usually accompanied by single or few lesions, prodromal itching, hyperesthesia, or dysesthesia in the affected area, and last from 5 to 7 days. Reactivation of HSV-2 may be completely asymptomatic such that about 1% of infected persons are shedding the virus at a given time.

C. Effects on Perinatal Outcome

1. Spontaneous miscarriage

   The medical literature provides conflicting evidence whether HSV-2 is associated with an increased risk for spontaneous miscarriage.[6]

2. Increased risk for PTL and delivery

   Primary infections in the second half of pregnancy have been associated with an increased risk of premature labor and delivery, and an increased risk for vertical transmission.[6]

3. Vertical transmission to the newborn

   About 70% to 85% of infections occur in infants in whom there is no history of maternal peripartum genital herpes infection. Transmission rates vary depending on whether viral shedding takes place with or without symptoms, or during an initial or recurrent infection. Mortality or neurologic impairment occurs in 40% of infected neonates. As noted earlier, the greatest risk for vertical transmission appears to be in late third-trimester primary herpes infections when women have not yet seroconverted. The rate of transmission is much lower in recurrent infections, estimated to be about 1 in 100.[5,6]

D. Diagnosis

1. Culture

   Culture of unroofed lesions remains the gold standard, although this test has a limited sensitivity because the herpes virus stops shedding before the lesion resolves; hence, the culture may have a false-negative result about 25% of the time. The yield of positive cultures on recurrent lesions is only 50%. The clinician should keep this mind when interpreting the culture results. This test has 100% specificity, that is, no false-positive results.

2. DNA PCR testing

   This is the emerging diagnostic test of choice because of its high sensitivity (95%) that can detect the presence of the virus as long as the ulcer is present. This modality also has a specificity of 90%. The higher cost of this test is limiting its use in primary care practices at this time.

3. Serologic testing

   Commercial tests can differentiate between HSV-1 and HSV-2 IgG antibodies. This testing can assist the clinician in diagnosing a case of primary herpes when the culture or PCR is positive and the serology for HSV-1 and HSV-2 IgG is negative.

E. Management during Pregnancy to Prevent Neonatal Herpes

1. Primary genital HSV

   a. Prenatal care: The initial prenatal assessment should include a careful history for genital lesions, specifically "blisters," ulcers, painful lesions, lesions associated with genital dysesthesias, and prodromal symptoms. Women with no known history of HSV whose partners have a history of recurrent herpes should be counseled to use condoms throughout pregnancy and to report symptoms suggestive of HSV.

   b. Primary HSV: Special attention must be given to women who may have contracted primary HSV during pregnancy, particularly if this has occurred in the late third trimester. Women at this stage of pregnancy with positive cultures or PCR testing and negative serologies are at high risk for vertical transmission of HSV to their newborn and should be comanaged with a perinatologist if possible.[7]

2. Recurrent genital HSV

   a. Routine third-trimester cultures: They are not indicated because of an inability to predict viral shedding at the time of delivery. RCT evidence reports that this practice has not decreased viral transmission rates.[8]

   b. Labor room assessment: This should include inquiries regarding recent lesions, even if the patient has no history of HSV. All patients with lesions or symptoms should be examined for herpes. Lesions that are distant from the vulva, vagina, and cervix are not a contraindication to vaginal delivery.[5] They should be covered with a dressing to prevent direct contact with the newborn.

   c. Indication for cesarean section: Cesarean intervention has been recommended for active herpes lesions or prodromal symptoms such as vulvar pain or burning. There appears to be no arbitrary time after rupture of the membranes when performing a cesarean section is not beneficial in preventing vertical transmission of the virus.[9] Some controversy exists as to the cost-effectiveness of performing cesarean section for patients with recurrent, active lesions because the neonatal transmission rate is low.[10]

   d. Acyclovir prophylaxis to prevent recurrent lesions: Several RCTs have investigated the use of acyclovir (400 mg orally three times a day from 36 to 40 weeks) to prevent the recurrence of symptomatic herpes.[11,12] This approach has been associated with decreased cesarean section rates without any increase in neonatal herpes infections. Acyclovir, a class C agent, appears to be safe in pregnancy.

3. Screening for herpes in women with no known history of genital HSV

Because most women with serologic evidence of chronic herpes infections have no knowledge of a previous infection, there has been interest in doing universal screening of women and their partners for types 1 and 2 HSV antibodies.[13] Universal screening would require treatment of 3849 women[14] and cost $4.1 million to prevent 1 case of neonatal death or disease with severe complications.[15] The US Preventive Services Task Force (USPSTF) does not recommend universal screening in pregnancy for this reason.[16]

F. Management of Neonatal Herpes

Clinicians should maintain a high risk of suspicion for neonatal herpes infection in infants who have signs or symptoms of sepsis such as irritability, lethargy, fever, or failure to feed.[17,18] Forty-five percent of neonatal herpes infections are localized to the skin, 25% are disseminated, and 30% have encephalitis. As described earlier, there may be no previous history of maternal infection. Diagnosis should be made using PCR testing of lesions and cerebrospinal fluid. Treatment consists of acyclovir (60 mg/kg/day) for 14 days for localized skin infections and 21 days for disseminated or central nervous system infections.

G. SOR A Recommendation

RECOMMENDATION	REFERENCE
Prophylactic use of acyclovir (400 mg three times a day) during the last 4 weeks of pregnancy reduces the risk for recurrence of herpes infection (NNT = 8) and subsequent need for cesarean section (NNT = 11).	12

REFERENCES

1. Fleming D, McQuillan G, Johnson R et al: Herpes simplex virus type 2 in the United States, 1976–1994, *N Engl J Med* 337:1105-1111, 1997.

2. Xu F, Sternberg MR, Kottiri BJ et al: Trends in herpes simplex virus type 1 and type 2 seroprevalence in the United States, *JAMA* 296:964-973, 2006.

3. Brown Z, Selke S, Zeh J et al: The acquisition of herpes simplex virus during pregnancy, *N Engl J Med* 337:509-515, 1997.

4. Hensleigh P, Andrews W, Brown ZA et al: Genital herpes during pregnancy: inability to distinguish primary and recurrent infections clinically, *Obstet Gynecol* 89:891-895, 1997.

5. ACOG practice bulletin: clinical management guidelines for obstetrician-gynecologists, Number 57, November 2004. Gynecologic herpes simplex virus infections, *Obstet Gynecol* 104:1111-1118, 2004.

6. Brown ZA, Benedetti J, Ashley R et al: Neonatal herpes simplex virus infection in relation to asymptomatic maternal infection at the time of labor, *N Engl J Med* 324:1247-1252, 1991.

7. Smith J, Cowan F, Munday P et al: The management of herpes simplex virus infection in pregnancy, *Br J Obstet Gynaecol* 105:255-260, 1998.

8. Arvin A, Hensleigh P, Prober C et al: Failure of antepartum maternal cultures to predict the infant's risk of exposure to herpes simplex virus at delivery, *N Engl J Med* 35:796-800, 1986.

9. Randolph A, Washington E, Prober C: Cesarean delivery for women presenting with genital herpes lesions: efficacy, risks, and costs, *JAMA* 270:77-82, 1993.

10. Gibbs R, Amstey M, Lezotte D: Role of cesarean delivery in preventing neonatal herpes virus infection, *JAMA* 270:94-95, 1993.

11. Watts DH, Brown ZA, Money D et al: A double-blind, randomized, placebo-controlled trial of acyclovir in late pregnancy for the reduction of herpes simplex virus shedding and cesarean delivery, *Am J Obstet Gynecol* 188:836-843, 2003.

12. Shefield JS, Hollier LM Hill JB et al: Acyclovir prophylaxis to prevent herpes simplex virus recurrence at delivery: a systematic review, *Obstet Gynecol* 102:1396-1403, 2003.

13. Baker D, Brown Z, Hollier LM et al: Cost effectiveness of herpes simplex virus type 2 serologic testing and antiviral therapy in pregnancy, *Am J Obstet Gynecol* 191:2074-2084, 2004.

14. Cleary KL, Pare E, Stamilio D et al: Type specific screening for asymptomatic herpes infection in pregnancy: a decision analysis, *BJOG* 112:731-738, 2005.

15. Thung SF, Grobman WA: The cost-effectiveness of routine antenatal screening for maternal herpes simplex virus-1 and -2 antibodies, *Am J Obstet Gynecol* 192:483-485, 2005.

16. US Preventive Services Task Force (USPSTF): Screening for genital herpes: recommended statement, Rockville, MD, 2005, Agency for Healthcare Research and Quality (AHRQ).

17. Sanchez PG: Perinatal infections and brain injury: current treatment options, *Clin Perinatol* 29:799-826, 2002.

18. Rudnick CM: Neonatal herpes simplex virus infections, *Am Fam Physician* 65:1138-1142, 2002.

X. HUMAN PAPILLOMAVIRUS
Amity Rubeor, DO

Human papillomavirus (HPV) infection is common in the United States with more than 20 million people, including pregnant women, being affected.[1]

A. Epidemiology

1. Prevalence

   The true prevalence of HPV is unknown, because it is not a reportable disease. Based on best estimates from office visits, it is likely the most common STD in the United States. About 5.5 million new cases are diagnosed every year.[1] Numerous studies have estimated prevalence in different age-groups. In 1997, Koutsky[2] estimated the prevalence of HPV among men and women 15 to 49 years of age to be 1% for genital warts, 4% for subclinical HPV detected by colposcopy or cytology, and 10% for subclinical HPV detected by DNA amplification. Prior infection was detected with antibodies to HPV in 60% of cases, and no prior infection was found 25% of the time.[2] Both Stone[3] in 2002 and Winer[4] in 2003 found that HPV-16 or other high-risk types were the most commonly detected HPV in women. Of women infected with HPV, most are infected in the first few years of becoming sexually active.[4]

2. Risk factors

   Young age is a major risk factor identified in HPV infections. Women younger than 25 years have a consistently higher prevalence, even after adjusting for other risk factors, such as number of sexual partners. The lifetime number of sexual partners remains the predominant risk factor for HPV infection.[5] Other weakly associated risk factors include oral contraceptive and tobacco use.[4] The use of oral contraceptives does not increase the prevalence of HPV but may increase the progression of the disease.[6] During pregnancy, a greater HPV viral load exists, likely secondary to relative immune suppression,[5] but results conflict whether this increases prevalence of HPV.[5,7,8] Patients who are immunocompromised, because of HIV or AIDS, also appear to have greater viral loads.[2]

B. Pathogenesis

HPVs are a group of closed-circular, double-stranded DNA viruses. They are transmitted through sexual contact with infected genital skin, mucous membranes, or body fluids from a partner with overt or subclinical HPV infection.[5] There are more than 80 subtypes of HPV, which are commonly classified as oncogenic (high risk) or non-oncogenic (low risk). Within the genome of HPV, some "early" genes (named for the timing and location of their expression) have been identified as oncoproteins (e.g., E6 and E7).[9] Their biochemical activity promotes cervical dysplasia, which may progress to malignancy. The most common oncogenic or high-risk subtypes are HPV-16 and -18. The most common non-oncogenic or low-risk subtypes are HPV-6 and -11.

C. Clinical Features

Most men or women exposed to HPV are asymptomatic; their immune system simply prevents expression of HPV at the cellular level. Some patients, as noted earlier, have a greater risk of expression. Those individuals exposed to low-risk or non-oncogenic subtypes will manifest infection as genital warts, most commonly identified as raised and "desiccated" lesions, resembling a small cauliflower.[9] In women, they can be found externally on the vulva, perineum, or surrounding the anus, or internally on the cervix, in the vagina, or within the anus. In men, common skin sites include the penis, the perineum, and perianal tissue; anal mucosa may also be involved. Lesions are usually individual but can be confluent. The clinical features of high-risk or oncogenic HPV subtypes are discussed in Section F in this chapter.

1. Maternal effects

   During pregnancy, rapid growth of condyloma can occur. These lesions may bleed, tear, cause discomfort, or lead to poor perineal healing after delivery.

2. Neonatal effects

   HPV transmission to the neonate is uncommon, and the route of transmission, whether transplacental, perinatal, or postnatal, has yet to be clearly identified.[10] A 1998 prospective study that used DNA polymerase testing observed the offspring of 112 infected women for 36 months after birth and found that, at the most, the transmission rate was 2.8%.[11] In a 1999 study, nasopharyngeal aspirates of neonates were tested at birth, 5 weeks, 6 months, 12 months, and 18 months. The rate of transmission of HPV was calculated at 30% when the birth aspirates were tested, but each subsequent aspirate was negative for HPV.[12] The rare disease of recurrent respiratory papillomatosis or laryngeal papillomatosis caused by HPV-6 and -11 has an incidence of 4 in 100,000 children; currently, prophylactic cesarean section for those women with genital warts is not recommended to prevent the disease.[13]

D. Diagnosis

1. Physical examination

   Diagnosis of low-risk, non-oncogenic HPV infection is done primarily by examination because the most common expression of low-risk HPV infection is genital warts. *Condylomata acuminata*, which resemble a small cauliflower, are the most common genital wart. However, there are less common presentations of genital warts. These include smooth, dome-shaped papules that are flesh colored and only about 1 to 4 mm in width, more keratotic genital warts that resemble a typical wart or seborrheic keratosis, and flat-topped papules that may be slightly raised.[14] Biopsy of these less common presentations may be warranted to rule out other infectious causative factors, such as syphilis and molluscum contagiosum.

2. Pap smear and HPV subtyping
Diagnosis of high-risk or oncogenic HPV is commonly done through routine Pap smear screening. Oncogenic HPV subtypes cause cervical dysplasia, which can appear as low- (LSILs) or high-grade squamous intraepithelial lesions (HSILs). In 2001, the American Society for Colposcopy and Cervical Pathology with the ACOG and 28 other participating professional and health organizations developed comprehensive evidence-based guidelines for management of cervical cytologic abnormalities.[5] Within these guidelines, identification of HPV subtypes through reflex HPV DNA subtyping was identified as an important management tool, specifically in the management of atypical squamous cells of undetermined significance (ASCUS). These guidelines are covered in greater depth in the cervical dysplasia section (see Section F).

E. Treatment

Management of high-risk HPV in pregnancy is discussed in Section F in this chapter. This section discusses treatment of low-risk HPV or genital warts. Regardless of whether a patient is pregnant, no treatment is 100% effective, and relapse can occur. Treatment cannot cure the viral infection but aims to remove bulky, unaesthetic lesions; smaller lesions may resolve spontaneously. Treatments can be administered by either the practitioner or patient; currently, no evidence suggests that any one treatment is better than another.

1. Practitioner-administered treatments
   a. Cryotherapy with liquid nitrogen (safe in pregnancy): Cryotherapy destroys the cellular tissue and active HPV within the cells of the wart. It frequently causes blisters of surrounding and underlying tissue, which can be painful. Overtreatment may lead to larger blisters and wound-care problems. It is effective for both external and vaginal/anal warts with clearance rates as great as 90% and recurrence rates of only 40%.[14]

   b. Electrodesiccation, laser or curettage (safe in pregnancy): Though expensive, these treatments offer clearance rates as great as 90%.[14] Typically, surgery or curettage is reserved for small numbers of larger warts, and laser and electrodesiccation are used on more widespread lesions that have been recalcitrant to other treatments. Specialized training is required.

   c. Trichloroacetic or bichloracetic acid (80-90%) application (safe in pregnancy): Apply trichloroacetic or bichloracetic acid to affected areas every 7 to 10 days. Apply only a small amount just to the warts themselves, allowing the solution to dry until a white "frosting" appears. These acids are caustic and destroy warts through chemical coagulation of proteins. If the acids contact adjacent normal tissue, talc, sodium bicarbonate, or liquid soap can be applied. Clearance rates have been as great as 60% to 80%, but repeated applications are frequently needed. Both acids can be applied to external and vaginal/anal warts, but generally the smaller and vaginal/anal warts respond better.[10]

   d. Podophyllin resin (5-25%) application (**contraindicated** in pregnancy): Podophyllin is an antimitotic agent that causes local tissue destruction. It is potentially fetotoxic. It should be applied only to affected areas (limit resin application to <0.5 ml or limit area treated to <10 cm²), allowed to dry, and can be repeated weekly. Four hours after application, the patient should wash the treated areas to decrease irritation.

2. Patient-administered treatments
   a. Imiquimod cream 5% (**contraindicated** in pregnancy): Imiquimod activates macrophages and dendritic cells to release interferon-α and other inflammatory cytokines killing HPV-infected cells through an immune response. It is applied once daily at bedtime, three times per week for up to 16 weeks. Six to 10 hours after application, the treated areas should be washed. Clearance rates range from 70% to 85%, and recurrence rates range from 5% to 20%.[5,14]

   b. Podofilox 0.5% solution or gel (**contraindicated** in pregnancy): Podofilox is a purified derivative of podophyllin that can be applied by a patient twice a day for 3 consecutive days, followed by 4 days of no application. Limit application amount of solution/gel to less than 0.5 ml or limit area to less than 10 cm². Clearance rates range from 45% to 90%, but recurrence can occur 30% to 60% of the time.[5,14]

With all treatments, some clearance should be noted in the first week. Growth during therapy is an indication for biopsy.[9] Warts that do not respond after 3 months of treatment should be reevaluated.[10] Hypopigmentation or hyperpigmentation can occur with all treatments. In the case of pregnancy, cesarean section may be necessary if lesions are extremely large and preclude safe vaginal delivery, but not because of transmission of infection.

F. Prevention

1. Non-oncogenic (low-risk) types

   Abstinence and monogamy with a single partner are two of the most effective ways to prevent transmission of HPV.[4,5] Limiting risk factors also effectively decrease rates of infection; this includes limiting number of sexual partners and limiting sexual partners to those with few sexual partners or those who have been abstinent for longer periods.[4,5] Theoretically, use of latex condoms should prevent transmission of virus particles, but not all areas of non-oncogenic HPV infection are covered by condoms, thus transmission can still occur.[5] Lacey and co-workers[15] studied the effect of a new vaccine against HPV-6 on 27 patients with genital warts, and 8 patients experienced complete clearing of warts with no recurrences.

   In phase II trials of Gardasil (Merck & Co., Whitehouse Station, NJ), the newly released quadrivalent vaccine composed of highly purified viruslike particles from the capsid proteins of HPV-6, -11, -16, and -18, the incidence of persistent HPV-6, -11, -16, or -18 infection at 35 months had decreased by 89% in women who received at least one dose of the vaccine compared with those who received placebo.[16] Vaccination with a quadrivalent vaccine such as this could significantly reduce the clinical manifestation of oncogenic and non-oncogenic HPV.[16] Currently, the Advisory Committee on Immunization Practices recommends administration of Gardasil via three injections (0, 2, and 6 months) to girls at 11 to 12 years of age, though it may be given starting at 9 years until 26 years of age. The vaccine is not yet recommended for men or pregnant women. Phase III trials are ongoing.

2. Oncogenic (high-risk) types

   As with non-oncogenic HPV, abstinence, monogamy, and limiting risk factors are some of the most effective ways to prevent transmission. Condom usage is still not proved to be an effective form of prevention of infection with high-risk HPV, as multiple studies have shown conflicting results.[5] However, vaccine development for high-risk HPV is advancing. In 2002, the *New England Journal of Medicine* published the results of a large clinical trial that randomized 2400 women to receive either a vaccine made with the L1 protein of HPV-16 or just the adjuvant. The vaccination schedule consisted of three injections at 0, 2, and 6 months. At follow-up in 18 months, there were no cases of HPV-16 persistent infection or HPV-16–related cervical dysplasia in those women who received the vaccine.[17] In 2006, a similar study concluded that an HPV-16 L1 vaccine could provide protection against persistent HPV-16 infection and related cervical dysplasia for at least 3.5 years after immunization, reducing the risk for cervical cancer.[18] It is estimated that although a vaccine against HPV-16 could prevent half of the cases of cervical cancer, a vaccine against HPV-16 and -18 would prevent two thirds of the cases of cervical cancer.[5] At the time of this publication, a bivalent vaccine against HPV-16 and -18 is undergoing clinical trials and may soon be released.

G. SOR A Recommendation

RECOMMENDATION	REFERENCES
The use of HPV vaccines composed of viruslike particles from HPV-16 with or without viruslike particles from HPV-6, -11, and -18 can decrease the incidence of HPV infection; however, the safety of these vaccines in pregnancy is not yet established.	16, 18

REFERENCES

1. Cates W: Estimates of the incidence and prevalence of sexually transmitted diseases in the United States, *Sex Transm Dis* 26(4):S2-S7, 1999.
2. Koutsky L: Epidemiology of genital human papillomavirus infection, *Am J Med* 102:3-8, 1997.
3. Stone K, Karem K, Sternberg M et al: Seroprevalence of human papillomavirus type 16 infection in the United States, *J Infect Dis* 186:1396-1402, 2002.
4. Winer R, Lee S, Hughes J et al: Genital human papillomavirus infections: incidence and risk factors in cohort of female university students, *Am J Epidemiol* 157(3):218-223, 2003.
5. Human papillomavirus, *ACOG Pract Bull* 61:1-22, 2005.
6. Negrini B, Schiffman M, Kurman R et al: Oral contraceptive use, human papillomavirus infection, and risk of early cytological abnormalities of the cervix, *Cancer Res* 50:4670-4675, 1990.

7. De Roda Husman A, Walboomers J, Hopman E et al: HPV prevalence in cytomorphologically normal cervical scrapes of pregnant women as determined by PCR: the age-related pattern, *J Med Virol* 46:97-102, 1995.

8. Morrison E, Gammon M, Goldberg G et al: Pregnancy and cervical infection with human papillomaviruses, *Int Fed Gynecol Obstet* 54:125-130, 1995.

9. Ault K: Human papillomavirus infections: diagnosis, treatment, and hope for a vaccine, *Obstet Gynecol Clin North Am* 30:809-817, 2003.

10. Centers for Disease Control and Prevention, Workowski KA, Berman SM: Sexually transmitted diseases treatment guidelines, 2006, *MMWR Recomm Rep* 55(RR-11):1-94, 2006.

11. Watts D, Koutsky L, Homes K et al: Low risk of perinatal transmission of human papillomavirus: results from a prospective cohort study, *Am J Obstet Gynecol* 178:365-373, 1998.

12. Tenti P, Zappatore R, Migliora P et al: Perinatal transmission of human papillomavirus from gravidas with latent infections, *Obstet Gynecol* 93:475-479, 1999.

13. Tasca RA, Clarke RW: Recur●nt respiratory papillomatosis, *Arch Dis Child* 91:689-691, 2006.

14. Evans R, Wiley D, Cole H: *External genital warts: diagnosis and treatment,* Chicago, 1997, American Medical Association.

15. Lacey C, Thompson H, Monteiro E et al: Phase IIa safety and immunogenicity of a therapeutic vaccine, TA-GW, in persons with genital warts, *J Infect Dis* 179:612-618, 1999.

16. Villa LL, Costa RL, Petta CA et al: Prophylactic quadrivalent human papillomavirus (types 6, 11, 16, and 18) L1 virus-like particle vaccine in young women: a randomized double-blind placebo-controlled multicentre phase II efficacy trial, *Lancet Oncol* 6:271-278, 2005.

17. Koutsky L, Ault K, Wheeler C et al: A controlled trial of a human papillomavirus type 16 vaccine, *N Engl J Med* 347:1645-1651, 2002.

18. Mao C, Koutsky LA, Ault K et al: Efficacy of human papillomavirus-16 vaccine to prevent cervical intraepithelial neoplasia, *Obstet Gynecol* 107(1):18-27, 2006.

XI. HEPATITIS B
Amity Rubeor, DO

The hepatitis B virus (HBV) is highly infectious and endemic in multiple countries, where chronic carriers of HBV serve as a primary reservoir of the virus.[1] The risk for development of chronic hepatitis after HBV infection is inversely related to the age at the time of acute infection. Thus, with perinatal exposure, neonates have a risk as great as 90% of becoming chronic carriers of HBV.[1]

A. Epidemiology
HBV is endemic in Africa, Eastern Europe, the Middle East, Central Asia, China, Southeast Asia, the Pacific Islands, and the Amazon basin of South America.[1] Prevalence in the United States is partially influenced by immigration from these endemic countries. In the United States, HBV accounts for 40% to

45% of all cases of hepatitis.[2] In 2002, the reported incidence of acute HBV infection in the United States was 8064 cases.[3] In pregnancy, the prevalence of acute HBV infection is 1 to 2 per 1000 pregnancies, and for chronic HBV infection, the prevalence is 5 to 15 per 1000 pregnancies.[2]

Individuals at risk for HBV infection include[4]:
1. Individuals with multiple sexual partners
2. Individuals with a sexual partner who has multiple sexual partners
3. Individuals with a history of sexually transmitted infections
4. Men who have sex with men
5. Unvaccinated health-care workers
6. Unvaccinated household members living with an HBV-infected individual
7. Intravenous drug users

B. Pathogenesis
HBV is an enveloped, double-stranded DNA virus that contains three principle antigens. The intact virus is known as the Dane particle. The surface antigen (HBsAg) is present on the envelope and circulates freely on infection. Its presence in an individual's serum indicates either an acute infection or chronic carriage. The middle portion of the Dane particle contains the core antigen (HBcAg); it does not circulate in the serum but is present only in infected hepatocytes. The hepatitis B e antigen (HBeAg) is found in the serum and indicates an extremely high inoculum and active viral replication.

Infected individuals do not need to be symptomatic to pass the virus to others. The virus spreads through percutaneous or mucosal exposure to infected blood or bodily fluids; blood contains the greatest concentration of HBV. Therefore, sharing needles with infected individuals, sexual contact with infected individuals, perinatal exposure, and even long-term household exposure to infected individuals can transmit the virus.[1] No evidence has been reported that breastfeeding poses an additional risk for transmission of HBV from lactating carriers to their infants.[5] All blood donors are screened for HBsAg; therefore, transmission through blood or blood product transfusion is rare.[6]

C. Clinical Course and Features
The clinical course of an HBV infection can be described in four phases[7,8]:
1. Immune tolerant
   The first phase, known as the *immune tolerant phase,* is the phase of viral incubation. HBV has an

incubation period of 45 to 180 days (1-6 months).[9] Without an immune response, HBV begins replication, shedding HBsAg and HBeAg into the serum. There is no acute liver inflammation and no increase in serum transaminase concentrations. In an infected neonate, this phase could last for years.[4]

2. Immune response

The next phase involves an "immune response"; when liver inflammation begins, transaminase concentrations become increased, and the immune system tries to develop antibodies against the different HBV antigens, including HBcAg found in the hepatocytes. Approximately 70% of adults and 90% of children younger than 5 years are asymptomatic in this phase.[4] Individuals who do experience development of acute hepatitis present with flu-like symptoms, including low-grade fever, malaise, fatigue, anorexia, and right upper quadrant or epigastric pain. On examination, the patient may exhibit jaundice, hepatomegaly, or upper abdominal tenderness to palpation.

A differential diagnosis for pregnant women with these signs and symptoms should include not only viral hepatitis but also acute fatty liver of pregnancy, cholestasis of pregnancy, and severe preeclampsia.[2] In 1% to 3% of individuals with acute hepatitis B, liver failure may occur. This can create life-threatening effects in a pregnant mother and her fetus. These women and those with chronic hepatitis B who have significant hepatic insufficiency should be comanaged with available high-risk or perinatology consultation. If a woman experiences development of acute HBV in the third trimester, she has a twofold to threefold increased risk for PTD, which may occur within 4 weeks of the onset of hepatitis.[10] No increased risk for intrauterine growth restriction, spontaneous abortion, or congenital abnormalities exists.[11]

If an individual remains in the "immune response" stage for longer than 6 months, he or she is given the diagnosis of chronic hepatitis B. Individuals who experience development of chronic hepatitis may also exhibit polyarteritis nodosa and/or membranous or membranoproliferative glomerulonephritis.[12]

3. Inactive carrier

In the next phase, known as the "inactive carrier" stage, active viral replication is thought to cease, and serum testing reveals antibodies to HBeAg. Most individuals, approximately 85% to 90%, enter this phase rapidly and eventually acquire lifelong immunity. However, some individuals, especially infected neonates and children, will not enter this phase rapidly but may continue to have intermittent episodes of HBV replication. Of these chronically infected individuals, 5% to 15% may seroconvert each year.[7] Individuals who continue to carry HBeAg are at increased risk for development of persistent hepatitis, cirrhosis, and hepatocellular carcinoma. The lifetime risk for death from cirrhosis or hepatocellular cancer in these individuals is 15% to 25%.[4]

4. Immune

The final phase is known as the "immune" stage. Individuals who reach this stage have antibodies against all of the antigens, which distinguish them from those who receive immunity from vaccination and have antibodies only to HBsAg. Approximately 3% of individuals infected with HBV pass from the inactive carrier to the immune stage each year.[12]

D. Diagnosis

With acute HBV, hepatic transaminases (aspartate [AST] and alanine transaminases [ALT]) are increased more than 10-fold, indicating hepatocellular injury. Often, this increase can precede signs of jaundice by approximately 1 to 2 weeks.[4] Bilirubin, alkaline phosphatase, and prothrombin time may also increase. The HBsAg has a sensitivity and specificity of 98% when testing for acute or chronic HBV infection.[13] With a positive HBsAg, one should then check for the HBeAg and IgM antibodies to HBcAg, both positive in active infection. A testing window may exist when the HBsAg is no longer positive and antibodies to HBsAg (indicating immunity) are not yet positive; positive IgM antibodies to the HBcAg will rule in HBV infection in these cases. Chronic carriers will always have HBsAg in their serum and IgG antibodies to HBcAg.

E. Treatment

1. Maternal treatment

Treatment of acute hepatitis B is largely supportive. Interferon-α and/or antiviral medications can be used in the treatment of chronic hepatitis B, but interferon-α is abortifacient and not considered safe in pregnancy.[2] A few studies have investigated the use of lamivudine (an antiviral) in pregnant women with chronic hepatitis B. Van Zonneveld and co-workers and colleagues measured the outcome of perinatal transmission in an observational study.[14] They found that using lamivudine decreased perinatal transmission, but more controlled studies need to be done before lamivudine can be recommended routinely.

2. Reducing perinatal transmission

Current management of acute and chronic hepatitis B in pregnancy focuses on reducing perinatal transmission. With acute HBV infection in the first trimester, the virus is transmitted to the newborn approximately 10% of the time.[6,15] Acute HBV infection in the third trimester can result in perinatal transmission about 80% to 90% of the time.[15] With immunoprophylactic intervention in the newborn, including hepatitis B immunoglobulin (0.5 ml HBIG given intramuscularly) and hepatitis B vaccination within 12 hours, the risk for transmission in both cases is reduced to less than 3%.[16] Infants should be bathed after birth, removing maternal blood, before either injection or vitamin K is given.[17] No evidence is available to support cesarean intervention to reduce the risk for congenital infection.

If the mother is a chronic carrier with only HBsAg in her serum, there is a 10% to 20% chance of vertical transmission, and immunoprophylaxis should be carried out in the same manner stated earlier.[2] If the mother is a chronic carrier with active viral replication and has HBeAg in her serum, then the risk for neonatal transmission is approximately 90%.[2] Without immunoprophylaxis, 85% of these infants could become chronic carriers, possibly experiencing development of chronic liver disease.[18]

If the maternal hepatitis B status is unknown on presentation to the labor and delivery suite, a woman should be screened by checking for HBsAg, and the neonate should receive the vaccine. Administration of HBIG can be delayed up to 7 days until results of maternal testing are known.

3. Breastfeeding

No evidence exists that breastfeeding poses any additional risk for transmission from HBV carrier mothers to infants. In a British study, Woo and coworkers[19] found similar rates of HBV transmission from HBsAg- and HBeAg-positive mothers to infants who were breastfed and those who were bottle-fed. Active and passive chemoprophylaxis with HBIG and the HBV vaccine should provide effective protection against congenital infection.

F. Prevention

Considered by many to be the first anticancer vaccine, the HBV vaccine is now being used in more than 100 countries as a routine immunization.[1] It has significantly decreased the prevalence of chronic hepatitis B and hepatocellular carcinoma. Between 1990 and 2004 in the United States, the greatest decline in incidence of HBV infection (94%) occurred in children and adolescents—the largest group targeted for HBV vaccination.[20]

1. Maternal

Since the publication of the previous edition of this book, the guidelines for HBV screening have changed. Now recommended by the CDC and ACOG, there is SOR level A evidence to screen all prenatal patients for HBV by testing for the HBsAg.[2,21] This is commonly done on patient presentation to her obstetrical provider and is repeated in the third trimester if her risk factors (see risk factors listed earlier) for HBV infection are high. ACOG also recommends that those women who are not immune to HBV but at risk for infection should start the vaccination series during pregnancy.[2] If an unvaccinated woman is exposed to HBV in her pregnancy, she should receive HBIG (dosed at 0.06 ml/kg) within 14 days of contact (she may need a second dose depending on the level of exposure) and then start the vaccination series.[2]

The vaccine is given in three doses at 0, 1, and 6 months. It is not necessary to restart the series if there has been a prolonged period between doses.[1] Ninety percent of healthy adults and 95% of infants, children, and adolescents have protective antibody concentrations to HBsAg after the vaccination series is completed.[22] Those individuals at risk for not developing appropriate immune response include individuals older than 30 years, obese individuals, and those who are immunodeficient.[1] By giving a booster dose of the vaccine, one can determine whether an individual just has waning immunity or if she did not develop immunity and needs an additional series.[1] Four to 12 weeks after administering the booster dose, check antibody levels to HBsAg. Those with waning immunity will have an HBs antibody level of at least 10 mIU/ml.[1]

2. Neonatal

After the administration of HBIG and the first HBV vaccine in the series, an infant born to a woman with positive HBsAg results needs to receive the additional two vaccinations at 1 to 2 and at 6 to 7 months of age. Then the infant needs to be screened at 9 to 15 months of age for antibodies to HBsAg.[20] If the infant is HBsAg negative and has an HBs antibody level of 10 mIU/ml or greater, he or she is protected and needs no further vaccination. If the infant is HBsAg negative and has a HBs antibody level less than 10 mIU/ml, he or she should be revaccinated with a second three-dose series and retested 1 to 2 months after administration of the final dose of vaccine. If the infant tests positive for HBsAg, the case should be reported to the local health department, and the infant should be observed for clearance or development of chronic HBV infection.[20]

G. SOR A Recommendation

EVIDENCE-BASED RECOMMENDATION	REFERENCES
All pregnant women should be screened for HBV by testing their serum for HBsAg.	2, 21

REFERENCES

1. Poland GA, Jacobson RM: Prevention of hepatitis B with the hepatitis B vaccine, *N Engl J Med* 351:2832-2388, 2004.
2. ACOG educational bulletin. Viral hepatitis in pregnancy. Number 248, July 1998 (replaces No. 174, November 1992). American College of Obstetricians and Gynecologists, *Int J Gynaecol Obstet* 63:195-202, 1998.
3. Incidence of acute hepatitis B—United States, 1990-2002, *MMWR Morbid Mortal Wkly Rep* 52:1252-1254, 2004.
4. Lin KW, Kirchner JT: Hepatitis B, *Am Fam Physician* 69:75-82, 2004.
5. Beasley RP, Stevens CE, Shiao IS et al: Evidence against breastfeeding as a mechanism for vertical transmission of hepatitis B, *Lancet* 2:740-741, 1975.
6. Centers for Disease Control: Protection against viral hepatitis. Recommendations of the Immunization Practices Advisory Committee (ACIP), *MMWR* 39:1-26, 1990.
7. Lee WM: Hepatitis B virus infection, *N Engl J Med* 337:1733-1745, 1997.
8. Lok AS, McMahon BJ: Chronic hepatitis B, *Hepatology* 34:1225-1241, 2001.
9. Gitlin N: Hepatitis B: diagnosis, prevention, and treatment, *Clin Chem* 43(8):1500-1506, 1997.
10. Gall SA: Maternal immunization, *Obstet Gynecol Clin North Am* 30:623-636, 2003.
11. Hieber JP, Dalton D, Shorey J et al: Hepatitis and pregnancy, *J Pediatr* 91:545-549, 1977.
12. Befeler AS, Di Bisceglie AM: Hepatitis B, *Infect Dis Clin North Am* 14:617-632, 2000.
13. McCready JA, Morens D, Fields HA et al: Evaluation of enzyme immunoassay (Eia) as a screening method for hepatitis B markers in an open population, *Epidemiol Infect* 107(3): 673-684, 1991.
14. Van Zonneveld M, van Nunen AB, Niesters HG et al: Lamivudine treatment during pregnancy to prevent perinatal transmission of hepatitis B virus infection, *J Viral Hepat* 10:294-297, 2003.
15. Sweet RL: Hepatitis B infection in pregnancy, *Obstet Gynecol Rep* 2:128-139, 1990.
16. Euler GL, Copeland JR, Rangel MC et al: Antibody response to postexposure prophylaxis in infants born to hepatitis B surface antigen-positive women, *Ped Infect Dis J* 22:123-129, 2003.
17. American Academy of Pediatrics: Hepatitis B and hepatitis C. In Peter G, editor: 1997 *Red Book: Report of the Committee on Infectious Diseases*, ed 24, Elk Grove Village, IL, 1997, American Academy of Pediatricians.
18. Sinatra FR, Shah P, Weissman JY et al: Perinatal transmitted acute icteric hepatitis B in infants born to hepatitis B surface antigen-positive and anti-hepatitis Be-positive carrier mothers, *Pediatrics* 70:557-559, 1982.
19. Woo D, Davies PA, Harvey DR et al: Vertical transmission of hepatitis B surface antigen in carrier mothers in two west London hospitals, *Arch Childhood Dis* 54:670-675, 1979.
20. A comprehensive immunization strategy to eliminate transmission of hepatitis B virus infection in the United States, Centers for Disease Control and Prevention, *MMWR Recomm Rep* 54(RR-16):1-34, 2005.
21. Kirkham C, Harris S, Grzybowski S: Evidence-based prenatal care: Part II. Third-trimester care and prevention of infectious diseases, *Am Fam Physician* 71(8):1555-1560, 2005.
22. Mast E, Mahoney F, Kane M et al: Hepatitis B vaccine. In: Plotkin SA, Orenstein WA, editors: *Vaccines*, Philadelphia, 2004, Saunders.

XII. HEPATITIS C IN PREGNANCY
Andrew Coco, MD, MS

After the ability to diagnose hepatitis C virus (HCV) was established in 1990, vertical transmission has been identified as the major source of infection in the pediatric population.[1] The objectives of this section are to discuss the selection of prenatal women for whom screening may be beneficial, the role of elective cesarean section in preventing perinatal transmission, and the role of breastfeeding in vertical transmission. The testing protocol for diagnosis of HCV in newborns also is discussed.

A. Epidemiology

The estimated global prevalence of HCV is 3%.[2] In the United States, about 1% of women of childbearing age are infected with HCV, which correlates to

40,000 births to HCV-positive women each year.[3] In the United States, 0.2% of children younger than 12 years have HCV infection.[4]

B. Pathogenesis

HCV does not cause fetal deformities or increase the rate of preterm birth.[5] The natural history of HCV does not appear to be affected by pregnancy.

C. Clinical Features

In this review, it is assumed that infected mothers and infants have asymptomatic chronic infection.

1. Diagnosis during pregnancy

   HCV in pregnant women is diagnosed as in nonpregnant patients. A standard HCV ELISA is confirmed by a supplementary antibody test such as the recombinant immunoblot assay. Because 15% of those with a positive antibody test will not have active infection, the reverse transcriptase PCR is used to detect HCV RNA to confirm active status.

2. Neonatal diagnosis

   In the first year of life the diagnosis of vertically acquired HCV is complicated by the presence of passively acquired maternal anti-HCV antibodies in exposed infants. Tests for the diagnosis of HCV in newborns of mothers who are positive for the HCV antibody have the following characteristics:

   a. Reliability of HCV RNA testing: HCV RNA is not reliable during the first month of life with a sensitivity of 22% and a specificity of 97%. In newborns older than 1 month, the sensitivity increases to 97%.[6]

   b. Maternal anti-HCV antibodies: These persist in infants up to 18 months of age, although more than 95% of noninfected infants will clear these antibodies by 1 year of age.[7]

3. Diagnosing vertical transmission

   Children are considered to be infected if they have two or more positive qualitative PCR results and/or are positive for anti-HCV antibodies beyond 18 months of age. Infection can be excluded when two or more qualitative PCR tests are negative or an anti-HCV antibody result is negative after 18 months of age. Therefore, the recommended sequence for testing is as follows[8]:

   a. Obtain two qualitative HCV PCRs between 2 and 6 months of age. If both are positive, then infection is presumed; if both are negative, then infection is excluded.

   b. In PCR-negative infants, the HCV antibody should be checked at 12 months to document clearance of maternal antibody. If positive, repeat after 18 months of age.

   c. In PCR-positive infants, obtain anti-HCV antibody test at 12 and 18 months of age to confirm infection.

   d. If results of the two initial PCR tests are mixed, then an anti-HCV antibody test is done at 12 and 18 months of age to determine the final status.

D. Treatment

Current medications used for treating HCV (interferon and ribavirin) are contraindicated in pregnancy.

E. Prevention

1. Screening in pregnancy

   The USPSTF, National Institutes of Health (NIH), CDC, and the American Association for the Study of Liver Diseases (AASLD) have their own recommendations for which adults should be screened for hepatitis C. They all recommend against screening low- to average-risk populations. The USPSTF also states that there is insufficient evidence for screening of high-risk populations.[9] The NIH, CDC, and AASLD have different definitions for who is considered to be a high-risk patient.[10-12] The combined recommendations of these groups for who merits screening are outlined in Table 9-4. No organization promotes the routine screening of pregnant women. Pregnant women should be screened the same as other adults, that is, based on risk factors as outlined in Table 9-4.

2. Vertical transmission

   Estimates of the risk for vertical transmission for HCV range from 3% to 10%.[13] This variation is due to the small size of most studies. The most precise estimates are obtained from two large, prospective, cohort studies of almost 2000 mother–infant pairs done in Europe and the United States.[14,15] The current best estimate from these studies is 5%, ranging from 3% to 7%.[8] Mother-to-child HCV transmission can occur before or during delivery. It is estimated that 40% of transmissions occur before delivery.[16] Table 9-5 lists potential risk factors for mother-to-child transmission of HCV. The major findings listed in Table 9-5, which have implications for pregnancy

TABLE 9-4 Risk Factors That Justify Screening (Based on Consensus Guidelines)

Injection drug use even once or twice many years ago

Receipt of blood transfusions or solid organ transplant before 1992

Receipt of clotting factor concentrates before 1987

Long-term hemodialysis

Individuals with multiple sexual partners

Spouses or household contacts of HCV-infected patients

Those who share instruments for intranasal cocaine use

Children born to mothers infected with HCV

Those with occupational exposure to HCV-positive blood

Patients with persistently abnormal alanine aminotransferase levels

Groups with Uncertain Risk Status: Other groups identified by the Centers for Disease Control and Prevention for whom routine screening is uncertain include recipients of transplanted tissue (not organs), those who use intranasal cocaine and other noninjection illegal drugs, individuals with a history of tattooing or body piercing, individuals with a history of multiple sex partners or sexually transmitted diseases, and long-term steady partners of hepatitis C virus (HCV)–positive persons. Therefore, these exposures were not included as risk factors that have screening recommendations.

management, are:

a. Elective cesarean section does not prevent vertical transmission.

b. Because HCV transmission may be related to length of time of membrane rupture and placement of fetal scalp electrode, it is prudent for clinicians to minimize these interventions with women positive for HCV antibodies.

c. Breastfeeding does not increase the risk for perinatal transmission.

F. SOR A Recommendations

RECOMMENDATIONS	REFERENCES
Elective cesarean section does not prevent vertical transmission of HCV.	*14, 15*
Breastfeeding does not transmit HCV infection.	*14, 17*

REFERENCES

1. Tovo PA, Lazier L, Versace A: Hepatitis B virus and hepatitis C virus infections in children, *Curr Opin Infect Dis* 18:261-266, 2005.
2. WHO. Global distribution of hepatitis A, B and C, *Wkly Epidemiol Rec* 77:45-47, 2002.
3. Alter MJ, Kruszon-Moran D, Nainan OV et al: The prevalence of hepatitis C virus infection in the United States, 1988 through 1994, *N Engl J Med* 341:556-562, 1999.

TABLE 9-5 Vertical Transmission Risk Factors

Risk Factor	Effect	References
Mode of delivery: vaginal compared with elective cesarean section	No difference	14, 15
Breastfeeding	No increase	14, 17
Maternal HIV coinfection	Twofold to threefold increase risk, but lessened with HAART	14, 18
Maternal HCV viral load	Increased risk with high viral load; transmission is remote with negative viremia	14, 15, 19
Sex of newborn	Twofold risk with female individuals	14
Prematurity	No effect	14, 20
Maternal injection drug use	Unclear	14, 20
Prolonged rupture of membranes	May increase risk	14, 15
Internal fetal monitoring	May increase risk	15

HIV, Human immunodeficiency virus; HAART, highly active antiretroviral therapy; HCV, hepatitis C virus.

4. Ruiz-Moreno M, Leal-Orozco A, Millan A et al: Hepatitis C virus infection in children, *J Hepatol* 1999;31(suppl 1):124-129.

5. Paternoster D, Santarossa C, Grella P et al: Viral load in HCV RNA-positive pregnant women, *Am J Gastroenterol* 96:2751-2754, 2001.

6. Gibb DM, Goodall RL, Dunn DT et al: Mother-to-child transmission of hepatitis C virus, *Lancet* 356:904-907, 2000.

7. England K, Pembrey L, Tovo PA et al: European Paediatric HCV Network. Excluding hepatitis C virus (HCV) infection by serology in young infants of HCV-infected mothers, *Acta Paediatr* 94(4):444-450, 2005.

8. Pemrey L, Newell ML, Tovo PA: The management of HCV infected pregnant women and their children European paediatric HCV network, *J Hepatol* 43:515-525, 2005.

9. U.S. Preventive Services Task Force. Screening for hepatitis C virus infection in adults: recommendation statement, *Ann Intern Med* 140(6):462-464, 2004.

10. National Institutes of Health. *Consensus development conference statement. Management of hepatitis C: 2002. June 10–12, 2002.* Available at: http://consensus.nih.gov/2002/2002hepatitisc2002116html.htm. Accessed February 5, 2005.

11. Recommendations for prevention and control of hepatitis C virus (HCV) infection and HCV-related chronic disease. Centers for Disease Control and Prevention, *MMWR Recomm Rep* 47(RR-19):1-39, 1998.

12. Strader DB, Wright T, Thomas DL et al: Diagnosis, management, and treatment of hepatitis C. AASLD Practice Guideline. Available at: https://www.aasld.org/eweb/docs/hepatitisc.pdf. Accessed February 5, 2005.

13. Pembrey L, Newell M-L, Peckham C: Is there a case for hepatitis C infection screening in the antenatal period? *J Med Screen* 10:161-168, 2003.

14. European Paediatric Hepatitis C Virus Network: A significant sex—but not elective cesarean section—effect on mother-to child transmission of hepatitis C virus infection, *J Infect Dis* 192:1872-1879, 2005.

15. Mast EE, Hwang LY, Seto DS et al: Risk factors for perinatal transmission of hepatitis C virus (HCV) and the natural history of HCV infection acquired in infancy, *J Infect Dis* 192:1880-1889, 2005.

16. European Paediatric HCV Network (Mok JYQ, Pembrey L, Tovo PA, Newell M-L): When does mother to child transmission of hepatitis C virus occur? *Arch Dis Child Fetal Neonatal Ed* 90:F156-F160, 2005.

17. European Paediatric HCV Network (Pembrey L, Tovo PA, Newell ML): Effects of mode of delivery and infant feeding on the risk of mother-to-child transmission of hepatitis C virus, *Br J Obstet Gynaecol* 108:371-377, 2001.

18. Tovo P-A, Palomba E, Ferraris G et al: Increased risk of maternal-infant hepatitis C virus transmission for women coinfected with human immunodeficiency virus type 1, *Clin Infect Dis* 25:1121-1124, 1997.

19. Okamoto M, Nagata I, Murakami J et al: Prospective re-evaluation of risk factors in mother-to-child transmission of hepatitis C virus: high virus load, vaginal delivery, and negative anti-NS4 antibody, *J Infect Dis* 182:1511-1514, 2000.

20. Resti M, Azzari C, Galli L et al: Maternal drug use is a preeminent risk factor for mother-to-child hepatitis C virus transmission: results from a multi-center study of 1372 mother–infant pairs, *J Infect Dis* 185:567-572, 2002.

XIII. HUMAN IMMUNODEFICIENCY VIRUS

Andrew Coco, MD, MS

Because management of HIV infection is rapidly changing, the reader is advised to consult the US Preventive Health Service website (http://aidsinfo.nih.gov) for more in-depth information and updates. Prevention of vertical transmission of HIV infection in developed countries is one of the greatest recent public health success stories. Unfortunately, the barriers to preventing vertical transmission are much more formidable in less well-developed areas of the world. This chapter focuses on management of pregnant women in the United States.

A. Epidemiology

An estimated 17.6 million women worldwide are living with HIV, and 640,000 children are newly infected each year, mostly from mother-to-child transmission.[1] In the United States, the annual number of perinatal transmissions had been dramatically reduced from a peak of 1000 to 2000 in the early 1990s to 280 to 370 in 2004.[2]

B. Pathogenesis

1. Timing of perinatal HIV transmission
   This likely occurs close to the time of or during childbirth.[3]

2. Effect of pregnancy on progression of HIV infection
   Studies in industrialized countries have failed to show an effect of pregnancy on HIV infection progression.[4,5] No evidence has been reported that HIV infection causes a fetal malformation syndrome or increases the rate of birth defects.[6,7]

3. Effect of maternal HIV RNA (viral load) level on perinatal transmission
   Data from large numbers of HIV-infected pregnant women treated with antiretroviral therapy show that viral load is strongly correlated with perinatal transmission.[8,9] Although rates of perinatal transmission are low when the viral load is undetectable on current assays, mother-to-child transmission has occurred among women with all levels of viral RNA.

4. Effect of cesarean delivery on progression of HIV infection
   Data from cohort studies have refuted earlier case–control studies that suggested a greater surgical

complication rate and demonstrated that the maternal risks of cesarean section are no different between HIV-positive and -negative women.[10,11] In other studies where it was evaluated, there was an increased number of minor complications in women with more advanced disease. The USPSTF concluded that complication rates were not of sufficient frequency or severity to outweigh the potential benefit of reduced transmission among women at heightened risk for transmission.[12]

C. Assessment of Disease Stage

Although most women diagnosed with HIV infection during pregnancy are asymptomatic, it is important to assess for signs of advanced disease and obtain additional baseline laboratory work. Women with CD4 lymphocyte counts less than 50/μl should have an ophthalmic examination for evidence of cytomegalovirus (CMV) retinitis. Additional laboratory tests include tuberculosis skin testing; *Toxoplasma gondii*, CMV, and hepatitis C antibody status if unknown; renal- and liver-function testing; lymphocyte subgroups (CD4 count); and plasma HIV RNA level (viral load).[13]

D. Diagnosis

1. Test options
   HIV infection in pregnancy can be diagnosed by the standard ELISA antibody test followed by a confirmatory Western blot assay. The rapid antibody test (results available in 10-30 minutes) is also an acceptable initial test option and would also require a Western blot to confirm.
2. Antepartum screening for HIV infection
   The USPSTF recommends that clinicians screen all pregnant women for HIV. This is grade A recommendation.[12] The USPSTF based their recommendation on several factors. It found good evidence that both standard and rapid HIV antibody tests accurately diagnose HIV in pregnancy. It also found fair evidence that universal counseling and voluntary testing increases the proportion of HIV-infected women that receive antiretroviral therapy before delivery. Other benefits of screening mentioned in the statement were that antiretroviral therapy is acceptable to pregnant women and leads to decreased rates of perinatal transmission. The American Academy of Family Physicians, CDC, American Medical Association, ACOG, Infectious Disease Society of America, AAP, and American College of Nurse-Midwives also have issued guidelines recommending that all pregnant women be routinely counseled and encouraged to have HIV testing. ACOG, AAP, and CDC extend these recommendations and state that HIV testing should be part of a routine battery of prenatal blood tests unless declined (the "opt-out" approach).

3. Retesting and testing in labor
   The CDC and ACOG are the only organizations to include recommendations for retesting for HIV in the third trimester in those with risk factors, as well as testing laboring women with unknown HIV status with the rapid test. Retesting in the third trimester would allow women who had seroconverted during the pregnancy the option of an elective cesarean section and antiretroviral therapy. Rapid testing of unidentified women in labor would allow those testing positive to receive intrapartum intravenous zidovudine (ZDU) and the option of cesarean section, whereas their newborns would receive treatment with oral ZDU prophylaxis for 6 weeks.
4. Resistance test (genotype) for detecting viral mutations to antiretroviral medications
   Recommendations for resistance testing for HIV-1–infected pregnant women are the same as for nonpregnant patients: acute HIV-1 infection, failure of antiretroviral regimen, suboptimal viral suppression after initiation of antiretroviral therapy, or high likelihood of exposure to resistant virus based on community prevalence or source characteristics.

E. Treatment

1. Preconception
   A large percentage of the HIV-infected women who become pregnant do so with a known diagnosis, and about 50% of these women are taking antiretroviral therapy in the first trimester.[14] Therefore, it is important to discuss pregnancy issues with all women of reproductive age who HIV positive. Issues to cover include selection of appropriate contraceptive method, education about perinatal transmission risks and the potential effect of antiretroviral therapy on pregnancy outcomes, avoiding agents with potential toxicity (efavirenz and hydroxyurea), administration of immunizations (influenza, hepatitis B, and pneumococcal), and enhancing maternal nutritional status.
2. Antepartum antiretroviral therapy (http://AIDSinfo.nih.gov)[15]

TABLE 9-6 Pediatric AIDS Clinical Trials Group (PACTG) 076 Zidovudine Regimen

Time of ZDV Administration	Regimen
Antepartum	Oral administration of 100 mg ZDV five times daily,* initiated at 14 to 34 weeks of gestation and continued throughout the pregnancy.
Intrapartum	During labor, intravenous administration of ZDV in a 1-hour initial dose of 2 mg/kg body weight, followed by a continuous infusion of 1 mg/kg body weight/hr until delivery.
Postpartum	Oral administration of ZDV to the newborn (ZDV syrup at 2 mg/kg body weight/dose every 6 hours) for the first 6 weeks of life, beginning at 8 to 12 hours after birth.†

*Oral zidovudine (ZDV) administered as 200 mg three times daily or 300 mg twice daily is currently used in general clinical practice and is an acceptable alternative regimen to 100 mg orally five times daily.

†Intravenous dosage for full-term infants who cannot tolerate oral intake is 1.5 mg/kg body weight intravenously every 6 hours. ZDV dosing for infants less than 35 weeks of gestation at birth is 1.5 mg/kg/dose intravenously, or 2.0 mg/kg/dose orally, every 12 hours, advancing to every 8 hours at 2 weeks of age if more than or equal to 30 weeks of gestation at birth or at 4 weeks of age if less than 30 weeks of gestation at birth.

All pregnant women should be offered antiretroviral therapy including ZDU (Table 9-6)[16] to decrease perinatal transmission. However, many factors are involved in deciding what other medications should be included in the regimen and when it should be started. Table 9-6 also provides the ZDU regimen for newborn prophylaxis. Because the long-term consequences of prenatal antiretroviral therapy, especially for exposed children, are unknown, ultimately, the decision to take medications must be made by the informed, expectant mother. The different scenarios and treatment recommendations are represented in Table 9-7, which is directly from the USPSTF guidelines.[15] Table 9-7 covers four common scenarios: pregnant women with HIV-1 infection who have not received prior antiretroviral therapy, women with HIV-1 infection receiving antiretroviral therapy during the current pregnancy, women with HIV-1 infection in labor who have had no prior therapy, and infants born to mothers who have received no antiretroviral therapy during pregnancy or after delivery.

Women receiving therapy should have HIV RNA levels monitored as in nonpregnant adults: monthly until undetectable, then every 3 months until 36 weeks for planning mode of delivery.

3. Mode of delivery

Before the era of viral load testing and combination antiretroviral therapy, several studies consistently showed that elective cesarean delivery before the onset of labor significantly reduced the rate of perinatal transmission by up to 80% compared with other modes of delivery.[17] As combination antiretroviral therapy has become the standard of care over the past few years, there have been no studies demonstrating any additional benefit of elective cesarean section compared with women who had a vaginal delivery if they were receiving antiretroviral therapy and had viral loads of less than 1000 copies/ml. Both modes of delivery resulted in vertical transmission rates of less than 2%. ACOG recommends the consideration of scheduled cesarean delivery for pregnant women with HIV-1 infection with viral loads of more than 1000 copies/ml.[18] The USPSTF has outlined four clinical scenarios with management recommendations regarding mode of delivery options in their guidelines (see Table 9-7).[15] Women electing cesarean section can be scheduled at 38 weeks instead of the customary 39 weeks to decrease the chance of rupture of membranes or labor onset because either would probably reduce the benefit of cesarean section considerably.

F. Prevention of Opportunistic Infections

Recommendations for prophylaxis are similar to nonpregnant adults and will not be covered here. Neonatal health-care providers of women receiving trimethoprim-sulfamethoxazole for *Pneumocystis carinii* or *T. gondii* prophylaxis should be informed that fetal exposure to this medication could lead to hyperbilirubinemia.

1. Immunizations

Hepatitis B, influenza, and pneumococcal immunizations may be administered during pregnancy,

TABLE 9-7 Clinical Scenarios and Recommendations for the Use of Antiretroviral Drugs to Reduce Perinatal Human Immunodeficiency Virus Type 1 Transmission

Scenario 1: pregnant women with HIV-1 infection who have not received prior antiretroviral therapy	• Pregnant women with HIV-1 infection must receive standard clinical, immunologic, and virologic evaluation. Recommendations for initiation and choice of antiretroviral therapy should be based on the same parameters used for persons who are not pregnant, although the known and unknown risks and benefits of such therapy during pregnancy must be considered and discussed.
	• The three-part ZDV chemoprophylaxis regimen, initiated after the first trimester, is recommended for all pregnant women with HIV-1 infection regardless of antenatal HIV RNA copy number to reduce the risk for perinatal transmission.
	• The combination of ZDV chemoprophylaxis with additional antiretroviral drugs for treatment of HIV-1 infection is recommended for infected women whose clinical, immunologic, or virologic status requires treatment or who have HIV-1 RNA >1000 copies/ml regardless of clinical or immunologic status and can be considered for women with HIV-1 RNA <1000 copies/ml.
	• Women who are in the first trimester of pregnancy may consider delaying initiation of therapy until after 10-12 weeks of gestation.
Scenario 2: women with HIV-1 infection receiving antiretroviral therapy during the current pregnancy	• Women with HIV-1 infection receiving antiretroviral therapy in whom pregnancy is identified after the first trimester should continue therapy. ZDV should be a component of the antenatal antiretroviral treatment regimen after the first trimester whenever possible, although this may not always be feasible.
	• For women receiving antiretroviral therapy in whom pregnancy is recognized during the first trimester, counseling regarding the benefits and potential risks for antiretroviral administration during this period should be provided, and continuation of therapy should be considered. If therapy is discontinued during the first trimester, all drugs should be stopped and reintroduced simultaneously to avoid the development of drug resistance.
	• Regardless of the antepartum antiretroviral regimen, ZDV administration is recommended during the intrapartum period and for the newborn.
Scenario 3: women with HIV-1 infection in labor who have had no prior therapy	• Several effective regimens are available. These include: 1. Intrapartum intravenous ZDV followed by 6 weeks of ZDV for the newborn 2. Oral ZDV and 3TC during labor, followed by 1 week of oral ZDV-3TC for the newborn 3. A single dose of nevirapine at the onset of labor followed by a single dose of nevirapine for the newborn at age 48 hours 4. The two-dose nevirapine regimen combined with intrapartum intravenous ZDV and 6-week ZDV for the newborn
	• In the immediate postpartum period, the woman should have appropriate assessments (e.g., CD4$^+$ count and HIV-1 RNA copy number) to determine whether antiretroviral therapy is recommended for her own health.
Scenario 4: infants born to mothers who have received no antiretroviral therapy during pregnancy or after delivery	• The 6-week neonatal ZDV component of the ZDV chemoprophylactic regimen should be discussed with the mother and offered for the newborn.
	• ZDV should be initiated as soon as possible after delivery, preferably within 6-12 hours of birth.
	• Some clinicians may choose to use ZDV in combination with other antiretroviral drugs, particularly if the mother is known or suspected to have ZDV-resistant virus. However, the efficacy of this approach for prevention of transmission has not been proved in clinical trials, and appropriate dosing regimens for neonates are incompletely defined for many drugs.
	• In the immediate postpartum period, the woman should undergo appropriate assessments (e.g., CD4$^+$ count and HIV-1 RNA copy number) to determine whether antiretroviral therapy is required for her own health. The infant should undergo early diagnostic testing so that HIV infection treatment can be initiated as soon as possible.

HIV, Human immunodeficiency virus; ZDV, zidovudine.

but it may be preferable to wait until HIV RNA has been suppressed to undetectable levels to avoid the theoretical increased risk for perinatal transmission that could occur with transient increases in the viral count after immunization.[10]

2. Antepartum care
   Women receiving therapy should have HIV RNA levels monitored as in nonpregnant adults: monthly until undetectable, then every 3 months until 36 weeks of gestation for planning mode of delivery.

3. Intrapartum care
   a. The final decision on elective cesarean section versus vaginal delivery should be made based on an HIV RNA level at 36 weeks of gestation.
   b. Intravenous ZDU (bolus of 2 mg/kg over 1 hour, then 1 mg/kg/hr throughout labor) should begin at the onset of labor, with rupture of membranes, or 3 hours before an elective cesarean section.
   c. Other oral antiretroviral medications should be continued per usual schedule during labor or before surgery.
   d. Artificial rupture of membranes should be avoided.
   e. Women with spontaneous rupture of membranes should have oxytocin (Pitocin) augmentation to decrease the interval from rupture to delivery.
   f. Scalp electrodes, fetal pH sampling, instrumental delivery, and episiotomy should be avoided.
   g. Midazolam (Versed) and ergot preparations (methylergonovine [Methergine]) should be avoided in women who have been receiving protease inhibitors because of potential delay in their metabolism.
   h. Infants should be washed before blood draws or injections.

4. Postpartum care
   a. Breastfeeding is not recommended because it is associated with an additional 15% to 20% risk for transmission of HIV.[19]
   b. Antiretroviral medications may be continued or discontinued depending on immune status and maternal choice. Women continuing therapy need to be carefully followed for adherence because the loss of incentive to prevent transmission may affect compliance.
   c. Contraception and safe sex practices should be discussed.

5. Newborn care[20]
   a. ZDU for 6 weeks (see Table 9-6) with baseline complete blood cell count
   b. *P. carinii* prophylaxis at 6 weeks after completion of ZDU (trimethoprim-sulfamethoxazole 40/200 per 5m @ 5-10 mg/kg/day trimethoprim divided every 12 hours)
   c. Determination of HIV-infection status with HIV DNA PCR testing at 1 to 2 days, 1 to 2 months, and 3 to 6 months of age; additional testing at age 14 days might allow for early detection of infection
   d. HIV infection can be reasonably excluded in nonbreastfed infants with two or more negative virologic tests performed at age older than 1 month, with one of those being performed at age older than 4 months

G. Pitfalls and Controversies

Regarding mode of delivery in women with a low or undetectable viral load, current USPSTF guidelines states that women with an HIV viral load less than 1000 copies/ml be offered the choice of an elective cesarean delivery or a vaginal delivery because at the time of publication in December 2004, it was unclear whether elective cesarean section provided any additional significant clinical benefit in reducing the rate of perinatal transmission. Since publication of these guidelines, an additional European prospective cohort study was published in a prominent journal showing that elective cesarean section may incur some additional benefit in women with undetectable viral loads.[21] However, when the analysis was controlled for receipt of antiretroviral therapy, no difference existed in perinatal transmission risk (adjusted OR, 0.52; 95% CI, 0.14-2.03; $p = 0.358$). Therefore, it remains appropriate to counsel women with viral loads less than 1000 copies/ml who are taking antiretroviral therapy that it is unlikely that elective cesarean section provides additional benefit in reducing perinatal transmission. These results also highlight the importance of ensuring that even women with a baseline viral load that is undetectable be treated with at least ZDV during their pregnancy to minimize the risk for perinatal transmission.

H. SOR A Recommendations

RECOMMENDATIONS	REFERENCES
Patients should undergo universal screening for HIV infection during pregnancy.	*13*
A benefit of antiretroviral therapy exists in preventing perinatal transmission from 25% to 8% with zidovudine monotherapy.	*16*
A decision on mode of delivery should be based on whether mother received antiretroviral therapy prenatally and viral load after 36 weeks of gestation.	*15, 21*

REFERENCES

1. Mofenson LM: Interaction between timing of perinatal human immunodeficiency virus infection and the design of preventive and therapeutic interventions, *Acta Paediatr Supp* 421:1-9, 1997.
2. UNAIDS/WHO-AIDS epidemic update–December 2004, Geneva, 2004, UNAIDS. Available at: http://www.unaids.org/epidemic-update.html. Accessed September 20, 2005.
3. Centers for Disease Control and Prevention: Revised recommendations for HIV screening of pregnant women, *MMWR Recomm Rep* 50(RR-19):63-85, 2001.
4. Saada M, Le Chenadec J, Berrebi A et al: Pregnancy and progression to AIDS: results of the French prospective cohorts, *AIDS* 14:2355-2360, 2000.
5. Burns DN, Landesman S, Minkoff H et al: The influence of pregnancy on human immunodeficiency virus type 1 infection: antepartum and post partum changes in human immunodeficiency virus type 1 viral load, *Am J Obstet Gynecol* 178:355-359, 1998.
6. Brocklehurst P, French R: The association between maternal HIV infection and perinatal outcome: a systematic review of the literature and meta-analysis, *Br J Obstet Gynaecol* 105:836-848, 1998.
7. Embree JE, Braddick M, Datta P et al: Lack of correlation of maternal human immunodeficiency virus infection with neonatal malformations, *Pediatr Infect Dis J* 8:700-704, 1989.
8. Mofenson LM, Lambert JS, Stiehm ER et al: Risk factors for perinatal transmission of human immunodeficiency virus type 1 in women treated with zidovudine. Pediatric AIDS Clinical Trials Group Study 185 Team, *N Engl J Med* 341:385-393, 1999.
9. Garcia PM, Kalish LA, Pitt J et al: Maternal levels of plasma human immunodeficiency virus type 1 RNA and the risk of perinatal transmission, *N Engl J Med* 341:394-402, 1999.
10. Watts DH, Lambert JS, Stiehm ER et al: Complications according to mode of delivery among human immunodeficiency virus-infected women with CD4 lymphocyte counts of < or = 500/microliter, *Am J Obstet Gynecol* 183:100-107, 2000.
11. Rodriquez EJ, Spann C, Jamieson D et al: Postoperative morbidity associated with cesarean delivery among human immunodeficiency virus-seropositive women, *Am J Obstet Gynecol* 184:1108-1111, 2001.
12. Screening for HIV: Recommendation Statement, U.S. Preventive Service Task Force, *Ann Intern Med* 143:32-37, 2005.
13. Watts DH: Management of human immunodeficiency virus infection in pregnancy, *N Engl J Med* 346:1879-1890, 2002.
14. Tuomala R, Shapiro D, Samelson R et al: Antepartum antiretroviral therapy and viral load in 464 HIV-infected women in 1998-1999, *Am J Obstet Gynecol* 182:285, 2000 (abstract).
15. Perinatal HIV Guidelines Working Group: Public Health Service Task Force recommendations for use of antiretroviral drugs in pregnant HIV-1 infected women for maternal health and interventions to reduce perinatal HIV-1 transmission in the United States, October 12, 2006, 1-65. Available at: http://aidsinfo.nih.gov/ContentFiles/PerinatalGL.pdf. Accessed November 7, 2006.
16. Connor EM, Sperling RS, Gelber R et al: Reduction of maternal-infant transmission of human immunodeficiency virus type 1 with zidovudine treatment, *N Engl J Med* 331:1173-1180, 1994.
17. The International Perinatal HIV Group. The mode of delivery and the risk of vertical transmission of HIV type 1—a meta-analysis of 15 prospective cohort studies, *N Engl J Med* 340:977-987, 1999.
18. ACOG Committee Opinion. Scheduled Cesarean delivery and the prevention of vertical transmission of HIV infection. Number 234, May 2000 (replaces number 219, August 1999), *Int J Gynaecol Obstet* 73:279-281, 2001.
19. Nduati R, John G, Mbori-Ngacha D et al: Effect of breastfeeding and formula feeding on transmission of HIV-1: a randomized clinical trial, *JAMA* 283:1167-1174, 2000.
20. Guidelines for the use of antiretroviral agents in pediatric HIV infection. Working Group on Antiretroviral Therapy and Medical Management of HIV-Infected Children convened by the National Resource Center at the François-Xavier Bagnoud Center, UMDNJ. The Health Resources and Services Administration (HRSA); and the National Institutes of Health (NIH). Available at: http://AIDSinfo.nih.gov. Accessed March 24, 2005.
21. European Collaborative Study: Mother-to-child transmission of HIV infection in the era of highly active antiretroviral therapy, *Clin Infect Dis* 40:458-465, 2005.

XIV. ASYMPTOMATIC BACTERIURIA AND URINARY TRACT INFECTION
Donna Cohen, MD, MSc

Asymptomatic bacteriuria (ASB) is defined as persistent bacterial colonization of the urinary tract in the absence of symptoms. The diagnosis is made by the growth of more than 100,000 colonies/ml of a single pathogen in a clean-voided, midstream urine sample.

A. Epidemiology

1. Prevalence
   ASB occurs in 2% to 10% of all pregnancies.[1]
2. Risk factors for ASB[2,3]
   a. Medical conditions such as diabetes, sickle cell trait, and obesity
   b. Women with a history of urinary tract infection
   c. Anatomic urinary tract or congenital abnormalities

d. Low socioeconomic status
e. Multiparity
3. Bacterial organisms
Escherichia coli is the most common pathogen, accounting for approximately 40% of positive cultures.[4] GBS, *Klebsiella, Proteus mirabilis, Enterobacter, Enterococcus,* and *Staphylococcus saprophyticus* account for the majority of the remaining positive urine cultures.

B. Pathogenesis

1. Physiologic changes of the urinary system in pregnancy
Pregnancy results in a number of physiologic changes that predispose a woman to urinary tract infections.[2,3]
   a. Hydroureter and hydronephrosis: This can begin as early as the 7th week of gestation and progress throughout the pregnancy.
   b. Hormonal changes: This can result in delaying ureteral peristalsis.
   c. Urinary retention
2. Upper urogenital tract infections
Vesicoureteral reflux may first appear or worsen in pregnancy, resulting in an increased risk for ascending infection. Obstruction to the flow of urine in pregnancy results in stasis and increases the risk for pyelonephritis complicating ASB.

C. Effects of Asymptomatic Bacteriuria on Perinatal Outcome

1. Pyelonephritis
Pyelonephritis occurs in 1% to 2% of all pregnancies. Undetected or untreated ASB in pregnancy, however, leads to acute pyelonephritis 20% to 30% of the time.[1]
2. PTL/LBW infants
A metaanalysis of many studies established that ASB is associated with an increased incidence of PTL and LBW infants.[5] Some controversy exists whether the ASB is merely a marker for low socioeconomic status, which is associated with LBW, or whether it is an independent predictor.

D. Symptomatic Urinary Tract Infections

Symptoms of lower urinary tract infections include varying degrees of dysuria, frequency, urgency, suprapubic pain, and sensation of pelvic pressure.

E. Pyelonephritis

Clinical signs of pyelonephritis include fever, chills, costovertebral tenderness, dysuria, frequency, anorexia, and nausea and vomiting. Complications include renal dysfunction, anemia, and acute respiratory insufficiency.[6]

F. Diagnosis

The diagnosis of ASB or urinary tract infections is made based on the growth of more than 100,000 colonies/ml of a single pathogen in a clean-voided, midstream sample. Lesser colony counts may be significant in catheterized specimens or when GBS bacteria are isolated. Urine culture is considered the gold standard for detection of ASB, compared with dipstick urinalysis or direct microscopy, which have poor positive and negative predictive values for detecting ASB. The USPSTF strongly recommends that all pregnant women be screened for ASB using urine culture at 12 to 16 weeks of gestation (grade A recommendation).[7] The ACOG further recommends routine screening for bacteriuria at the first prenatal visit.[8] Routine screening and treatment of ASB in pregnancy has been shown to be cost-effective and is recommended because of the association of ASB with pyelonephritis.[9]

G. Treatment for Asymptomatic Bacteriuria and Symptomatic Lower Urinary Tract Infection

A recent Cochrane review of 14 trials demonstrated that the treatment of ASB is associated with a reduction in the incidence of PTL or LBW (OR, 0.60; 95% CI, 0.45-0.80; NNT = 20) and a reduction in the incidence of pyelonephritis (OR, 0.24; 95% CI, 0.19-0.32; NNT = 7).[1]
1. Antibiotic regimens[3,10]
The following antibiotic regimens are recommended for 3- or 7-day courses:
   a. Ampicillin, 250 mg four times daily
   b. Amoxicillin, 500 mg three times daily
   c. Cephalexin, 250 mg four times daily
   d. Nitrofurantoin, 100 mg two or four times daily
   e. Trimethoprim-sulfamethoxazole, 1 double-strength tablet twice daily (avoid in first trimester and use with caution in late pregnancy)
   f. Other cephalosporins
   Ampicillin has traditionally been the antibiotic of choice for treatment; however, recently, *E. coli* has become increasingly resistant to ampicillin.[11,12]

2. Duration of treatment

Current standard treatment for ASB in pregnant women involves 3- or 7-day antibiotic regimens. Single-dose treatment is associated with a decrease in side effects, such as nausea, vomiting, or diarrhea.[13] However, a recent Cochrane review of 10 studies concluded that there is insufficient evidence to determine whether single-dose antibiotic therapy is as effective as 4- to 7-day therapy in treating ASB in pregnancy.[13]

3. Follow-up

a. A TOC urine culture: This should be performed within 4 weeks after treatment to ensure clearance of bacteriuria. Patients should undergo repeat surveillance cultures during pregnancy.

b. Persistent ASB or infection: If ASB persists, then retreatment based on sensitivities is indicated.

c. Patients with more than one relapse or reinfection: These patients should be placed on bacterial suppression therapy. Ampicillin, amoxicillin, nitrofurantoin, and cephalexin are all appropriate choices for suppression.

H. Treatment for Pyelonephritis

1. Outpatient treatment

Recent evidence has demonstrated that outpatient management of pyelonephritis is a reasonable option in women who are able to tolerate oral medications with no evidence of sepsis, PTL, or respiratory insufficiency.[14,15] Those patients who are medically stable can be treated with antibiotic regimens (ampicillin, amoxicillin, cephalexin, nitrofurantoin, other cephalosporins) for 10 to 14 days, with therapy adjusted based on urine culture sensitivities.[3,4,10]

2. Inpatient treatment

Patients who are unable to tolerate oral medications or who are medically unstable require hospitalization. Management should include close monitoring of vital signs, intravenous fluids, laboratory evaluation including complete blood cell count, serum creatinine, electrolytes, and urine studies. A chest radiograph should be obtained if any tachypnea or dyspnea develops. Patients should also be monitored for any evidence of contractions or PTL. The following intravenous antibiotic regimens are recommended initially and may be adjusted once urine sensitivities return[3,4]:

a. Ampicillin 2 g every 6 hours *plus* gentamicin 3 to 5 mg/kg daily

b. Ceftriaxone 1 to 2 g every 12 to 24 hours

c. Cefotaxime 1 to 2 g every 8 hours

3. Duration of treatment

Parenteral antibiotics should be continued until patients remain afebrile for 24 to 48 hours. Oral therapy is then continued to complete a 10- to 14-day course.

4. Patient response

Patients should respond and demonstrate improvement to the above management within 48 hours. Any patient who fails to improve should undergo evaluation for obstruction, stone, or abscess, which is most often visualized by renal ultrasound.

5. Follow-up

After completing a course of antibiotic therapy for acute pyelonephritis, clinicians can either follow the patient with serial urine cultures or initiate daily antibiotic suppression therapy. Amoxicillin, a cephalosporin, or nitrofurantoin can all be used depending on the urine culture sensitivities. Recurrent bacteriuria develops in 30% to 40% of women after completion of antibiotic therapy.[16] Patients who receive suppression therapy do demonstrate lower rates of persistent bacteriuria, although suppression therapy has not be shown to significantly alter the rate of recurrent pyelonephritis.[17]

I. Group B Streptococcus

Patients with GBS isolated from urine in any concentration during their current pregnancy should receive intrapartum chemoprophylaxis for the prevention of perinatal GBS disease.[18] Women with symptomatic GBS urinary tract infections or ASB with colony counts greater than 100,000 colony-forming units/ml during pregnancy should be treated with penicillin or amoxicillin as per above management guidelines. However, the management of low colony counts of asymptomatic GBS bacteriuria remains controversial with no existing protocol. A recent survey of expert senior obstetricians at US training programs indicated that a majority of respondents (65/85 respondents) treat low colony counts of asymptomatic GBS bacteriuria during pregnancy.[19]

J. SOR A Recommendations

RECOMMENDATIONS	REFERENCES
All pregnant women should be screened for ASB using urine culture at 12 to 16 weeks of gestation or the first prenatal visit.	7, 8
Patients identified with ASB should receive antibiotic treatment to reduce the risk for pyelonephritis (NNT = 7) and LBW babies (NNT = 20).	1
Patients with group B streptococcus isolated from urine in any concentration during their current pregnancy should receive intrapartum chemoprophylaxis.	18

REFERENCES

1. Smaill F, Vazquez JC: Antibiotics for asymptomatic bacteriuria in pregnancy, *Cochrane Database Syst Rev* (2):CD000490, 2007.
2. Patterson T, Andriole V: Detection, significance, and therapy of bacteriuria in pregnancy: update in the managed health care era, *Infect Dis Clin North Am* 11:593-608, 1997.
3. Sheffield J, Cunningham FG: Urinary tract infection in women, *Obstet Gynecol* 106:1085-1092, 2005.
4. Millar L, Cox S: Urinary tract infections complicating pregnancy, *Infect Dis Clin North Am* 11:13-26, 1997.
5. Romero R, Oyarzun E, Mazor M et al: Meta-analysis of the relationship between asymptomatic bacteriuria and preterm delivery/low birth weight, *Obstet Gynecol* 73:576-582, 1989.
6. Hill JB, Sheffield JS, McIntire DD et al: Acute pyelonephritis in pregnancy, *Obstet Gynecol* 105:18-23, 2005.
7. U.S. Preventive Services Task Force (USPSTF). Screening for asymptomatic bacteriuria: recommendation statement, Rockville, MD, 2004, Agency for Healthcare Research and Quality (AHRQ).
8. American Academy of Pediatrics and American College of Obstetricians and Gynecologists: *Guidelines for prenatal care*, ed 5, Elk Grove Village, IL, 2002, American Academy of Pediatrics; Washington, DC, 2002, American College of Obstetricians and Gynecologists.
9. Rouse D, Andrews W, Goldenberg R et al: Screening and treatment of asymptomatic bacteriuria of pregnancy to prevent pyelonephritis: a cost-effectiveness and cost-benefit analysis, *Obstet Gynecol* 86:119-123, 1995.
10. Cunningham FG, Leveno KJ, Bloom SL et al: Renal and urinary tract disorders. In Cunningham FG, Leveno KJ, Bloom SL et al, editors: *Williams obstetrics*, ed 22, New York, 2005, McGraw-Hill.
11. Peddie BA, Bailey RR, Wells JE: Resistance of urinary tract isolates of *Escherichia coli* to cotrimoxazole, sulphonamide, trimethoprim and ampicillin: an 11-year survey, *NZ Med J* 100:341-342, 1987.
12. Sanders CC, Sanders WE Jr: Beta-lactam resistance in gram-negative bacteria: global trends and clinical impact, *Clin Infect Dis* 15:824-839, 1992.
13. Villar J, Widmer M, Lydon-Rochelle MT et al: Duration of treatment for asymptomatic bacteriuria during pregnancy, *Cochrane Database Syst Rev* (2):CD000491, 2000.
14. Millar LK, Wing DA, Paul RH et al: Outpatient treatment of acute pyelonephritis in pregnancy: a randomized controlled trial, *Obstet Gynecol* 86:560-564, 1995.
15. Wing DA, Hendershott CM, Debuque L et al: Outpatient treatment of acute pyelonephritis in pregnancy after 24 weeks, *Obstet Gynecol* 94:683-688, 1999.
16. Cunningham FG, Morris GB, Mickal A: Acute pyelonephritis of pregnancy: a clinical review, *Obstet Gynecol* 42:112-117, 1973.
17. Lenke R, VanDorsten J, Schifrin B: Pyelonephritis in pregnancy: a prospective randomized trial to prevent recurrent disease evaluating suppressive therapy with nitrofurantoin and close surveillance, *Am J Obstet Gynecol* 146:953-957, 1983.
18. Prevention of perinatal group B streptococcal disease revised. Centers for Disease Control and Prevention, *MMWR Morb Mortal Wkly Rep* 51(RR-11):1-22, 2002.
19. Aungst M, King J, Steele A et al: Low colony counts of asymptomatic group B streptococcus bacteriuria: a survey of practice patterns, *Am J Perinatol* 21:403-407, 2004.

XV. PNEUMONIA IN PREGNANCY

For a detailed discussion of pneumonia in pregnancy, see Chapter 8, Section A.

XVI. RUBELLA
Rachel Elizabeth Hall, MD, FAAFP

A. Epidemiology
Maternal and fetal rubella infections were common 40 years ago. Mass rubella vaccination began in 1969, and in 2005, the CDC was able to announce the elimination of endemic rubella and congenital rubella syndrome (CRS) in the United States, with less than 25 cases per year of reported rubella since 2001.[1] However, rubella remains endemic in other areas of the world; therefore, vigilance to immunize should continue. Two main risk factors for CRS remain: US immigrants and travel outside the United States during early pregnancy.[2]

B. Natural History
1. Acute rubella infection

   Acute rubella infection consists of a maculopapular rash lasting up to 3 days, generalized lymphadenopathy including posterior auricular and occipital nodes, and transient arthritis and arthralgia. About 50% to 70% of infections are symptomatic.

2. Transmission/incubation

   The incubation period is 14 to 21 days. Transmission occurs via respiratory droplets. Patients are most infectious in the prodromal phase preceding the rash.

3. Immunity

   Immunity to rubella is documented by serology with declining complement fixation titers. This pattern is common after naturally acquired infections and vaccination. Reinfection can occur in previously infected individuals and can result in fetal transmission in about 5% of the cases that occur during the first trimester.[3,4] There are rare case reports of CRS due to reinfection despite immune level titers[5,6]; however, the risk for reinfection with documented immunity is less than 5%, and the risk for resultant CRS is extremely low.[7]

4. Vertical transmission[8,9]

   Rubella infections occurring during the first 11 weeks of gestation are associated with a 90% risk for congenital defects. After 16 weeks of gestation, this risk is negligible. Typically, infections between 12 and 16 weeks have only newborn hearing loss as sequelae.

C. Effects on Perinatal Outcome: Congenital Rubella Syndrome

Effects on perinatal outcome of CRS include[9,10]:

1. Transient effects (newborn to 6 months old)

   These include hepatosplenomegaly, pneumonia, jaundice, hemolytic anemia, and thrombocytopenic purpura.

2. Permanent abnormalities

   These include sensorineural deafness (may be profound), congenital heart defects (especially patent ductus arteriosus), cataracts, microphthalmia, and encephalopathy.

3. Late-onset effects

   These include endocrine dysfunction (diabetes, thyroid disease, and growth hormone deficiency), ocular and auditory damage, progressive encephalopathy, vascular sclerosis, and hypertension. About 50% to 70% of infants may appear normal at birth and develop manifestations after the neonatal period.

D. Management Guidelines

Management guides for CRS include[11]:

1. Routine screening

   Routine screening for rubella immunity should occur at or before the onset of prenatal care. A recent Canadian study indicated that routine screening for rubella during pregnancy was occurring 94% of the time.[9]

2. Potential exposure of the nonimmune patient

   Immediate serologic evaluation of the nonimmune patient should occur with potential exposure to rubella. Hemagglutination inhibition antibodies are followed by complement-fixation antibodies within several days after onset of rash.

3. Patient with acute rubella infection during early pregnancy

   Patients who have a diagnosis of acute rubella in the first 16 weeks of pregnancy should be offered counseling and consideration of termination of pregnancy. Immunoglobulin does not prevent congenital rubella infection but may modify its clinical course. If therapeutic abortion is declined, intramuscular immunoglobulin is given at a dose of 55 ml/kg.[12]

E. Prevention

The prevention of congenital rubella remains one of the most significant successful public health stories of the twentieth century. Vaccine efficacy is estimated to be greater than 97%.[7] About 30% of women of childbearing age who have the two-dose measles, mumps, and rubella (MMR) vaccine develop low antibody levels within 15 years of vaccination.[10] Thus, clinicians must maintain vigilance as to which of their patients should be revaccinated in the preconceptional period or during the postpartum period. In addition, vaccination needs to be offered to nonpregnant immigrants when they seek medical care to reduce this infection source.[3,8] Inadvertent vaccination during pregnancy is generally associated with no adverse fetal effect, although rare subclinical neonatal rubella cases have been reported.[13] The theoretical risk for CRS caused by vaccination during pregnancy is estimated to be from 0.5% to 1.6%.[14,15] In 2001, the CDC changed the recommended period in which not to conceive after receiving a rubella-containing vaccination from 3 months to 28 days.[14,16] In addition, inadvertent vaccination during pregnancy is no longer a consideration for termination.[16,17]

REFERENCES

1. Centers for Disease Control and Prevention: Achievements in public health: elimination of rubella and congenital rubella syndrome—United States, 1969-2004, *MMWR* 54:279-282, 2005.

2. Mehta NM, Thomas RM: Antenatal screening for rubella—infection or immunity, *BMJ* 325:90-91, 2002.
3. Banerji A, Ford-Jones EL, Kelly E et al: Congenital rubella syndrome despite maternal antibodies, *CMAJ* 173:1678-1681, 2005.
4. Coulter C, Wood R, Robson J: Rubella infection in pregnancy, *Commun Dis Intell* 23:93-96, 1999.
5. Aboudy Y, Barnea B, Yosef L et al: Clinical rubella re-infection during pregnancy in a previously vaccinated woman, *J Infect* 41:187-189, 2000.
6. Ushida M, Katow S, Furukawa S: Congenital rubella syndrome due to infection after maternal antibody conversion with vaccine, *Jpn J Infect Dis* 56:68-69, 2003.
7. Weir E, Sider D: A refresher on rubella, *CMAJ* 172:1680-1681, 2005.
8. Danovaro-Holliday MC, Zimmerman L, Reef SE: Preventing congenital rubella syndrome (CRS) through vaccination of susceptible women of childbearing age, *J Womens Health Gend Based Med* 10:617-619, 2001.
9. Gyorkos TW, Tannenbaum TN, Abrahamowicz M et al: Evaluation of rubella screening in pregnant women, *CMAJ* 159:1091-1094, 1998.
10. Davidkin I, Peltola H, Leinikki P et al: Duration of rubella immunity induced by two-dose measles, mumps and rubella (MMR) vaccination: a 15-year follow-up in Finland, *Vaccine* 18:3106-3112, 2000.
11. Centers for Disease Control and Prevention: Control and prevention of rubella: evaluation and management of suspected outbreaks, rubella in pregnant women, and surveillance for congenital rubella syndrome, *MMWR* 50:1-23, 2001.
12. American Academy of Pediatrics: Rubella. In Pickering LK, Baker CJ, Long SS et al, editors: *Red book: 2006 report of the committee on infectious diseases,* ed 27, Elk Grove Village, IL, 2006, American Academy of Pediatrics, pp 574-579.
13. Hofmann J, Kortung M, Pustowoit B et al: Persistent fetal rubella vaccine virus infection following inadvertent vaccination during early pregnancy, *J Med Virol* 61:155-158, 2000.
14. Centers for Disease Control and Prevention: Notice to readers: revised ACIP recommendation for avoiding pregnancy after receiving a rubella-containing vaccine, *MMWR* 50:1117, 2001.
15. Stegmann BJ, Carey JC: TORCH infections, *Curr Womens Health Rep* 2:253-258, 2002.
16. Sur DK, Wallis DH: Vaccinations in pregnancy, *Am Fam Physician* 68:299-304, 2003.
17. Bar-Oz B, Levicheck Z, Moretti ME et al: Pregnancy outcome following rubella vaccination, *Am J Med Genet* 130A:52-54, 2004.

XVII. VARICELLA ZOSTER
Stephen D. Ratcliffe, MD, MSPH

A. Epidemiology
1. Immune status

   Most pregnant women are immune to varicella because of previous infection. History of infection is highly predictive of immunity.[1] Eighty percent of adult women with a negative history have serologic evidence of immunity. Adult immigrants from tropical countries may have a much lower rate of immunity.[2]

2. Incidence

   The incidence of varicella in pregnancy is 5 to 10 in 10,000.[3]

B. Natural History
1. Transmission

   Infection is transmitted by direct contact (droplet, aerosol from vesicular fluid of skin lesions) or respiratory secretions.

2. Significant exposure

   This occurs by face-to-face contact with an infected person for at least 5 minutes, contact indoors with an infected person for longer than 1 hour, or living in the same household as an infected person. Infectivity extends from 1 to 2 days before onset of rash until the lesions are crusted, usually 4 to 5 days after onset of rash. The incubation period is 10 to 21 days.[2]

C. Effects on Perinatal Outcome
Prospective data from a 1994 British study[4] suggest that the varicella in gravidas may not be more severe than in nonpregnant adults.

1. Maternal pneumonia

   It is uncertain whether chickenpox pneumonitis is more common or severe in pregnancy. Retrospective data may represent reporting bias of hospitalized cases, according to the above study. Risk factors of pregnancy associated with increased severity of varicella pneumonia are third-trimester occurrence, smoking, chronic obstructive pulmonary disease, systemic steroids, and severity of the rash.[5]

2. Fetal varicella embryopathy

   This fetal infection is similar to CRS with limb hypoplasia, encephalomyelitis, cataracts, chorioretinitis, microphthalmia, and intrauterine growth restriction.[6] There is a 1% chance of embryopathy if infection occurs in the first trimester, 2.2% chance if between 13 and 20 weeks of gestation, and 0% if infection occurs later in pregnancy, according to prospective data from a large 1994 study.[4] Ultrasound findings for fetal infection include polyhydramnios, limb and ventricular abnormalities, fetal hydrops, and liver hyperechogenicities.[7,8]

3. Association with spontaneous abortion

   No evidence has been reported that the rate of spontaneous abortion is increased.[9]

4. Vertical transmission

Perinatal transmission, and subsequent congenital disseminated varicella, is likely if maternal varicella rash occurs in the critical period between 5 days before and 2 days after delivery.[10,11]

a. Infants exposed by maternal infection from 28 to 7 days before delivery: These infants receive the transplacental maternal antibody. If neonatal chickenpox ensues, it usually follows a benign course.

b. Exposure 7 to 3 days before delivery: Progressively fewer newborns have varicella antibodies when the mother's rash occurs 7 to 3 days before delivery.

c. Exposure less than 3 days before delivery: No antibody is detected in babies born less than 3 days after onset of the mother's rash.[4]

d. Neonatal varicella infections: Varicella infections occasionally occur in the critical period without the patient receiving the recommended immunoglobulin. The clinical attack rate in infants whose mothers developed rash between 7 days before and 7 days after delivery is 60%.[5]

e. Herpes zoster in infancy: This has been reported in those born to mothers with varicella in the second half of pregnancy.[4] No evidence exists that maternal herpes zoster causes intrauterine infection.

D. Management Guidelines

1. Nonimmune pregnant women

These women should avoid contact with those who have varicella or zoster infections. Risk for exposure may be unavoidable in the prodromal phase (before lesions erupt).

2. Determination of immunity

Immunity is determined by enzyme-linked or latex agglutination; complement-fixation titers are not sensitive enough.[4]

3. Significant exposure in a nonimmune pregnant woman

This exposure should be treated with varicella-zoster immunoglobulin (VZIG) 125 units/10 kg. The minimum dose is 125 units, and the maximum dose is 625 units intramuscularly, given within 96 hours of exposure.

The previous producer of VZIG ceased production of this immunoglobulin in 2004 and supplies are essentially depleted. A new form of VZIG, called *VariZIG,* is available under an investigational new drug application submitted to the Food and Drug Administration.[12] VariZIG is administered by FFF Enterprises (24-hour telephone, 800-843-7477) and can usually be obtained by the clinician within 24 hours. The new VariZIG has been shown to be comparable with the previous VZIG product in terms of safety and efficacy.[13]

If an institution anticipates that it will commonly need the use of VZIG, it is recommended that its local institutional review board preapprove the use of this agent to expedite its delivery because of its status as an investigational new drug.

If it is not possible to obtain VZIG for the postexposure patient, the administration of 400 mg/kg immunoglobulin intravenous can be used.

4. Maternal varicella infections

Antiviral therapy should be administered for varicella pneumonia and severe varicella in pregnancy; acyclovir, at 10 mg/kg IV three times daily for a minimum of 5 days, has been recommended.[3]

5. Herpes zoster

Herpes zoster does not require treatment.

6. Infants with perinatal exposure

Exposure resulting from maternal infection in which the rash occurs 5 days before until 2 days after birth should receive VZIG, 1.25 ml intramuscularly, immediately after birth. These infants must be monitored closely for 14 to 16 days (the end of any possible incubation period) and may still need intravenous or oral acyclovir at 10 to 15 mg/kg/dose every 8 hours should congenital varicella ensue.[3] Maternal VZIG primarily attenuates the disease course in infants. There is some indication that the clinical attack rate of perinatal varicella may be modified by its use.[4]

E. Prevention

1. Vaccination

This is indicated for immunocompetent children older than 12 months without a history of varicella. In persons older than 12 years, two doses of vaccine administered 4 to 8 weeks apart are recommended.

2. Preconception

Question all women of childbearing age regarding chickenpox history. Those with negative replies should be offered the varicella vaccine or serologic testing followed by vaccination of susceptible patients. Pregnancy should be avoided for 1 month after each vaccine dose.[2] The Varivax manufacturer has established a Pregnancy Registry accessed by phone (800-986-8999) to monitor the outcome of women receiving the vaccine 3 months before or at any time during pregnancy.

3. Pregnancy

Question all women regarding their chickenpox history. Obtain a varicella IgG level for women with a negative/unknown history of previous infection or who have not completed a Varivax immunization series.

4. After delivery

The varicella vaccine may be considered for a nursing mother.[2] The first dose could be given on discharge from the hospital, and the second dose at the 2-month well-child check.

Acknowledgment

I acknowledge the contribution of Jennifer Bell, M.D., who authored this section in the second edition of *Family Practice Obstetrics*.

REFERENCES

1. Rouse D, Gardner M, Allen SJ et al: Management of the presumed susceptible varicella (chickenpox)-exposed gravida: a cost-effectiveness/cost-benefit analysis, *Obstet Gynecol* 87: 932-936, 1996.
2. CDC: Prevention of varicella updated recommendations of the Advisory Committee on Immunization Practices (ACIP), *MMWR* 48(RR-06):1-5, 1999.
3. Nathwani D, Maclean A, Conway S et al: Varicella infections in pregnancy and the newborn, *Br J Infect* 36:59-71, 1998.
4. Enders G, Miller E, Cradock-Watson J et al: Consequences of maternal varicella and herpes zoster in pregnancy: prospective study of 1739 cases, *Lancet* 343:1547-1550, 1994.
5. Inocencion G, Loebsein R, Lalkin A et al: Managing exposure to chickenpox during pregnancy, *Can Fam Physician* 4: 745-747, 1998.
6. Brunell PA: Fetal and neonatal varicella-zoster infections, *Semin Perinatol* 7:47-56, 1983.
7. Pretorius DH, Hayward I, Jones KL et al: Sonographic evaluation of pregnancies with maternal varicella infection, *J Ultrasound Med* 11:459-463, 1992.
8. Meyberg-Solomayer GC, Fehm T, Muller-Hansen I et al: Prenatal ultrasound diagnosis, follow-up and outcome of congenital varicella syndrome, *Fetal Diagn Ther* 21:296-301, 2006.
9. Pastuszak AL, Levy M, Schick B et al: Outcome after maternal varicella infection in the first 20 weeks of pregnancy, *N Engl J Med* 330:901-905, 1994.
10. Miller E, Cradock-Watson JE, Ridehalgh MS: Outcome in newborn babies given anti-varicella-zoster immunoglobulin after perinatal maternal infection with varicella-zoster virus, *Lancet* 12:371-373, 1989.
11. Tan MP, Koren G: Chickenpox in pregnancy: revisited, *Reprod Toxicol* 21:410-420, 2006.
12. CDC: A new product (VariZIG) for postexposure prophylaxis of varicella available under an investigational new drug application expanded access protocol, *MMWR* 55:209-210, 2006.
13. Koren G, Money D, Boucher M et al: Serum concentrations, efficacy, and safety of a new, intravenously administered varicella zoster immune globulin in pregnant women, *J Clin Pharmacol* 42:267-274, 2002.

XVIII. CYTOMEGALOVIRUS
Stephen D. Ratcliffe, MD, MSPH

A. Epidemiology

CMV is a herpes virus that commonly infects young adults. It is transmitted via respiratory droplets, urine, sexual activity, breastfeeding, and blood transfusions. Women who reside or work with young children as teachers, day-care workers, or health-care workers are at particular risk for contracting this viral infection. Rates of young children who are infected with CMV vary between 15% and 25% in day-care settings, and carriers shed this virus in urine and other secretions for up to 14 months after primary infection.[1] It is estimated that up to 25% of all congenital CMV infections are related to day-care exposure. CMV transmission in child-care homes occurs at a rate comparable with day-care centers.[2] Preterm infants less than 32 weeks of gestation are at increased risk for contracting CMV infection via breastfeeding.[3]

Higher socioeconomic groups have a lower seroprevalence of CMV, and thus are at increased risk for contracting a primary infection during pregnancy. Primary maternal infections occur in 0.7% to 4% of pregnancies, with 30% to 40% of these infections resulting in congenital infection. Recurrent infection occurs more commonly (1-14%) but results in congenital infection only 0.2% to 2% of the time. CMV is the most common congenitally acquired infection, affecting approximately 45,000 fetuses per year in the United States (0.2-2.2% of all neonates) and causing symptomatic infections in the newborns of between 8% and 14% of these infections.[1] Because of the subtle or asymptomatic presentation of CMV infections, clinicians underdiagnose this infection both during pregnancy and after childbirth. Congenital CMV infections are the leading infectious cause of hearing loss and developmental delay.

B. Natural History

1. Maternal

CMV infections are usually subclinical, occasionally associated with a "mononucleosis"-like illness with pharyngitis, lymphadenopathy, and fever.

These infections may be accompanied by hepatitis, pneumonia, and thrombocytopenia. Primary maternal infections that occur in the preconception or periconceptional periods have a lower risk for fetal infection (10-20%) than primary CMV infections acquired during pregnancy (40-50%).[4,5] Maternal CMV infections may occur in women with preexisting immunity.[6]

2. Fetal
   Fetal structural effects are most pronounced after first-trimester infections and are characterized by microcephaly and periventricular echodensities. Other fetal ultrasonographic features include intrauterine growth restriction, ventriculomegaly, and hepatosplenomegaly.

3. Neonatal
   a. Symptomatic (CMV inclusion disease): The newborn presents with hepatosplenomegaly (60-74%), petechiae (76-79%), jaundice (63-67%), and microcephaly (50%). Abnormal laboratory studies include thrombocytopenia, hyperbilirubinemia, abnormal liver function tests, and increased cerebrospinal fluid protein. Abnormal computed tomography (CT) findings, including ventricular enlargement and intracranial calcifications, occur in more than 50% of infected newborns. More than 90% of infants who survive the initial infection experience long-term complications such as sensorineural hearing loss, chronic neurologic dysfunction (seizures, developmental delay, mental retardation), and visual impairment.[7]
   b. Asymptomatic: These infants have the congenital infection but are asymptomatic in the newborn period. They experience many of the long-term complications listed earlier but at a lower incidence. Hearing loss is the most common impairment affecting about 15% of those infected, although two thirds of this sensory hearing loss may not be detected with the newborn hearing screen.[8] This impairment may be detected by audio-evoked response testing as early as 2 to 3 months of age and may progress to profound hearing loss by 3 to 4 years of age. Developmental delay and/or mental retardation affect about 15% of this group.

C. Diagnosis

1. Prenatal
   The presence of specific ultrasonographic abnormalities (e.g., periventricular or intestinal echodensities, ascites, ventriculomegaly) identifies fetuses that are more severely affected. Amniotic fluid or fetal blood can be analyzed for CMV by culture, PCR testing, or using the shell vial assay.[9] The latter test has a sensitivity/specificity that approaches 100% and is considered the gold standard.[1]

2. Neonatal
   The standard diagnostic tools include culture and PCR testing of the neonatal urine. The advantage of the latter method is its more rapid reporting. PCR testing followed by dot-blot hybridization is again the test of choice.[4] The shell vial assay is also utilized for this purpose.

D. Treatment Guidelines

Preliminary RCT evidence exists that treatment of symptomatic congenital CMV infection with ganciclovir 6 mg/kg every 12 hours for 6 weeks results in improved hearing at 6 months and no improvement in hematologic or hepatic function; it is also associated with neutropenia in the majority of patients.[10,11] Family physicians will need to refer symptomatic neonates to receive this treatment after a discussion of the risks and benefits have been explained to the infant's parents. Because of the progressive nature of hearing impairment, infected infants should undergo audiologic screening every 6 months until 10 years of age.[1]

E. Prevention

1. Patient education
   Women at increased risk for contracting CMV during pregnancy, such as day-care workers and mothers with a toddler in day care, should know their CMV antibody status. Those women who are seronegative should be counseled how to decrease the risk for acquiring this infection. This counseling should consist of frequent hand washing and the use of gloves while changing diapers or having extensive contact with saliva. This regimen has been shown in an RCT to be effective in preventing the acquisition of CMV during pregnancy.[12] Another important group at increased risk for acquiring CMV during pregnancy is the subset of young women with a history of STDs. These women should be counseled to use condoms throughout their pregnancy and to avoid new sexual partners.

2. Provider education
   Clinicians have not been adequately informed about the silent epidemic of CMV. The three at-risk

groups identified earlier should undergo serologic testing for the presence of CMV IgM and IgG antibodies at the onset of pregnancy. If seronegative, they should have reenforced counseling throughout pregnancy to minimize potential contact with sources of CMV.[13]

3. Primary prevention with active immunization: Towne vaccine

The Towne vaccine has been shown in RCTs to prevent transmission of CMV in kidney transplant recipients. This vaccine has been tested in women of childbearing age and has been shown to induce cellular immunity that persisted for the 6 months of monitoring. This vaccine offers the potential for primary prevention of this devastating congenital infection.[14,15]

4. Primary prevention with passive immunization

Patients who acquire primary CMV infection during pregnancy have the greatest risk (about 25%) for having infants with symptomatic congenital infection. A large, prospective, nonrandomized trial demonstrated that treatment with hyperimmune CMV immunoglobulin markedly decreased risk for congenital infection to 3% (OR, 0.02; $p < 0.001$).[16] The need to confirm the effectiveness and safety of passive immunization with RCTs is clear.

REFERENCES

1. Bale J, Miner L, Petheram S: Congenital cytomegalovirus infection, *Curr Treat Options Neurol* 4:225-230, 2002.
2. Bale J, Zimmerman B, Dawson J et al: Cytomegalovirus transmission in child care homes, *Arch Pediatr Adolesc Med* 153: 75-79, 1999.
3. Vochem M, Hamprecht K, Jahn G et al: Transmission of cytomegalovirus to preterm infants through breast milk, *Pediatr Infect Dis J* 12:53-58, 1998.
4. Revello M, Gerna G: Diagnosis and management of human cytomegalovirus infection in the mother, fetus, and newborn infant, *Clin Microbiol Rev* 15:680-715, 2002.
5. Boppana S, River L, Fowler K et al: Intrauterine transmission of cytomegalovirus to infants of mothers with preconceptional immunity, *N Engl J Med* 344:36-71, 2001.
6. Daiminger A, Bader U, Enders G: Pre- and periconceptional primary cytomegalovirus infection: risk of vertical transmission and congenital disease, *BJOG* 112:116-126, 2005.
7. Noyola D, Demmler G, Nelson C et al: Early predictors of neurodevelopmental outcome in symptomatic congenital cytomegalovirus infection, *J Pediatr* 138:325-331, 2001.
8. Fowler K, Dahle A, Boppana S et al: Newborn hearing screening: will children with hearing loss caused by congenital cytomegalovirus infection be missed? *J Pediatr* 135:60-64, 1999.
9. Bodeus M, Hubinont C, Bernard P et al: Prenatal diagnosis of human cytomegalovirus by culture and polymerase chain reaction: 98 pregnancies leading to congenital infection, *Prenat Diagn* 19:314-317, 1999.
10. Kimberlin D, Lin C, Sanchez P et al: Ganciclovir treatment of symptomatic congenital cytomegalovirus infection: results of a phase III randomized trail. Abstract presented at the 40th International Conference on Antimicrobial Agents and Chemotheryapy, Toronto, September 17-20, 2000.
11. Whitley R, Cloud G, Bruber W et al: Ganciclovir treatment of symptomatic congenital cytomegalovirus infection: results of a phase II study, *J Infect Dis* 175:1080-1086, 1997.
12. Adler S, Finney J, Manganello A et al: Prevention of child-to-mother transmission of cytomegalovirus by changing behaviors: a randomized controlled trial, *Pediatr Infect Dis J* 15: 240-241, 1996.
13. Griffiths P: Strategies to prevent CMV infection in the neonate, *Semin Neonatol* 7:293-299, 2002.
14. Adler S, Hempfling S, Starr S et al: Safety and immunogenicity of the Towne strain cytomegalovirus vaccine, *Pediatr Infect Dis J* 17:2058-2061, 1998.
15. Fowler K, Stagno S, Pass R: Maternal immunity and prevention of congenital cytomegalovirus infection, *JAMA* 289:1108-1111, 2003.
16. Nigo G, Adler SP, La Torre R et al: Passive immunization during pregnancy for congenital cytomegalovirus infection, *N Engl J Med* 353:1350-1362, 2005.

XIX. TOXOPLASMOSIS
Amity Rubeor, DO

Congenital toxoplasmosis can cause significant morbidity and mortality in the fetus or developing child.[1] A primary infection with *T. gondii* during a woman's pregnancy puts the fetus at greatest risk.

A. Epidemiology

According to the 1999-2000 NHANES, 15.8% of women in the United States between the ages of 12 and 49 have serologic evidence of previous *T. gondii* infection.[2] Nevertheless, congenital toxoplasmosis is a rare occurrence in the United States, with an incidence of about 1 to 10 in 10,000 live births.[3] The incidence is greater in countries such as France and Austria, where the consumption of undercooked meat is greater.

B. Pathogenesis

T. gondii is an obligate intracellular protozoan that can be found in raw meat (as a tissue cyst) and cat feces (as an oocyst). When a pregnant woman ingests either of these forms, her digestive system breaks down the cyst wall and releases the infective form of *T. gondii*. From here the infective form invades the intestinal lumen cells and transforms into the metabolically active tachyzoite form; tachyzoites easily disseminate through the circulatory system and infect many organs, including the placenta. Through the placenta, the tachyzoite can be transmitted to the fetus.

First-trimester infections are transmitted to the fetus in only about 15% of cases.[4] However, these congenital infections tend to be more severe, with an overall mortality rate of 5%.[5] Third-trimester infections are transmitted to the fetus in about 60% of cases, but the majority of these infants are born with subclinical infections.[4] Severe congenital toxoplasmosis has been rarely reported with maternal third-trimester infection.[1]

C. Clinical Features

1. Maternal

   Of those women who are exposed and acquire a primary *T. gondii* infection during pregnancy, 90% will be asymptomatic.[4] Women who do show signs of infection usually present with "flu-like" symptoms, including general malaise, a low-grade fever, or lymphadenopathy. A solitary enlarged cervical lymph node is the most common clinical presentation.[1] Immunocompromised individuals may experience more extensive pulmonary and central nervous system involvement. Chorioretinitis, causing maternal photophobia and blurry vision, is a rare clinical presentation with acute infection, but it is associated with greater fetal risk for congenital disease if not recognized and treated.

2. Fetal and neonatal

   Because women can be asymptomatic with infection, the diagnosis of toxoplasmosis may not be entertained until fetal abnormalities are identified via ultrasound or when the infant presents with symptoms suggestive of congenital disease. Sonographic findings of ventriculomegaly, brain or hepatic calcifications, splenomegaly, ascites, or a thickened placenta should raise concerns for toxoplasmosis. Daffos and colleagues studied 746 pregnant women at risk for congenital toxoplasmosis.[7] Sixty percent of those women at greatest risk for having severe fetal infection (i.e., those with infections at <16 weeks of gestation) had sonographic evidence of fetal infection.[1] Infants with congenital infection may demonstrate chorioretinitis, abnormal spinal fluid, anemia, splenomegaly, jaundice, fever, lymphadenopathy, intracerebral calcifications, or hydrocephalus. However, most infants with congenital infection are asymptomatic at birth.

D. Diagnosis

1. Maternal infection

   Serology is the primary method of diagnosis. Tests most frequently used include ELISA, indirect fluorescent antibody test, and an immunosorbent agglutination assay.[8] During an infected individual's immune response, IgM appears earlier and declines more rapidly than IgG. However, IgM levels can persist for years in an exposed individual, complicating diagnosis. Even though the sensitivity and specificity of the above tests range between 93.3% and 100% and 77.5% and 100%, respectively,[9] unacceptable false-positive test results do occur. This erroneous test result may lead some patients with presumed toxoplasmosis early in pregnancy to terminate a normal pregnancy. Therefore, it is recommended that positive IgM serology be further evaluated at the preferred reference laboratory, Toxoplasma Serology Laboratory, Palo Alto Medical Foundation (PAMF-TSL; http://www.pamf.org/serology; 415-326-8120).[10] At this laboratory, a *Toxoplasma* serological profile, which includes the "gold standard" Sabin–Feldman dye test, IgM ELISA, IgA ELISA, IgE ELISA, and a differential agglutination test, can be done to better elucidate an acute versus previous *Toxoplasma* infection.

2. Fetal congenital infection

   The preferred test for diagnosing congenital toxoplasmosis is the highly sensitive (>98%) and specific (>98%) PCR analysis of amniotic fluid.[11] This should be done about 4 weeks after the diagnosis of the acute maternal infection to prevent the possibility of false-negative results.[12] However, the testing should be avoided at less than 18 weeks of gestation because of the lower sensitivity and greater risk for fetal injury.[13] Monthly fetal ultrasounds are also recommended for pregnant women with suspected or diagnosed acute toxoplasmosis.[4]

3. Neonatal congenital infection

   When infection is suspected in the newborn, peripheral blood samples from the mother and neonate should be taken, looking for the presence of IgM and IgA antibodies.[5] Other viral congenital infections, notably herpes, CMV, and rubella, should also be ruled out. Neonatal cerebrospinal fluid studies (including PCR for *T. gondii* DNA), head imaging, and an indirect funduscopic examination for chorioretinitis should be performed.

E. Treatment

1. Maternal toxoplasmosis

Spiramycin is the recommended treatment for toxoplasmosis acquired in the first and early second trimesters (Table 9-8). Spiramycin can only be obtained through the Food and Drug Administration (301-827-2127); it is available at no cost after consultation with the Toxoplasma Reference Laboratory (PAMF-TSL). Spiramycin acts by decreasing transmission to the fetus and has been shown to decrease transmission rates by 60%.[14]

TABLE 9-8 **Treatment of *Toxoplasma gondii* Infection in Pregnant Women and Neonates**

Patient	Medication(s) and Dosage	Duration of Therapy
Pregnant woman diagnosed with acute toxoplasmosis during the first 21 weeks of gestation	Spiramycin: 1 g every 8 hours with food	**If** fetal infection highly suspected or diagnosed, stop spiramycin at 18 weeks and change to the regimen of pyrimethamine, sulfadiazine, and folinic acid; continue until delivery (see below). **If** no sonographic evidence of fetal infection exists and amniotic fluid PCR testing is negative for infection, continue spiramycin until delivery.
Pregnant woman diagnosed with acute toxoplasmosis acquired in the late second trimester or third trimester + Pregnant woman with a diagnosed or highly suspected fetal infection	Pyrimethamine: 100 mg/day divided BID for 2 days, then 50 mg/day + Sulfadiazine: 75 mg/kg/day divided BID (maximum 4 g/day) for 2 days, then 100 mg/day divided BID (maximum 4 g/day) + Folinic acid: 10-20 mg/day	**If** fetal infection is highly suspected or diagnosed, continue the regimen until delivery. **If** no sonographic evidence of fetal infection exists and amniotic fluid PCR testing is negative for infection, may consider change to spiramycin and continue until delivery but would consult a reference laboratory. **Continue** folinic acid for 1 week after cessation of pyrimethamine.
Newborn with highly suspected or diagnosed congenital toxoplasmosis	Pyrimethamine: 2 mg/kg/day divided BID for 2 days, then 1 mg/kg/day for 2 or 6 months, then 1 mg/kg every Monday, Wednesday, and Friday +	Continue therapy for 1 year.
	Sulfadiazine: 100 mg/kg/day divided BID +	Continue therapy for 1 year.
	Folinic acid: 10 mg three times per week +	Administer while dosing pyrimethamine and for 1 week after pyrimethamine discontinued.
	Prednisone (when CSF protein is >1 g/dl and/or when active chorioretinitis threatens vision): 1 mg/kg/day divided BID	Continue until CSF protein elevation ceases and/or when active chorioretinitis no longer threatens vision.

Adapted from Montoya JG, Rosso F: Diagnosis and management of toxoplasmosis, *Clin Perinatol* 32:705-726, 2005; and Remington JS, McLeod R, Thullierz P et al: Toxoplasmosis. In Remington JS, Klein JO, Wilson CB et al, editors: *Infectious diseases of the fetus and newborn infant,* ed 6, St. Louis, 2006, Saunders.

PCR, Polymerase chain reaction; BID, twice a day; CSF, cerebrospinal fluid.

It concentrates in the placenta but does not cross and should be continued even when PCR testing on amniotic fluid is negative because of possible later fetal infection.[1] If pregnant women are suspected of acquiring the infection late in the second trimester or during the third trimester, pyrimethamine, sulfonamides, and folic acid should be used for treatment because the ability of spiramycin to decrease vertical transmission wanes late in the second trimester[4] (see Table 9-8).

2. Confirmed in utero congenital toxoplasmosis
When amniotic fluid PCR for *T. gondii* confirms an active fetal or congenital infection, the recommended treatment regimen consists of pyrimethamine, sulfadiazine, and folinic acid (see Table 9-8). Clinicians should obtain pharmacologic and perinatal consultations to balance treatment efficacy with the avoidance of bone-marrow suppression.

3. Neonates with congenital toxoplasmosis
The most widely accepted treatment regimen for neonates with congenital toxoplasmosis includes sulfadiazine, pyrimethamine, and folinic acid (see Table 9-8). Currently, the Chicago Collaborative Treatment Trial at the University of Chicago is studying appropriate management of congenital toxoplasmosis. (Contact Dr. Rima McLeod for information and to enroll patients in the study [773-834-4152].[15])

F. Prevention

Routine screening is not recommended in the United States because of the low prevalence of the disease. As a result, the positive predictive value of abnormal maternal serology is less than 1%. It is, however, recommended to screen women with HIV disease for this infection. In a high-prevalence area in Belgium, a risk reduction program that emphasized hygienic precautions with cats and the proper preparation of meat resulted in a 60% reduction in seroconversion.[16] In the United States, consuming a tissue cyst in undercooked meat is the primary means of infection, but ingestion of oocysts in cat feces has been implicated in some epidemics.[1]

The ACOG recommends that all pregnant women be counseled in methods to prevent acquisition of toxoplasmosis.[17] Therefore, family physicians should counsel their prenatal patients to avoid eating undercooked meat (including beef, pork, lamb, and venison)[1] and suggest to those women with cats to avoid cleaning litter boxes or to wear gloves (with subsequent hand washing) when cleaning them. If the cats are strictly "indoor cats," and their only food source is manufactured cat food, then these suggestions could be loosened.[17] It is also suggested that pregnant women where gloves when working with soil and subsequently wash their hands.[17]

REFERENCES

1. Remington JS, McLeod R, Thullierz P et al: Toxoplasmosis. In Remington JS, Klein JO, Wilson CB et al, editors: *Infectious diseases of the fetus and newborn infant,* ed 6, St Louis, 2006, Saunders.
2. Jones JL, Kruszon-moran D, Wilson M: *Toxoplasma gondii* infection in the United States, 1999-2000, *Emerg Infect Dis* 9:55-62, 2003.
3. Lopez A, Dietz VJ, Wilson M et al: Preventing congenital toxoplasmosis, *MMWR Recomm Rep* 49:59-68, 2000.
4. Montoya JG, Rosso F: Diagnosis and management of toxoplasmosis, *Clin Perinatol* 32:705-726, 2005.
5. Mittendorf R, Pryde P, Herschel M et al: Is routine antenatal toxoplasmosis screening justified in the United States? Statistical considerations in the application of medical screening tests, *Clin Obstet Gynecol* 42:163-175, 1999.
6. Dunn D, Wallon M, Peyron F et al: Mother-to-child transmission of toxoplasmosis: risk estimates for clinical counseling, *Lancet* 353:1829-1833, 1999.
7. Daffos F, Forestier F, Capella-Pavlovsky M et al: Prenatal management of 746 pregnancies at risk for congenital toxoplasmosis, *N Engl J Med* 318:271-275, 1988.
8. Andrews JI, Diekema DJ, Yankowitz J: Prenatal testing for infectious disease, *Clin Lab Med* 23:295-315, 2003.
9. Wilson M, Remington JS, Clavet C et al: Evaluation of six commercial kits for detection of human immunoglobulin M antibodies to *Toxoplasma gondii.* The FDA Toxoplasmosis Ad Hoc Working Group, *J Clin Microbiol* 35(12):3112-3115, 1997.
10. U.S. Public Health Service, Department of Health and Human Services and Food and Drug Administration: *FDA public health advisory: limitations of toxoplasma IgM commercial test kits,* Rockville, MD, 1997, Department of Health and Human Services, Food and Drug Administration.
11. Forestier F, Hohlfeld P, Sole Y et al: Prenatal diagnosis of congenital toxoplasmosis by PCR: extended experience (letter), *Prenat Diagn* 18:405-415, 1998.
12. Hohfeld P, Daffos F, Costa JM et al: Prenatal diagnosis of congenital toxoplasmosis with a polymerase-chain reaction test on amniotic fluid, *N Engl J Med* 331(11):695-699, 1994.
13. Romand S, Wallon M, Franck J et al: Prenatal diagnosis using polymerase chain reaction on amniotic fluid for congenital toxoplasmosis, *Obstet Gynecol* 97:296-300, 2001.
14. Mombro M, Perathoner C, Leone A et al: Congenital toxoplasmosis: 10-year follow up, *Eur J Ped* 154(18):635-639, 1995.
15. McAuley J, Boyer KM, Patel D et al: Early and longitudinal evaluations of treated infants and children and untreated historical patients with congenital toxoplasmosis: the Chicago Collaborative Treatment Trial, *Clin Infect Dis* 18:38-72, 1994.
16. Foulan W, Naessens A, Derde M: Evaluation of the possibilities for preventing toxoplasmosis, *Am J Perinatol* 11:57-61, 1994.
17. Perinatal viral and parasitic infections, *ACOG Pract Bull* 20: 1-21, 2000.

XX. PARVOVIRUS B19
Amity Rubeor, DO

Although there is no conclusive evidence that parvovirus B19 is teratogenic, maternal infection with vertical transmission of the virus has been associated with spontaneous abortion, hydrops fetalis, and stillbirth.[1,2]

A. Epidemiology
Parvovirus B19 was first identified as a cause of nonimmune hydrops fetalis in 1984.[3] It is endemic in the winter and spring, and primarily infects children. Approximately 50% of women of childbearing age are immune.[4] Nonimmune women at greatest risk for infection are pregnant women with children ages 6 to 7, pregnant women with a number of children at home, and school teachers.[5] The annual incidence in the United States of acute parvovirus B19 infection in pregnancy is estimated to be 1 in 400 pregnancies.[6]

B. Pathogenesis
Parvovirus B19 is a small, nonenveloped, single-stranded DNA virus. It is primarily transmitted via contact with nasal or oral secretions and appears to survive on plates and utensils. With infection, the virus will reach peak viremia within the first 2 days; viremia can last 7 to 10 days.[1] The virus invades human erythroid-progenitor lineage cells or other cells with the P antigen, including placental, fetal liver, and fetal heart cells.[7] Its pathogenesis includes lysis of red blood cell precursors, which may lead to severe anemia.[8,9] The risk for vertical transmission to the fetus is estimated to be 33%, with fetal outcomes dependent on gestational age.[9,10]

C. Clinical Features
1. Childhood infection
   In children, infection causes a time-limited viral syndrome, known as *erythema infectiosum* or "the fifth disease." This is manifested as the hallmark exanthem of "slapped cheeks," which spreads to the trunk with a lacy, reticular appearance. The rash appears 2 to 3 weeks after the initial period of viremia, when a child may have flu-like symptoms. It is during the viremic stage that a child is contagious, not when the rash is observed.
2. Maternal infection
   The most common adult presentation is polyarthralgias, primarily in the knees and proximal interphalangeal joints.[1] This also occurs after the viremic phase.[9] Rarely do adults present with a rash; only approximately one third of pregnant women manifest a rash.[11] Commonly, pregnant women present with flu-like symptoms, including low-grade fever, sore throat, malaise, and headache.[9] However, 25% of women will be asymptomatic.[9] Although uncommon, a maternal aplastic crisis can result from parvovirus infection.
3. Fetal infection
   Congenital infection can manifest as miscarriage in the first trimester and as fetal anemia, myocarditis, high-output cardiac failure, fetal hydrops, or stillbirth in the second or third trimesters.[9,10] Still, the neonatal outcome of pregnancies affected with maternal parvovirus is normal in 90% to 95% of cases.[12,13] Nonimmune hydrops fetalis occurs in only about 3% to 8% of maternal infections, and it spontaneously resolves in about one third of cases.[14] The incidence of fetal demise among women with proven acute parvovirus B19 infection ranges between 2% and 9%, and is greatest before 22 weeks of gestation.[2]

D. Diagnosis
1. Maternal infection
   The preferred serologic test in the diagnosis of acute maternal parvovirus B19 infection is the mμ-capture EIA; it detects IgM without competitive binding of IgG.[9,15] It has a sensitivity of 89.1% and specificity of 99.4%.[9] IgM antibodies are detected late in the viremic stage of the virus, between days 7 and 10 after infection.[1] They remain detectable for about 3 to 5 months.[16] IgG may be detected within 10 to 12 days and persist to provide lifelong immunity.[1] After maternal exposure, if initial antibody screens are negative, repeat testing should be done at 3 to 4 weeks to rule out seroconversion.[9]
2. Fetal infection
   Fetal IgM antibodies do not appear in the fetal circulation until after 22 weeks of gestation, and thus are not acceptable as a testing modality for congenital infection.[2] PCR testing of fetal tissue or fluids is highly sensitive for congenital infection.[1] However, because it does require invasive sampling, more commonly fetal surveillance is done through ultrasonography. When acute maternal infection is confirmed with positive IgM titers, the majority of perinatal practitioners will monitor the fetus with weekly ultrasounds for 8 to

10 weeks, assessing for any evidence of evolving fetal hydrops.[2] This will manifest as abnormal fluid collections in the fetus, including scalp edema, pericardial or pleural effusions, or ascites. In 2002, Cosmi and colleagues[10] reported that fetal anemia could be detected through noninvasive Doppler velocimetry. Middle cerebral artery peak velocity values found to be greater than 1.50 multiples of the median for gestational age are generally associated with fetal anemia and warrant invasive testing to confirm anemia.[9]

E. Treatment

Currently, no antiviral treatments are available for maternal or childhood infections. However, if serial ultrasounds show evidence of fetal hydrops, intervention may be warranted. There are two approaches to the management of fetal hydrops. The active approach consists of intrauterine fetal transfusions when fetal anemia is confirmed.[9] The second approach is more conservative and involves continued close monitoring without intervention. To date, retrospective studies have found conservative management to be comparable with the active approach.[13,17] However, with future prospective RCTs, clinicians will be able to approach treatment in a more evidence-based manner.

F. Prevention

At preconception and early prenatal visits, clinicians should instruct those women at increased risk for exposure to parvovirus B19 to use frequent hand washing at home and work. Currently, no recommendations have been made to remove pregnant women who work in schools or day cares from their workplace during parvovirus outbreaks because the typical rash does not occur until after the viremic period has passed.[2] Clinicians should encourage their maternity patients to report any flu-like illnesses, especially if they are accompanied with rash or polyarthralgias. Parvovirus B19 vaccinations may be available in the future for those women without childhood immunity.[9]

REFERENCES

1. Andrews JI, Diekema DJ, Yankowitz, J: Prenatal testing for infectious disease, *Clin Lab Med* 23:295-315, 2003.
2. Perinatal viral and parasitic infections, *ACOG Pract Bull* 20:1-21, 2000.
3. Brown T, Anaud A, Ritchie L et al: Intrauterine parvovirus infection associated with hydrops fetalis, *Lancet* 2:1033-1034, 1984.
4. Hedrick J: The effects of human parvovirus B19 and cytomegalovirus during pregnancy, *J Perinat Neonat Nurs* 10:30-39, 1996.
5. Valeur-Jensen AK, Pedersen CB, Westergaard T et al: Risk factors for parvovirus B19 infection in pregnancy, *JAMA* 281(12):1099-1105, 1999.
6. Murphy J, Jones DC: Managing the gravida with parvovirus, *Obstet Gynecol Manag* 1-7, 2000.
7. Brown KE, Anderson SM, Young NS: Erythrocyte P antigen: cellular receptor for B19 parvovirus, *Science* 262(5130):114-117, 1993.
8. Torok TJ, Qi-yun W, Gary Jr W et al: Prenatal diagnosis of intrauterine infection with parvovirus B19 by the polymerase chain reaction, *J Infect Dis* 14:149-155, 1995.
9. Ramirez MM, Mastrobattista JM: Diagnosis and management of human parvovirus B19 infection, *Clin Perinatol* 32:697-704, 2005.
10. Cosmi E, Mari G, Chiaie LD et al: Noninvasive diagnosis by Doppler ultrasonography of fetal anemia resulting from parvovirus infection, *Am J Obstet Gynecol* 187:1290-1293, 2002.
11. Hager JH, Alder SP, Koch WC et al: Prospective evaluation of 618 pregnant women exposed to parvovirus B19: risk and symptoms, *Obstet Gynecol* 91:412-420, 1998.
12. Guidozzi F, Ballot D, Rothberg A: Human B19 parvovirus infection in an obstetric population: a prospective study determining fetal outcome, *J Reprod Med* 39:36-38, 1994.
13. Levy R, Weissman A, Blomberg G et al: Infection by parvovirus B19 during pregnancy: a review, *Obstet Gynecol Surv* 52:254-259, 1997.
14. Rodis JF, Borgida AF, Wilson M et al: Management of parvovirus infection in pregnancy and outcomes of hydrops: a survey of members of the Society of Perinatal Obstetricians, *Am J Obstet Gynecol* 179:985-988, 1998.
15. Jordan JA: Diagnosing human parvovirus B19 infection: guidelines for test selection, *Mol Diagn* 6(4):307-312, 2001.
16. Anand A, Gray ES, Brown T et al: Human parvovirus infection in pregnancy and hydrops fetalis, *N Engl J Med* 316(4):183-186, 1987.
17. Sheikh A, Ernest J, O'Shea M: Long-term outcome in fetal hydrops from parvovirus B19 infection, *Am J Obstet Gynecol* 167:337-341, 1992.

SECTION B Abdominal Pain and Gastrointestinal Illness

Ellen L. Sakornbut, MD

Common obstetric-related causes of abdominal pain, such as round ligament pain and heartburn, are covered in Chapter 4, Section E. This section covers causes of abdominal pain and other gastrointestinal illnesses that are commonly seen in pregnant women. Blunt abdominal trauma is covered in Section C of this chapter.

I. DIAGNOSTIC TESTING

A. Abdominal Pain in Pregnancy

Pregnant women presenting with acute abdominal pain during pregnancy present several considerations that may increase diagnostic difficulty. Many clinicians hesitate to use imaging modalities for diagnosis fearing an exposure of the pregnancy to ionizing radiation, although failure to diagnose an acute abdomen may lead to disastrous consequences for the pregnant woman, her unborn child, or both.

B. Laboratory Tests

Minor increase of the white blood cell count is frequently seen in normal pregnancy, which may increase diagnostic difficulty. An observational study of 76 women operated on for acute appendicitis during a total of 40,000 pregnancies found only 50% accuracy in prediction of acute appendicitis. Women discovered to have a normal appendix did not differ significantly with regard to gestational age at presentation, signs of peritoneal irritation, body temperature, or leukocyte count.[1]

Other laboratory tests that change in normal pregnancy include liver function tests. Albumin and γ-glutamyl transpeptidase levels decrease; total, free, and conjugated bilirubin decrease; and AST level remains the same. ALT level shows small increases in the second trimester but stays in a normal range, whereas alkaline phosphatase level increases throughout pregnancy, peaking in the third trimester.[2]

C. Use of Magnetic Resonance Imaging

MRI has been evaluated as diagnostic modality for appendicitis, intraabdominal or pelvic abscess, and miscellaneous other diagnoses in most patients,[3,4] and current knowledge does not indicate any adverse effects of pregnancy exposure.[5]

D. Computed Tomography Imaging

CT of the abdomen carries the disadvantage of a small dose of ionizing radiation to the fetus but has demonstrated efficacy in the diagnosis of appendicitis[6] and multiple other causes of acute abdomen seen in pregnancy. It is more widely available and quicker, and thus may be more advantageous in some situations, than MRI.

E. Ultrasound

Ultrasound is safe, widely available, and has been used effectively in diagnosis of multiple intraabdominal conditions during pregnancy. It is the procedure of choice for suspected biliary tract disease and should be first line for diagnosis of pelvic masses. Coupled with color-flow Doppler, two-dimensional ultrasound can be effective in imaging for suspected ovarian torsion. It has been widely used for diagnosis of appendicitis in the pediatric population with only limited experience in pregnancy.[7]

II. APPENDICITIS IN PREGNANCY

Appendicitis does not have an increased or decreased incidence during pregnancy, but delays in diagnosis and resultant increase in perforation may increase morbidity as compared with the nonpregnant state. Appendicitis occurs in approximately 0.1% of all pregnancies without predilection for any trimester. Perforation occurs in 14% to 33% of cases, is more common if surgery occurred more than 24 hours after the onset of symptoms, and is more common in the second half of pregnancy (presumably because of delayed diagnosis). Accuracy of diagnosis ranges from 56% to 81%.

A. Perinatal Outcomes

Fetal mortality rate is about 35% with perforation. In one study, fetal losses occurred in 9% of negative laparotomies but increased to 17% if a diseased appendix was found and 75% if perforated.[8] In a series of 52 cases, fetal mortality was 10% overall with a 5% preterm birth incidence.

B. Clinical Findings

Clinical findings in pregnancy may vary with up to 50% of all patients presenting in the second trimester with atypical presentation,[9] but the majority of patients present with right lower quadrant pain. It has been proposed that the position of the appendix usually changes during pregnancy with rotation from the right lower quadrant to the right upper quadrant as the pregnancy advances. However, a prospective study comparing appendiceal location in term gravidas undergoing elective cesarean, pregnant women in the second half of pregnancy with appendicitis, and nonpregnant women with appendicitis failed to confirm this variance in location,[10] and another study comparing incisional location in gravidas

TABLE 9-9 Differential Diagnosis of Right Lower Quadrant Pain in Pregnancy

Diagnosis	Characteristic Findings	Diagnostic Testing
Ectopic pregnancy	Usually differentiated by history and physical examination (see Chapter 6)	Pelvic ultrasound, hCG level
Ovarian cyst	Large unruptured cysts may cause pain, but rupture is usually accompanied by abrupt onset of pain	Pelvic ultrasound
Torsion of adnexa	May be intermittent if twisting and untwisting occur but is usually severe; pain location variable; nausea, vomiting, leukocytosis, and peritoneal signs may be present	Pelvic ultrasound with color-flow Doppler, MRI
Degenerating fibroid	Red degeneration or bionecrosis, caused by fibroid growing beyond its blood supply, usually second trimester, accompanied by uterine tenderness, vomiting, low-grade fever	Pelvic ultrasound, MRI

Adapted from Chambers JT, Thiagarajah S, Kitchin JD: Torsion of the normal fallopian tube during pregnancy, *Obstet Gynecol* 54:487-489, 1979.
hCG, Human chorionic gonadotropin; MRI, magnetic resonance imaging.

concluded that McBurney's point was optimal as an incision site even in the third trimester.[11]

C. Differential Diagnosis

The differential diagnosis of RLQ pain in pregnancy is presented in Table 9-9.

D. Treatment

Laparoscopic surgery has been used extensively during pregnancy for cholecystectomy and appendectomy[12]; it appears to be safe and is technically feasible in all trimesters of pregnancy.[13] Laparoscopic surgery results in shorter hospital stays[14] than open appendectomy. Premature labor occurs in up to 83% of third-trimester patients with appendicitis[15,16]; therefore, consideration should be given to transfer of patients to a setting with increased perinatal capabilities, weighing delay in treatment and possible inaccuracy of diagnosis against the risk for perforation and its attendant morbidity.

III. NEPHROLITHIASIS

Healthy pregnant women excrete more calcium in their urine than during the nonpregnant state, but they are relatively protected from stone formation by the concomitant excretion of increased amounts of endogenous thiosulfate.[17] The presentation of nephrolithiasis is similar during pregnancy to the nonpregnant state, with costovertebral angle, flank, or abdominal pain. This may be accompanied by hematuria, nausea, vomiting, urgency, dysuria, and frequency. Large observational studies find an incidence of nephrolithiasis between 1 in 244 and 1 in 3300 pregnancies, more commonly in whites than blacks.[18] Most studies confirm presentation commonly in the second or third trimester. One series confirmed an increased incidence of preterm rupture of membranes.[17]

Nephrolithiasis should be suspected if there is a history of renal calculi, preexisting urologic problems, fever persisting in pyelonephritis greater than 48 hours after institution of parenteral antibiotics, or more severe pain than is usually encountered with pyelonephritis.

A. Diagnosis

Ultrasonography carries a diagnostic accuracy from 60%[19] to 95%.[20] If ultrasound is negative, single-shot intravenous pyelography should be considered next, although CT or MRI may also be used.

B. Management

Conservative management results in passage of the stone between 70% and 80% of cases, but surgical interventions, including cystoscopy with placement of stent, percutaneous nephrostomy, or ureteroscopy with extraction may be used as necessary.[21]

IV. CHOLELITHIASIS AND CHOLECYSTITIS

A. Epidemiology

Pregnancy is associated with an increased incidence of cholelithiasis. Increased estrogen and progesterone levels predispose to the formation of lithogenic bile and bile stasis. The incidence of symptomatic biliary disease is not increased (1/1500), although the diagnosis may be made or reported on a less frequent basis owing to numerous abdominal complaints common to pregnancy. The rate of cholecystectomy in pregnancy is between 1 and 6 per 10,000 pregnancies.

B. Complications of Cholecystitis

Pancreatitis is a possible complication of cholelithiasis. Maternal and fetal mortality rates have been reported to be high but appear to be decreased with the use of total parenteral nutrition.

C. Options for Treatment

1. Conservative management
   This is generally pursued because resolution of symptoms may occur after the pregnancy. In large case series, about 40% of patients do not respond to conservative therapy and require intervention, and the need for intervention in the early postpartum/peripartum period is common.[22,23]
2. Endoscopic treatment with stone extraction[24,25]
3. Laparoscopic cholecystectomy
   This can be performed for recurrent or intractable symptoms, including acute cholecystitis and gallstone pancreatitis. Results of these studies demonstrate safety and efficacy of laparoscopic cholecystectomy with possible limitations in late pregnancy.[26-28]
4. Open cholecystectomy
   This operation is performed for intractable cases in which laparoscopic procedures may not be desirable.

V. GASTROENTERITIS

Gastroenteritis presents as in the nonpregnant patient and can be managed in a similar fashion, with oral hydration preferable if the patient tolerates fluids. The patient's hydration should be monitored more closely because of the risk for PTL with dehydration.

VI. ACUTE HEPATIC DISORDERS IN PREGNANCY

A. Intrahepatic Cholestasis of Pregnancy

Intrahepatic cholestasis of pregnancy (ICP) has a variable incidence depending on ethnic factors; its incidence rate is less than 2% in the general population in the United States but occurs more commonly in Chile and Sweden. This condition is characterized by intense pruritus, occasionally mild jaundice and dark urine, mild-to-moderate increases of transaminases, and marked increase of alkaline phosphatase. Serum bile acid levels and sulfated metabolites of progesterone are increased, and bile acid transport across the placenta is abnormal. The syndrome is more common in the third trimester and resolves after delivery. It is associated with increased rates of stillbirth, fetal distress, and prematurity. An increased risk for maternal coagulopathy exists, possibly because of the use of therapies such as cholestyramine, which affects absorption of fat-soluble vitamin K.[29] Ursodeoxycholic acid (UDCA) when compared with cholestyramine or with placebo is effective in improving bile acid transport across the placenta[30] and increasing biliary excretion of sulfated progesterone metabolites.[31] It decreases serum bile acids, serum bilirubin, and serum transaminases; decreases symptoms of pruritus; and increases average birth weight of infants and term birth rates.[32,33]

B. Acute Fatty Liver of Pregnancy

Acute fatty liver of pregnancy is a rare but catastrophic illness that occurs more commonly during first pregnancies and pregnancies with multiple gestations, usually late in the third trimester or within a few days of delivery.[34] The onset of the disease is heralded by anorexia, nausea, vomiting, malaise, and headache, followed by epigastric and right upper quadrant abdominal pain with jaundice, polyuria-polydipsia (in the absence of diabetes), and thrombocytopenia. The patient may become comatose with hepatic encephalopathy, bleeding diatheses, and metabolic acidosis. This illness occurs in pregnancies where the fetus is homozygous for a deficiency in long-chain 3-hydroxyacyl-coenzyme A-dehydrogenase (a disorder of mitochondrial fatty acid oxidation) and the mother is a carrier (heterozygote).[35] Maternal disease occurs when the ability of the maternal liver to metabolize free fatty acids is overwhelmed by the production of free fatty acids from the homozygous fetus.

Some features of acute fatty liver of pregnancy are common to both acute fatty liver and preeclampsia: mild hypertension, proteinuria, and edema. Maternal mortality rates are high if diagnosis and delivery are delayed, but are reported as 12% in a multisite study of teaching hospitals.[33]

C. Preeclampsia- and Eclampsia-Associated Hepatic Changes

Preeclampsia- and eclampsia-associated hepatic changes include nausea, vomiting, and epigastric and right upper quadrant pain, with liver abnormalities present in 50% of patients with eclampsia. The HELLP (hemolysis, elevated liver enzymes, and low platelets) syndrome is characterized by microangiopathic hemolytic anemia and increased AST, ALT, and thrombocytopenia. Another cause of increased liver enzymes in pregnancy-induced hypertension is subcapsular or intrahepatic hematoma, which may lead to catastrophic rupture (see Chapter 16, Section H).

D. Fulminant Hepatitis

Fulminant hepatitis, an inflammation of the liver usually of viral origin, presents with increases in transaminases and bilirubin, coagulopathy, encephalopathy, and renal failure. Although serologic studies are pending, there may be some difficulty in distinguishing this catastrophic illness from acute fatty liver. Delivery of the fetus is indicated in acute fatty liver and may be necessary for fetal survival in fulminant hepatitis.

VII. SUMMARY AND SOR A RECOMMENDATIONS

Abdominal complaints are common in pregnancy and may represent nonthreatening conditions. However, failure to diagnose serious causes of nonobstetric abdominal pain may have severe consequences for the well-being of mother or fetus, or both. Most causes of the acute abdomen are treated in a similar manner during pregnancy as in the nonpregnant state. Providers should be aware of the risks for PTL with serious abdominal conditions in the second half of pregnancy.

RECOMMENDATION	REFERENCES
Treatment with UDCA decreases symptoms of pruritus, increases term birth rates, and increases birth weight.	31, 32

REFERENCES

1. Maslovitz S, Gutman G, Lessing JB et al: The significance of clinical signs and blood indices for the diagnosis of appendicitis during pregnancy, *Gynecol Obstet Invest* 56(4):188-191, 2003.
2. Bacq Y, Zarka O, Brechot JF et al: Liver function tests in normal pregnancy: a prospective study of 103 pregnant women and 103 matched controls, *Hepatology* 23(5):1030-1034, 1996.
3. Birchard KR, Brown MA, Hyslop WB et al: MRI of acute abdominal and pelvic pain in pregnant patients, *Am J Roentgenol* 184(2):452-458, 2005.
4. Oto A, Ernst RD, Shah R et al: Right-lower-quadrant pain and suspected appendicitis in pregnant women: evaluation with MR imaging-initial experience, *Radiology* 234(2):445-451, 2005.
5. Leyendecker JR, Gorengaut V, Brown JJ: MR imaging of maternal diseases of the abdomen and pelvis during pregnancy and the immediate postpartum period, *Radiographics* 24(5):1301-1316, 2004.
6. Ames Castro M, Shipp TD, Castro EE et al: The use of helical computed tomography in pregnancy for the diagnosis of acute appendicitis, *Am J Obstet Gynecol* 184(5):954-957, 2001.
7. Barloon TJ, Brown BP, Abu-Yousef MM et al: Sonography of acute appendicitis in pregnancy, *Abdom Imaging* 20:149-151, 1995.
8. Al-Mulhim AA: Acute appendicitis in pregnancy: a review of 52 cases, *Int Surg* 81:2995-2997, 1996.
9. Ueberrueck T, Koch A, Meyer L et al: Ninety-four appendectomies for suspected acute appendicitis during pregnancy, *World J Surg* 28(5):508-511, 2004.
10. Hodjati H, Kazerooni T: Location of the appendix in the gravid patient: a re-evaluation of the established concept, *Int J Gynaecol Obstet* 81(3):245-247, 2003.
11. Popkin CA, Lopez PP, Cohn SM et al: The incision of choice for pregnant women with appendicitis is through McBurney's point, *Am J Surg* 183(1):20-22, 2002.
12. Rollins MD, Chan KJ, Price RR: Laparoscopy for appendicitis and cholelithiasis during pregnancy: a new standard of care, *Surg Endosc* 18(2):237-241, 2004.
13. Ahmad TA, Shelbaya E, Razek SA et al: Experience of laparoscopic management in 100 patients with acute abdomen, *Hepatogastroenterology* 48(39):733-736, 2001.
14. Lyass S, Pikarsky A, Eisenberg VH et al: Is laparoscopic appendectomy safe in pregnant women? *Surg Endosc* 15(4):377-379, 2001.
15. Mourad J, Elliott JP, Erickson L et al: Appendicitis in pregnancy: new information that contradicts long-held clinical beliefs, *Am J Obstet Gynecol* 182(5):1027-1029, 2000.

16. Visser BC, Glasgow RE, Mulvihill KK et al: Safety and timing of nonobstetric abdominal surgery in pregnancy, *Dig Surg* 18(5):409-417, 2001.
17. Yatzidis H: Gestational urinary hyperthiosulfaturia protects hypercalciuric normal pregnant women from nephrolithiasis, *Int Urol Nephrol* 36(3):445-449, 2004.
18. Lewis DF, Robichaux AG 3rd, Jaekle RK et al: Urolithiasis in pregnancy. Diagnosis, management and pregnancy outcome, *J Reprod Med* 48(1):28-32, 2003.
19. Butler EL, Cox SM, Eberts EG et al: Symptomatic nephrolithiasis complicating pregnancy, *Obstet Gynecol* 96(5 pt 1): 753-756, 2000.
20. Parulkar BG, Hopkins TB, Wollin MR et al: Renal colic in pregnancy: a case for conservative management, *J Urol* 159:365-368, 1998.
21. Butler EL, Cox SM, Eberts EG et ai: Symptomatic nephrolithiasis complicating pregnancy, *Obstet Gynecol* 96(5 pt 1):753-756, 2000.
22. Davis A, Katz VL, Cox R: Gallbladder disease in pregnancy, *J Reprod Med* 40:759-762, 1995.
23. Glasgow RE, Visser BC, Harris HW et al: Changing management of gallstone disease during pregnancy, *Surg Endosc* 12:241-246, 1998.
24. Barthel JS, Chowdhury T, Miedema BW: Endoscopic sphincterotomy for the treatment of gallstone pancreatitis during pregnancy, *Surg Endosc* 12:394-399, 1998.
25. Nesbitt TH, Kay HH, McCoy MC et al: Endoscopic management of biliary disease in pregnancy, *Obstet Gynecol* 87:806-809, 1996.
26. Barone JE, Bears S, Chen S et al: Outcome study of cholecystectomy during pregnancy, *Am J Surg* 177(3):232-236, 1999.
27. Sungler P, Heinerman PM, Steiner H et al: Laparoscopic cholecystectomy and interventional endoscopy for gallstone complications during pregnancy, *Surg Endosc* 14(3):267-271, 2000.
28. Lu EJ, Curet MJ, El-Sayed YY et al: Medical versus surgical management of biliary tract disease in pregnancy, *Am J Surg* 188(6):755-759, 2004.
29. Reyes H: The enigma of intrahepatic cholestasis of pregnancy: lessons from Chile, *Hepatology* 2:87-90, 1982.
30. Serrano MA, Brites D, Larena MG et al: Beneficial effects of ursodeoxycholic acid on alterations induced by cholestasis of pregnancy in bile acid transport across the human placenta, *J Hepatol* 25:829-839, 1998.
31. Meng LJ, Reyes H, Palma J et al: Effects of ursodeoxycholic acid on conjugated bile acids and progesterone metabolites in serum and urine of patients with intrahepatic cholestasis of pregnancy, *J Hepatol* 127:1029-1040, 1997.
32. Kondrackiene J, Beuers U, Kupcinskas L: Efficacy and safety of ursodeoxycholic acid versus cholestyramine in intrahepatic cholestasis of pregnancy, *Gastroenterology* 129(3):894-901, 2005.
33. Zapata R, Sandoval L, Palma J et al: Ursodeoxycholic acid in the treatment of intrahepatic cholestasis of pregnancy. A 12-year experience, *Liver Int* 25(3):548-554, 2005.
34. Fesenmeier MF, Coppage KH, Lambers DS et al: Acute fatty liver of pregnancy in 3 tertiary care centers, *Am J Obstet Gynecol* 192(5):1416-1419, 2005.
35. Bellig LL: Maternal acute fatty liver of pregnancy and the associated risk for long-chain 3-hydroxyacyl-coenzyme a dehydrogenase (LCHAD) deficiency in infants, *Adv Neonatal Care* 4(1):26-32, 2004.

SECTION C Trauma in Pregnancy

Mark Deutchman, MD

Traumatic injury is the leading nonobstetric cause of death in women of childbearing age.[1] Maternal survival is a good predictor of fetal survival but does not guarantee fetal survival. Fetal death rates in pregnancy exceed maternal death rates threefold to ninefold.[2] The objectives of this section are as follows:
1. To understand the frequency and causes of traumatic injuries that may occur during pregnancy
2. To understand how physiologic changes in pregnancy affect the pathogenesis, evaluation, and treatment of the pregnant trauma patient
3. To describe an evidence-based approach to evaluation of the traumatized pregnant patient

I. EPIDEMIOLOGY AND RISK FACTORS

About 6% to 7% of women suffer some type of trauma during pregnancy. The most common causes of injury during pregnancy are motor vehicle accidents, domestic violence, and falls. Motor vehicle accidents cause most of the episodes of trauma during pregnancy. In one retrospective study based on birth certificate data, 2.8% of pregnant women were involved in a motor vehicle accident as the driver.[3] An unknown additional number were involved in motor vehicle accidents as the passenger.

A. Seat Belt Use
Pregnant women may mistakenly assume that it is inadvisable for them to wear seatbelts or may wear them improperly. When advising pregnant women about restraint use, be alert to these risk factors for nonuse[3]:
1. Younger women
2. Smokers
3. Alcohol users
4. Those who have not completed high school
5. Those who did not receive prenatal care in the first trimester

B. Domestic Violence
Domestic violence has been reported in 3% to 29% of pregnant women depending on population and study method.[4] Common indicators of domestic

violence include[5]:
1. Depression
2. Substance abuse
3. Frequent emergency department visits

It is important to remember that domestic violence spans all ages, races, and socioeconomic groups.[5] Victims frequently conceal their situation. A history of abuse must be sought out by clinicians, and victims should be encouraged to seek help. Pregnant women who have been victims of domestic violence have an increased incidence of PTL and chorioamnionitis.[6]

C. Falls

The risk for falls increases during pregnancy because of awkwardness of movement and orthostatic hypotensive episodes.

II. PATHOGENESIS

Trauma during pregnancy can inflict the same types of direct injury to mother or fetus as may occur in nonpregnant patients. In addition, the pregnant state creates risk for some additional unique injuries. The following sections list unique injuries in the pregnant trauma patient.

A. Premature Rupture of Membranes

B. Placental Abruption

C. Fetomaternal Hemorrhage

Fetomaternal hemorrhage may cause fetal anemia or result in Rh sensitization in Rh-negative women.

D. Uterine Rupture

E. Amniotic Fluid Embolism

F. Placental Abruption

Placental abruption is the leading cause of fetal death in trauma survived by the mother. Direct trauma to the maternal abdomen as may occur in motor vehicle accidents or domestic violence is the main mechanism of injury causing abruption. Abruption may occur as the result of direct injury and shearing forces or as a result of the effects of maternal shock.[7] Abruption can occur up to 4 or 5 days after trauma[11] but more commonly occurs within the first 6 hours.[8,9] Although the risk for abruption

increases with the severity of the trauma,[10] even minor trauma can produce abruption; therefore, all patients should be evaluated. Pregnant women involved in automobile accidents at speeds greater than 30 miles/hour are at greatest risk for abruption.[10,11] PTL is much more common than abruption, occurring 10 times more often in some studies. PTL is also a potential marker for abruption.[12]

G. Massive Maternal Injuries

Severe maternal head or chest injury significantly increases the risk for maternal death and accompanying fetal death.[7] Maternal pelvic fracture may produce direct fetal injury but is more likely to cause fetal injury or death because of maternal shock resulting from massive retroperitoneal hemorrhage. Direct fetal injury is most likely to occur from penetrating trauma such as gunshot or stab wounds.

III. CLINICAL FEATURES

Physiologic changes in pregnancy may alter the woman's response to injury. These changes are displayed in Table 9-10. These changes complicate the clinical diagnosis of the severity of shock in the pregnant woman because 30% of blood volume may be lost before clinical signs of hypovolemia appear. In addition, direct assessment of the status of the second patient—the fetus—is difficult.

Because the physiologic changes of pregnancy may mask the usual clinical signs of shock, laboratory tests may be helpful. Sensitive indicators of tissue hypoperfusion include serum bicarbonate levels less than 19 to 25 mEq/L and increased serum lactate levels. These laboratory findings have been correlated with poor fetal outcome, as have fluid resuscitation with large amounts of intravenous fluids and decreased maternal pH and Po_2.[12] Clinical features of trauma in pregnancy that have prognostic value for the fetus are listed in the following sections.

A. Minor Maternal Injury

The fetal death rate in cases of minor maternal injury is less than 2%.

B. Maternal Blood Flow

Maternal blood flow is maintained at the expense of uteroplacental blood flow.[13] Therefore, the fetus may be severely compromised even when maternal vital signs are normal.

TABLE 9-10 **Physiologic Effects of Pregnancy Related to Evaluation of the Trauma Patient**[14]

Parameter	Change
Uterine location	Becomes intraabdominal
Supine hypotension	Common
Signs of peritoneal irritation	Diminished
Gastric emptying	Delayed
Diaphragm location	Elevated
Airway	Edematous
Blood pressure	Decreases
Hemoglobin	Decreases 20%
Respiratory rate	Increases 20%
Serum bicarbonate and P_{CO_2}	Decreases 15%
Blood volume	Increases 35-50%
Cardiac output	Increases 40%
Heart rate	Increases 15%
Fibrinogen and clotting factors	Increases 50-200%
White blood cell count	Increase
Arterial pH	Increase
Plasma volume	Increases 45%

C. Maternal Survival

The most sensitive indicator of fetal survival is maternal survival. The leading cause of fetal death is maternal death.

D. Major Trauma

Major trauma resulting in long-bone fractures, rib fractures, and life-threatening maternal injury is associated with a 40% incidence of fetal death.

E. Uterine Rupture

Uterine rupture is rare but is associated with nearly 100% fetal mortality.[15]

F. Mother Ejected from Vehicle[16]

G. Mother as Motorcycle Rider or Pedestrian[16]

H. Unrestrained Mother Involved in a Motor Vehicle Accident[16]

IV. DIAGNOSIS

Initial diagnosis of the severely injured pregnant trauma patient is the same as that of any trauma patient.

A. Airway: Secure the Airway

B. Breathing: Administer Oxygen and Assist Ventilation

C. Circulation: Control Bleeding, Establish Intravenous Access, and Administer Volume Replacement

D. Disability or Neurologic Deficits

E. Exposure: Environment

After assessing and supporting the woman's vital signs, the well-being of the fetus is assessed. PTL and placental abruption are the primary conditions that threaten the fetus and are the conditions that maternal evaluation protocols are designed to detect. Maternal observation, electronic fetal monitoring, and limited laboratory testing are the primary methods used.

F. Placental Abruption

Most abruptions are evident using fetal monitoring in the first few hours. PTL can accompany even minor trauma. The presence of contractions should increase the clinical suspicion of abruption.[12] Signs and findings associated with abruption include[15,17]:
1. More than six to eight uterine contractions per hour
2. Vaginal bleeding
3. Uterine tenderness
4. Signs of maternal hypovolemia
5. Fetal heart rate pattern abnormalities

G. Electronic Monitoring to Detect Maternal/Fetal Injury

In the case of major trauma, some authors recommend 24 hours of continuous electronic fetal monitoring to detect placental abruption and PTL.[18] In the case of minor trauma, a short period of monitoring (nonstress test) is recommended.[12,19] A prospective series found that a 4-hour monitoring period and a Kleihauer–Betke (K-B) test were able to detect all patients with trauma-related poor pregnancy outcome who would not otherwise have been hospitalized because of the severity of their trauma. Frequent preterm contractions (>8/hour) were associated with abruption.[15] Extended monitoring or more extensive evaluation is not warranted unless there is evidence of abruption, fetal compromise, or frequent preterm contractions.[12]

Electronic fetal monitoring may detect fetal heart rate abnormalities with or without accompanying uterine contractions. Late fetal heart decelerations should be assumed to represent fetal compromise. A sinusoidal fetal heart rate pattern is associated with fetal anemia from fetomaternal hemorrhage or abruption.

H. Vaginal Examination

If vaginal examination reveals fluid, fern testing and pH testing (Nitrazine testing) for amniotic fluid should be performed to determine whether membranes have been ruptured. If vaginal examination reveals bleeding, abruption or another severe event such as uterine rupture should be assumed. The absence of vaginal bleeding does **not** exclude abruption because concealed hemorrhage has been found to be more likely in abruption caused by trauma.[7,17] In one study of pregnant motor vehicle trauma victims, vaginal bleeding was seen only in those later found to have abruption.[10]

I. Role of Ultrasound

Ultrasonography may be used to examine for abruption, but a negative test does **not** exclude placental abruption. Ultrasonography provides additional significant information, including gestational age, placental location, and can diagnose uterine rupture.

J. Coagulation Studies

Routine use of coagulation tests has not been shown to help in evaluation or management.[17]

K. Abdominal Pain/Tenderness

Subjective reports of abdominal pain and objective findings of abdominal tenderness have not been shown to help predict which patients are at greater risk for PTD.[20]

V. TREATMENT

Treatment of the pregnant trauma patient focuses first on support of maternal vital signs and treatment of maternal injuries because the best predictor of fetal survival is maternal survival. Any clinically indicated diagnostic tests usually used in trauma evaluation should be performed including radiographs, blood counts and typing, and peritoneal lavage or ultrasound to rule out intraperitoneal hemorrhage. The threshold for sonographic diagnosis of hemoperitoneum is probably about 200 ml in nonpregnant patients; the threshold in pregnant patients is unknown. Special considerations in the resuscitation of pregnant women are listed in the following sections.[21]

A. Aspiration

Pregnant women are at increased risk for vomiting and subsequent aspiration. Rapid sequence intubation and gastric emptying are preferred.

B. Vena Cava Compression

Position the patient in the left lateral rather than supine position to avoid vena cava compression and resultant maternal supine hypotension. Avoid lower extremity intravenous lines because vena cava compression by the gravid uterus may prevent infused fluids from reaching the maternal central circulation.

C. Fluid Resuscitation

Replace estimated blood loss 3:1 with lactated Ringer's solution.

D. Use of Vasopressors

The vasopressors norepinephrine and epinephrine should be avoided because they decrease uterine blood flow. Ephedrine increases both maternal blood pressure and uterine blood flow. Dopamine increases uterine blood flow in dosages up to 5 μg/kg/min.

E. Placement of Chest Tubes

Chest tubes placement should be higher than usual because of diaphragm elevation in pregnancy.

F. Rh Immunoglobulin

Rh immunoglobulin should be administered to Rh-negative women who have trauma.[22] The $Rh_o(D)$ immunoglobulin (RhoGAM) dosage for Rh-negative mothers is based on K-B testing. One fetal cell per 1000 maternal cells represents a 5-ml hemorrhage (assuming a maternal blood volume of 5 L). Rh-negative mothers can be sensitized by as few as 1 to 3 fetal cells per 500,000 maternal cells. Rh-negative mothers should receive 300 μg $Rh_o(D)$ immunoglobulin (RhoGAM) for each 15 ml of estimated fetal cells in their circulation. The minimum Rho(D) immunoglobulin (Rho-GAM) dose should be 300 μg.

G. Tocolysis

Tocolysis is recommended by some authors if the fetus is stable, and they note that it is usually successful.[18] If tocolysis is to be used, magnesium sulfate is preferable to β-mimetics because the latter causes both maternal and fetal tachycardia and may mask signs of shock.

H. Duration of Monitoring

The duration of observation and period of monitoring continue to be a matter of physician judgment. Electronic uterine activity monitoring should be initiated on mothers at or beyond 20 weeks of gestation. Patients with minor trauma may be monitored for 4 hours,[15] whereas those with more severe trauma should be monitored for 24 hours.[12] Uterine contractions occurring at a frequency of 6 to 8 per hour or more indicate increased risk for abruption and premature delivery. These discharge criteria are prudent based on available evidence:

1. Resolution of uterine contractions
2. Reassuring fetal heart rate pattern
3. Confirmation that membranes are not ruptured
4. No vaginal bleeding or uterine tenderness
5. If patient is Rh negative, appropriate dose of $Rh_o(D)$ immunoglobulin (RhoGAM) has been given
6. Patient understands discharge instructions and follow-up plans

I. Perimortem Cesarean Delivery

Perimortem cesarean delivery should be considered because fetal survival is impossible for more than a few minutes after maternal death. In its Advanced Cardiac Life Support program, the American Heart Association recommends that all physicians be prepared to perform perimortem cesarean delivery of a viable fetus whose mother has not responded to 4 to 5 minutes of cardiopulmonary resuscitation.[23] This procedure is also recommended by the ACOG, although no time criteria are specified.[11] Longer arrest-to-delivery times are associated with increased neurologic deficits in surviving infants. Perimortem cesarean delivery is also recommended

as an aid to maternal resuscitation because emptying the uterus dramatically increases cardiac output by relieving uterine compression of the aorta and vena cava. When perimortem cesarean delivery is performed, the attending team should be prepared to provide resuscitation care for the newborn.

VI. CLINICAL COURSE AND PREVENTION

The clinical course of an unrestrained pregnant woman involved in motor vehicle accident is serious, as shown in Table 9-11. Some pregnant women mistakenly assume that it is dangerous for them to wear seatbelts, shoulder harnesses, or both, but lap and shoulder belt restraints are safer than the risk for collision with the dashboard or other parts of the interior of the car.[24] Airbags should *not* be disabled during pregnancy.[11] All clinicians should have a high index of suspicion for domestic violence when treating trauma during pregnancy.[22]

VII. PITFALLS AND CONTROVERSIES

The value of testing for fetomaternal hemorrhage using the K-B test (except in Rh-negative mothers) is controversial, but K-B testing is still recommended by some authors for all patients.[15,19] One trial found that a positive K-B test identified all pregnant women who developed PTL after trauma.[25] The value and safety of tocolysis for the pregnant trauma patient having contractions is controversial as well.

TABLE 9-11 Odds Ratios for Adverse Outcomes for an Unrestrained Pregnant Woman in a Motor Vehicle Accident

Outcome	*Odds Ratio*
Low birth weight infant	1.3
Excessive bleeding during delivery	2.1
Fetal death	3.0

From Hyde LK, Cook LJ, Olson LM et al: Effect of motor vehicle crashes on adverse fetal outcomes, *Obstet Gynecol* 102:279-286, 2003.

VIII. SOR RECOMMENDATIONS

The following recommendations are based on level C evidence:

1. Pregnant women riding in automobiles should use three-point restraints and should **not** disable airbags.[4,11]

2. Domestic violence should be considered when taking the history in cases of trauma in pregnancy.[22]

3. Changes in maternal physiology complicate evaluation of trauma in pregnant women, making careful evaluation necessary.[14]

4. Care and support of maternal vital signs take precedence over that of the fetus.[2]

5. Vaginal bleeding is a powerful indicator of placental abruption.[10]

6. Uterine contractions are associated with placental abruption and early delivery.[15,17]

7. K-B testing may be helpful to identify patients at low risk for PTL after trauma.[25]

8. Ultrasonography is not helpful to rule OUT abruption.[10]

9. Perimortem cesarean delivery performed within 5 minutes of maternal cardiac arrest improves the likelihood of intact survival of a fetus that has reached a viable gestational age.[11,23]

10. Perimortem cesarean delivery performed within 5 minutes of maternal cardiac arrest improves chances of successful maternal resuscitation.[11,23]

REFERENCES

1. Fildes J, Reed L, Jones N et al: Trauma: the leading cause of maternal death, *J Trauma* 32:643-645, 1992.
2. Kissinger DP, Rozycki GS, Morris JA et al: Trauma in pregnancy: predicting pregnancy outcome, *Arch Surg* 126:1 079-1086, 1991.
3. Hyde LK, Cook LJ, Olson LM et al: Effect of motor vehicle crashes on adverse fetal outcomes, *Obstet Gynecol* 102: 279-286, 2003.
4. McFarlane J, Parker B, Soeken K et al: Assessing for abuse during pregnancy: severity and frequency of injuries and associated entry into prenatal care, *JAMA* 267:3176-3178, 1992.
5. Poole GV, Martin JN, Perry KG et al: Trauma in pregnancy: the role of interpersonal violence, *Am J Obstet Gynecol* 174:1873-1876, 1996.
6. Berenson AB, Wiemann CM, Wilkinson GS et al: Perinatal morbidity associated with violence experienced by pregnant women, *Am J Obstet Gynecol* 170:760-769, 1994.
7. Kettel LM, Branch DW, Scott JR: Occult placental abruption after maternal trauma, *Obstet Gynecol* 71:449-453, 1988.
8. Stone KI: Trauma in the obstetric patient, *Obstet Gynecol Clin North Am* 26(3):459-467, 1999.
9. Shah KH, Simons RK, Holbrook T et al: Trauma in pregnancy: maternal and fetal outcomes, *J Trauma Injury Crit Care* 45(1):83-86, 1998.
10. Reis PM, Sander CM, Pearlman MD: Abruptio placentae after auto accidents, *J Reprod Med* 45:6-10, 2000.
11. ACOG educational bulletin. Obstetric aspects of trauma management. Number 251, September 1998 (replaces Number 151, January 1991, and Number 161, November 1991). American College of Obstetricians and Gynecologists, *Int J Gynaecol Obstet* 64:8794, 1999.
12. Rosenfeld JA: Abdominal trauma in pregnancy: when is fetal monitoring necessary? *Postgrad Med* 88:89-94, 1990.
13. Greiss FC: Uterine vascular response to hemorrhage during pregnancy, *Obstet Gynecol* 27:549-554, 1966.
14. Kuczkowski KM: Trauma in the pregnant patient, *Curr Opin Anaesthesiol* 17:145-150, 2004.
15. Pearleman MD, Tintinalli JE, Lorenz RP: A prospective, controlled study of outcome after trauma during pregnancy, *Am J Obstet Gynecol* 162:1502-1510, 1990.
16. Curet MJ, Schermer CR, Demarest GB et al: Predictors of outcome in trauma during pregnancy: identification of patients who can be monitored for less than 6 hours, *J Trauma* 49:18-25, 2000.
17. Dahmus MA, Sibai BM: Blunt abdominal trauma: are there any predictive factors for abruptio placentae or maternal-fetal distress? *Am J Obstet Gynecol* 169:1054-1059, 1993.
18. Williams JK, McClain L, Rosemurgy AS et al: Evaluation of blunt abdominal trauma in the third trimester of pregnancy: maternal and fetal considerations, *Obstet Gynecol* 75:33-37, 1990.
19. Goodwin TM, Breen MT: Pregnancy outcome and fetomaternal hemorrhage after noncatastrophic trauma, *Am J Obstet Gynecol* 162:665-671, 1990.
20. Pak LL, Reece EA, Chan L: Is adverse pregnancy outcome predictable after blunt abdominal trauma? *Am J Obstet Gynecol* 1998;179:1140-1144.
21. Coleman MT, Trianfo VA, Rund DA: Nonobstetric emergencies in pregnancy: trauma and surgical conditions, *Am J Obstet Gynecol* 177:497-502, 1997.
22. Davis JW, Parks SN, Kaups KL et al: Victims of domestic violence on the trauma service: unrecognized and underreported, *J Trauma* 54:352-355, 2003.
23. American Heart Association: Advanced cardiac life support 2005: cardiac arrest associated with pregnancy, *Circulation* 112: IV-150-IV-153, 2005. Available at: http://circ.ahajournals.org/cgi/reprint/112/24_suppl/IV-150. Accessed September 16, 2007.
24. Moorcroft DM, Stitzel MD, Duma GG et al: Computational model of the pregnant occupant: predicting the risk of injury in automobile crashes, *Am J Obstet Gynecol* 189:540-544, 2003.
25. Muench M, Baschat A, Reddy U et al: Kleihauer-Betke testing is important in all cases of maternal trauma, *J Trauma* 57:1094-1098, 2004.

SECTION D Dermatoses of Pregnancy

Stephen T. Olin, MD

I. BACKGROUND

The "dermatoses of pregnancy" is a daunting subject largely as a result of overlapping, archaic, confusing, and misleading terminology based on anecdotes and case reports leading to a myriad of eponyms. More importantly, pregnant women are subject to the same dermatologic problems that affect men and nonpregnant women. Compounding the confusion is the lack of knowledge about the dermatoses associated with pregnancy on the part of obstetricians and gynecologists, primary care physicians, and many dermatologists.

Beginning in 1982, several clinicians attempted to reclassify the dermatoses of pregnancy based on immunofluorescence microscopy, laboratory findings, and distinct clinical characteristics via retrospective studies of pregnant women and evidenced-based systematic reviews. Currently, two main classification schemes are used, the first having been proposed by Holmes and Black in 1982,[1] which included pemphigoid gestationis (PG; herpes gestationis), polymorphic eruption of pregnancy (PEP), pruritic urticarial papules and plaques of pregnancy (PUPPP), prurigo of pregnancy, and pruritic folliculitis of pregnancy. In 1998, Shornick[2] outlined the second classification representing a further simplification and consisting of PG, PEP, prurigo of pregnancy, and ICP. Shornick suggested that pruritic folliculitis of pregnancy belonged in the group of prurigo of pregnancy because only a few more cases of pruritic folliculitis of pregnancy have been described since the original report in 1981.[3] Some authors, however, still consider this condition to be a separate entity because of histopathologic features of sterile folliculitis.

Subsequently, Kroumpouzos and Cohen[4] provided an evidence-based, systematic review in 2003 representing an analysis of the literature on specific dermatoses of pregnancy from January 1962 to January 2002. They followed the classification as outlined by Holmes and Black[1] and Shornick[2]: ICP, herpes gestationis, PUPPP, prurigo of pregnancy, and pruritic folliculitis of pregnancy (believed by these authors to represent a separate entity).

More recently, Ambros-Rudolph and colleagues[5] presented an algorithm that facilitates discrimination of the various pruritic dermatoses of pregnancy, pointing to appropriate diagnostic and therapeutic measures through analysis of the various clinical characteristics observed in 505 patients from 1994 to 2004 based on clinical findings, onset of presentation, hematoxylin and eosin (H&E) pathologic stains; immunofluorescence microscopy; laboratory investigation; and fetal risk (Figure 9-1).

II. SPECIFIC DERMATOSES

The following four entities represent a "rationalized" classification of the specific dermatoses of pregnancy: PG, PEP, atopic eruption of pregnancy, and ICP.

A. Pemphigoid Gestationis

1. Synonyms
   a. Gestational pemphigoid
   b. Herpes gestationis
2. Incidence
   The incidence of PG is 1 in 50,000.
3. Key features
   a. These are intensely pruritic vesiculobullous eruptions on urticated erythema with periumbilical involvement developing during late pregnancy or the immediate postpartum period. Lesions typically begin on abdomen, often within or immediately adjacent to the umbilicus.
   b. Possible subepidermal blisters may be evident on H&E stain.
   c. Linear C3 depositions along dermal-epidermal junction demonstrated on immunofluorescence microscopy.
   d. Increased risk of small-for-gestational age births and risk for prematurity.
   e. Spontaneous resolution over weeks to months after delivery.
4. Pathophysiology
   Currently, PG is believed to be caused by the production of an autoantibody with potential cross-reactivity between placental tissue and skin. Immunogenetic studies have revealed a 100% incidence rate of anti-human leukocyte antigen (HLA) antibodies in patients with a history of gestational pemphigoid.
5. Clinical course
   The classic presentation of PG is late pregnancy with abrupt onset of intensely pruritic urticarial

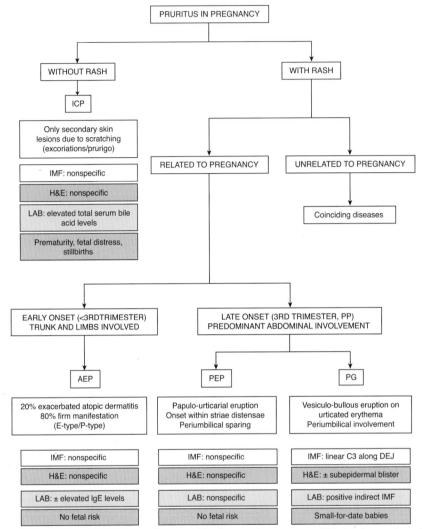

FIGURE 9-1. Algorithm for differential diagnosis of pruritic skin diseases in pregnancy. AEP, Atopic eruption of pregnancy; DEJ, dermoepidermal junction; H&E, hematoxylin and eosin; ICP, intrahepatic cholestasis of pregnancy; IMF, immunofluorescence microscopy; LAB, laboratory investigations; PEP, polymorphic eruption of pregnancy; PG, pemphigoid gestationis; PP, postpartum.

lesions on the trunk progressing in generalized fashion spreading along the face, mucous membranes, palms, and soles (Figures 9-2 and 9-3). A flare at the time of delivery is a notable feature that is seen in 75% of cases. Gestational pemphigoid typically recurs with subsequent pregnancies, menstruation, and use of oral contraceptive. Most women experience complete resolution over weeks to months after delivery, whereas there are rare instances of continued involvement late in the postpartum period.

6. Treatment/management
   Most women respond to systemic corticosteroids tapering to the lowest effective dose. Refractive cases have been treated with cyclophosphamide, pyridoxine, dapsone, cyclosporine, gold, methotrexate, and plasmapheresis. However, because of the rare nature of this disorder, no controlled therapeutic trials have been conducted.

7. Sequelae/follow-up
   Women with a history of PG appear to be at increased risk for the development of Graves' disease.

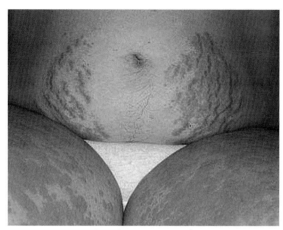

FIGURE 9-2. Pemphigoid gestationis (see Color Plates).

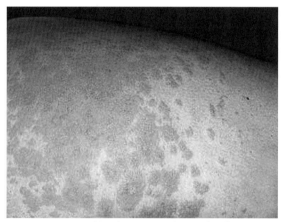

FIGURE 9-3. Pemphigoid gestationis (see Color Plates).

B. Polymorphic Eruption of Pregnancy (Pruritic Urticarial Papules and Plaques of Pregnancy)

1. Key features
   a. Papular urticarial eruption, usually developing during late-term pregnancy
   b. Most frequently occurs in primiparous women
   c. Onset typically begins within abdominal striae, sparing umbilicus
   d. Resolves spontaneously and rapidly after delivery
   e. No identified maternal or fetal risk
   f. Rarely recurs

2. Incidence
   PEP/PUPPP is the most common of the pregnancy-related dermatoses with an estimated incidence of 1 in 160 pregnancies.

3. Causative factors
   Although uncertain, a recent metaanalysis confirmed a previously suggested association with multiple gestation, suggesting that rapid, late stretching of abdominal skin may be a predisposing factor.[4]

4. Pathophysiology
   Immunofluorescence microscopy, H&E staining, and laboratory findings are nonspecific or negative. HLA typing shows no variation from normal control samples.

5. Clinical presentation
   Intensely pruritic urticarial papules and plaques begin in the latter part of the third trimester and the immediate postpartum period. For a matter of days, lesions spread sparing face, palms, and soles. Lesions usually begin in the abdominal striae and typically spare the periumbilical area (Figures 9-4 and 9-5).

6. Treatment
   Treatment is symptomatic utilizing potent topical corticosteroids and oral antihistamines with resolution typically occurring 7 to 10 days after delivery.

C. Atopic Eruption of Pregnancy

1. Key features
   a. Eczematous papular dermatitis appearing early in pregnancy
   b. Associated with exacerbation of previously diagnosed or new-onset atopic dermatitis
   c. Existing pathology nonspecific; laboratory evaluation normal (increased IgE detected in two studies)[6]; immunofluorescence negative

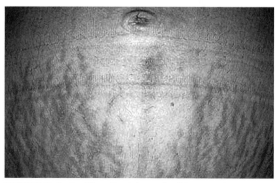

FIGURE 9-4. Pruritic urticarial papules/plaques of pregnancy (PUPPP) (see Color Plates).

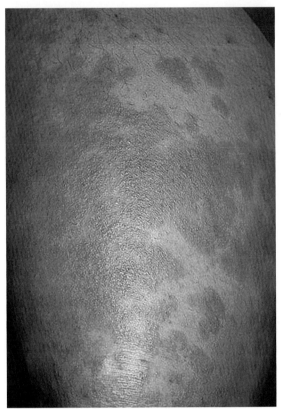

FIGURE 9-5. Pruritic urticarial papules/plaques of pregnancy (PUPPP) (see Color Plates).

2. Incidence
   Incidence varies from 1 in 300 to 450 pregnancies.
3. Causative factors
   The cause of atopic eruption of pregnancy is unknown, aside from reported cases of increased IgE and other patients having been reported to have cholestasis.
4. Clinical course
   Onset occurs during second or third trimester with discrete, excoriated papules, predominately on extensor surfaces and occasionally on the abdomen. Disease process may last for weeks to months after delivery with variable recurrence during subsequent pregnancies.
5. Treatment
   The condition remains symptomatic responding to topical corticosteroids, ultraviolet B light therapy, or benzoyl peroxide.

6. Impact on pregnancy
   No cases of maternal or fetal risk have been reported, as is the case with PEP/PUPPP.

D. Intrahepatic Cholestasis of Pregnancy

1. Key features
   a. Pruritus without primary lesions
   b. Only secondary excoriations/prurigo nodularis
   c. Biochemical cholestasis without identifiable cause
   d. Spontaneous resolution after delivery
   A positive family history is seen in up to 50% of those affected, and incidence is greater in association with twin pregnancies.
2. Incidence
   Incidence of ICP is 1 in 100 to 150 pregnancies.
3. Clinical course
   ICP typically manifests in the third trimester by intense pruritus and secondary excoriations. As with most pruritic conditions, symptoms are worse at night; in addition, pruritus is more pronounced on the trunk, palms, and soles. Pruritus without treatment tends to persist for the duration of the pregnancy.
   Jaundice, clay-colored stools, or dark urine may develop in 20% to 50% of patients. Jaundice may be complicated by steatorrhea with subsequent vitamin K deficiency and prolongation of the prothrombin time, increasing risk for hemorrhage. There have been some reports of increased incidence of cholelithiasis, although this risk remains debatable.[4] The most sensitive laboratory finding in ICP is postprandial increase of serum bile acid levels (cholic acid, deoxycholic acid, and chenodeoxycholic acid). There appears to be no maternal morbidity or mortality, other than the potential for malabsorption or prolonged prothrombin time caused by vitamin K deficiency, leading to subsequent bleeding abnormalities. However, ICP fetal risks include distress, still birth, and PTD believed to result from placental anoxia from vasoconstriction of placental chorionic veins from toxic bile acids and meconium. Fetal complications can be reduced by treatment and delivery between 36 and 38 weeks with favorable lung maturity and cervix.
4. Treatment
   Mild ICP responds to symptomatic treatment with emollients and topical antipruritics. Systemic antihistamines are of minimal effectiveness. Ultraviolet

B phototherapy has been reported to be effective.[2] Several small uncontrolled studies have reported that cholestyramine may be effective in up to 50% of patients; in addition, cholestyramine may precipitate vitamin K, leading to coagulopathy.[4] UDCA has been shown in four randomized trials to be effective in the control of the pruritus and serologic abnormalities.[3] UDCA is a naturally occurring hydrophilic bile acid that enhances the excretion of hydrophobic bile acids, other hepatotoxic compounds, and sulfated progesterone metabolites. UDCA has been shown to reduce bowel acid levels in cord blood, amniotic fluid, and colostrum. UDCA works faster than cholestyramine, has been shown to be safe for mother and fetus, and may result in decreased fetal mortality associated with ICP.[4]

5. Outcome/sequelae

Recurrence in subsequent pregnancies occurs in 60% to 70% of cases or with use of oral contraceptives. The condition usually resolves within the first month after delivery.

III. CONCLUSION

Most clinicians caring for pregnant women should recognize the normal physiologic changes that are quite common, such as hyperpigmentation (chloasma/melasma), postpartum telogen effluvium, striae, spider angiomas, palmar erythema, and varicosities. In addition, one should never lose cognizance that pregnant women are not immune to most dermatoses that affect their nonpregnant counterparts.

As a result of the reviews by Ambros-Rudolph and colleagues,[5] Kroumpouzos and Cohen,[4] and Shornick,[2] a previous hodgepodge of ill-defined, overlapping, confusing, and misleading disorders, the dermatoses of pregnancy have been condensed into an understandable group of disorders that typically occur early in pregnancy (atopic eruption of pregnancy) or late in pregnancy (PEP or PG). ICP presents with pruritus, and only secondary skin lesions manifested as excoriations or prurigo nodularis. PEP and PG, where not clinically obvious, can be easily differentiated by the typical immunofluorescence findings found in PG. ICP presents the greatest risk to the fetus with PG resulting in risk for prematurity and small-for-gestational age births. Roger and colleagues have suggested that a skin biopsy with direct immunofluorescence be obtained when presented with an otherwise unexplained pruritic disease of pregnancy if skin eruption is present; otherwise, obtain serum liver function tests and bile acids, if only pruritis without primary lesions is presented.[7]

REFERENCES

1. Holmes RC, Black MM: The specific dermatoses of pregnancy: a reappraisal with specific emphasis on a proposed simplified clinical classification, *Clin Exp Dermatol* 7:67-73, 1982.
2. Shornick J: Dermatoses of pregnancy, *Semin Cut Med Surg* 17:172-181, 1998.
3. Zoberman E, Farmer ER: Pruritic folliculitis of pregnancy, *Arch Dermatol* 117:20-22, 1981.
4. Kroumpouzos G, Cohen L: Specific dermatoses of pregnancy: an evidenced-based systemic review, *Am J Obstet Gynecol* 188:1083-1092, 2003.
5. Ambros-Rudolph C, Mullegger R, Vaughn Jones S et al: The specific dermatoses of pregnancy revisited and reclassified: a retrospective 2-center study in 505 pregnant patients, *J Am Acad Dermatol* 54:395-404, 2006.
6. Holmes RC, Black MM: The specific dermatoses of pregnancy, *J Am Acad Dermatol* 8:405-412, 1983.
7. Roger D, Vaillant L, Fignon, A et al: Specific pruritic diseases of pregnancy. A prospective study of 3192 pregnant women, *Arch Dermatol* 130:734-739, 1994.

SECTION E Acute Neurologic Conditions

Ellen L. Sakornbut, MD

I. CARPAL TUNNEL SYNDROME

A. Epidemiology/Natural History

Nocturnal hand pain is a common symptom during late pregnancy, but a much smaller number of pregnant women demonstrate nerve conduction or electromyographic abnormalities of carpal tunnel syndrome (CTS). A Danish population-based study found an incidence rate of 16% of women with hand symptoms during pregnancy, about one third with median nerve symptoms and one fourth with ulnar nerve symptoms.[1] Symptoms are more common in older primiparous women with generalized edema.[2]

B. Differential Diagnosis

Differential diagnosis of CTS should include acroparesthesia caused by kinking of blood vessels in the thoracic outlet. Median nerve distribution is important in making the diagnosis.

C. Treatment

Treatment is usually successful with wrist splints, reducing pain and improving grip strength.[3] If symptoms are more persistent, steroid injection into the carpal tunnel may be used. The majority of cases resolve after delivery. If the onset of carpal tunnel symptoms occurs in the first two trimesters of pregnancy or if the patient has a positive Phalen test within 30 seconds and abnormal two-point discrimination at the fingertips (>6 mm), she is more likely not to respond to conservative therapy and require surgery after delivery.[4] Surgery during pregnancy has been recommended by some authors for patients with sensory symptoms and motor latency more than 5 milliseconds.[5] Patients with CTS in pregnancy are more likely to experience development of CTS in the nonpregnant state.[6]

II. BELL'S PALSY

Bell's palsy is three times more common during pregnancy than in nonpregnant women of the same age. It is most common in the third trimester. Treatment with steroids is indicated if onset is earlier than the late third trimester and facial nerve paralysis is complete.[7] Prognosis is good in most cases.

III. MERALGIA PARESTHETICA

Meralgia paresthetica (MP) presents with numbness, pain, and paresthesias in the anterolateral thigh. Entrapment of the lateral femoral cutaneous nerve beneath the inguinal ligament as the uterus enlarges is the most common cause of the condition during pregnancy, although MP may also be caused by a neuroma. If the diagnosis is in doubt, it may be confirmed by infiltration of local anesthetic where the nerve passes under the inguinal ligament with subsequent relief of pain. The condition is more common in the third trimester.[8] A population-based study in the Netherlands found an incidence of 4 per 10,000 people with strong associations to pregnancy and CTS, although MP may be seen in other conditions.[9] Most patients do not require treatment and the condition resolves spontaneously, although a trial of local corticosteroid injection in the area of the nerve entrapment might be considered in a highly symptomatic patient.[10]

IV. OBSTETRIC PALSY

A. Pathophysiology

An obstetric palsy is caused by compression of lumbosacral nerve plexus and individual nerves against the pelvic bones by the fetal head. Alternatively, nerve compression may occur with forceps rotation. The incidence of obstetric palsy has decreased because of modern obstetric practices.

B. At-Risk Patients

The patients at increased risk for an obstetric palsy are short primigravidas with cephalopelvic disproportion or patients with occiput posterior presentation or other reasons for midforceps delivery. The patient may have experienced a protracted second stage. The patient may remember onset of sharp pain during the second stage.

C. Footdrop Palsy

A large observational study of more than 6000 women delivering at a university hospital determined the incidence rate of obstetric palsy to be approximately 0.9%. The most common risk factors associated with obstetric palsy were nulliparity and prolonged second stage of labor.[11] The most common palsy is footdrop associated with compression of the L4 and L5 roots against the sacrum.[12] L4, L5, and S1 roots may be compressed in the pelvis close to the sciatic notch presenting a picture similar to typical sciatica. Footdrop palsy may also be caused by peroneal nerve compression between leg holders and the head of the fibula, although this is less commonly encountered with usual precautions. Most patients recover within 8 weeks because the injury usually involves only distortion of the myelin sheath (neurapraxic lesion). If recovery takes longer, an electromyogram can be performed to diagnose axonal degeneration.

V. PSEUDOTUMOR CEREBRI OR BENIGN INTRACRANIAL HYPERTENSION

Benign intracranial hypertension is associated with increases in estrogen levels but remains an infrequent condition in pregnancy. Clinical presentation is usually a diffuse, unremitting headache not responding to pain modalities and not explained by other findings or conditions. In contrast, migraine headaches generally improve with sedation or sleep and may recur but occur episodically. Benign intracranial hypertension usually begins in the second trimester and lasts 1 to 3 months or may last until the postpartum period. The dual goals of treatment during pregnancy include relief of symptoms (headache) and preservation of vision. Treatment modalities include analgesia, weight control, diuretics (acetazolamide),[13,14] steroids, and serial lumbar punctures. Rarely, surgical treatment may be necessary, specifically optic nerve sheath fenestration, lumboperitoneal shunting, or both.

REFERENCES

1. de la Fuente Fonnest I, Ellitsgaard V: [Hand symptoms and pregnancy], *Ugeskr Laeger* 160(40):5791-5794, 1998.
2. Ekman-Ordeberg G, Salgeback S, Ordeberg G: Carpal tunnel syndrome in pregnancy: a prospective study, *Acta Obstet Gynaecol Scand* 66:233-235, 1987.
3. Courts RB: Splinting for symptoms of carpal tunnel syndrome during pregnancy, *J Hand Ther* 8:31-34, 1995.
4. Stahl S, Blumenfeld Z, Yarnitsky D: Carpal tunnel syndrome in pregnancy: indications for early surgery, *J Neurol Sci* 136:182-184, 1996.
5. Assmus H, Hashemi B: [Surgical treatment of carpal tunnel syndrome in pregnancy: results from 314 cases], *Nervenarzt* 71(6):470-473, 2000.
6. Al-Qattan MM, Manktelow RT, Bowen CV: Pregnancy-induced carpal tunnel syndrome requiring surgical release longer than 2 years after delivery, *Obstet Gynecol* 84:249-251, 1994.
7. Walling A: Bell's palsy in pregnancy and the puerperium, *J Fam Pract* 36:559-563, 1993.
8. Jones RK: Meralgia paresthetica as a cause of leg discomfort, *Can Med Assoc J* 111:541-542, 1974.
9. van Slobbe AM, Bohnen AM, Bernsen RM et al: Incidence rates and determinants in meralgia paresthetica in general practice, *J Neurol* 251(3):294-297, 2004.
10. Grossman MG, Ducey SA, Nadler SS et al: Meralgia paresthetica: diagnosis and treatment, *J Am Acad Orthop Surg* 9(5):336-344, 2001.
11. Wong CA, Scavone BM, Dugan S et al: Incidence of postpartum lumbosacral spine and lower extremity nerve injuries, *Obstet Gynecol* 101(2):279-288, 2003.
12. Whittaker WG: Injuries to the sacral plexus in obstetrics, *J Can Med Assoc* 79:622-627, 1978.
13. Tang RA, Dorotheo EU, Schiffman JS et al: Medical and surgical management of idiopathic intracranial hypertension in pregnancy, *Curr Neurol Neurosci Rep* 4(5):398-409, 2004.
14. Lee AG, Pless M, Falardeau J et al: The use of acetazolamide in idiopathic intracranial hypertension during pregnancy, *Am J Ophthalmol* 139(5):855-859, 2005.

SECTION F Cervical Cytology in Pregnancy

Richard Hudspeth, MD

Cytologic screening of the uterine cervix has become an important part of prenatal care. Little evidence-based information is available to support testing during pregnancy; nonetheless, it is a part of routine care to perform a Papanicolaou test during a woman's pregnancy. New technologies, such as liquid-based cytology and HPV testing, have added an additional element of decision making. In addition, no trials exist, or ever will, that compare management strategies of abnormal cytology specifically in pregnant women. In the United States, cervical cancer rates continue to decrease, whereas our ability to intervene with diagnostic and therapeutic interventions continues to increase. However, the primary goal in evaluating cervical cytology during pregnancy has not changed: to rule out the presence of cervical cancer.[1]

I. EPIDEMIOLOGY AND RISK FACTORS

A. Morbidity and Mortality

The American Cancer Society estimates that in 2006 about 9710 cases of invasive cervical cancer will be diagnosed and about 3700 women will die of cervical cancer in the United States.[2] The worldwide burden of disease is much greater, with cervical cancer estimated to be the second most common cancer among women. Worldwide, there were more than 493,000 new cases diagnosed and 273,500 deaths from cervical cancer in 2000. Approximately 85% of these deaths occurred in developing countries, and in some parts of the world, cervical cancer claims the lives of more women than do pregnancy-related causes.[3]

B. Age-Related Risks

Half of women diagnosed with cervical cancer are between the ages of 35 and 55 with it rarely occurring in women younger than 20. About 20% of women with cervical cancer are diagnosed when they are older than 65.[2] The mean age of pregnant women with cervical cancer has been estimated at 33.8 years.[4] Approximately 50% of all women newly diagnosed with cervical cancer had never had a Pap test, and an additional 10% had not been adequately screened in the last 5 years.[5]

C. Ethnic Factors

Cervical cancer occurs most often in Hispanic women; the rate for Hispanic women is more than twice that of non-Hispanic white women. Black women develop this cancer about 50% more often than do non-Hispanic white women.[2]

D. Cervical Dysplasia in Pregnancy

The risk for cervical dysplasia in pregnant women is similar to that of nonpregnant women, with an incidence rate on Pap smear of 1.2% to 2.2%. The incidence of cervical intraepithelial neoplasia (CIN) in pregnant women ranges from 3.4% to about 10%, but carcinoma of the cervix is uncommon occurring in only 1 to 10 of every 10,000 pregnancies.[6-10] Cervical cancer comprises 25% of all malignancies during pregnancy, yet only 3% of all cervical cancers are identified during pregnancy.[4] Few health-care providers will diagnose a pregnant woman with cervical cancer.

E. Role of Human Papillomavirus Infection

HPV is the most certain risk factor for CIN and cervical cancer. HPV is a necessary factor of cervical cancer given that more than 99% of cervical cancers are associated with specific "high-risk" types of HPV.[11] The most prevalent high-risk types detected in cervical cancer are HPV-16 (53%), -18 (15%), -45 (9%), -31 (6%), and -33 (3%).[12]

F. Other Risk Factors

Other risk factors for invasive cervical cancer include early age at sexual initiation (initiation before 16 years of age carries twice the risk for those who wait until after age 20),[13,14] multiple sexual partners in the last 5 years,[15] multiparity,[16] and the presence of other cofactors such as smoking,[17,18] HIV,[19] and *C. trachomatis*.[20-24] Oral contraceptive pills also show a moderate association with increased risk for squamous cell carcinoma (OR, 1.4)[25] and invasive adenocarcinoma of the cervix,[26,27] although the risk for CIN with oral contraceptive pill use is less clear. Sexual intercourse with an uncircumcised male individual has also been identified as increasing a woman's risk for cervical cancer.[28]

II. PATHOGENESIS

A. Progression of Disease

Previous thinking suggested that all identification of disease represented a progression on a continuum to cervical cancer. A recent change in how we understand the regression, progression, and persistence of HPV and the relation to CIN has led to the view that CIN grade 1 (CIN 1) may be better characterized as an acute transient infection, whereas CIN 2 or 3 may be more accurately characterized as a precancerous lesion. The presence of high-risk HPV and not simply the presence of CIN 1 determines the risk for a precancerous lesion.[29-31] This change in view has certainly lessened the aggressiveness for treatment of CIN 1 in management protocols, perhaps even more so in pregnant women given that the likelihood of cancer is low.

B. Natural History of Human Papillomavirus Infection

Numerous studies have elicited the natural history of an acquired HPV infection and subsequent intraepithelial lesions.[32-35] In one of these studies, the median duration of 70% of the new infections was 8 months, with another 19% cleared by 18 months, and only 9% persisting at 24 months.[32] Ostor's[30] comprehensive review of published studies since 1950 showed CIN 1 regressing 60% of the time, persisting 30% of the time, and progressing to CIN 3 in 10% of patients; CIN 1 progressed to cancer about 1% of the time.[30] Since publication of the Ostor article, the ALTS Trial information has confirmed progression of CIN 1 to CIN 2/3 at about 13%.[31]

It has been estimated to take in excess of 6 years from HPV infection to development of CIN 3 and 13 years from normal cytology to the development of cervical cancer.[36] The lesson to be learned is that most HPV infections are transient and benign. It is persistence of infection with high-risk HPV that puts the woman at risk for progression of CIN and the development of cervical cancer.[37]

III. CLINICAL FEATURES

The identification of cervical dysplasia may present challenges to a clinician who may be unfamiliar, and indeed, even those familiar with the changes to the cervix during pregnancy.[38]

A. Chadwick's Sign in Early Pregnancy

Early in pregnancy the cervix softens, becomes cyanotic, and appears with a bluish hue (Chadwick's sign) because of increased vascularity and edema.

B. Changes in Cervical Appearance

Greater estrogen levels during early pregnancy cause cervical glands and stroma to undergo squamous metaplasia and endocervical gland hyperplasia with subsequent endocervical eversion onto the ectocervix. Early in pregnancy these hormonal changes are less pronounced, but as the pregnancy progresses these changes, such as the eversion by 16 to 18 weeks, can actually aid in an evaluation resulting in a satisfactory colposcopy.

C. Cervical Mucus

Endocervical glands produce increased amounts of thick, tenacious mucus. Application of acetic acid (3-5%), use of a ringed forceps to carefully remove excess mucus, or simply moving the mucus with a small cotton-tipped applicator may aid in fully examining the cervix.

D. Changes in Vaginal Dimensions

As the pregnancy progresses, vaginal walls become redundant and lax secondary to hyperemia. The vagina also lengthens and undergoes epithelial thickening. Using a speculum placed through a condom or the thumb of a latex glove with the tip of the thumb portion of the glove removed may act as a vaginal side wall retractor to aid in unobstructed access to the cervix.

E. Pregnancy-Related Changes on Cervical Cytology

Decidual cells with variably staining cytoplasm and large nuclei may mimic a HSIL as they degenerate and shed from the endometrium.[39] In addition, these physiologic metaplastic changes of the cervix during pregnancy can easily resemble CIN, and the enhanced vascularity may accentuate existing vascular patterns, suggesting that the lesions are of a higher grade than in reality.[6,40] However, underdiagnosis at colposcopy has been documented during pregnancy as well.[41] Care must be exercised when undertaking evaluation of the cervix in pregnancy.

IV. DIAGNOSIS

A. Pap Smears/Human Papillomavirus Testing

It has been well established that the Pap smear has reduced the incidence of cervical cancer by early recognition of cervical abnormalities. Although no separate evidence-based guidelines exist for pregnant women, the current recommendations suggest following the same guidelines for the pregnant woman as one would for the nonpregnant woman, with some slight modifications as outlined later. The current published guidelines are widely available but are currently being revised, and new guidelines may be published soon.[42,43]

Liquid-based cytology offers the clinician a choice of collection methods. This technology is commonly used, although some question exists as to the "improvement" over conventional cytology. A recent study in *Lancet* questioned whether liquid-based cytology is better than conventional cytology, with conventional cytology more likely to detect high-grade cervical lesions.[44]

The introduction of HPV testing now serves as an adjunct for interpreting Pap smear results. Guidelines have been released to help clinicians best use HPV testing.[45] Since the release of HPV testing, numerous studies have been published (see later) that may affect the way clinicians continue to use HPV testing. Regardless of the collection method, conventional or liquid based, HPV reflex testing can be utilized at the time of the initial Pap smear sampling. With a liquid-based collection, reflex testing can be performed from the sample obtained. With conventional cytology, a co-collection method must be used in addition to the conventional slide preparation.

Other methods of cervical cancer detection and prevention are used in developing countries or other low-resource settings such as the "see and treat" programs that use visual inspection with acetic acid application and treat immediately without delay. These methods are not addressed in this text.

No algorithmic protocol can anticipate every clinical situation or possible scenario. When faced with confusing or conflicting information, pregnant women should expect to have the same degree of correlation with cytology, colposcopic impression, and histology that nonpregnant women have. If poor correlation exists, then a reexamination of all components should be initiated.

Currently accepted protocols from possible initial cytological samples are below.

1. Normal

   It is common to repeat cytology at about 6 weeks after delivery. However, in women with no risk factors for CIN and a normal initial Pap smear, the rate of SIL on the postpartum Pap smear was only 1 in 1000. The postpartum Pap smear has a greater rate of detection of endocervical cells. It may be possible to recommend women have their Pap smear repeated at the recommended interval rather than always at 6 weeks.[46]

2. Atypical squamous cells of undetermined significance (ASCUS)

   Multiple studies have confirmed the risk for ≥ CIN 2 at initial colposcopy after ASCUS with HPV high-risk positive (HR+) is about 15% to 20%, whereas HPV high-risk negative (HR−) is approximately 1%.[47-49] Therefore, HPV testing is useful information in the management of ASCUS. However, the likelihood that a pregnant woman with ASCUS has HPV HR (84%) is similar to a result of HPV HR in LSIL.[50]

3. LSIL

   Colposcopy is the current recommendation. The ALTS Trial showed that a LSIL result is too high of a marker for HPV HR to make HPV testing useful, especially in young women.[51] However, some authors suggest that LSIL or ASCUS would not require evaluation until the postpartum period.[52,53]

4. ASC-H

   About 10% of all ASC will return with this result.[54,55] Currently, colposcopy is the current recommendation. Some information suggests that a significant percentage, 70% to 86% of these smears, regardless of collection method, will be positive for HPV HR and CIN 2/3 found in 27% to 40%.[31,55] Recent studies have begun to question the wisdom of automatic referral of ASC-H for colposcopy without using HPV testing, especially in those women older than 30.[56-58] However, generalizing this to pregnant women can be challenging given that a small study looking specifically at pregnant women showed that ASC-H in pregnant women may have a lower predictive value for a HSIL and a positive HPV may have a lower positive predictive value in this population.[59]

5. Second ASCUS

   A prepregnant ASCUS followed by an ASCUS in pregnancy should be followed by colposcopy.

6. HSIL or cancer

   Colposcopy is indicated with referral to or co-management with gynecologic oncology.

B. Further Diagnosis with Colposcopy: Management and Treatment of Abnormal Cytology during Pregnancy

No trials exist that compare management strategies in pregnant women. However, it is important to remember that endocervical curettage (ECC) is not acceptable in pregnancy. Although no evidence through direct trial will ever exist concerning the use of ECC in pregnancy, given the potential harm of perforation of amniotic membranes, placental injury such as bleeding, infection risk, or possible loss of the pregnancy, it is reasonable to assume the harm outweighs the benefit of ECC.[60]

Biopsy is deemed safe and accurate in pregnancy.[41,61] Biopsy in pregnancy has not contributed to pregnancy loss, whereas biopsy improves diagnostic accuracy.[1] Cervical biopsy during pregnancy is often accompanied by brisk bleeding. Simple *immediate* pressure and application of Monsel's solution almost always stops any bleeding. Rarely, a suture may be required.

Currently accepted protocols from possible colposcopic and histological findings are as follows:

1. Normal

   If the correlation of the colposcopy, histology, and cytology is appropriate, then repeating cytology at 6 weeks after delivery is acceptable.

2. Unsatisfactory colposcopy

   This was most likely performed in early pregnancy. Repeating colposcopy at a later gestational age (>20 weeks) may afford a satisfactory colposcopy.

3. LSIL

   A postpartum examination with cytology, colposcopy with biopsy and ECC, is an acceptable option. Some may prefer to monitor these with examinations each trimester (without an ECC). A discussion with the patient, consideration of follow-up, and availability of resources may be necessary to determine the best choice for an individual patient.

4. HSIL

   Repeating cytology, colposcopy with biopsy but no ECC, each trimester to monitor for progression is recommended. No treatment is necessary. Most cases (80%) will persist, some will regress, and rarely will a high-grade lesion progress to cancer by the postpartum period.[62]

5. Microinvasive disease or invasive cervical carcinoma

In either case, consultation with a gynecologist oncologist is necessary. In cases of suspected microinvasive disease, a conization may be undertaken. This is a diagnostic procedure only and is not therapeutic. Conization has known potential complications including risk for pregnancy loss, substantial hemorrhage, and PTD. The variables associated with decision making in these cases are many, including but not limited to gestational age, staging of the patient's cancer, and patient preference. A discussion of all of these factors is beyond the scope of this chapter.

V. CLINICAL PREVENTION

Certainly decreasing risk factors can aid in the prevention of cervical cancer. In addition, development of adequate screening programs for women at greatest risk could go a long way toward cervical cancer prevention. The Cochrane Database has only one study directly related to successful programs for cervical cancer prevention screening programs. This study states: "There was sufficient evidence from good quality RCTs to support the use of invitation letters in increasing the uptake of Pap smears. There was also some evidence to suggest that educational materials may increase Pap smear uptake. Thus, attempts to increase the informed uptake of screening should be pursued alongside initiatives to increase actual uptake, but until such evidence becomes available no implications for how this should be implemented can be given."[63] Most clinicians understand the complexities of this task.

The most recent development in prevention is the release of a quadrivalent HPV recombinant vaccine (types 6, 11, 16, 18), marketed as Gardasil. This appears to be a highly effective vaccine (achieving nearly 100% efficacy).[64] Current recommendations suggest vaccinating 11- to 12-year-old girls, but it can be used in women aged 9 to 26. The course is three injections given, with the second and third given at 2 and 6 months after the first dose. The published price of the dose is approximately $119.75 per dose. Check with your local agencies for insurance coverage of this vaccine.

VI. SOR A RECOMMENDATIONS

RECOMMENDATIONS	REFERENCES
Cervical biopsy is safe in pregnancy.	*41, 61*
Vaccinate against HPV.	*64*
Work toward community screening programs to reach women at high risk for cervical cancer.	*63*

REFERENCES

1. LaPolla JP, O'Neill C, Wetrich D: Colposcopic management of abnormal cervical cytology in pregnancy, *J Reprod Med* 33:301-306, 1988.
2. American Cancer Society: *Detailed guide: cervical cancer. What are the key statistics about cervical cancer?* Available at: http://www.cancer.org/docroot/CRI/content/CRI_2_4_1X_What_are_the_key_statistics_for_cervical_cancer_8.asp?sitearea. Accessed October 2006.
3. World Health Organization: *Planning and implementing cervical cancer prevention & control programs. A manual for managers.* Available at: http://www.who.int/reproductive-health/cancers/cervical_cancer_prevention_control_programs_intro.pdf. Accessed October 2006. [Original source: Alliance for Cervical Cancer Prevention (ACCP): *Planning and implementing cervical cancer prevention & control programs. A manual for managers,* Seattle, 2004, ACCP.
4. Hacker NF, Berek JS, Lagasse LD et al: Carcinoma of the cervix associated with pregnancy, *Obstet Gynecol* 59:735-746, 1982.
5. Ferris DG, Cox JT, O'Connor DM et al: *Modern colposcopy textbook and atlas,* Dubuque, IA, 2004, Kendall/Hunt Publishing Co.
6. Apgar BS, Zoschnick LB: Triage of the abnormal Papanicolaou smear in pregnancy, *Prim Care* 25:483-500, 1998.
7. Baltzer J, Regenbrecht ME, Kopcke W et al: Carcinoma of the cervix and pregnancy, *Int J Gynaecol Obstet* 31:317-323, 1990.
8. Patsner B: Management of low-grade cervical dysplasia during pregnancy, *South Med J* 83:1405-1412, 1990.
9. Bertini-Oliveira AM, Keppler MM, Luisi A et al: Comparative evaluation of abnormal cytology, colposcopy and histopathology in preclinical cervical malignancy during pregnancy, *Acta Cytol* 26:636-644, 1982.
10. Hannigan EV: Cervical cancer in pregnancy, *Clin Obstet Gynecol* 33:837-845, 1990.
11. Bosch FX, Lorincz A, Munoz N et al: The causal relationship between human papillomavirus and cervical cancer, *J Clin Pathol* 55:244-265, 2002.
12. Bosch FX, Manos MM, Munoz N et al: Prevalence of human papillomavirus in cervical cancer: a worldwide perspective. International biological study on cervical cancer (IBSCC) Study Group, *J Natl Cancer Inst* 87:779-780, 1995.
13. Herrero R, Brinton LA, Reeves WC et al: Sexual behavior, venereal diseases, hygiene practices, and invasive cervical cancer in high risk population, *Cancer* 65:380-386, 1990.
14. La Vecchia C, Franceschi S, DeCarli A et al: Sexual factors, venereal diseases, and the risk of intraepithelial and invasive cervical neoplasia, *Cancer* 58:935-941, 1986.

15. Svare EI, Kjaer SK, Worm AM et al: Risk factors for HPV infection in women from sexually transmitted disease clinics: comparison between two areas with different cervical cancer incidence, *Int J Cancer* 75:1-8, 1998.

16. Munoz N, Franceschi S, Bosetti C et al: Role of parity and human papillomavirus in cervical cancer: the IARC multicentric case-control study, *Lancet* 359:1093-1101, 2002.

17. Castellsague X, Bosch FX, Munoz N: Environmental cofactors in HPV carcinogenesis, *Virus Res* 89:191-199, 2002.

18. Szarewski A, Cuzick J: Smoking and cervical neoplasia: a review of the evidence, *J Epidemiol Biostat* 3:229-256, 1998.

19. Mandelblatt JS, Kanetsky P, Eggert L et al: Is HIV infection a cofactor for cervical squamous cell neoplasia? *Cancer Epidemiol Biomarkers Prev* 8:97-106, 1999.

20. Wallin KL, Wiklund F, Luostarinen T et al: A population-based prospective study of *Chlamydia trachomatis* infection and cervical carcinoma, *Int J Cancer* 101:371-374, 2002.

21. Schachter J, Hill EC, King EB: *Chlamydia trachomatis* and cervical neoplasia, *JAMA* 248:2134, 1982.

22. Koskela P, Anttila T, Bjorge T et al: *Chlamydia trachomatis* infection as a risk factor for invasive cervical cancer, *Int J Cancer* 85:35-39, 2000.

23. Smith JS, Munoz N, Herrero R et al: Evidence for *Chlamydia trachomatis* as a human papillomavirus cofactor in the etiology of invasive cervical cancer in Brazil and the Philippines, *J Infect Dis* 185:324-331, 2002.

24. Anttila T, Saikku P, Koskela P et al: Serotypes of *Chlamydia trachomatis* and risk for development of cervical squamous cell carcinoma, *JAMA* 285:47-51, 2001.

25. Moreno V, Bosch FX, Munoz N et al: International Agency for Research on Cancer. Multicentric Cervical Cancer Study Group. Effect of oral contraceptives on risk of cervical cancer in women with human papillomavirus infection: the IARC multicentric case-control study, *Lancet* 359:1085-1092, 2002.

26. Thomas DB, Ray RM: Oral contraceptives and invasive adenocarcinoma and adenosquamous carcinomas of the uterine cervix. The World Health Organization Collaborative Study of Neoplasia and Steroid Contraceptives, *Am J Epidemiol* 144:281-289, 1996.

27. Peters RK, Chao A, Mack TM et al: Increased frequency of adenocarcinoma of the uterine cervix in young women in Los Angeles County, *J Natl Cancer Inst* 76:423-428, 1986.

28. Castellsague X, Bosch FX, Munoz N et al: The International Agency for Research on Cancer Multicenter Cervical Cancer Study Group. Male circumcision, penile human papillomavirus infection, and cervical cancer in female partners, *N Engl J Med* 346:1105-1112, 2002.

29. Koutsky LA, Homes KK, Critchlow CW et al: Cohort study of risk of cervical intraepithelial neoplasia grade 2 or 3 associated with cervical papillomavirus infection, *N Engl J Med* 327:1272-1278, 1992.

30. Ostor AG: Natural history of CIN: a critical review, *Int J Gynecol Path* 12:186-192, 1993.

31. Cox JT, Schiffman M, Soloman D: ASCUS-LSIL Triage Study (ALTS) Group. Prospective follow-up suggests similar risk of subsequent cervical intraepithelial neoplasia grade 2 or 3 among women with cervical intraepithelial neoplasia grade 1 or negative colposcopy and directed biopsy, *Am J Obstet Gynecol* 188:1406-1412, 2003.

32. Ho GYF, Bierman R, Beardsley L et al: Natural history of cervicovaginal papillomavirus infection in young women, *N Engl J Med* 338:423-428, 1998.

33. Bauer HM, Ting Y, Greer CE et al: Genital human papillomavirus infection in female university students as determined by PCR-based method, *JAMA* 265:472-477, 1991.

34. Melnikow J, Nuovo J, Willan AR et al: Natural history of cervical squamous intraepithelial lesions: a meta-analysis, *Obstet Gynecol* 92:727-735, 1998.

35. Einstein MH, Burk RD: Persistent human papillomavirus infection: definitions and clinical implications, *Papillomavirus Report* 12:119-123, 2001.

36. Teale G: The prevention of cervical intraepithelial neoplasia, *Obstet Gynecol* 5:21-27, 2003.

37. Koliopoulos G, Martin-Hirsch P, Paraskevaidis E et al: HPV testing versus cervical cytology for screening for cancer of the uterine cervix, *Cochrane Database of Systemic Reviews* 2003, Issue 4. Art. No.: CD004709. DOI: 10.1002/14651858. CD004709.

38. Fowler WC, Walton LA, Edelman DA: Cervical intraepithelial neoplasia during pregnancy, *South Med J* 73:1180-1185, 1980.

39. Michael CW, Esfahani FM: Pregnancy-related changes: a retrospective review of 278 cervical smears, *Diagn Cytopathol* 17:99-107, 1997.

40. Ostergard DR, Nieberg RK: Evaluation of abnormal cervical cytology during pregnancy with colposcopy, *Am J Obstet Gynecol* 134:756-758, 1979.

41. Economos K, Veridiano NP, Delke I et al: Abnormal cervical cytology in pregnancy: a 17-year experience, *Obstet Gynecol* 81:915-918, 1993.

42. Wright TC, Cox JT, Massad LS et al: 2001 consensus guidelines for the management of women with cervical cytological abnormalities, *JAMA* 287:2120-2129, 2002.

43. American Society for Coloscopy and Cervical Pathology: *Consensus guidelines.* Available at: www.asccp.org/consensus.shtml. Accessed September 4, 2007.

44. Davey E, Barratt A, Irwig L et al: Effect of study design and quality on unsatisfactory rates, cytology classification, and accuracy in liquid-based versus conventional cervical cytology: a systematic review, *Lancet* 367:122-132, 2006.

45. Wright TC, Schiffman M, Solomon D et al: Interim guidance for the use of human papillomavirus DNA testing as an adjunct to cervical cytology for screening, *Obstet Gynecol* 103(2):304-309, 2004.

46. Jazayeri A, Heffron JA, Harnety P et al: Antepartum and postpartum Papanicolaou smears: are both necessary? *J Reprod Med* 44:879-882, 1999.

47. Cox JT, Lorincz AT, Schiffman MH et al: HPV testing by hybrid capture appears to be useful in triaging women with a cytologic diagnosis of ASCUS, *Am J Obstet Gynecol* 172:946-954, 1995.

48. Manos MM, Kinney WK, Hurley LB et al: Identifying women with cervical neoplasia: using human papillomavirus DNA testing for equivocal Papanicolaou results, *JAMA* 281:1605-1610, 1999.

49. Solomon D, Schiffman MH, Tarone R: Comparison of three management strategies for patients with atypical squamous cells of undetermined significance: baseline results from a randomized trial, *J Natl Cancer Inst* 93:293-299, 2001.

50. Lu DW, Pirog EC, Zhu X et al: Prevalence and typing of HPV DNA in atypical squamous cells in pregnant women, *Acta Cytol* 47:1008-1016, 2003.

51. ASCUS-LSIL Triage Study (ALTS) Group: A randomized trial on the management of low-grade squamous intraepithelial lesion cytology interpretations, *Am J Obstet Gynecol* 188:1393-1400, 2003.

52. Jain AG, Higgins RV, Boyle MJ: Management of low-grade squamous intraepithelial lesions during pregnancy, *Am J Obstet Gynecol* 177:298-302, 1997.

53. Murta EFC, de Andrade FC, Adad SJ et al: Low-grade cervical squamous intraepithelial lesion during pregnancy: conservative antepartum management, *Eur J Gynaecol Oncol* 25:600-602, 2004.

54. Selvaggi SM: Reporting of atypical squamous cells cannot exclude a high-grade squamous intraepithelial lesion (ASC-H) on cervical samples: is it significant? *Diagn Cytopathol* 29:38-41, 2003.

55. Alli PM, Ali SZ: Atypical squamous cells of undetermined significance—rule out high-grade squamous intraepithelial lesion: cytopathologic characteristics and clinical correlates, *Diagn Cytopathol* 28:308-312, 2003.

56. Wu HH, Allen SL, Kirkpatrick JL et al: Reflex high-risk human papilloma virus DNA test is useful in the triage of women with atypical squamous cells cannot exclude high-grade squamous intraepithelial lesion, *Diagn Cytopathol* 34(10):707-710, 2006.

57. Liman AK, Giampoli EJ, Bonfiglio TA: Should women with atypical squamous cells, cannot exclude high-grade squamous intraepithelial lesion, receive reflex human papillomavirus-DNA testing? *Cancer (Cancer Cytopathology)* 105(6):457-460, 2005.

58. Srodon M, Parry Dilworth H, Ronnett BM: Atypical squamous cells, cannot exclude high-grade squamous intraepithelial lesion: diagnostic performance, human papillomavirus testing, and follow-up results, *Cancer* 108(1):32-38, 2006.

59. Onuma K, Saad RS, Kanbour-Shakir AI et al: Clinical implications of the diagnosis "atypical squamous cells, cannot exclude high-grade squamous intraepithelial lesion" in pregnant women, *Cancer* 108(5):282-287, 2006.

60. Massad SL, Wright TC, Cox TJ et al: Managing abnormal cytology results in pregnancy, *J Lower Genital Tract Dis* 9:146-148, 2005.

61. Cristoforoni PM, Gerbaldo DL, Philipson J et al: Management of the abnormal pap smear during pregnancy: lessons for quality improvement, *J Lower Genital Tract Dis* 3:225-230, 1999.

62. Coppola A, Sorosky J, Casper R et al: The clinical course of cervical carcinoma in situ diagnosed during pregnancy, *Gynecol Oncol* 67:162-165, 1997.

63. Forbes C, Jepson R, Martin-Hirsch P: Interventions targeted at women to encourage the uptake of cervical screening, *Cochrane Database Syst Rev* (3):CD002834, 2002.

64. Mao C, Koutsky LA, Ault KA et al: Efficacy of human papillomavirus-16 vaccine to prevent cervical intraepithelial neoplasia, *Obstet Gynecol* 107:18-27, 2006.

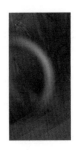

CHAPTER 10

Treatment of Psychiatric Disorders in Pregnancy

Ellen L. Sakornbut, MD

SECTION A Affective Disorders

I. UNIPOLAR DEPRESSION

The epidemiology, natural history, diagnosis, and management of unipolar depression are discussed in the following sections.

A. Epidemiology and Natural History of Depression in Pregnancy

Although the incidence of depression is cited to be as common as 1 in 10 people, the prevalence of women with this diagnosis is greater. Depression during pregnancy has been associated with poor pregnancy outcome, including low birth weight, premature birth, and delivery of a small-for-gestational-age infant.[1] The incidence of depressive symptoms during pregnancy has been noted to be as high as 26% in an inner-city prenatal clinic.[2] Pregnancy is not protective for depression or relapses of previously diagnosed depression, and women who discontinue treatment before conception or at discovery of pregnancy are at increased risk for relapse compared with women who maintain medication regimen (hazard ratio, 5.0; 95% confidence interval, 2.8-9.1; $p < 0.001$).[3]

Special groups of patients deserve consideration for continuance of medication or treatment of affective disorder if diagnosed. The rate of recurrence of bipolar disorder during pregnancy with discontinuance of lithium is greater than 50%, similar to nonpregnant

control subjects observed over a 40-week period. The rate of recurrence of bipolar disorder is even greater (relative risk, 2.9) in women after delivery compared with nonpregnant control subjects observed in weeks 41 to 64 after discontinuance of lithium.[4] Some authors support a link between postpartum psychosis and bipolar disorder.[5] In addition, some studies have found increased rates of depression in pregnant women being treated for substance abuse[6]; those who have been victims of sexual, verbal, or physical abuse[7]; and assault victims.[8] Whether depressive symptoms represent normal grieving or clinical depression, women who have experienced stillbirth in the previous pregnancy are at greater risk than control subjects for depressive symptoms during and after the next pregnancy, especially in pregnancies occurring less than 1 year after the stillbirth.[9]

If untreated, clinical depression will generally not improve in the postpartum period when the incidence of depressive disorders increases. During the postpartum period, the mother–infant dyad may be further at risk for poor bonding and other difficulties in adaptation to family life (see Chapter 21, Section A).

B. Diagnosis of Depression

The diagnostic criteria for depression during pregnancy do not differ from the nonpregnant state. Clinicians may feel more comfortable in using screening instruments, such as the Beck Depression Inventory or Zung Depression Scale, to identify patients who warrant further assessment. They should recognize that screening instruments have a 20% false-positive rate, and application of standard diagnostic criteria is advisable. The *Diagnostic and Statistical Manual of*

Mental Disorders, Fourth Edition (DSM-IV) is the current U.S. standard for psychiatric diagnosis. A primary care (PC) version has been developed that focuses on symptomatic presentations common in this setting.[10] The DSM-IV PC uses the same symptom-driven diagnostic criteria as the original DSM-IV.

C. Nonpharmacologic Treatment

Psychotherapy may be chosen for women with mild-to-moderate depression, particularly those who are reluctant to try medication during pregnancy or the postpartum period. Two forms of psychotherapy have emerged as particularly beneficial in the treatment of depression. Cognitive-behavioral therapy (CBT) focuses on the negativistic, self-defeating thoughts common in depressive states. It theorizes that negative thoughts (experienced as automatic and self-deprecating) often create feelings of depression and have as their enduring source irrational beliefs about self, surroundings, and the future. Patients using CBT learn to monitor themselves and stop automatic thoughts with negative affective valence (e.g., "I'm so stupid," "I can't do anything right," "Nothing will ever change") and rationally examine the evidence for these thoughts as truth statements. Patients then learn to substitute rational thinking for irrational thoughts. In this way, they restructure the inaccurate and usually negative, pessimistic, and devaluing beliefs that serve as sources or reinforcement of the negative thinking.[11] Interpersonal therapy (IPT) focuses on role identity, transitions, and conflicts that often surround the psychosocial triggers of syndromes or episodes of illness. IPT has been shown to be effective in the maintenance treatment of major depression alone and in combination with medication.[12]

D. Pharmacologic Treatment during Pregnancy

1. Deciding whether to use antidepressant medication

   Although some physicians may hesitate to use antidepressant medication during pregnancy, the risk of untreated depression often outweighs the risks of medication. The use of medication to treat depression during pregnancy involves an informed consent process weighing risks and benefits. Similarly informed women may make widely divergent decisions. Specific considerations that should be weighed include previous history of mood disorders, postpartum depression and/or psychosis, severity of symptoms, and other risk factors for poor obstetric outcome.

2. Evidence about teratogenicity of selective serotonin reuptake inhibitors (SSRIs)

   Most of the studies available regarding newer antidepressant medications are of prospective cohort design and enrolled more than 100 women for each of the medications studied. Most of these are from the Motherisk Program in Toronto. None of the older SSRIs or newer antidepressant medications has been associated with an increased risk for major malformations in these study populations. Medications studied include fluoxetine, fluvoxamine, paroxetine, sertraline, venlafaxine, citalopram, escitalopram, trazodone, nefazodone, and bupropion. Two unpublished, non–peer-reviewed studies from the manufacturer have recently caused issuance of alerts about a possible association of paroxetine and cardiac defects, but the nature of these defects has not been clarified and neither has the level of risk. This is in contrast with existing metaanalyses that do not demonstrate increased malformations above the background rate of 1% to 3%.[13] A possible consideration may be not to use paroxetine during the period of organogenesis, but discontinuance of the medication should be considered carefully in the total context of benefits and possible risks.

   Tricyclic antidepressants (TCAs) do not appear to increase the rate of fetal malformations, increase the rate of intrauterine death, or alter postnatal development, although the quality and quantity of studies are insufficient.[14,15] Given the increased side-effect profile associated with tricyclic use and the lack of clinical data proving safety, there does not appear to be an advantage to the use of TCAs in pregnancy versus newer antidepressants. They are classified as FDA category D.

3. Neonatal adaptation problems

   Multiple reports are available that link some SSRIs to poor neonatal adaptation and increased admission rates to the special care nursery. Case reports indicate some difficulty in determining whether effects on infants were caused by withdrawal or by direct toxicity of the medication.[16] One report appears to suggest a withdrawal syndrome.[17] Early reports of fluoxetine suggest increased risk for prematurity and low birth weight, but 30% of these patients were taking multiple psychotropic medications during pregnancy.[18] It is difficult to know what part other medications or comorbidity may have contributed to these outcomes.

The neonatal discontinuation syndrome includes respiratory distress, jitteriness, poor feeding, hypoglycemia, increased need for admission to a special care nursery, and even convulsions. SSRIs associated with the neonatal discontinuation syndrome include paroxetine, fluoxetine, sertraline, and citralopram.[19] Reports of neonates demonstrating symptoms associated with SSRI exposure in the third trimester sometimes include other psychopharmacologic agents but generally demonstrate benign course of the syndrome.[20] Paroxetine use in the third trimester is associated with a high rate of poor neonatal adaptation or discontinuation syndrome.[21]

The incidence of neonatal discontinuation syndrome is unknown. Infants exposed in the third trimester to SSRIs demonstrated transient symptoms of mild respiratory distress and, less commonly, hypotonia in 30% of cases compared with 9% of nonexposed infants in a prospective cohort study. This study found an increased rate of infants (39%) experiencing symptoms when exposed to maternal paroxetine and clonazepam, and symptomatic infants had greater paroxetine levels compared with asymptomatic infants, suggesting an interaction of paroxetine and clonazepam.[22] A population-based, retrospective study comparing neonatal outcomes in SSRI-exposed pregnancies, pregnancies in depressed women not treated with SSRIs, and control subjects found a lower rate of respiratory symptoms, 13.9% versus 7.8%, comparing exposed and nonexposed infants.[23] Caution must be exercised in comparing outcomes of pregnancies in all nonrandomized studies because it is possible that pregnancy risks could vary in women treated with one or two psychopharmacotherapeutic agents and women who were not treated.

An uncommon (2/1000 live births) but more serious syndrome associated with SSRI exposure in late pregnancy is persistent pulmonary hypertension in the newborn. Preliminary evidence from a case–control study suggests a twofold increase in the incidence of primary pulmonary hypertension in neonates with SSRI use in late pregnancy.[24] Comparisons of serotonergic symptom scores between exposed and nonexposed infants show a fourfold increase in pregnancies with fluoxetine or citalopram third-trimester exposure and inversely proportionate decreases in 5-hydroxyindoleacetic acid concentrations.[25] This finding suggests an underlying mechanism for observed symptoms.

4. Medication-specific information

Information about individual antidepressants is listed in Table 10-1. A pilot study of maternal serum and neonatal cord blood levels of SSRIs, including paroxetine, fluoxetine, sertraline, and venlafaxine, showed cord blood to maternal blood ratios of approximately 0.5 to 1.0; only fluoxetine and its metabolite (norfluoxetine) persisted with measurable neonatal blood levels at 5 days after delivery.[26]

II. BIPOLAR DISORDER

A. Bipolar Disorder and Pregnancy

Patients with bipolar illness, whether type I or II, may experience acute worsening during pregnancy or in the immediate postpartum period. Bipolar women are at greater risk for reproductive cycle events that trigger symptomatic episodes. Women with a history of bipolar disorder should be strongly considered for prophylaxis with a mood-stabilizing agent in the immediate postpartum period based on a high rate of relapse in untreated women.[3,4] Postpartum psychosis, rare compared with postpartum depression, is considered by many authorities to be a bipolar spectrum condition. Dysphoric manias accompanied by Schneiderian first-rank psychotic symptoms (e.g., hallucinations, thought broadcasting) may be seen.

B. Diagnosis of Bipolar I and Bipolar II Disorders

Bipolar I disorder is differentiated from bipolar II disorder by the presence of mania. Bipolar II illness (hypomania with major depression) is considered the most common presentation of the illness. The current DSM-IV criteria for hypomanic episodes require 4 days of expanded mood. However, 1- to 3-day episodes are more typical. Thus, the DSM-IV criteria lack sensitivity for the diagnosis. National Institute of Mental Health prospective data point to several temperamental/personality determinants that may be more associated with bipolar (usually bipolar II) outcome.[27] These are mood lability, the presence of mental or physical energy/activity existing concurrently with the depressed mood, social anxiety, and intense daydreaming. Clinicians may be

TABLE 10-1 Safety Information on Individual Antidepressant Medications

Antidepressant	Congenital Malformations	Preterm Birth or Low Birth Weight	Neonatal Adaptation Syndrome	References
Fluoxetine	No increased risk		Reported to cause poor neonatal adaptation	42
Venlafaxine	No increased risk	No increased risk		43
Citalopram	No increased risk	No increased risk	Relative risk of 4.2 (95% confidence interval, 1.71-10.26) of neonatal adaption syndrome	44, 45
Escitalopram	No increased risk			44
Fluvoxamine	No increased risk			46
Paroxetine	No increased risk	No increased risk	High risk for poor neonatal adaptation	18-22
Sertraline	No increased risk		Reports of poor neonatal adaptation	45
Mirtazapine	No increased risk			44
Bupropion	No increased risk			47
Trazodone	No increased risk	No increased risk		48
Nefazodone	No increased risk	No increased risk		47

less comfortable making a diagnosis of bipolar illness. Its prevalence is greater than previously believed, and hypomanic episodes are recurrent (to be distinguished from normal happiness that does not occur in this recurrent manner). Clinicians also fail to consider family history, longitudinal course, and problematic treatment responses to antidepressant therapy (refractory, erratic, premature, or short-lived).[28] Affected children of patients with bipolar I pursue a predominantly depressive course, and cyclic temperamental presentations often precede syndromal episodes.

C. Nonpharmacologic Treatment

Psychotherapy may be chosen by patients with mild-to-moderate symptoms. Sleep hygiene and avoidance of mood-altering substances (including caffeine) and third-shift work may be helpful.

D. Pharmacologic Treatment

Risk–benefit decisions regarding the treatment of bipolar illness during pregnancy are similar to those in unipolar depression, with the exception that mood stabilizers such as lithium, valproate, and

carbamazepine are known risks as teratogens in first-trimester exposures. These are discussed in the following section.

E. Impact of Pharmacologic Treatment on Pregnancy

Five mood-stabilizing agents are summarized below with respect to their use in pregnancy.
1. Lithium (FDA category D)
   Early studies suggest a strong link between Epstein's anomaly of the heart and lithium exposure.[29,30] Although the relative risk of this rare defect calculated in these studies was estimated to be as much as 400, more recent prospective and retrospective cohort studies demonstrate a relative risk of 1.5 to 3.0 and 1.2 to 7.7, respectively, for cardiac malformations.[31,32] Furthermore, during an 8-year regional study of congenital heart disease in the Baltimore-Washington area, approximately 1% of children with congenital heart disease had Epstein's anomaly, with a prevalence of 5.2 per 100,000 births. Of the 47 children with Epstein's anomaly, the only factor that was associated with this anomaly was benzodiazepine exposure.[33]

Neonatal complications associated with antepartum exposure to lithium include goiter,[34] hypotonia, respiratory distress syndrome, cyanosis, lethargy, and weak suck and Moro reflexes in the neonatal period,[35] but these problems have been noted to be reversible. A study of maternal and infant serum lithium levels found uniform passage of lithium across the placenta with increasing rates of neonatal adaptation problems noted with greater infant serum levels (0.64 mEq/L) and significant reduction of levels when maternal doses were held 24 to 48 hours before delivery.[36] These authors propose such a strategy to reduce newborn adaptation problems.

2. Valproic acid (FDA category D)
Fetal levels of valproic acid are the same or greater than maternal levels. Neural tube defects (especially spina bifida) occur in 2.5% of infants exposed to valproic acid during the first trimester. Maternal serum α-fetoprotein and targeted ultrasound examinations are indicated. Recent information suggests that valproate teratogenicity is dose related. Doses greater than 1000 mg/day are associated with greater risk for major congenital malformations than pregnancies exposed to lower daily doses.[37] Other malformations include cardiac defects, oral clefts, hypospadias, and limb reduction defects. The overall risk for fetal defects appears to be between 5% and 8%. Breast milk levels are 2% of maternal serum levels; hence, there are no contraindications to breastfeeding.

3. Carbamazepine (FDA category C)
Carbamazepine has been associated with craniofacial defects, fingernail hypoplasia, and developmental delays.[38] Breast milk levels are 40% of maternal serum levels and there are no contraindications to breastfeeding.

4. Atypical antipsychotics
Atypical antipsychotics include quetiapine, risperidone, clozapine (Clozaril), and olanzapine. To date, these agents do not demonstrate any teratogenic effects based on data from the Motherisk Program in Toronto and the Israeli Teratogen Information Service. This prospective cohort trial did find an increased risk for low birth weight, 10% versus 2%, in exposed infants when compared with nonexposed infants.[39]

5. Lamotrigine
An ongoing multicenter observational study comparing four antiepileptic drugs (AEDs), lamotrigine, valproic acid, carbamazepine, and phenytoin (Dilantin), has found low serious adverse effects associated with lamotrigine as compared with the other AEDs.[40] The use of lamotrigine is associated with a low rate of major congenital malformations, but a positive dose–response relation has been established with this AED.[41]

F. Electroconvulsive Therapy

Refractory and psychotic depression has been treated with electroconvulsive therapy (ECT) in all trimesters of pregnancy. A review of 300 case reports covering 5 decades found a complication rate of less than 10%. Complications included transient fetal arrhythmias, uterine contractions, abdominal pain, and mild vaginal bleeding.[27] An additional report of abdominal pain, maternal hypertension, and vaginal bleeding with recurrent ECT speculates that these episodes represented recurrent mild abruption.[33]

Recommendations for precautions with ECT during pregnancy include pelvic examination, discontinuance of nonessential anticholinergic medication, uterine and fetal monitoring, intravenous hydration and administration of a nonparticulate antacid before the procedure, intubation during the procedure, and elevation of the pregnant woman's right hip to reduce caval compression.[27] In addition, because it appears that abruption may occur with ECT,[33] the authors recommend that the procedure not be performed in women with hypertensive disorders, and that it be discontinued if the procedure results in vaginal bleeding, severe hypertension, or abdominal pain.

G. Summary of Treatment for Depressive Disorders in Pregnancy

Mood disorders are commonly encountered in pregnancy and are associated with increased risk for poor pregnancy outcome. Discontinuation of medication during or before pregnancy is associated with a high rate of relapse and carries risk to both mother and infant. Use of SSRIs and other newer antidepressants in pregnancy appears to be safe with respect to congenital malformations. Depending on specific medication and dosage, a significant percentage of those infants exposed to SSRIs will experience transient difficulties with adaptation to extrauterine life and a much smaller percentage appear to be at risk for persistent pulmonary hypertension. Treatment of bipolar disorder in pregnancy remains a challenging concern because of an increased incidence of major congenital malformations with use of many mood-stabilizing agents (AEDs) and limited information about atypical antipsychotic medications. These women experience a high rate of relapse for depression during and immediately after pregnancy; therefore, possible strategies include no mood-stabilizing agent during pregnancy with institution of medication immediately after delivery or the use of the lowest effective dose during pregnancy with avoidance, where possible, of valproic acid during the first trimester.

In addition, women who abuse substances; women who have experienced sexual, verbal, or physical abuse; and women who have experienced a previous stillbirth comprise a subset of patients who experience increased rates of depression during pregnancy. Programs that address these specific problems and methods of increasing social support may be useful in addition to any considerations of pharmacotherapy.

Informed consent should be obtained for use of any pharmacotherapy for mood disorders during pregnancy. Risks and benefits should be explored on an individual basis, and monitoring during the pregnancy should be ongoing to determine the efficacy of nonpharmacologic and pharmacologic interventions.

REFERENCES

1. Orr ST, Miller CA: Maternal depressive symptoms and the risk of poor pregnancy outcome, *J Clin Epidemiol* 17:165-171, 1995.
2. Kim HG, Mandell M, Crandall C et al: Antenatal psychiatric illness and adequacy of prenatal care in an ethnically diverse inner-city obstetric population, *Arch Womens Ment Health* 9(2):103-107, 2006.
3. Cohen LS, Altshuler LL, Harlow BL et al: Relapse of major depression during pregnancy in women who maintain or discontinue antidepressant treatment, *JAMA* 295(5):499-507, 2006.
4. Viguera AC, Nonacs R, Cohen LS et al: Risk of recurrence of bipolar disorder in pregnant and non-pregnant women after discontinuing lithium maintenance, *Am J Psychiatry* 157:1179-1184, 2000.
5. Chaudron LH, Pies RW: The relationship between postpartum psychosis and bipolar disorder: a review, *J Clin Psychiatry* 64(11):1284-1292, 2003.
6. Hans SL: Demographic and psychological characteristics of substance-abusing pregnant women, *Clin Perinatol* 26:55-74, 1999.
7. Hedin LW, Janson PO: The invisible wounds: the occurrence of psychological abuse and anxiety compared with previous with previous experience of physical abuse during the childbearing years, *J Psychosom Obstet Gynecol* 20:136-144, 1999.
8. Nayak MB, Al-Yattama M: Assault victim history as a factor in depression during pregnancy, *Obstet Gynecol* 94:204-208, 1999.
9. Hughes PM, Turton P, Evans CD: Stillbirth as a risk factor for depression and anxiety in the subsequent pregnancy: a cohort study, *BMJ* 318:1721-1724, 1999.
10. American Psychiatric Association (APA): *Diagnostic and statistical manual of mental disorders, primary care edition,* ed 4, Washington, DC, 1995, APA.
11. Wright JH, Becke AT: Cognitive therapy. In Hales RE, Yudofsky SC, Talbott JA, editors: *Textbook of psychiatry,* ed 2, Washington, DC, 1994, The American Psychiatric Press.
12. Frank E, Grochocinski VJ, Spanier CA et al: Interpersonal psychotherapy and antidepressant medication: evaluation of a sequential treatment strategy in women with recurrent major depression, *J Clin Psychiatry* 61:51-57, 2000.
13. Einarson A, Koren G: Counseling pregnant women treated with paroxetine. Concern about cardiac malformations, *Can Fam Physician* 52:593-594, 2006.
14. Nulman I, Rovet J, Stewart DE et al: Neurodevelopment of children exposed in utero to antidepressant drugs, *N Engl J Med* 336:258-262, 1997.
15. Wisner KL, Gelenberg AJ, Leonard H et al: Pharmacologic treatment of depression during pregnancy, *JAMA* 282:1264-1269, 1999.
16. Haddad PM, Pal BR, Clarke P et al: Neonatal symptoms following maternal paroxetine treatment: serotonin toxicity or paroxetine discontinuation syndrome? *Psychopharmacology* 19(5):554-557, 2005.
17. de Moor RA, Mourad L, ter Haar J et al: Withdrawal symptoms in a neonate following exposure to venlafaxine during pregnancy, *Ned Tijdschr Geneeskd* 147:1370-1372, 2003.
18. Chambers CD, Johnson KA, Dick LM et al: Birth outcomes in pregnant women taking fluoxetine, *N Engl J Med* 335:1010-1015, 1996.
19. Sanz EJ, De-las-Cuevas C, Kiuru A et al: Selective serotonin reuptake inhibitors in pregnant women and neonatal withdrawal syndrome: a database analysis, *Lancet* 365(9458):482-487, 2005.
20. Cissoko H, Swortfiguer D, Giraudeau B et al: Neonatal outcome after exposure to selective serotonin reuptake inhibitors late in pregnancy, *Arch Pediatr* 12(7):1081-1084, 2005.
21. Costei AM, Kozer E, Ho T et al: Perinatal outcome following third trimester exposure to paroxetine, *Arch Pediatr Adolesc Med* 156(11):1129-1132, 2002.
22. Oberlander TF, Misri S, Fitzgerald CE et al: Pharmacologic factors associated with transient neonatal symptoms following prenatal psychotropic medication exposure, *J Clin Psychiatry* 65(2):230-237, 2004.
23. Oberlander TF, Warburton W, Misri S et al: Neonatal outcomes after prenatal exposure to selective serotonin reuptake inhibitor antidepressants and maternal depression using population-based linked health data, *Arch Gen Psychiatry* 63(8):898-906, 2006.
24. Chambers CD, Hernandez-Diaz S, Van Marter LJ et al: Selective serotonin-reuptake inhibitors and risk of persistent pulmonary hypertension of the newborn, *N Engl J Med* 354(6):579-587, 2006.
25. Laine K, Heikkinen T, Ekblad U et al: Effects of exposure to selective serotonin reuptake inhibitors during pregnancy on serotonergic symptoms in newborns and cord blood monoamine and prolactin concentrations, *Arch Gen Psychiatry* 60(7):720-726, 2003.
26. Rampono J, Proud S, Hackett LP et al: A pilot study of newer antidepressant concentrations in cord and maternal serum and possible effects in the neonate, *Int J Neuropsychopharmacol* 7(3):329-334, 2004.

27. Akiskal HS, Maser JD, Zeller PJ et al: Switching from unipolar to bipolar II: an 11-year prospective study of clinical and temperamental predictors in 559 patients, *Arch Gen Psychiatry* 52:114-123, 1995.

28. Manning JS, Haykal RF, Akiskal HS: The role of bipolarity in depression in a family practice setting, *Psychiatric Clin North Am* 22:689-703, 1999.

29. Sipek A: Lithium and Epstein's anomaly, *Cor Vasa* 31:149-156, 1989.

30. Zalstein E, Koren G, Einarson T et al: A case-control study on the association between first trimester-exposure to lithium and Epstein's anomaly, *Am J Cardiol* 65:817-818, 1990.

31. Cohen LS, Friedman SM, Jefferson JW et al: A re-evaluation of the risk of in-utero exposure to lithium, *JAMA* 271:146-150, 1994.

32. Jacobson SJ, Jones K, Johnson K et al: Prospective multicentre study of pregnancy outcome after lithium exposure during the first trimester, *Lancet* 339:530-533, 1992.

33. Correa-Villasenor A, Ferenz C, Neill CA et al: Epstein's anomaly of the tricuspid valve: genetic and environmental factors. The Baltimore-Washington Infant Study Group, *Teratology* 50:137-147, 1994.

34. Frassetto F, Tourneur Martel F, Barjhoux CE et al: Goiter in a newborn exposed to lithium in utero, *Ann Pharmacother* 36(11):1745-1748, 2002.

35. Kozma C: Neonatal toxicity and transient neurodevelopmental deficits following prenatal exposure to lithium: another clinical report and a review of the literature, *Am J Med Genet A* 132(4):441-444, 2005.

36. Newport DJ, Viguera AC, Beach AJ et al: Lithium placental passage and obstetrical outcome: implications for clinical management during late pregnancy, *Am J Psychiatry* 162(11):2162-2170, 2005.

37. Bradai R, Robert E: Prenatal ultrasonographic diagnosis in epileptic mothers on valproic acid: retrospective study of 161 cases in central eastern France register of congenital malformations, *J Gynecol Obstet Biol Reprod (Paris)* 27:413-419, 1998.

38. Jones KL, Lacro RV, Johnson BA et al: Pattern of malformations in children of women treated with carbamazepine during pregnancy, *N Engl J Med* 320:1661-1666, 1989.

39. McKenna K, Koren G, Tetelbaum M et al: Pregnancy outcome of women using atypical antipsychotic drugs: a prospective comparative study, *Clin Psychiatry* 66(4):444-449; quiz 546, 2005.

40. Meador KJ, Baker GA, Finnell RH et al: NEAD Study Group. In utero antiepileptic drug exposure: fetal death and malformations, *Neurology* 67(3):407-412, 2006.

41. Morrow J, Russell A, Guthrie E et al: Malformation risks of antiepileptic drugs in pregnancy: a prospective study from the UK Epilepsy and Pregnancy Register, *J Neurol Neurosurg Psychiatry* 77(2):193-198, 2006.

42. Addis A, Koren G: Safety of fluoxetine during the first trimester of pregnancy: a meta-analytical review of epidemiological studies, *Psychol Med* 30(1):89-94, 2000.

43. Einarson A, Fatoye B, Sarkar M et al: Pregnancy outcome following gestational exposure to venlafaxine: a multicenter prospective controlled study, *Am J Psychiatry* 158(10):1728-1730, 2001.

44. Sivojelezova A, Shuhaiber S, Sarkissian L et al: Citalopram use in pregnancy: prospective comparative evaluation of pregnancy and fetal outcome, *Am J Obstet Gynecol* 193(6):2004-2009, 2005.

45. Einarson TR, Einarson A: Newer antidepressants in pregnancy and rates of major malformations: a meta-analysis of prospective comparative studies, *Pharmacoepidemiol Drug Saf* 14(12):823-827, 2005.

46. Kulin NA, Pstuzak A, Sage SR et al: Pregnancy outcome following maternal use of the new selective serotonin reuptake inhibitors: a prospective, controlled multi-center study, *JAMA* 279:659-661, 1998.

47. Chun-Fai-Chan B, Koren G, Fayez I et al: Pregnancy outcome of women exposed to bupropion during pregnancy: a prospective comparative study, *Am J Obstet Gynecol* 192(3):932-936, 2005.

48. Einarson A, Bonari L, Voyer-Lavigne S et al: A multicentre prospective controlled study to determine the safety of trazodone and nefazodone use during pregnancy, *Can J Psychiatry* 48(2):106-110, 2003.

SECTION B   Anxiety Disorders

The anxiety disorders addressed in this section include panic attacks, generalized anxiety disorder, agoraphobia, and obsessive-compulsive disorder (OCD).

I. PANIC ATTACKS

Evidence about panic disorder in pregnancy comes from retrospective studies, with some women experiencing relief of panic symptoms during pregnancy and others experiencing exacerbation or onset in the postpartum period.[1]

A. Nonpharmacologic Treatment

Psychotherapy of panic disorder is generally cognitive based with particular attention to exposure–response control strategies, controlled breathing techniques, and other methods.

B. Pharmacologic Treatment

1. Antidepressants

   Most patients with panic disorder should be considered for treatment with SSRIs or serotonin noradrenaline reuptake inhibitors (SNRIs). The risks and benefits of these medications are covered extensively in the previous section. Given the amount of safety information available, there seems no benefit to the use of TCAs for this indication.

2. Benzodiazepines (FDA category D)

   Although some earlier studies suggest a possible link of benzodiazepine use and congenital defects, an Israeli study including approximately

600 women using benzodiazepines during pregnancy did not find any increase in congenital defects[2] and a large matched case–control study found no increased association between congenital abnormalities and use of benzodiazepines in the second and third month of pregnancy.[3] Neonatal abstinence syndrome and "floppy baby" may occur in infants who received benzodiazepines during the third trimester with withdrawal symptoms, sedation, hypotonia, poor suck, apneic spells, and impaired response to cold stress.[4] Studies of cord blood levels of diazepam administered to women in labor demonstrate almost double the concentration in cord blood as compared with maternal levels, resulting in significant increases in respiratory depression and muscle tone inhibition.[5] Neurobehavioral effects have been studied up to 4 years of age with variable results.[2,6]

This information suggests considerable caution be exercised if benzodiazepines are administered extensively during the end of the third trimester or during labor. If benzodiazepines are to be used, some authors suggest the smallest possible dose that controls symptoms with more frequent dosing intervals and the avoidance of polytherapy.[7]

II. GENERALIZED ANXIETY DISORDER

Generalized anxiety disorder responds to TCAs, SSRIs, SNRIs, and buspirone. TCAs and SSRIs have been summarized earlier (see Section A). No published reports exist of buspirone use in humans during pregnancy.

III. AGORAPHOBIA

The treatment of agoraphobia entails control of panic attacks and anticipatory anxiety with psychotherapy (cognitive) aimed at regaining a sense of mastery of one's environment.

IV. OBSESSIVE-COMPULSIVE DISORDER

Prospective studies are lacking on the influence of pregnancy and postpartum events as a result of OCD. Some women with postpartum flares of OCD have reported aggressive obsessions directed toward the newborn.[8] Another retrospective interview study reported 29% of women with worsening in the postpartum period, but the majority of women remained stable during pregnancy.[9] Nonpharmacologic options include close monitoring with the addition of techniques such as "thought-stopping."[10] Treatment medications have included SSRIs and clomipramine. Clomipramine has been observed with adverse effects in the newborn[11] and with an increase in congenital malformations[12]; therefore, its use in pregnancy should be avoided.

REFERENCES

1. Hertzberg T, Walbrbeck K: The impact of pregnancy and puerperium on panic disorder: a review, *J Psychosom Obstet Gynecol* 20:59-64, 1999.
2. Ornoy A, Arnon J, Shectman S et al: Is benzodiazepine use in pregnancy really teratogenic? *Reprod Toxicol* 12:511-515, 1998.
3. Eros E, Czeizel AE, Rockenbauer M et al: A population-based case-control teratologic study of nitrazepam, medazepam, tofisopam, alprazolam and clonazepam treatment during pregnancy, *Eur J Obstet Gynecol Reprod Biol* 101(2):147-154, 2002.
4. McElhatton PR: The effects of benzodiazepine use during pregnancy and lactation, *Reprod Toxicol* 8:461-475, 1994.
5. Pan B, Lu Y, Wang D: Determination of diazepam concentration in maternal and fetal serum after intravenous administration during active phase of labor and its effects on neonates, *Chung Hua Fu Chan Ko Tsa Chih* 30:707-710, 1995.
6. Viggedal G, Hagberg BS, Laegreid L et al: Mental development in late infancy after prenatal exposure to benzodiazepines, a prospective study, *J Child Psychol Psychiatry* 34:295-305, 1993.
7. Iqbal MM, Sobhan T, Ryals T: Effects of commonly used benzodiazepines on the fetus, the neonate, and the nursing infant, *Psychiatr Serv* 53(1):39-49, 2002.
8. Maina G, Albert U, Bogetto F et al: Recent life events and obsessive-compulsive disorder (OCD): the role of pregnancy/delivery, *Psychiatry Res* 89:49-58, 1999.
9. Williams KE, Koran LM: Obsessive-compulsive disorder in pregnancy, the puerperium, and the premenstruum, *J Clin Psychiatry* 58:330-334, 1997.
10. Chelmow D, Halfin VP: Pregnancy complicated by obsessive-compulsive disorder, *J Matern Fetal Med* 6(1):31-34, 1997.
11. Schimmell MS, Katz EZ, Shaag Y et al: Toxic neonatal effects following maternal clomipramine therapy, *J Clin Toxicol* 29(4):479-484, 1991.
12. Tango R, Berney P, Schulz P: [Selective serotonin reuptake inhibitors (SSRIs) in pregnancy] [Article in French], *Rev Med Suisse* 2(61):981-985, 2006.

SECTION C Schizophrenia

Schizophrenia occurs in approximately 1% of 1.5% of the general population. Community mental health centers treat many of these patients living in the community setting. Although fertility rates may be diminished among patients with anovulatory cycles because of neuroleptic medication, functional issues diminish the ability of patients with schizophrenia to effectively use contraception.

I. EFFECT OF SCHIZOPHRENIA ON PREGNANCY

A recent metaanalysis of available studies documents overall problems in study design but at least a two-fold risk for stillbirth or fetal death in pregnancies of women with schizophrenia.[1] A large cohort study of women with schizophrenia and affective disorders in Australia compared with women without psychiatric diagnosis found significantly greater incidences of placental abruption, low birth weight, and congenital cardiac abnormalities in the offspring of women with schizophrenia.[2] Another large cohort study of women with schizophrenia in Sweden found similar increases in low birth weight, prematurity, stillbirth, and small-for-gestational age size with odds ratios more than doubled, even controlling for other social risk factors.[3]

II. TREATMENT OF SCHIZOPHRENIA IN PREGNANCY

The majority of patients with a diagnosis of schizophrenia or schizophreniform-like psychosis need adequate pharmacologic management during pregnancy to allow normal function in activities of daily living and cooperation with pregnancy care. The minimum effective dose should be used, keeping in mind the possibility of exacerbation during the intrapartum and postpartum periods.

A. Teratogenicity

Little high-quality information exists about the use of atypical antipsychotics and potential for producing congenital malformations. A joint study conducted by the Motherisk Program in Toronto and the Israeli Teratogen Information Service found no increase in congenital abnormalities or low birth weight, but the number of pregnant women observed was limited (olanzapine: n = 60; risperidone: n = 49; quetiapine: n = 36; and clozapine: n = 6).[4]

B. Effects on Fetal Monitoring

Older neuroleptic agents may diminish fetal heart rate reactivity and may confound interpretation of antepartum testing. No information is available on newer agents and their effect on heart rate reactivity.

REFERENCES

1. Webb R, Abel K, Pickles A et al: Mortality in offspring of parents with psychotic disorders: a critical review and meta-analysis, *Am J Psychiatry* 162(6):1045-1056, 2005.
2. Jablensky AV, Morgan V, Zubrick SR et al: Pregnancy, delivery, and neonatal complications in a population cohort of women with schizophrenia and major affective disorders, *Am J Psychiatry* 162(1):79-91, 2005.
3. Nilsson E, Lichtenstein P, Cnattingius S et al: Women with schizophrenia: pregnancy outcome and infant death among their offspring, *Schizophr Res* 58(2-3):221-229, 2002.
4. McKenna K, Koren G, Tetelbaum M et al: Pregnancy outcome of women using atypical antipsychotic drugs: a prospective comparative study, *J Clin Psychiatry* 66(4):444-449, 2005.

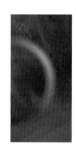

Antenatal Testing for Fetal Surveillance and Management of the Postterm Pregnancy

SECTION A Overview of Antenatal Testing

Stephen D. Ratcliffe, MD, MSPH

I. USE OF A SCREENING INSTRUMENT

Antenatal screening tests are used to assess the health of the fetus. Many factors need to be considered in interpreting the results of these tests:

What is the condition that warrants additional fetal surveillance?

Given this condition, what is the likelihood or probability that the fetus is at considerable risk for hypoxemia or acidosis?

What is the gestational age?

Are there other factors that could be causing the apparent abnormal test, such as the use of medication or the presence of maternal dehydration?

However, before clinicians begin to take these factors into account, they should strive to understand the underlying concepts that are essential to the accurate interpretation of antenatal screening tests.

A. Sensitivity

Sensitivity refers to the percentage of tests that are abnormal when the fetus is compromised (i.e., a true-positive test result). As shown in Table 11-1, when applying the nonstress test (NST) to various maternal conditions, the sensitivity of this test (true positive) to accurately identify compromised fetuses is 56%.[1]

B. Specificity

Specificity refers to the percentage of tests that are normal when the fetus is normal or not compromised (true-negative result). Commonly used antenatal tests, such as the NST or contraction stress test (CST), have a specificity of more than 95%. These reassuring results often allow clinicians additional time to observe high-risk conditions.

C. Positive Predictive Value

The positive predictive value refers to the diagnostic accuracy of an abnormal test result to predict a compromised fetus. As the pretest probability of a given disease condition decreases, the positive predictive value of the test also decreases. For this reason, antenatal testing should be used selectively to assess high-risk pregnancies and not applied routinely to low-risk pregnancies. Using data from Table 11-1, the positive predictive value of a nonreactive NST in predicting a compromised fetus in a postterm pregnancy is only 15%. For this reason, an abnormal NST is followed up by a CST or biophysical profile (BPP), either of which has a greater positive predictive value.

D. Negative Predictive Value

The negative predictive value refers to the diagnostic accuracy of a normal test result to predict a healthy fetus. Antenatal testing, when used to assess the postterm pregnancy, has a negative predictive value greater than 99% in predicting fetal viability or the prevention

TABLE 11-1 Use of the Nonstress Test as a Screening Test

Condition	Sensitivity (%)	Positive Predictive Value (%)
Postterm pregnancy	44	15
IUGR	56	69
Hypertension	31	44
Diabetes mellitus	53	31

From Devoe LD: The nonstress test, *Obstet Gynecol Clin North Am* 17:111-128, 1990.
IUGR, Intrauterine growth restriction.

of a fetal demise within 1 week. Table 11-2 summarizes the negative predictive value of four common tests of fetal well-being.

II. INDICATIONS FOR ANTENATAL TESTING

A. Selected Maternal Conditions That Warrant Antenatal Testing

Selected maternal conditions that warrant antenatal testing include:
1. Diabetes mellitus (all forms)
2. Chronic renal disease
3. Hypertensive disorders
4. Systemic lupus erythematosus
5. Antiphospholipid syndrome
6. Cyanotic heart disease
7. Maternal substance abuse
8. Hemoglobinopathies

B. Selected Pregnancy-Related Conditions That Warrant Antenatal Testing

Selected pregnancy-related conditions that warrant antenatal testing include:
1. Rh sensitization
2. Intrauterine growth restriction (IUGR)
3. Pregnancy-induced hypertension
4. Postterm pregnancy
5. Decreased fetal movement
6. Previous fetal demise
7. Oligohydramnios
8. Multiple gestation
9. Polyhydramnios

III. EFFECT OF GESTATIONAL AGE ON ANTENATAL TESTING

Many situations arise in caring for the *preterm* prenatal patient in which assessment of fetal well-being is helpful before deciding whether further intervention is warranted. Fetal reactivity and heart rate acceleration patterns are less pronounced in the preterm fetus. This section focuses on how to adapt antenatal testing for the preterm fetus between 24 and 34 weeks of gestation.

A. Effect of Gestational Age on Diagnostic Criteria

Castillo and colleagues[2] conducted a cohort of women with prolonged NST (90-minute testing periods) every 2 weeks beginning at 24 weeks of gestation to compile the following normative data for the preterm fetus:
1. Baseline fetal heart rate
   The baseline fetal heart rate decreases steadily as a function of advancing gestational age.

TABLE 11-2 Reassurance of Normal Fetal Surveillance Tests: Prevention of Fetal Demise

Type of Fetal Surveillance	Number Studied in Case Series	Stillbirth Rate*	Negative Predictive Value (%) within 1 Week of Normal Test
Nonstress test	5,861	1.9/1000	99.8
Contraction stress test	12,656	0.3/1000	99.97
Biophysical profile	44,617	0.8/1000	99.92
Modified biophysical profile	54,617	0.8/1000	99.92

*The stillbirth rate is corrected for lethal congenital anomalies and unpredictable causes of demise.
Data from ACOG practice bulletin. Antepartum fetal surveillance. Number 9, October 1999 (replaces Technical Bulletin Number 188, January 1994). Clinical management guidelines for obstetrician-gynecologists, *Int J Gynaecol Obstet* 68:175-185, 2000.

2. Frequency of fetal heart rate accelerations
   Fetal heart rate accelerations occur less often at earlier gestational ages and tend to be of lesser amplitude.
3. Frequency of fetal heart rate decelerations
   An association exists between periodic or episodic decelerations during the late second trimester and an increased risk for preterm premature rupture of membranes (PPROM)[3] and small-for-gestational-age infants.[4]
4. Effect of gestational age on NST interpretation
   As a result of their study, Castillo and colleagues[2] recommend extending the period of evaluation from 30 to 60 minutes and reduce the amplitude of heart rate accelerations for NST reactivity from 15 to 10 beats/min to evaluate gestations between 24 and 32 weeks.

B. Use of Antenatal Testing with Preterm Premature Rupture of the Membranes

PPROM is a particularly challenging condition to manage (see Chapter 12, Section H). The two major complications of this condition are chorioamnionitis and oligohydramnios. Referral to a tertiary care center at an early gestational age may be advised because of availability of neonatal intensive care services. Situations exist, however, when this is not feasible.

1. Monitoring for infection
   Neither the NST (sensitivity 39%) nor the BPP (sensitivity 25%) has been shown to be a sensitive predictor of chorioamnionitis in the setting of PPROM, although both tests are commonly used in this setting for this purpose.[5,6]

IV. MONITORING FOR DECREASED AMNIOTIC FLUID

Oligohydramnios, often associated with abnormal fetal heart rate tracings and adverse neonatal outcomes, occurs more frequently with PPROM. The clinician can monitor this condition directly by obtaining an amniotic fluid index (AFI). The AFI varies daily with PPROM.

V. WHEN TO BEGIN ANTENATAL SURVEILLANCE

Antenatal fetal surveillance is initiated when a maternal or pregnancy-related condition is suspected to be exerting harmful effects on fetal health. For example, once a diagnosis of IUGR has been made, serial antenatal testing is started regardless of the gestational age.

REFERENCES

1. Devoe LD: The nonstress test, *Obstet Gynecol Clin North Am* 17:111-128, 1990.
2. Castillo RA, Devoe LD, Arthur AM et al: The preterm nonstress test: effects of gestational age and length of study, *Am J Obstet Gynecol* 160:172-175, 1989.
3. Yanagihara T, Ueta M, Hanaoka U et al: Late second-trimester nonstress test characteristics in the preterm delivery before 32 weeks of gestation, *Gynecol Obstet Invest* 51:32-35, 2001.
4. Yanagihara T, Hata T: Comparison of late-second-trimester nonstress test characteristics between small for gestational age and appropriate for gestational age infants, *Obstet Gynecol* 94:921-924, 1999.
5. Lewis DF, Adair CD, Week JW: A randomized controlled trial of daily nonstress testing versus biophysical profile in the management of preterm premature rupture of the membranes, *Am J Obstet Gynecol* 181:1495-1499, 1999.
6. Del Valle GO, Joffe GM, Izquierdo LA et al: The biophysical profile and the nonstress test: poor predictors of chorioamnionitis and fetal infection in prolonged preterm premature rupture of membranes, *Obstet Gynecol* 80:106-110, 1992.

SECTION B Types of Antenatal Testing

Stephen D. Ratcliffe, MD, MSPH

I. NONSTRESS TEST

The NST,[1] developed in the early 1970s, remains a mainstay in assessing the presence or lack of fetal well-being. A NST is reactive, or normal, when fetal heart rate accelerations occur in conjunction with perceived fetal movement. Accelerations take place through stimulation of the cardioaccelerator fibers from the upper thoracic spinal cord and are affected by activity in the brainstem and cortex. These neurologic pathways are influenced by numerous intrinsic and extrinsic factors: sympathetic discharge and adrenergic receptors, behavioral state, circadian rhythms, gestational age and maturation, intrinsic rate and myocardial contractility, baroreceptor and chemoreceptor reflexes, exogenous dietary substrates, and drugs.

A reactive NST generally indicates that the fetal autonomic nervous system is intact and that its oxygenation status is satisfactory. A reactive NST correctly identifies a healthy fetus 99.8% of the time (negative predictive value, see Table 11-2). The duration of this healthy prognosis varies depending on the maternal or fetal condition undergoing surveillance. Pregnancies with PPROM may undergo fetal surveillance using NSTs on a daily basis, whereas in the prolonged or postterm pregnancy, twice weekly testing is generally recommended.

A. Technique and Interpretation

1. Indications and contraindications
   The NST generally is used as the primary screening test when there is an increased index of suspicion for IUGR, fetal hypoxemia, or placental insufficiency. Additional maternal and fetal conditions prompting consideration of an NST are included in Table 11-1. Although there are no major contraindications to the administration of the NST, interpretation must take into consideration potentially confounding situations. Concurrent maternal illnesses, use of sedative medications, and caloric deprivation are some of the conditions that can result in a nonreactive NST when the fetus is not compromised.[1]

2. Administration of the NST
   The NST should be administered under stable, predictable circumstances. Factors to be considered include the following:
   a. Dietary state: NST testing should be conducted 1 to 2 hours after eating.
   b. Medications/drug use: Drug use or smoking that occurs shortly before testing should be avoided.
   c. Maternal position: A semi-Fowler position, with hip displacement, should be used to avoid vena caval compression that can occur when the gravid woman lies flat on her back.
   d. Gestational age: Different testing criteria should be applied at a gestational age of less than 34 weeks, as addressed in Section A.
   e. Testing time: Testing usually requires 30 minutes but may be extended to 60 to 90 minutes.

3. Criteria for a reactive or normal NST
   An NST is considered to be reactive when 2 accelerations of greater than 15 beats/min occur in a 20-minute span. The *long* criteria state that the accelerations should remain above the 15 beats/min rate for 15 seconds; the *short* criteria suggest accelerations should initially exceed 15 beats/min and should take longer than 10 seconds to return to the baseline. The two criteria are comparable in predicting fetal compromise.[2]

4. Improving diagnostic accuracy
   Depending on the condition being evaluated, Table 11-1 shows that the false-positive rate of a nonreactive NST varies from six of every seven tests for the postterm pregnancy to one of every three tests for IUGR. Many strategies have been developed for use as an adjunct to the NST to improve its accuracy.
   a. Fetal heart rate decelerations: The clinician should be alerted to the presence of variable decelerations, with or without contractions, that may occur during the course of an NST. These suggest the possibility of cord compression, which may be caused by maternal positioning or oligohydramnios. In this situation, an amniotic fluid index (AFI) should be obtained, particularly if a prolonged deceleration occurs (i.e., lasting >1 minute and <90 beats/min or 40 beats less than the baseline rate).[3] Labor induction may be indicated in this situation based on maternal and fetal well-being factors.
   b. Amniotic fluid volume: The importance of adequate amniotic fluid has been established.[4] Some centers routinely combine the NST and AFI, particularly in the evaluation of the postterm pregnancy. This combining of these testing factors is called the *modified biophysical profile* (MBPP), which is detailed later in this section.
   c. Vibroacoustic stimulation (VAS): VAS is a method of fetal stimulation that uses a single 1- to 2-second sound stimulus applied to the lower maternal abdomen with an artificial larynx. The healthy fetus should respond to this stimulation with fetal heart rate accelerations. One group has used VAS extensively in conjunction with NST and AFI, and has experienced no fetal deaths among 5973 women.[5] A Cochrane review involving 9 trials and 4838 participants demonstrated that VAS safely reduced the incidence of nonreactive NSTs (relative risk [RR] 0.62; 95% confidence interval [CI], 0.53-0.74; number needed to treat [NNT] = 20) and the overall testing time by about 10 minutes.[6]

B. Management of the Nonreactive Nonstress Test

The physician should take into account multiple factors in evaluating a nonreactive NST (e.g., risk status of the patient, gestational age). The main points of a decision-making algorithm for this situation are summarized as follows:

1. Assess for concurrent maternal conditions that could lead to a nonreactive NST.
2. Extend the testing period, when possible, to 60 to 90 minutes or use VAS to attempt to obtain a reactive tracing.
3. Evaluate other parameters of the fetal tracing. Obtain an AFI, particularly if variable decelerations are present.
4. Conduct a CST or BPP if the NST remains nonreactive.
5. Consider induction, consultation, or both if the CST is positive or if the BPP score is 6 or less.

C. Evidence to Support Use of Nonstress Testing

Retrospective case reviews in which the NST has been used as the initial test of fetal surveillance for high-risk pregnancies have been associated with a sixfold reduction in perinatal mortality compared with unscreened groups of patients at low risk.[1] However, the four randomized controlled trials (RCTs) that studied the efficacy of this screening test do not support its use alone in assessing future fetal well-being.[7] This test conveys useful information regarding immediate fetal health and also appears to provide limited prognostic information regarding future fetal or placental reserve.

II. CONTRACTION STRESS TEST

The CST, developed by Ray and Freeman[8] in the early 1970s, measures the fetal response to maternal contractions. Late decelerations after a contraction may indicate fetal hypoxia as a result of uteroplacental insufficiency.

A. Administration of Contraction Stress Test

Uterine contractions, at a rate of three in 10 minutes, should occur with a low-dose oxytocin infusion (0.5 mU/min) or as a result of nipple stimulation. The patient should remain in a semi-Fowler position for both of these techniques to prevent aortocaval compression and maternal hypotension. Both techniques to achieve uterine contractions have comparable efficacy, with the nipple stimulation CST being more cost-effective.[9]

B. Indications

CSTs usually are performed when fetal compromise is suspected and the NST has been nonreactive or nonreassuring.

C. Contraindications

CSTs should not be performed in situations in which vaginal delivery is contraindicated, including the following:

1. Previous classical cesarean section
2. Preterm labor (actual or threatened)
3. PPROM
4. Known placenta previa

D. Interpretation

A CST is *positive* when greater than 50% of the contractions are followed by late decelerations. Uterine hyperstimulation, defined as contractions occurring more often than every 2 minutes or lasting longer than 90 seconds, should not be present. An *equivocal* CST occurs in the setting of hyperstimulation or when occasional late decelerations are noted. A *negative* CST is one in which no decelerations are noted.

E. Management of a Positive Contraction Stress Test

Every attempt should be made to correct any underlying maternal condition that may be contributing to the positive CST.[10] For example, correction of severe maternal dehydration with vigorous intravenous hydration may correct uterine hypoperfusion and an abnormal CST.

Attention to the reactivity of the fetal tracing also is an important factor.

1. Nonreactive NST/positive CST
   A nonreactive NST coupled with a positive CST often indicates fetal compromise and should be acted on in an expeditious fashion, usually in the form of labor induction or cesarean delivery.
2. Reactive NST/positive CST
   This often represents a false-positive test result and may not require immediate delivery as long as a plan for further assessment is delineated. A BPP may be used in this to provide additional information.
3. Reactive NST/negative CST
   This combination is reassuring, and the recommended follow-up for fetal surveillance

depends on the severity of the condition being monitored.

4. If variable decelerations are noted in an otherwise reassuring test, an AFI should be done to assess for oligohydramnios.

F. Evidence to Support Use of the Contraction Stress Test

Table 11-2 demonstrates a case series analysis that compares the use of CST with other forms of fetal surveillance indicating its use is associated with the lowest incidence of fetal demise within 7 days of a reassuring test result.[11] An RCT comparing CST versus umbilical artery Doppler velocimetry (DV) in the setting of confirmed IUGR indicated that DV performs in a superior fashion.[12] DV is discussed later.

III. FETAL MOVEMENT COUNTING

A. Natural History of Fetal Movement

Cataloging a mother's perception of fetal movement is a technique for assessing fetal well-being that has been used for more than a century.[13] Studies using real-time ultrasonography have shown that the fetus has frequent gross body movements, up to an average of 17 movements in 20 minutes.[14] A periodicity and diurnal variation in fetal body movements have been noted, with the number of fetal movements being less in the morning and more in the evening. It is common for women to perceive a relative decrease in the intensity of fetal movement as pregnancy progresses, largely as a result of increasing fetal size and decreasing amniotic fluid. The number of fetal movements and overall pattern of activity should not markedly diminish as a woman approaches her due date.[15]

In one retrospective study of women at low risk, expectant mothers presenting to labor and delivery with the chief complaint of decreased fetal movement have a compromised fetus 8% to 12% of the time.[16] However, there are conflicting studies as to the gravity of this presenting complaint. Over a 20-month period, Harrington and colleagues[17] demonstrated that women who presented with a complaint of decreased fetal movement did not have worse perinatal outcomes than did the general population. Dubiel and colleagues[18] studied the outcomes of 599 low-risk pregnancies presenting with a complaint of decreased fetal movement. The overall perinatal mortality of this cohort was 3.8%. The authors of both studies agreed that it is prudent to counsel patients to be aware of fetal movements and to agree on a formal surveillance plan when a marked decrease in movement is noted. In Dubiel and colleagues' study,[18] the NST was a more sensitive test than DV in evaluating these patients.

B. Testing Regimens

In the 1970s, investigators attempted to develop fetal movement counting testing regimens. None of the regimens presented in this section has been shown in RCTs to decrease perinatal mortality. Many different regimens for counting fetal movements have been developed. Patient convenience factors often have affected compliance with these regimens. Despite the lack of supporting evidence, these methods may be used on a selective basis to complement other types of antenatal tests.

The count to 10 method is popular and has a high patient acceptance rate.[19] The patient chooses a 2-hour period when she can quietly monitor fetal movements. Fetal movement is defined as any kick, flutter, swish, or roll. In one cohort study, the mean time to perceive the 10 movements was 20.9 minutes, and 99.5% of patients had counted 10 movements within 90 minutes.[20] The authors recommended fetal movement counting only in the evening because of the increased movements associated with diurnal variation, although in other studies, the patient was allowed to choose the best time to perform the test.

Other methods use discrete time periods (i.e., 60 minutes repeated three times a week). The Sadovsky method[21] has patients counting four movements three times a day after meals. This method requires greater time and organizational commitment than the count to 10 method.

C. Evidence to Support the Use of Fetal Movement Counting

Grant and co-workers[22] demonstrated in a RCT that enrolled more than 68,000 women that the use of routine fetal movement counting in low-risk populations did not reduce perinatal mortality, although findings from a cohort study[20] linked the count to 10 method with a decrease in perinatal mortality in low-risk populations.

IV. BIOPHYSICAL PROFILE

The BPP, first reported by Manning in 1980, uses a combination of high-resolution ultrasonography and the NST to assess for evidence of fetal hypoxemia or compromise.[23] When applied to known high-risk conditions, such as IUGR, the use of BPP is associated with a reduction in perinatal mortality to less than that of low-risk populations.[24]

A. Indications and Contraindications

The BPP is used to assess the status of the fetus in high-risk pregnancies, usually when the primary test of surveillance, the NST, is equivocal or nonreactive.

B. Test Administration

A clinician or technician skilled at ultrasonography spends 30 minutes observing fetal breathing movements, gross body movements, and tone, using defined standards. The AFI is calculated, and an NST is performed. Some centers omit the NST if the other four testing parameters are judged to be normal. Each of these five areas of surveillance has objective criteria that must be met, and a score of either a 0 or 2 (i.e., no partial score of 1) is assigned.[23] Although 30 minutes of observation has been allowed to complete the BPP, the average time to record the sonographic aspects of the test is 8 minutes, and fewer than 2% of tests require 30 minutes of observation.

C. Test Interpretation

BPPs that are 8 of 8 (NST excluded) or 10 of 10 are viewed as reassuring and have a lower false-positive rate (higher specificity) than the NST or CST (see Table 11-2). In this situation, the clinician can avoid intervention in the setting of prematurity or an immature cervix. A low BPP score of 0 to 2 has a strong correlation to fetal hypoxemia and should be viewed as an indication for immediate delivery with the availability of neonatal resuscitation. A score of 4 usually warrants immediate action, whereas a score of 6 is more equivocal and requires serial testing to determine the most appropriate course of action.

D. Evidence to Support Use of Biophysical Profile

The BPP has been used widely as a screening test for fetal well-being, based on cohort studies and case series. Only two RCTs in a Cochrane Review have studied its efficacy in improving perinatal outcomes.[25] These RCTs do not support its use as a superior test of fetal well-being over its counterpart, the NST. The Cochrane Library states that "the data are insufficient to reach any definite conclusion about the benefit or otherwise of the BPP as a test of fetal well being."

V. MODIFIED BIOPHYSICAL PROFILE

The MBPP takes two of the most sensitive components of the BPP, the NST and AFI, to create a test of fetal surveillance.[26] It is less time-consuming and expensive than the BPP, and it provides an evaluation of immediate fetal health and uteroplacental function.

A. Indications and Contraindications

The MBPP is used in many settings as an initial test of fetal well-being for maternal and pregnancy-related conditions. The MBPP has no contraindications, although clinicians should be aware of factors, such as maternal sedation or illness, that can result in an abnormal NST with a healthy fetus.

B. Test Administration/ Interpretation

The NST is administered in the manner described earlier. The AFI is determined using bedside ultrasound and is the sum of the measurements of the deepest vertical pockets of amniotic fluid found in each of the four abdominal quadrants. The measured fluid pockets must be free of umbilical cord. The MBPP is abnormal if the NST is abnormal (nonreactive, presence of deep or prolonged variable decelerations, presence of late decelerations) or if the AFI is less than 5 cm. AFIs of 5 to 8 cm are considered *low normal* and may require follow-up scanning at more frequent intervals. As discussed earlier, nonreactive NSTs may be handled by prolonging testing or by the administration of VAS.

C. Evidence to Support the Use of Modified Biophysical Profile

The MBPP has not been studied in a randomized, prospective fashion. Miller and colleagues[26] reported on a series of 15,482 high-risk pregnancies in which 54,617 MBPPs were performed as an initial test of fetal surveillance. This study provides evidence of how this test can be viewed with respect to other forms of antenatal testing. It has been further validated with a comparative analysis of the MBPP versus CST in performing antenatal surveillance of high-risk pregnancies in a cohort of more than 5500 women.[27] Evidence to date suggests that the use of the MBPP instead of the NST in assessing the postterm pregnancy results in a 50% decrease in rate of fetal demise in the week after a normal test result (0.8 vs 1.9 fetal deaths per 1000).[11]

TABLE 11-3 Positive Predictive Value of Components of the Modified Biophysical Profile for Prediction of Fetal Compromise in Labor

Components	Positive Predictive Value (%)
Nonreactive NST plus AFI > 5 plus no decelerations	50
Nonreactive NST plus AFI < 5 plus no decelerations	57
Nonreactive NST plus AFI < 5 plus decelerations	64
Complete biophysical profile < 8	59
Nonreactive NST	57
AFI < 5	37
Presence of deceleration	39
Prolonged decelerations	63
Variable decelerations	37
Late decelerations	34

From Miller D, Rabello Y, Paul R: The modified biophysical profile: antepartum testing in the 1990s, *Am J Obstet Gynecol* 174:812-817, 1996.
NST, Nonstress test; AFI, amniotic fluid index.

1. Positive predictive value of MBPP
   The positive predictive values in Table 11-3 were generated with the application of MBPP to selected high-risk conditions. When this test is applied to low-risk patients, the positive predictive value of this test decreases dramatically. The false-positive rate is lowest when both aspects of the MBPP, the AFI and NST, are abnormal.
2. Negative predictive value of MBPP
   The negative predictive value of the MBPP is comparable with that of the BPP and CST, and is greater than the NST alone (see Table 11-1).

D. Further Modification of the Modified Biophysical Profile: Use of the Single-Deepest Pocket

Preliminary RCT evidence exists that the identification of an adequate single-deepest pocket of amniotic fluid instead of using the four-quadrant AFI may decrease the need for induction whereas not having any adverse effects on perinatal outcomes.[28]

VI. UMBILICAL ARTERY DOPPLER VELOCIMETRY

Umbilical artery DV is a test of antenatal surveillance that became widely available in the 1990s. It uses ultrasound technology to observe umbilical artery blood flow during systole and diastole. Fetuses developing uteroplacental insufficiency show decreased velocity, absent flow, or in severely affected states, a reversal of flow. This new technology has been studied using RCTs more than any other form of fetal surveillance.[29-31]

A. Indications and Contraindications

The major indication for DV is to evaluate the umbilical vascular status in pregnancies complicated by IUGR and moderate-to-severe hypertensive disorders.[29] Umbilical artery DV has been studied in other pregnancy-related and maternal conditions, such as postdates pregnancy, and has not been found to be superior to other existing forms of fetal surveillance.[32] It offers no benefit when applied to low-risk populations.[33] There are no contraindications for performing this noninvasive test.

B. Test Administration and Interpretation

DV measures flow indices of the umbilical artery peak waveform during systole (S), the end-diastolic frequency shift (D), and the mean peak frequency shift over the cardiac cycle (A) that result in the following measurements[11]:
1. Systolic/diastolic ratio (S/D)
2. Resistance index (S-D/S)
3. Pulsatility index (S-D/A)

Abnormal umbilical artery DV has been defined as absent end-diastolic flow or a flow index greater than 2 standard deviations above the mean for gestational age. Reversed end-diastolic flow, an uncommon finding, is associated with poor perinatal outcomes and is viewed as an ominous finding.[34]

C. Evidence to Support the Use of Doppler Velocimetry

A previous metaanalysis published in the Cochrane Library concluded that the use of umbilical artery DV as a means of surveillance in pregnancies complicated by IUGR was associated with a decrease in perinatal mortality.[35] Concern arose over data accuracy in one of the trials included in the previous metaanalysis. A more recent Cochrane review excludes this study, and the outcome of improved perinatal mortality narrowly misses statistical significance (odds ratio [OR], 0.71; 95% CI, 0.50-1.01).[29] Currently, there is insufficient power in the number of study participants to make a definitive statement about the ability of DV to improve perinatal mortality. The outcomes that are improved with the use of DV versus NST in the evaluation of IUGR include the following:

1. Decreased number of antenatal admissions (NNT = 8)
2. Decreased number of inductions (NNT = 25)
3. Decreased number of elective deliveries (inductions plus elective cesarean deliveries) (NNT = 30)
4. Decreased number of cesarean deliveries for abnormal fetal heart rate tracings (NNT = 14)

D. Uses of Fetal Doppler Technology in Maternity Care

The Society of Obstetricians and Gynecologists of Canada has recently released evidence-based guidelines with respect to newer study modalities.[36] These recommendations include:

1. Umbilical artery DV should be available for the assessment of the fetal circulation in pregnancies with suspected severe placental insufficiency.
2. Reduced, absent, or reversed umbilical artery end-diastolic flow is an indication for enhanced fetal surveillance or delivery.
3. Umbilical artery DV should not be used as a screening tool in healthy pregnancies because it has not been shown to be of benefit in low-risk populations.

E. Use of Doppler Study of Middle Cerebral Artery

An emerging potential tool to provide antenatal surveillance of severe placental insufficiency is the use of Doppler technology to study fetal middle cerebral artery (MCA) flow. The theoretic underpinning of this approach is that increased MCA flow is indicative of physiologic shunting indicating increased fetal stress. Several studies have shown an association between increased MCA flow and adverse perinatal outcomes when umbilical artery flow studies have been normal.[37,38] RCTs are needed to determine whether increased MCA flow, indicative of shunting, will have the sensitivity and specificity to improve clinical outcomes.

VII. SOR A RECOMMENDATIONS

RECOMMENDATIONS	REFERENCES
VAS may be safely used to shorten the time required to administer an NST.	6
In the setting of severe IUGR, umbilical artery DV is the superior form of antenatal fetal surveillance. Its use in this setting is associated with a near-statistical decrease in perinatal mortality and reductions in inductions rates (NNT = 25), decreased number of elective deliveries (NNT = 30), and cesarean delivery for nonreassuring fetal tracings (NNT = 14).	29

REFERENCES

1. Devoe L: The nonstress test, *Obstet Gynecol Clin North Am* 17:111-128, 1990.
2. Willis D, Blanco J, Hamblen K et al: The nonstress test: criteria for the duration of fetal heart rate acceleration, *J Reprod Med* 35:901-903, 1990.
3. Bourgeois F, Thiagarajah S, Harbert G: The significance of fetal heart rate decelerations during nonstress testing, *Am J Obstet Gynecol* 150:213-216, 1984.
4. Locatelli A, Vergani P, Toso L et al: Perinatal outcome associated with oligohydramnios in uncomplicated term pregnancies, *Arch Gynecol Obstet* 269:130-133, 2004.
5. Clark S, Sabey P, Jolley K: Nonstress testing with acoustic stimulation and amniotic fluid volume assessment: 5973 tests without unexpected fetal death, *Am J Obstet Gynecol* 160:694-697, 1989.
6. Tan K, Smyth R: Fetal vibroacoustic stimulation for facilitation of tests of fetal wellbeing, *Cochrane Database Syst Rev* (1): CD002963, 2001.
7. Pattison N, McCowan L: Cardiotocography for antepartum assessment, *Cochrane Database Syst Rev* (2):CD001968, 2000.
8. Ray M, Freeman R: Clinical experience with the oxytocin challenge test, *Am J Obstet Gynecol* 114:1-8, 1972.
9. Rosenzweig B, Levy J, Schipiour P et al: Comparison of nipple stimulation and exogenous oxytocin contraction stress tests: a randomized prospective study, *J Reprod Med* 34:950-954, 1989.
10. Lagrew D: The contraction stress test, *Clin Obstet Gynecol* 38:11-25, 1995.
11. ACOG practice bulletin. Antepartum fetal surveillance. Number 9, October 1999 (replaces Technical Bulletin Number 188, January 1994). Clinical management guidelines for obstetrician-gynecologists, *Int J Gynaecol Obstet* 68:175-185, 2000.
12. Soregaroli M, Bonera R, Danti L et al: Prognostic role of umbilical artery Doppler velocimetry in growth-restricted fetuses, *J Matern Fetal Neonatal Med* 11:199-203, 2002.
13. Velazquez M, Rayburn W: Antenatal evaluation of the fetus using fetal movement monitoring, *Clin Obstet Gynecol* 45:993-1003, 2002.

14. Rayburn W: Fetal body movement monitoring, *Obstet Gynecol Clin North Am* 17:129-145, 1990.

15. Olesen A, Svare J: Decreased fetal movements: background, assessment, and clinical management, *Acta Obstet Gynecol Scand* 83:818-826, 2004.

16. Whitty J, Garfinkel D, Divon M: Maternal perception of decreased fetal movement as an indication of antepartum testing in a low-risk population, *Am J Obstet Gynecol* 165:1084-1088, 1991.

17. Harrington K, Thompson O, Jordan L et al: Obstetric outcome in women who present with a reduction in the fetal movements in the third trimester of pregnancy, *J Perinat Med* 26:77-82, 1998.

18. Dubiel M, Gudmundsson S, Thuring-Jonsson A et al: Doppler velocimetry and nonstress test for predicting outcome of pregnancies with decreased fetal movements, *Am J Perinatol* 14:139-144, 1997.

19. Smith C, Davis S, Rayburn W: Patients' acceptance of monitoring fetal movement: a randomized comparison of charting techniques, *J Reprod Med* 37:144-146, 1997.

20. Moore T, Piacquadio K: A prospective evaluation of fetal movement screening to reduce the incidence of antepartum fetal death, *Am J Obstet Gynecol* 160:1075-1079, 1989.

21. Sadovsky E, Weinstein F, Even Y: Antepartum fetal evaluation by assessment of fetal heart rate and fetal movements, *Int J Gynaecol Obstet* 19:21-26, 1981.

22. Grant A, Elbourne D, Valentin L et al: Routine formal fetal movement counting and risk of antepartum late death in normally formed singletons, *Lancet* 2(8659):345-349, 1989.

23. Manning F: The fetal biophysical profile score: current status, *Obstet Gynecol Clin North Am* 17:147-162, 1990.

24. Manning F, Morrison I, Harman C et al: Fetal assessment based on fetal biophysical profile scoring: experience in 19,221 referred high-risk pregnancies, *Am J Obstet Gynecol* 157:880-884, 1987.

25. Alfirevic Z, Neilson J: Biophysical profile for fetal assessment in high risk pregnancies, *Cochrane Database Syst Rev* (2):CD000038, 2000.

26. Miller D, Rabello Y, Paul R: The modified biophysical profile: antepartum testing in the 1990s, *Am J Obstet Gynecol* 174:812-817, 1996.

27. Nageotte MP, Towers CV, Asrat T: The value of a negative antepartum test: contraction stress test or modified biophysical profile, *Obstet Gynecol* 84:231-234, 1994.

28. Chauhan SP, Doherty DD, Magann EF et al: Amniotic fluid index vs single deepest pocket technique during modified biophysical profile: a randomized controlled trial, *Am J Obstet Gynecol* 191:661-667, 2004.

29. Neilson JP, Alfirevic Z: Doppler ultrasound in high risk pregnancies, *Cochrane Database Syst Rev* (2):CD000073, 2000.

30. Nienhuis S, Vles J, Gerver W et al: Doppler ultrasonography in suspected intrauterine growth retardation: a randomized clinical trial, *Ultrasound Obstet Gynecol* 9:6-13, 1997.

31. Westergaard H, Langhoff-Roos J, Lingman G et al: A critical appraisal of the use of umbilical artery Doppler ultrasound in high-risk pregnancies: use of meta-analyses in evidence-based obstetrics, *Ultrasound Obstet Gynecol* 17:464-476, 2001.

32. Pearce J McFarland P: A comparison of Doppler flow velocity waveforms, amniotic fluid columns, and the nonstress test as a means of monitoring post-dates pregnancies, *Obstet Gynecol* 77:204-208, 1991.

33. Mason G, Lilford R, Porter J et al: Randomised comparison of routine versus highly selective use of Doppler ultrasound in low risk pregnancies, *Br J Obstet Gynaecol* 100:130-133, 1993.

34. Karsdorp V, van Vugt J, van Geijn H et al: Clinical significance of absent or reversed end diastolic velocity waveforms in umbilical artery, *Lancet* 344:1664-1668, 1994.

35. Neilson JP: Doppler ultrasound in high risk pregnancies. In Enkin MW, Keirse MJNC, Renfrew MJ, Neilson JP, editors: *Pregnancy and childbirth module, Cochrane Database of Systematic Reviews: review No 03881. Cochrane updates on disk,* Oxford, 1994, Update Software.

36. Gagnon R, Van den Hof M, Bly S et al: The use of fetal Doppler in obstetrics, *J Obstet Gynaecol Can* 25:601-607, 2003.

37. Sterne G, Shields LE, Dubinsky TJ: Abnormal fetal cerebral and umbilical Doppler measurements in fetuses with intrauterine growth restriction predicts the severity of perinatal morbidity, *J Clin Ultrasound* 29:146-151, 2001.

38. Hershkovitz R, Kingdom JCP, Geary M et al: Fetal cerebral blood flow redistribution in late gestation: identification of compromise in small fetuses with normal umbilical artery Doppler, *Ultrasound Obstet Gynecol* 15:209-212, 2000.

S E C T I O N C Management of the Postterm Pregnancy

Richard Hudspeth, MD

Although the percentage of women with posterm pregnancies continues to decline, clinicians are still faced with the challenge of providing recommendations to families encountering a patient whose pregnancy passes the expected due date. This section provides information why pregnancies become postterm, why postterm pregnancies are a potential dilemma, and what current evidence-based recommendations suggest to prevent and manage postterm pregnancies.

I. EPIDEMIOLOGY AND RISK FACTORS

Postterm pregnancy is defined as lasting beyond 294 days, or 42 weeks, since the onset of the last menstrual period (LMP). *Prolonged* pregnancy is defined as lasting beyond 287 days, or 41 weeks, since the onset of the LMP. The use of the term *postdates* should be discouraged.

Compared with data from 1990, the National Vital Statistics Reports for 2002 indicates a dramatic national trend toward fewer deliveries beyond 42 weeks, with an even sharper decline in deliveries going beyond 40 weeks of gestation.[1] Approximately

6.7% of deliveries in 2002 were postterm, compared with 11.3% in 1990, representing a 40% decline. In addition, the number of births at, or beyond, 40 weeks declined from 48% in 1990 to 37% in 2002, with a concurrent increase in births between 37 and 39 weeks.

Although inaccurate dating plays a major role in the occurrence of postterm pregnancies, other factors have also been cited. Menstrual dating can be unreliable. In one retrospective analysis of approximately 25,000 pregnancies, nearly 72% of patients induced for this indication were not postterm if ultrasound dates alone, rather than LMP, were used to calculate gestational age.[2] Another study reported a positive predictive value of LMP estimates of gestational age at only 0.119 for postterm pregnancies.[3]

Some fetal malformations, such as anencephaly or fetal adrenal hyperplasia, have been associated with prolonged pregnancy.[4] Metabolic deficiencies such as nitric oxide in cervical fluid,[5] placental sulfatase, or abnormal persistence of 15-hydroxy-prostaglandin dehydrogenase (PGDH) have also been implicated.[4] Both maternal and paternal genetic factors may also play a role.[6] Women with previous prolonged pregnancy are at increased risk for recurrence in a subsequent birth,[7,8] whereas male sex fetuses are more often encountered in postterm pregnancies than female fetuses.[9]

II. PATHOGENESIS

Ballantyne[10] in the early 1900s first described the postmature infant as one who has stayed too long, whereas McClure-Browne[11] in the 1960s published data to show that perinatal mortality increases with gestational age. Although the perinatal mortality rate is much lower today, it still falls within 1 to 2 per 1000 in postterm pregnancies (excluding fetal malformations), despite antenatal testing. Table 11-1 illustrates the link between advancing gestational age and stillbirth risk.[12] Other more recent studies of varying design continue to confirm that advancing gestational age puts the family at risk for stillbirth.[13,14] What remains unknown is the reason for this increase in perinatal mortality. Uteroplacental insufficiency has long been thought to play a major role, though it is not clear whether this is an inevitable result of advancing gestational age, or whether failure to achieve spontaneous labor is somehow a marker for uteroplacental insufficiency.[12]

III. CLINICAL FEATURES

Complications of postterm pregnancy can be considered to fall into two categories: maternal and fetal. Fetal complications are more likely to be associated with smaller fetuses, whereas maternal complications are more common with larger fetuses.

A. Fetal Complications
Features of the dysmature infant are characteristic: meconium-stained skin; long nails; and a withered-appearing, small, and fragile placenta. These features occur in 20% of postterm pregnancies. Other risks associated with the postterm infant may include asphyxia, hypoglycemia, and temperature instability. Oligohydramnios incidence increases with advancing gestational age.[15]

Perinatal mortality rates are greater among low-birth-weight infants, who are also more likely to have nonreassuring fetal heart tracings, a significantly greater incidence of low pH (<7.2), and require cesarean delivery more often than those infants of normal or high birth weights.[13,16,17] However, birth complications can also occur among macrosomic postterm infants, including brachial plexus injury or even death.

B. Maternal Complications
Maternal morbidity—dysfunctional and prolonged labor; genital tract trauma such as vaginal side wall tears, cervical lacerations, and third- and fourth-degree perineal extensions; wound infection; postpartum hemorrhage; fistula formation; and greater cesarean delivery rates—occurs at greater rates in postterm pregnancies, typically associated with fetal macrosomia.[17] In addition, maternal morbidity may include psychological factors related to carrying a pregnancy beyond term and the physical discomforts experienced at later gestational ages.

IV. MANAGEMENT

The choice facing provider and patient when encountering a postterm pregnancy becomes one of expectant management versus induction. Risks associated with expectant management should be explained to the patient and her family to help guide the conversation. Strong evidence supports the choice of induction beginning at 41 weeks over expectant management, based on a reduction in perinatal mortality.[12,18,19] A Cochrane review of

19 RCTs concluded that routine induction after 41 weeks reduces perinatal mortality (OR, 0.20; 95% CI, 0.06-0.70) with a NNT of approximately 500 to prevent 1 stillbirth.[18] A more recent meta-analysis showed a similar, but not statistically significant, reduction in perinatal mortality for labor induction compared with expectant management (0.09% vs 0.33%; OR, 0.41; 95% CI, 0.14-1.18).[19]

Although some studies have shown a reduction in cesarean delivery rates (20.1% vs 22.0%; OR, 0.88; 95% CI, 0.78-0.99),[20] there is no evidence to support that induction of labor increases the likelihood of cesarean delivery.[18] An Agency for Healthcare Research and Quality report concurs with similar findings.[12]

Options for antenatal testing have not been adequately studied with RCTs among postterm pregnancies. Given the 1 to 2 per 1000 perinatal mortality rate in postterm fetuses, an RCT would need to enroll more than 40,000 women in each arm to determine a twofold difference in risk for stillbirth between two competing methods of antepartum surveillance.[12] One study that compared perinatal losses with antenatal surveillance beginning at 41 versus 42 weeks suggests that beginning testing at 41 weeks may result in reduced perinatal morbidity and mortality, as well as lower rates of intrapartum fetal heart rate abnormalities.[21] Tests for antenatal risk assessment have lower sensitivity than specificity, but greater negative predictive values than positive predictive values. It is the low risk for adverse outcomes that is the main "driver" of this high negative predictive value (i.e., the likelihood that a fetus with a normal test will have a normal outcome). False-negative results of antenatal testing, therefore, increase with advancing gestational age."[12] No single method of antenatal testing has been shown to be superior to another. A 2004 ACOG Practice Bulletin nonspecifically states that "many practitioners use twice-weekly testing" and "assessment of amniotic fluid volume appears to be important."[22]

V. CLINICAL COURSE AND PREVENTION

A. Routine Ultrasound to Establish Accurate Dating

Data from four RCTs that assessed the impact of routine versus indicated ultrasound in early pregnancy found that routine early pregnancy ultrasound reduces the number of labor inductions required for management of postterm pregnancy (OR, 0.68; 95% CI, 0.57-0.82; absolute risk reduction = 1%) with a NNT of 100 ultrasounds to prevent a postterm induction.[23] An additional RCT done after publication of that Cochrane review supported that a program of routine first-trimester ultrasound resulted in a significant reduction in inductions for postterm pregnancy.[24] Expected variation for ultrasound dating is ±7 days up to 20 weeks of gestation, ±14 days between 20 and 30 weeks of gestation, and ±21 days beyond 30 weeks of gestation.[22]

B. Routine Membrane Sweeping

Membrane sweeping is accomplished by placing the gloved index finger approximately 2 cm into the cervix and making a circular, sweeping motion. This maneuver is performed on a weekly basis, beginning at 38 to 40 weeks of gestation, in an attempt to reduce the number of patients who develop postterm pregnancy requiring induction. The Cochrane Library analyzed 12 RCTs of this intervention and found that risk for cesarean delivery was similar between groups (RR, 0.90; 95% CI, 0.70-1.15).[25] Sweeping of the membranes was associated with reduced duration of pregnancy and reduced frequency of pregnancy continuing beyond 41 (RR, 0.59; 95% CI, 0.46-0.74) and 42 weeks (RR, 0.28; 95% CI, 0.15-0.50). Membrane sweeping must be performed in eight women (NNT = 8) to avoid one formal induction of labor. No evidence of maternal or neonatal risk has been reported. Patient discomfort was measured in only one study, but results indicate that this is an important factor for the provider to weigh.

VI. PITFALLS AND CONTROVERSIES

Sixty-eight percent of all pregnant women in the United States receive at least one ultrasound, according to 2002 data.[12] An early ultrasound for every pregnancy may be an unrealistic, or even an unnecessary, goal. However, based on studies that indicate a reduction in postterm inductions when early pregnancy ultrasound is used, its routine use should be strongly considered.

Use of membrane sweeping in all pregnant women, in an effort to reduce postterm pregnancy, may be controversial. The Cochrane review on this subject notes that the "rationale for performing routinely an intervention with the potential to induce labor in women with an uneventful pregnancy at

38 weeks of gestation is, at least, questionable."[25] Obviously, the final decision rests with the patient after a balanced discussion with her provider.

Few studies have examined the cost of the various interventions covered in this chapter. In those that have, there is no consensus, and results are based on unique clinical settings with limited generalizability.[20,26] Questions to consider when determining costs include: What is available in the community? What is the price differential for induction versus expectant management? Who bears the cost of the different interventions?

VII. SOR A SUMMARY RECOMMENDATIONS

RECOMMENDATIONS	REFERENCES
Early ultrasound to accurately date the pregnancy reduces the number of women who require induction for a postterm pregnancy (NNT = 100).	23
Sweeping of the membranes beginning at 38 weeks of gestation reduces the number of inductions for postterm pregnancies (NNT = 8).	25
Induce patients at 41+ weeks to reduce perinatal mortality. This will not increase the cesarean section rate, and may actually reduce it.	19, 20

REFERENCES

1. Martin JA, Hamilton BE, Sutton PD et al: Births: final data for 2002, *Natl Vital Stat Rep* 52(10):16-19, 2003.
2. Gardosi J, Vanner T, Francis A: Gestational age and induction of labour for prolonged pregnancy, *Br J Obstet Gynaecol* 105(2):247-248, 1998.
3. Kramer M, McLean F, Boyd M et al: the validity of gestational age estimation by menstrual dating in term, preterm and postterm gestations, *JAMA* 260(22):3306-3308, 1988.
4. Resnik R, Calder A: Post-term pregnancy. In Creasy RK, Resnik R, editors: *Maternal-fetal medicine*, ed 4, Philadelphia, 1999, W.B. Saunders.
5. Vaisanen-Tommiska M, Nuutila M, Ylikorkala O: Cervical nitric oxide release in women postterm, *Obstet Gynecol* 103(4):657-662, 2004.
6. Laursen M, Bille C, Oleson AW et al: Genetic influence on prolonged gestation: a population-based Danish twin study, *Am J Obstet Gynecol* 190(2):489-494, 2004.
7. Oleson AW, Basso O, Olsen J: Risk of recurrence of prolonged pregnancy, *BMJ* 326(7387):476, 2003.
8. Mogren I, Stenlund H, Hogberg U: Recurrence of prolonged pregnancy, *Int J Epidemiol* 28(2):253-257, 1999.
9. Divon MY, Ferber A, Nisell H et al: Male gender predisposes to prolongation of pregnancy, *Am J Obstet Gynecol* 187(4):1081-1083, 2002.
10. Ballantyne JW: The problem of the postmature infant, *J Obstet Gynaecol Br Emp* 2:36, 1902.
11. McClure-Browne J: Postmaturity, *Am J Obstet Gynecol* 85:73-78, 1963.
12. Myers ER, Blumrick R, Christian AL et al: Management of prolonged pregnancy. Evidence Report/Technology Assessment No. 53 (prepared by Duke Evidence-based Practice Center, Durham, NC, under contract No. 290-97-0014). AHQR Publication No. 02-E018. Rockville, MD, May 2002, Agency for Healthcare Research and Quality (AHQR).
13. Caughey AB, Musci TJ: Complications of term pregnancies beyond 37 weeks of gestation, *Obstet Gynecol* 103(1):57-62, 2004.
14. Olesen AW, Westergaard JG, Olsen J: Perinatal and maternal complications related to postterm delivery: a national register-based study, 1978-1993, *Am J Obstet Gynecol* 189(1):222-227, 2003.
15. Sarno A, Ahn M, Phelan J: Intrapartum amniotic fluid volume at term: association of ruptured membranes, oligohydramnios and increased fetal risk, *J Reprod Med* 35:719-723, 1990.
16. Divon MY, Haglund B, Nisell H et al: Fetal and neonatal mortality in the postterm pregnancy: the impact of gestational age and fetal growth restriction, *Am J Obstet Gynecol* 178:726-731, 1998.
17. Sylvestre G, Fisher M, Westrean M et al: Nonreassuring fetal status in the prolonged pregnancy: the impact of fetal weight, *Ultrasound Obstet Gynecol* 18:244-247, 2001.
18. Crowley P: Interventions for preventing or improving the outcome of delivery at or beyond term, *Cochrane Database of Systemic Reviews,* 2006, Issue 4, Art No.: CD000170. DOI: 10.1002/14651858. CD000170.pub2.
19. Sanchez-Ramos L, Olivier F, Delke I et al: Labor induction versus expectant management for postterm pregnancies: a systematic review with meta-analysis, *Obstet Gynecol* 101:1312-1318, 2003.
20. Hannah M, Hannah W, Hellman J et al: Induction of labor as compared with serial antenatal monitoring in post-term pregnancy, *N Engl J Med* 326:1587-1592, 1992.
21. Bouchner C, Williams J, Castro L et al: The efficacy of starting postterm antenatal testing at 41 weeks as compared with 42 weeks of gestational age, *Am J Obstet Gynecol* 159:550-554, 1988.
22. ACOG Practice Bulletin: management of postterm pregnancy, *Obstet Gynecol* 104(3):639-645, 2004.
23. Neilson JP: Ultrasound for fetal assessment in early pregnancy, *Cochrane Database Syst Rev* (2):CD000182, 2000.
24. Bennett KA, Crane JM, O'Shea P et al: First trimester ultrasound screening is effective in reducing postterm labor induction rates: a randomized controlled trial, *Am J Obstet Gynecol* 190(4):1077-1081, 2004.
25. Boulvain M, Stan C, Irion O: Membrane sweeping for induction of labour, *Cochrane Database Syst Rev* (1):CD000451, 2005.
26. Fonseca L, Monga M, Silva J: Postdates pregnancy in an indigent population: the financial burden, *Am J Obstet Gynecol* 155(5):1214-1216, 2003.

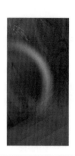

Preterm Labor

Preterm labor (PTL) and subsequent preterm delivery (PTD) of infants before 37 weeks of gestation are among the most vexing problems in obstetrics. Although neonatal mortality and morbidity have improved with advances in neonatal medicine, the incidence of PTD in the United States has increased from 9.4% of births in 1984 to 11% in 2000.[1] The very preterm birth rate (<32 completed weeks) was 1.9% in 2000. Complications of prematurity are responsible for at least a third of infant deaths in the United States.[2] The results of large-scale programs for the reduction of PTD have been inconsistent at best.

Birth weight is an important predictor of neonatal outcome. Low-birth-weight (<2500 g) infants account for two thirds of neonatal deaths in the United States; very-low-birth-weight infants (<1500 g) account for half of neonatal deaths. Very-low-birth-weight infants have a 95 times greater risk for death than infants born weighing greater than 2500 g at birth and a 7 times greater risk for death than infants weighing 1500 to 2499 g at birth. Intrauterine growth restriction accounts for a significant percentage of low-birth-weight infants and may reduce the birth weight of 30% of infants born prematurely.

This chapter advocates a clinical approach that seeks to identify patients who are most likely to deliver prematurely and to identify interventions aimed to decrease these risks. Once a patient presents with symptoms suggestive of PTL, rapid diagnosis of this disorder is important. Using the best evidence available, the clinician first must decide whether treatment is indicated, then decide on therapy.

REFERENCES

1. Martin JA, Hamilton BE, Ventura SJ et al: Births: final data for 2000, *Natl Vital Stat Rep* 50(5):1-101, 2002.

2. Callaghan WM, MacDorman MF, Rasmussen SA et al: The contribution of preterm birth to infant mortality rates in the United States, *Pediatrics* 118:1566-1573, 2006.

SECTION A Risk Factors for Preterm Delivery

William Gosnell Sayres, Jr., MD

Half of PTDs are the result of spontaneous onset of labor with intact membranes. One fourth of PTDs are considered medically indicated. Neonatal outcomes for indicated PTDs are no different than outcomes for spontaneous PTD.[1] One fourth of PTDs occur after preterm premature rupture of membranes (PPROM).

Accurate assessment of risk for PTD allows for the focusing of resources and interventions on patients most likely to benefit. The variable results of carefully studied PTD prevention programs may be the result of inaccurate antenatal risk assessment or ineffective interventions.[2] Table 12-1 presents odds ratios *for PTD* associated with selected *historical items* and antenatal screening tests. Rather than presenting the opportunity for primary prevention of PTL, some of these tests may reflect an ongoing *irreversible* pathologic process.[3]

I. DEMOGRAPHIC AND HISTORICAL RISK FACTORS

Multiple demographic and historical risk factors for PTD have been identified.[4,5] Table 12-2 lists patient characteristics frequently associated with PTD. The impact of individual risk factors varies among populations and individuals. Previous PTD is the

TABLE 12-1 Clinical Indicators and Risk for Preterm Delivery

Clinical Indicator	PTD OR	References
History of PTD	2.5-3.6	7
Interpregnancy interval < 6 months	1.4	11
Smoking	1.3-1.4	7
Periodontal disease	2.0	22
BMI < 19.8		
Nullipara	2.3	2
Multipara	1.8	2
Bleeding after 20 weeks	5.3	4
Manual cervical examination	1.43 per unit Bishop score	23
Cervical ultrasound		23
40 mm	1.98	
35 mm	2.35	
30 mm	3.79	
26 mm	6.19	
22 mm	9.49	
13 mm	13.99	
Fetal fibronectin		25
Symptomatic, delivery within 7-10 days		
Positive	5.42	
Negative	0.25	
Asymptomatic, delivery < 34 weeks		
Positive	4.01	
Negative	0.78	

PTD, Preterm delivery; OR, odds ratio; BMI, body mass index.

most predictive historical risk factor. Women with a history of one previous PTD carry a 17% to 37% risk of recurrence.[6] Risk increases with subsequent PTDs. The risk for recurrence of PTD is increased the earlier the prior delivery occurred.[7] The odds ratios (ORs) for interpregnancy interval of less than 6 months associated with birth at 24 to 32 weeks is 2.2, birth at 33 to 36 weeks is 1.6,[8] and overall preterm birth is 1.6.[9] A history of loop electrical

excision procedure (LEEP) or laser cone treatments for cervical intraepithelial neoplasia is associated with PPROM.[10] The effect of stress is greatest if there is an increase during the pregnancy.[11] Physically strenuous work worsens the prognosis of low socioeconomic groups in particular.[12]

II. MATERNAL INFECTION

Maternal genitourinary infection is an important risk factor for PTD (Table 12-2).[13,14]

A. Asymptomatic Bacteriuria

Treatment of asymptomatic bacteriuria (ASB) reduces the incidence of pyelonephritis and may decrease incidence of PTD.[15]

B. Lower Genitourinary Infection

Infections with syphilis, gonorrhea, and chlamydia are all associated with PTD and low birth weight.[16]

C. Maternal Group B Streptococcal Infection

Maternal group B streptococcal infection is significantly associated with increased neonatal morbidity and mortality. There is an inconsistent association of maternal group B streptococcal infection with PTL, although it appears to be associated with PPROM.[17]

D. Bacterial Vaginosis

Bacterial vaginosis (BV) is a polymicrobial infection by anaerobic bacteria, *Gardnerella vaginalis* and *Mycoplasma hominis,* replacing the normal lactobacillus-predominant flora of the vagina. BV is associated with an increased risk for PTD (OR, 1.4-1.8).[18-21]

E. Maternal Periodontal Disease

An evolving literature has established an association between maternal periodontal disease and increased risk for PTD.[22]

III. ESTABLISHMENT OF RISK

A. Manual Cervical Examination

Safe and inexpensive, a digital cervical examination offers an immediate assessment of risk. A *cervical score* (cervical length [cm] − cervical dilation [cm]) of less than 0 is predictive of PTD. A Bishop score of greater than or equal to 6 indicates high risk.[23]

TABLE 12-2 Risk Factors for Preterm Delivery

Demographic and Psychosocial Characteristics	Pregnancy History	Medical/Gynecologic History	Current Pregnancy
Low SES	History of PTD	Uterine anomalies: bicornuate uterus, cervical changes resulting from DES exposure	Maternal infection: bacteriuria, syphilis, gonorrhea, chlamydia, GBS infection, bacterial vaginosis
Maternal age <18 and >35		Cervical incompetence: history of cervical conization or multiple abortions	First- or second-trimester vaginal bleeding
Black race			Uterine enlargement: multiple pregnancy, polyhydramnios
Psychosocial stress			Cervical change
Physically strenuous work			Uterine activity
Substance abuse: tobacco, cocaine, alcohol			Short interpregnancy interval
Poor nutritional status: BMI < 19.8, poor pregnancy weight gain			
Domestic violence			
Maternal depression			

SES, Socioeconomic status; PTD, preterm delivery; DES, diethylstilbestrol; GBS, group B streptococcus; BMI, body mass index.

TABLE 12-3 Preterm Labor Risk Assessment

One or More Major Factors*		Two or More Minor Factors*	
History	This Pregnancy	History	This Pregnancy
Previous preterm delivery	Multiple gestation	1 second-trimester abortion	Bleeding after week 12
Previous cone biopsy	Uterine anomaly	>2 first-trimester abortions	Pyelonephritis
Diethylstilbestrol exposure in utero	Cervix effaced > 80% at 28- or 32-week examination		Smoking >10 cigarettes/day
>1 second-trimester abortion	Cervix dilated > 1 cm at 28- or 32-week examination		Febrile illness (temperature > 39°C)
	Uterine irritability		
	Abdominal surgery		
	Cervical cerclage		
	Polyhydramnios		

Data from Yawn BP, Yawn RA: Preterm birth prevention in rural practice, *JAMA* 262:230-233, 1989.
*Patient is considered "high risk" for preterm labor when these conditions are present.

Cervical dilation greater than or equal to 1 cm and effacement greater than or equal to 30% also indicates risk.[24]

B. Ultrasound Examination of the Cervix

Because the results of the cervical examination vary between examiners, ultrasound has been advocated as offering a more reproducible cervical evaluation. As ultrasound cervical length shortens to less than 30 mm at 24 and 28 weeks of gestation, risk for PTD progressively increases.[23,24] Table 12-1 quantifies these risks.

C. Fetal Fibronectin Testing

Fetal fibronectin is a fetal basement membrane protein. Presence of fetal fibronectin in cervical or vaginal secretions after 20 weeks of gestation indicates disruption of the maternal-fetal interface, possibly the result of upper genital tract inflammation. The predictive value of this test varies with patient presentation and increases with symptoms or history of PTD. Low likelihood of PTD with a negative test result makes this test useful for ruling out true PTL in a symptomatic patient.[25]

Cervicovaginal mucus must be collected from the ectocervix or posterior vaginal fornix before digital examination. Test accuracy is confounded by recent coitus, vaginal bleeding, rupture of membranes, vaginal lubricants or disinfectants, and abnormal vaginal flora.[25]

REFERENCES

1. Owen J, Baker SK, Hauth JL: Is indicated or spontaneous preterm delivery more advantageous for the fetus? *Am J Obstet Gynecol* 163:868-872, 1990.
2. Iams JD, Goldenberg RL, Mercer BM et al: The preterm prediction study: recurrence risk of spontaneous preterm birth, *Am J Obstet Gynecol* 178:1035-1040, 1998.
3. Goldenberg RL, Rouse DJ: Prevention of premature birth, *N Engl J Med* 339:313-320, 1998.
4. Gjerdingen DK: Premature labor, part I: risk assessment, etiologic factors, and diagnosis, *J Am Board Fam Pract* 5:495-509, 1992.
5. American College of Obstetricians and Gynecologists (ACOG): Assessment of risk factors for preterm birth. Practice bulletin No. 31, Washington, DC, 2001, ACOG.
6. American College of Obstetricians and Gynecologists (ACOG): Preterm labor. Technical bulletin No. 206, Washington, DC, 1995, ACOG.
7. Adams MM, Elam-Evans LD, Wilson HG et al: Rates of and factors associated with recurrence of preterm deliver, *JAMA* 283:1591-1596, 2000.
8. Smith GCS, Pell JP, Dobbie R: Interpregnancy interval and risk of preterm birth and neonatal death: retrospective cohort study, *BMJ* 327:313-316, 2003.
9. Conde-Agudelo A, Rosas-Bermudez A, Fafury-Goeta AC: Birth spacing and risk of adverse perinatal outcomes: a meta-analysis, *JAMA* 295:1809-1823, 2006.
10. Sadler L, Saftlas A, Wang W et al: Treatment for cervical intraepithelial neoplasia and risk of preterm delivery, *JAMA* 291:2100-2106, 2004.
11. Williamson HA, LeFevre M, Hector M: Association between life stress and serious perinatal complications, *J Fam Pract* 29:489-496, 1989.
12. Simpson JL: Are physical activity and employment related to preterm birth and low birth weight? *Am J Obstet Gynecol* 168:1231-1238, 1993.
13. McGregor JA, French JI, Parker R et al: Prevention of premature birth by screening and treatment for common genital tract infections: results of a prospective controlled trial, *Am J Obstet Gynecol* 173:157-167, 1995.
14. Meis PJ, Goldenberg RL, Mercer B et al: The preterm prediction study: significance of vaginal infections, *Am J Obstet Gynecol* 173:1231-1235, 1995.
15. Smaill F: Antibiotics for asymptomatic bacteriuria in pregnancy, *Cochrane Database Syst Rev* (2):CD000490, 2001.
16. Andrews WW, Goldenberg RL, Mercer B et al: The preterm prediction study: association of second-trimester genitourinary chlamydia infection with subsequent preterm birth, *Am J Obstet Gynecol* 183:662-668, 2000.
17. Regan J, Klebanoff M, Nugent R et al: Colonization with group B streptococci in pregnancy and adverse outcome: VIP Study Group, *Am J Obstet Gynecol* 174:1354-1360, 1996.
18. Flynn CA, Helwig AL, Meurer LN: Bacterial vaginosis in pregnancy and role of prematurity: a meta-analysis, *J Fam Pract* 48:885-892, 1999.
19. Hauth JC, Goldenberg RL, Andrews WW et al: Reduced incidence of preterm delivery with metronidazole and erythromycin in women with bacterial vaginosis, *N Engl J Med* 333:1732-1736, 1995.
20. Hillier SL, Nugent RP, Eschenbach DA et al: Association between bacterial vaginosis and preterm delivery of a low-birth-weight infant, *N Engl J Med* 333:1737-1742, 1995.
21. Meis PJ, Goldenberg RL, Mercer B et al: The preterm prediction study: significance of vaginal infections, *Am J Obstet Gynecol* 173:1231-1235, 1995.
22. Offenbacher S, Boggess KA, Murtha AP et al: Progressive periodontal disease and the risk of very preterm delivery, *Obstet Gynecol* 107:29-36, 2006.
23. Iams JD, Goldenberg RL, Meis PJ et al: The length of the cervix and the risk of spontaneous premature delivery, *N Engl J Med* 334:567-572, 1996.
24. Stubbs TM, Van Dorsten JP, Miller MC: The preterm cervix and preterm labor: relative risks, predictive values, and change over time, *Am J Obstet Gynecol* 155:829-834, 1986.
25. Ramsey PS, Andrews WW: Biochemical predictors of preterm labor: fetal fibronectin and salivary estriol, *Clin Perinatol* 30:701-733, 2003.

S E C T I O N B Antenatal Interventions for Prevention of Preterm Delivery

William Gosnell Sayres, Jr., MD

I. PSYCHOSOCIAL INTERVENTIONS FOR THE PREVENTION OF PRETERM DELIVERY

A. Antenatal Education

The primary focus of antenatal education efforts is on the early recognition of symptoms of PTL. The premise behind this educational effort is that women who recognize their contractions present to their providers in earlier stages of PTL and have a greater likelihood of successful tocolysis.[1] Educational programs also have been aimed at the providers of prenatal care, particularly the varied personnel interacting with the patient as she negotiates the system. Before evaluation by her provider, the patient encounters medical receptionists, telephone triage personnel, nursing staff, and others. If these staff members are not alerted to the symptoms of PTL, inappropriate delay between onset of symptoms and clinical evaluation may occur. Prenatal providers are challenged by the variability of symptoms that may precede PTL, including vaginal discharge, bleeding, backache, and diarrhea.[2] Not only do patients often present with atypical symptoms, but the literature suggests that 50% of women do not feel their contractions at all or do not perceive them as painful.[2] It is critical to the success of education-based programs that clinicians and their support staff maintain a high level of suspicion when the patient has these symptoms.

B. Psychosocial Support

An enhanced social and emotional environment has positive psychological and behavioral effects, and also may be reflected in better physical health. A metaanalysis of prospective studies of social support in pregnancy failed to show a decreased incidence of PTD.[3] A high suspicion for psychosocial duress should be maintained and these issues explored with the patient. Women who suffer a drastic increase in personal stress during pregnancy should be identified as having greater potential for adverse pregnancy outcome.[4]

C. Lifestyle Modification

Educational and behavior modification efforts should focus on at-risk aspects of a patient's lifestyle. Smoking and other substance abuse should be addressed aggressively. Continued smoking in the face of active counseling may serve as an indicator of other psychosocial stresses.

D. Nutritional Support

Nutritional support has been studied among large groups of pregnant women from lower socioeconomic groups. Patients who present with low weight and experience poor weight gain during pregnancy are at high risk for PTD.[5] Among these women, many of whom may be malnourished and at risk for PTL and low birth weight, dietary supplements of calories and protein increase birth weights 40 to 60 g on average but do not extend gestations.[6] Although gestations may not be extended by dietary supplements, increasing birth weight can be expected to improve prognosis (see Chapter 4, Section A). Calcium supplementation (2 g/day) in at-risk populations (low socioeconomic status, lactose intolerance) has been associated with a lower incidence of PTD and with lower rates of hypertension and proteinuric preeclampsia.[7]

E. Activity Restriction

The use of prophylactic bed rest has not been shown to prevent PTD in high-risk pregnancies and in one trial of twin pregnancies was associated with an increased rate of PTD.[8] Once a diagnosis of PTL or early cervical change has been established, however, activity restriction becomes important. For various reasons, many patients are poorly compliant with activity restriction. It is critical that the patient's psychosocial background be explored carefully in the context of PTD. Creative use of community and family resources may be required for compliance.

F. Sexual Activity

Sexual activity in itself does not increase the risk for PTD.[9] Self-palpation for uterine contractions after sexual activity is recommended for patients thought to be at increased risk for PTL. Patients diagnosed with PTL or early cervical change should maintain pelvic rest.

G. Regular Nursing Contact

Patients at increased risk for PTL and PTD benefit from intense nursing contact.[10]

II. MEDICAL INTERVENTIONS

A. Screening for Infection

1. Gonorrhea, syphilis, and chlamydia

   Clinicians should perform routine screening for gonorrhea, syphilis, and chlamydia at the onset of prenatal care. Patients who have positive results should undergo a test of cure at a subsequent appointment. The Centers for Disease Control and Prevention recommends that at the beginning of the third trimester clinicians consider rescreening patients considered at increased risk for contracting one of these sexually transmitted diseases during pregnancy (see Chapter 9, Section A).

2. Group B streptococcus

   Guidelines for universal prenatal screening are discussed in Chapter 9, Section A. For patients at risk for PTD, screening could be considered at earlier than 35 to 37 gestational weeks.[11]

3. Bacterial vaginosis (BV)

   The incidence of PTD may be reduced by screening for and treatment of BV in patients already considered high risk for prematurity because of previous PTD,[12-15] although one metaanalysis has concluded that treatment does not improve pregnancy outcome.[16] Screening and treatment of BV in asymptomatic low-risk women does *not* reduce the incidence of PTD. Criteria for diagnosis of BV have been developed by Nugent and co-workers[17] and Amsel and colleagues.[18] Treatment of diagnosed infection includes either clindamycin (300 mg orally twice daily for 7 days) or metronidazole (500 mg orally twice daily for 7 days).[12] Vaginal administration of antibiotics is not effective.

4. Treatment of periodontal disease

   Treatment of periodontal disease with scaling and root planing in one large trial did not decrease the incidence of birth before 37 weeks.[19]

5. Home uterine activity monitoring

   Patients may not experience contractions that may presage the onset of PTL. Asymptomatic uterine contractions may be detected with a home uterine activity monitor. Women considered high risk for PTD typically are monitored for 1 hour twice daily from gestational weeks 24 to 36. Monitor recordings are then transmitted electronically to a central location, possibly hundreds of miles away. Patients are contacted daily by a nurse. Although contractions are associated with an increased risk for PTD, outcomes of monitored patients do not show a consistent beneficial effect, whereas use of prophylactic tocolytics and unscheduled visits increase.[10,20]

6. Progestational agents

   Antenatal administration of 17-α-hydroxyprogesterone caproate appears to improve pregnancy outcome in patients with a history of preterm birth[21,22] (Figure 12-1). Weekly intramuscular injections of 250 mg 17-α-hydroxyprogesterone caproate from 16 to 20 weeks of gestation until 36 weeks result in fewer deliveries before 37 weeks (number needed to treat [NNT] = 6).[23] Incidence of birth weight less than 2500 g is decreased (NNT = 7), as well as other complications of prematurity. Injections begin at 16 to 20 weeks and continue until 36 weeks. Other than injection-site discomfort, few adverse effects occur. Alternatively, daily vaginal 100-mg progesterone suppositories given from 24 to 34 weeks of gestation also improve outcome.[24] Optimal route of

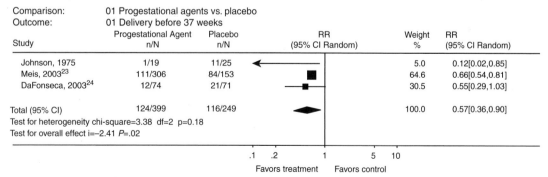

FIGURE 12-1. Progestational agent versus placebo in women at high risk for delivery at less than 37 weeks of gestation. CI, Confidence interval; RR, relative risk. (From Mackenzie R, Walker M, Armson A, Hannah ME: Progesterone for the prevention of preterm birth among women at increased risk: a systematic review and meta-analysis of randomized controlled trials, *Am J Obstet Gynecol* 194:1234-1242, 2006, with permission.)

administration and dose of progesterone and long-term safety have not yet been established.

REFERENCES

1. Yawn BP, Yawn RA: Preterm birth prevention in a rural practice, *JAMA* 262:230-233, 1989.
2. Katz M, Goodyear K, Creasy RK: Early signs and symptoms of preterm labor, *Am J Obstet Gynecol* 162:1150-1153, 1990.
3. Hodnett ED, Fredericks S: Support during pregnancy for women at increased risk of low birthweight babies, *Cochrane Database Syst Rev* (3):CD000198, 2003.
4. Williamson HA, LeFevre M, Hector M: Association between life stress and serious perinatal complications, *J Fam Pract* 29:489-496, 1989.
5. Goldenberg RL, Rouse DJ: Prevention of premature birth, *N Engl J Med* 339:313-320, 1998.
6. Kramer MS, Kakuma R: Energy and protein intake in pregnancy, *Cochrane Database Syst Rev* (4):CD000032, 2003.
7. Hofmeyr GJ, Atallah AN, Duley L: Calcium supplementation during pregnancy for preventing hypertensive disorders and related problems, *Cochrane Database Syst Rev* (3):CD001059, 2006.
8. Sanders MC, Dick JS, Brown I: The effects of hospital admission for bed rest on the duration of twin pregnancy: a randomized trial, *Lancet* i:793-795, 1985.
9. Read JS, Klebanoff MA: Sexual intercourse during pregnancy and preterm delivery: effects of vaginal microorganisms, *Am J Obstet Gynecol* 163:514-519, 1993.
10. Dyson DC, Danbe KH, Bamber JA et al: Monitoring women at high risk for preterm labor, *N Engl J Med* 338:15-19, 1998.
11. Centers for Disease Control and Prevention: Prevention of perinatal group B streptococcal disease: a public health perspective, *MMWR Recomm Rep* 45(RR-7):1-24, 1996.
12. Hauth JC, Goldenberg RL, Andrews WW et al: Reduced incidence of preterm delivery with metronidazole and erythromycin in women with bacterial vaginosis, *N Engl J Med* 333:1732-1736, 1995.
13. Hillier SL, Nugent RP, Eschenbach DA et al: Association between bacterial vaginosis and preterm delivery of a low-birth-weight infant, *N Engl J Med* 333:1737-1742, 1995.
14. Meis PJ, Goldenberg RL, Mercer B et al: The preterm prediction study: significance of vaginal infections, *Am J Obstet Gynecol* 173:1231-1235, 1995.
15. McDonald H, Brocklehurst P, Parsons J: Antibiotics for treating bacterial vaginosis in pregnancy, *Cochrane Database Syst Rev* (1):CD000262, 2005.
16. Okun N, Gronau KA, Hannah ME: Antibiotics for bacterial vaginosis or *Trichomonas vaginalis* in pregnancy: a systematic review, *Obstet Gynecol* 105:857-868, 2005.
17. Nugent RP, Krohn MA, Hillier SL: Reliability of diagnosing bacterial vaginosis is improved by a standardized method of Gram stain interpretation, *J Clin Microbiol* 29:297-301, 1991.
18. Amsel R, Totten PA, Spiegel CA et al: Nonspecific vaginitis: diagnostic criteria and microbial and epidemiologic associations, *Am J Med* 74:14-22, 1983.
19. Michalowicz BS, Hodges JS, DiAngelis AJ et al: Treatment of periodontal disease and the risk of preterm birth, *N Engl J Med* 355:1885-1894, 2006.
20. Corwin MJ, Mou SM, Sunderji SG et al: Multicenter randomized clinical trial of home uterine activity monitoring: pregnancy outcomes for all women randomized, *Am J Obstet Gynecol* 175:1281-1285, 1996.
21. Ables AZ, Chauhan SP: Preterm labor: diagnostic and therapeutic options are not all alike, *J Fam Pract* 54:245-252, 2005.
22. Dodd JM, Flenady V, Cincotta R, Crowther CA: Prenatal administration of progesterone for preventing preterm birth, *Cochrane Database Syst Rev* (1):CD004947, 2006.
23. Meis PJ, Klebanoff M, Thom E et al: Prevention of recurrent preterm delivery by 17 alpha-hydroxyprogesterone caproate, *N Engl J Med* 348:2379-2385, 2003.
24. Da Fonseca EB, Bittar RE, Carvalho MHB et al: Prophylactic administration of progesterone by vaginal suppository to reduce the incidence of spontaneous preterm birth in women at risk: a randomized placebo-controlled double-blind study, *Am J Obstet Gynecol* 188:419-424, 2003.

SECTION C Diagnosis of Preterm Labor

William Gosnell Sayres, Jr., MD

Early diagnosis of PTL is critical to tocolytic success. Tocolysis is less effective when initiated after the cervix has reached 3 cm dilation and 50% effacement.[1] Distinguishing true PTL from clinically unimportant symptoms often is difficult. Use of contractions as the sole criterion for diagnosis may result in error in 40% to 70% of cases.[2]

Labor is defined as regular uterine contractions accompanied by descent of the presenting fetal part and progressive dilation and effacement of the cervix. Cervical effacement of 80% or dilation of greater than or equal to 2 cm in the presence of regular uterine contractions would indicate PTL. Patients often present without all the features mentioned previously. The clinician is then faced with the difficult task of identifying women who *are truly in premature labor,* while avoiding inappropriate treatment of those *who are not.*

I. INITIAL EVALUATION OF THE SYMPTOMATIC PATIENT

Initial evaluation of the patient symptomatic for PTL includes the following procedures (Figure 12-2).

A. Establish Integrity of Fetal Membranes

The clinician should use a sterile speculum examination to evaluate pooling, ferning, and Nitrazine reaction. In this setting, an initial digital cervical examination should be avoided because of the risk of PPROM.

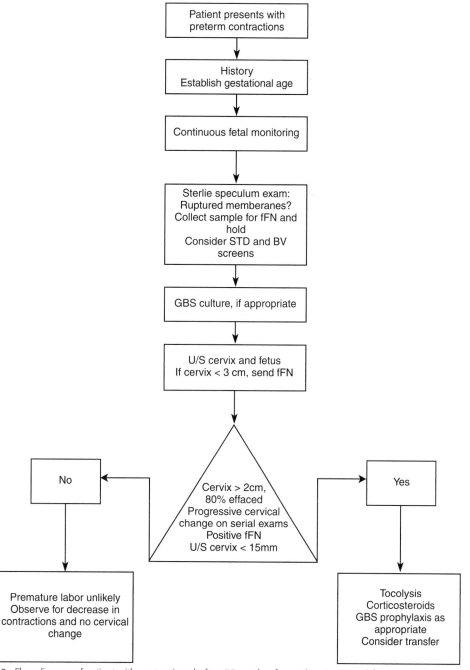

FIGURE 12-2. Flow diagram of patient with contractions before 35 weeks of gestation. BV, Bacterial vaginosis; fFN, fetal fibronectin; GBS, group B streptococcus; STD, sexually transmitted disease; U/S, ultrasound.

B. Infectious Disease Surveillance

Cervical cultures for gonorrhea and chlamydia are indicated, if not already done. Unless the patient is a known carrier, perineal and perirectal culture for group B streptococcus should be obtained.

C. Urinalysis

A "clean-catch" or catheter-obtained urine analysis is indicated to rule out infection, renal disease, and hypertensive disorders. Test results suggestive of infection should be sent for culture and sensitivity.

D. Fetal Fibronectin

Women presenting with painful, regular contractions can undergo fetal fibronectin testing before having a digital cervical examination. Clinical performance of the fetal fibronectin test is outlined in Table 12-1. The high negative predictive value of this test is useful in ruling out PTL. Confounders include previous digital cervical examination, coitus within 48 hours, vaginal bleeding, rupture of the membranes, abnormal vaginal flora, and the use of vaginal lubricants or disinfectants.[3]

E. Serial Digital Cervical Examinations

Serial cervical examinations are required to detect progressive changes in cervical effacement and dilation. Having one clinician perform these examinations tends to minimize differences in examination techniques.

F. Ultrasound Examination

Ultrasound examinations are useful for confirmation of gestational age, follow-up fetal growth, amniotic fluid volume, and placental location. An example of normal cervical length is shown in Figure 12-3. The dating accuracy of a third-trimester ultrasound is ±3 weeks, making this aspect of limited utility. A short cervix has been variably defined as 15 to 18 mm with likelihood ratios of PTD ranging from 6.7 to 14.3. For an example of shortened cervical length, refer to Figure 12-4. On the other hand, a 30-mm cervix yields a likelihood ratio of 0.2. A positive fetal fibronectin result increases the predictive value of a short cervix.[4]

G. Other Medical Conditions

Other concurrent conditions, such as pneumonia, cholecystitis, appendicitis, and viral gastroenteritis, may precipitate PTL. A thorough review of systems and physical examination should identify these conditions.

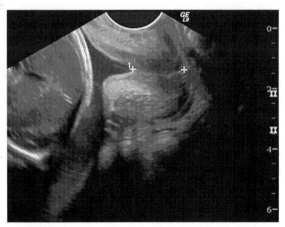

FIGURE 12-3. Sonogram of a normal cervical length. (Courtesy Donald Cubberly, MD)

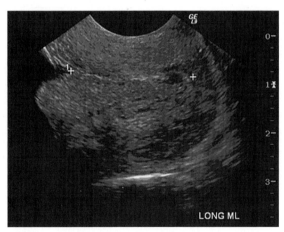

FIGURE 12-4. Sonogram of a shortened cervix. (Courtesy Donald Cubberly, MD)

II. DISTINGUISHING FALSE FROM TRUE LABOR

For the symptomatic patient who presents *without cervical changes* noted earlier, tocolytic therapy should be delayed until true labor is diagnosed.

A. Serial Examinations

Repeated gentle digital cervical examinations, after intact fetal membranes have been established, provide the clinician with the necessary information to make a diagnosis of true PTL.

B. Single-Dose Terbutaline

One dose of 0.25 mg terbutaline subcutaneously may abolish false contractions and shorten triage time.[5]

III. FETAL PROGNOSIS

A decision to treat PTL reflects the clinician's assessment that the risk to the fetus being delivered immediately is greater than the risk to fetus and mother of tocolysis. Tocolysis may delay delivery only 24 to 48 hours, time enough for glucocorticoid administration and potential maternal transport. With advancing gestational age, fetal prognosis improves, and incremental gains in prognosis decrease. Neonatal survival improves to 90% at 29 weeks, after which mortality decreases by 1% per week gained. Morbidity improves significantly until 35 weeks, after which delaying delivery exerts less of an effect.[6] The birth weight at which mortality ceases to improve significantly is 1600 gm, whereas morbidity improves significantly until 1900 g.[7]

REFERENCES

1. Yawn BP, Yawn RA: Preterm birth prevention in a rural practice, *JAMA* 262:230-233, 1989.
2. American College of Obstetricians and Gynecologists (ACOG): Management of preterm labor. Practice bulletin No. 43, Washington, DC, 2003, ACOG.
3. Ramsey PS, Andrews WW: Biochemical predictors of preterm labor: fetal fibronectin and salivary estriol, *Clin Perinatol* 30:701-733, 2003.
4. Gomez R, Romero R, Medina L et al: Cervicovaginal fibronectin improves the prediction of preterm delivery based on sonographic cervical length in patients with preterm uterine contractions and intact membranes, *Am J Obstet Gynecol* 192:350-359, 2005.
5. Guinn DA, Goepfert AR, Owen J et al: Management options in women with preterm uterine contractions: a randomized clinical trial, *Am J Obstet Gynecol* 177:814-818, 1997.
6. Copper RL, Goldenberg RL, Creasy RK et al: A multicenter study of preterm birth weight and gestational age-specific neonatal mortality, *Am J Obstet Gynecol* 168:78-84, 1993.
7. Goldenberg RL, Nelson KG, Davis RO et al: Delay in delivery: influence of gestational age and the duration of delay on perinatal outcome, *Obstet Gynecol* 64:480-484, 1984.

SECTION D Pharmacologic Management of Preterm Labor

William Gosnell Sayres, Jr., MD

Once the diagnosis of PTL has been established and expected improvement in fetal prognosis is believed to justify medical interventions to delay delivery, tocolysis should be considered. The data supporting the use of tocolytics are equivocal,[1] whereas the potential severe side effects of these agents affecting mother and fetus are well documented. Because the identification of true premature labor remains problematic, study inclusion decisions will affect outcome. For example, studies before 1990 might not have included administration of antenatal corticosteroids. PTL is the end result of a cascade of events. With the exception of the nonsteroidal antiinflammatory agents, all of the treatments discussed are aimed simply at inhibiting uterine contractions. Most future research will be aimed at elucidating the cause of premature labor and then at interventions earlier in the chain of causation, rather than at the drugs we currently use.

I. CONTRAINDICATIONS TO TOCOLYSIS

Contraindications to tocolysis are presented in Table 12-4, together with contraindications to individual tocolytic agents. Clinicians must consider conditions that may predispose the mother to complications of pharmacologic tocolysis. Conditions of pregnancy that threaten fetal viability, such as chorioamnionitis, also must be considered (see Chapter 16, Section C).

TABLE 12-4 Contraindications to Tocolysis

General	Relative	β-Sympathomimetics	Magnesium sulfate
Fetal distress	Preterm premature rupture of membranes	Maternal organic heart disease	Hypocalcemia
Chorioamnionitis		Poorly controlled diabetes, thyrotoxicosis, hypertension	Myasthenia gravis
Maternal medical instability			Renal failure

II. LABORATORY STUDIES

If use of tocolytics is to be considered, admission laboratory studies should include complete blood counts, serum electrolytes, glucose, and urinalysis. An admission electrocardiogram also may be considered for patients who have a history of organic heart disease.

III. β-SYMPATHOMIMETICS

A. Mechanism of Action

β-Sympathomimetics cause smooth muscle relaxation through activation of uterine β_2 receptors. Intracellular cyclic adenosine monophosphate levels are increased, reducing availability of intracellular free calcium. The affinity of myosin light-chain kinase for calmodulin also is decreased, reducing the sensitivity of the myosin-actin contractile unit for calcium.[2]

B. Metabolism

Excretion occurs primarily through the kidney. Half-life varies greatly among patients. Terbutaline and ritodrine cross the placenta.[3]

C. Efficacy

The use of β-sympathomimetics delays delivery of patients in PTL for approximately 48 hours. Outcome studies that measure neonatal morbidity (respiratory distress syndrome) and mortality have shown inconsistent results.[4] Once labor has been stopped with the parenteral administration of β-mimetic agents, oral agents commonly are prescribed.[5] This practice does not improve outcome and has high rates of maternal side effects. No demonstrated benefit exists for the prophylactic use of β-mimetics for patients judged to be *at risk* for PTL.[4]

The use of these drugs has done little to reduce the national rates of premature delivery. This lack of consistent research support for the use of β-mimetic agents provides a contrast with well-documented adverse drug effects and indicates a thoughtful and considered approach to their use. β-Mimetic tocolytics may prolong a pregnancy long enough to transport the patient to a center that is better equipped to manage a premature neonate. Prolongation of preterm pregnancy for 48 hours allows for the administration of corticosteroids before 34 weeks of gestation.

D. Adverse Drug Effects

1. Maternal
   a. Cardiovascular: The hemodynamic changes of pregnancy exacerbate the cardiovascular side effects of β-mimetic drugs. In particular, maternal plasma volume is increased (especially in multiple gestations, which present more frequently in PTL). Baseline cardiac output is increased in pregnancy. The more severe side effects generally occur during parenteral therapy. Patients with preexisting heart disease (i.e., valvular heart disease, coronary heart disease, and hypertension) are at particular risk for potentially disastrous complications, such as congestive heart failure and myocardial ischemia.

   Maternal tachycardia (average maximum increase in pulse of 40 beats/min) occurs in more than 80% of patients. Increase in maternal pulse is predictable enough that it can be used as a basis for dosage of tocolytics. Hypertension, hypotension, and an increase in pulse pressure may occur with β-mimetic agents. Nodal and ventricular cardiac arrhythmias may occur in 2% of patients treated parenterally.

   Congestive heart failure is the most common serious cardiovascular side effect of these agents.[6] Predisposing conditions include multiple gestation, persistent tachycardia (>130 beats/min), maternal infection, and iatrogenic fluid overload. There may be an association between antepartum glucocorticoid use and maternal congestive heart failure as well.[2]

   b. Metabolic effects: Glucose intolerance is believed to be secondary to increased gluconeogenesis. The use of β-mimetic drugs should be avoided in women with insulin-dependent diabetes because frank diabetic ketoacidosis may occur.[2] Hypokalemia occurs secondary to potassium influx into cells and does not represent overall depletion of stores. Potassium therapy is not necessary unless levels decline to less than 2.5 mEq/L.[2]

   c. Symptomatic side effects: Women frequently suffer from nervousness, restlessness, and anxiety. Although not necessarily medically significant, these symptoms may lead to noncompliance. Nausea, vomiting, and flushing may occur.

2. Fetal side effects

   Effects on the fetus appear to be less drastic than maternal effects and consist of tachycardia, hypoglycemia, hypocalcemia, and hypotension.[3]

E. Dosage and Monitoring of Therapy

For dosage and monitoring of β-sympathomimetic therapy, see Table 12-5.

TABLE 12-5 Administration and Dosage of Tocolytics

Tocolytic	Infusion Rate	Oral Dosage	Comments
Ritodrine	Initiate at 50-100 μg/min Increase infusion by 50 μg/min every 10 minutes until labor is inhibited, side effects occur, or a maximal infusion rate of 350 μg/min is reached Sustain infusion for 12-24 hours	Initial dose of 10 mg 30 minutes before stopping infusion, 10 mg every 2 hours or 20 mg every 4 hours for 24 hours Maintenance: 10-20 mg every 4-6 hours Maximum dose: 120 mg/day	Use caution in employing this agent. Assess for maternal and fetal contraindications. Monitor for maternal adverse effects, such as congestive heart failure.
Terbutaline	Continuous infusion: 250 μg/min loading dose intravenously over 1-2 minutes; 10-25 μg/min for 12 or more hours Intermittent subcutaneous dosage: 250 μg subcutaneously every 4 hours	2.5-5 mg every 4 hours	Apply same precautions as with ritodrine.
Magnesium sulfate	Loading dose: 4-6 g intravenously over 20 minutes Maintenance: 1-4 g/hr for 8-12 hours		
Nifedipine		Loading dose: 10-20 mg sublingually every 20 minutes for up to 3 doses Maintenance: 10-20 mg orally every 6 hours	
Indomethacin		Loading dose: 50 mg orally or 50-100 mg rectally Maintenance: 25-50 mg every 4-6 hours	Secondary agent used in gestations <34 weeks. Duration of use not to exceed 24-48 hours.
Glucocorticoids	Betamethasone phosphate or acetate: 6 mg intramuscularly, repeat in 24 hours Dexamethasone phosphate: 5 mg intramuscularly every 12 hours up to a maximum dose of 20 mg		Evidence strongly supports its use with PTL or PPROM before 34 weeks of gestation to reduce neonatal respiratory distress syndrome and mortality.

PPROM, Preterm premature rupture of membranes; PTL, preterm labor.

IV. MAGNESIUM SULFATE

A. Mechanism of Action

Smooth muscle relaxation occurs secondary to the reduction of acetylcholine released at the motor end plate or by direct effects through competition with calcium at the motor end plate or in the cell membrane.[2]

B. Metabolism

The kidney primarily excretes magnesium. Caution is indicated for patients with potential renal disease.[2]

C. Efficacy

Although in widespread use as a tocolytic, metaanalysis of available randomized controlled trials (RCTs) showed no effect on prolonging pregnancy, decreasing neonatal respiratory distress syndrome, or improving neonatal survival.[7] Early placebo-controlled studies of magnesium sulfate ($MgSO_4$) used lower doses than are now commonly in use, and this may explain lack of benefit in these trials.[8] $MgSO_4$ does show equal effectiveness as a tocolytic, however, in comparative studies with β-mimetics.[9] Compared with β-mimetics, side effects are less severe, and therapeutic drug levels can be monitored. Addition of this agent to ritodrine may increase the efficacy of the former, but the risk for negative side effects, particularly pulmonary edema, may be increased.[2] Magnesium levels of 4 to 8 mEq/L are thought to be associated with tocolysis.[8] Oral magnesium is ineffective in the treatment and prevention of PTL, and it is ineffective for maintenance therapy after acute treatment.

D. Adverse Drug Effects

$MgSO_4$ can have adverse effects on both the mother and the fetus.

1. Maternal

   Magnesium toxicity is dose dependent and can be anticipated by monitoring maternal magnesium levels and by neurologic examination. With proper precautions, magnesium is probably safer for tocolysis than ritodrine or terbutaline. Calcium is available for reversal of magnesium toxicity.[2]

2. Fetal

   Newborns do not appear to excrete magnesium as rapidly as adults and may show drowsiness and hypotonia. These effects are more pronounced when magnesium is administered for longer than 24 hours.[2] It is possible that use of high-dose $MgSO_4$ (50 g) may be associated with neonatal intraventricular hemorrhage.[10]

E. Dosage

Table 12-5 provides dosage information for $MgSO_4$.

V. CALCIUM CHANNEL BLOCKERS

A. Mechanism of Action

Through the blockade of membrane-bound calcium channels, influx of calcium ions, which usually occurs with cell excitation, does not occur, and contraction is inhibited. Nifedipine, which has few cardiac side effects, has been the agent primarily studied.

B. Efficacy

Calcium channel blockers prolong pregnancy. The NNT for prolongation of pregnancy by 7 days is 11. Delivery after 34 weeks is also increased. Although mortality is not affected, several measures of newborn morbidity are improved.[11]

C. Side Effects

Maternal flushing, headache, dizziness, and nausea are due to transient hypotension, which might be severe with sublingual administration of nifedipine.

Animal studies have shown a decrease in uterine blood flow with a corresponding decline in fetal arterial oxygen pressure and oxygen saturation. These potential effects do not appear to be important in humans. Blood pressure must be monitored closely.[2,8]

D. Dosage

Table 12-5 provides dosage information for nifedipine.

VI. PROSTAGLANDIN SYNTHETASE INHIBITORS

A. Mechanism

Prostaglandins appear to play a role in the processes of cervical ripening, gap junction formation, and uterine contractions, all of which are necessary for labor. Prostaglandin synthetase allows the conversion of arachidonic acid to active metabolites, including prostaglandins $F_2\alpha$ and E. It is postulated by some authors that PTL may be stopped by blocking this conversion.[13]

B. Efficacy

As with calcium channel blockers, large prospective studies of efficacy are not available for analysis. Prostaglandin synthetase inhibitors used for the treatment of PTL include indomethacin, sulindac, and ketorolac. Efficacy is similar to other tocolytics.[12,13] Maternal reactions requiring cessation of treatment are less than for other tocolytics.[14]

C. Adverse Drug Effects

Maternal effects are mild and consist mainly of gastritis. Renal effects must be kept in mind, especially in the presence of dehydration. Fetal effects are most concerning. Premature closure of the ductus arteriosus has been shown. It appears to be reversible and more significant at more mature gestations. Oligohydramnios can occur secondary to decreased fetal urine output, and it resolves with discontinuation of the drug. By potentially decreasing amniotic fluid volume, prostaglandin synthetase inhibitors may be relatively effective in the context of polyhydramnios. Primary fetal pulmonary hypertension and necrotizing enterocolitis have been noted with therapy of greater than 2 days' duration.[2,12] Because of these potential adverse side effects, family physicians should use these agents to treat PTL in gestations less than 34 weeks and for periods not to exceed 24 to 48 hours.

D. Dosage

Table 12-5 provides dosage information for indomethacin.

VII. ANTIBIOTICS

A. Group B Streptococcal Prophylaxis

PTL is an indication for group B streptococcal antibiotic prophylaxis.[15] Assuming a maternal colonization rate of 19%, the overall risk ratio for early-onset neonatal group B streptococcal disease is 1:100 in infants delivered before 35 weeks of gestation.[16]

VIII. GLUCOCORTICOIDS FOR FETAL LUNG MATURATION

A. Mechanism

Fetal lung maturation appears to be accelerated through the stimulation of surfactant release in alveoli.

B. Efficacy

Evidence from large, prospective RCTs is strong that glucocorticoids given before 34 weeks of gestation, at least 24 hours and not longer than 7 days before delivery, improve neonatal outcomes.[17,18] This intervention decreases the incidence and severity of respiratory distress syndrome and improves neonatal survival rates (Figure 12-5). Glucocorticoid administration also improves neonatal morbidity in the setting of PTL with ruptured membranes before 34 weeks of gestation. Table 12-6 shows the number needed to treat with glucocorticoids to prevent these devastating neonatal outcomes. Data on efficacy at less than 27 weeks of gestation are scant.[19] Repeat doses of glucocorticoids do not improve outcome.[20]

C. Side Effects

Maternal diabetes and hypertension may potentially deteriorate with glucocorticoid administration. Betamethasone used in conjunction with β-sympathomimetic agents has been associated with maternal pulmonary edema, although it (and dexamethasone) has minimal mineralocorticoid activity.[21]

D. Dosage

Table 12-5 provides dosage information for glucocorticoids.

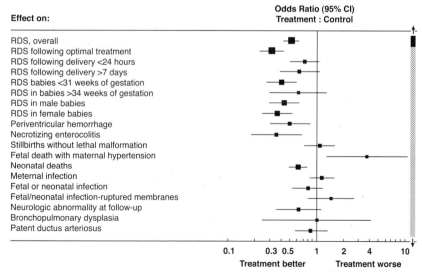

FIGURE 12-5. Effects of corticosteroids on fetal maturation given before preterm delivery (15 trials reviewed). CI, Confidence interval; RDS, respiratory distress syndrome. (From Crowley P: Corticosteroids prior to preterm delivery. In Enkin MW, Keirse MNC, Renfrew MJ, Neilson JP, editors: *Pregnancy and childbirth module. Cochrane Database of Systematic Reviews, Review No. 02955. Cochrane updates on disk,* Oxford, 1994, Update Software.)

TABLE 12-6 Corticosteroids before Preterm Delivery

Improved Perinatal Outcomes	Number Needed to Treat to Achieve Outcome
Decreased incidence of respiratory distress syndrome	11
Decreased incidence of neonatal intraventricular hemorrhage	9
Decreased incidence of neonatal death	25

IX. SOR A RECOMMENDATIONS

RECOMMENDATIONS	REFERENCES
β-Mimetics decrease the number of women in PTL giving birth within 48 hours (NNT = 7). They are associated with significant side effects.	1, 4
Administration of corticosteroids in PTL from 26 to 34 weeks reduces incidence of neonatal death, respiratory distress syndrome, and intraventricular hemorrhage in preterm infants. Corticosteroids are effective in PTL with intact membranes, PPROM, and hypertensive disorders of pregnancy (see Table 12-6).	17, 18

REFERENCES

1. Gyetvai K, Hannah ME, Hodnett ED et al: Tocolytics for preterm labor: a systematic review, *Obstet Gynecol* 94:869-877, 1999.
2. Besinger RE, Niebyl JR: The safety and efficacy of tocolytic agents for the treatment of preterm labor, *Obstet Gynecol Surv* 45:415-439, 1990.
3. Hearn AE, Nagey DA: Therapeutic agents in preterm labor: tocolytic agents, *Clin Obstet Gynecol* 43:787-801, 2000.
4. Anotayanonth S, Subhedar NV, Garner P et al: Betamimetics for inhibiting preterm labour, *Cochrane Database Syst Rev* (4): CD004352, 2004.
5. Macones GA, Berlin M, Berlin JA: Efficacy of oral beta-agonist maintenance therapy in preterm labor: a meta-analysis, *Obstet Gynecol* 85:313-317, 1995.
6. Higby K, Xenakis EM-J, Pauerstein CJ: Do tocolytic agents stop preterm labor? A critical and comprehensive review of efficacy and safety, *Am J Obstet Gynecol* 168:1247-1259, 1993.
7. Crowther CA, Hiller JE, Doyle LW: Magnesium sulphate for preventing preterm birth in threatened preterm labour, *Cochrane Database Syst Rev* (4):CD001060, 2002.
8. Lewis DL: Magnesium sulfate: the first-line tocolytic, *Obstet Gynecol Clin North Am* 32:485-500, 2005.
9. Berkman ND, Thorp JM, Lohr KN et al: Tocolytic treatment for the management of preterm labor: a review of the evidence, *Am J Obstet Gynecol* 188:1648-1659, 2003.
10. Mittendorf R, Dammann O, Lee K-S: Brain lesions in newborns exposed to high-dose magnesium sulfate during preterm labor, *J Perinatol* 26:57-63, 2006.
11. King JF, Flenady VJ, Papatsonis DNM et al: Calcium channel blockers for inhibiting preterm labour, *Cochrane Database Syst Rev* (1):CD002255, 2003.
12. Hearne AE, Nagey DA: Therapeutic agents in preterm labor: tocolytic agents, *Clin Obstet Gynecol* 43:787-801, 2000.
13. American College of Obstetricians and Gynecologists (ACOG): Management of preterm labor. Practice bulletin No. 43, Washington, DC, 2003, ACOG.
14. King J, Flenady V, Cole S et al: Cyclo-oxygenase (COX) inhibitors for treating preterm labour, *Cochrane Database Syst Rev* (2):CD001992, 2005.
15. Centers for Disease Control and Prevention: Prevention of perinatal group B streptococcal disease: a public health perspective, *MMWR Recomm Rep* 45(RR-7):1-24, 1996.
16. Regan J, Klebanoff M, Nugent R et al: Colonization with group B streptococci in pregnancy and adverse outcome: VIP Study Group, *Am J Obstet Gynecol* 174:1354-1360, 1996.
17. Liggins GC, Howie RN: A controlled trial of antepartum glucocorticoid treatment for prevention of the respiratory distress syndrome on premature infants, *Pediatrics* 50: 515-525, 1972.
18. Roberts D, Dalziel S: Antenatal corticosteroids for accelerating fetal lung maturation for women at risk of preterm birth, *Cochrane Database Syst Rev* (3):CD004454, 2006.
19. Morrison JJ, Rennie JM: Clinical, scientific and ethical aspects of fetal and neonatal care at extremely preterm periods of gestation, *Br J Obstet Gynaecol* 104:1341-1350, 1997.
20. Guin DA, Atkinson MW, Sullivan L et al: Single vs. weekly courses of antenatal corticosteroids for women at risk of preterm delivery, *JAMA* 286:1581-1587, 2001.
21. Gonik B, Creasy RK: Preterm labor: its diagnosis and management, *Am J Obstet Gynecol* 154:3-8, 1986.

SECTION E Incompetent Cervix

William Gosnell Sayres, Jr., MD

I. EPIDEMIOLOGY

Cervical incompetence plays an independent but related role with uterine contractions in PTD. The incidence of incompetent cervix has been reported to be 1 in 500 to 2000 pregnancies.[1] Although this area has not been studied thoroughly, it is likely that this condition does not exist as a single entity. Many other factors (i.e., preterm contractions) contribute to the premature dilation of the cervix. The diagnostic challenge is assessing the contribution of cervical incompetence to PTD together with the contribution of other factors. The role of other factors in this disorder explains the high rate (70%) of pregnancy success without intervention in women with a previous diagnosis of an incompetent cervix and the failure of some trials to show a benefit from cervical cerclage.[2] Because surgical intervention often is the treatment of choice, correct diagnosis is crucial.

II. PATHOPHYSIOLOGY

The cause of this disorder can be divided into congenital conditions and cervical trauma. In utero exposure to diethylstilbestrol (DES) is most commonly associated with congenital incompetent cervix, as well as with other female reproductive tract abnormalities. Visible abnormalities, such as the coxcomb or hood appearance of the cervix, should raise the suspicion of cervical incompetence resulting from DES exposure.[3] Trauma to the cervix may result in incompetence, although the effects are highly variable and depend on extent of trauma and maternal factors. Common sources of cervical trauma include precipitous delivery, overzealous mechanical dilation, recurrent induced abortions, and cervical conization.[4]

III. DIAGNOSIS OF INCOMPETENT CERVIX

A. Preconception

Although incompetent cervix may be suggested by historical factors, diagnosis is made on a functional basis. As cervical cerclage is commonly used, it is crucial to exclude other reasons for preterm cervical dilation (e.g., preterm contractions or infection) before making this diagnosis. Recurrent second-trimester pregnancy loss, especially with a history of rapid, painless cervical effacement and dilation, strongly suggests an incompetent cervix. Preconceptual diagnosis remains problematic because cervical anatomy and function are different in the pregnant state. A hysterosalpingogram may show cervical abnormalities and other reproductive tract abnormalities, which might explain recurrent second-trimester pregnancy loss.

B. Prenatal

Once pregnancy has been established, this diagnosis can be made on the basis of preterm cervical effacement and dilatation without other causes (i.e., uterine contractions or infection). Recently, ultrasound criteria for cervical incompetence have been suggested. At 20 to 28 weeks of gestation, 35 mm is the median ultrasound cervical length with a cervical length of 25 mm at the 10th percentile. Any findings of early effacement such as funneling are considered abnormal.[5]

IV. MANAGEMENT

Treatment of incompetent cervix is bed rest, together with close monitoring of cervical status and uterine activity. Elimination of risk factors for PTL should be pursued as much as possible. Ultrasound may be used to follow cervical status.[6] Trials evaluating the efficacy of cerclage placement for women judged to be at high risk for PTL and PTD have had variable results. There has been a statistically nonsignificant trend to prolong pregnancies but with an accompanying increase in hospital admissions, frequency of tocolysis, and puerperal sepsis.[2] A review of two RCTs of cervical cerclage for a sonographically shortened cervix failed to demonstrate improved outcomes.[7]

REFERENCES

1. Parisi VM: Cervical incompetence and preterm labor, *Clin Obstet Gynecol* 31:585-598, 1988.
2. Drakeley AJ, Roberts D, Alfirevic Z: Cervical stitch (cerclage) for preventing pregnancy loss in women, *Cochrane Database Syst Rev* (1):CD003253, 2003.
3. Kaufman RH, Adam E, Binder GL et al: Upper genital tract changes and pregnancy outcome in offspring exposed in utero to diethylstilbestrol, *Am J Obstet Gynecol* 137:299-306, 1980.
4. Jones JM, Sweetnam P, Hibbard BM: The outcome of pregnancy after cone biopsy of the cervix: a case-control study, *Br J Obstet Gynaecol* 86:913-916, 1979.
5. Harger JH: Cerclage and cervical insufficiency: an evidence based approach, *Obstet Gynecol* 100:1313-1327, 200.
6. American College of Obstetricians and Gynecologists (ACOG): Cervical insufficiency. Practice bulletin No. 48, Washington, DC, ACOG, 2003.
7. Beleh-Rak T, Okun N, Windrim R et al: Effectiveness of cervical cerclage for a sonographically shortened cervix: a systematic review and meta-analysis, *Am J Obstet Gynecol* 189: 1679-1687, 2003.

SECTION F Management of Preterm Delivery

William Gosnell Sayres, Jr., MD

I. MATERNAL TRANSFER

Intensive perinatal and neonatal care has improved the prognosis of preterm infants, especially those born before 32 weeks of gestation.[1] Maternal transfer is a necessary consideration when PTD is considered unavoidable and neonatal intensive care services are not available.

II. FETAL SURVEILLANCE

The decision to monitor the preterm fetus should be made with the consideration that the low-birth-weight infant is more susceptible to the deleterious effects of asphyxia and acidosis. In particular, asphyxia leads to a greater incidence of respiratory disorders and intraventricular hemorrhage.[2] Given the catastrophic consequences of prolonged asphyxia before delivery of the preterm infant, continuous direct fetal monitoring is recommended. Preterm fetal heart tracings are more likely to appear nonreactive than those of term gestations, presumably because of fetal central nervous system immaturity. Diagnosis of fetal asphyxia indicates immediate delivery.[3]

III. ROUTE AND METHOD OF DELIVERY

The debate surrounding the method of delivery of the preterm infant centers on the risk for intraventricular hemorrhage from decompression of the fetal head as it is delivered over the perineum. It is not entirely clear whether such a mechanism for intraventricular hemorrhage exists. The greatest influence on intraventricular hemorrhage is the birth weight and gestational age of the infant.[4] Prophylactic cesarean delivery of the vertex infant does not necessarily allow for a wider route of delivery in the preterm gestation and has potentially more complications than cesarean at term. Prophylactic forceps has been advocated as a way to avoid trauma to the fetal head but appears to have little therapeutic effect on the basis of retrospective studies.[4] Generous episiotomy has been recommended but also has failed to show improved outcomes in retrospective studies.[5] The lack of prospective randomized trials in this area calls for a commonsense approach. Prophylactic forceps cannot be recommended. Vacuum extraction is contraindicated in premature delivery. Use of episiotomy can be justified when obstruction at the perineum significantly delays delivery.

IV. ANESTHESIA

Management of pain in PTL is complicated by the enormous psychosocial stress the laboring mother might be experiencing. Because of potential depression of the neonate, narcotic analgesia should be used with caution, just as in a term delivery. Epidural anesthesia may offer the theoretic advantage of a relaxed perineum, although the potential fetal malposition and increased rates of forceps deliveries also must be considered. No prospective trials are available to recommend one method of anesthesia over another.

REFERENCES

1. Hauth JC, Goldenberg RL, Andrews WW et al: Reduced incidence of preterm delivery with metronidazole and erythromycin in women with bacterial vaginosis, *N Engl J Med* 333: 1732-1736, 1995.
2. Westgren LM, Malcus P, Svenningsen N: Intrauterine asphyxia and long-term outcome in preterm fetuses, *Obstet Gynecol* 67:512-516, 1986.
3. Bottoms S: Delivery of the premature infant, *Clin Obstet Gynecol* 38:780-789, 1995.
4. Barrett JM, Boehm FH, Vaughn WK: The effect of type of delivery on neonatal outcome in singleton infants of birth weight of 1000 gm or less, *JAMA* 250:625-629, 1983.
5. Platek D, Chazotte C, Schulman M: Episiotomy does not protect against intraventricular hemorrhage in the very-low-birth-weight neonate, *Am J Obstet Gynecol* 168:371-376, 1993.

Section G Programs Aimed at Identifying Patients at Risk for Preterm Labor and Subsequent Patient Care

Stephen D. Ratcliffe, MD, MSPH

I. BACKGROUND

Women who do not seek prenatal care are at significant risk for PTD. Provision of routine prenatal care, however, does not prevent those poor outcomes. Modeled after programs developed in France by Papiernik and later adopted by Creasy and colleagues, *enhanced*[1] prenatal care seeks first to identify patients at greatest risk for PTD. Patients then are observed closely in hopes of diagnosing PTL in its early stages and improving the chance of delaying delivery.[2] These programs have met with mixed results but overall have not been shown to reduce the incidence of preterm births. At a minimum, the adoption of a system such as presented subsequently would provide a framework in which newer developments might be adopted.

Continuous quality improvement (CQI) techniques have been used in medical settings since the early 1990s in an attempt to decrease variation in clinician practices and aim for improvements in care processes and clinical outcomes. CQI uses a Plan/Do/Study/Act (PDSA) model that provides continual measured feedback to members of the care delivery team that often results in an improvement in translating evidence into practice.[3] This approach has been successfully applied to a low-birth-weight prevention program in an urban setting and is currently being piloted in a family medicine practiced-based network in the northeastern United States.[4,5]

II. PROVIDER EDUCATION

All hospital, paramedical, and office personnel (i.e., receptionists, nurses, paramedics) with potential contact with pregnant patients receive an educational program aimed at improving knowledge of PTL. The purpose of this education is to streamline the evaluation and treatment of patients potentially suffering from PTL. Depending on the scope of the educational program and the community in which it is developed, community-wide awareness of PTL is increased as well.

III. CONTINUOUS QUALITY IMPROVEMENT PROGRAM DESIGN/ IMPLEMENTATION

The prevention of premature/low-birth-weight infants encompasses a range of biomedical and psychosocial interventions. Many clinicians serve medically underserved populations where the incidence of low-birth-weight infants is much greater than the community norm. These settings are particularly well suited to the design and implementation of prevention programs. The following basic requirements should be met before proceeding with program development.

A. Institutional Support
CQI takes time and financial resources. This effort must have the sustained support of top program leadership.

B. Program Leadership
Members of the CQI team should represent various members of the health-care team including clinical, nursing, front office, health education, finance, and other administration, and patients. Strong team leadership and team building increase the chances of success.

C. Obtain Baseline Measurements
It is essential to compile baseline measurements of existing care processes and clinical outcomes such as the incidence of prematurity and low-birth-weight outcomes.

D. Identify Interventions/ Process Measurements
The team collaborates on how to improve and modify existing care processes. Data collection tools to measure adherence to the new care processes are developed, and mechanisms to compile these measurements are implemented.

E. Enact Plan/Do/Study/ Act Cycle
Process measurements are collected and disseminated to the team members on an ongoing basis. On the basis of this feedback, the CQI can institute additional refinements and improvements to the care model.

Ultimately, the incidence of premature and low-birth-weight babies will determine the overall effectiveness of the model.

IV. PRENATAL INTERVENTIONS

The following evidence-based interventions can be used in part or as a whole to construct the low-birth-weight prevention program.

A. Baseline Urine Culture

Baseline urine cultures are obtained to screen for ASB. Patients with ASB are treated, and subsequent urine cultures are obtained at a follow-up visit for a test of cure.

B. Sexually Transmitted Disease Screening

Screening for sexually transmitted diseases is done at the onset of prenatal care and should be repeated at 28 weeks for high-risk patients.

C. Bacterial Vaginosis Screening

BV screening should be done at onset of care and at 24 to 28 weeks of gestation for patients with previous history of PTD.

D. Drug Screening

Drug screening should be considered for high-risk patients.

E. Periodontal Disease

Clinicians conduct systematic assessment for periodontal disease. When feasible, patients receive basic dental interventions to treat existing periodontal disease.

F. Smoking

Patients undergo serial assessments for smoking status.

G. Depression

Patients undergo depression screening at the onset of prenatal care, at 28 weeks of gestation, and in the postpartum period using a validated depression screen such as the Edinburgh Post Partum Depression Screen.

H. Domestic Violence

Patients undergo domestic violence screening and appropriate interventions.

I. Increasing Interpregnancy Spacing

Family physicians work with their clinical teams to increase patient knowledge and access to affordable contraceptive methods.

J. Use of Progesterone

Patients with a history of spontaneous PTD are candidates to receive progesterone 17 hydroxyprogesterone caproate, 250 mg intramuscularly weekly between weeks 20 and 34.

V. PATIENT MANAGEMENT

All patients undergo special surveillance for many of the conditions listed earlier. Other patients with increased risk for prematurity/low birth weight may undergo more extensive interventions such as the weekly progesterone injections. An attempt should be made to provide the appropriate level of ongoing level of risk assessment and screening to each patient by some member of the health-care team. This is quite compatible with recommendations of the Future of Family Medicine Project, which advocates elements such as chronic disease management using team structures.

REFERENCES

1. Goldenberg RL, Rouse DJ: Prevention of premature birth, N Engl J Med 339:313-320, 1998.
2. Yawn BP, Yawn RA: Preterm birth prevention in a rural practice, JAMA 262:230-233, 1989.
3. Eddy DM: Investigational treatments: how strict should we be? JAMA 278:179-188, 1997.
4. Ratcliffe SD, Horwood K, Kerber R: Using Geographic Information Systems (GIS) techniques to measure the impact of a low birth weight prevention program in a medically underserved urban setting. Presented at the North American Primary Care Research Group, April 1992, San Diego.
5. Ratcliffe SD, Coco A, Anderson J: The IMPLICIT (Interventions to Minimize Preterm Labor using Continuous Quality Improvement Techniques) FamNet: analysis of two years of baseline data. North America Primary Care Research Group Distinguished Paper, October 2006, Tucson, AZ.

SECTION H Preterm Premature Rupture of the Membranes

William Gosnell Sayres, Jr., MD

I. DEFINITION

PPROM is the rupture of the fetal membranes before the onset of labor before 37 weeks of gestation.

II. EPIDEMIOLOGY

One third of preterm deliveries are the result of PPROM. Risk factors for PPROM include infection, lower socioeconomic status, cigarette smoking, sexually transmitted infections, prior cervical conization, prior PTD, prior PTL in the current pregnancy, uterine distention (e.g., twins, hydramnios), cervical cerclage, amniocentesis, and vaginal bleeding in pregnancy.[1]

III. NATURAL HISTORY

The later in pregnancy the membranes rupture, the greater likelihood that delivery will ensue within 24 hours. Although the principal threat to the fetus in PPROM is prematurity, infection contributes to fetal and maternal morbidity, while playing a role in the initiation of labor. The principle threats to the fetus are complications of prematurity. Risk for sepsis is increased. Intrauterine complications include umbilical cord compression, placental abruption, infection, and pulmonary developmental problems. Maternal complications include infections and placental abruption.

IV. MANAGEMENT

A. Diagnosis and Initial Assessment

During the initial examination of the patient with PPROM, the clinician should never perform a digital cervical examination. A digital vaginal examination shortens the latency between rupture of membranes and onset of labor, and increases the chance of intrauterine infection.

1. Sterile speculum examination
   Direct observation of fluid from the cervical canal is the most reliable method of diagnosis. Having the patient cough or the application of fundal pressure may promote flow of fluid. Fluid in the vaginal vault may be tested for ferning and reaction with Nitrazine paper, although the latter test loses accuracy if the fluid is contaminated by blood, urine, or antiseptic solutions. Observation of blue fluid after transuterine amnioinfusion of indigocarmine dye confirms diagnosis.

2. Accurate dating of the pregnancy must be obtained
   Ultrasound evaluation should be considered in all cases of PPROM. Oligohydramnios supports the diagnosis of PPROM. Dating of the pregnancy and estimated fetal weight and presentation are important information to obtain as well, although these estimates are likely to be affected by oligohydramnios. Information obtained includes degree of oligohydramnios, fetal weight, and presence of anomalies.

3. Testing for fetal lung maturity
   Testing should be considered at 32 to 34 weeks. Vaginal amniotic fluid may be used to assess fetal lung maturity using the phosphatidyl glycerol test. Routine amniocentesis remains controversial, but it allows a more complete fetal lung evaluation and a chance to culture the amniotic fluid.

4. Screening for infection
   Cervical cultures for *Chlamydia trachomatis* and *Neisseria gonorrhoeae,* as well as distal vaginal and anal cultures for group B streptococcus, should be obtained.

5. Fetal monitoring
   Umbilical cord compression and infection may lead to fetal compromise. Nonstress tests and amniotic fluid indices are the mainstays of fetal surveillance (see Chapter 11, Section A).

B. Management

As in the management of PTL, the clinician is faced with balancing the risks and benefits of pregnancy prolongation versus early delivery when treating PPROM (Figure 12-6). Risks for prolonged ruptured membranes include chorioamnionitis and umbilical cord compression. Delay of delivery may allow for fetal lung maturation and administration of corticosteroids. The benefits of expectant management versus active induction of labor can be expected to be greater earlier in the gestation. The "conservative" management algorithm is based on publications by Mercer[1] and is predicated on gestational age. Prolongation of pregnancy after 34 weeks may result in

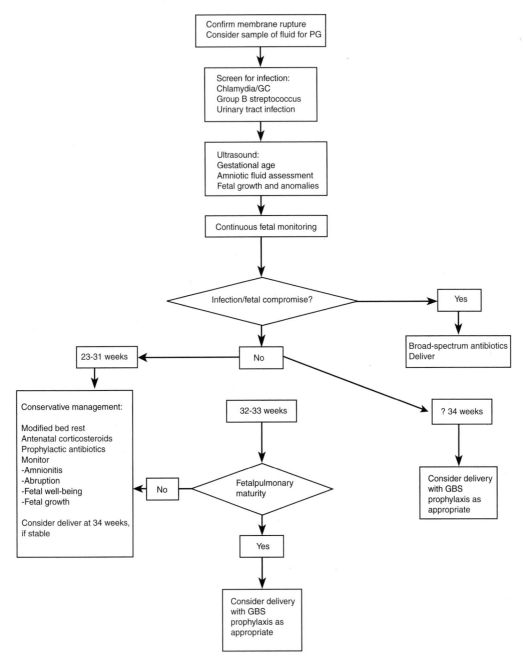

FIGURE 12-6. Preterm premature rupture of membranes at 24 to 34 weeks of gestation. (Based on Mercer BM: Preterm premature rupture of the membranes: diagnosis and management, *Clin Perinatol* 31(4):765-782, 2004.)

worse outcome.[2] Management of previable gestations is not presented.

1. Fetal monitoring
Nonstress testing is performed to identify fetal compromise and maternal contractions. Amniotic fluid index reflects oligohydramnios (see Chapter 11, Section A). The biophysical profile may be helpful in early gestation when nonstress testing is less specific.

2. Monitoring for infection
Maternal temperature, uterine tenderness, and fetal tachycardia are indications of intrauterine infection. Routine leukocyte counts or other parameters (such as C-reactive protein) have not been found to offer consistently any advantage in early diagnosis (see Chapter 16, Section C).

3. Antibiotic therapy
Antibiotic therapy has been shown to prolong pregnancy and decrease perinatal infections, neonatal intraventricular hemorrhage, and respiratory distress syndrome, whereas not reducing perinatal mortality (Table 12-7).[3] Ampicillin and erythromycin given intravenously for 48 hours followed by an additional 5 days of oral therapy was used in one large trial.[4]

4. Group B streptococcus prophylaxis
Unless cultures are negative and there is no previous history of group B streptococcus infection, intrapartum prophylactic antibiotics should be given.

5. Corticosteroids
Corticosteroids result in a decrease in respiratory distress syndrome and intraventricular hemorrhage in infants born prematurely as a result of PPROM.[5] Mercer[1] recommends treatment up to 32 weeks and in suspected cases of fetal pulmonary immaturity up to 34 weeks.

6. Tocolysis
Tocolysis does not improve pregnancy outcome.[6]

V. SOR A RECOMMENDATION

RECOMMENDATION	REFERENCE
Administration of antibiotics after PPROM results in delay in delivery and reduction of neonatal morbidity (see Table 12-7).	3

TABLE 12-7 Antimicrobial Therapy in Expectant Management of Preterm Premature Rupture of the Membranes

Improved Outcome	Number Needed to Treat to Achieve Outcome
Prolonged gestation more than 48 hours	9
Prolonged gestation more than 1 week	18
Decreased incidence of chorioamnionitis	12.5
Decreased incidence of neonatal infection	14
Decreased incidence of neonatal RDS	10
Decreased incidence of IVH	20

Data from Kenyon SL, Taylor DJ, Tarnow-Mordi W et al: Broad-spectrum antibiotics for preterm, prelabour rupture of fetal membranes: the ORACLE I randomized trial, *Lancet* 357:979-988, 2001; and Mercer BM, Miodovnik M, Thurnau GR et al: Antibiotic therapy for reduction of infant morbidity after preterm premature rupture of the membranes: a randomized controlled trial, *JAMA* 278:989-995, 1997.

IVH, Intraventricular hemorrhage; RDS, respiratory distress syndrome.

REFERENCES

1. Mercer BM: Preterm premature rupture of the membranes, *Obstet Gynecol* 101:178-193, 2003.
2. Naef RW, Allbert JR, Ross EL et al: Premature rupture of membranes at 34-37 weeks' gestation: aggressive versus conservative management, *Am J Obstet Gynecol* 178:126-130, 1998.
3. Kenyon S, Boulvain M, Neilson J: Antibiotics for preterm rupture of membranes, *Cochrane Database Syst Rev* (2): CD001058, 2003.
4. Mercer BM, Miodovnik M, Thurnau GR et al: Antibiotic therapy for reduction of infant morbidity after preterm rupture of the membranes: a randomized trial, *JAMA* 278:989-995, 1997.
5. Harding JE, Pang J-M, Knight DM et al: Do antenatal corticosteroids help in the setting of preterm rupture of membranes? *Am J Obstet Gynecol* 184:131-139, 2001.
6. How HY, Cook CR, Cook VD et al: Preterm premature rupture of membranes: aggressive tocolysis versus expectant management, *J Matern Fetal Med* 7:8-12, 1998.

S E C T I O N I # Conclusion

William Gosnell Sayres, Jr., MD

The prevention of premature birth remains a major challenge in U.S. obstetrics. Recognition of infectious, endocrine, anatomic, and most recently genetic factors in the cause of PTL have led to primary interventions such as antenatal treatment of BV. Rates of PTD nevertheless are increasing. Once true PTL has started, we can at best delay delivery for 48 hours to allow for administration of corticosteroids and possible transfer to higher level care. It is likely that PTL in many cases is the result of a complex, multifactorial process. Family physicians are uniquely positioned to intervene at all levels of the natural history of PTL from preconception and prenatal care to the posthospital care of the premature infant.

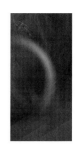

CHAPTER 13

Birth Crisis: Caring for the Family Experiencing Perinatal Death or the Birth of a Child with Medical Complications

Elizabeth G. Baxley, MD

For most people, the birth of a child is eagerly anticipated. Family members will be eager to see the new baby and, in most cases, will have developed expectations that the infant will be in good physical condition. Any significant variation from a healthy birth outcome is likely to trigger feelings of loss. In these situations, parents, family members, friends, and health-care providers all grieve this loss, often in separate and distinct processes of emotional adaptation. This chapter discusses strategies that health-care providers can use to support families who experience the birth of a child who is stillborn, premature, born with congenital anomalies, or has any other significant medical problem. A perinatal crisis can occur any time after the period of viability. Although issues of grief related to miscarriage earlier in pregnancy are relevant, they are discussed elsewhere (see Chapter 6, Section C).

I. PREPARATION FOR A BIRTH CRISIS

Perinatal death and the birth of infants with significant problems are inevitable aspects of maternity care. Preplanning for these types of crises by hospital staff is essential so that families receive optimal care and support when complications occur. Many factors affect how a birth crisis is handled. If parents are aware of complications during the pregnancy and have had some opportunity, even a few hours, to prepare for the possibility of an adverse outcome, they are likely to deal with it more easily than if

the problem comes as a complete surprise at the time of birth. In addition, problems that follow a relatively short and easy labor may be perceived differently than those that occur after an arduous and prolonged labor or a cesarean delivery. The social supports available to the delivering woman, as well as the woman's cultural background, substantially impact the manner in which the family experiences grief after a perinatal tragedy.

II. IMPACT ON FAMILIES

A. Maternal Reactions

Prenatal experiences often influence the intensity of the grief that a mother feels in the event of an adverse pregnancy outcome. This influence is related to the strength of the prenatal attachment that the mother has experienced. Lederman[1] defines behaviors indicative of attachment as "recognizing the individuality and attributes of the fetus, imaginative role rehearsal, thoughts about giving of oneself to the child, and fantasy about interactions with the child." Many mothers have a specific sense of the child after quickening, and often indicate this through use of affectionate names for the fetus.

Women are generally concerned about the health of their child during pregnancy and may feel responsible for a fetal demise or the birth of a child with significant disabilities. This feeling of responsibility is enhanced when there are preexisting conditions that may have affected the pregnancy, such as hypertension or diabetes, or if the mother made lifestyle choices that are associated with poor birth outcomes, such as smoking, alcohol or substance use, or poor nutrition. Remorse about lack of commitment to prenatal care or adherence to regularly scheduled appointments may also play a role in the grief reaction.

The fact that this psychological bereavement occurs simultaneously with the physiologic recovery from pregnancy and delivery can further complicate the postpartum course. Risk factors for more intense or complicated grief reactions include loss at a later gestational age, preloss feelings of low self-esteem and a sense of inadequacy, preexisting psychiatric symptoms, and absence of other living children.[2] Women with these risk factors will often benefit from referral for professional support after a pregnancy loss. Chronic posttraumatic stress disorder as a result of childbirth may develop in up to 1.5% of women.[3]

When a diagnosis of a severe anomaly is made during pregnancy, many women are faced with the heartbreaking decision of whether to continue or terminate the pregnancy. This situation often prompts a reevaluation of values and religious beliefs. A decision to terminate a pregnancy often is associated with feelings of guilt, in addition to the grief of losing a child. Because of the controversial nature of such a decision, many women keep the termination a secret outside of a trusted few family members and friends. This secrecy may lead to a feeling of profound isolation during the grief period.[4] When a prenatal diagnosis is made that is incompatible with life, a perinatal hospice approach may provide a meaningful alternative to termination of pregnancy for some women.[5]

B. Paternal Reactions

Fathers experience a sense of loss and responsibility at the time of a perinatal crisis, the severity of which may be influenced by their involvement in the pregnancy, the mental image they had of the infant and its future, or their perception of how the situation will affect their partner and their relationship.[6] Many men are emotionally involved in the pregnancy from the outset, anticipating the new baby, accompanying the mother to prenatal and ultrasound appointments, hearing fetal heart tones, feeling fetal movements, and participating in preparations for the nursery at home.

Expressions of sympathy from family members, employers, or friends that occur during the immediate bereavement period are frequently directed at how the mother is doing. Many men feel a sense of powerlessness to help their partner or infant at the time of birth crisis, which may be manifest in their becoming critical of or angry with medical personnel caring for their partners.[7]

Although fathers experience sadness, they also feel that they have to be strong to support their wives. Fathers typically find a role in handling the concrete tasks of caring for siblings, notifying family and friends of the crisis, and making funeral arrangements when necessary.[8] Some fathers experience a *double-bind* situation, worrying that discussing their feelings with their partner will upset her, yet being aware that not sharing feelings makes them appear uncaring.[9]

Fathers report that the social support they receive is markedly different than that directed toward the mother. They often perceive a lack of social acceptance for their own grieving, even though they may experience difficulty returning to their normal work and family routines, and adapt by developing an external appearance impression of composure.[7] Fathers report feeling a mixture of need for isolation and opportunities for appropriate support in their grieving.

C. Siblings

The grieving response of siblings to the loss of a baby may vary depending on the meaning of the newborn and his or her death to the sibling and the family. The intensity of sibling grief often correlates with the level of parental distress. Grieving parents may have a period in which their ability to be emotionally available to their remaining children is reduced. They may feel uncertain as to how to discuss the loss with surviving siblings, believing in some cases that they should shield them from their sadness and pain. A reluctance to talk about the dead infant may then be interpreted by young children as an indication of blame.

Young children do not have a clear concept of time and will often have difficulty understanding the permanency of death. As they experience the grief of other family members, their own feelings of separation, abandonment, and threat to security will need attention and reassurance. Toddlers through early school-age children may have concrete questions about death (i.e., "How can Johnny eat when he is dead?"). Preadolescents and teenagers may act out their feelings through behavior changes.[10]

Children need open and direct communication when faced with a death in the family. In the setting of fetal demise, young children need to hear clearly that the fetus or infant has died, avoiding the confusion that can accompany euphemisms such as "God took the baby away" or "The baby is in an eternal sleep." Encouraging siblings of all ages to discuss their understanding of and feelings about the death of the infant is important in helping children deal with the experience of loss. Books and stories about the death of pets or animals can be helpful in explaining the concept of death and associated feelings that can occur. Well-intentioned statements to older children that they must be strong for their parents may encourage them to deny their own feelings of sadness and should be avoided.[9]

D. Caregiver Reactions

Throughout a pregnancy, maternity providers and their staff also develop close relationships with the pregnant woman, her family or support persons, and the unborn baby. Physicians have characterized their response to a fetal demise or birth of a child with significant handicapping conditions as following the same continuum of grief as that experienced by parents.[11]

Complicating this grief response, providers are also faced with questioning their own care and management decisions during the pregnancy and labor. This questioning often leads them to feeling some measure of responsibility for the outcome, regardless of whether it is warranted. Physicians caring for patients for whom there is a sudden, unexpected death of an infant report fear that they missed something and that they might be blamed for the death. Nurses have reported similar concerns while caring for the laboring patient, often wondering if quicker recognition of potential problems might have resulted in a better outcome. These personal experiences of caregivers have a significant impact on their grief experience and the empathy they feel with the affected family.

E. Extended Family

Extended family may include aunts, uncles, grandparents, and close friends of the expectant couple. These individuals often share the parent's eagerness for the new baby to be incorporated into the family. The loss of an infant through fetal demise, or the perceived inability of the child to participate in usual family activities because of a disability, may generate expressions of loss and grief among extended family members. As with fathers, working through this grief process can be submerged or delayed as they support the parents of the deceased or handicapped child.[12] For these family members, expressions of grief often are not expressed fully until several months have passed.

III. MEDICAL MANAGEMENT

Medical management of the birth crisis must first focus on the medical stability of the infant and the mother. If an intensive resuscitation effort is required, some member of the staff should be assigned to provide support and information to the parents. It is essential that parents have the opportunity to see and, preferably, to touch their infant before it is taken from the birthing room. Only in cases of absolute emergency should this step be omitted. Absence of contact with the infant only generates more fear and anxiety, and opens the door for questions about the care that was provided. If the infant has to be moved to another unit, at least one family member should be invited to accompany the infant, recognizing that families may deal with this situation differently. For example, fathers may feel torn between staying with their partner at this time of mutual crisis and leaving to be with the newborn.

IV. PSYCHOLOGICAL MANAGEMENT

A. Timing, Location, and Participants

As soon as possible after birth, the health-care provider needs to meet with the parents. It is important that the meeting be held in a quiet, private room without interruptions so that everyone can focus on the issues being discussed. Anyone whom the couple wishes to be present should be included in the discussion, including older siblings of the infant, extended family members, and other social supports as identified.

Parents should never be placed in the position of solo decision making on issues that may have long-term implications. Grief reactions can become more complicated if the clinician unwittingly separates the parents. Talking with the couple together starts the process of open communication between them that can continue in the future.

B. Conveying Information

Parents often report knowing that there is a problem with their infant before or at the same time as the health-care providers. Therefore, a sensitive, open, and direct approach to communication is most likely to be successful. Trout[13] suggests that the first aspect of this interaction be the "facilitation of the love relationship" between the baby and parents. During the meeting with the parents, it is important to maintain a positive tone that emphasizes the infant's personhood and positive attributes, whereas realistically portraying the problems that exist. Information about an infant's death, or about the diagnosis of a child with significant medical problems, should be conveyed in a nonjudgmental, empathic tone.

It is necessary to balance conveying complete information to the parents at the initial encounter with not overwhelming them. Although it is essential that complete information about the infant's condition, treatment, and prognosis be given, parents may not be able to fully retain some, or even most, of what is said at the initial meeting. Care providers should acknowledge this early in the conversation and assure parents that they will return later to answer additional questions that arise.

Parents may differ in the ways that they process information and make decisions. Some are more comfortable with thorough explanations that include all the possible outcomes. These parents often are immediately prepared to take an active role in decision making. Others may wish the provider to emphasize what is most likely to happen without exploration of every conceivable occurrence. They may wish to defer to the physician or health-care provider's judgment in most decisions. Health-care providers should avoid making assumptions about what people prefer; instead, they should inquire about the level of information that is desired at the initial meeting. Addressing the process of communication early makes this an open topic for future discussions as parents adapt over time.

One of the most challenging things for parents to deal with is the uncertainty that typically exists in birth crisis situations. Health-care providers need to be sensitive to conflicting information that parents may receive from other professionals and from family members about what has occurred and what should be done. The quality and amount of education provided to a family involved in a birth crisis is a major factor in determining which families go on to function well and which families experience chaos and dysfunction.[14] Decisions that must be made should be framed in terms of the parents' own family values, whenever possible.

During the first meeting, it is important to review emotionally laden issues with parents. Physicians must be willing to hear a range of emotions, including anger, sadness, disbelief, or denial, that parents may express at the time of crisis. This catharsis is important in enabling them to proceed through the remainder of the grief process and to adapt to the situation. Mothers often wonder if their actions were responsible for the outcome and express guilt about perinatal problems but may be reluctant to voice those concerns aloud. A gentle, open-ended inquiry (i.e., "Is there anything you are wondering about that might have caused or contributed to this?") is helpful in getting parents to air their concerns and allowing an opportunity for the provider to reassure parents that they did not cause the poor outcome. Parents should be counseled about the range of emotional responses they may experience over time and be assured that the feelings that they have are normal and can be managed realistically.

Virtually every parent asks the question "Why me?" This question should be understood as a complex expression of emotion, in addition to being a request for information. Health-care providers thoughtfully respond to this question by considering both levels. Medical explanations should be labeled as offering a scientific answer to the question, and providers should differentiate between what is well-established factual information and what is informed judgment or conjecture. At the same time, providers should acknowledge that such explanations do not address fully the range of emotions that parents usually have and should ask about personal, spiritual, or religious beliefs. Parents should be encouraged to explore their values with trusted family members, friends, clergy, or professionals as a key element of working through grief. The acknowledgment that "you didn't deserve this" and "this isn't fair" can be a helpful initial response to the existential question of "Why me?"[15]

Important principles to remember when communicating with families include the following:
1. Avoid use of medical jargon.

   Understanding can be facilitated by avoiding the use of medical jargon and abbreviations, and by physically demonstrating equipment or showing pictures that depict relevant findings. It often is helpful to review the labor and delivery course, and to give positive feedback to the parents for their own actions and decisions when appropriate. When describing known medical syndromes, using common lay terms in conjunction with technical language is a helpful educational technique.
2. Provide written information.

   Whenever possible, parents should be provided with written information about birth crisis, the normal grief response, and any medical or social information that would help them deal with ongoing disabilities in the newborn. Preprinted materials, diagrams, and videotapes can help parents to process complex information accurately after a discussion has taken place.

3. Be realistic and hopeful.

In their discussion, providers should balance presentation of a realistic picture without eliminating hope for the best possible outcome. They should be willing to say "I don't know" when this is an appropriate response. Predictions should be avoided, as an individual infant's course can often prove these predictions wrong.

C. Examination

When an infant has died, it is important to suggest that family members see and hold the deceased infant for as long as they wish. If the parents refuse or are reluctant to see or hold the infant, it may be helpful to ask what they would like to hear about the infant. Positive regard for the individual child and family can be communicated by calling the child by name or, if the child has not yet been named, using the terms "your daughter" or "your son." Many hospitals photograph the infant, and some offer a lock of hair or newborn cap for the family to keep in memory of the lost child. The ability to hold, see, and touch the dead infant or the infant with disabilities often decreases parental fears and fantasies about these abnormalities.

Parents need to be made aware of any anomalies, even when a fetal demise has occurred. When family members view the body of an infant who has obvious physical abnormalities, it is suggested that the infant be dressed or draped initially in a manner that focuses on the normal-appearing body parts. Subsequently, the provider can examine the infant in the presence of the parents, gradually revealing and explaining areas of deformity. Positive comments on the normal aspects of the infant are important at this time, with statements such as "what perfect little hands." In the case of a child with disabilities, hearing that the infant has strong lungs, a lusty cry, or beautiful eyes helps the parents focus on their child as an individual.

Postmortem examination is recommended when there is no obvious cause of demise, and chromosomal studies should be obtained when there is a physical anomaly. The option of an autopsy should be presented in a respectful way that emphasizes the care that the body will receive and the benefits of this procedure to surviving and future family members.

D. Available Resources

Parents face significant adaptive tasks in caring for infants with medical problems or disabilities.[13] As the integral caregivers for the child, parents must have a sense of competence and strength before the child leaves the hospital. If a child is born with significant disabilities, parents may express concern about the child's future independence. An approach that balances realism, without eliminating hope, is appropriate. Helping parents to realize that a disability may not be as much of an impediment to future independence as initially perceived can help in their acceptance of the disability. Interactions always should end with a review of the information presented, a mutually agreed-on plan of action, and a specifically scheduled time to meet again.

Information should be given about the varieties of social supports and services available. These parents are faced with managing a child with disabilities whereas at the same time dealing with the accompanying economic decisions that will affect the whole family.[16] Health-care providers need to be knowledgeable about key community resources so that they can make prompt, appropriate referrals. Parent-to-parent support services can be particularly useful, filling a role that complements the work of health-care professionals. Families consistently report that contact with other parents who have been in similar situations, or have children with similar diagnoses, is extraordinarily helpful in providing emotional support, technical information, and resource guidance. Some hospitals and community organizations have established formal parent-matching systems. In other settings, this is done on a more informal basis. Names of parents should not be given to infant bereavement groups without permission. Likewise, professional or paraprofessional support agencies should not be contacted before receiving parental approval.

E. Coping

Parents may feel a sense of personal failure and fear that both they and their child will not be accepted as integral components of the family structure. They may worry that there will be extraordinary stresses within their marriage, and often seek reassurance about the impact of perinatal crisis on marital and family relationships. Support and assistance in dealing with family issues should be offered, while avoiding false reassurance, because marital and family disruption often do occur in these situations. This support is best accomplished by not assuming how parents or family members will react, but rather by being forthright and inquiring directly about such concerns and offering information about counseling resources.

Parents who have a child with a disability or chronic illness often struggle to accept and incorporate that child into their lives. They need to develop a sense of control in dealing with the child's needs and the changes necessary in their own lives. There is a potential for prolonged or recurrent feelings of grief among parents and other family members. These can occur at unexpected times and may be manifest in a variety of emotional forms. The coping process required in adapting to the birth of a child with a medical complication or disability requires the adjustment of internal values to allow reattachment after the loss of the idealized child. This adjustment typically takes place as family members strive to normalize life and progress through the child's developmental milestones. It is important for the provider to provide some anticipatory guidance to the parents about what to expect as they proceed through the grief process. Discussion of these feelings and the importance of being open to the support of others can be helpful. Informing couples that it is common for partners to be at different stages of grief at different times may reduce conflict and misunderstanding in the relationship.

F. Discharge Planning

Families who have a child with special health-care needs should have well-organized plans developed before hospital discharge. Parents should leave the hospital with concrete information provided about professional services, in-home supports, parent-to-parent contacts, and access to emergency care. Isolation often is the most significant factor in poor parental adaptation. As part of the emergence of empowerment, parents need to develop a sense of confidence about their ability to meet their child's needs before they leave the hospital.

Parents of very premature or extremely low-birth-weight infants may experience emotional confusion immediately after birth, often followed by a period of joy, and then reappearance of the negative feelings at the end of a long period of care.[17] Providers should be aware of this potential for a delayed crisis reaction and plan close follow-up care to assess parental coping. Active involvement of parents in the care of their premature infants can be helpful in alleviating the anxiety related to loss and impairment.[18] An intervention program that combines early crisis intervention, psychological aid through the infant's hospitalization, and intense support at critical times has been shown to reduce emotional trauma related to premature birth.[19]

Early and frequent follow-up must be scheduled at the time of discharge to assist in the family's ongoing adaptation. Postpartum depression is a possible manifestation of family stresses and inadequate supportive relationships.[20] Referrals to family-centered services in the community, including early intervention programs, parent organizations, and other resources, can be an effective way of ensuring that families receive the support they need.

Couples often inquire about how long they should wait before attempting another pregnancy. Although time should be allowed for parents to grieve the pregnancy loss, at least one prospective study has shown that early repeat pregnancy after a *miscarriage* significantly lessened feelings of grief for many women.[21] Rather than giving advice on the ideal timing of the next pregnancy, it is prudent for the provider to explore the parents' own feelings about timing of subsequent pregnancies, to answer questions they may have, and to relay information on feelings that might arise during the next pregnancy. These feelings include happiness, fear, or anxiety. Exploring ways of coping with these feelings in advance may be useful.

G. Provider Reactions

It is important for providers to be aware of their own feelings of loss when a birth crisis occurs. It is unreasonable to expect that professionals do not react emotionally to difficult situations. Families generally are quite accepting of care providers' expressions of emotion.

Providers should look to colleagues, friends, and their own family for continuing support. One study reviewed ethical decision-making processes among nurses and physicians, and found that there are significant differences in values, motivations, and expectations.[22] Nurses often place the highest value on a caring perspective, which entails responsiveness and sensitivity to the patient's wishes. Physicians may place greater emphasis on a patient's rights and a scientific approach that implies a major concern with disease and its cure. These differences may lead to communication gaps among health-care professionals and have the potential to interfere unnecessarily with the support provided to parents or families in crisis situations. Professionals need to communicate openly with each other to ensure that this interference does not occur. One effective way to do this is to approach the birth crisis as a sentinel event and conduct a multidisciplinary, systems-based approach to reviewing the care provided to reduce preventable complications in the future.[23]

Fears about malpractice litigation or professional review when unfavorable birth outcomes occur may undermine open and honest communication at a time when it is most important. Fear of blame, anxiety over the medical management of a case, or identification with a parent's grief must not result in provider avoidance behavior with parents, family members, or staff. A commitment to being present for parents at the time of and after a birth crisis is a critical role for the primary care provider.

V. CONCLUSION

For everyone involved in a birth crisis, the grief process is a necessary step in the healing process and, as such, is psychologically adaptive. Individuals move through a range of emotional responses based on their own individual needs. Recognition of these needs may affect the medical management and follow-up that is necessary. Variables that affect individual grief reactions relate to previous losses experienced, the meaning of the pregnancy to each family member, cultural influences that dictate accepted patterns of mourning behaviors, and the manner in which the birth crisis is explained and supported by health-care providers.

Considerable work has been done on the general principles of crisis intervention. The basic tenets include providing care based on individuals' needs; breaking down large problems into smaller, more manageable components; pointing out assets as well as problems; focusing on short-term goals; linking people in crisis with reliable supports; and planning frequent follow-up contacts. These principles apply well to the management of birth crises.

Acknowledgments

I acknowledge previous significant contributions from Ita M. Killeen, MD, Maureen Van Dinter, RN, FNP, CPNP, and William E. Schwab, MD.

REFERENCES

1. Lederman RP: *Psychosocial adaptation in pregnancy: assessment of seven dimensions of maternal development,* Englewood Cliffs, NJ, 1984, Prentice-Hall.
2. Hunfeld JAM, Wladimiroff JW, Passchier J: The grief of late pregnancy loss, *Patient Educ Couns* 31:57-64, 1997.
3. Ayers S, Pickering AD: Do women get posttraumatic stress disorder as a result of childbirth? A prospective study of incidence, *Birth* 28(2):111-118, 2001.
4. Bryar SH: One day you're pregnant and one day you're not: pregnancy interruption for fetal anomalies, *J Obstet Gynecol Neonatal Nurs* 25:559-566, 1997.
5. Calhoun BC, Reitman JS, Hoeldtke NJ: Perinatal hospice: a response to partial birth abortion for infants with congenital defects, *Issues Law Med* 13:125-143, 1997.
6. Theut SK, Pedersen FA, Zaslow MJ et al: Perinatal loss and parental bereavement, *Am J Psychiatry* 146:635-639, 1989.
7. Johnson MP, Puddifoot JE: The grief response in the partners of women who miscarry, *Br J Med Psychol* 69:313-327, 1966.
8. Worth NJ: Becoming a father to a stillborn child, *Clin Nurs Res* 6:71-89, 1997.
9. Puddifoot JE, Johnson MP: The legitimacy of grieving: the partner's experience at miscarriage, *Soc Sci Med* 45:837-845, 1997.
10. Gibbons MB: A child dies, a child survives: the impact of sibling loss, *J Pediatr Health Care* 6:65-72, 1992.
11. Mandell F, McCain M, Reece R: Sudden and unexpected death, *Am J Dis Child* 141:748-750, 1987.
12. Parks RM: Parental reactions to the birth of a handicapped child, *Health Soc Work* 2:51-66, 1977.
13. Trout MD: Birth of a sick or handicapped infant: impact on the family, *Child Welfare* 62:337-348, 1983.
14. Canam C: Common adaptive tasks facing parents of children with chronic conditions, *J Adv Nurs* 18:46-53, 1993.
15. Kushner HS: *When bad things happen to good people,* New York, 1981, Avon.
16. Kandel I, Merrick J: The birth of a child with disability. Coping by parents and siblings, *Scientific World Journal* 3:741-750, 2003.
17. Eriksson BS, Pehrsson G: Emotional reactions of parents after the birth of an infant with extremely low birth weight, *J Child Health Care* 9(2):122-136, 2005.
18. Mayes LC: Child mental health consultation with families of medically compromised infants, *Child Adolesc Psychiatr Clin N Am* 12(3):401-421, 2003.
19. Jotzo M, Poets CF: Helping parents cope with the trauma of premature birth: an evaluation of a trauma-preventive psychological intervention, *Pediatrics* 115(4):915-919, 2005.
20. O'Sullivan SB: Infant-caregiver interaction and the social development of handicapped infants, *Phys Occup Ther Pediatr* 5: 1-12, 1985.
21. Cuisinier M, Janssen H, de Graauw C et al: Pregnancy following miscarriage: course of grief and some determining factors, *J Psychosom Obstet Gynecol* 17:168-174, 1966.
22. Grundstein-Amado R: Differences in ethical decision-making processes among doctors and nurses, *J Adv Nurs* 17:129-137, 1992.
23. Nusbaum MRH, Helton MR: A birth crisis, *Fam Med* 34(6):423-425, 2002.

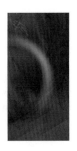

Management of Labor

Kent Petrie, MD, and Walter L. Larimore, MD

Family-centered birthing defines the birth process as a normal physiologic process that should be observed expectantly, positively, and conservatively with the expectation of a good outcome until proven otherwise and with the understanding that birth is a vital life event for the family experiencing it. The World Health Organization defines normal birth as "spontaneous in onset, low-risk at the start of labor and remaining so throughout labor and delivery… the infant is born spontaneously in the vertex position between 37 and 42 completed weeks of pregnancy…after birth the mother and infant are in good condition."[1] The aim of care and caring during normal birth is "to achieve a healthy mother and child with the least possible level of intervention that is compatible with safety."[1]

This chapter assumes that there must be a valid, evidence-based reason to interfere in any way with the normal, natural, physiologic process of birth. Birth attendants who practice evidence-based maternity care need to review critically the potential risks, benefits, safety, effectiveness, and cost of each tradition, practice, procedure, or intervention selected by them or the family. The effect on the encouragement and empowerment of the childbearing family unit, particularly the woman giving birth, must be assessed critically. Each intervention must be evaluated as part of the entire birth event, with the understanding that small, seemingly insignificant interventions may have a cascade effect on the entire birth and family.

Family- and person-centered birth attendants must understand that the *"maximin"* strategy and *worst-case scenario* approach practiced by many

obstetric providers,[2] when applied to low-risk labors, may not be as safe or satisfying for the mother, unborn child, or birth attendant as is a less interventional approach. The goal of family-centered birthing must include not only safety for the mother and child, but also the provision of the birthing experience as a positive stepping-stone into parenthood and family life. Childbirth may be experienced as a natural physiologic family-oriented event or as a *high-tech* medical procedure, an approach that has been referred to as "the industrialization of childbirth."[3] The experience often has much more to do with the attitude and approach of the laboring patient's medical and nursing attendants than with the mother's clinical condition. In most low-risk populations, more than 90% of women should be able to have a healthy birthing outcome without medical intervention.[4] The approach to the miracle of birth discussed in this chapter is one that should foster the normal physiologic processes and gain maximum benefit from the childbearing couple's inherent physical, psychosocial, relational, and spiritual resources. Any balanced approach to the birth process requires attentiveness to possible complications and an ability to respond to them appropriately.

This chapter bases its recommendations, whenever possible, on randomized controlled trial (RCT) data but, secondary to space constraints, references only the most important studies. When lacking firm evidence on which to base beliefs or practices, birth attendants should allow their patients to decide among the available options for those aspects of their birth care for which benefits have not been proved.

REFERENCES

1. World Health Organization: *Care in normal birth: a practical guide. Report of a technical working group,* Publication no. WHO/FRH/HSM/96.24, Geneva, 1996, WHO.
2. Brody H, Thompson JR: The maximin strategy in modern obstetrics, *J Fam Pract* 12:977-985, 1981.
3. Odent M: *The Farmer and the obstetrician,* London, 2002, Free Association Books Limited.
4. Scherger JE, Levitt C, Acheson LS et al: Teaching family-centered perinatal care in family medicine (educational research and methods). Parts I and II, *Fam Med* 24:288-298, 368-374, 1992.

SECTION A Normal Labor

Kent Petrie, MD,
and Walter L. Larimore, MD

I. DEFINITIONS

Labor is a process by which contractions of the pregnant uterus progressively dilate the cervix, then expel the fetus. *Term pregnancy* is 37 to 42 weeks of gestation. *Preterm labor* occurs before 37 weeks of gestation. *Abortion* is either spontaneous or iatrogenic termination of pregnancy before 20 weeks of gestation. A *prolonged pregnancy* occurs after 41 weeks of gestation. Pregnancy is considered *postterm* or *postdates* after 42 weeks of gestation (see Chapter 11, Section C).

II. CAUSES OF LABOR

The precise physiologic cause of labor is not completely understood. Decreased secretion of progesterone by the placenta appears to be one factor. As the placenta shifts from producing more progesterone to producing more estrogen, prostaglandin production (prostaglandin $F_2\alpha$ and prostaglandin E_2) appears to be stimulated, and these prostaglandins, produced by the uterine endometrium, decidua, and fetal membranes, are strong stimulants of uterine contractions. Activation of the fetal hypothalamic-pituitary-adrenal axis appears to play an additional role in initiation of labor.[1] It appears less likely that oxytocin of maternal or fetal origin plays an active or essential role in the spontaneous onset of labor. The most potent stimulant to the myometrium during labor appears to be prostaglandin $F_2\alpha$ from the decidua.[2]

III. ONSET OF LABOR

True labor is defined as progressive dilation of the cervix with uterine contractions. *False labor* is defined as uterine contractions that do not lead to cervical dilation. False labor contractions are often, but not always, irregular, of brief duration, and limited in discomfort to the lower abdomen or back. *Show* or *bloody show* is a small amount of blood-tinged mucus from the vagina and is thought to represent the extrusion of the mucus plug from the cervical canal and to be a dependable sign of the impending onset of labor, provided that the patient has not been examined. The blood loss is minimal; more significant bleeding must be considered an abnormal condition.

The classic definition of labor as it appears in *Williams Obstetrics*[3] is "uterine contractions that bring about demonstrable effacement and dilation of the cervix." This definition may be difficult to apply in patients in early labor with painful contractions but little detectable change in the cervix. A second approach is to define the onset of labor as beginning at the time of admission to the labor unit. Based on observations at the National Maternity Hospital in Dublin, Ireland, O'Driscoll and colleagues[4] state that, in the nulliparous patient, a diagnosis of labor and admission to the labor unit require uterine contractions accompanied by bloody show, spontaneous rupture of membranes, or complete effacement of the cervix (not necessarily with any dilation). In both the U.S. and Irish definitions, painful contractions alone are not sufficient evidence to make the diagnosis of true labor.

IV. STAGES OF LABOR

A. Dilation
Dilation of the cervix describes the degree of opening of the cervical os. The cervix can be described as undilated or closed (0 cm), fully dilated (10 cm), or any point in between.

B. Effacement
Effacement of the cervix describes the process of thinning (or decreasing thickness) that the cervix undergoes before and during labor. The normal nonpregnant cervix is approximately 2 to 3 cm long (or thick) and is said to be uneffaced or to have 0% effacement. A 3-cm-thick cervix that has thinned to 2 cm in thickness would be said to be about 30%

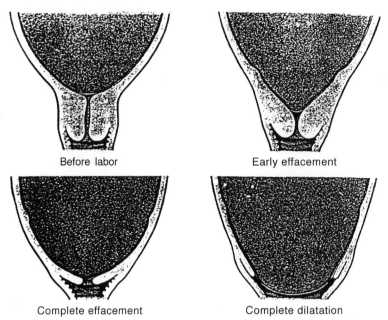

Before labor

Early effacement

Complete effacement

Complete dilatation

FIGURE 14-1. Cervical effacement and dilation in the primigravida. (From Mechanism of normal labor, Ross clinical education aid, no. 13, Columbus, OH, 1975, Ross Laboratories, 1975.)

effaced, thinning to 1.5 cm in thickness would be 50% effaced, and so forth. With complete, or 100%, efface-ment, the cervix is paper-thin. Effacement is said to occur from above downward, as the internal os mus-cle fibers are drawn upward toward the lower uterine segment. As a general rule, nulliparas undergo nearly complete cervical effacement before dilation begins. In contrast, multiparas can undergo dilation before significant effacement begins (Figure 14-1).

C. Bishop's Scores
The Bishop's and Modified Bishop's cervical scoring systems (Table 14-1) are quantitative measurements for cervical dilation, effacement, station, consistency, and position. In 1964, Bishop developed this scoring system, which quantified that the state of the cervix is closely related to the success of induction of labor. Bishop concluded that a score of 9 or more indicated that the chance of a vaginal delivery after induction was not statistically different from that observed with spontaneous labor. The American College of Obstetricians and Gynecologists (ACOG) still recog-nizes these criteria and suggests cervical ripening be accomplished before induction in patients with lower scores (≤4).[5]

TABLE 14-1 Calculating Bishop's Score

	0	1	2	3
Dilatation	0	1-2	3-4	5-6
Effacement	0-30	45-50	60-70	80
Station	−3	−2	−1	+1, +2
Consistency	Firm	Medium	Soft	—
Position	Posterior	Mid	Anterior	

Inducibility: 5 = multipara; 7 = primipara.

D. Stages and Phases of Labor
Traditionally, labor has been defined as having three stages.

1. First stage
   Prelabor is a term used by some clinicians as a period of increased uterine activity that occurs for a few weeks before labor. This uterine activity is believed to initiate softening of the cervix, some cervical effacement, or some cervical dilation. The first stage of labor begins when uterine contrac-tions are of sufficient frequency, intensity, and

duration to initiate and sustain cervical effacement and dilation, and it ends when the cervix is
fully dilated. The first stage of labor is divided into
latent (prodromal) and active phases.

a. Latent phase: The latent phase, first described
   by Friedman,[6] precedes active labor by a variable duration (1-20 hours), usually is characterized by less intense and less regular contractions of shorter duration, and can be difficult
   to distinguish from false labor. A prolonged
   latent phase is defined as being greater than or
   equal to 20 hours in nulliparas and greater
   than or equal to 14 hours in multiparas.

b. Active phase: The active phase of labor is characterized by regular, intense contractions lasting at least 60 seconds. The active phase of
   labor is more rapid and predictable than the
   latent phase, yet there is still considerable individual variation. In general, the active phase
   begins when the cervix is dilated to 4 or 5 cm.
   The 95th percentile for the minimum slope of
   cervical dilation for active labor in nulliparas is
   1.2 cm dilation per hour, and in multiparas
   is 1.5 cm dilation per hour. During the active
   phase, the fetal head should descend progres-

sively in the pelvis; however, failure for the fetal
head to descend should not be considered abnormal until the cervix is fully dilated.

   i. Duration of first stage: The average du-
      ration of first-stage labor in nulliparas is
      8 hours and in multiparas 5 hours. The
      duration of the latent phase varies con-
      siderably, with little impact on the prog-
      nosis for delivery. The rate of cervical
      dilatation in the active phase correlates
      with the outcome of labor.

  ii. Friedman curve: From observation of the
      progress of normal labors, Friedman
      described a graphic representation of pro-
      gressive cervical dilation for nulliparous
      and multiparous patients. Comparing a
      laboring patient's rate of cervical dilation
      with Friedman's average curves can detect
      abnormal labor patterns (Figure 14-2).
      Friedman divided the active phase of
      the first stage of labor into three stages:
      (1) acceleration phase, (2) phase of maxi-
      mum slope, and (3) deceleration phase.

c. Engagement: The fetal head can become engaged before or during labor. Practically speaking,

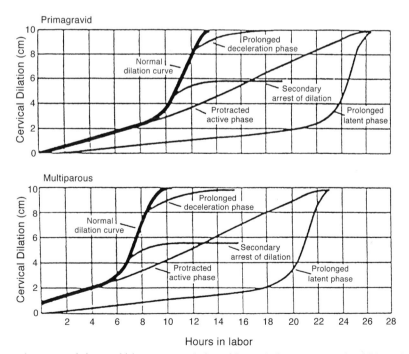

FIGURE 14-2. Composite curves of abnormal labor progress. (Adapted from Friedman EA: Disordered labor: objective evaluation and management, *J Fam Pract* 2:167-172, 1975.)

engagement occurs when the presenting part has reached the ischial spines (0 station). Engagement in the vertex presentation refers to the descent of the biparietal diameter, the greatest transverse diameter of the fetal head to or through the pelvic inlet (Figure 14-3).

d. Transition phase: Transition is the period of active labor just before the cervix reaches full dilation. Contraction pains tend to be most intense at this time and may be most difficult to handle. Transition often is associated with nausea and a premature urge to push.

2. Second stage
Second-stage labor begins when dilation of the cervix is complete, and it ends with the birth of the infant. Average duration is 50 minutes in nulliparous women and 20 minutes in multiparous women. Second stage is considered prolonged at or beyond 2 hours for nulliparas and at or beyond 1 hour for multiparas, if no regional anesthesia is being used. Second stage involving the use of regional anesthesia can be 1 hour longer (3 hours for nulliparas and 2 hours for multiparas). If progress is being made, most birth attendants need not intervene during a prolonged second stage, provided that the mother and fetus are stable, except to monitor the situation carefully and to encourage position changes. If there is continued progress, longer times are not associated with increased morbidity.

a. Cardinal movements of labor: The cardinal movements of labor, occurring in the first and second stages of labor, are shown in Figure 14-4.

   i. Engagement and flexion of the head
   ii. Internal rotation
   iii. Delivery by extension of the head
   iv. External rotation
   v. Delivery of the anterior shoulder
   vi. Delivery of the posterior shoulder

3. Third stage
The third stage of labor begins after delivery, and it ends when the placenta is expelled. The third stage has been divided into the phase of placental separation and the phase of placental extrusion. Retention of the placenta for greater than 30 minutes is generally considered a prolonged third stage and intervention is necessary.

E. Palpation of the Presenting Part

1. Identification
On initial assessment of the cervix, the presentation of the infant should be identified. Initial palpation of the cervix is contraindicated if there is a history of bleeding or rupture of membranes without labor. Vertex presentation usually is confirmed by palpation of suture lines or fontanel. Palpation that cannot confirm the identity of the presenting part with reasonable certainty should cause one to consider a transabdominal ultrasound examination.

2. Station
The relation between the fetal presenting part and the pelvic landmarks is defined by station. When the presenting part is at 0 station, it is at the level of the ischial spines (the major landmarks for the

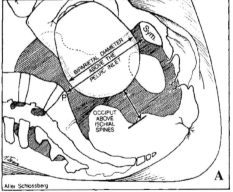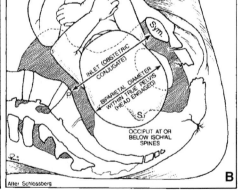

FIGURE 14-3. **A,** When the lowermost portion of the fetal head is above the ischial spines, the biparietal diameter of the head is not likely to have passed through the pelvic inlet and is not engaged. **B,** When the lowermost portion of the fetal head is at or below the ischial spines, it is usually engaged. Exceptions occur when there is considerable molding or caput formation, or both. *P,* Sacral promontory; *Sym,* symphysis pubis; *S,* ischial spine.

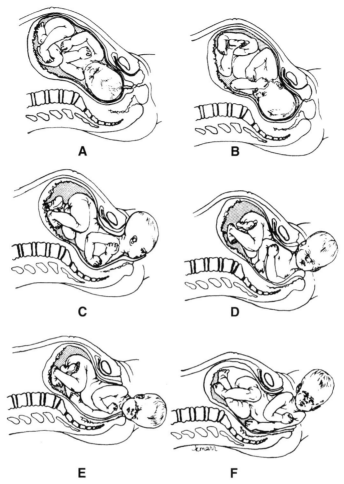

FIGURE 14-4. Mechanism of labor in the left occiput anterior position. **A,** Engagement and flexion of the head. **B,** Internal rotation. **C,** Delivery by extension of the head. **D,** External rotation. **E,** Delivery of the anterior shoulder. **F,** Delivery of the posterior shoulder. (From Niswander K: *Obstetric and gynecologic disorders: a practitioner's guide.* Flushing, NY, 1975, Medical Examination, with permission.)

midpelvis). If the presenting part is 1 or 2 cm below the spines, it is described as +1 or +2 station. If it is 1 or 2 cm above the spines, it is described as −1 or −2 station. The presenting part is defined as floating when it is palpated at −3 station or above. The presenting part is said to be ballotable when it can be pressed easily out of the pelvis and *float* up into the uterus. At +3 station, the presenting part is typically *crowning* (distending the perineum during contractions) (Figure 14-5).

3. Position
The position of the presenting part describes the relation between a certain portion of the presenting part and the surrounding pelvis. Anterior is closest to the symphysis, posterior is closest to the coccyx, and transverse is closest to the sidewall (Figure 14-6). The index landmark for the vertex presentation is the occiput, for the breech presentation is the sacrum, and for a face presentation is the mentum (or chin). For example, *occiput posterior* defines the occiput as being closest to the maternal coccyx, and *left occiput anterior* implies that the occiput is directed toward the left side of the maternal symphysis (Figure 14-7).

4. Asynclitism
Although the fetal head tends to rest in the transverse axis of the pelvic inlet during labor, the sagittal suture, although remaining parallel to that

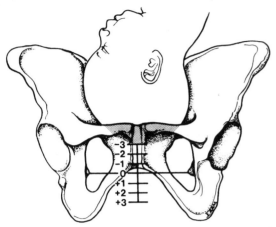

FIGURE 14-5. Estimation of descent of fetal head into the pelvis. Zero station is diagnosed when the fetal vertex has reached the level of the ischial spines. (From Niswander K: *Obstetrics: essentials of clinical practice,* ed 2, Boston, 1981, Little, Brown.)

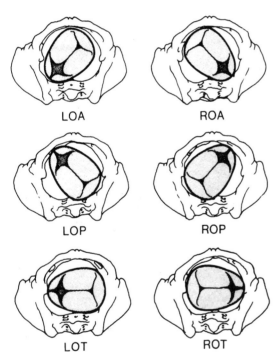

LOA   ROA

LOP   ROP

LOT   ROT

FIGURE 14-6. Vaginal palpation of the large and small fontanels and the frontal, sagittal, and lambdoidal sutures determines the position of the vertex. LOA, Left occiput anterior; LOP, left occiput posterior; LOT, left occiput transverse; ROA, right occiput anterior; ROP, right occiput posterior; ROT, right occiput transverse. (From Niswander K: *Obstetric and gynecologic disorders: a practitioner's guide,* Flushing, NY, 1975, Medical Examination.)

axis, may not lie midway between the sacral promontory and the symphysis pubis. The lateral deflection of the fetal head anteriorly or posteriorly is called *asynclitism.* Posterior asynclitism is deflection of the sagittal suture toward the sacrum or coccyx. Anterior asynclitism is deflection toward the symphysis. Moderate degrees of asynclitism can result in dysfunctional labor, and position changes in labor that reduce the degree of asynclitism are those positions that allow the fetal head to find or take advantage of the roomiest areas of the pelvic cavity.

5. Fetal head changes
   a. Caput succedaneum: During normal labor, the fetal head undergoes a variety of changes when in the vertex position. If the part of the fetal scalp overlying the cervical os becomes edematous before the complete dilation of the cervix, this swelling is known as *caput* or *caput succedaneum.*
   b. Molding: Movement of the fetal skull secondary to the flexibility of the suture lines is critical to the fetus during labor and delivery. Usually the margins of the occipital bones (and less frequently the margins of the frontal bone) are pressed under the margins of the parietal bones, or the parietal bones may overlap one another. This process, called *molding,* is quite important, especially in the contracted pelvis, because it may account for a reduction in the biparietal diameter of the fetal skull by 0.5 to 1.0 cm.

F. Evaluation of Pelvic Adequacy

Even in the most experienced hands, clinical pelvimetry and x-ray and computed tomography pelvimetry have limited application. Pelvic adequacy is proved only by a trial of labor.

1. Clinical pelvimetry

Clinical pelvimetry is the clinical estimation of pelvic adequacy. Clinically, the anteroposterior diameter of the inlet of the true pelvis is estimated by determining the diagonal conjugate measurement, the distance from the sacral promontory to the inner inferior surface of the pubis, which is measured clinically (Figure 14-8). A measurement of greater than 11.5 cm suggests but does not confirm adequacy. The interspinous diameter is estimated by palpating the distance between the ischial spines (Figure 14-9). This clinical estimate of the midpelvis requires experience. A distance of 9 cm

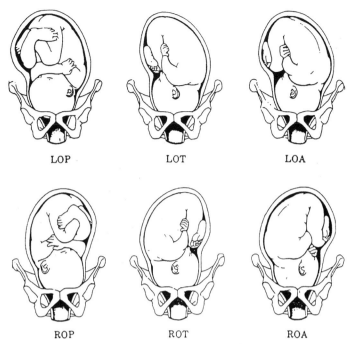

FIGURE 14-7. Various vertex presentations. LOA, Left occiput anterior; LOP, left occiput posterior; LOT, left occiput transverse; ROA, right occiput anterior; ROP, right occiput posterior; ROT, right occiput transverse. (From *Obstetrical presentation and position,* Columbus, OH, 1975, Ross Laboratories.)

or less suggests possible contracture. The arch of the pubis is the clinical measurement of use in determining the pelvic outlet. A contracted outlet with a pelvic angle of less than 90 degrees may contribute to obstructed labor. Prognosis for vaginal delivery in these cases often depends on the posterior sagittal diameter of the pelvis (the distance from the sacrum to a right angle intersection with a line between the ischial tuberosities).[7] Pubic angles greater than 90 degrees may decrease outlet dystocia.

G. Care in Early Labor

1. The "maximin" approach
   Birth attendants trained in high-risk tertiary centers often develop a *"maximin" approach* to labor, whereby they "choose the alternative that makes the best of the worst possible outcome, regardless of the probability that that outcome will occur."[8] This is also called the *worst-case analysis,* whereby "one accepts the least favorable interpretation of intelligence reports concerning the enemy's forces and intentions, and directs one's own strategy toward

the worst possible contingencies."[8] In the hands of clinicians who care for women at low risk, however, this strategy may be illogical, unsatisfying, expensive, and potentially harmful. The evolution of the management of normal labor in the United States into one that is increasingly interventional appears more often than not to have occurred without the support of RCT data. This chapter examines the data that support or refute many traditional labor and delivery interventions, practices, and procedures used to manage normal labor.

2. Family-centered birthing
   Many birth attendants approach the management of labor using principles of family-centered birthing and following a philosophy of avoiding unnecessary medical interventions and of fostering maximum involvement of patients in decisions about their care.[9] The elements of family-centered birthing are discussed in this chapter. The major goal of family-centered birthing is safe childbirth for the mother and the infant. Secondary goals include enhancement of the childbearing woman's social support systems, facilitation of parent–child

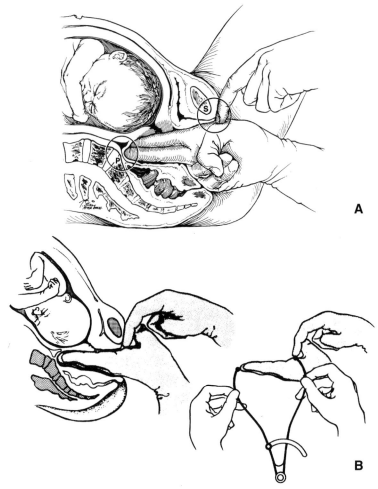

FIGURE 14-8. A, Vaginal examination to determine the diagonal conjugate. *P,* Sacral promontory; *S,* symphysis pubis. **B,** Estimation of diagonal conjugate measurement. Vaginal fingers reach for the promontory of the sacrum, with note taken of the point at which the symphysis pubis touches the metacarpal bone *(left)*. The distance is measured with the calipers *(right)*. (From Niswander K: *Obstetrics: essentials of clinical practice,* ed 2, Boston, 1981, Little, Brown.)

bonding, and equipping and empowering the childbearing family.[10-14]

3. The *P*s

In the past, many physicians viewed labor as a process that can and must be managed for pregnant patients. Standard maternal care text books discuss the three *P*s of labor management: *p*ower, *p*assage, and *p*assenger. Some have expanded these basic three to include two other *P*s: either *p*ositions (meaning position changes during labor and delivery) or *p*syche (meaning psychosocial preparation and support).

A case can be made that most labor does not need to be interventionally managed, and that knowing when and how not to intervene may be a higher order skill than routinely intervening.[15] Simply stated: "If you mess around with a process that works well 98% of the time, there is potential for much harm."[16] "In populations where medical intervention is used only when clearly necessary, more than 90% of women will have a healthy birth outcome without any intervention."[17] Asking the question "What then can maternity care providers do to keep normal labor normal?" has

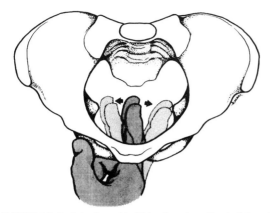

FIGURE 14-9. Palpation of ischial spines to estimate interspinous diameter. (From Niswander K: *Obstetrics: essentials of clinical practice,* ed 2, Boston, 1981, Little, Brown.)

led to the development of the 10 *P*s of keeping normal labor normal: (1) philosophy, (2) partners, (3) providers, (4) pain control, (5) procedures, (6) patience, (7) preparation, (8) positions, (9) payment mechanisms, and (10) prayer or spirituality.[18]

A considerable and growing literature suggests that there are interventions and noninterventions that maternity caregivers, payers, and institutions could consider, delete, or provide that would increase their likelihood of keeping normal labor normal. Many of these are discussed in this chapter.

4. Sterile vaginal examination on admission
Use of sterile gloves during all vaginal examinations during pregnancy, labor, and delivery is recommended.[19] Repeated or frequent vaginal examinations, especially by more than one caregiver, should be avoided as much as possible. Rectal examinations have virtually no place in the birth setting.

If rupture of the membranes is suspected in the patient at term but cannot be confirmed with perineal observation, the cervix can be visualized by using a sterile speculum, carefully inserted, so as to visualize any fluid in the posterior vaginal fornix. A digital examination should be avoided if the patient does not appear to be in active labor. Vernix or meconium, when observed, confirms the rupture of the membranes and the presence of amniotic fluid. If the fluid present is still in question, a sample may be collected for testing. If no fluid is seen, the fetus may be pushed out of the pelvis with a hand placed above the pubis,

externally, by an assistant, and the cervix visualized during this process for leakage of fluid. If none is seen, fluid from the os can be collected for testing.

a. Nitrazine test: The basis for the Nitrazine test is that the normal pH of the vaginal secretions is 2.5 to 4.5 (acidic), and the pH of the amniotic fluid is usually 7.0 to 7.5 (neutral). Nitrazine test papers can be used to evaluate secretion pH colorimetrically. A sterile swab can be used to collect the secretions or fluid, which is touched to the Nitrazine paper, and the color obtained is compared with a color chart. Ruptured membranes can be indicated by a pH of 6.5 to 7.5 (blue/green, blue/gray, or deep blue). Intact membranes can be indicated by a pH of less than 4.5 (yellow, olive/yellow, or olive/green). False-positive Nitrazine readings may occur with a bloody show, with cervical mucus, or in the presence of semen.

b. Ferning: Amniotic fluid if placed on a microscope slide and allowed to air-dry can be examined under a microscope and is seen to look like the fronds of a Boston fern. Normal vaginal secretions produce a granular pattern when dried on a microscope slide.

5. Subsequent vaginal examinations during labor
Although there is no standard frequency of vaginal examinations during labor, examinations should be kept to a minimum to avoid intraamniotic infection.[1] Examinations should be performed only at the following times:

a. On admission

b. At 1- to 4-hour intervals in the first stage and at 1-hour intervals in the second stage depending on the patient's progress

c. At rupture of membranes to evaluate cord prolapse

d. Before intrapartum administration of analgesia

e. With the patient's urge to push to document complete dilation

f. If problems occur, such as nonreassuring fetal heart rate (FHR) patterns

H. Labor Interventions

1. Nothing by mouth (NPO) and intravenous (IV) fluids
NPO, the tradition of routinely withholding food and drink during labor, has been practiced widely in the past. As recently as 1985, one obstetric textbook states, "In essentially all circumstances, food

and oral fluids should be withheld during active labor and delivery."[20] The traditional rationale is to prevent aspiration; however, the risk appears to be low, and aspiration has not been reported as a significant cause of maternal morbidity and mortality. Birth attendants using NPO policy typically use IV fluids. Routine NPO and IV fluid policies lack supporting scientific evidence and may pose risks, such as immobilization, fluid overload, and maternal hyperglycemia.[7,9,21] When given the choice, most women prefer taking oral liquids in labor. A reasonable alternative for a woman who does not want or need IV fluids, but may desire IV access later in labor (i.e., for pain medications), is a heparin lock.

2. Enemas

Enemas in early labor have traditionally been used in the belief that they shorten labor, reduce pain, and reduce fecal contamination. No studies have shown a difference in duration of labor of women who did or did not receive an enema. No data have been reported of increased neonatal infection or increased perineal wound infections in women who do not have an enema. In fact, no medical evidence supports the routine use of enemas in laboring women.[21] One metaanalysis states, "There is insufficient evidence to recommend the use of enemas during labor. Enemas generate discomfort and generate costs and unless there is evidence to promote their use, this should be discouraged."[22]

3. Perineal shaving

Perineal shaves or shaving the pubic hair in labor is commonly used in some settings. Traditionally, shaving was performed to reduce wound infections and to improve wound approximation. Shaving the skin does not diminish surgical wound infections, however, and preoperative cleaning without shaving results in less likelihood of infection. Shaving can lead to increased postpartum discomfort. Routine shaving of the perineum in laboring women is neither desirable nor necessary.[1,5,23] In cases in which the perineal hair is long or dense, these hairs can be clipped shorter if necessary for laceration repair. When given the choice, most women prefer avoiding routine perineal shaving.

4. Amniotomy

Amniotomy, or deliberate rupture of the fetal membranes, is a well-established tradition of labor in the United States. Reported purposes for amniotomy include evaluation of the amniotic fluid for meconium, ease in applying internal monitoring devices, and reduction of time in labor. Potential adverse effects have been suggested, however, including cord prolapse, maternal or fetal infection, fetal laceration or scalp infection, fetal cephalohematoma, increased caput, and increased malalignment of fetal cranial bones. Animal studies report greater force of cervical dilation with the head alone than when fetal membranes are intact. Most of the RCTs show that amniotomy performed between 3 and 6 cm dilation shortens labor by 1 to 2 hours and show a trend toward reduction in the use of oxytocin and 5-minute Apgar score of less than 7.[24] One RCT showed that amniotomy reduced the incidence of dystocia, defined as a period of at least 4 hours, after 3 cm dilation, with a mean rate of dilatation of less than 0.5 cm/hr.[25] Most RCTs on amniotomy occurred in centers where a large percentage of the mothers received epidural anesthesia.[24,26]

The Cochrane review states:

The trend toward an increase in caesarean section rate seen in the metaanalysis, combined with the (unpublished) evidence of an increase in the hourly rate of fetal heart abnormalities, and the increase in the frequency of caesarean section for fetal distress observed in one multicenter trial suggest that we should temper our enthusiasm for a policy of routine early amniotomy. Adverse effects of amniotomy (on FHR tracings, and consequently, on the risk of caesarean section for fetal distress) are likely to be greatest in centers where electronic fetal monitoring (EFM) is routinely used without fetal scalp blood sampling as an adjunct. These effects would likely be attenuated by fetal blood sampling, by amnioinfusion in the presence of worrisome variable decelerations, or by a combination of both. In essence, this implies providing interventions to minimize the secondary effects of a previous routine intervention. Given the current state of knowledge, it would seem to be a reasonable approach to reserve amniotomy for labors which are progressing slowing.[24]

If amniotomy is to be performed during labor, the following criteria should be met:

a. Vertex presentation

b. Engagement in the pelvis; if there is polyhydramnios or an unengaged presenting part, it is prudent to puncture the membranes with a small-gauge needle to avoid cord prolapse

c. Adequate cervical dilatation to allow an atraumatic procedure but at least 3 cm dilatation

d. Evaluation of fetal heart tones immediately before and after the procedure

5. Active management of labor (AML)

O'Driscoll and colleagues[4] in the early 1970s introduced the practice of AML in primigravidas at National Maternity Hospital in Dublin, Ireland. The original goal of AML was to ensure delivery of every patient within 12 hours of admission for labor. AML now is recognized as a nulliparous labor management regimen that has kept primary cesarean delivery rates low (5-7%) and stable over 30 years at the National Maternity Hospital. During this same time frame, the cesarean delivery rate in the United States has seen a sixfold increase. There has been considerable interest in adapting aspects of AML to settings in the United States.

The Irish AML protocol applies to nulliparous patients with a singleton fetus in the vertex position; in the absence of fetal distress, meconium, macrosomia, malposition, and major bleeding; includes the presence of a midwife throughout labor; and includes extensive prenatal education. Outcome data from four RCTs in the United States currently do not show strong support that the routine use of AML confers clear benefits for nulliparous patients. Most centers in the United States using the AML protocol do not provide the labor support services listed in the Irish studies; therefore, the results obtained may not be equally beneficial. The key elements of AML used at the National Maternity Hospital in Dublin are as follows:

a. Standard antenatal education program: Nulliparous patients are taught that once a diagnosis of labor is made, they will most likely deliver within 12 hours and will receive constant supportive care by a nurse-midwife.

b. Precise diagnosis of labor: Applying the labor criteria of regular, painful contractions in the presence of complete cervical effacement, rupture of membranes, or bloody show, an attempt is made to keep this diagnosis precise.

c. Amniotomy: An amniotomy is performed after diagnosing labor.

d. Continuous emotional support: A nurse-midwife provides constant nursing and emotional support throughout the labor process.

e. Intermittent fetal auscultation and movement in labor: Patients are encouraged to ambulate during labor and are monitored on an intermittent basis using fetal auscultation.

f. Prompt diagnosis and treatment of ineffective uterine contractions: Progress of labor that is not making approximately 1 cm/hr of cervical dilation is treated with the institution of oxytocin augmentation using an initial rate of 4 to 6 mU/min and increased in those increments until a maximum infusion rate of 34 to 40 mU/min. These doses would be considered high, excessive, or dangerous in most U.S. hospitals. Patients in Dublin often are allowed to be off the monitor (intermittent auscultation [IA] is used) and out of bed while on oxytocin, likely affecting outcomes. Oxytocin is also commonly started in the second stage when progress and descent are slow.

g. Continuous Internal Medical Audit: Every nulliparous labor record is reviewed on a weekly basis to monitor for compliance with the labor management protocol.

The largest American trial of AML that attempted to replicate the entire Irish model did not demonstrate a decrease in cesarean delivery rate.[27] Major differences existed in continuous electronic FHR monitoring, ambulation in labor, and in the second stage management, where cesarean rates were eight times greater than in the Irish studies. Initiation of oxytocin in the second stage was a key factor. A metaanalysis of the three best North American studies of AML did show a decrease in primary cesarean delivery rate by 34% (odds ratio [OR], 0.66; 95% confidence interval [CI], 0.54-0.81), making the components of AML worthy of consideration in family-centered maternity care.[28]

V. ALTERNATIVES IN DELIVERY SITES

In the United States, the options for delivery sites have expanded from conventional hospital obstetric units to in-hospital birthing units, freestanding birth centers, home birth centers, and the family's home. Traditional labor care in the United States assumes that hospitals are the safest place for every birth. Proponents of nonhospital alternatives emphasize their ability to identify high-risk women with intrapartum complications at an early, not yet serious, stage and rapidly transfer patients who need immediate hospital care. Skeptics point to the impreciseness of risk prediction for labor, however.

Proponents of out-of-hospital delivery believe that hospital complications appear to arise without warning because few hospital care providers remain with their patients throughout the entire labor. Early signs and symptoms of complications may remain unrecognized until the *apparent-sudden* emergency. Proponents also point out the risks of being in a hospital in general, including iatrogenic complications, negative side effects to medications, negative side effects to technology, nosocomial infections, and iatrogenic cesarean birth rate.

Many reports have been published on the outcomes of nonhospital childbirth practices. Most of these have been retrospective and limited to states or intrastate regions. Accumulation of these data cannot resolve the safety questions because outpatient practices that experience poor outcomes rarely publish their results, and small retrospective studies on almost any topic skew toward success. In 2000, the Cochrane Library, in its metaanalysis on home versus hospital birthing, concluded: "There is no strong evidence to favor either home or hospital birth for selected, low-risk pregnant women. In countries and areas where it is possible to establish a home birth service backed up by a modern hospital system, all low-risk pregnant women should be offered the possibility of considering a planned home birth and they should be informed about the quality of the available evidence to guide their choice."[29]

A more recent Cochrane review in 2005 found benefits for "homelike" versus conventional institutional settings for birth.[30] Six trials of in-hospital low-intervention birthing room deliveries of 8677 women were reviewed and the investigators concluded: "Home-like birth settings are intended for women who prefer to avoid medical intervention during labor and birth, but who either do not wish or cannot have a home birth. The results of six trials suggest modest benefits, including decreased medical intervention and higher rates of spontaneous vaginal birth, breastfeeding, and maternal satisfaction."[30]

This chapter confines its discussion primarily to in-hospital care. The principles and practices suggested can be applied equally by the maternity caregiver in any labor setting.

VI. SUMMARY

After initially admitting and evaluating a woman in labor, routine procedures, protocols, or practices that lack evidence of benefit to the mother or to the fetus should remain the choice of the childbearing family. Birth attendants need to be aware of data that affect these decisions to manage laboring women with a more flexible and individual plan. Clinicians who adhere to routine plans and traditions, the safety or efficacy of which is not substantiated in the medical literature, do so only to comfort themselves. The low-risk laboring woman should have the right to decide the aspects of care for which benefits are small or unproved.

VII. SOR A RECOMMENDATIONS

RECOMMENDATIONS	REFERENCES
No evidence has been reported to support routine enemas or perineal shaving during labor.	22, 23
A homelike in-hospital birth setting increases the rates of spontaneous vaginal delivery, breastfeeding, and maternal satisfaction with the birth experience.	30
Routine early amniotomy shortens labor but is associated with a trend toward increased cesarean delivery for fetal distress. Amniotomy should therefore be reserved for patients with abnormal labor progress.	24
AML, particularly initiation of oxytocin in the second stage for lack of labor progress, can reduce cesarean delivery rates.	28

REFERENCES

1. Funai EF, Norwitz ER: Normal labor and delivery, *UpTodate Online* 1:1-20, 2007. Available at: www.uptodate.com.
2. Cunningham FG, editor: Parturition theories. In *Williams obstetrics,* ed 21, Norwalk, CT, 2001, McGraw-Hill.
3. Cunningham FG, editor: Normal labor. In *Williams obstetrics,* ed 21, Norwalk, CT, 2001, McGraw-Hill.
4. O'Driscoll K, Foley M, MacDonald D: Active management of labor as an alternative to cesarean section for dystocia, *Obstet Gynecol* 63:485-490, 1984.
5. ACOG practice bulletin. Induction of labor, number 10, 1999, Washington, DC, 1999, American College of Obstetricians and Gynecologists.

6. Friedman EA: *Labor: clinical evaluation and management,* ed 2, New York, 1978, Appleton, Century, Crofts.

7. Enkin MW, Keirse MJNC, Renfrew MJ, Neilson J: *A guide to effective care in pregnancy and childbirth,* ed 2, Oxford, 1995, Oxford University Press.

8. Brody H, Thompson JR: The maximin strategy in modern obstetrics, *J Fam Pract* 12:977-985, 1981.

9. Scherger JE, Levitt C, Acheson LS et al: Teaching family-centered perinatal care in family medicine (educational research and methods). Parts I and II, *Fam Med* 24:288-298, 368-374, 1992.

10. Larimore WL: Family-centered birthing: history, philosophy, and need, *Fam Med* 27:140-146, 1995.

11. Larimore WL: Family-centered birthing: a niche for family physicians, *Am Fam Physician* 47:1365-1366, 1993.

12. Larimore WL: Family-centered birthing: a style of obstetrics for family physicians, *Am Fam Physician* 48:725-728, 1993.

13. Larimore WL: The role of the father in childbirth, *Midwifery Today* 51:15-17, 1999.

14. Larimore WL, Reynolds JL: Future of family practice maternity care in America: ruminations on reproducing an endangered species—family physicians who deliver babies, *J Am Board Fam Pract* 7:478-488, 1994.

15. Midmer DK: Does family-centered maternity care empower women? The development of the woman-centered childbirth model, *Fam Med* 24:216-221, 1992.

16. Hon E: Crisis in obstetrics-the management of labor, *Int J Childbirth Educ* 13-15, 1987.

17. Scherger JE: Management of normal labor and birth, *Prim Care* 20:713-719, 1993.

18. Larimore WL, Cline MK: Keeping normal labor normal, *Prim Care* 27:221-236, 2000.

19. Schutte M, Treffers P, Kloostermen G et al: Management of premature rupture of membranes: the risk of vaginal examination to the infant, *Am J Obstet Gynecol* 146:395-400, 1983.

20. Pritchard JA, MacDonald PC, Gant NF, editors: *Williams obstetrics,* ed 17, Norwalk, CT, 1985, Appleton-Century-Crofts.

21. Smith MA, Ruffin MT, Green LA: The thoughtful management of labor, *Am Fam Physician* 45:1471-1481, 1993.

22. Cuervo LG, Rodríguez MN, Delgado MB: Enemas during labor, *Cochrane Database Syst Rev* (2):CD000330, 2000.

23. Basevi V, Lavender T: Routine perineal shaving on admission in labour, *Cochrane Database Syst Rev* (1):CD001236, 2001.

24. Fraser WD, Turcot L, Krauss I et al: Amniotomy for shortening spontaneous labour, *Cochrane Database Syst Rev* (2): CD000015, 2000.

25. Fraser WD, Marcoux S, Moutquin JM et al: Effect of early amniotomy on the risk of dystocia in nulliparous women. The Canadian Early Amniotomy Study Group, *N Engl J Med* 168:1145-1149, 1993.

26. Parisi VM: Amniotomy in labor—how helpful is it? *N Engl J Med* 328:1193-1194, 1993.

27. Frigoletta F, Leiberman E, Long J et al: A clinical trial of active management of labor, *N Engl J Med* 333:745-750, 1994.

28. Glantz J, McNanley T: Active management of labor: a meta-analysis of cesarean delivery rates for dystocia in nulliparas, *Obstet Gynecol Surv* 52:497-505, 1997.

29. Olsen O, Jewell MD: Home versus hospital birth, *Cochrane Database Syst Rev* (2):CD000352, 2000.

30. Hodnett ED, Downe S, Edwards N et al: Home-like versus conventional institutional settings for birth, *Cochrane Database Syst Rev* (1):CD000012, 2005.

SECTION B Ambulation and Positions in Labor

Kent Petrie, MD,
and Walter L. Larimore, MD

I. HISTORY AND TRADITIONS

For the last century in most industrialized nations, the labor position chosen by most physicians has been the supine position. The traditional dorsal lithotomy position in the labor and delivery rooms was developed primarily to benefit the birth attendant by allowing adequate access to the perineum for examination during labor and for operative delivery. When women are allowed to choose their own position of labor, however, they seldom choose the supine position. In latent and early active stage labor, women almost never choose the dorsal lithotomy position. One quote in the medical literature from 1882 sums up the commonsense reasons for avoiding the supine or dorsal lithotomy positions: "The care with which the parturient women of uncivilized people avoid the dorsal decubitus, the modern obstetric position at the termination of labor, is sufficient evidence that it is a most undesirable position for ordinary cases of confinement."[1] Women choose vertical positions (sitting, standing, squatting, kneeling) or nonsupine horizontal positions (side-lying or knee chest). When women are allowed or encouraged to change or choose positions while in labor and without instruction, the typical woman frequently changes positions, with an average of seven to eight position changes.[1]

II. PHYSIOLOGIC EFFECTS OF THE SUPINE POSITION IN LABOR

No evidence has been reported in the literature that the supine position in labor is advantageous, and much evidence suggests that the dorsal position may result in a cascade effect of problems (Figure 14-10).[2] Some women are adversely affected in the supine position because of decreased blood pressure, decreased uterine blood flow, and increased catecholamines. These problems often can be prevented or alleviated by position changes and avoidance, whenever possible, of the supine position.[1,3,4]

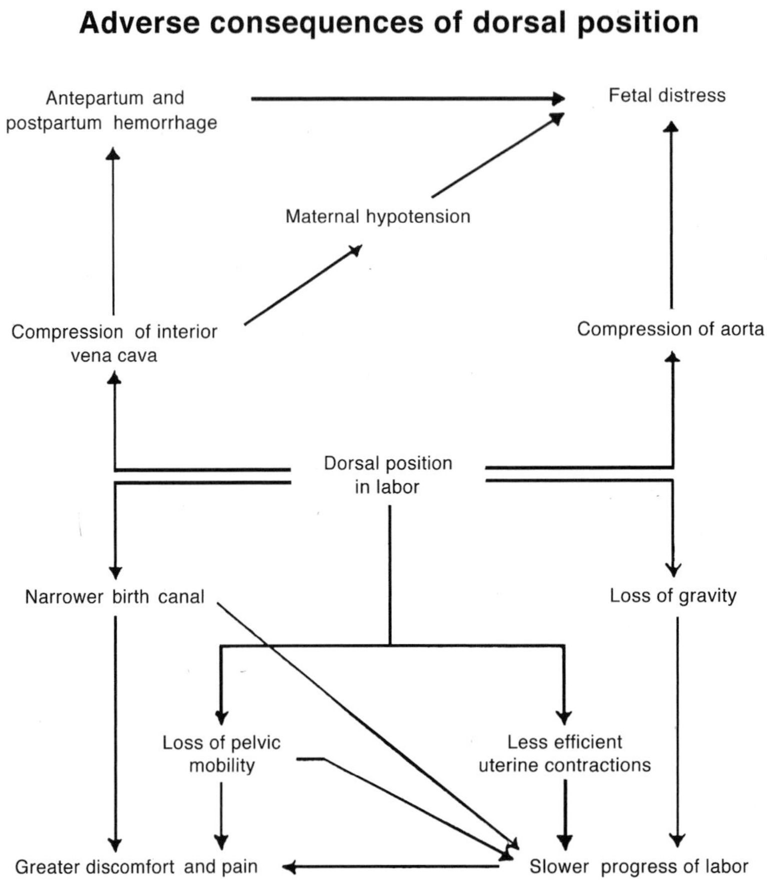

Adverse consequences of dorsal position

FIGURE 14-10. Dorsal recumbency, although convenient for vaginal examinations, intravenous fluids, and electronic fetal monitoring, does not hasten labor. (From McKay S, Mahart CS: Laboring patients need more freedom to move, *Contemp OB/GYN* 90-119, July 1984.)

III. AMBULATION IN LABOR

Before institutionalized labor and delivery, walking was commonly practiced in the latent and active stages of labor. General agreement exists in the literature that many women desire mobility during labor. However, the possible benefits of walking on the progress and outcomes of labor and delivery remain inconclusive.

A. Ambulation in Labor without Epidural Analgesia

Reports of ambulation in labor have been encouraging, stating that walking could reduce the duration of the first stage of labor, reduce the need for labor augmentation with oxytocin, reduce the need for analgesia, reduce the requirement for episiotomies and instrumental deliveries,[5] reduce incidence of cesarean births,[5] increase patient satisfaction,[5-9] and decrease the incidence of fetal distress.[5,9] No studies have shown any risk for fetal compromise in women allowed to ambulate during labor.[10] Other studies found no benefit of standing or walking.[11,12]

The most often quoted RCT on the effect of walking on labor and delivery concludes that it does not provide any particular benefit or negative consequence.[12] This study was done in an institution with an epidural rate of approximately 6%, a cesarean rate of approximately 6%, and a forceps rate of approximately 4%. The study claims it is likely that these rates are not going to be improved by "walking, talking, partying, jumping up and down, or whatever. There is almost no room to demonstrate the study effect."[13] Position change may be more important than simply walking or assuming any single *best* position.[14]

B. Ambulation in Labor with Epidural Analgesia

The evaluation of walking in many studies has been limited in duration, with ambulation being stopped when IV or epidural analgesia was required. There has been a recent trend to reduce the motor block associated with epidural analgesia, thus allowing patients to continue ambulation after the epidural is administered. Two RCTs of nulliparas with epidural anesthesia and combined spinal-epidural analgesia found no detectable effect of walking on any outcome of labor and delivery.[15,16] In these studies, the time spent walking was short (<15% of the duration of the first stage of labor) and sitting in a chair was permitted as "upright" time.

In a more recent RTC, the mean ambulation time was longer (29% of the first stage of labor). Although the duration of labor and pain relief was unaffected by walking, the ambulatory group required smaller doses of anesthetic and oxytocin, suggesting ambulation during labor with epidural analgesia may be advantageous.[17] A recent meta-analysis of five RCTs of first-stage ambulation with epidural demonstrated no clear benefit to delivery outcomes or satisfaction with analgesia, but confirmed no adverse outcomes.[18]

IV. ADVANTAGES OF POSITION CHANGE IN LABOR

Because the positions chosen by women to relieve pain may improve the progress of labor, pain may be a biologically useful stimulus to their seeking the most advantageous labor position. Position change has been reported to make labor more comfortable and efficient through a variety of mechanisms.

1. Uterine contractions are often stronger in intensity but lower in pain.[6]
2. Positions other than the dorsal supine may improve the uterospinal axis.[19]
3. Position change away from the dorsal lithotomy may improve maternal blood pressure and placental flow.[6]
4. Multiple positions present a variety of head angles to the pelvis.[19]
5. The uterine drive axis may be improved with position changes.[19]
6. The pelvis can be physically enlarged in certain positions. For example, the squatting position may open the pelvic outlet by as much as 28%.[20]

V. LABOR IN WATER

Labor in water and water birth are discussed in Section C as methods of nonpharmacologic pain control in labor and delivery.

VI. SUMMARY

If women are to use the many positions available to them in labor successfully to maximize comfort and improve labor progress and efficiency, they must be instructed in these types of positions by their care provider and encouraged to practice them. Birth attendants need to gain comfort and experience with ambulation and different labor positions to provide maximum assistance to laboring patients.[21] An excellent, well-illustrated resource is the *Labor Progress Handbook* by Simkin and Ancheta.[4]

VII. SOR A RECOMMENDATION

RECOMMENDATION	REFERENCES
Ambulation and position change in labor with or without epidural analgesia causes no adverse maternal or fetal consequences. Although metaanalysis reports of benefits are mixed, a patient who chooses an upright labor position should not be discouraged from walking or assuming alternative labor positions.	*18, 22*

REFERENCES

1. Roberts J: Maternal position during the first stage of labour. In Chalmers I, Eakin MW, Keirse MJ, editors: *Effective care in pregnancy and childbirth,* Oxford, 1989, Oxford University Press.
2. McKay S, Mahart CS: Laboring patients need more freedom to move, *Contemp OB/GYN* 90-119, 1984.
3. Smith MA, Ruffin MT, Byrd JE et al: A critical review of labor and birth care (clinical review). Obstetric Interest Group of the North American Primary Care Research Group, *J Fam Pract* 33:281-292, 1991.
4. Simkin P, Ancheta R: *The labor progress handbook,* London, 2000, Blackwell Science, Ltd.
5. Albers L, Anderson D, Cragin L et al: The relationship of ambulation in labor to operative delivery, *J Nurse-Midwifery* 42:1-8, 1997.
6. Mendez-bauer C, Arroyo J, Garcia Ramos C et al: Effects of standing position on spontaneous uterine contractility and other aspects of labor, *J Perinat Med* 3:89-100, 1977.
7. Stewart P, Calder AA: Posture in labour: patients' choice and its effect on performance, *Br J Obstet Gynaecol* 91:1091-1095, 1984.

8. Read JA, Miller FC, Raul RH: Randomized trial of ambulation versus oxytocin for labor enhancement: a preliminary report, *Am J Obstet Gynecol* 139:669-672, 1981.

9. Flynn AM, Kelly J, Hollins G et al: Ambulation in labour, *Br Med J* 2:591-593, 1978.

10. Kelly FW, Terry R, Naglieri R: A review of alternative birthing positions, *J Am Osteopath Assoc* 99:470-474, 1999.

11. McManus TJ, Calder AA: Upright posture and the efficacy of labor, *Lancet* 1:72-74, 1978.

12. Bloom SL, McIntire DD, Kelly MA et al: Lack of effect of walking on labor and delivery, *N Engl J Med* 339:76-79, 1998.

13. Klein MC: Walking in labor, *J Fam Pract* 48:229, 1999.

14. Fenwick L: Birthing: techniques for managing the physiologic and psychological aspects of childbirth, *Perinat Nurs* 51-62, 1984.

15. Vallejo MC, Firestone LL, Mandell GL et al: Effect of epidural analgesia with ambulation on labor duration, *Anesthesiology* 95:857-861, 2001.

16. Collis RE, Harding SA, Morgan BM: Effect of maternal ambulation on labour with low-dose combined spinal-epidural analgesia, *Anesthesia* 54:535-539, 1999.

17. Frenea S, Chirossel C, Rodriguez R et al: The effects of prolonged ambulation on labor with epidural analgesia, *Anesth Analg* 98:224-229, 2004.

18. Roberts CL, Algert CS, Olive E: Impact of first-stage ambulation on mode of delivery among women with epidural analgesia, *Aust N Z J Obstet Gynaecol* 44:489-494, 2004.

19. Fenwick L, Simkin P: Maternal positioning to treat dystocia, *Clin Obstet Gynecol* 30:83-99, 1987.

20. Russell JGB: Molding of the pelvic outlet, *J Obstet Gynaecol Br Commonw* 76:817-820, 1969.

21. Smith MA, Ruffin MT, Green LA: The thoughtful management of labor, *Am Fam Physician* 45:1471-1481, 1983.

22. Lupe PJ, Gross TL: Maternal upright posture and mobility in labor—a review, *Obstet Gynecol* 67:727-734, 1986.

Section C Intrapartum Pain Management

Kent Petrie, MD,
and Walter L. Larimore, MD

Relief of pain in labor provides the patient with the comfort needed to experience her birth process as positively as possible, whereas avoiding fetal compromise or causing other harm. Options available in the United States include psychoprophylaxis; parenteral opioid analgesic; and inhaled, local, and regional analgesia. Any medication given during labor has potential side effects for the mother or infant; therefore, none should be administered as a matter of routine.[1] Ideal pain relief should provide good analgesia, be safe for the mother and infant, be predictable and constant in its effects, be reversible if necessary, be easy to administer, and be under the control of the mother. It should not interfere with uterine contractions or interfere with the mother's mobility. A method that fulfills all of these criteria does not yet exist.[1]

The ACOG and the American Society of Anesthesiologists have issued a joint position statement that reflects the prevailing viewpoint on pain management in labor: "Labor results in severe pain for many women. There is no other circumstance where it is considered acceptable for a person to experience untreated severe pain, amenable to safe intervention, while under a physician's care. Maternal request is a sufficient medical indication for pain relief during labor."[2]

I. PSYCHOPROPHYLAXIS

A. History

In the 1940s, physicians recognized the relation between fear and the intensity of pain in labor. Since the 1970s, a variety of psychoprophylactic methods have been used by laboring patients.[3,4] These techniques of relaxation, positive imagery, and breathing generally are mastered by the patient during the prenatal period. Prenatal education that includes relaxation skills and focusing on positive outcomes has been shown to be more successful than those that solely teach breathing techniques. The effect of prenatal education can vary depending on the teaching ability of the individual instructor and the receptiveness of the patient and her labor companion.

1. Prenatal education classes

    An increased sense of control by use of nonpharmacologic methods of pain management can be a matter of great importance to some patients. The least formal of these methods is the removal of anxiety through educating the woman and a trusted companion who will be present at the birth. The Lamaze and Bradley methods are two popular methods that commonly are taught in prenatal education classes that use psychoprophylaxis to control fear and anxiety and increase tolerance to pain. Women routinely should be encouraged to participate in classes that offer education in these or similar methods.[5,6]

    It should be noted, however, that women who strongly expect that psychoprophylaxis, when performed correctly, will prevent all pain may respond with disappointment, anger, or guilt if the pain is greater than expected. Although decreasing anxiety and fear does increase tolerance for labor pain, it is important to realize that there are women who benefit from pain medication during labor.[6-8] Furthermore, surveys show that a patient's level of satisfaction with her birth experience may depend more on her sense of control over decisions regarding pain management than her overall level of pain.[9,10] Women should be educated about their pain relief options and encouraged to actively participate in decisions regarding pain management in labor.

II. NONPHARMACOLOGIC PAIN CONTROL TECHNIQUES

A. Relaxation Techniques

Nonpharmacologic methods of pain relief during labor include massage and relaxation techniques. Other methods that promote relaxation are discussed elsewhere in this chapter and include support from labor attendants, position changes, physical contact, and ambulation. Approximately 90% of women find relaxation and massage to be good for pain relief. Its effectiveness depends on the compliance of the woman, the stage of labor at which it is used, and the availability of the partner to help.[1] Hypnosis has been shown to be beneficial for managing labor pain in highly motivated patients.[11] Nonpharmacologic techniques are generally well accepted by laboring women and have no demonstrated adverse effects.[6] An excellent systematic review of these nonpharmacologic measures by Simkin and O'Hara lends support to their use for temporary relief of pain in labor.[12]

B. Transcutaneous Electrical Nerve Stimulation

Transcutaneous electrical nerve stimulation (TENS) units for labor pain have received mixed reviews in the literature. In the United Kingdom, about 5.5% of women use TENS in labor. A quarter of these women thought that it gave good pain relief, but another quarter did not find it helpful.[1] Other surveys have confirmed that TENS provides no or limited benefits.[13] Modifications of equipment or technique may increase the usefulness of this technique.

C. Herbal and Alternative Therapies

Complementary and alternative therapies are increasingly used in pregnancy and labor (for an in-depth discussion, see Chapter 3, Section I).[14] A Cochrane metaanalysis supports the effectiveness of acupuncture and hypnosis for pain relief in labor but finds no evidence for benefits of music, white noise, aromatherapy, biofeedback, massage, reflexology, herbal medicines, homeopathy, or magnets.[15]

D. Hydrotherapy

Studies of hydrotherapy in labor have investigated only immersion in warm water, not showers.[16] Although birth attendants may be divided about hydrotherapy, women in labor like to use warm-water baths in the first and early second stages of labor.[16] Women report that the heat is analgesic, and the buoyancy of water is relaxing.[17] One RCT of hydrotherapy showed an association with a slower increase in pain, quicker increases in Bishop's score, less labor augmentation, and greater patient satisfaction.[18] A recent Cochrane review reports similar positive outcomes: "Water immersion during the first stage of labour significantly reduces epidural/spinal analgesia requirements and reported maternal pain, without adversely affecting labour duration, operative delivery rates, or neonatal wellbeing. Immersion in water during the second stage of labour increased women's reported satisfaction with pushing."[16]

E. Intradermal Sterile Water Injections

A promising technique for first-stage "back labor" pain is the use of intradermal sterile water injections. Four 0.1-ml intradermal injections of sterile water with a 25- or 27-gauge needle form small blebs in the skin. Two injection sites are over the posterior superior iliac spines; two are 2 to 3 cm below and 1 to 2 cm medial to the first points; see Figure 14-11 for injection points. The injections cause intense stinging for 15 to 30 seconds, followed within 2 minutes by partial to complete relief of back pain lasting 45 to 90 minutes.[20] The injections can be repeated as needed. Three published RCTs have reported similar results.[20-23]

III. PHARMACOLOGIC PAIN CONTROL TECHNIQUES

A. Narcotic Pain Control

Parenteral narcotics (opioids) are popular and commonly used labor analgesics that can be given by oral, intramuscular, or IV routes.[6,7,24] The most commonly prescribed parenteral opioids worldwide for labor pain are meperidine and morphine. Their use in the United States has been reduced by the availability of less toxic and more efficacious opioids (fentanyl). Opioids with

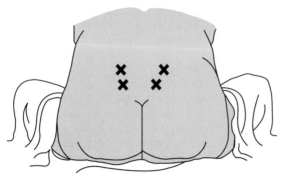

FIGURE 14-11. Intradermal injections of 0.1 ml sterile water in the treatment of women with back pain during labor. Sterile water is injected into four locations on the lower back, two over each posterior superior iliac spine (PSIS) and two 3 cm below and 1 cm medial to the PSIS. The injections should raise a bleb below the skin. Simultaneous injections administered by two clinicians will decrease the pain of the injections.

mixed agonist-antagonist properties (nalbuphine, butorphanol) have gained popularity because of their "dose ceiling" effect with regard to maternal respiratory depression. Butorphanol, for example, at doses greater than 10 mg, continues to intensify analgesia without increasing respiratory depression. Table 14-2 lists popular parenteral opioids and their doses for labor pain. IV doses are preferred to avoid variable absorption with intramuscular injection.[25]

Patient-controlled analgesia with opioids is a dosing option that provides rapid onset of pain relief, excellent control of pain, and a sense of control and independence for the patient. Fentanyl is a commonly used agent with a loading dose of 50 to 100 μg, a basal rate of 100 μg/hr, and intermittent doses of 50 to 100 μg every 5 to 10 minutes.[26]

As a class, opioid side effects include sedation and respiratory depression of the mother or neonate, reduced newborn sucking reflex, and reduced newborn social interaction. Other potential adverse effects include maternal hypotension, nausea, vomiting, dizziness, and decreased gastric motility. Parenteral opioids also reduce FHR variability and may limit the birth attendants' ability to interpret FHR tracings.[27]

When compared with epidural anesthesia, women receiving opioid analgesia are more likely to have a shorter first and second stage of labor, have a reduced risk for operative vaginal delivery, and have a reduced risk for fever during labor (see discussion of epidural analgesia in Section B.III.B). Epidural analgesia provides significantly better pain relief than parenteral opioids.

B. Inhaled Analgesia

Inhaled analgesia with a nitrous oxide and oxygen mixture has been used in the United States since the 1950s.[6] The patient self-administers the nitrous oxide with a handheld face mask. It is used in about 60% of deliveries in Great Britain, where about 85% of users find it helpful.[1] One report suggests that nitrous oxide shortens labor. Excellent pain relief is reported nearly 75% of the time, but a major disadvantage is occasional nausea and vomiting.[6] A systematic review has concluded that nitrous oxide is inexpensive, easy to

TABLE 14-2 **Parenteral Opioids for Labor Pain**

Agent	Usual Dosage	Frequency	Onset	Neonatal Half-life
Meperidine (Demerol)	25-50 mg (IV)	Every 1-2 hr	5 min (IV)	13-22.4 hr
	50-100 mg (IM)	Every 2-4 hr	30-45 min (IM)	63 hr for active metabolites
Fentanyl	50-100 μg (IV)	Every 1 hr	1 min	5.3 hr
Nalbuphine (Nubain)	10 mg (IV or IM)	Every 3 hr	2-3 min (IV)	4.1 hr
				15 min (IM)
Butorphanol (Stadol)	1-2 mg (IV or IM)	Every 4 hr	1-2 min (IV)	Not known
			10-30 min (IM)	Similar to nalbuphine in adults
Morphine	2-5 mg (IV)	Every 4 hr	5 min (IV)	7.1 hr
	10 mg (IM)			30-40 min (IM)

From ACOG Practice Bulletin, Obstetric anesthesia and analgesia, Number 36, July 2002, Washington, DC, 2002, American College of Obstetricians and Gynecologists.
IV, Intravenously; IM, intramuscularly.

use, safe for mother and fetus, and more effective than opioids but less effective than epidural analgesia.[28]

C. Regional Analgesia

A variety of techniques and anesthetic agents are available for peripheral or regional blocks. Each approach has risks and benefits, which should be reviewed with the childbearing couple preferably during prenatal counseling.

1. Paracervical block

Paracervical block is effective in relieving the discomfort of uterine contractions during the first stage of labor.[7] With proper technique, up to 75% of patients report effective analgesia.[29,30] Practiced much more commonly in the 1950s and 1960s, its use decreased with reports of fetal bradycardia (mean incidence, 15%). Studies report a significantly greater incidence of postparacervical block fetal bradycardia when the FHR pattern is nonreassuring before the block is administered. It is recommended to restrict the use of paracervical blocks to patients with reassuring FHR patterns.[6] The technique of administering the paracervical block appears to affect the incidence of fetal bradycardia. Submucous applications of local anesthetics result in significantly fewer bradycardia episodes than deeper injections. Once fetal bradycardia occurs, the effect may last 90 minutes; however, bradycardia occurs, on average, 7 minutes after paracervical block is administered and usually lasts 8 minutes. Paracervical anesthesia is easy to learn, is easy to administer, and results in good analgesia but should be administered in a shallow injection (see Chapter 18, Section B for technique).

2. Pudendal block

Bilateral pudendal nerve blocks relieve pain arising from the distention of the vagina and perineum in the second stage of labor. Health-care providers may supplement an epidural analgesia if the sacral nerves are inadequately blocked, and may provide analgesia for low and outlet forceps. A pudendal block provides anesthesia only to the lower portion of the vagina and the introitus (see Chapter 18, Section B for technique).

3. Topical lidocaine gel application

Vulvar application of 2% lidocaine jelly during the second stage of labor has been shown to reduce perceived pain at delivery when compared with placebo. Patients also reported less immediate postpartum pain. The application had no effect on the incidence of perineal laceration.[31]

4. Epidural block

Compared with other methods, epidural block provides the most effective pain relief in labor. Epidural analgesia has grown in popularity as laboring women's expectations for pain control in childbirth have increased.[32] Epidural analgesia has a high acceptance rate, with greater than 90% of women reporting it to be good or very good and 85% indicating they would choose it again.[1] Epidural analgesia may not confer greater satisfaction with the birth experience, however, and it involves many risks.[7,33]

a. Risks of epidural block: Epidural blocks require the services of an individual skilled and practiced in the technique, and significantly increase the cost of labor and delivery. Multiple potential maternal-fetal complications can occur. Because of the following potential adverse effects on labor progress and morbidity, the maternity caregivers should be prepared to intervene as necessary with oxytocin or operative delivery.

   i. Sudden hypotension and resultant fetal stress
   ii. Spinal headache
   iii. Epidural space hematoma or infection
   iv. Inadvertent intravascular injection of anesthetic resulting in maternal seizures or cardiac arrest
   v. Maternal respiratory depression resulting from "high" spinal block
   vi. Urinary retention and the need for bladder catheterization

b. Absolute contraindications to epidural block[7]

   i. Refractory maternal hypotension
   ii. Maternal coagulopathy
   iii. Maternal use of once-daily dose of low-molecular-weight heparin within 12 hours
   iv. Untreated maternal bacteremia
   v. Skin infection over site of needle placement
   vi. Increased intracranial pressure caused by mass lesion

c. Effects of epidural block on labor and maternal and infant outcomes

The growth in popularity of epidural analgesia has been accompanied by much controversy in the literature about the effects of epidural block on the course and conduct of labor and on maternal and infant outcomes. In May 2001, a group of family physicians, obstetrician-gynecologists, anesthesiologists, nurse-midwives, and childbirth educators met at the Nature and Management of Labor Pain symposium sponsored by the Maternity Center Association and the New York Academy of Medicine.[24,34] Participants analyzed two systematic reviews on epidural analgesia.[35,36] These reviewers and another recent metaanalyses draw similar conclusions[33]:

   i. Epidural analgesia provides more effective pain relief during labor than alternative methods.

   ii. Epidural analgesia increases the duration of the second stage of labor, the use of oxytocin, the rates of instrument-assisted vaginal deliveries, and the incidence of third- and fourth-degree perineal lacerations.

   iii. Epidural analgesia increases the likelihood of maternal fever and increases the incidence of neonatal sepsis evaluation and neonatal antibiotic treatment. There is no significant difference, however, in newborn Apgar scores or cord pH levels.

   iv. Epidural analgesia has not been consistently shown to increase rates of cesarean delivery compared with use of parenteral opioids. Some authors suggest such an association, and studies are ongoing that should strengthen the evidence.[37] ACOG currently states that "the question of whether [epidural] use is associated with an increased risk of cesarean delivery remains controversial."[7]

Table 14-3 summarizes the available evidence.[24] An excellent "summary" statement in a recent Cochrane review seems quite accurate: "Given evidence of the effects of epidural analgesia on the dynamics of labor, a mother receiving

---

TABLE 14-3 **Effects of Epidural Analgesia on Labor and Maternal and Infant Outcomes**

Labor Factors	*Outcome*	*P*
Effects on Labor		
Duration of first stage	Increased by 26 minutes	NS
Duration of second stage	Increased by 15 minutes	<0.05
Pain score (100 mm VAS)		
First stage	40 mm lower	<0.0001
Second stage	29 mm lower	<0.001
Use of oxytocin (Pitocin) after analgesia	Increased (OR, 2.8; 95% CI, 1.89-4.16)	<0.05
Third- or fourth-degree perineal laceration	Increased (OR, 1.7-2.7)	N/A
Instrument-assisted delivery	Increased (OR, 2.1; 95% CI, 1.48-2.93)	<0.05
Cesarean delivery	OR, 1.0; 95% CI, 0.77-1.28	NS
Maternal outcomes		
Fever >38°C (100.4°F)	Increased (OR, 5.6; 95% CI, 4.0-7.8)	<0.001
Low backache		
At 3 months	OR, 1.0; 95% CI, 0.6-1.6	NS
At 12 months	OR, 1.4; 95% CI, 0.9-2.3	NS
Urinary incontinence	No increase	NS
Breastfeeding success at 6 weeks	No difference	NS
Infant outcomes		
5-minute Apgar score <7	No difference	NS
Low umbilical cord pH	No difference	NS
Neonatal sepsis evaluation	Increased	N/A
Neonatal antibiotic treatment	Increased	N/A

From Leeman L, Fontaine P, King V et al: The nature and management of labor pain: part II. Pharmacologic pain relief, *Am Fam Physician* 68:1115-1120, 2003. Data from Leighton BL, Halpern SH: The effects of epidural analgesia on labor, maternal and neonatal outcomes: a systematic review, *Am J Obstet Gynecol* 186(suppl 5):S69-S77, 2002; and Lieberman E, O'Donoghue C: Unintended effects of epidural analgesia during labor: a systematic review, *Am J Obstet Gynecol* 186(suppl 5):S31-S68, 2002.
NS, Not significant; VAS, visual analog scale; OR, odds ratio; CI, confidence interval; N/A, not applicable.
Outcomes compared with control groups that primarily received parenteral opioids.

epidural analgesia may not be considered to be having a 'normal' labor."[33]

d. Reducing the adverse effects of epidural analgesia on labor

Epidural analgesia has become almost routine in many hospitals and is requested by increasing numbers of women. Rates of epidural analgesia use have been shown to decrease with increased prenatal education, increased support during labor, and increased availability of alternative pain control methods in the birthing environment.[12] The literature suggests the following measures to reduce the adverse effects of epidural analgesia on the labor process:

  i. Changes in epidural drugs and techniques have been developed to optimize pain control whereas minimizing negative side effects.[24] Low doses of bupivacaine (Sensorcaine) and ropivacaine (Naropin) have replaced lidocaine (Xylocaine) to reduce motor blockade and improve a patient's ability to push in the second stage of labor.[32]

  ii. Although the current data are controversial, it appears that delayed placement of epidural analgesia may reduce the risk for cesarean delivery.[24] "After weighing this conflicting data, the ACOG Task Force on Cesarean Delivery Rates recommended that, when feasible, obstetric practitioners should delay the administration of epidural analgesia in nulliparous women until cervical dilation reaches 4 to 5 cm and that other forms of analgesia be used until that time."[27]

  iii. Low-dose, continuous infusion and intermittent bolus, patient-controlled epidural analgesia have not been shown to be superior to standard epidural techniques.[7]

  iv. Combined spinal epidural (CSE) analgesia, or the "walking epidural," is gaining popularity. An intrathecal opioid is administered before the continuous epidural infusion. Compared with epidural alone, CSE provides faster onset of effective pain relief and increases maternal satisfaction, but it is associated with more maternal itching. No difference, however, has been found in maternal mobility after CSE, and no differences have been found in forceps delivery, cesarean delivery rates, or admissions of infants to the neonatal unit.[38] An advantage of CSE may be the potential for the intrathecal medication to suffice as the sole analgesic in patients who are likely to deliver within 2 or 3 hours after injection.[39]

  v. Delayed pushing in nulliparous women with epidurals (waiting 1-3 hours after complete dilation), sometimes called allowing the patient to "labor down," has been shown to reduce the risk for difficult operative vaginal deliveries or cesarean deliveries.[40] Women with a high fetal station or occiput transverse position were most likely to benefit from delayed pushing. Cord pH levels were lower in infants born after delayed pushing, but no differences in neonatal morbidity were noted.

5. Spinal anesthesia

Spinal anesthesia is used for operative procedures, including cesarean section, instrumental delivery, and manual removal of the placenta. The local anesthetic is injected into the cerebrospinal fluid through a fine (25-gauge) atraumatic needle. The onset of action is rapid, and the effect lasts for about 2 hours. Indications, complications, and contraindications are similar to those for epidural block discussed previously, with the exception that the risk for spinal headache is greater than with epidural anesthesia.

6. Intrathecal narcotics for labor analgesia

Intrathecal analgesia is an effective technique for relief of first-stage labor pain. The procedure is safe and can be learned easily by family physicians currently performing diagnostic lumbar puncture. It is particularly useful in practices where continuous lumbar epidural anesthesia is not available.[41]

a. Actions of intrathecal narcotics

  i. Small doses of narcotic injected into the subarachnoid space bind selectively with opioid receptors, promoting effective analgesia (not anesthesia) without significant motor or autonomic blockade.

  ii. Intrathecal narcotics provide more effective analgesia for visceral pain than somatic pain and are more useful in early first-stage labor than in the second stage of labor. A pudendal block or local infiltration may be needed for second-stage perineal pain and repair of episiotomy or tears.

iii. Intrathecal narcotics do not prolong first- or second-stage labor. The more water-soluble narcotics (morphine) are slower in onset (15-60 minutes) but longer acting (6-10 hours). They remain in the cerebrospinal fluid longer and are more likely to circulate to higher centers and cause adverse side effects. The more lipid-soluble narcotics (fentanyl and sufentanil) are faster in onset (5-10 minutes) and shorter in duration of activity (1.5-3.5 hours).

b. Procedure for intrathecal narcotic administration[39]

i. Position the patient near the edge of the bed in the lateral recumbent or sitting position determined by comfort.

ii. Flex spine anteriorly as much as possible.

iii. Identify the L3-4 interspace at the level of the iliac crests.

iv. Prepare and drape the L3-4 interspace area and anesthetize the skin and interspinous ligament with 1% lidocaine.

v. Perform lumbar puncture with a narrow-gauge spinal needle (24G to 27G) using an introducer (18G to 19G), and document free flow of cerebrospinal fluid.

vi. Inject intrathecal narcotic mixture. Common preservative-free preparations include:
(a) Fentanyl citrate (Sublimaze), 15-25 mcg
(b) Sufentanil citrate (Sufenta), 3-15 μg
(c) Morphine sulfate (Duramorph), 0.2-0.5 mg

vii. Combination of fentanyl or sufentanil plus morphine is commonly administered.

viii. Remove needle and monitor maternal blood pressure and FHR for 30 to 60 minutes.

ix. The patient may ambulate when stable.

c. Side effects of intrathecal narcotics
i. Pruritus (50%)
ii. Nausea and vomiting (30-50%)
iii. Urinary retention (30%)
iv. Delayed respiratory depression (rare but more common with morphine)
v. Spinal headache (related to technique)

d. Side effects of intrathecal narcotics can be minimized or treated with:
i. Naltrexone (ReVia): A single dose of 12.5 to 50 mg orally is given immediately after delivery.
ii. Nalbuphine (Nubain): This is a synthetic narcotic agonist-antagonist analgesic. A dose of 5 to 10 mg intravenously is given immediately after delivery.
iii. Naloxone (Narcan): A dose of 0.4 mg bolus or 0.6 mg/hr infusion is given for more serious side effects (e.g., urinary retention and respiratory depression).

IV. CONCLUSIONS

Women in the United States today have fewer options for labor pain management than women in countries such as Canada[42] and the United Kingdom.[1] Studies to discover the factors responsible for limited choice have yielded few data.[43] It has been postulated that the growing popularity of epidural analgesia in the United States may be in part because the only other option presented to patients is parental opioids. Family physicians are in an excellent position to understand and offer a wider variety of nonpharmacologic and pharmacologic methods of pain relief to their patients in labor.

V. SOR A RECOMMENDATIONS

RECOMMENDATIONS	REFERENCES
Among many alternative therapies, acupuncture and hypnosis have been shown to be effective for pain relief in labor.	*15*
Water immersion during the first stage of labor reduces epidural use and maternal reports of labor pain.	*16*
Epidural analgesia increases the duration of the second stage of labor, rates of instrument-assisted vaginal delivery, and maternal fever.	*33*
Delayed pushing in patients with epidural analgesia reduces the risk for difficult vaginal or cesarean deliveries.	*40*

REFERENCES

1. Findley I, Chamberlain G: ABC of labour care. Relief of pain, *BMJ* 318:927-930, 1999.
2. ACOG committee opinion. Pain relief during labor. No. 295, July 2004, *Obstet Gynecol* 104:213, 2004.
3. Dick-Read G, Wessel H, Ellis F: *Childbirth without fear: the original approach to natural childbirth,* ed 5, New York, 1984, Harper & Row.
4. Fenwick L: Birthing: techniques for managing the physiologic and psychosocial aspects of childbirth, *Perinat Nurs* May/June:51-62, 1984.
5. Enkin MW, Keirse MJNC, Renfrew MJ et al: *A guide to effective care in pregnancy and childbirth,* ed 2, Oxford, 1995, Oxford University Press.
6. Smith MA, Acheson LS, Byrd JE et al: A critical review of labor and birth care (clinical review). Obstetrical Interest Group of the North American Primary Care Research Group, *J Fam Pract* 33:281-292, 1991.
7. ACOG practice bulletin. Obstetric anesthesia and analgesia, number 36, Washington, DC, July 2002, American College of Obstetricians and Gynecologists.
8. Melzack R, Taenzer P, Feldman P et al: Labour is still painful after prepared childbirth training, *Can Med Assoc J* 125:357-359, 1981.
9. Goodman P, Mackey MC, Tavakoli AS: Factors related to childbirth satisfaction, *J Adv Nurs* 46:212-219, 2004.
10. McCrea BH, Wright ME: Satisfaction in childbirth and perceptions of personal control in pain relief during labour, *J Adv Nurs* 29:877-881, 1999.
11. Cyna AM, McAuliffe GL, Andrew MI: Hypnosis for pain relief in labour and childbirth: a systematic review, *Br J Anaesth* 93:505-509, 2004.
12. Simkin PP, O'Hara M: Nonpharmacologic relief of pain during labor: systematic review of five methods, *Am J Obstet Gynecol* 186(suppl 5):S131-S159, 2002.
13. Carroll D, Tramer M, McQuay H et al: Transcutaneous electrical nerve stimulation in labour pain: a systematic review, *Br J Obstet Gynaecol* 104:169-175, 1997.
14. Huntley AL, Coon JT, Ernst E: Complementary and alternative medicine for labor pain: a systematic review, *Am J Obstet Gynecol* 191:36-49, 2004.
15. Smith CA, Collins CT, Cyna AM et al: Complementary and alternative therapies for pain management in labour, *Cochrane Database Syst Rev* (4):CD003521, 2006.
16. Cluett E R, Nikodem VC, McCandlish RE et al: Immersion in water in pregnancy, labour and birth, *Cochrane Database Syst Rev* (2):CD000111, 2004.
17. Woodward J, Kelly SM: A pilot study for a randomized trial of waterbirth versus land birth, *Br J Obstet Gynecol* 111:537-542, 2004.
18. Cammu H, Clasen K, Van Wettenu L: Is having a warm bath during labor useful? *Acta Obstet Gynaecol Scand* 73:468-472, 1994.
19. Reynolds JL: Intracutaneous sterile water for back pain in labor, *Can Fam Physician* 40:1785-1792, 1994.
20. Ader L, Hasson B, Wallin G: Parturition pain treated by intracutaneous injections of sterile water, *Pain* 41:133-138, 1990.
21. Martensson L, Wallin G: Labour pain treated with cutaneous injections of sterile water: a randomized controlled trial, *Br J Obstet Gynaecol* 106:633-637, 1999.
22. Martensson L, Nyberg K, Wallin G: Subcutaneous versus intracutaneous injections of sterile water for labor analgesia: a comparison of perceived pain during administration, *Br J Obstet Gynaecol* 107:1248-1251, 2000.
23. Trolle B, Moller M, Kronborg H et al: The effect of sterile water blocks on low back pain, *Am J Obstet Gynecol* 164:1277-1281, 1990.
24. Leeman L, Fontaine P, King V et al: The nature and management of labor pain: part II. Pharmacologic pain relief, *Am Fam Physician* 68:1115-1120, 2003.
25. Bricker L, Lavender T: Parenteral opioids for labor pain relief: a systematic review, *Am J Obstet Gynecol* 186(suppl 5):S94, 2002.
26. Grant GJ: Management of pain during labor and delivery, *UpToDate Online* 13.2, 2005. Available at: www.uptodate.com.
27. American College of Obstetricians and Gynecologists (ACOG): *Task Force on Cesarean Delivery Rates. Evaluation of cesarean delivery.* Washington, DC, 2000, ACOG.
28. Rosen MA: Nitrous oxide for relief of labor pain: a systematic review, *Am J Obstet Gynecol* 186(suppl 5):S110, 2002.
29. Ranta P, Jouppila P, Spalding M et al: Paracervical block—a viable alternative for labor pain relief? *Acta Obstet Gynecol Scand* 74:122-125, 1995.
30. Rosen MA: Paracervical block for labor analgesia: a brief historic review, *Am J Obstet Gynecol* 186(suppl 5):S127-S130, 2002.
31. Collins MK, Porter KB, Brooke E et al: Vulvar application of lidocaine for pain relief in spontaneous vaginal delivery, *Obstet Gynecol* 84:335-337, 1994.
32. Caton D, Frolich MA, Euliano TY: Anesthesia for childbirth: controversy and change, *Am J Obstet Gynecol* 186(suppl 5): S25-S30, 2002.
33. Howell CJ: Epidural versus non-epidural analgesia for pain relief in labour, *Cochrane Database Syst Rev* (2):CD000331, 2000.
34. Leeman L, Fontaine P, King V et al: The nature and management of labor pain: part I. Nonpharmacologic pain relief, *Am Fam Physician* 68:1109-1112, 2003.
35. Leighton BL, Halpern SH: The effects of epidural analgesia on labor, maternal and neonatal outcomes: a systematic review, *Am J Obstet Gynecol* 186(suppl 5):S69-S77, 2002.
36. Lieberman E, O'Donoghue C: Unintended effects of epidural analgesia during labor: a systematic review, *Am J Obstet Gynecol* 186(suppl 5):S31-S68, 2002.
37. Lieberman E, Lang JM, Frigoletto F et al: Epidurals and cesareans: the jury is still out, *Birth* 26:196-199, 1999.
38. Hughes D, Simmons SW, Brown J et al: Combined spinal-epidural versus epidural analgesia in labour, *Cochrane Database Syst Rev* (4):CD003401, 2003.
39. Fontaine P, Adam P, Svendsen KH: Should intrathecal narcotics be used as a sole labor analgesic? A prospective comparison of spinal opioids and epidural bupivicaine, *J Fam Pract* 51: 630-635, 2002.
40. Fraser WD, Marcoux S, Krauss I et al: Multicenter, randomized, controlled trial of delayed pushing for nulliparous women in the second stage of labor with continuous epidural analgesia. The PEOPLE (Pushing Early or Pushing Late with Epidural) Study Group, *Am J Obstet Gynecol* 182:1165-1172, 2000.
41. Herpolsheimer A, Schretenthaler J: The use of intrapartum intrathecal narcotic analgesia in a community-based hospital, *Obstet Gynecol* 84:931-936, 1994.
42. Levitt C: *Survey of routine maternity care and practices in Canadian hospitals.* Ottawa, 1995, Canadian Institute of Child Health.
43. Marmor TR, Krol DM: Labor pain management in the United States: understanding patterns and the issue of choice, *Am J Obstet Gynecol* 186(suppl 5):S173-S180, 2002.

SECTION D Support in Labor

Kent Petrie, MD,
and Walter L. Larimore, MD

Historically, mothers have labored in an environment of supportive family and companions.[1] This was most recently evident in the early twentieth century when western women labored at home. However, by the mid-twentieth century, birthing practices shifted to hospital birth in large labor wards, isolating women from family and friends. It was not until the 1960s, with the growth of prepared childbirth classes, that fathers were invited back into the labor and birth rooms.[2] Today, women are returning to the concept of continuous intrapartum support by companions and fathers. Hospitals have embraced this concept with the design of comfortable birthing rooms for single-room maternity care.

RCTs consistently have shown that the presence of a companion during labor results in many favorable outcomes, including a decrease in the incidence of meconium-stained amniotic fluid, reduced use of oxytocin, and reduced cesarean birth. A reduction in low Apgar scores, fetal and maternal morbidity, and operative deliveries has also been noted.[3-5] Table 14-4 shows some of the combined outcome data from the RCTs on labor support.[3,6] Birth attendants are encouraged to respect a woman's choice of companions during labor and birth and her desire for empathetic support by caregivers.

I. DOULA MODEL

One of the most remarkable developments in continuous birthing support is the development of doula services. Doulas are women who are trained and experienced in childbirth, although they may or may not have given birth themselves. As reviewed by Penny Simkin,[7] the elements of continuous labor support include the following:

1. Attention to physical comfort (touch and massage; assistance with positioning, bathing, grooming; applying heat and cold)
2. Emotional support for the laboring woman (praise, reassurance, encouragement, and continuous presence)

TABLE 14-4 Evidence for Continuous Support During Labor

Outcome	Relative Risk	95% Confidence Interval	NNT*	ARR (%)†
Use of any analgesia (all types of support providers)	0.87	0.79 to 0.96	16	6
Use of any analgesia (doulas or other nonhospital staff)	0.72	0.49 to 1.05	N/A	N/A
Operative vaginal delivery (all types of support providers)	0.89	0.83 to 0.96	50	2
Operative vaginal delivery (doulas or other nonhospital staff)	0.59	0.42 to 0.81	32	3
Cesarean delivery (all types of support providers)	0.90	0.82 to 0.99	100	1
Cesarean delivery (doulas or other nonhospital staff)	0.74	0.61 to 0.90	22	4
Birth not satisfactory to mother (all types of support providers)	0.73	0.65 to 0.83	50	2
Birth not satisfactory to mother (doulas or other nonhospital staff)	0.67	0.58 to 0.78	7	14

NNT, Number needed to treat; ARR, absolute risk reduction; N/A, not applicable.
* NNT is the number of women who will need to receive the intervention to prevent a single case of the outcome.
† ARR is the absolute risk reduction in the intervention group compared with the control group.
Information from reference 3. Table from reference 6.

3. Guidance and emotional support for the laboring woman's partner and loved ones

4. Information sharing (nonmedical advice, explanation of policies and procedures, anticipatory guidance)

5. Advocacy (facilitation of communication between the laboring woman and hospital staff to assist in making informed decisions)[2]

Doulas specialize in nonmedical skills and do not perform clinical tasks, diagnose medical conditions, offer second opinions, or give medical advice. The doula's goal is to help the woman have a safe and satisfying childbirth as the woman defines it. When a doula is present, some women feel less need for pain medications or may postpone them until later in labor. It is not the role of the doula to discourage the mother from her choices. The doula helps the mother become informed about various options, including the risks, benefits, and accompanying precautions or interventions for safety. Doulas can help maximize the benefits of pain medications while minimizing their undesirable side effects. The comfort and reassurance offered by the doula are beneficial regardless of the use of pain medications.

According to the Doulas of North America, the terminology describing labor support can be confusing.[8] When a person uses any of the following terms to describe herself, she may need to clarify what she means by the term. The word *doula* is derived from Greek, meaning "woman's servant." In labor support terminology, "doula" refers to a supportive companion (not a friend or loved one) professionally trained to provide labor support. "Doula" also refers to laywomen who are trained or experienced in providing postpartum care (mother and newborn care, breastfeeding support and advice, cooking, childcare, errands, and light cleaning) for the new family. To distinguish between the two types of doulas, one may refer to "birth doulas" and "postpartum doulas." *Monitrice* is a French word originally used by Fernand Lamaze to refer to a specially trained nurse or midwife who provides nursing care and assessment in addition to labor support. Today, *monitrice* is often used as a synonym for "birth assistant" or "labor assistant." "Labor support professional," "labor support specialist," and "labor companion" are synonyms of "birth doula." "Birth assistant" and "labor assistant" are sometimes used as synonyms for "doula" but also may refer to laywomen who are trained to assist a midwife (e.g., vaginal examinations, set up for the birth, fetal heart checks) and provide some labor support.

II. BENEFITS OF CONTINUOUS SUPPORT IN LABOR

Benefits of continuous emotional support in labor have been clearly demonstrated in two large metaanalyses.[2] The first impressive study in 1996, a metaanalysis of four RTCs[5] conducted on young, low-income, nulliparous women, demonstrated that continuous support by a doula had the following results:

1. Shorter duration of labor by 2.8 hours (95% CI, 2.2-3.4)

2. Twice the rate of spontaneous vaginal birth (relative risk [RR], 2.01; 95% CI, 1.5-2.7)

3. Half the frequency of oxytocin use (RR, 0.46; 95% CI, 0.4-0.7)

4. Half the frequency of forceps use (RR, 0.46; 95% CI, 0.3-0.7)

5. Half the frequency of cesarean birth (RR, 0.54; 95% CI, 0.4-0.7)

A more recent metaanalysis[3] of 15 RTCs of labor support including almost 13,000 women showed significant but more modest benefits, including:

1. Reduced need for pain medication (74% vs. 77%)

2. Reduced operative vaginal delivery (16% vs. 18%)

3. Reduced cesarean delivery (11.4% vs. 13.1%)

4. Increased spontaneous vaginal birth (72% vs. 69%)

5. More satisfactory childbirth experience (93% vs. 91%)

6. Fewer Apgar scores less than 7 at 5 minutes (0.8% vs. 2.0%)

7. Fewer neonatal sepsis evaluations (4.5% vs. 9.5%)

A recent North American trial[9] was conducted in hospitals with high rates of routine medical interventions (EFM, oxytocin use, and epidural anesthesia). In this setting, serving primarily highly educated white women receiving continuous support by labor nurses, significant difference in cesarean delivery rate, duration of labor, use of regional anesthesia, and neonatal outcomes were not demonstrated. It has been postulated that benefits of continuous labor support may be greatest for young disadvantaged women who would otherwise labor alone.[2]

Regardless of the clinical outcomes noted earlier, these and other studies demonstrate significant psychological benefits of continuous labor support.[10-12] Doulas help women cope with the labor experience, and almost all women prefer continuous support during their labors.[9] Doulas impact the woman's psychological adjustment to motherhood beyond the intrapartum experience. Studies show improved breastfeeding and reduced postpartum depression among women who receive doula care.[12,13]

III. INCORPORATING CONTINUOUS LABOR SUPPORT IN HOSPITAL SETTINGS

It is now considered inappropriate for hospitals to exclude any category of support person from labor and birth. If women have preferences for who should be with them at this time, these preferences should be respected and, if possible, accommodated.

The Cochrane evaluation of labor support states, "Given the clear benefits and no known risks associated with intrapartum support, every effort should be made to ensure that all laboring women receive continuous support. This support should include continuous presence, the provision of hands-on comfort, and encouragement."[3] Depending on the circumstances, ensuring the provision of continuous support may require the following:

1. Alterations in the current work activities of midwives and nurses, such that they are able to spend less time on ineffective activities and more time providing support
2. Continuing education programs that teach the art and science of labor support
3. Changes to more flexible methods of staffing labor wards, which permit the staff census to match more closely the patient census
4. Adoption of hospital policies encouraging the presence of experienced laywomen, including female relatives

The constant attendance provided by midwives may represent a doula effect. It has been suggested that the constant or increased attendance of a labor nurse may render a doula effect. One study comparing family physicians and midwives found few differences in the management of labor and birth; however, nulliparous women managed by family physicians were more likely to undergo cesarean birth (14% vs. 8%) resulting from a diagnosis of dystocia. The authors hypothesized that the time spent in continuous support provided by the midwives, as opposed to the physicians, may have explained this observed difference. At the very least, in situations in which continuous family or nursing support is not available, the provision of a female companion would be likely to improve maternal

well-being. Birth attendants would be wise to consider such an intervention. Maternity care providers and facilities that do not currently provide continuous labor support may be wise to consider training or supporting a doula program. The national organization, Doulas of North America, is located in Jasper, Indiana (888-788-DONA).

IV. LABOR NURSES AND CONTINUOUS SUPPORT

Studies of continuous labor support provided solely by labor nurses fail to show the dramatic outcomes demonstrated in the doula studies,[14] especially in high-risk centers.[9] Nurses may be less able to provide effective emotional and physical support than a doula because they adhere to their institutional patterns and protocols for pain relief, fetal surveillance, and labor and delivery policies.[2]

V. THE FATHER OR SIGNIFICANT OTHER

The presence of the father during labor and birth, based on RCTs, appears to increase strongly the mother's satisfaction with the birthing experience. No evidence of harm exists from allowing fathers to be involved actively in labor and birth or to attend cesarean births with an awake mother.[4] In multivariate models, emotional support from a mate during labor and birth accounts for the largest portion of variance.[15] As compared with labor nurses, fathers are significantly more likely to be present in the labor room, offer comforting items, and touch their partner. Mothers consistently rate the father's presence as significantly more helpful than that of the nurses.

Additional studies show that the impact of fathers who attend labor and birth is greater than that of fathers who attend only early labor. Women whose partners were involved in the entire birth process report less pain, receive less medication, and report more positive experiences. The higher the level of support from the father, the less likely women were to use epidural anesthesia. A caution concerning these findings would be that preexisting differences or selection criteria may exist between the groups of fathers studied. There appears to be no risk associated with the father's attendance at labor and birth, and several positive benefits have been reported; every effort should be made to encourage and allow the father to participate actively in the labor and birth.[15]

VI. SIBLINGS

Allowing and encouraging the presence of siblings at all or part of their mother's labor and birth is a more recent and growing trend. The few reports available represent self-selected families. No significant negative effects have been shown in any children studied who have attended labor or delivery. Reports by parents indicate a significant increase in caretaking and mothering behaviors in the birth-attending group, but no studies to date have controlled for selection or reporting bias.[4] The scant evidence existing concerning sibling presence at labor or birth indicates no short-term harm to the children and suggests the possibility of increased nurturing behavior.

VII. SUMMARY

RCTs show multiple clear benefits and no significant risks associated with labor support. Every effort should be made to ensure that all laboring women receive support. This is especially true for trained support personnel and should include the provision of encouragement, hands-on care, position change, and ambulation assistance.

VIII. SOR A RECOMMENDATION

RECOMMENDATION	REFERENCES
Women receiving continuous support during labor experience reduced use of analgesia (NNT = 16), reduced operative vaginal delivery (NNT = 32-50), reduced cesarean delivery (NNT = 22-100), and increased satisfaction with the birth experience (NNT = 7-50).	3, 6

REFERENCES

1. Rosenberg K, Trevathan W: Birth, obstetrics and human evolution, *BJOG* 109:1199-1200, 2002.
2. Stuebe A, Ponkey S, Barbieri RL: Continuous intrapartum support, *UpToDate Online* 13.2, 2005. Available at: www.suptodate.com.
3. Hodnett ED, Gates S, Hofmeyer GJ et al: Continuous support for women during childbirth, *Cochrane Database Syst Rev* (3): CD003766, 2003.
4. Smith MA, Acheson LS, Byrd JE et al: A critical review of labor and birth care (clinical review). Obstetrical Interest Group of North American Primary Care Research Group, *J Fam Pract* 33:281-292, 1991.
5. Zhang J, Bernasko JW, Leybovich E et al: Continuous labor support from labor attendant for primiparous women: a meta-analysis, *Obstet Gynecol* 88:739, 1996.
6. Leeman L, Fontaine P, King V et al: The nature and management of labor pain: part I. Nonpharmacologic pain relief, *Am Fam Physician* 68:1109-1112, 2003.
7. Simkin PP, O'Hara MA: Nonpharmacologic relief of pain during labor: systemic reviews of five methods, *Am J Obstet Gynecol* 186:S131, 2002.
8. Simkin PP, Way P: The doulas' contribution to modern maternity care. Doulas of North America position paper. Seattle, WA, 1998, DONA International. Available at: www.dona.org.
9. Hodnett ED, Lowe NK, Hannah ME et al: Effectiveness of nurses as providers of birth labor support in North American hospitals: a randomized controlled trial, *JAMA* 288:1373-1380, 2002.
10. Campero L, Garcia C, Diaz C et al: "Alone, I wouldn't have known what to do": a qualitative study on social support during labor and delivery in Mexico, *Soc Sci Med* 47:395-399, 1998.
11. Gordon NP, Walton D, McCadam E et al: Effects of providing hospital based doulas in health maintenance organization hospitals, *Obstet Gynecol* 93:422-427, 1999.
12. Hofmeyr GJ, Nicodem VC, Wolman WL et al: Companionship to modify the clinical birth environment: effects on progress and perceptions of labour, and breastfeeding, *Br J Obstet Gynaecol* 98:756-760, 1991.
13. Wolman WL, Chalmers B, Hofmeyr GL et al: Postpartum depression and companionship in the clinical birth environment: a randomized controlled study, *Am J Obstet Gynecol* 168:1388-1392, 1993.
14. Gagnon AJ, Waghorn K, Covel C: A randomized trial of one-on-one nurse support of women in labor, *Birth* 24:71-74, 1997.
15. Larimore WL: The role of the father in childbirth, *Midwifery Today* 51:15-17, 1999.

S E C T I O N   E   Intrapartum Fetal Heart Rate Monitoring

Kent Petrie, MD,
and Walter L. Larimore, MD

Fetal compromise resulting in intrapartum fetal asphyxia or fetal demise can be reduced with appropriate evaluation of fetal well-being. The goal of FHR monitoring should be to detect with the highest predictive value possible signs that warn of fetal compromise in time to prevent or correct adverse outcome, causing as little unnecessary intervention as possible. Continuous EFM (with or without procedures such as fetal scalp pH sampling, fetal pulse oximetry, fetal scalp stimulation, or fetal vibroacoustic stimulation, which are discussed in Chapter 16, Section A) and intermittent auscultation (IA) of the fetal heart are the methods most commonly used for intrapartum fetal surveillance.

I. CONTINUOUS ELECTRONIC FETAL MONITORING

A. Background

Continuous EFM is a technology that dates back to the 1960s and became routine in most labor units before evidence from RCTs showed efficacy or safety. EFM is the most prevalent maternity care procedure in the United States. EFM is routinely performed without informed consent taking place.[1]

RCTs in a variety of delivery settings for low-risk mothers show no improvement in neonatal outcome with EFM.[2] The use of EFM increased from 44.6% of live births in 1980 to 62.2% in 1988 to 73.7% in 1992. By 1997, 83% of all live births had EFM, and this number has been stable since then. According to a *National Vital Statistics Report* article, EFM use is likely underreported.[3]

Expert panels in the United States and Canada have advised against routine EFM in low-risk pregnancies and have found weak evidence for inclusion or exclusion for routine use in high-risk pregnancies.[4] This change in attitude among policy makers in clinical medicine was the result primarily of a series of RCTs that documented the benefits and risks of EFM. By 1995, ACOG stated that although all women in labor needed some form of fetal monitoring, the choice of technique (EFM or IA) was based on a variety of factors and should be left to the judgment of the individual birth attendant and patient.[2]

Technologies such as EFM need to be developed carefully and tested in limited settings, usually academic centers, before widespread adoption. Their efficacy and safety need to be shown before they become routine practice. RCTs of EFM versus IA prompted Roger Freeman,[5] author of popular textbooks of fetal monitoring, to reflect: "Clearly, the hoped-for benefit from intrapartum electronic fetal monitoring has not been realized. It is unfortunate that randomized, controlled trials were not carried out before this form of technology became universally applied. Before we discard the electronic fetal monitor, however, we must realize that the randomized trials all had dedicated nurses assigned to the auscultation groups." It is evident from the experience with EFM that such widespread adoption of a technology can lead to misuse, misinterpretation, misunderstanding, and unnecessary concerns with malpractice and litigation.

B. Study Results

1. Retrospective studies

   Early large, retrospective studies using historical controls suggested that EFM resulted in fewer infants with low Apgar scores, reduced neonatal mortality, and improved neurologic outcome.[6,7] It was simply assumed that continuous EFM would be more accurate than IA in detecting FHR patterns, which would be sensitive in predicting the potential for actual fetal compromise. This assumption led to many experts recommending or urging continuous EFM for all women in labor.

2. Prospective RCTs

   The Cochrane Library has summarized the data from nine RCTs and found that, with the exception of a small reduction in the rate of neonatal seizures in high-risk subgroups, the use of routine EFM has no measurable impact on morbidity and mortality.[8] The only two follow-up studies to date have indicated that the long-term neurologic effects of these seizures have been minimal. No significant differences were observed in 1-minute Apgar scores less than 4 or 7, rate of admissions to neonatal intensive care units, perinatal deaths, or cerebral palsy. An increase associated with the use of EFM was observed in the rate of cesarean delivery (RR, 1.41; 95% CI, 1.23-1.61) and operative vaginal delivery (RR, 1.20; 95% CI, 1.11-1.30).[8]

   a. EFM versus IA: Of the RCTs that have now investigated EFM, seven have compared EFM with IA.[8] An early Cochrane review compared IA with EFM plus optional fetal scalp pH sampling in preterm labor and reported no differences in perinatal outcomes, cesarean birth rate, or 18-month psychomotor development.[9] Another review compared a monitored group with an IA group, and a third group with EFM and optional fetal scalp pH sampling.[10] Although fetal scalp pH sampling reduced the increased frequency of cesarean birth, no differences in perinatal morbidity or mortality could be detected in any of the groups.

   b. EFM plus scalp pH sampling versus IA: At least six RCTs have compared EFM plus scalp pH sampling with IA. These data suggest no benefit to EFM on neonatal outcome other than the measure of neonatal seizure when EFM is backed by scalp pH. Secondary review of these data shows that the reduced risk for seizures was limited to induced, augmented, or prolonged labors.[10] This effect has not been shown in trials with premature infants, EFM without scalp pH, and liberal versus restricted EFM.[2,8]

c. EFM in low-risk populations: Nine RCTs of EFM have been conducted in low-risk populations. All show clearly no difference in neonatal outcome except that assisted deliveries were more common in the EFM group.[8] These studies revealed inconsistent results on the influence of EFM on the frequency of cesarean birth.[11] Two RCTs have examined liberal versus restrictive use of EFM in labor and showed no significant difference in the outcomes measured.[12,13]

C. Electronic Fetal Monitoring as a Screening Test

The positive predictive value of abnormal FHR patterns is low with continuous EFM. Only about 20% of *nonreassuring* EFM tracings are associated with a low 5-minute Apgar score. Multiple studies have shown that normal FHR tracings predict good 5-minute Apgar scores in more than 99% of monitored pregnancies indicating a high negative predictive value (ability to predict the absence of disease). When applied to the population of laboring women in most family practice settings with a low incidence of uteroplacental insufficiency, EFM has a high incidence of false-positive results with a resulting low positive predictive value. EFM is, by itself, a poor screening test. In addition, it is not a diagnostic test. A diagnostic test should confirm or reject a possible diagnosis, a criterion not met by EFM alone.[2,4]

D. Indications for Electronic Fetal Monitoring

Although current standards in many hospital settings dictate the use of continuous EFM for most patients at high risk (including thick meconium staining, oxytocin use, twins, medically complicated pregnancies, use of prostaglandin gel, abnormal FHR by auscultation, dysfunctional labor, vaginal breech delivery), ACOG recommendations state that "intermittent auscultation of the fetal heart…is equivalent to continuous EFM in the assessment of fetal condition."[2] The recommendations recognize, however, that intrapartum fetal assessment by monitoring of the heart rate is only one parameter of fetal well-being, and that, in certain situations, the

limited number of nurses available may preclude the capacity to monitor the FHR by auscultation.[2] In addition, the individual physician's medicolegal concerns, the physician's skills in using and interpreting the technology, and the community standard of practice each contribute to an individual clinician's decision to use EFM despite the data or the risks of using EFM.

E. Medicolegal Considerations

Physicians often cite malpractice fears as a reason to continue using EFM, despite a lack of demonstrated effectiveness. It is paradoxical that monitor strips are as easily *overread* in the courtroom as the labor room. Interpreter reliability is variable. EFM recordings have the potential to become more harmful than helpful during malpractice litigation defense and may increase the malpractice suit risk for providers.[2,8]

F. Risks of Electronic Fetal Monitoring

1. Suboptimal maternal fetal perfusion
   EFM has the tendency to keep the mother in a supine position with the potential result of a *cascade effect* secondary to aortocaval compression and poor labor mechanics (see figure in Section B in this chapter). Telemetry monitoring has the potential to allow women to be upright and walking but has not been studied to compare outcomes with women who remained monitored in bed.
2. False-positive results lead to unnecessary interventions
   Abnormal FHR tracings have a low positive predictive value, which often leads to a cascade of unnecessary interventions and accompanying morbidities to the mother and infant.
3. Scalp lead complications
   A less common complication of internal EFM (occurring in <2% of the deliveries) is scalp infection secondary to the scalp electrode. Rarer complications with an internal scalp electrode include sepsis, cerebrospinal fluid leakage, meningitis, and cranial osteomyelitis.
4. False-negative results lead to missed fetal distress
   The most dramatic risk of EFM is inaccurate pattern interpretation, allowing a true fetal distress to go unrecognized or causing unneeded intervention for a healthy fetus. Definitions of FHR patterns are reviewed in detail in Chapter 16, Section A.

II. INTERMITTENT AUSCULTATION OF THE FETAL HEART RATE

RCTs have shown that IA is at least as effective as EFM in detecting fetuses in need of medical intervention.[8,11] It imparts no direct risk to the fetus. Although it has been alleged that significant variable decelerations and evidence of uteroplacental insufficiency could escape diagnosis using periodic auscultation, no studies have yet confirmed this fear. RCTs comparing EFM with IA show no clear effect on analgesic use or the mother's perception of pain, but some differences in maternal perceptions do surface.[12,13] The EFM group felt too restricted in labor. Although these women tended to be left alone more often, there was no apparent difference in their perceptions of the labor as being unpleasant. In two RCTs, the method of monitoring was less important to women than was the support they received from staff and companions.[12,13] Regular auscultation by a personal attendant, as used in these studies, seems to be the practice of choice for the physiologic labor.

A. American College of Obstetricians and Gynecologists Guidelines

ACOG guidelines for patients at low risk recommend that the FHR may be monitored by either IA or continuous EFM. The standard practice is to evaluate and record the FHR at least every 30 minutes after a contraction in the active stage of labor and at least every 15 minutes in the second stage of labor.[2] ACOG has issued guidelines for intermittent FHR auscultation when risk factors are present during labor or when intensified monitoring is deemed to be appropriate. These guidelines, although not evidence based, recommend during the active phase of the first stage of labor, the FHR should be evaluated by auscultation every 15 minutes. During the second stage of labor, the FHR should be evaluated and recorded at least every 5 minutes.[2] In both low- and high-risk patients, the auscultation is performed during a contraction and for at least 30 seconds thereafter.

B. Nursing Requirements

If FHR auscultation is to be used as the primary method of fetal monitoring in labor, a 1:1 nurse-to-patient ratio is required, at least during the second stage of labor. It has been suggested that this staffing requirement is too vigorous for some labor and delivery units. ACOG guidelines for continuous EFM recommend that the FHR record should be evaluated at least every 5 minutes when EFM is used.[2] The staffing needs for either method, based on these guidelines, may actually be similar.

III. THE "ADMISSION MONITOR TEST STRIP"

Many institutions that use IA include an initial continuous EFM period of 15 to 20 minutes. If the initial strip is normal, the patient has the option of continuous or intermittent FHR monitoring. The poor positive predictive value of nonreassuring FHR patterns in RTCs, however, makes one skeptical that "admission strips" would be any better. ACOG guidelines do not mention the concept of an admission test strip,[2] and the Society of Obstetrics and Gynecology of Canada guidelines specifically discourage its use.[8] If performed, the "admission strip" may at best serve as a baseline on which change can be measured.

A. Evidence for Routine Admission Test Strip

A 2001 RCT (N = 3751) comparing Doppler auscultation with an admission test strip showed no differences in terms of fetal outcomes (acidosis, seizures, low Apgar scores, and NICU admissions). In the group that received the admission test strip, there was an increase in augmentation of labor, epidural use, and operative delivery (number needed to harm [NNH] = 18 for vaginal operative delivery; NNH = 67 for cesarean delivery).[14]

A subsequent, larger RCT (N = 8628), published in 2003, also found no benefit to the admission test strip for the fetus. However, this study found no increase in operative delivery (either vaginal or cesarean), likely because of widespread use of scalp pH (9.3% of population had at least one scalp pH determination).[15]

B. Conclusion

"Admission monitor test strips" provide no demonstrable benefit, although they may increase operative vaginal delivery or cesarean delivery unless widespread use of adjunctive measures such as scalp pH is added to ascertain their findings. An ongoing RTC currently is being sponsored by the Cochrane Collaborative.[16]

C. Summary

Continuous EFM alone is not a good screening tool for the population of laboring women in most family practice settings regardless of risk status. It offers no advantage over standard nursing care and

IA of the FHR for most laboring women at low risk. The routine use of continuous EFM for all women in labor appears to increase the risk for instrumental and cesarean delivery with no improvement in fetal outcome. Although EFM provides reassurance for some women and many birth attendants, it is no substitute for the personal support and attendance of laboring women by supportive and caring health-care personnel. All childbearing women need some form of fetal monitoring to detect developing problems. The monitoring type to be used should be individualized for each childbearing family, based on a variety of location, resource, medicolegal, and birth attendant factors. The benefits once claimed for EFM are minimal. The risks associated with the use of EFM, especially the risk for cesarean delivery, warrant the critical scrutiny of each clinician as how best to use this form of fetal surveillance. The ACOG's current position, which leaves the decision to the woman and her birth attendant, is appropriate.[2]

IV. SOR A RECOMMENDATIONS

RECOMMENDATIONS	REFERENCES
Continuous EFM is associated with increased rates of operative vaginal and cesarean delivery without improvements in perinatal outcomes.	*8*
An admission monitor test strip shows no demonstrable fetal benefits but may be associated with increased operative vaginal and cesarean delivery rates.	*14, 15*

REFERENCES

1. Larimore WL, Cline MK: Keeping normal labor normal, *Prim Care* 27:221-236, 2000.
2. American College of Obstetricians and Gynecologists: Fetal heart rate patterns: monitoring, interpretation and management. ACOG technical bulletin no. 207, Washington, DC, 1995, ACOG.
3. Ventura SJ, Mathews TJ, Curtin SC: Declines in teenage birth rates, 1991-97: national and state patterns, *Natl Vital Stat Rep* 47:1-17, 1998.
4. Liston R, Crane J, Hamilton E et al: Fetal health surveillance in labour, *J Obstet Gynaecol Can* 24:250-262, 2002.
5. Freeman R: Intrapartum fetal monitoring—a disappointing story, *N Engl J Med* 322(9):624-626, 1990.
6. Smith MA, Acheson LS, Byrd JE et al: A critical review of labor and birth care (clinical review). Obstetrical Interest Group of the North American Primary Care Research Group, *J Fam Pract* 33:281-292, 1991.
7. Smith MA, Ruffin MT, Green LA: The thoughtful management of labor, *Am Fam Physician* 45:1471-1481, 1993.
8. Thacker SB, Stroup D, Chang M: Continuous electronic heart rate monitoring for fetal assessment during labor, *Cochrane Database Syst Rev* (2):CD000063, 2001.
9. Grant AM: EFM plus scalp sampling vs intermittent auscultation in labour. In Eakin MW, Keirse MJNC, Renfrew MJ, Neilson JP, editors: *Pregnancy and childbirth module. Cochrane Database Systematic Reviews, Cochrane Updates on Disk,* Oxford, 1993, Update Software.
10. Grant AM: Fetal blood sampling as adjunct to heart rate monitoring. In Chambers I, editor: *Oxford database of perinatal trials,* Oxford, 1992, Update Software.
11. Grant AM: EFM alone vs intermittent auscultation in labor. In Eakin MW, Keirse MJNC, Renfrew MJ, Neilson JP, editors: *Pregnancy and childbirth module. Cochrane Database Systematic Reviews, Cochrane Updates on Disk,* Oxford, 1993, Update Software.
12. Grant AM: Liberal vs restrictive use of EFM in labour. In Eakin MW, Keirse MJNC, Renfrew MJ, Neilson JP, editors: *Pregnancy and childbirth module. Cochrane Database Systematic Reviews, Cochrane Updates on Disk,* Oxford, 1993, Update Software.
13. Grant AM: Liberal vs restrictive use of EFM in low-risk labour. In Eakin MW, Keirse MJNC, Renfrew MJ, Neilson JP, editors: *Pregnancy and childbirth module. Cochrane Database Systematic Reviews, Cochrane Updates on Disk,* Oxford, 1993, Update Software.
14. Mires G, William F, Howie P: Randomized controlled trial of cardiotocography versus Doppler auscultation of fetal heart at admission in labour in low risk obstetric population, *BMJ* 322:1457-1462, 2001.
15. Impey L, Reynolds M, MacQuillan K et al: Admission cardiotocography: a randomized controlled trial, *Lancet* 361:465-470, 2003.
16. Devane D, Lalor JG, Daly S et al: Cardiotocography versus intermittent auscultation of fetal heart on admission to labour ward for assessment of fetal wellbeing, *Cochrane Database Syst Rev* (1):CD005122, 2005.

S E C T I O N F Normal Delivery and Birthing Positions

Kent Petrie, MD,
and Walter L. Larimore, MD

I. PREPARATION FOR DELIVERY

The delivery most often attended by family physicians is the spontaneous vaginal delivery. Before delivery and toward the end of the second stage of labor, preparation should be made for delivery. Most birth attendants begin these preparations when the multiparous patient is at near or complete dilation, or when the nulliparous patient begins to crown.

Crowning is the term used to describe the appearance of the fetal scalp between the dilating introitus. As the second stage begins to near its end, the perineum bulges with each contraction and each time the woman bears down. The vaginal opening becomes more dilated by the fetal head with each contraction. During this process, the perineum begins a thinning process.

Some birth attendants assist the process with perineal massage. The birth attendant may place his or her thumb on the outside of the perineum and the index or index and middle finger on the inside of the perineum, gently massaging the perineum from midline laterally on each side. The method has been described in case studies as being soothing to the patient, reducing the length and depth of perineal tears, reducing the need for episiotomy, and by some authors, being pain relieving.[1] A RCT from the midwifery literature, however, did not find the practice to increase the likelihood of an intact perineum, but it was associated with fewer third-degree tears.[2]

Two RCTs of antepartum perineal massage report reduced perineal trauma in primips who practice the technique.[3,4] In the Canadian Perineal Massage Trial, the intervention group of pregnant women was instructed in the daily manual stretching of the perineal muscles for 10 minutes starting at 34 to 35 weeks of gestation. Patients or their partners were advised to insert their thumbs into the vaginal opening and gently pull down for 2 minutes at each of the 4, 6, and 8 o'clock positions. The study showed that the prenatal perineal massage helped preserve an intact perineum without damaging a gravida's future sexual satisfaction or increasing her risk for urinary incontinence. Of the intervention group, 24% of primiparas delivered over an intact perineum compared with 15% of the control group.[3]

II. POSITIONING FOR DELIVERY

The patient is placed in a delivery position or, preferably, allowed to assume the most comfortable delivery position for her delivery. The traditional dorsal lithotomy position on the delivery room table was developed almost primarily to benefit the birth attendant by allowing adequate access to the perineum for operative delivery. Increasing numbers of family physicians and midwives are avoiding this delivery position, however, which has been implicated in increased delivery pain, increased perineal tears, increased extensions of episiotomies, and possibly increased fetal distress. At least 11 RCTs have evaluated delivery positions.[5] The combined data suggest that an upright position during the second stage reduces intolerable pain, difficulty bearing down, instrumented vaginal delivery, and episiotomy rate.[6,7]

The lateral side-lying or Sims' position for birth is one that many family physicians have less experience in using.[8] This position adapts readily to almost any hospital bed, delivery bed, or delivery table (with the exception of the birthing chair), and has been reported in several case series to be associated with reduced blood loss, reduced hypotension, reduced fetal distress, decreased perceived maternal pain, and reduced numbers of episiotomies when compared with the lithotomy position. The side-lying position may not be adequate for deliveries requiring large episiotomies, operative deliveries, or regional anesthesia.[7,8]

Regarding the hands-and-knees position, the Cochrane Library suggests, "The best position for babies during birth is head down, with the back of their head facing forward. When babies lie with the back of their head towards the mothers' side (lateral) or towards the mothers' back (posterior), the labor may be longer and more painful. Although assuming the hands-and-knees posture in late pregnancy does not improve pregnancy outcomes, the use in labor is worth further investigating."[9] Case studies have likewise suggested the hands-and-knees position as quite useful in accomplishing rotation of an occiput posterior position, and it is a useful maneuver for reducing shoulder dystocia.

Many of the management paradigms traditionally used with the delivering woman include positions, policies, protocols, and procedures that lack evidence of benefit to the mother or the fetus. The birth attendant needs to be aware of these data and to become more comfortable with an individualized, flexible delivery plan. Labor and delivery positions, policies, or protocols with no proven scientific basis and no indication of clear superiority for the mother or fetus should be left to the discretion of the delivering parents.

A. The Birthing Bed
Birthing beds have gained increasing popularity and use in the United States. These beds combine the advantages of the birthing chair (mobility, ease of position change, decreased pain in second stage, improved bearing down) with the advantages of a traditional delivery table (at least for the birth attendant), while being much more comfortable than

either the chair or the table. Although expensive to purchase, they are increasingly incorporated into birthing units in hospital and nonhospital settings. These multiposition beds allow a delivering patient to assume a variety of positions and facilitate upright positioning. They have the advantage of equal usability for nontraditional and traditional or operative deliveries.

B. Immersion in Water during Delivery

Delivery in water is a controversial issue.[10] On one hand, midwives and other maternity caregivers report that it is a relaxing and satisfying environment in which to birth.[11] On the other hand, there is a dearth of evidence as to the safety and effectiveness of this option. Its promotion as a therapeutic tool for laboring women began to appear in the English medical literature in the 1980s. The first published account of a birth in water in the United Kingdom occurred in 1987.[12] Although much more commonly practiced in the United Kingdom than the United States, its use in the United States appears to be growing.[13,14] Labor and birth in water is actively promoted as helpful and safe. Birthing pools for hire or for institutional purchase are widely advertised. It is not known how widespread water labor and delivery is in the United States. Some birthing centers and hospitals are responding to this demand by providing pools in birthing suites, whereas others allow pool rental. Many of these centers have developed guidelines for this practice; however, opinions differ as to what constitutes safe practice.

Many possible benefits are suggested for the mother and infant including nonpharmacologic pain relief, acceleration of labor, reduction of maternal blood pressure, increased maternal control over the birth environment, reduced perineal trauma, improved psychosocial outcomes, improved maternal satisfaction with labor and delivery, and avoidance of nonindicated interventions.[1,13,14]

Possible hazards that have been suggested for the mother include increased risk for infection, reduction of effective contractions, increased perineal trauma, increased risk for postpartum hemorrhage, risk for water embolism, and restriction of mobility. Possible hazards that have been suggested for the infant include increased risk for infection, increased admission to special care nurseries, risk for trauma resulting from inability to breath at birth, and water aspiration.[1,13,14]

Limited data are available from two published and two ongoing RCTs, three nonrandomized cohort studies, and several case series. These data indicate that water labor is prolonged compared with traditional care (690 vs. 552 minutes) and most marked in primiparas (767 vs. 632 minutes); women are more likely to have second-degree tears but are less likely to need augmentation. No differences were seen in episiotomy use, Apgar scores, perineal infection, or postpartum fever.[1,10] A Cochrane review of available data in 2004 concluded:

> There is evidence that water immersion during the first stage of labor reduces the use of analgesia and reported maternal pain, without adverse outcomes on labor duration, operative delivery or neonatal outcomes. The effects of immersion in water during pregnancy or in the third stage are unclear. One trial explores birth in water, but is too small to determine the outcomes for women or neonates.[14]

Case reports are available of infant deaths after delivery in water, but few details have been published. In most of these cases, the infant was held under water for some considerable time after birth.[15]

Given past maternity care experiences with interventions becoming widely accepted before being adequately evaluated (i.e., continuous EFM, routine IV lines in labor, routine episiotomy), it seems reasonable for evidence-based maternity caregivers to insist on adequate evaluation of labor and birth in water before widespread implementation.

III. DELIVERY MANEUVERS

As crowning progresses and after the delivery position has been achieved, appropriate drapes may be placed under the woman and the perineum prepared. Most birth attendants use an iodine solution and attempt to cleanse the vulvovaginal and rectal areas, despite any RCT data concerning the safety or risk of doing so. Delivery anesthesia, if used, is chosen at this time; most deliveries can be performed without anesthesia if that is the patient and birth attendant's preference.

A. Delivery of the Head

Many physicians have been taught to perform the modified Ritgen maneuver to deliver the fetal head (Figure 14-12). This maneuver consists of exerting pressure on the chin of the fetus through the perineum, just in front of the coccyx, with one hand,

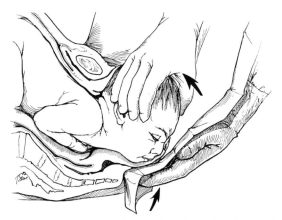

FIGURE 14-12. Near completion of the delivery of the fetal head by the modified Ritgen maneuver. Moderate upward pressure is applied to the fetal chin by the posterior hand, while the suboccipital area of the fetal head is held against the symphysis.

while the other hand exerts pressure superiorly against the occiput. Historically, the Ritgen maneuver accomplished the same maneuver by inserting a finger into the rectum. Classically, these maneuvers have been thought to control delivery and extend the head to allow it to be delivered through the smallest diameter. It is now recognized that extending the head on the perineum presents not the smallest diameter (the occipitobregmatic) but the largest diameter (the occipitofrontal) to the perineum (Figure 14-13). The Ritgen maneuver or modified Ritgen maneuver may increase the risk for

tearing or episiotomy. Although the Ritgen and modified Ritgen maneuvers can accelerate the delivery process, they may be considerably more traumatic to the maternal perineum.

Midwives have practiced the exact opposite for several centuries. As the flexed head passes through the vaginal introitus, the smallest head diameter (the occipitobregmatic) is preserved if the vertex is maintained in a state of flexion. As flexion is maintained, the perineum can be massaged slowly over the face, under the chin and around the ears, before the head is allowed to extend. This method is less traumatic to the maternal perineum and reduces the need for episiotomy or resultant perineal tearing.

Only one RCT has tested this hypothesis. The HOOP trial (Hands On Or Poised) in England was designed to compare the effect of two methods of perineal management used during spontaneous vaginal delivery on the prevalence of perineal pain reported at 10 days after birth. At the end of the second stage of labor, women were allocated to either the *hands-on* method, in which the midwife's hands put pressure on the infant's head and support *(guard)* the perineum, and then lateral flexion was used to facilitate delivery of the shoulders, or the *hands poised* method, in which the midwife kept her hands poised, not touching the head or perineum and allowing spontaneous delivery of the shoulders.[16] Of the women in the *hands poised* group, 34% reported pain in the previous 24 hours at 10 days after delivery compared with 31% in the hands-on group (RR, 1.10; 95% CI, 1.01-1.18; $p = 0.02$). The rate of episiotomy was significantly lower in

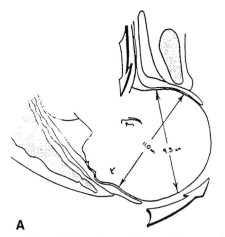
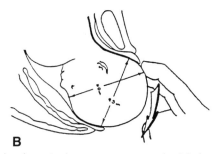

A   **B**

FIGURE 14-13. A, In occipitoanterior positions, pushing extends the head, causing it to present a greater (occipitofrontal) diameter. **B,** Flexing of head presents the smallest (suboccipitobregmatic) diameter.

the hands poised group (RR, 0.79; 99% CI, 0.65-0.96; $p = 0.008$), but the rate of manual removal of placenta was significantly greater (RR, 1.69; 99% CI, 1.02-2.78; $p = 0.008$). The researchers concluded that the reduction in pain observed in the hands-on group potentially could affect a substantial number of women.

B. Pushing at Delivery

Tradition in the United States is to have the laboring mother use Valsalva pushing at the end of the second stage of labor, wherein the mother holds her breath and bears down to *push the baby out,* as opposed to expiration pushing or exhalant bearing down, wherein the mother breathes (*breathes the baby out*) while bearing down in the second stage of labor, which is practiced by many midwives. The available data from RCTs suggest that second-stage pushing or bearing-down efforts involving the Valsalva maneuver, although resulting in a slightly shorter second stage of labor, may compromise maternal-fetal gas exchange, which can result in FHR abnormalities or reduced Apgar scores. RCTs suggest that the practice of sustained (Valsalva) bearing down at delivery may have a deleterious fetal effect unless any potential shortening of the second stage is mandatory.[17,18]

Another age-old pushing tradition is for the birth attendant to ask another attendant to apply fundal pressure at the end of the second stage. This is a practice for which insufficient evidence exists to support a clear recommendation supporting or opposing the practice. It should be avoided in the setting of shoulder dystocia. It should be used with caution otherwise until further research clarifies the issue.

Another common practice is to have patients begin pushing as soon as the cervix reaches complete dilation. RCTs support delaying pushing until the presenting part descends.[19-21] According to the PEOPLE (Pushing Early or Pushing Late with Epidural) Study, this policy has been shown to reduce second-stage cesarean birth and difficult operative vaginal deliveries in nulliparous women, particularly in those with epidural analgesia.[20]

C. Oropharyngeal Suctioning

After the delivery of the head, the nostrils and mouth usually are suctioned with a *bulb syringe.* A finger may be passed over the neck of the fetus to determine whether it is encircled by the umbilical cord. A nuchal cord or cord around the neck occurs in 10% to 15% of all deliveries. If the cord is loose, it may be slipped over the infant's head. If extremely tight, the cord may be cut between two clamps and released, or alternatively, the infant may be delivered between the nuchal loop.

D. Meconium Staining

If meconium staining was present during labor or delivery, the nasooropharynx may be suctioned thoroughly with a DeLee suction device, using a suction apparatus or wall suction instead of oral suction, before delivery of the shoulders. This technique has been shown to reduce the incidence of meconium aspiration or pneumonitis; however, care must be taken to reduce stimulation to the posterior pharynx. If the posterior pharynx is stimulated too vigorously, a vagal response may be stimulated, resulting in fetal bradycardia.

Some birth attendants differentiate between thick meconium and thin meconium. The presumption clinically is that thin meconium is *watered down* with amniotic fluid or reduced in amount when compared with thick meconium and is less caustic to the fetal lung if aspirated.

Four RCTs have addressed the problem of endotracheal intubation of vigorous meconium-stained infants born at term. No evidence from these data support that endotracheal intubation and aspiration of the airways in nonasphyxiated, meconium-stained infants is of any benefit. One review suggests that this procedure is associated with a 1.2% increased risk for acquiring meconium aspiration syndrome, or that for every 83 vigorous meconium-stained infants born at term who are exposed to routine endotracheal intubation and aspiration at birth, 1 case of meconium aspiration syndrome is caused. A Cochrane review concludes: "Routine endotracheal intubation at birth in vigorous term meconium-stained babies has not been shown to be superior to routine resuscitation including oro-pharyngeal suction. This procedure cannot be recommended for vigorous infants until more research is available."[22]

E. Delivery of the Shoulders

After the head is born, it typically turns toward one of the maternal thighs, assuming a transverse position. Often the shoulders are born spontaneously, with little effort. If not, the sides of the head may be grasped between two hands. With gentle downward traction, only in the vertical plane, the anterior shoulder typically can be delivered easily. Often, clinicians then attempt to deliver the posterior shoulder before completely delivering the anterior arm (Figure 14-14). Midwives have long taught that after delivering the anterior shoulder, failure to deliver completely the anterior arm may increase

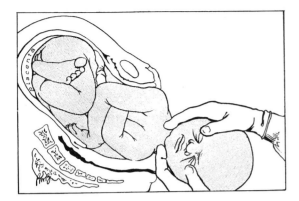

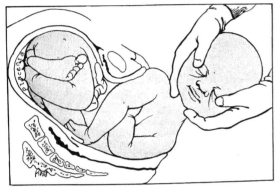

FIGURE 14-14. Gentle downward traction to bring about descent of anterior shoulder *(top)*. Delivery of anterior shoulder is completed; gentle upward traction is applied to deliver the posterior shoulder *(bottom)*.

periurethral and vaginal tearing. Although tested in no RCTs to date, some recommend that birth attendants, after delivering the anterior shoulder, attempt to deliver the anterior arm completely.

After delivery of the anterior shoulder and arm, an upward movement of the head typically accomplishes delivery of the posterior shoulder and arm. The movements to deliver the shoulders by applying traction to the fetal head are only in a vertical plane, with as little traction as possible, to reduce any increased risk for brachial plexus, neck, or clavicle injury.

F. Delivery of the Body
After delivery of both shoulders through the introitus, the remainder of the delivery requires little or no assistance. At this point, the birth attendant can allow the parents to reach down to the perineum, grasping the infant under the arms, around the trunk, and facilitating the parent's completing the birth of the baby onto the maternal abdomen, which facilitates early skin-to-skin contact between the mother and newborn baby.

G. After Delivery
The infant's airway should be cleared completely and the umbilical cord clamped after delivery. At this point, one of the labor support persons may wish to cut the cord. Ongoing RCTs in term infants are evaluating early versus late cord clamping in the third stage of labor.[23] No evidence has been reported of a significant effect in the timing of cord clamping on the incidence of postpartum hemorrhage or fetomaternal transfusion. The effects on neonatal grunting, neonatal respiratory distress, or neonatal jaundice are inconclusive.

Evidence does exist that delayed clamping of the cord in preterm infants by 30 to 120 seconds, rather than early clamping, seems to be associated with less need for transfusion and less intraventricular hemorrhage. There are no clear differences in other outcomes.[24]

The infant should be dried, wrapped warmly, and if stable, allowed to bond with the mother (or parents). An exception to drying off the infant is often made for mothers who desire that the infant be delivered to their chest for bonding or breastfeeding. These infants can be covered with warm blankets. No RCT data speak against this approach, and some anecdotal data speak to increased breastfeeding success with this maneuver.

H. Bonding
Although few data exist to document a maternal-infant bonding effect, no data indicate any harm from this time together, and several case series document increased maternal satisfaction with this time of bonding. A time of bonding, similar to so many other labor and delivery traditions, may be left to the discretion of the mother and should not be discouraged or prevented without indication.

IV. SOR A RECOMMENDATIONS

RECOMMENDATIONS	REFERENCES
In nulliparous patients with epidural analgesia, delayed pushing in the second stage of labor reduces difficult operative vaginal and cesarean deliveries.	20

| Routine endotracheal intubation at birth of vigorous term meconium-stained infants should be avoided. | 23 |
| Delayed clamping of the cord in preterm infants reduces the need for transfusion and the incidence of intraventricular hemorrhage. | 24 |

REFERENCES

1. Cammu H, Clasen K, Van Wettenu L: Is having a warm bath during labor useful? *Acta Obstet Gynaecol Scand* 73:468-472, 1994.
2. Stamp G, Kruzins G, Crowther C: Perineal massage in labour and prevention of perineal trauma: a randomized controlled trial, *BMJ* 322:1277-1280, 2001.
3. Labrecque M, Eason E, Marloux S et al: Randomized controlled trial of prevention of perineal trauma by perineal massage during pregnancy, *Am J Obstet Gynecol* 180:593-600, 1999.
4. Shipman MK, Boniface DR, Tefft ME et al: Antenatal perineal massage and subsequent perinatal outcomes: a randomized controlled trial, *Br J Obstet Gynaecol* 104:787-791, 1997.
5. Gupta JK, Hofmyer GJ: Position of women during second stage of labor, *Cochrane Database Syst Rev* (1):CD002006, 2004.
6. Smith MA, Acheson LS, Byrd JE et al: A critical review of labor and birth care (clinical review). Obstetrical Interest Group of the North American Primary Care Research Group, *J Fam Pract* 33:281-292, 1991.
7. Smith MA, Ruffin MT, Green LA: The thoughtful management of labor, *Am Fam Physician* 45:1471-1481, 1993.
8. Kirkwood CR, Clark L: Lateral Sims deliveries: a new application for an old technique, *J Fam Pract* 17:101-115, 1983.
9. Hofmeyr GJ, Kulier R: Hands and knees posture in late pregnancy or labour for fetal malposition (lateral or posterior), *Cochrane Database Syst Rev* (2):CD001063, 2005.
10. McCandlish R, Renfrew M: Immersion in water during labor and birth: the need for evaluation, *Birth* 20:79-85, 1993.
11. Kitzinger S: Sheila Kitzinger's letter from England, *Birth* 18:170-171, 1991.
12. Stacey L: Splash baby Charlie makes medical history, *Chat*, November 7, 1987.
13. Findley I, Chamberlain G: ABC of labour care. Relief of pain, *BMJ* 318:927-930, 1999.
14. Nikodem VC, Cluett ER, McCandlish RE et al: Immersion in water in pregnancy, labour and birth, *Cochrane Database Syst Rev* (2):CD000111, 2004.
15. Kitzinger S: *Homebirth and other alternatives to hospital*, London, 1991, Dorling Kindersley.
16. McCandlish R, Bowler U, van Asten H et al: A randomized controlled trial of care of the perineum during second stage of normal labour, *Br J Obstet Gynaecol* 105:1262-1272, 1998.
17. Petersen L, Besuner P: Pushing techniques in labor: issues and controversies, *J Obstet Gynecol Neonat Nurs* 26:719-726, 1997.
18. Roberts JE: The "push" for evidence: management of the second stage, *Midwifery Women's Health* 47:2-15, 2002.
19. Fraser WD, Marcoux S, Krauss I, et al: Multicenter, randomized, controlled trial of delayed pushing for nulliparous women in the second stage of labor with continuous epidural anesthesia. The PEOPLE (Pushing Early or Pushing Late with Epidural) Study Group, *Am J Obstet Gynecol* 182:1165-1172, 2000.
20. Petrou S, Coyle D, Fraser WD: Cost-effectiveness of a delayed pushing policy for patients with epidural anesthesia. The PEOPLE (Pushing Early or Pushing Late with Epidural) Study Group, *Am J Obstet Gynecol* 182:1158-1164, 2000.
21. Vause S, Congdon HM, Thornton JG: Immediate and delayed pushing in the second stage of labour for nulliparous women with epidural anesthesia: a randomized controlled trial, *Br J Obstet Gynaecol* 105:186-188, 1998.
22. McDonald SJ, Abbott JM: Effect of timing of umbilical cord clamping of term infants on maternal and neonatal outcomes. (Protocol), *Cochrane Database Syst Rev* (1):CD004074, 2003.
23. Halliday HL: Endotracheal intubation at birth for preventing morbidity and mortality in vigorous, meconium-stained infants born at term, *Cochrane Database Syst Rev* (1):CD005000, 2001.
24. Rabe H, Reynolds G, Diaz-Rossello J: Early versus delayed umbilical cord clamping in preterm infants, *Cochrane Database Syst Rev* (4):CD003248, 2004.

S E C T I O N   G   Management of the Second Stage

Matthew K. Cline, MD

I. BACKGROUND AND DEFINITIONS

The second stage of labor begins with complete dilatation of the cervix and ends with delivery of the fetus. The second stage can be divided into two portions: an initial latent phase involving passive descent of the presenting part, and a later active phase in which the patient experiences a significant urge to push when the presenting part reaches the pelvic floor. This section examines traditional approaches to the second stage together with evidence that can help guide the physician in its management.

II. DURATION OF THE SECOND STAGE

A. Background

Traditionally, the second stage in nulliparas has followed a "2-hour rule" that is thought to have originated from an article by Hamilton, who published a series of papers from 1853 to 1871 that illustrated apparent benefits by using forceps to shorten the second stage. In his 1861 article, Hamilton states, "Whenever the os has become fully dilated, so that an ear can be felt, I hold that the danger to the child usually becomes imminent if allowed to remain undelivered much more than 2 hours."[1] This article was referenced in a 1952 case series report by Hellman and Prystowsky,[2] which showed increasing adverse neonatal and maternal outcomes when the second stage was longer than 2.5 hours. The ACOG defines a prolonged second stage as 2 hours in nulliparas and 1 hour in multiparas, adding an additional hour in cases where the patient has an epidural.[3]

B. Current Evidence

Albers[4] observed 2511 women in labor who did not receive epidural analgesia or oxytocin and found that the mean length of the second stage in nulliparas was 54 minutes, with the 95th percentile being 146 minutes. For multiparas, the mean duration of the second stage was 18 minutes, with the 95th percentile of 64 minutes. Neither maternal nor fetal morbidity was increased with longer duration of the second stage.[4]

Mentiglou and colleagues[5] evaluated a group of more than 6000 women and found that there was no significant relation between the length of the second stage and decreased 5-minute Apgar score, neonatal seizures, or neonatal ICU admissions. In another cohort, Myles and Santolaya[6] note similar stable neonatal outcomes for patients with a second-stage duration less than 2 hours compared with those whose stage lasted more than 4 hours. In addition, they found that 80% of patients with a second stage longer than 2 hours still delivered vaginally; this decreased to 65% delivering vaginally at 4 hours.[6]

C. Risk Factors for Prolonged Duration of the Second Stage

Cohort data support the following risk factors for a prolonged second stage:
1. Nulliparity
2. Use of epidural analgesia
3. Diabetes (even when controlling for the presence of macrosomia)
4. Macrosomia
5. Preeclampsia
6. Chorioamnionitis
7. Persistent occiput posterior position[7]

D. Conclusion

Based on the above information, it is reasonable to continue the second stage beyond any specific time frame as long as progress is being made and fetal monitoring is reassuring.

III. POSITIONS

Numerous authorities have discussed the shortcomings of the supine or dorsal lithotomy position for the second stage of labor; it is generally preferred, however,

by clinicians because of the full access it provides to the perineum. A Cochrane review[8] evaluated 19 studies that compared outcomes based on delivery position (total of 5764 patients) and found that the upright or lateral position (compared with lithotomy position) was associated with the following results:
1. Decreased duration of the second stage
2. Slight reduction in rates of assisted delivery
3. Reduction in episiotomy
4. Small decrease in second-degree perineal lacerations
5. Increase in the estimated blood loss of more than 500 ml
6. Reduced severe pain during the second stage
7. Lower rates of abnormal FHR patterns

IV. MANAGEMENT OF SECOND STAGE WITH EPIDURAL

A. "Rest and Descend"

One traditional pushing method involves beginning to push with complete dilatation, at the onset of the second stage, regardless of whether the patient feels the urge to bear down. In patients without epidural analgesia, the urge to push may coincide with complete dilatation; in patients with epidural, however, studies suggest possible benefit in allowing the head to descend until it distends the pelvic floor.

In an RCT of 1862 nulliparous women with epidural, the study group waited at least 2 hours after reaching complete dilatation to begin pushing compared with immediate pushing when completely dilated with the control group. Difficult delivery and midpelvic procedures were decreased in the delayed pushing group (NNT = 22), with a slightly greater rate of spontaneous delivery and no differences in neonatal morbidity scores. The authors concluded that delayed pushing is an effective strategy to reduce difficult deliveries in nulliparas; those with a transverse or posterior fetal position at full dilatation seemed to benefit the most (NNT to avoid 1 difficult delivery was 8 in this subgroup).[9] Overall neonatal morbidity was not increased. Other similar studies have also noted no difference in cord pH, Apgar scores, perineal injury, or endometritis.[10,11]

B. Discontinuation of Epidural Analgesia for the Second Stage

In many sites, it is common practice to discontinue epidural analgesia at a predetermined point (such as the onset of the second stage) to potentially decrease the possibility of dystocia or instrumental delivery.

The Cochrane metaanalysis of this topic contains 5 studies, with 462 patients. Although each study used a different medication or administration protocol, there was no difference noted in patients with full epidural analgesia in the second stage versus those who discontinued the epidural medication with regard to rate of instrumental delivery rate, cesarean delivery rate, or any neonatal outcome evaluated. However, those patients whose epidural was stopped experienced a significant increase in levels of pain relief reported as "inadequate."[12]

V. PUSHING TECHNIQUES

Several small studies comparing open glottis with closed glottis (Valsalva) pushing during the second stage reported that recurrent Valsalva maneuvers were associated with slightly lower Apgar scores and cord blood pH in the neonate. In 1993, Parnell and colleagues[13] compared these two methods directly and found that there were no significant differences in measured duration of the second stage or neonatal outcomes such as Apgar scores or cord pH. A more recent RCT of 320 nulliparas without epidural analgesia who were randomized to "coached" (instructed to perform closed glottis pushing) versus "uncoached" (patients told to "do what comes naturally") did show a slight shortening of the second stage of labor by 13 minutes in the "coached" group, but no change in fetal outcomes, cesarean delivery, or assisted vaginal delivery rates.[14] Based on these small studies, there is no clearly preferred method of pushing for the second stage of labor.[15]

VI. MANAGEMENT OF PERINEAL PAIN

The discomfort experienced by the patient during the second stage includes sources of pain experienced throughout the active first stage of labor (uterine and cervical pain) in addition to pain experienced through the somatic nerves of the lower vagina and perineum caused by distention and stretching of the tissue as the presenting part descends. Methods for management of the pain of labor are discussed in Section C of this chapter.

VII. EPISIOTOMY

A 1997 systematic review of RCTs of management that could prevent perineal trauma during delivery yielded 80 articles, 16 of which were analyzed in detail. Five potential factors affected perineal integrity: episiotomy, third-trimester perineal massage, mother's position in the second stage, method of pushing, and use of epidural analgesia. Of these, only limiting episiotomy was found to be well supported by the existing literature on limiting perineal trauma at birth.[16]

A Cochrane review[17] of episiotomy includes 6 studies, with a total of 4850 patients. In the routine episiotomy group, the rate of episiotomy was 72.7% compared with 27.6% in the restrictive group.[17] Compared with routine use, restrictive episiotomy yielded the following results:

1. Less posterior trauma (RR, 0.74)
2. Decreased need for suturing (RR, 0.69)
3. Fewer healing complications (RR, 0.69)
4. No difference in severe vaginal or perineal trauma
5. No difference in dyspareunia, urinary incontinence, or pain measures
6. Higher rates of anterior perineal laceration (RR, 1.79)

VIII. MANAGEMENT OF THE PERINEUM

As the vertex crowns and comes beneath the symphysis pubis, many practitioners have been traditionally taught to perform a Ritgen maneuver to deliver the fetal head, which consists of exerting pressure on the chin of the fetus through the perineum to extend the head and effect delivery. However, this extension of the fetal head actually presents the occipitofrontal diameter of the head to the perineum, which is considerably larger than the occipitobregmatic, or smallest diameter of the fetal head. The use of pressure on the fetal occiput to maintain flexion during crowning can potentially result in less extensive perineal laceration (see Section H in this chapter).

The HOOPs trial was designed to compare two methods of perineal management. In the *hands-on* method, the delivery attendant puts pressure on the infant's head and supports the perineum using lateral flexion to deliver the shoulders; in the *hands poised* group, the attendant does not touch the head or perineum and allows spontaneous delivery of the head and shoulders. There was a small but significant increase in reported pain in the hands poised group, though the rate of episiotomy was lower in this group. The researchers conclude the reduction in pain was clinically significant (NNT = 33).[18] Thus, there are small but significant benefits to having the clinician assist in managing the perineum. Maintaining the fetal head in flexion can assist by providing the smallest diameter for delivery.

IX. OXYTOCIN AUGMENTATION IN THE SECOND STAGE

A randomized trial of the use of oxytocin at the onset of the second stage in 226 nulliparas with an epidural and no previous use of oxytocin during labor revealed lower rates of operative vaginal delivery and cesarean delivery with similar infant outcomes in the group that received augmentation.[19] Oxytocin was started at 2 mU/min and doubled every 20 minutes to a maximum of 16 mU/min unless fetal decelerations occurred or the period between contractions became less than 1 minute. Of note is that in patients with a fetus in an occiput posterior or occiput transverse position at the onset of the second stage, there was no change in the need for operative delivery, just those in occiput anterior positions. Treated patients had a second stage that was an average of 17 minutes shorter, and had 13% fewer episiotomies or second-degree tears (NNT to prevent 1 laceration was 5.7).

X. USE OF A PARTOGRAM

Is it possible to predict the progress of the second stage at the time of complete dilatation? Although Friedman suggested and pioneered graphical representations of labor (both dilatation and descent), these generally stop at complete dilatation. A prospective cohort of 1413 women (nulliparas and multiparas) was evaluated with standard partographs to the point of complete dilatation, then with a newly devised second-stage partogram that

TABLE 14-5 Assigning Second-Stage Partogram Score

Points	Station	Position
0	Above +1	LOP, OP, or ROP
1	At +1	LOT or ROT
2	Below +1	LOA, OA, or ROA

LOA, Left occiput anterior; LOP, left occiput posterior; LOT, left occiput transverse; OA, occiput anterior; OP, occiput posterior; ROA, right occiput anterior; ROP, right occiput posterior; ROT, right occiput transverse.

was developed for the study.[20] The position of the fetal head and the station were determined to calculate the patient's "score" (see Table 14-5). A score of 5 is assigned if the fetus was crowning and anal dilatation present (imminent delivery), and a score of 6 indicates delivery.

Normograms were created for nulliparas (n = 744) and multiparas (n = 669); nulliparas started the second stage with an average score of 3 and reached 6 at 90 minutes; multiparas started with a score of 3 and reached 6 at 60 minutes. The data for nulliparas in terms of predicting the outcome of the second stage are given in Table 14-6. The clinical utility of assessing the score at the onset of the second stage could include predicting those patients who are at greater risk for a difficult second stage (facilitating early intervention): Consider the use of oxytocin in the second stage in multiparas who begin the second stage with a score less than 3 or nulliparas with a score less than 2. A prospective application of this scoring system in an RCT has not been done.

TABLE 14-6 Outcome of the Second Stage Compared with Initial Second-Stage Partogram Score for Nulliparas

Initial Score	Rate of Vaginal Delivery	Rate of Instrumental Vaginal Delivery	Rate of Caesarean Delivery
0	25%	63%	12%
1	23%	70%	7%
2	42%	53%	5%
3	55%	45%	0%
4	65%	35%	0%
5	98%	2%	0%

XI. SOR A RECOMMENDATIONS

RECOMMENDATIONS	REFERENCES
With continued progress and reassuring fetal monitoring, the second stage may be allowed to continue up to 4 hours or more.	4-6
In patients with epidural analgesia, use of a "rest and descend" period at the onset of the second stage can shorten the period of active pushing and reduce maternal exhaustion without neonatal morbidity.	9-11
Avoid discontinuation of epidural analgesia in the second stage; it is not associated with improved outcomes but does lead to increased patient reports of inadequate pain relief.	12
Adopt a restrictive approach to use of episiotomy because this decreases posterior trauma, need for suturing, and healing complications.	17

REFERENCES

1. Hamilton G: Classical observations and suggestions in obstetrics, *Edinburgh Med J* 7:313, 1861.
2. Hellman l, Prystowsky H: The duration of the second stage of labor, *Am J Obstet Gynecol* 63:1223-1233, 1952.
3. American College of Obstetrics and Gynecology Committee on Practice Bulletins-Obstetrics: ACOG Practice Bulletin Number 49, December 2003: Dystocia and augmentation of labor, *Obstet Gynecol* 102:1445-1453, 2003.
4. Albers LL: The duration of labor in healthy women, *J Perinatol* 19:114-119, 1999.
5. Mentiglou S, Manning F, Harman C et al: Perinatal outcome in relation to second stage: perinatal outcome in relation to second-stage duration, *Am J Obstet Gynecol* 173:906-912, 1995.
6. Myles T, Santolaya J: Maternal and neonatal outcomes in patients with a prolonged second stage, *Obstet Gynecol* 102: 52-58, 2003.
7. Fitzpatrick M, McQuillan K, O'Herlihy C: Influence of persistent occiput posterior position on delivery outcome, *Obstet Gynecol* 98:1027-1031, 2001.
8. Gupta JK, Nikodem VC: Woman's position during second stage of labour, *Cochrane Database Syst Rev* (2):CD002006, 2000.
9. Fraser WD: Multicenter, randomized, controlled trial of delayed pushing for nulliparous women in the second stage of labor with continuous epidural analgesia. The PEOPLE (Pushing Early or Pushing Late with Epidural) Study Group, *Am J Obstet Gynecol* 182(5):1165-1172, 2000.
10. Hansen SL, Clark SL, Foster JC: Active pushing versus passive fetal descent in the second stage of labor: a randomized controlled trial, *Obstet Gynecol* 99:29-34, 2002.
11. Plunkett B, Lin A, Wong C et al: Management of the second stage of labor in nulliparas with continuous epidural anesthesia, *Obstet Gynecol* 102:109-114, 2003.

12. Torvaldsen S, Roberts CL, Bell JC et al: Discontinuation of epidural analgesia late in labour for reducing the adverse delivery outcomes associated with epidural analgesia, *Cochrane Database Syst Rev* (4):CD004457, 2004.
13. Parnell C, Langhoff-Roos J, Iverson R et al: Pushing method in the expulsive phase of labor: a randomized trial, *Acta Obstet Gynecol Scand* 72:31-35, 1993.
14. Bloom SL, Casey BM, Schaffer JI et al: A randomized trial of coached versus uncoached pushing during the second stage of labor, *Am J Obstet Gynecol* 194:10-13, 2006.
15. Parnell C, Langhoff-Roos J, Iverson R et al: Pushing method in the expulsive phase of labor: a randomized trial, *Acta Obstet Gynecol Scand* 72:31-35, 1993.
16. Flynn P, Franiek J, Janssen P et al: How can second-stage management prevent perineal trauma? A critical review, *Can Fam Physician* 43:73-84, 1997.
17. Corroli G, Belizan J: Episiotomy for vaginal birth, *Cochrane Database Syst Rev* (2):CD000081, 2000.
18. McCandlish R, Bowler U, van Asten H et al: A randomized controlled trial of care of the perineum during second stage of normal labour, *Br J Obstet Gynaecol* 105:1262-1272, 1998.
19. Saunders NJ, Spiby H, Gilbert L et al: Oxytocin infusion during second stage of labor in primiparous women using epidural analgesia: a randomized double blind placebo controlled trial, *BMJ* 299:1423-1426, 1989.
20. Sizer AR, Evans J, Bailey SM et al: A second-stage partogram, *Obstet Gynecol* 96:678-683, 2000.

SECTION H Management of the Perineum

Valerie J. King, MD, MPH

Perineal trauma during childbirth is common. More than 85% of women who have a vaginal birth sustain some sort of perineal trauma, and 60% to 70% receive stitches to repair perineal trauma.[1] Perineal trauma is any damage to the genitalia during childbirth that occurs spontaneously or intentionally by surgical incision (episiotomy). Episiotomy is an incision into the perineal musculature to enlarge the vaginal outlet for birth. Perineal trauma affects women's well-being immediately after birth and can lead to long-term consequences as well. In the United Kingdom, where better data are available than in the United States, 23% to 42% of women continue to have perineal discomfort for 10 to 12 days after delivery, and 7% to 10% of women have prolonged pain when measured at 3 to 18 months after delivery. Almost 25% report dyspareunia at 3 months after delivery, and 3% to 10% report fecal incontinence at that time after birth. Perineal discomfort disrupts normal adjustment to motherhood, family life, and breastfeeding.[1]

I. EPIDEMIOLOGY

A. Incidence

The episiotomy rate in 1980 was approximately 64% in the United States, whereas in 2002, the rate had decreased to approximately 27%. This means that episiotomy was performed on more than 750,000 women during that year. More than 42% of U.S. women who did not have an episiotomy in 2002 were reported to have required repair of an obstetric laceration.[2]

B. Wide Variation in Episiotomy Rates

The episiotomy rate is less than 10% in the Netherlands where a substantial proportion of births are at home and midwives attend most births. In the United Kingdom, most vaginal births are attended by midwives and the episiotomy rate is about 13%. The rate approaches 100% in some eastern European countries.[1]

C. Factors Associated with Increased Perineal Trauma

In observational studies, factors associated with increased perineal trauma include previous perineal trauma[3]; use of oils, lubricants, lithotomy position, and epidural anesthesia[4]; perineal compresses and water-based lubricants[5]; short duration of labor and unemployment[6]; older maternal age, greater birth weight, shoulder dystocia, and edema of the perineum[7]; nulliparity, greater birth weight, perineal edema, manual perineal protection, inadequate visualization of the perineum, and a long duration of bearing down during second stage.[8]

D. Factors Associated with Lower Rates of Perineal Trauma

In observational studies, protective factors associated with lower rates of perineal trauma include warm compresses, flexion of the fetal head, and lateral birth positions[4]; regular maternal exercise[6]; and less pushing instruction.[9] Low socioeconomic status and higher parity are associated with less perineal trauma among multiparous women, whereas lower socioeconomic status, kneeling or hands-and-knees position at delivery, and manual support of the perineum appear to be protective factors for nulliparas.[10]

II. DIAGNOSIS

Visual inspection is the mainstay of diagnosing the location and extent of genital tract damage related to childbirth. A good visual inspection and complete examination are facilitated by appropriate patient position, adequate exposure, excellent lighting, and sufficient analgesia or patient comfort with the examination. After a thorough visual inspection, the clinician should gently examine the anterior and posterior genital structures, including the anal sphincter, for evidence of laceration, bleeding, or other damage. Anterior perineal trauma is injury to the labia, anterior vagina, urethra, or clitoris, and is usually associated with little morbidity. Posterior perineal trauma is any injury to the posterior vaginal wall, perineal muscles, or anal sphincter. In addition to the location of the trauma, the clinician should note the extent of damage. The conventional categorization system ranks genital tract trauma from first through fourth degree. First-degree tears involve only skin; second-degree tears involve the underlying perineal musculature; third-degree tears partially or completely disrupt the anal sphincter; and fourth-degree tears completely disrupt the external and internal anal sphincter and the rectal mucosa.

III. TREATMENT

A substantial evidence base exists from RCTs to guide repair and treatment of perineal trauma associated with childbirth. This summary focuses on materials and methods of repair, as well as interventions to promote comfort and healing of perineal trauma. Section H.V addresses the many things that can be done to help prevent and reduce the severity of perineal trauma.

A. Suturing versus Nonsuturing of Perineal Trauma

Although the available trials are small and have methodologic weaknesses, there is some evidence that not suturing low-grade perineal trauma can be harmful. It is not possible to isolate first- from second-degree trauma in these studies. As a practical matter, many clinicians do not suture hemostatic first-degree trauma. Perineal trauma should have the benefit of suturing until there are trials large enough to definitively exclude harms such as those found in these studies.[11,12]

B. Type of Suture Material for Repair

Clinicians must decide which type of suture material to use in performing a repair. Substantial evidence is available to guide this choice, including a Cochrane review of absorbable synthetic suture versus catgut suture material for perineal repair.[12] The review contains 8 RCTs of variable quality and includes a total of 3681 primiparous and multiparous women. The metaanalysis found that the use of synthetic absorbable suture compared with catgut suture was associated with less pain in the first 3 days (OR, 0.62; 95% CI, 0.54-0.71), less need for analgesics up to 10 days after birth (OR, 0.63; 95% CI, 0.52-0.77), and less suture dehiscence (OR, 0.45; 95% CI, 0.29-0.70). The Cochrane review also found that there was more need for removal of suture material in the absorbable suture group (OR, 2.01; 95% CI, 1.56-2.58) and no significant differences in long-term pain (OR, 0.81; 95% CI, 0.61-1.08). However, one of the larger RCTs (N = 793) included in the metaanalysis evaluated women at 1 year after delivery and found more dyspareunia in the catgut group (8% vs. 13%; NNT = 20) together with fewer women who had resumed pain-free intercourse (8% vs. 14%; NNH = 16).[13]

Three RCTs have compared rapidly absorbed polyglactin 910 with standard polyglactin 910, with a total of 2003 women enrolled in these trials.[1,12] Rapidly absorbed polyglactin suture generally had improved outcomes over standard polyglactin 910 including less pain with walking in first 2 weeks after delivery, less need for suture removal, and no significant differences in overall perineal pain, pain on sitting, or dyspareunia.

C. Method of Repair of Perineal Trauma

Clinicians must also decide on the most appropriate method of suturing trauma to reduce pain and improve healing. No high-quality evidence exists to support a particular method of suturing except for the issue of how to approximate the perineal skin during a repair. The Ipswich Childbirth Study, a randomized trial including 1780 women, compared a two-stage closure with a three-stage closure.[14] In the two-stage closure, the skin edges were closely approximated (<0.5-cm gap), but subcuticular sutures were not placed. The three-stage repair was the same except that subcuticular stitches were placed to bring the skin

edges together. No significant differences in pain at 24 and 48 hours or 10 days after delivery were found in the Ipswich trial. Women allocated to two-stage repair were less likely to report tight stitches (14% vs. 18%; RR, 0.77; 95% CI, 0.62-0.96; NNT = 25), less likely to have pain at 3 months after delivery, and more likely to have resumed pain-free intercourse. Among those who had resumed intercourse, there was significantly less dyspareunia (15% vs. 19%; RR, 0.80; 95% CI, 0.65-0.99; NNT = 25). Women in the two-stage repair group were also less likely to report needing to have suture material removed (7% vs. 12%; RR, 0.61; 95% CI, 0.45-0.83; NNT = 20). A 1-year follow-up study found women allocated to the two-stage repair were also less likely to report that perineum felt different than before delivery (30% vs. 40%; RR, 0.75; 95% CI, 0.61-0.91; NNT = 10).[13] No other clear differences were evident between groups at 1 year after delivery.

D. Topical Anesthetics to Treat Immediate Postpartum Perineal Pain

A Cochrane review of topically applied anesthetic agents to treat perineal pain after childbirth included 8 RCTs and a total of 976 women.[15] Five of the trials measured pain and need for additional analgesia in the first 1 to 3 days after birth. All five of these studies compared the topical anesthetic agent with placebo, and one also compared a topical agent with a vaginal indomethacin suppository. The various topical agents included 2% lidocaine gel, 5% lidocaine spray and ointment, 5% lidocaine with 2% cinchocaine, and 1% pramoxine with 1% hydrocortisone acetate foam (Epifoam). There were no significant differences in pain at 24 or 72 hours after birth. One trial with 97 women did find that use of Epifoam was significantly associated with lower need for other analgesics (OR, 0.58 [0.40-0.84]).

E. Therapeutic Ultrasound to Treat Postpartum Perineal Pain and Dyspareunia

Another modality less commonly used in the United States is therapeutic ultrasound for the treatment of postpartum perineal pain and dyspareunia. A Cochrane review includes 4 RCTs and a total of 659 women.[16] Two of the trials were placebo-controlled studies in the immediate postpartum period. Based on these two trials, women who received ultrasound for acute perineal pain were more likely to report improvement (OR, 0.37;

95% CI, 0.19-0.69). One RCT (N = 76) compared pulsed electromagnetic energy with ultrasound for acute perineal pain up to 4 days after delivery. Those treated with ultrasound had more perineal bruising at 10 days after delivery (OR, 1.64; 95% CI, 1.04-2.60) but were less likely to report perineal pain at 10 days (OR, 0.56; 95% CI, 0.34-0.92) and 3 months (OR, 0.43; 95% CI, 0.22-0.84) after delivery. The fourth trial (N = 69) evaluated women treated with ultrasound for persistent (at least 2 months after childbirth) perineal pain and/or dyspareunia, and found that those who received ultrasound were less likely to report pain with sexual intercourse compared with the placebo group (OR, 0.31; 95% CI, 0.11-0.84). Based on these studies, there is good evidence to recommend ultrasound therapy as beneficial, particularly for women with persistent perineal pain after childbirth. Little evidence is available on potential harms or costs of this intervention.

IV. CLINICAL COURSE AND PREVENTION

Many interventions can be used to prevent perineal trauma during childbirth including perineal massage, avoidance of episiotomy, and operative vaginal delivery. This section explores each of the interventions that have been studied with an eye toward preventing damage to the genital tract during childbirth. It is probable that many routine interventions used in childbirth may increase the risk for perineal trauma. Judicious rather than routine use of most interventions is likely to improve outcomes for healthy childbearing women.

A. Antenatal Perineal Massage
Massage of the perineum in the last weeks of pregnancy has been well studied in two RCTs. Nearly 2400 women were studied in the Labrecque[17] and Shipman[18] trials. Labrecque and colleagues' study[17] of 1527 women compared a policy of perineal massage from 34 or 35 weeks until delivery with no massage control group. Among women having a vaginal delivery who had not had a previous vaginal delivery, 24.3% of massage group and 15.1% of control group had intact perineum (NNT = 11). Women who had greater adherence to the program of perineal massage were even more likely to have an intact perineum. Differences among women with prior vaginal delivery were not statistically significant. No differences were found in women's sense of control, satisfaction, or the incidence of need for suturing of vulvar or vaginal trauma.

Labrecque and colleagues[19] also assessed the views of women in the intervention arm of this study. Women in the trial generally found perineal massage to be an acceptable and positive experience. Participants would favor using it again in another pregnancy and would recommend it to another pregnant woman. They viewed the effect on their relationship with their partner to be either positive or negative depending on whether the partner participated with performing the massage.

The smaller RCT of 861 women by Shipman and colleagues[18] found that antenatal perineal massage had some benefit in reducing second- and third-degree tears, episiotomies, and instrumental deliveries after adjusting for maternal age and infant birth weight. The perineal tear rates were 69.0% versus 75.1% (p = 0.024; NNT = 16), and the operative delivery rates were 34.6% versus 40.9% (p = 0.034; NNT = 16). Analysis stratified for mother's age found a greater benefit in women older than 30.

B. Intrapartum Perineal Massage in Labor
If perineal massage before labor has benefits in terms of reducing perineal trauma, then the obvious next question is whether massage carried on during labor can also reduce perineal trauma. Because observational studies have found that use of oils, lubricants, and compresses are associated with greater perineal trauma, it was also critical that this question be evaluated with a well-designed RCT. Stamp and her colleagues[20] conducted a large trial that randomized 1340 women to massage and stretching of the perineum with a water-based lubricant with each contraction during second stage or usual care. The trial enrolled approximately equal numbers of multiparous and primiparous women cared for in labor by midwives in three large Australian hospitals.

No differences were found between the perineal massage intervention and usual care groups in terms of intact perineum, episiotomy use, first- and second-degree tears, pain at 3 and 10 days after birth, or pain at 3 months after birth. However, there was a lower risk for third-degree tears in the massage group (RR, 0.47 [0.23-0.93]). Twelve of 708 in the massage group versus 23 of 632 in the control group had third-degree tears (NNT = 51). The length of second stage among primiparous women averaged 10 minutes less in the massage group (84.0 vs. 94.6 minutes; p = 0.05). The trial did not report women's views on having perineal massage during the second stage of labor.

C. Warm Compresses

Albers and colleagues[21] conducted a randomized trial that included 1211 women. Women were allocated to warm compresses to the perineum during the second stage of labor, massage with a water-based lubricant, or no touch to the perineum during the second stage until crowning of the infant's head. No statistically significant differences were reported in genital tract trauma among the three groups, even when controlling for parity, use of epidural anesthesia, or birth weight greater than 4000 g. A logistic regression analysis of all predictors of genital tract trauma among trial participants found that nulliparity (OR, 4.59; 95% CI, 3.29-6.64), birth weight greater 4000 g (OR, 1.87; 95% CI, 1.17-3.37), being a non-Hispanic white woman (OR, 1.34; 95% CI, 1.06-1.73), and having more than a high-school education (OR, 1.27; 95% CI, 1.01-1.62) were associated with greater rates of trauma. Predictors of less perineal trauma were sitting upright for delivery (OR, 0.68; 95% CI, 0.50-0.91) and having the head born between contractions (OR, 0.82; 95% CI, 0.67-0.99). It appears that neither perineal massage nor application of warm compresses to the perineum during second stage is likely to reduce perineal trauma over a "no touch" policy. However, this trial provides some evidence that upright sitting positions for delivery and delivery of the head between contractions reduce the risk for genital tract trauma.

D. Epidural Anesthesia

Epidural anesthesia provides excellent analgesia for most women; however, its use is not without certain adverse effects. Use of epidural anesthesia is associated with greater rates of operative vaginal delivery. Lieberman and O'Donoghue's[22] systematic review identified seven observational studies that reported perineal lacerations as an outcome. Across these studies it appears that epidural anesthesia increases the risk for severe perineal trauma by approximately twofold. It appears that the mechanism for this increase is not the epidural per se, but rather increased use of instrumented vaginal delivery and episiotomy. The use of epidural analgesia is known to increase the risk for operative vaginal delivery that, in turn, increases the risk for severe perineal injury. Avoidance of epidural analgesia may also contribute to greater rates of intact perineum and decrease incidence of more severe perineal injury during childbirth.

E. Restrictive versus Liberal Use of Episiotomy

Although episiotomy rates have been decreasing in the United States, more than one fourth of American women continue to receive episiotomy. Episiotomy is arguably the single intervention most associated with perineal damage and particularly with third- and fourth-degree tears. Despite this, many routine episiotomies continue to be done, likely because of provider preference.[23]

A Cochrane review of episiotomy in vaginal birth includes 6 RCTs of generally sound quality with more than 4800 patients.[24] It found that a policy of restrictive episiotomy use is associated with less posterior trauma (RR, 0.88 [95% CI, 0.84-0.92]; NNT = 10) and less need for suturing (RR, 0.74 [95% CI, 0.71-0.77]; NNT = 4). Women allocated to the restrictive groups did experience more anterior trauma (RR, 1.79 [95% CI, 1.55-2.07]) but had overall fewer healing complications (RR, 0.69 [95% CI, 0.56-0.85]). No differences in severe vaginal or perineal (third- or fourth-degree) trauma, dyspareunia, urinary incontinence, or postpartum pain were found.

F. Episiotomy and the Risk for Severe Perineal Trauma

Despite the fact that the above metaanalysis of RCTs of routine versus restricted use of episiotomy did not demonstrate a significant difference in the risk for severe perineal or vaginal trauma, there is a substantial body of observational study data that suggests that episiotomy is associated with more severe perineal outcomes. Multiple large retrospective cohort studies have also found that there is a strong association between episiotomy and the risk for severe perineal trauma. This association appears to be found in situations in which median episiotomy is the dominant type of episiotomy used.[25,26] This provides further evidence to recommend that a restrictive policy of episiotomy should be used.

G. Median versus Mediolateral Episiotomy

No trials directly comparing median versus mediolateral episiotomy are included in the Cochrane review of routine versus restrictive use of episiotomy because the studies were of poor quality. Only one of the RCTs in the Cochrane review used median episiotomy, whereas the remainder used mediolateral episiotomy. In the one trial that used median episiotomy,[27] nearly all cases of third- and fourth-degree perineal trauma were associated with median episiotomy. The trial enrolled 703 women. There were 52 cases of severe perineal trauma (46/47 severe lacerations among primiparous women and 6/6 among multiparous women), with all but one occurring in the episiotomy group.

H. Maternal Position at Birth

A Cochrane review on positions for women during second stage of labor contains 19 RCTs of variable quality with a total of 5764 participants.[28] The use of any upright or lateral position, compared with supine or lithotomy positions, was associated with increased risk for second-degree perineal tears (RR, 1.23; 95% CI, 1.09-1.39) and increased risk for estimated blood loss greater than 500 ml (RR, 1.68; 95% CI, 1.32-2.15), but fewer episiotomies (RR, 0.84; 95% CI, 0.79-0.91), shorter second stage of labor (weighted mean difference, 4.29 minutes [2.95-5.64 minutes]), fewer reports of severe pain during second stage of labor (RR, 0.73; 95% CI, 0.60-0.90), fewer abnormal FHR patterns (RR, 0.31; 95% CI, 0.08-0.98), and fewer assisted deliveries (RR, 0.84; 95% CI, 0.73-0.98). There are trade-offs between greater rates of second-degree perineal trauma and lower rates of episiotomy with upright birth positions. Upright positions are associated with less use of assisted vaginal delivery, and this is associated with less perineal damage over spontaneous birth. However, there might be more postpartum blood loss with upright positions. Women should be offered the choice of birth position based on these and other considerations such as maternal preference and ability to assume an upright position.

I. Method of Pushing during Second Stage

A prospective cohort study by Benyon[29] found a much greater rate of sutured perineal trauma among women who were coached to push in the traditional manner (63%) compared with women who were given no exhortation to push (39%). Insufficient evidence exists to recommend a particular style of pushing during the second stage. There may, however, be other reasons to encourage physiologic pushing over directed Valsalva pushing.

J. Manual Techniques for Delivery of the Infant

The HOOP Study was a multicenter RCT conducted in the United Kingdom by McCandlish and colleagues.[30] It enrolled 5471 women to compare the manual techniques of hands-on (pressure on the baby's head with guarding of the perineum followed by lateral flexion to deliver the shoulders) versus hands poised (not touching head, perineum, or shoulders) methods for delivery of the infant.

Fewer women in the hands-on group reported perineal pain at 10 days after birth (RR, 1.10; 95% CI, 1.01-1.18). Episiotomy rates were lower in the hands poised group (RR, 0.79; 95% CI, 0.65-0.96), and incidence of manual removal of placenta was greater in hands poised group (RR, 1.69; 95% CI, 1.02-2.78). No significant differences were found in the extent or severity of trauma between the two groups. Although this trial provides reasonable evidence to support standard manual procedures to encourage flexion of the fetal head and guarding of the perineum during uncomplicated vaginal birth, the benefits are modest. Women should be allowed a choice in the matter, and if they feel strongly about wanting a hands poised delivery, birth attendants should try to accommodate their wishes.

K. Forceps versus Vacuum Extractor for Operative Vaginal Delivery

A Cochrane review containing 10 RCTs of reasonable quality found that use of a vacuum extractor (VE) was associated with less trauma for the mother.[31] Compared with forceps, use of a VE resulted in 60% less maternal genital tract trauma (OR, 0.41; 95% CI, 0.33-0.50) and less severe perineal pain at 24 hours (OR, 0.54; 95% CI, 0.31-0.93). However, VE use was associated with greater numbers of cephalohematomas among the infants (OR, 2.38; 95% CI, 1.68-3.37). Although there is good evidence to support the use of vacuum extraction over forceps for an assisted vaginal delivery to limit maternal trauma and pain, there are some trade-offs in terms of fetal injury. However, these types of fetal injuries do not seem to increase the need for follow-up or readmission of the infant. The use of forceps may be indicated on other grounds in specific situations. The concurrent use of episiotomy and instrumental delivery increases the risk for significant perineal trauma. Therefore, use of episiotomy should be limited for spontaneous and assisted vaginal births.

V. PITFALLS AND CONTROVERSIES

The diffusion of high-quality evidence into practice is often slow. Most physicians and other health professionals continue to practice in the way they were trained, and the pace of change is generational. Geographic patterns of care and training may account for some of the slow diffusion of newer ideas and techniques, and resistance to adoption of evidence in practice. Most of the high-quality evidence about prevention and treatment of perineal damage in childbirth does not originate from North American studies. For example, the use of episiotomy in many countries, including the United States, is still more frequent than in many other industrialized countries with similar or better birth outcomes. Few U.S. clinicians appear to have heard of or tried the two-stage technique and continue to perform a repair that includes subcuticular stitches. Many clinicians persist in using chromic suture because it was the material they used in training and they are more comfortable with it.

In addition, there may be less willingness on the part of U.S. physicians to adopt some of these evidence-based care practices because they were studied by midwives in settings where midwives provide the majority of care. Nurse-midwives in Great Britain and the areas of the former British Commonwealth are responsible for most of the world's literature on the care of normal childbearing women. In the U.S. setting, where midwives do not care for the majority of laboring women, most research efforts are directed at studying care practices that are applicable to smaller subsets of women. In addition, common care practices such as confining women to bed for labor and delivery, using supine positions for delivery, and coached pushing may contribute to situations in which genital tract trauma in childbirth is more common. Changing these types of routines requires multidisciplinary effort from birth attendants, nursing staff, and childbearing women.

Some of the care practices summarized earlier do not have strong or sufficient evidence behind them. Clinicians often have to care for women with suboptimal evidence to guide them, but should not fall into the trap of disregarding high-quality evidence that is likely to be valid across settings. There are also always patients who do not fit neatly into the types of subjects who are included in particular studies. The clinical setting of a particular study may also influence its findings and generalizability. For example, when antepartum perineal massage was first studied, it did not appear effective until it was studied in settings with lower episiotomy rates.

Nearly all of the outcomes that have been studied in this body of literature are short-term; consequently, there is little to guide clinicians about the effects of alternative care practices outside of the most immediate postpartum period. There are unintended consequences of many commonly used childbirth procedures. For example, although the majority of women in the United States now receive epidural analgesia during childbirth, it is not known whether information about increased need for operative vaginal delivery and greater risk for perineal damage are part of the counseling that women receive before electing epidural analgesia.

VI. SOR A RECOMMENDATIONS

RECOMMENDATIONS	REFERENCES
The use of a synthetic absorbable suture material versus catgut for perineal repair results in less pain at 3 and 10 days and a decreased incidence of wound dehiscence. Rapidly absorbed polyglactin 910 (e.g., Vicryl Rapide) is superior to standard polyglactin 910 (e.g., Vicryl).	12
The use of a two- versus a three-stage perineal repair is associated with decreased postpartum pain at 3 months and decreased incidence of dyspareunia (NNT = 25). This technique omits subcuticular suturing. The skin should be apposed but left unsutured.	13
The use of therapeutic ultrasound is effective for the treatment of both acute and prolonged postpartum perineal discomfort.	16
Antenatal perineal massage for the nulliparous patient beginning at 34 to 35 weeks is associated with an increased likelihood of having an intact perineum after delivery (NNT = 11).	19
Routine episiotomy offers no advantages. A restrictive versus routine policy of episiotomy use is associated with decreased posterior trauma (NNT = 10) and need for suture repair (NNT = 4).	24
Upright birth positions are associated with less perineal trauma and use of assisted vaginal delivery. However, there may be more postpartum blood loss with upright positions. Women should be offered the choice of birth position based on these and other considerations such as maternal preference and ability to assume an upright position.	28

Continued

Use of standard manual procedures to encourage flexion of the fetal head and guarding of the perineum during uncomplicated vaginal birth versus a "hands poised" approach results in less perineal pain at 10 days after delivery. However, the benefits of this intervention are small and should not outweigh a woman's preference.	30
Vacuum devices offer advantages over forceps for an uncomplicated assisted vaginal delivery in terms of maternal trauma and pain. Women should be informed of the potential risks and benefits of the use of either type of instrument for both themselves and their infants.	31

REFERENCES

1. Kettle C: Perineal care, *Clin Evid* 13:1-19, 2005.
2. Kozak LJ, Owings MF, Hall MJ: National Hospital Discharge Survey: 2002 annual summary with detailed diagnosis and procedure data. National Center for Health Statistics, *Vital Health Stat* 13(158):1-199, 2005.
3. Martin S, Labrecque M, Marcoux S et al: The association between perineal trauma and spontaneous perineal tears, *J Fam Pract* 50:333-337, 2001.
4. Albers LL, Anderson D, Cragin L et al: Factors related to perineal trauma in childbirth, *J Nurse Midwifery* 41:269-276, 1996.
5. Lydon-Rochelle MT, Albers L, Teaf D: Perineal outcomes and nurse-midwifery management, *J Nurse Midwifery* 40:13-18, 1995.
6. Klein MC, Janssen PA, MacWilliam L et al: Determinants of vaginal-perineal integrity and pelvic floor functioning in childbirth, *Am J Obstet Gynecol* 176:403-410, 1997.
7. Parnell C, Langhoff-Roos J, Moller H: Conduct of labor and rupture of the sphincter ani, *Acta Obstet Gynaecol Scand* 80:256-261, 2001.
8. Samuelsson E, Ladfors L, Wennerholm UB et al: Anal sphincter tears: prospective study of obstetric risk factors, *BJOG* 107:926-931, 2000.
9. Greenshields W, Hulme H, Oliver S, editors: *The perineum in childbirth: a survey of women's experiences and midwives practices,* London, 1993, National Childbirth Trust.
10. Aikins Murphy P, Feinland JB: Perineal outcomes in a home birth setting, *Birth* 25:226-234, 1998.
11. Fleming EM, Hagen S, Niven C: Does perineal suturing make a difference? The SUNS trial, *BJOG* 110:684-689, 2003.
12. Kettle C, Johanson RB: Absorbable synthetic versus catgut suture material for perineal repair, *Cochrane Database Syst Rev* (2):CD000006, 2000.
13. Grant A, Gordon B, Mackrodt C et al: The Ipswich childbirth study: one year follow up of alternative methods used in perineal repair, *BJOG* 108:34-40, 2001.
14. Gordon B, Mackrodt C, Fern E et al: The Ipswich Childbirth Study: 1. A randomized evaluation of two stage postpartum perineal repair leaving the skin unsutured, *BJOG* 105:435-440, 1998.
15. Hedayati H, Parsons J, Crowther, CA: Topically applied anaesthetics for treating perineal pain after childbirth, *Cochrane Database Syst Rev* (2):CD004223, 2005.
16. Hay-Smith EJC: Therapeutic ultrasound for postpartum perineal pain and dyspareunia, *Cochrane Database Syst Rev* (2): CD000495, 2000.
17. Labrecque M, Eason E, Marcoux S et al: Randomized controlled trial of prevention of perineal trauma by perineal massage during pregnancy, *Am J Obstet Gynecol* 180:593-600, 1999.
18. Shipman MK, Boniface DR, Tefft ME et al: Antenatal perineal massage and subsequent perineal outcomes: a randomized controlled trial, *BJOG* 104:787-791, 1997.
19. Labrecque M, Eason E, Marcoux S: Women's views on the practice of prenatal perineal massage, *BJOG* 108:499-504, 2001.
20. Stamp G, Kruzins G, Crowther C: Perineal massage in labour and prevention of perineal trauma: randomized controlled trial, *BMJ* 322:1277-1280, 2001.
21. Albers LL, Sedler KD, Bedrick EJ et al: Midwifery care measures in the second stage of labor and reduction of genital tract trauma at birth: a randomized trial, *J Midwifery Womens Health* 50:365-372, 2005.
22. Lieberman E, O'Donoghue C: Unintended effects of epidural analgesia during labor: a systematic review, *Am J Obstet Gynecol* 186(5):S31-S68, 2002.
23. Graham ID, Carroli G, Davies C et al: Episiotomy rates around the world: an update, *Birth* 32(3):219-223, 2005.
24. Carroli G, Belizan J: Episiotomy for vaginal birth, *Cochrane Database Syst Rev* (2):CD000081, 2000.
25. Labrecque M, Maillargeon L, Dallaire M et al: Association between median episiotomy and severe perineal lacerations in primiparous women, *CMAJ* 156:797-802, 1997.
26. Bansal RK, Tan WM, Ecker JL et al: Is there a benefit to episiotomy at spontaneous vaginal delivery? A natural experiment, *Am J Obstet Gynecol* 175:897-901, 1996.
27. Klein MC, Gauthier RJ, Jorgensen SH et al: Does episiotomy prevent perineal trauma and pelvic floor relaxation? *Online J Curr Clin Trials* Doc No 10, July 1, 1992.
28. Gupta JK, Hofmeyr GJ: Position for women during second stage of labour for women without epidural anaesthesia, *Cochrane Database Syst Rev* (1), 2004.
29. Benyon CL: Normal second stage of labour: a plea for reform in its conduct, *J Obstet Gynaecol Br Commonwealth* 64:815-820, 1957.
30. McCandlish R, Bowler U, van Asten H et al: A randomized controlled trial of care of the perineum during second stage of normal labour, *BJOG* 105:1262-1272, 1998.
31. Johanson RB, Menon V: Vacuum extraction versus forceps for assisted vaginal delivery, *Cochrane Database Syst Rev* (2): CD000224, 2000.

S E C T I O N I Management of Third-Stage Labor

Kent Petrie, MD, and Walter L. Larimore, MD

Third-stage labor begins after delivery of the fetus and ends with delivery of the placenta and membranes. After delivery of the infant and cutting of the umbilical cord, the placenta usually separates spontaneously from the uterine wall within 5 to 10 minutes.

There are two approaches to the clinical management of the third stage: expectant management and active management. *Expectant management* involves waiting for signs of separation and allowing the placenta to deliver spontaneously or be aided by gravity or nipple stimulation. Expectant management is also known as conservative or physiologic management and is popular in some northern European countries and in some maternity units in the United States and Canada. It is also the usual practice in home deliveries.

In contrast, with *active management,* the birth attendant chooses to intervene in this process by using one or more of the following interventions:

- Administration of a prophylactic oxytocic after delivery of the infant
- Early cord clamping and cutting
- Free bleeding of the maternal end of the cord
- Controlled cord traction of the umbilical cord
- Upward kneading pressure on the anterior uterine wall

The active management of the third stage is virtually standard practice in the United Kingdom and Australia.

I. DELIVERY OF THE PLACENTA

A. Free Bleeding of the Cord

Cord drainage in the third stage involves unclamping the previously clamped and separated umbilical cord and allowing the blood from the placenta to drain freely into an appropriate receptacle. Two small RCTs have been included in a Cochrane review that showed a reduction in length of the third stage and a reduced incidence of retained placenta at 30 minutes.[1] Free bleeding of the cord also provides a theoretic reduction of risk for fetal-maternal transfusion.

B. Spontaneous Placental Separation

While waiting for the placenta to separate, the fundus may be checked frequently to ensure that the uterus does not become atonic and filled with blood. It is important to wait for signs of placental separation before applying traction to the umbilical cord. Excessive traction may result in tearing of the umbilical cord, tearing of the placenta, or inversion of the uterus.

Although placenta separation typically occurs within 5 to 10 minutes after delivery, 30 minutes is considered normal. Classically, spontaneous separation of the placenta is indicated by the uterus becoming a globular shape. The fundus firms and appears to rise in the abdomen. A sudden gush of blood is followed by the cord appearing to lengthen as the placenta moves into the vagina.

C. Assisted Placental Separation

After partial or complete separation has occurred, gentle fundal massage and firm, steady traction on the umbilical cord usually effects delivery of the placenta. The Brandt–Andrews maneuver, a cephalad shearing motion exerted with the abdominal hand on the uterus while applying traction to the umbilical cord simultaneously with the other hand (Figure 14-15), has been said to effect removal of the placenta easily without increasing risk for uterine inversion. One RCT has compared patients managed with this maneuver (plus 10 units oxytocin administered intramuscularly with delivery of the newborn's anterior shoulder) with patients managed with minimal intervention (no traction or fundal massage or oxytocin).[2] Those managed with the Brandt–Andrews maneuver had a significantly lower risk for postpartum hemorrhage, retained placenta (>30 minutes), and need for additional

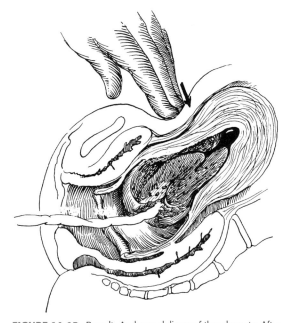

FIGURE 14-15. Brandt–Andrews delivery of the placenta. After the fundus is firm, moderate tension is exerted on the umbilical cord, whereas the other hand *shears off* the placenta from the uterine wall by upward kneading pressure on the anterior uterine wall. (From Wilson JR: *Atlas of obstetric technic,* ed 2, St. Louis, 1969, Mosby. Daisy Stilwell, medical illustrator.)

uterotonic agents to control hemorrhage. Another intervention that has been shown to assist placental separation is the injection of 1 ml oxytocin diluted in 9 ml normal saline injected into the umbilical vein through an IV catheter.[3] The technique significantly reduced the need for manual removal of the placenta (NNT = 8).

D. Manual Extraction of the Placenta

If the placenta has not separated after 20 to 30 minutes, and cannot be removed by the maneuvers described previously, and if the patient is appropriately anesthetized, manual removal or extraction of the placenta may be performed to reduce potential excessive blood loss. Intrauterine bacterial contamination and postpartum endometritis are rare complications of this procedure, and prophylactic antibiotics are generally recommended.[4]

The procedure is accomplished by using one hand abdominally to grasp the fundus and hold it downward firmly. The other hand reaches into the uterine cavity to gently peel off the placenta using a rotatory or circumferential sweep of the hands to separate the placenta (Figure 14-16). One must attempt to achieve a clean plane of separation. The placenta, after separation, may normally be easily removed. After removal, vigorous fundal massage and administration of uterotonic agents minimize subsequent bleeding.

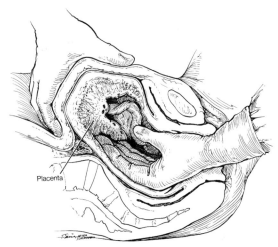

Placenta

FIGURE 14-16. Manual removal of the placenta. The fingers are alternately abducted, adducted, and advanced until the placenta is detached completely.

E. Active Third-Stage Management of the Placenta

In a Cochrane review, the active management of the third stage of labor when compared with expectant management was associated with reduced maternal blood loss, reduced postpartum hemorrhage of more than 500 ml, and reduced length of the third stage.[5] Active management was associated with an increased risk for maternal nausea, vomiting, and hypertension (when ergotamine was used). No advantages or disadvantages were noted for the neonate. The reviewers conclude, "Routine active management is superior to expectant management in terms of blood loss, postpartum hemorrhage, and other serious complications of the third stage of labor. Active management should be the routine management of choice for women expecting to deliver a baby by vaginal delivery in a maternity hospital."[5]

F. Examination of the Placenta

After removal, the placenta, its membranes, and the umbilical cord should be examined. If missing cotyledons or segments of the placenta are noted, manual exploration of the intrauterine cavity or curettage may be indicated. No data support the routine manual exploration of the uterus after delivery.[6]

The membranes should be evaluated for vessels that end blindly at the edge of membranes. Such a finding may suggest a succenturiate lobe, which may need to be removed manually or by curettage. The umbilical cord should be examined for the presence of two arteries and one vein. The absence of one umbilical artery may suggest congenital anomalies of the newborn. Whenever abnormalities of the placenta are suspected, formal pathologic evaluation of the placenta is indicated.

II. ACTIVE PROPHYLAXIS OF POSTPARTUM ATONY AND HEMORRHAGE

In addition to their use to facilitate placenta separation, oxytocics are widely used *after* delivery of the placenta to avoid excessive postpartum hemorrhage secondary to uterine atony. After the placenta delivers, gentle fundal massage to check for firmness should be part of routine postpartum management. The Cochrane review of prophylactic oxytocin in the third stage demonstrated reduced blood loss, postpartum hemorrhage, and need for therapeutic oxytocics.[7] Prophylactic use of ergotamine-oxytocin in combination is associated with a small but statistically significant reduction of postpartum hemorrhage over oxytocin alone, but the small advantage is outweighed by the increase in maternal side effects, including increase of diastolic blood pressure and nausea and vomiting.[8] Prostaglandins have generally been reserved for treatment of postpartum hemorrhage when other measures fail. Metaanalyses of prostaglandins as prophylactic agents in the third stage show less effectiveness than oxytocin or ergotamines in preventing postpartum hemorrhage. Both oral misoprostol and injectable prostaglandins cause significantly more nausea, vomiting, diarrhea, increase of maternal temperature, and shivering. The Cochrane reviewers conclude, "Neither intramuscular prostaglandins nor oral misoprostol are preferable to conventional injectable uterotonics as part of the active management of the third stage of labor especially for low-risk women."[9]

Routine postpartum hemorrhage prophylaxis practice in the United States is to use 5 or 10 units of oxytocin intramuscularly or 20 units of oxytocin in 1 L run at 10 ml/min until bleeding is controlled, then at 1 to 2 ml/min. The IV drip (as opposed to IV bolus or intramuscular injection) generally is preferred due to the tendency of IV bolus therapy to cause marked hypertension. On occasions when oxytocin is insufficient, postpartum hemorrhage may occur. Treatment of this condition is discussed in detail in Chapter 16, Section E.

III. REPAIR OF LACERATIONS OF THE BIRTH CANAL

Iatrogenic or spontaneous lacerations of the birth canal may be repaired before or after delivery of the placenta. The cervix, vagina, and perineum must be thoroughly inspected after delivery. Conditions resulting in more spontaneous lacerations or extensions of episiotomies include precipitous deliveries, forceps or vacuum-assisted deliveries, large infant deliveries, and upright deliveries accompanied by perineal edema. Lacerations that are large or do not stop bleeding spontaneously should be repaired. Abrasions or superficial lacerations that do not bleed actively generally do not require suturing.

A. First-Degree Lacerations

First-degree lacerations are normally superficial lacerations that have minimal bleeding. They are most commonly found on the fourchette, perineal skin, or vaginal mucous membranes, but not the underlying fascia or muscle.

B. Second-Degree Lacerations

Second-degree tears include the subcutaneous tissue and fascia of the perineal body, but not the rectal sphincter. Most require careful repair.

C. Third-Degree Lacerations

Third-degree tears extend through the skin, mucous membranes, and perineal body, and involve fibers of the rectal sphincter. Meticulous layer closure is required.

D. Fourth-Degree Lacerations

Fourth-degree tears extend through the rectal sphincter and expose the lumen of the rectum. Careful inspection of all large lacerations should look for extension of the tears up the vaginal side walls and in the periurethral areas (Figure 14-17).

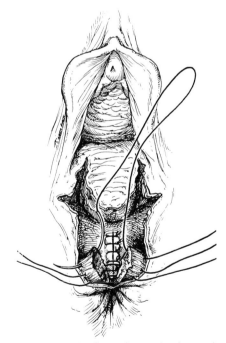

FIGURE 14-17. Repair of complete perineal tear. The rectal mucosa has been repaired with interrupted, fine chromic catgut sutures. The torn ends of the sphincter ani are next, approximated with two or three interrupted chromic catgut sutures. The wound is then repaired, as in a second-degree laceration or an episiotomy.

E. Suture Materials and Repair Techniques

Because the repair of perineal tears is virtually the same as that of episiotomy incisions, the choice of suture materials and repair techniques are discussed in that section (see Chapter 18, Section E).

IV. SOR A RECOMMENDATION

RECOMMENDATION	REFERENCE
Prophylactic oxytocin in the third stage given as the anterior shoulder is delivered, in conjunction with controlled traction on the umbilical cord (active management of stage three), is associated with reduced blood loss, postpartum hemorrhage, and need for therapeutic oxytocics.	5

REFERENCES

1. Soltani H, Dickson F, Symonds I: Placenta cord drainage after spontaneous vaginal delivery as part of the management of the third stage of labor, *Cochrane Database Syst Rev* (4): CD004665, 2005.
2. Khan GO, John IS, Wani S et al: Controlled cord traction versus minimal intervention techniques in delivery of the placenta: a randomized controlled trial, *Am J Obstet Gynecol* 177:770-774, 1997.
3. Carroli G, Bergel G: Umbilical vein injection for management of retained placenta, *Cochrane Database Syst Rev* (4): CD001337, 2001.
4. Tandberg A, Albrecht S, Iversen OE: Manual removal of the placenta. Incidence and clinical significance, *Acta Obstet Gynecol Scand* 78:33-36, 1999.
5. Prendiville WJ, Elbourne D, McDonald S: Active versus expectant management of the third stage of labour, *Cochrane Database Syst Rev* (3):CD000007, 2000.
6. Epperly TD, Fogarty JP, Hodges SG: Efficacy of routine postpartum uterine exploration and manual sponge curettage, *J Fam Pract* 28:172-176, 1989.
7. Cotter A, Ness A, Tolosa J: Prophylactic oxytocin for the third stage of labor, *Cochrane Database Syst Rev* (4):CD001808, 2001.
8. McDonald S, Abbott JM, Higgins SP: Prophylactic ergotamine-oxytocin versus oxytocin for the third stage of labour, *Cochrane Database Syst Rev* (1):CD000201, 2004.
9. Gulmezoglu AM, Forna F, Villar J et al: Prostaglandins for the prevention of postpartum hemorrhage, *Cochrane Database Syst Rev* (1):CD000494, 2004.

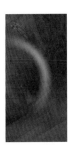

CHAPTER **15**

Management of Labor Abnormalities

S E C T I O N A Dystocia
in the Nulliparous Patient

Matthew K. Cline, MD

From the 1960s to the early 2000s, the cesarean section rate in the United States increased more than fourfold, peaking at a rate of 22.8% in 1989 and then slowly declining to 20.7% in 1997. This decline reversed with the subsequent reduction in vaginal birth after cesarean deliveries and the increase in the incidence of primary cesarean sections, such that the overall cesarean section delivery rate increased to 27.6% by 2003. The primary cesarean section rate for 1997 was 14.6% of births, with 6.1% of births occurring by repeat cesarean section; by 2003, the primary cesarean delivery rate had climbed to 19.1%, with 8.5% of births occurring by repeat cesarean.[1] Although this increase is due to multiple factors, nearly 50% of cesarean sections occur because of dystocia or difficult labor in women experiencing their first labors. After reviewing the diagnosis and potential causes of dystocia, methods of prevention and treatment options will be discussed.

I. DIAGNOSIS OF DYSTOCIA

The diagnosis of dystocia is made when the laboring woman is not making continual progress in cervical dilatation or fetal descent during the *active* phase of labor.

II. CAUSES OF DYSTOCIA

A. Inaccurate Diagnosis of Labor

When a nulliparous patient presents with regular, painful contractions, the clinician is faced with the question: "Is this labor?" One leading text defines labor as "progressive dilatation of the uterine cervix in association with repetitive uterine contractions."[2] The vagueness of this definition can allow the diagnosis of labor to be made when the patient is still experiencing the latent phase of labor. One of the essential components of the active management of labor (AML), in use at National Maternity Hospital in Dublin, Ireland, since the mid-1960s, is a more specific diagnosis of labor. In the Irish model, the diagnosis of labor for the nulliparous patient requires not only painful, regular contractions, but also the presence of either complete cervical effacement, spontaneous rupture of membranes, or bloody show.

Another approach to a specific diagnosis of labor is illustrated by McNiven and colleagues,[3] who evaluated the use of a specific diagnosis of labor (presence of regular, painful contractions together with cervical dilatation greater than 3 cm) in nulliparous women presenting to a hospital labor and delivery unit. Patients were randomly allocated to an "early labor assessment" group (sent home with reassurance if less than 3 cm dilated) or to usual care on the labor ward. The study found that the group with the specific diagnosis of labor had a decrease in cesarean section rates from 10.6% to 7.6%, as well as lower rates of use of oxytocin augmentation, use of any pain medications or epidurals, shorter times spent in labor, and a shortened second stage of labor by nearly 20 minutes. Women in the experimental group also had significantly higher satisfaction scores.[3]

A large observational study (N = 8818) at Case Western Reserve University over 8 years evaluated patients who presented with contractions and intact membranes and were admitted to the hospital; the local definition of "active phase" was cervical dilatation of 4 cm or greater with regular contractions. When comparing the outcomes of nulliparas admitted in latent versus active phase of labor, those who were admitted in latent labor had a cesarean delivery rate of 14.2% versus a rate of 6.7% for those admitted in the active phase. While suggesting the need for a randomized large trial to assess possible causes, one reason suggested by the authors was that early admission (in the latent phase) to the labor and delivery suite increases the chance of dystocia.[4]

B. Inadequate Contractions

Inadequate contractions account for greater than 80% of instances of dystocia. This condition must be appropriately managed before arriving at a diagnosis of cephalopelvic disproportion (CPD). In a review of indications for cesarean section at the University of Wisconsin, more than 35% of cesarean deliveries done for the diagnosis of CPD were reclassified as being done secondary to inefficient uterine contractions.[5]

C. Cephalopelvic Disproportion

In retrospect, the diagnosis of CPD is often inaccurate; 65% to 85% of women successfully deliver vaginally with a trial of labor after a primary cesarean section for the diagnosis of CPD.[6] Some of the reasons for a clinical diagnosis of CPD include the following:

1. Persistent occiput posterior (OP) position (see Chapter 17, Section F)
   OP is the most common malposition encountered in the laboring patient, with about 15% of fetuses in this position at the onset of labor. The OP malposition increases the rates of operative vaginal delivery and cesarean section, especially in the subset that remains in the OP position (about 5% of deliveries).[7]
2. Fetal macrosomia
   Incidence of cesarean section increases as a function of increasing fetal weight.[8]

3. Abnormal maternal pelvis
   A maternal pelvis that is narrowed in the anteroposterior dimension (android or platypoid) is associated with an increased risk for dystocia and diagnosis of CPD. Data from the National Maternity Hospital (Dublin, Ireland) support that CPD caused by maternal pelvis abnormalities is uncommon, occurring in about 1 in 250 primigravidas.
4. Other fetal malpresentations
   See Chapter 17 for a discussion of other fetal malpresentations.
5. Congenital anomalies
   Anomalies that distort the anatomy of the presenting part, such as hydrocephalus or a large cystic hygroma of the fetal neck, can prevent delivery of the fetus through an otherwise adequate pelvis. Although this affects only a small percentage of deliveries, it can result in CPD.

III. FACTORS ASSOCIATED WITH DYSTOCIA

A. Prolonged Latent Phase of Labor

Many authors define a prolonged latent phase of labor as a period of regular contractions without significant cervical dilatation lasting longer than 20 hours in the primigravida and longer than 12 hours in the multipara. Although previously thought to contribute only to maternal exhaustion, a retrospective study has shown that a prolonged latent phase is associated with subsequent dystocia and an increased rate of cesarean delivery.[9]

B. Contemporary Labor Management

1. Continuous electronic fetal monitoring (EFM)
   As discussed in Chapter 14, Section E, continuous EFM became the standard before any randomized controlled trials (RCTs) were conducted to determine whether this technology was beneficial in low-risk women in labor. Subsequent studies have revealed that the use of continuous EFM in low-risk populations is associated with an increased incidence of dystocia and cesarean section when compared with monitoring with intermittent auscultation.[10]
2. Ambulation in labor
   Settings that use continuous EFM or have high rates of epidural use often restrict the freedom of

the laboring mother to move about and change position during labor.

3. Use of regional anesthesia

In many obstetric units, the use of epidural (often referred to as "regional") analgesia has increased since the late 1980s. During this time, an association between epidural use and increased dystocia and cesarean section rates has been noted, with one recent retrospective trial of 1733 low-risk term nulliparas with spontaneous labor showing that the risk for cesarean section was 3.7 times greater in patients who received an epidural (1 additional cesarean section noted for every 7.7 epidurals).[11]

Although many maternity care providers have observed a prolonged or difficult labor in the presence of an epidural, more recent metaanalyses have come to different conclusions. Halpern and co-workers[12] report on data from 10 trials (2369 patients) that showed that there was no increase in cesarean section rates associated with epidural use, though patients with epidural had longer first stages (prolonged by 42 minutes) and second stages (prolonged by 14 minutes) of labor. Women with epidurals had lower pain scores during labor and had decreased rates of dissatisfaction when compared with patients receiving parenteral opioids. A recent Cochrane review of 3157 patients (11 studies) found similar results, with the first stage of labor prolonged by 140 minutes, the second stage prolonged by 12 minutes, an increased use of oxytocin augmentation (odds ratio [OR], 1.99) and instrumented vaginal delivery (OR, 1.93), but no increase in cesarean section rates associated with epidural anesthesia.[13] However, within this metaanalysis, the studies are heterogeneous; in those with early epidural (3 cm dilated or less), there was an increase in cesarean delivery, whereas those with delayed epidural analgesia to 4 cm dilation or later showed no significant effect on labor outcome. Additional support of this contention comes from Lieberman and colleagues'[14] retrospective review of more than 1700 nulliparas in spontaneous labor, which found that the risk for cesarean section was greatest in patients who received epidural anesthesia before dilating to 5 cm or descending to −1 station,[14] suggesting that delaying the use of regional anesthesia when possible may decrease the risk for dystocia. Although this area remains controversial, possible methods of minimizing the effects on the progress of labor are discussed in Section IV.F.

4. Premature rupture of membranes (PROM) at term without onset of labor

This entity is discussed in greater detail in Section B of this chapter.

5. Management of the second stage of labor

This area is discussed in greater detail in Chapter 14, Section G.

IV. PREVENTION OF DYSTOCIA

A. Antenatal Education

Expectations of labor and delivery events among primigravidas and their families can be influenced by appropriate prenatal education. In one randomized study, a 10-minute educational meeting with a clinic nurse that centered on when to come to the hospital for labor cut the rate of outpatient hospital visits for false labor from 57% of primigravidas to 30% (number needed to treat [NNT] = 3.6, meaning 1 patient visit to the hospital for false labor would be prevented by having 3.6 patients receive the "treatment" of an educational nurse meeting).[15]

B. Diagnosis of Labor

See earlier (see Section A.II.A) for a discussion of inaccurate diagnosis of labor.

C. Maternal Support during Labor

Cochrane data reveal multiple benefits of the use of an experienced labor support person (or "doula") accompanying women in labor. With the metaanalysis including 13 trials with more than 4900 patients, the presence of a doula was associated with a reduced need for medication for pain relief (OR, 0.60; NNT = 9.3), operative vaginal delivery (OR, 0.78; NNT = 32), reduced cesarean delivery (OR, 0.77; NNT = 38), and reduced number of neonates with Apgar scores less than 7 at 5 minutes (OR, 0.50; NNT = 83). Maternal satisfaction also was improved.[16]

D. Position Changes during Labor

An RCT involving 1067 women in active labor at 36 to 41 weeks of gestation concluded that there was no evidence of harm in allowing patients to ambulate throughout labor.[17] However, many authors have discussed the multiple benefits that can occur when the laboring patient is allowed to modify her position based on comfort. Smith and co-workers[18] claim, "There is good evidence that position change is useful in achieving good progress in labor, is well tolerated, and can be accomplished safely. Position change may be more important than a single 'best' position."

Although many labor units still use the dorsal lithotomy position for delivery (mainly because of caregiver convenience), there is evidence to suggest significant benefits of other positions. Upright delivery reduces the lumbar lordosis and directs the fetal head toward the outlet of the pelvis rather than directly into the posterior aspect of the pubis. In addition, gravity can add up to 35 mmHg to the pressure exerted by the presenting part when the mother is upright during delivery.[19]

E. Intermittent Monitoring during Labor

The Cochrane review of trials involving more than 50,000 patients comparing intermittent monitoring with continuous fetal monitoring made the following conclusions: compared with intermittent auscultation, routine EFM was associated with a decreased risk for a 1-minute Apgar score less than 4 (relative risk [RR], 0.82; 95% confidence interval [CI], 0.65-0.98; NNT = 167) and a decreased risk for neonatal seizures (RR, 0.50; 95% CI, 0.30-0.82; NNT = 500). However, results from different studies were heterogeneous, and the increases in neonatal seizures were noted only in the setting of use of oxytocin. No significant differences were seen in 1-minute Apgar scores less than 7, rate of admissions to neonatal intensive care units (NICUs), and perinatal death. Continuous EFM was associated with an increased rate of cesarean delivery (RR, 1.33; 95% CI, 1.08-1.59; number needed to harm [NNH] = 42) and total operative delivery (RR, 1.23; 95% CI, 1.15-1.31; NNH = 50).[10]

F. Analgesia

The controversy that exists in the medical literature concerning epidural use and increased rates of cesarean section is discussed earlier in Section A.III.B.3. However, the metaanalyses that show no increase in the cesarean section rate with regional anesthesia do reveal that epidural use is associated with prolonged first and second stages of labor and an increase in the rate of assisted vaginal delivery. For patients who request pharmacologic methods of pain relief, patient satisfaction is greater and pain scores during labor are lower with epidural analgesia compared with parenteral opioid analgesia.[13] With this in mind, are

there specific steps that can be taken to minimize the potential for dystocia and cesarean delivery with epidural use? As noted earlier in Section A.III.B.3, delaying the use of regional anesthesia until the patient is at least 4 cm dilated may decrease the risk for dystocia.

G. Persistent Occiput Posterior Position

One factor identified in spontaneous rotation of the OP is the levator sling, which can enhance flexion and thus the likelihood of rotation as the fetus descends. With epidural analgesia, motor blockade can occur, thus decreasing the possibility of spontaneous rotation of the fetal head. Manual rotation techniques generally attempt to replicate the forces provided by the levator sling and pelvic floor while adding a rotational component.

What can be done in labor to enhance spontaneous rotation? When the fetus is in the OP position, supine maternal positions encourage extension of the fetal head into the hollow of the sacrum (see Chapter 17, Section F). Having the mother curl forward at the hips will increase the force encouraging flexion of the head and present the smaller suboccipitobregmatic diameter of the fetal head to the pelvic outlet. Pelvic rocking (tilting the pelvis back and forth with the mother on her hands and knees) also can help rotate the OP fetus, as well as the use of an exaggerated lateral Sims' position with the fetal spine positioned upward.[19]

H. Role of Hydration

One small study by Garite and colleagues[20] is worthy of review, as it raises a question about current labor management. A total of 195 nulliparas in spontaneous active labor at 2 to 5 cm dilated were randomized to receive either 125 or 250 ml/hr intravenous (IV) fluid during labor. The two groups were comparable; the occurrence rate of labors longer than 12 hours was lower in the high-IV rate group (13% vs. 26%; NNT = 8), and the duration of the first stage was 70 minutes shorter in this group. The rates of oxytocin administration for inadequate labor progress was lower in the high-rate group (49% vs. 65%) and the rate of cesarean delivery was also lower (9.9% vs. 17.0%), though both narrowly missed statistical significance. These results suggest that hydration status during labor in nulliparas can play a role in contributing to dysfunctional labor and, if replicated, could potentially lead to a change in labor management.

V. TREATMENT

A. Prolonged Latent Phase

Women experiencing a prolonged latent phase (defined as more than 20 hours in nulliparas) often respond best to therapeutic rest. Choices for this include morphine sulfate or other narcotics given in sufficient dose to allow the patient to sleep. Most patients will awaken in active labor, whereas about 10% to 15% will have stopped contracting and were in false labor.[21] The Irish model uses an antepartum ward where patients contracting but not in labor can be observed and treated for 12 hours before being sent home.

B. Stage One Management

1. Amniotomy

   Amniotomy as an intervention has been evaluated in a Cochrane review[22] and noted to decrease the incidence of dystocia (OR, 0.33; NNT = 9) and the use of oxytocin in labor (OR, 0.79; NNT = 25) but has also been associated with a near-statistical increase in the rate of cesarean delivery (OR, 1.26; NNH = 85). The decrease in dystocia was most pronounced in patients dilated 3 cm or more at the time of amniotomy.[23] Although the incidence of cord prolapse has not been reported to be increased in the trials of amniotomy, it is reasonable to balance its benefit in decreasing oxytocin use and dystocia with the possible risk for increasing cesarean delivery rate in choosing to use this intervention.

2. Oxytocin augmentation

   Table 15-1 compares current low-, intermediate-, and high-dose oxytocin protocols. The low- and high-dose protocols are those that the American College of Obstetricians and Gynecologists (ACOG) suggested in their technical bulletin[24]; the high-dose regimen is similar to the standard oxytocin protocol used at the National Maternity Hospital in Dublin. Two trials of low- versus high-dose oxytocin (Pitocin) support the benefit of a high dose in the setting of induction. In the larger study, Satin and co-workers[25] show that high-dose oxytocin (Pitocin; starting dose 6 mU/min, increasing by 6 mU/min every 20 minutes) was associated with a 9% cesarean rate, a spontaneous delivery rate of 75%, and a forceps delivery rate of 12% in 944 patients. In the low-dose group of 732 patients, the cesarean rate was 12%, the spontaneous delivery rate was 68%, and the forceps delivery rate was 16%. Although another study by Xenakis and colleagues[26] was smaller, it revealed a cesarean rate of 10.4% in the high-dose group (n = 154) and of 25.7% in the low-dose group (n = 156). Both studies showed slightly greater rates of hyperstimulation in the high-dose groups, but equivalent Apgar scores and NICU admission rates. Based on these data, high-dose Pitocin appears to offer advantages in the setting of augmentation of labor. Of note is that the ACOG also states that during augmentation with oxytocin, fetal well-being "should be assessed electronically or by auscultation and recorded every 15 minutes during the first stage of labor and every 5 minutes during the second stage of labor."[24]

3. Fetal heart rate monitoring

   As discussed in Chapter 14, Section E, use of continuous EFM in low-risk populations is associated with an increased incidence of dystocia and cesarean section. Unless there are specific indications for continuous monitoring, intermittent auscultation should be encouraged for all women in labor.

4. Monitoring the progress of labor

   Most authorities consider active-phase labor arrest to occur when the cervix has not dilated despite 2 hours of active labor. This 2-hour "magic number" may indeed need revision, based on a

TABLE 15-1 **Oxytocin Protocols**

Regimen	Initial Dose	Increase Increment	Dosage Interval	Maximum Dose
Low-dose	0.5-1 mU/min	1 mU/min	30-40 minutes	20 mU/min
Intermediate	2 mU/min	2 mU/min	15 minutes	None
High-dose	6 mU/min	3-6 mU/min	20-40 minutes	42 mU/min

Adapted from Dystocia and augmentation of labor. ACOG practice bulletin, Number 49, December 2003, *Obstet Gynecol* 102:1445-1454, 2003.

study of active-phase labor arrest. Rouse and colleagues[27] treated 542 women diagnosed with arrest (cervix at least 4 cm dilated with less than 1 cm of change in 2 hours) with oxytocin using a goal of obtaining at least 200 Montevideo units for at least 4 hours before considering cesarean delivery. Ninety-seven percent of parous women and 88% of nulliparas delivered vaginally (overall vaginal delivery rate, 92%). In this population, the cesarean section rate would have been 26% if all patients had been operatively delivered when active-phase arrest was diagnosed. Based on the use of the 4-hour protocol, the overall cesarean section rate was 8%. In this population, the epidural rate was 96% in nulliparas and 89% in primiparas; patients were delivered by cesarean for failure to progress after the 4 hours of oxytocin, for nonvertex presentation, or for nonreassuring fetal heart tones.[27]

C. Stage Two Management

For more information on stage two management, see Chapter 14, Section G.

1. Persistent OP position
   a. Position changes: Encouraging position changes increases the chance of rotation.
   b. Manual rotation: Generally, this maneuver is attempted after the cervix is completely dilated with the presenting part on or near the pelvic floor; the goal of the operator is to recreate the forces of the levator sling whereas adding a slight rotational force. Refer to Chapter 17, Section F for a detailed description of the technique of manual rotation.
   c. Vaginally assisted delivery: Attempt a vacuum-assisted or forceps-assisted delivery when the presenting part is below +2 station if maternal exhaustion occurs. Assisted vaginal deliveries can attempt to deliver the infant in an OP position (see Chapter 18, Section D), although the potential for a failed operative vaginal delivery is greater than with an occiput anterior position.
   d. Rotational forceps: Use of forceps for rotation to OA is possible *but should be limited to operators with sufficient skill and experience with the technique of midforceps rotation.* Cesarean section is often the preferred method of delivery for a persistent OP in the presence of failure to descend during the second stage.

2. Pushing strategies
   a. Delay pushing until the fetal head is on the pelvic floor or until the urge to push is felt.[28]
   b. Vary maternal pushing positions.
   c. Avoid pushing in the dorsal lithotomy position.
3. Use of oxytocin
   Theoretical concerns have been raised about the ability of epidural analgesia to block certain neural reflexes that enhance pushing during the second stage (most notably Ferguson's reflex, whereby vaginal distention during the second stage increases oxytocin secretion). Observational studies using intrauterine pressure catheters have demonstrated decreased intrauterine pressures during the second stage when regional anesthesia is used.[29] In an RCT of starting oxytocin in the second stage of patients laboring with an epidural in place, Saunders and co-workers[30] note lower rates of operative vaginal delivery (NNT = 12) in the oxytocin group together with lower cesarean section rates (NNT = 65) and fewer second-degree lacerations. Infant outcomes were similar.[30]

D. Cephalopelvic Disproportion

Clinicians should have a high index of suspicion for a greater incidence of dystocia with macrosomia infants, particularly if a contracted maternal pelvis is present. Neither x-ray nor computed tomography pelvimetry has been shown to be a reliable predictor of CPD. In the setting of appropriate use of oxytocin to rule out dysfunctional labor, CPD can be diagnosed when there is lack of fetal descent to a station of +1 or lower despite complete (or near-complete) cervical dilatation in the absence of malrotation.

VI. EVIDENCE TO SUPPORT ACTIVE MANAGEMENT OF LABOR

Several early trials of various portions of active management showed decreased rates of dystocia and cesarean intervention, but did not evaluate the entire protocol. The largest U.S. trial of AML involved nearly 2000 patients and attempted to incorporate all aspects of the Irish model. This study failed to show a significant difference in cesarean section rates, although labors were nearly 2 hours shorter in the study group.[31] This study, however, did use continuous EFM and epidural analgesia, and lacked a specific review policy. A metaanalysis of the three best North American studies of AML shows a decrease in primary cesarean section rate of 34% (OR, 0.66; 95% CI, 0.54-0.81) without adverse fetal outcome. Together with subsequent decreases in patients who choose repeat cesarean rather than vaginal birth in their next pregnancy, widespread use of AML would be expected to decrease total cesarean section rate by 13%.[32]

It is useful to revisit the experience in Dublin as it has unfolded over the 1990s. From 1989 to 2000, the nulliparous cesarean delivery rate at National Maternity Hospital has increased from 8.1% to 16.6%, with the largest portion of the increase occurring in induced labors (and the rate of induction has increased from 17% to 40%). For those patients presenting in spontaneous labor, however, the cesarean delivery rate for those managed with an AML protocol has been stable at 5%. Perinatal outcomes have remained unchanged, and the second-stage cesarean rate for those who present in labor has remained stable at 0.5% in nulliparas.[33]

VII. SUMMARY

As dystocia in the nulliparous patient is a common problem, clinicians should have focused strategies for its management when it occurs. Awareness of factors that can cause dystocia can allow their avoidance in certain instances. A comprehensive understanding of the recognition, treatment, and prevention of dystocia in the primigravid patient should increase the probability of a safe vaginal delivery.

VIII. SOR A RECOMMENDATIONS

RECOMMENDATIONS	REFERENCES
Use of a specific diagnosis for admission for labor in nulliparas (such as 3-4 cm dilated and complete cervical effacement) decreases cesarean delivery rates, reduces use of pain medications, and improves patient satisfaction.	*3, 4*
Involve a doula whenever possible to decrease the risk for operative vaginal delivery, cesarean delivery, and Apgar score less than 7 at 5 minutes, and to improve maternal satisfaction.	*16*
In nulliparas with epidural analgesia, delay onset of pushing until the head is on the perineum or the urge to push is perceived by the patient to enhance the likelihood of spontaneous vaginal birth.	*28*

REFERENCES

1. Hamilton BE, Marin JA, Sutton PD: Births: preliminary data for 2003, *Natl Vital Stat Rep* 53:1-17, 2004.
2. Gabbe SG, Niebyl JR, Simpson JL, editors: *Obstetrics: normal and problem pregnancies,* ed 3, New York, 1996, Churchill Livingstone.
3. McNiven PS, Williams JI, Hodnett E et al: An early labor assessment program: a randomized, controlled trial, *Birth* 25: 5-10, 1998.
4. Bailit JL, Dierker L, Blanchard MH et al: Outcomes of women presenting in active versus latent phase of spontaneous labor, *Obstet Gynecol* 105:77-79, 2005.
5. Byrd JE, Lytton DE, Vogt SC et al: Diagnostic criteria and the management of dystocia, *J Fam Pract* 27:595-599, 1988.
6. Duff P, Southmayd K, Read JA: Outcome of trial of labor in patients with a single previous low transverse cesarean section for dystocia, *Obstet Gynecol* 71:380-383, 1988.
7. Gardberg M, Laakkonen E, Salevaara M: Intrapartum sonography and persistent occiput posterior position: a study of 408 deliveries, *Obstet Gynecol* 91:746-749, 1998.
8. Turner MJ, Rasmussen MJ, Turner JE et al: The influence of birth weight on labor in nulliparas, *Obstet Gynecol* 76: 159-163, 1990.
9. Chelmow D, Kilpatrick SJ, Laros RK: Maternal and neonatal outcomes after prolonged latent phase, *Obstet Gynecol* 81: 486-491, 1993.
10. Thacker SB, Stroup DF, Chang M: Continuous electronic heart rate monitoring for fetal assessment during labor. *Cochrane Database of Systematic Reviews* 2006, Issue 3. Art. No.: CD000063.
11. Lieberman E, Lang JM, Cohen A et al: Association of epidural analgesia with cesarean delivery in nulliparas, *Obstet Gynecol* 88:993-1000, 1996.
12. Halpern SH, Leighton BL, Ohlsson A et al: Effect of epidural's parenteral opioid analgesia on the progress of labor, *JAMA* 280:2105-2110, 1998.
13. Howell CJ: Epidural versus non-epidural analgesia for pain relief in labour, *Cochrane Database Syst Rev* (4):CD000331, 2000.
14. Lieberman E, Lang JM, Cohen A et al: Association of epidural analgesia with cesarean delivery in nulliparas, *Obstet Gynecol* 88:993-1000, 1996.
15. Bonovich L: Recognizing the onset of labor, *J Obstet Gynecol Neonat Nurs* 19:141-145, 1990.
16. Hodnett ED: Caregiver support for women during childbirth, *Cochrane Database Syst Rev* (1):CD000199, 2002.
17. Bloom SL, McIntire DD, Kelly MA et al: Lack of effect of walking on labor and delivery, *N Engl J Med* 339:76-79, 1998.
18. Smith MI, Acheson LS, Byrd JA et al: A critical review of labor and birth care, *J Fam Pract* 33:281-292, 1991.
19. Fenwick L, Simkin P: Maternal positioning to prevent or alleviate dystocia in labor, *Clin Obstet Gynecol* 30:83-89, 1987.
20. Garite TJ, Weeks J, Peters-Phair K et al: A randomized controlled trial of the effect of increased intravenous hydration on the course of labor in nulliparous women, *Am J Obstet Gynecol* 183:1544-1548, 2000.
21. Cohen WR, Acker DB, Friedman EA, editors: *Management of labor,* ed 2, Rockville, MD, 1989, Aspen Publishers.

22. Fraser WD, Turcot L, Krauss I et al: Amniotomy for shortening spontaneous labour, *Cochrane Database Syst Rev* (2): CD000015, 2000.

23. Fraser WD, Marcoux S, Moutquin MM et al: Effect of early amniotomy on the risk of dystocia in nulliparous women, *N Engl J Med* 328:1145-1149, 1993.

24. American College of Obstetricians and Gynecologists Committee on Practice Bulletins-Obstetrics: ACOG Practice Bulletin Number 49, December 2003. Dystocia and augmentation of labor, *Obstet Gynecol* 102:1445-1454, 2003.

25. Satin A, Leveno K, Sherman M et al: High-versus low-dose oxytocin for labor stimulation, *Obstet Gynecol* 80:111-116, 1992.

26. Xenakis E, Langer O, Piper J et al: Low-does versus high-dose oxytocin augmentation of labor a randomized trial, *Am J Obstet Gynecol* 173:1874-1878, 1995.

27. Rouse DJ, Owen J, Hauth JC: Active-phase labor arrest: oxytocin augmentation for a least 4 hours, *Obstet Gynecol* 93: 323-328, 1999.

28. Fraser WD, Marcoux S, Krauss I et al: Multicenter, randomized, controlled trial of delayed pushing for nulliparous women in the second stage of labor with continuous epidural analgesia. The PEOPLE (Pushing Early or Pushing Late with Epidural) Study Group, *Am J Obstet Gynecol* 182(5):1165-1172, 2000.

29. Seitchik J, Holden AE, Castillo M: Amniotomy and oxytocin treatment of functional dystocia and the route of delivery, *Am J Obstet Gynecol* 155:585-592, 1986.

30. Saunders NJ, Spiby H, Gilbert L et al: Oxytocin infusion during second stage of labour in primiparous women using epidural analgesia: a randomised double-blind placebo controlled trial, *BMJ* 299:1423-1426, 1989.

31. Frigoletto F, Leiberman E, Long J et al: A clinical trial of active management of labor, *N Engl J Med* 333:745-750, 1995.

32. Glantz JC, McNanley TJ: Active management of labor: a meta-analysis of cesarean delivery rates for dystocia in nulliparas, *Obstet Gynecol Surv* 52:497-505, 1997.

33. Foley ME, Alarab M, Daly L et al: The continuing effectiveness of active management of first labor, despite a doubling in overall nulliparous cesarean delivery, *Am J Obstet Gynecol* 191:891-895, 2004.

S E C T I O N   B Term

Premature Rupture of the Membranes

Wendy Brooks Barr, MD, MPH, MSCE

Term PROM is a common obstetric event, occurring in 8% of term pregnancies.[1,2] It is defined as the rupture of the amniotic membranes before the onset of labor at more than 37 weeks gestational age. Although the diagnosis of this condition is straightforward, the management has been controversial for decades, with clinicians continuing to debate the proper management of this condition for optimal maternal and neonatal outcomes.

I. EPIDEMIOLOGY AND RISK FACTORS

Term PROM occurs in approximately 8% of term pregnancies with a stable incidence reported over last several decades. There are no definitive risk factors for this condition, and it occurs equally in low- and high-risk populations. One study in Poland notes that, in their patient population, the condition occurs more commonly in primigravidas compared with multigravidas.[3] A case–control study looking for associations between vaginal infections and term PROM report that women with PROM were more commonly colonized with *Candida albicans* and *Klebsiella pneumonia* compared with women without PROM.[4] This study did not find an association between colonization with *Gardnerella vaginalis* and PROM.

II. CLINICAL FEATURES AND DIAGNOSIS

A. History

Term PROM is a clinical diagnosis that can be confirmed using several techniques. Women typically report having a gush of clear fluid or will report feeling like they urinated on themselves without needing to go to the bathroom. Patients can sometimes confuse PROM with normal urinary stress incontinence during pregnancy. Therefore, PROM should be confirmed by a clinician either in the office or in the labor suite if the symptoms are at all unclear.

B. Physical Findings

PROM can be confirmed on physical examination by performing a sterile speculum examination:

1. Once the speculum is placed, the clinician is looking for pooling of amniotic fluid in the vaginal vault.
2. Vaginal discharge/fluid can also be tested with Nitrazine paper, with a blue color indicating a high likelihood that there is amniotic fluid present.
3. Finally, if PROM is not obvious on physical examination, some vaginal fluid should be placed on a slide to dry for at least 10 minutes to be examined under the microscope for ferning (fern test).

III. TREATMENT

Treatment strategies for term PROM are discussed in the following sections (Table 15-2).

TABLE 15-2 Summary of Risks and Benefits of Induction with Oxytocin, Induction with Vaginal Prostaglandin, and Conservative Management for Term Premature Rupture of Membranes

Induction	Benefits	Risks
Oxytocin vs. conservative	Shorter time to delivery Shorter labor Greater maternal satisfaction Decreased chorioamnionitis Decreased endometritis Decreased maternal antibiotics Decreased neonatal infection (weak association) Decreased neonatal antibiotics Decreased neonatal intensive care unit (NICU) admission	Increased epidural analgesia
Prostaglandin vs. conservative	Shorter time to delivery Greater maternal satisfaction Decreased chorioamnionitis Decreased maternal antibiotics Decreased neonatal antibiotics Decreased NICU admission	Increased maternal diarrhea
Oxytocin vs. prostaglandin	Shorter time to delivery Shorter labor Decreased chorioamnionitis Decreased maternal nausea/vomiting Decreased neonatal infection (weak association) Decreased neonatal antibiotics Decreased NICU admission	Increased epidural analgesia

A. Avoidance of Early Digital Examinations

The treatment for term PROM has been controversial. Clinicians must weigh the risks for infection associated with prolonged rupture of membranes, in particular, early-onset group B streptococcus (GBS) infections (OR, 11.5),[5] with the risks associated with labor induction. This risk for infection is particularly associated with doing an initial digital cervical examination.[2] Because of this strong association between early digital examinations in PROM and neonatal infection, ACOG gives a level A recommendation not to perform digital examinations in patients with PROM who are not in labor and not planning on undergoing immediate induction of labor.[6]

B. Management Strategies

Management strategies for term PROM include:
1. Conservative management for 24 to 72 hours until onset of spontaneous labor, followed by induction if no spontaneous labor
2. Immediate induction with oxytocin
3. Immediate induction with vaginal prostaglan-

dins (e.g., prostaglandin E_2 [PGE_2]), if cervix unfavorable
4. Immediate induction with misoprostol (vaginal or oral)

C. Results of Studies

1. TermPROM Study[7]
   This was a large, multicenter RCT involving more than 5000 patients. The study compared four different management strategies:
   a. Immediate induction with oxytocin
   b. Immediate induction with vaginal PGE_2
   c. Conservative management up to 4 days followed by induction with oxytocin
   d. Conservative management for up to 4 days followed by induction with vaginal PGE_2
   The study investigators reported the following results:
   a. Most women who are conservatively managed will deliver spontaneously without complications after term PROM, with 78% of the women in the conservative management group going into spontaneous labor within the 4-day observation period.

b. There were no differences in cesarean rates or neonatal infections between all the management strategies.

c. Women with immediate induction with oxytocin were less likely to have infants who required NICU stays longer than 24 hours compared with mothers in the conservative management followed by oxytocin induction group.

d. Infants born to mothers in the immediate induction with oxytocin group were less likely to receive antibiotics compared with those in the immediate induction with prostaglandins or conservative management followed by oxytocin induction group.

e. Women in the immediate induction with oxytocin group were less likely to experience development of chorioamnionitis compared with all other treatment groups.

f. Mothers in the immediate induction groups were more satisfied with their management experiences than those in the comparable conservative management followed by induction groups.

2. Large metaanalysis

Mozurkewich and Wolf[1] conducted a metaanalysis involving more than 7000 women. They compared three management schemes:

a. Immediate induction with oxytocin

b. Immediate induction with intravaginal prostaglandin

c. Conservative management with delayed induction with oxytocin

They reported the following results:

a. No differences were found in cesarean rates or neonatal infections among all the management strategies.

b. Immediate oxytocin induction had fewer cases of chorioamnionitis and endometritis compared with conservative management.

c. Immediate induction with vaginal prostaglandins resulted in more cases of chorioamnionitis compared with immediate induction with oxytocin, but fewer cases when compared with conservative management. They did not find any significant differences between management schemes for cesarean delivery or neonatal infections.

3. Cochrane reviews

Database of Systematic Reviews has several metaanalyses examining term PROM management. One analysis evaluated immediate oxytocin compared with expectant management,[6] whereas a second analysis compared prostaglandin versus oxytocin induction.[7] The results are as follows:

a. No differences were found in cesarean section rate between immediate oxytocin induction compared with expectant management or prostaglandin induction.[8]

b. Lower rates of chorioamnionitis and endometritis occurred with immediate oxytocin induction compared with expectant management.[8]

c. A significant reduction occurred in serious neonatal infections with immediate oxytocin induction compared with expectant management (this analysis included studies with infants between 34 and 36 weeks of gestation, which could have biased the results).[8]

d. There was increased epidural use, internal fetal heart rate monitoring, and cesarean section for failed induction with immediate oxytocin induction compared with conservative management.[8]

e. Prostaglandin induction was associated with an increase in neonatal infections, chorioamnionitis, NICU admissions, and neonatal antibiotic therapy compared with oxytocin induction.[9]

f. The role of misoprostol in PROM inductions remains unclear. Several small studies were underpowered for patient-oriented outcomes but found that the admittance–delivery intervals with women who were managed with misoprostol were shorter than with expectant management but longer than with oxytocin induction.[10,11]

D. Issues with Conservative Management

1. Setting: home versus hospital observation

The TermPROM Study Group found that observation at home was associated with an increased risk for maternal predelivery antibiotics in nulliparas, for cesarean sections, and for neonatal infections in women not colonized with GBS.[12] Overall, they found no clinical advantage for women to be observed at home rather than in the hospital.

2. Duration of observation

The TermPROM Study and most other RCTs comparing labor induction and conservative management allowed for observation up to 96 hours, although many patients in these groups were induced before 96 hours. Shalev and colleagues[13] performed a nonrandomized prospective study comparing 12- versus 72-hour conservative management followed by oxytocin induction, if necessary, in 566 women with term PROM. They found no differences in the rates of cesarean delivery, neo-natal infections, or chorioamnionitis. The only advantage found for the shorter observation period was a shorter length of stay (5 vs. 6 days; $p < 0.01$), and also that patients who underwent induction after the 72-hour expectant management period had an increased risk for cesarean delivery compared with those who required induction after the 12-hour expectant management period.

IV. SOR A RECOMMENDATIONS

RECOMMENDATIONS	REFERENCES
Immediate induction with oxytocin is the preferred management strategy for term PROM given the benefits of decreased maternal infections (chorioamnionitis [NNT = 37] and endometritis [NNT = 125]) likely outweigh the risks for increased epidural use (NNH = 33).	*1, 7, 8*
Although given that several metaanalyses show no differences in cesarean section, neonatal infection rates, or mortality, conservative management followed by oxytocin induction, if needed, remains an acceptable strategy if the patient and provider prefer this strategy.	
Induction with oxytocin is preferred over induction with prostaglandin (for either immediate or delayed induction) with lower rates of neonatal infections (NNT = 83), chorioamnionitis (NNT = 50), NICU admission longer than 24 hours (NNT = 38), and neonatal antibiotic therapy (NNT = 29).	*9*

REFERENCES

1. Mozurkewich EL, Wolf FM: Premature rupture of membranes at term: a meta-analysis of three management schemes, *Obstet Gynecol* 89:1035-1043, 1997.
2. Mozurkewich E: Management of premature rupture of membranes at term: an evidence-based approach, *Clin Obstet Gynecol* 42:749-756, 1999.
3. Semczuk-Sikora A, Sawulicka-Oleszczuk H, Semczuk M: Management in premature rupture of the membranes (PROM) at term—own experiences, *Ginekol Pol* 72:759-764, 2001.
4. Kovavisarach E, Sermsak P, Kanjanahareutai S: Aerobic microbiological study in term pregnant women with premature rupture of the membranes: a case-control study, *J Med Assoc Thai* 84:19-23, 2001.
5. Benitz WE, Gould JB, Druzin ML: Risk factors for early-onset group B streptococcal sepsis: estimation of odds ratios by critical literature review, *Pediatrics* 103:e76, 1999.
6. Morgan Ortiz F, Baez Barraza J, Quevedo Castro E et al: Misoprostal and oxytocin for induction of cervical ripening and labor in patients with term pregnancy and premature membrane rupture, *Ginecol Obstet Mex* 70:469-476, 2002.
7. Hannah ME, Ohlsson A, Farine D et al: Induction of labor compared to expectant management for prelabor rupture of the membranes at term, *N Engl J Med* 334:1005-1010, 1996.
8. Tan BP, Hannah ME: Oxytocin for prelabour rupture of membranes at or near term, *Cochrane Database Syst Rev* (3), 2005.
9. Tan BP, Hannah ME: Prostaglandins versus oxytocin for prelabour rupture of membranes at term, *Cochrane Database Syst Rev* (2):CD000159, 2000.
10. Butt KD, Bennett KA, Crane JM et al: Randomized comparison of oral misoprostal and oxytocin for labor induction in term prelabor membrane rupture, *Obstet Gynecol* 94:994-999, 1999.
11. Ozden S, Delikara MN, Avci A et al: Intravaginal misoprostal vs. expectant management in premature rupture of membranes with low Bishop scores at term, *Int J Gynaecol Obstet* 77:109-115, 2002.
12. Hannah ME, Hodnett ED, Willan A et al: Prelabor rupture of the membranes at term: expectant management at home or in hospital? *Obstet Gynecol* 96:533-538, 2000.
13. Shalev E, Peleg D, Eliyahu S et al: Comparison of 12 and 72 hour expectant management of premature rupture of membranes in term pregnancies, *Obstet Gynecol* 85:766-768, 1995.

SECTION C Induction of Labor

James M. Nicholson, MD, MSCE

Induction of labor is the process of stimulating contractions in a pregnant woman to produce progressive cervical dilatation and delivery. Ideally, labor induction is done when the benefits of this intervention outweigh its risks. However, high-quality data are limited regarding the benefits and risks of labor induction as compared with expectant management, or the benefits and risks of new types of labor induction as compared with more traditional means of labor induction. Despite these limitations, labor induction rates in the United States currently are increasing.[1,2] Labor induction remains an important part of modern maternity care.

I. INDICATIONS

A. Standard Maternal Indications

The following conditions are associated primarily with an increased risk for maternal mortality or significant maternal morbidity,[3,4] but most maternal indications also pose significant risk to the fetus:

1. Severe preeclampsia, eclampsia
2. Term PROM (>12 hours) or suspected chorio-amnionitis
3. Maternal medical conditions (diabetes mellitus, chronic hypertension, renal disease, chronic pulmonary disease)
4. Risk for precipitous labor (cervical dilatation ≥4 cm) or significant distance of the mother from the delivering hospital (geographic or social)
5. Psychological distress from fetal demise during current pregnancy

B. Standard Fetal Indications

The following conditions are associated with an increased risk for uteroplacental insufficiency and fetal death if delivery is delayed.[3,4] Antenatal surveillance is often conducted in the weeks before labor induction to ensure fetal well-being pending delivery (see Chapter 11, Section B).

1. Postterm pregnancy (≥42 weeks 0 days of gestation)
2. Oligohydramnios (amniotic fluid index ≤5)
3. Intrauterine growth restriction (fetal size <10% for gestational age)
4. Rh sensitization
5. Prior term stillborn infant

C. Preventive Labor Indications

Although controversial, a growing body of research has associated delivery midway through the term period of pregnancy with the lowest rates of a variety of adverse birth outcomes.[5-7] A recent systematic review concluded that a routine policy of labor induction after 41 weeks of gestation, as compared with expectant management until 42 weeks of gestation, provides lower cesarean delivery risk and a trend toward decreased neonatal mortality.[8] The routine delivery of women at 39 to 40 weeks of gestation has not been studied using prospective RCTs. However, preventive labor induction has been used in several settings to encourage their patients to deliver early in the term period, with the timing of preventive labor induction based on each woman's pattern of obstetric risk.[9,10] Retrospective studies of this activity report better rates of adverse birth outcomes than groups treated with the current standard of care. Indications for preventive term labor induction include impending cephalopelvic disproportion, impending uteroplacental insufficiency, early preeclampsia, and increasing maternal dysphoria.

II. RELATIVE CONTRAINDICATIONS TO INDUCTION OF LABOR

A variety of conditions exists that make attempted vaginal delivery unacceptably dangerous.[3,4]

A. Maternal Contraindications

Absolute maternal contraindications to labor induction include placenta previa, prior classic cesarean section, prior non–lower uterine segment uterine scar (e.g., myomectomy), more than one low-transverse cesarean delivery, invasive cervical cancer, and hypersensitivity to induction agent. Relative maternal contraindications include one prior low-transverse cesarean delivery, narrow pelvis, or significant maternal medical condition (cardiac, pulmonary, or neurologic disease).

B. Fetal Contraindications

Absolute fetal contraindications to labor induction include the presence of active maternal genital herpes, untreated human immunodeficiency virus infection, transverse lie, vasa previa, significant hydrocephalus, and severe intrauterine growth restriction with abnormal Doppler studies. Breech presentation is a strong relative contraindication to labor induction.

III. ISSUES RELATED TO LABOR INDUCTION

A. Definition of Success

Successful labor induction is defined as an intervention leading to progressive cervical dilatation and simple vaginal delivery. Some investigators have used time limits, such as delivery by 24 or 12 hours, to further define induction success.[11] However, the importance of identifying and tolerating a relatively long latent phase, to safely maximize vaginal delivery rates, has been described in the literature.[12,13]

B. Induction and Measured Outcomes

Despite historical concerns,[14-18] induction of labor is not as hazardous as once thought. Two systematic reviews conclude that labor induction, as compared with expectant management, does not adversely affect rates of common birth outcomes (e.g., mode of delivery, degree of maternal perineal trauma, type of nursery admission, and neonatal Apgar scoring).[8,19] Maternal satisfaction with labor induction has not been adequately studied. Cost-effectiveness analyses are highly impacted by time interval between admission and delivery, by group cesarean delivery rates, and by NICU admission rates.

C. Obstetric Risk, Gestational Age, and Confounding by Indication

The impact of common obstetric risk factors on adverse birth outcomes increases with increasing gestational age during the final weeks of pregnancy.[7] Attempts to compare the outcomes of women who are induced with those who enter spontaneous labor often ignore both the reason(s) that the induction was initiated (prevention of maternal/fetal mortality or increased obstetric risk) and the impact of increasing gestational age on birth outcomes.[9,15] Adjustment for these issues has been shown to reduce or eliminate the apparent association between labor induction and greater rates of adverse birth outcomes.[20]

D. Cervical Readiness

The state of the cervix is an important factor in the success or failure of labor induction. A firm, rigid, unripe cervix may require three to four times the amount of uterine contractility to produce dilatation as a soft, compliant cervix.[21] A variety of scoring systems exists to assess the state of the cervix,[22,23] but the most popular remains the Bishop's score (Table 15-3). Clinical history, gestational age, and parity are also important predictive factors.

IV. CERVICAL RIPENING

Before the onset of spontaneous labor, the uterine cervix usually softens, thins out, dilates, and moves anteriorly. If these changes have not occurred before the start of the induction of labor, then cervical ripening is needed. Attempts to soften the cervix pharmacologically or mechanically before the initiation of labor induction are based on the assumption that artificial ripening will provide the same or similar benefits as physiologic ripening. This assumption may not always be correct because cervical ripening involves not only dilatation, as occurs readily with the use of a Foley catheter, but chemical changes in the collagen and proteoglycan matrix, increase in edema and vascularity, and increase in leukocytes and macrophages.[21] Despite these concerns, a variety of methods are currently used for cervical ripening before labor induction (Table 15-4).

TABLE 15-3 Calculating the Bishop's Score

	0	1	2	3
Dilatation	0	1-2	3-4	5-6
Effacement	0-30	45-50	60-70	80
Station	−3	−2	−1	+1,+2
Consistency	Firm	Medium	Soft	—
Position	Posterior	Mid	Anterior	—

Inducibility: 5 = multipara, 7 = primipara.

A. Prostaglandins and Cervical Ripening

Conclusive evidence now exists that the use of prostaglandins, as compared with placebo or no agent, promotes cervical ripening and increases the likelihood of successful labor induction.[24,25] The two commonly used prostaglandins are Prostaglandin E_1 (PGE_1) and Prostaglandin E_2 (PGE_2). A significant portion of women treated with prostaglandins develop effective labor and do not require additional augmentation (4-7% with PGE_2, 40% with PGE_1).[24-26]

1. Types of prostaglandins, dosage, and route of administration

   PGE_2 (dinoprostone), in both vaginal gel form and vaginal insert form, is approved for preinduction cervical ripening by the Federal Drug Administration (FDA). Although PGE_1 (misoprostol) in pill-fragment form is also used throughout the United States for cervical ripening, this specific usage has not been approved by the FDA. Dosages of these medications are listed in Table 15-4. The vaginal route of administration appears to be optimal for all prostaglandins. An advantage to the PGE_2 vaginal insert is the ability to remove it by its string if hyperstimulation occurs. Attempts to wash out PGE_2 vaginal gel or PGE_1 pill fragments are often ineffective.

2. Efficacy and cost

   Women receiving PGE_1 or PGE_2 for preinduction cervical ripening, as compared with women who receive placebo, are much more likely to have an adequate Bishop's score at the time their induction is started. The two types of prostaglandins are probably equally effective in promoting cervical ripening, although PGE_1 is much less expensive and its use is associated with shorter median time to delivery.[25]

TABLE 15-4 Cervical Ripening and Labor-Induction Agents

Induction Agent	Ripening	Induction	Dose	Comments
Membrane stripping	++	+	Membrane stripping, or cervical massage, weekly starting at 38 weeks of gestation	Membrane stripping is usually uncomfortable. Group B streptococcus colonization is a relative contraindication.
PGE$_1$: misoprostol (Cytotec)	+++	+++++	25-μg pill fragment (1/4 of 100-μg tablet) placed vaginally every 4-6 hours for a maximum of 6 doses in 24 hours	Misoprostol should be used only in an inpatient setting because of increased risk for uterine hyperstimulation. Fetal monitoring before, during, and after administration allow for the rapid diagnosis of fetal intolerance and for the treatment of uterine tetany.
PGE$_2$: dinoprostone—vaginal insert (Cervidil), vaginal gel (Prepidil)	++++	++	Vaginal insert: 10-mg dinoprostone pledget, inserted vaginally, for 12 hours; repeated doses do not carry FDA approval Vaginal gel: 0.5 mg PGE$_2$ placed in 2.5-ml gel, placed vaginally every 6-8 hours for maximum of 3 uses	PGE$_2$ products provide a gentler ripening process than PGE$_1$, but hyperstimulation can occur. Monitoring before, during, and after insertion is recommended. The vaginal insert is easily removable by its "tail."
Foley bulb catheter	+++	+	14F-16F catheter inflated with 30 ml fluid; larger catheters (24F, 80-ml bulb) have been used; Foley catheter may be placed at traction, and instillation of fluid (saline or dilute PGE$_2$ solution) may be used	The Foley bulb catheter is primarily a ripening agent, but it causes uterine contractions and can cause uterine hyperstimulation. Fetal monitoring after insertion is recommended. Physiologic ripening may lag behind Bishop's scoring. Additional induction agents are usually required (oxytocin or amniotomy).
Early amniotomy	N/A	+	N/A	The use of early amniotomy as a primary induction agent should be limited to multiparous women.
Late amniotomy	N/A	++	N/A	Late amniotomy is usually used as an adjunct to other methods of labor induction, such as prostaglandins or oxytocin.
Oxytocin (Pitocin)	+	+++++		

PGE$_1$, Prostaglandin E$_1$; PGE$_2$, prostaglandin E$_2$; FDA, Federal Drug Administration; N/A, not applicable.
Vertex presentation should be confirmed before the start of either cervical ripening or labor induction.

3. Side effects and safety issues
   The use of all prostaglandins is associated with rare symptoms of fever, nausea, vomiting, diarrhea, and abdominal pain (<1%). Uterine hypertonus and hyperstimulation occur more often in prostaglandin-treated women than in women with placebo or no treatment. Until fur-

ther studies evaluating the safety of outpatient ripening protocols are published, prostaglandins should be administered in a hospital setting followed by careful observation of both fetal heart tones and uterine contractility. Fetal heart rate abnormalities and passage of thick meconium occur more frequently after the use of

PGE$_1$ compared with placebo, PGE$_2$, or the Foley catheter.[25]

B. Foley Catheter and Cervical Ripening

The use of a transcervical Foley catheter to promote cervical ripening gained popular support in the United States in the late 1990s.[26] Foley catheters cause mechanical cervical dilatation.

1. Foley catheter protocols

   Most protocols use a 14F or a 16F Foley catheter with a 30-ml balloon, although some investigators have used catheters as large as 24F and balloon volumes as high as 80 ml.[27] The catheters are inserted by blind digital guidance or using direct visualization. Some protocols have included an extraamniotic infusion of either saline or dilute PGE$_2$ solution through the Foley catheter.

2. Efficacy

   Women receiving Foley catheters, as compared with women who receive prostaglandin medications, are provided with equivalent change in Bishop's score.[26]

3. Side effects and safety issues

   Identification of the placenta by prenatal ultrasound, and avoidance of this organ during Foley bulb placement, reduces the likelihood of iatrogenic placental separation and resultant bleeding. Rarely, artificial rupture of membranes can occur during placement. Foley bulb placement increases maternal discomfort, and epidural analgesia can be initiated before placement. Importantly, there appears to be no increased risk for preterm birth in subsequent pregnancies after use of a Foley catheter for cervical ripening.[28]

C. Other Methods of Cervical Ripening

Estrogen, relaxin, and laminaria have been used previously for cervical ripening but are currently not recommended. Breast stimulation has been tested but has been linked to unacceptable rates of fetal death.[29] Studies of the impact of sexual intercourse on cervical ripening have provided conflicting results. Similarly, amniotic membrane stripping has not been determined to provide a clear-cut improvement in cervical Bishop's score, although it does reduce the average gestational age of labor onset.[31] Two methods of treatment that currently are under investigation include the use of acupuncture[30] and the use of isosorbide mononitrate. The latter method appears to provide cervical ripening without promoting uterine contractions, and it may therefore be a method that can be used safely in the outpatient setting.

V. METHODS OF INDUCTION

Labor induction, in contrast with cervical ripening, is directed at causing uterine contractions, progressive cervical dilatation, and eventual delivery. A variety of effective methods has been developed to accomplish this goal. The safety of labor induction from the neonate's perspective may be enhanced by refraining from initiating an induction until the 39th week of pregnancy has started or until fetal lung maturity has been confirmed via amniocentesis. Pregnancy dating by early (6-20 weeks) ultrasound improves induction safety.[3] Induction methods are listed in Table 15-4.

A. Alternative Medicine

A variety of alternative methods is used to promote labor induction. Cochrane reviews of homoeopathy[29] and acupuncture[30] both concluded that there is insufficient evidence to guide women and their providers in a discussion of risks and benefits of these methods. The uses of both breast stimulation and cohosh tea have been linked with fetal demise and are currently not recommended means of labor induction.

B. Amniotic Membrane Stripping

Amniotic membrane stripping results in increased prostaglandin production proportional to the area of detachment and a shorter interval to the onset of labor. A recent review[31] estimated that a protocol involving the weekly stripping of membranes starting at 38 weeks of gestation would need to be performed on eight women to avoid one indicated induction. As compared with other methods of labor induction, cesarean delivery rates and rates of other adverse birth outcomes were not changed after membrane stripping. Potential complications of membrane stripping include significant maternal discomfort, iatrogenic rupture of membranes (with risk for cord prolapse, other cord impingement, or fetal hemorrhage from vasa previa), and promotion of chorioamnionitis. However, these complications are rare.

C. Amniotomy

High-quality data concerning the benefits and risks of amniotomy as a primary induction agent currently are not available. Recent reviews of this intervention[32] reflect that, when compared with oxytocin infusion or intravaginal prostaglandins, amniotomy is less effective in promoting the rapid onset of labor. Amniotomy carries a small risk for umbilical cord prolapse and fetal intolerance (because of umbilical cord rearrangement after the loss of amniotic fluid), and these risks are heightened if the presenting part is above −2 station. Early amniotomy (e.g., before 3-4 cm dilatation) leads to greater cesarean delivery rates and febrile morbidity. Other than in situations of multiparity linked with a high Bishop's score, amniotomy is probably best used as an adjunct to other induction methods.

D. Foley Catheters with and without Other Methods

Although Foley catheters are primarily used to promote cervical ripening, their use occasionally precipitates both cervical ripening and the onset of labor. Approximately 5% of women receiving Foley catheters alone required no other uterine stimulant before delivery.[26] This was not significantly different from the 7% of women who developed labor after receiving PGE_2 gel.

As labor induction agents, Foley catheters are often used together with other induction modalities. Extraamniotic saline infusion has not been found to be highly effective at altering the course of labor, but the addition of oxytocin, PGE_1, and PGE_2 (dinoprostone gel or solution) all promote faster delivery with minimal impact on other birth outcomes.[33]

E. Prostaglandins

The first studies describing the use of prostaglandins for labor induction were highly optimistic about the potential to improve labor induction outcomes in patients of mixed parity, various indications, and variable cervical Bishop's scores.[34,35] However, because of subsequent concerns about a possible association between labor induction and both cesarean delivery (possibly caused by confounding by indication) and neonatal jaundice (probably caused by dilute oxytocin solutions, iatrogenic prematurity, or both), labor induction activity became increasingly limited to specific indications.[3] Since the early 1990s, different types, doses, routes of administration, and schedules have been developed and tested. However, birth outcomes after labor induction have improved only marginally during this time.

1. PGE_2 (dinoprostone)

A recent review of 57 studies evaluated PGE_2, as compared with placebo or oxytocin alone, and concluded that PGE_2 products increase the likelihood of delivery within 24 hours of the start of labor induction and decrease cesarean delivery rates.[24] However, oxytocin augmentation and/or

amniotomy are usually needed after the use of PGE_2 products. PGE_2 medications appear to be relatively safe for labor induction, and they cause less uterine hyperstimulation and are less likely to cause the passage of thick meconium than PGE_1. However, PGE_2 medications are relatively expensive compared with other modern methods of labor induction, and the interval between first dosage and delivery is longer than that for either PGE_1 or Foley catheters. Both forms of PGE_2 can be used for labor induction in the setting of PROM, although the dosage of the gel form should be reduced from 0.5 to 0.25 mg. The use of multiple doses of PGE_2 (vaginal insert form) was associated, in one retrospective study, with increased rates of febrile morbidity and fetal intolerance. However, this study did not consider the issue of confounding by indication, for example, that women requiring multiple doses of PGE_2 were different from women who did not require multiple doses of PGE_2.

2. PGE_1 (misoprostol)

Misoprostol is an attractive agent because of its low cost, excellent efficacy compared with other induction agents, and ease of administration.

a. Dosage, route of administration, and efficacy: A review of 17 studies[36] suggests that the preferred dosage regimen is the vaginal application of an initial dose of 25 μg PGE_1 followed by additional 25-μg doses every 4 to 6 hours for a maximum of 6 doses within 24 hours. Buccal or oral administration is still under active study and should be used with caution. A larger review evaluating 62 trials[37] concluded that, as compared with conventional methods of labor induction such as vaginal pGE_2 and oxytocin, PGE_1 usage was associated with less need for epidural analgesia and fewer failures to achieve vaginal delivery within 24 hours. However, overall rates of cesarean delivery were not changed after the use of PGE_1.

b. Safety issues: Based on multiple studies and reviews,[25,36,37] PGE_1 is clearly associated with greater rates of uterine hyperstimulation and passage of thick meconium before delivery. After the use of PGE_1 for labor induction, many studies report greater rates of cesarean delivery for fetal intolerance of labor, but lower rates of cesarean delivery for failure to progress. Its use in women with prior history of uterine wall surgery is contraindicated.[38] Anecdotal reports of uterine rupture in women without prior cesarean delivery exist, but the combined strength of the available studies does not provide the power to address this unusual and serious outcome. Although PGE_1 is used by the majority of hospitals in the United States for labor induction, and although its use is endorsed by ACOG, it has not been officially approved by the FDA as either a cervical ripening agent or a labor induction agent. Full written informed consent and specific discussion of off-label usage are recommended before the use of misoprostol for either cervical ripening or labor induction.

F. Oxytocin Protocols

Despite the significant advances that have been made over the past few decades in cervical ripening techniques and labor induction protocols, oxytocin (Pitocin) remains the workhorse of labor induction. Oxytocin may be added after any cervical ripening agent, although a 1-hour delay is required after discontinuance of PGE_2 vaginal insert, and a 4-hour delay is required after the last dose of PGE_2 gel or PGE_1. Many protocols for labor induction call for rapid increases in the oxytocin dosage at 15-minute intervals until an adequate contraction pattern is obtained. However, this rapid increase can result in uterine hyperstimulation and fetal intolerance of labor. Studies of the in vitro activity of oxytocin have led to recommendations for lower-dose protocols with longer intervals between dose increments from 30 to 60 minutes. Use of these protocols may result in unacceptable delays in reaching a therapeutic response.

ACOG guidelines currently call for oxytocin to be administered in a controlled IV infusion of a diluted solution by a secondary administration set into a primary infusion of physiologic electrolyte solution.[3] ACOG recommends initial doses of 0.5 to 1 mU/min, with increases every 30 to 60 minutes by increments of 1 to 2 mU/min, until satisfactory labor is achieved or a maximum of 20 to 40 mU/min is reached. Local and institutional preferences should be considered in developing procedures for the administration of oxytocin. Pulsed infusions at 10-minute intervals may also decrease the amount of medication and fluid given. Oxytocin can often be reduced, or even discontinued, after rupture of membranes in a woman in the active phase of labor.

ACOG recommends electronic fetal and uterine monitoring for patients receiving oxytocin. Initial and periodic examinations monitoring cervical progress are important to ongoing management of the oxytocin infusion. As with other patients in labor, maternal vital signs must be monitored carefully and appropriately modified for other complications (e.g., hypertension or infection). Attention to the amount and type of fluids that the patient receives is particularly important in any long-term administration of oxytocin. Using concentrations of 20 units oxytocin/L, rather than 10 units/L, and limitation of the total dose to 40 mU/min help to prevent complications related to fluid overload.

Medical and nursing staff attending patients receiving oxytocin must be trained to recognize signs of maternal or fetal complications of the drug and begin emergent therapy (discontinuance of the drug, oxygen, change in maternal position, use of tocolytics) as indicated. Provision for abdominal delivery should be confirmed before initiating oxytocin therapy because complications could require this option.

VI. FAILED LABOR INDUCTION AND FUTURE POSSIBILITIES

Unfortunately, not all women who require or request cervical ripening and/or labor induction achieve a simple vaginal delivery. Some women never achieve cervical dilatation despite the use of modern ripening techniques. However, it is not always clear whether these women have been given adequate time to move through the latent phase of the first stage of labor.[12] Women induced for suspected fetal macrosomia often require cesarean delivery for cephalopelvic disproportion, but it is likely that this indication would have become apparent after the eventual onset of spontaneous labor. Similarly, women induced for borderline intrauterine growth retardation or borderline oligohydramnios often require cesarean delivery for fetal intolerance of labor, but it is likely that this indication would have become apparent after the eventual onset of spontaneous labor.

Recent advances in cervical ripening and labor induction have not been able to reduce U.S. rates of cesarean delivery, which reached an all-time high of 29.3% in 2004. The likelihood of cephalopelvic disproportion and uteroplacental insufficiency, the two most common indications for primary cesarean delivery, both increase as a function of increasing gestational age. In addition, various demographic and clinical factors risk factors for cesarean delivery are increasing within the U.S. population (e.g., obesity, advanced maternal age, gestational diabetes, chronic hypertension). One potential solution to the increasing U.S. cesarean delivery rates would be to offer preventive labor induction relatively early in the term period of pregnancy, with a strong emphasis on adequate cervical ripening (e.g., PGE_2 for nulliparous women and Foley catheters for multiparous women), tolerance of a long latent phase, and an individualized approach to labor induction. Hence, women with an isolated risk for cephalopelvic disproportion might receive PGE_1/Foley catheter/high-dose oxytocin/late amniotomy, whereas women with significant risk for uteroplacental insufficiency might receive serial doses of PGE_2/low-dose oxytocin/late amniotomy. Reasonable criteria for the diagnosis of failure to progress during the active phase of the first stage would also be helpful. Hence, optimal birth outcomes might be obtained only if the timing of labor induction, the choice of cervical ripening medications, and the methods of labor induction are individualized and carefully applied. Such an approach has been reported from two different settings[7,9] and is currently being studied in randomized controlled format.

VII. SUMMARY

Labor induction should be used to improve birth outcomes and when the potential benefits outweigh the potential risks. Labor induction, when based on one or more of the standard indications, reduces maternal and neonatal mortality.[3] Elective induction of labor earlier in the term period increases the likelihood of a low Bishop's score on admission,[9] but because of the availability of cervical ripening agents, elective term labor induction appears safe for both mother and infant.[39] Term labor induction for preventive indications, between 38 and 41 weeks of gestation, is not yet part of standard practice. Ongoing RCTs comparing term labor induction versus standard practice will determine whether this practice reduces rates of common adverse birth outcomes including cesarean delivery and NICU admission.[5-7,40,41] Labor induction before 39 weeks 0 days of gestation may be associated with increased risk for fetal lung immaturity and should be attempted only when potential benefits outweigh potential risks (e.g., in the presence of preeclampsia, oligohydramnios, or fetal growth restriction). In summary, labor induction should be performed for an established indication, in the setting of established pregnancy dating, and after documented informed consent has been obtained.

VIII. SOR A RECOMMENDATIONS

RECOMMENDATIONS	REFERENCES
Routine labor induction beginning after 41 weeks of gestation, as compared with expectant management beyond this gestational age, has been associated with lower rates of cesarean delivery and reduced passage of thick meconium.	8, 19
In the setting of a labor induction complicated by an unfavorable uterine cervix (modified Bishop's score <6), pretreatment with prostaglandin medications (e.g., PGE_1 and PGE_2) and/or a Foley bulb catheter provides better birth outcomes than either cervical ripening with laminaria or induction without any method of ripening.	24, 25
Labor induction for ACOG-approved indications reduces maternal and neonatal mortality.	3

Acknowledgment

I acknowledge the contributions made by Janis Byrd, MD, the author of this section in the second edition of *Family Practice Obstetrics*.

REFERENCES

1. Rayburn WF, Zhang J: Rising rates of labor induction: present concerns and future strategies, *Obstet Gynecol* 100(1):164-167, 2002.
2. Martin JA, Hamilton BE, Sutton PD et al: Births: final data, *Natl Vital Stat Rep* 54(2):1-116, 2003.
3. American College of Obstetrics and Gynecologists (ACOG): Induction of labor. ACOG Practice bulletin 10, Washington, DC, 1999, ACOG.
4. Hadi H: Cervical ripening and labor induction: clinical guidelines, *Clin Obstet Gynecol* 43(3):524-536, 2000.
5. Caughey AB, Musci TJ: Complications of term pregnancies beyond 37 weeks gestation, *Obstet Gynecol* 103(1):57-61, 2004.
6. Caughey AB, Washington A, Laros RK: Neonatal complications of term pregnancy: rates by gestational age increase in a continuous, not threshold, fashion, *Am J Obstet Gynecol* 192:185-190, 2005.
7. Nicholson JM, Kellar LC, Kellar GM: The impact of the interaction between increasing gestational age and obstetrical risk on birth outcomes: evidence of a varying optimal time of delivery, *J Perinatol* 26:392-402, 2006.
8. Sanchez-Ramos L, Olivier F, Delke I et al: Labor induction versus expectant management for postterm pregnancies: a systematic review with meta-analysis, *Obstet Gynecol* 101(6):1312-1318, 2003.
9. Nicholson JM, Kellar LC, Cronholm PF et al: Active management of risk in pregnancy at term in an urban population: an

association between a higher induction of labor rate and a lower cesarean delivery rate, *Am J Obstet Gynecol* 191:1516-1528, 2004.

10. Nicholson JM, Yeager DL, Macones GA: A preventive approach to obstetric care in a rural hospital: association between higher rates of preventive labor induction and lower rates of cesarean delivery, *Ann Fam Med* 5:310-319, 2007.

11. Vahratian A, Zhang J, Troendle JF et al: Labor progression and risk of cesarean delivery in electively induced nulliparas, *Obstet Gynecol* 105(4):698-704, 2005.

12. Rouse DJ, Owen J, Hauth JC: Criteria for failed labor induction: prospective evaluation of a standarized protocol, *Obstet Gynecol* 96(5):671-677, 2000.

13. Simon CA, Grobman WA: When has an induction failed, *Obstet Gynecol* 105(4):705-709, 2005.

14. Ben-Haroush A, Yogev Y, Glickman H et al: Indicated labor induction with vaginal prostaglandin E2 increases the risk of cesarean delivery in multiparous women with no previous cesarean section, *J Perinatal Med* 32(1):31-36, 2004.

15. Yeast JD, Jones A, Poskin M: Induction of labor and the relationship to cesarean delivery: a review of 7001 consecutive inductions, *Am J Obstet Gynecol* 180(3):628-633, 1999.

16. Prysak M, Castronova FC: Elective induction versus spontaneous labor: a case-control analysis of safety and efficacy, *Obstet Gynecol* 92:47-52, 1998.

17. Maslow AS, Sweeny AL: Elective induction of labor as a risk factor for cesarean delivery among low-risk women at term, *Obstet Gynecol* 95:917-922, 2000.

18. Cammu H, Martens G, Ruyssinick G et al: Outcomes after elective labor induction in nulliparous women: a matched cohort study, *Am J Obstet Gynecol* 186:240-249, 2002.

19. Crowley P: Elective induction of labour at < 41 weeks gestation. In Enkin MW, Keirse MJNC, Renfew MJ, Neilson JP, editors: *Pregnancy and childbirth module, Cochrane Database of Systematic Reviews, review no. 04143, April 1992,* Cochrane updates on disk, Disk Issue 1, Oxford, 1994, Update Software.

20. Alexander JM, McIntire DD, Leveno KJ: Prolonged pregnancy: induction of labor and cesarean births, *Obstet Gynecol* 97(6):911-915, 2001.

21. Bryd JE: Labor induction. In Ratcliffe S, et al, editors: *Family practice obstetrics,* ed 2, Philadelphia, 2001, Hanlety & Belfus.

22. Bishop EH: Pelvic scoring for elective induction, *Obstet Gynecol* 24:266-268, 1964.

23. Bujold E, Blackwell SC, Hendler I et al: Modified Bishop's score and induction of labor in patients with a previous cesarean delivery, *Am J Obstet Gynecol* 191:1644-1648, 2004.

24. Kelly AJ, Kavanaugh J, Thomas J: Vaginal prostaglandin (PGE$_2$ and PGF$_{2a}$) for induction of labour at term, *Cochrane Database Systematic Rev* (4):CD003101, 2003.

25. Hofmeyr GJ, Gulmezoglu AM: Vaginal misoprostol or cervical ripening and induction of labour, *Cochrane Database Syst Rev* (1):CD000941, 2003.

26. Sciscione AC, McCullough H, Manley JS et al: A prospective, randomized comparison of Foley catheter insertion versus intracervical prostaglandin E2 gel or preinduction cervical ripening, *Am J Obstet Gynecol* 180(1 pt 1):55-59, 1999.

27. Levy R, Kanengiser B, Furman B et al: A randomized trial comparing a 30-mL and an 80-mL Foley catheter balloon for preinduction cervical ripening, *Am J Obstet Gynecol* 191: 1632-1636, 2004.

28. Sciscione A, Larkin M, O'Shea A et al: Preinduction cervical ripening with the Foley catheter and the risk of subsequent preterm birth, *Am J Obstet Gynecol* 190:751-754, 2004.

29. Kavanagh J, Kelly AJ, Thomas J: Breast stimulation for cervical ripening and induction of labor, *Cochrane Database Syst Rev* (3): CD003392, 2005.

30. Smith CA: Acupuncture for induction of labour, *Cochrane Database Syst Rev* (1):CD002963, 2004.

31. Bouvain M, Stan C, Irion O: Membrane sweeping for induction of labour, *Cochrane Database Syst Rev* (1):CD000451, 2005.

32. Bricker L, Luckas M: Amniotomy alone for induction of labour, *Cochrane Database Syst Rev* (4):CD002862, 2000.

33. Sherman DJ, Frenkel E, Pansky M et al: Balloon cervical ripening with extra-amniotic infusion of saline or prostaglandin E2: a double-blind, randomized controlled study, *Obstet Gynecol* 97(3):375-380, 2001.

34. Shepherd JH, Bennett MJ, Laurence D et al: Prostaglandin vaginal suppositories: a simple and safe approach to the induction of labor, *Obstet Gynecol* 58:596-600, 1981.

35. O'Herlihy C, Macdonald HN: Influence of pre-induction prostaglandin E2 vaginal gel on cervical ripening and labor, *Obstet Gynecol* 54:708-710, 1979.

36. Bartusevicius A, Barcaite E, Nadisauskiene R: Oral, vaginal and sublingual misoprostol for induction of labor, *Int J Gyneacol Obstet* 91:2-9, 2005.

37. Hofmeyr GJ: Induction of labour with misoprostol, *BJOG* 106:798-803, 1999.

38. Lyndon-Rochelle M, Holt VL, Easterline TR et al: Risk of uterine rupture during induction of labor among women with a prior cesarean delivery, *N Engl J Med* 345:3-8, 2001.

39. Santana W, Flake D: What are the risks and benefits of elective induction for uncomplicated term pregnancies? *J Fam Pract* 55(11):983-985, 2006.

40. Caughey AB, Nicholson JM, Cheng YW et al: Induction of labor and cesarean delivery by gestational age, *Am J Obstet Gynecol* 195(3):700-705, 2006.

41. Nicholson JM, Kellar LC, Kellar GM: The impact of the interaction between increasing gestational age and obstetrical risk on birth outcomes: evidence of a varying optimal time of delivery, *J Perinatol* 26(7):392-402, 2006.

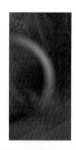

Intrapartum Complications

SECTION A Fetal Intolerance of Labor

Kent Petrie, MD

Continuous electronic fetal monitoring (EFM) is a technology that is commonly used to assess fetal well-being during labor. Despite lack of evidence that outcomes are improved with its use (see Chapter 14, Section E), EFM is still applied to 75% of laboring patients in the United States.[1-3] In many hospitals, it is routinely used, especially in patients at high risk. This section discusses the definitions for the interpretation of EFM tracings and suggests strategies for dealing with nonreassuring patterns that may reduce unnecessary interventions.

I. ELECTRONIC FETAL HEART RATE MONITORING PROTOCOLS

In North America, both the American College of Obstetrics and Gynecology (ACOG) and the Society of Obstetricians and Gynecologists of Canada (SOGC) have issued policy statements regarding the use of EFM. Their recommendations do not distinguish between external and internal fetal heart rate (FHR) monitoring.[3,4] Modern computerized external Doppler monitor tracings have high signal quality, making external FHR tracings almost indistinguishable from internal fetal scalp electrode tracings.

A. The "Low-Risk" Patient

The low-risk patient may be monitored by continuous EFM or intermittent auscultation (IA). IA utilizes a Doppler or DeLee stethoscope to listen to the FHR for at least 1 minute after a uterine contraction at the following frequency:
1. Every 30 minutes during the first stage of labor
2. Every 15 minutes during the second stage of labor

A patient whose status is determined to be low risk at the time of admission can become high risk at any time. Regular surveillance is important to recognize if/when this change occurs. These recommendations, and those to follow, are consistent with ACOG recommendations.[3]

B. The "High-Risk" Patient

Common high-risk conditions for which increased intrapartum surveillance is appropriate include:
1. Oxytocin induction or augmentation
2. Twin gestation
3. Hypertension/preeclampsia
4. Dysfunctional labor
5. Meconium staining
6. Diabetes
7. Prematurity
8. Intrauterine growth restriction (IUGR)
9. Oligohydramnios
10. Abnormal FHR by auscultation

Patients at high risk may be monitored by IA, but at an increased frequency as compared with women at low risk. The FHR is still recorded for 1 minute after uterine contractions:
1. Every 15 minutes during the first stage of labor
2. Every 5 minutes during the second stage of labor

Alternatively, these women can be monitored with continuous EFM (external or internal), with evaluation of the tracing at least every 15 minutes during the first stage of labor and every 5 minutes during the second stage of labor. Careful documentation of the evaluation is important.

C. Electronic Fetal Monitor Interpretation

Every EFM tracing should be read thoroughly and consistently, accurately assessing the following features:

- Baseline:
    Rate
    Variability
- Periodic:
    Accelerations
    Early decelerations
    Late decelerations
    Variable decelerations

Pattern recognition of FHR tracings is outlined in Table 16-1 and is demonstrated in FHR tracing examples (Figures 16-1, 16-2, and 16-3).

1. FHR variability

    FHR baseline variability, defined as variation of successive beats in the FHR, is central to the assessment of fetal well-being. It is an important index of cardiovascular function and is regulated by the fetal autonomic nervous system.

    The presence of normal FHR baseline variability (6-25 beats/min) predicts a vigorous fetus at the time of measurement. FHR variability has typically been described on internal fetal scalp electrode tracings, but modern external monitors with computer autocorrelation produce tracings that mirror internal monitor quality.

2. FHR classification systems (Table 16-2)

    The currently accepted classification scheme for FHR patterns divides patterns into two categories: reassuring and nonreassuring.[3,5]

    a. Reassuring FHR patterns show an absence of nonreassuring patterns. Reassuring tracings are quite reliable in predicting an infant with normal oxygenation and acid-base status (i.e., few false-negative results, excellent high negative predictive value).

    b. Nonreassuring FHR patterns are quite nonspecific. They cannot reliably predict whether a fetus is well oxygenated, depressed, or acidotic (i.e., many false-positive results, low positive predictive value).

    c. "Fetal distress" is an imprecise and nonspecific term. In a 2004 Committee Opinion, the ACOG[6] recommends that the term *fetal distress* be replaced by *non-reassuring fetal status*. It is far more clinically relevant, however, to describe the "non-reassuring FHR pattern" and outline management plans accordingly, rather than assume the "fetal status" is compromised.[6]

3. National Institutes of Health (NIH) guidelines

    In 1997, the NIH published their Research Guidelines for the Interpretation of EFM, proposing standardized and unambiguous definitions for FHR tracings on which future research could be based.[5] These guidelines state that a full description of any FHR tracing requires a qualitative and quantitative description of the following factors:

    a. Baseline rate
    b. Baseline FHR variability
    c. Presence of accelerations
    d. Periodic or episodic decelerations
    e. Changes or trends of FHR patterns over time

4. Variability patterns

    The only "new" definitions in the 1997 guidelines pertain to FHR variability. The guidelines eliminated the older distinction between "short-term" variability (beat-to-beat) and "long-term" variability (variation over time, such as a sinusoidal pattern), but defined FHR variability categories as follows:

    a. "Absent" variability = undetectable FHR variability
    b. "Minimal" variability = variability ≤ 5 beats/minute
    c. "Moderate" variability = variability 6 to 25 beats/minute
    d. "Marked" variability = variability ≥ 25 beats/minute

5. Advanced Life Support and Obstetrics (ALSO) mnemonic for EFM interpretation[7]

    To sum up the important features of EFM interpretation, the ALSO course includes the following mnemonic:

DR C BRAVADO

Define **R**isk	low or high
Contractions	comment on frequency
Baseline **RA**te	bradycardia, normal, or tachycardia
Variability	at least 5-10 beats/min (persistent reduced variability is a particularly ominous sign)
Accelerations	present or absent (at least 15-beat change from baseline lasting 15 seconds)
Decelerations	early, variable, or late
Overall	assessment (reassuring or nonreassuring) and plan of management

TABLE 16-1 Nomenclature for Fetal Heart Rate Interpretation

Baseline rate	The approximate mean FHR rounded to 5 beats/min during a 10-minute segment, excluding periodic or episodic changes, periods of marked variability, or segments that differ by >25 beats/min. In any 10-minute window, the baseline duration must be at least 2 minutes or the baseline is described as indeterminate for that period. In such cases, one may need to refer to previous 10-minute windows to assess baseline rate.
Tachycardia	Baseline FHR >160 beats/min
	Maternal conditions:
	Fever
	Dehydration
	Medications
	Anxiety
	Thyroid disease
	Fetal/intrauterine conditions:
	Chorioamnionitis
	Hypoxia/acidosis
	Dysrhythmia
Bradycardia	Baseline FHR <110 beats/min
	Possible cause: uteroplacental insufficiency or cord compression
	Hypoxic causes:
	Cord prolapse/compression
	Maternal hypotension
	Uterine hyperstimulation
	Abruptio placenta
	Uterine rupture
	Nonhypoxic causes:
	Bradydysrhythmia
	Vagal stimulation during second stage
	Hypothermia (fetal dive reflex)
Baseline variability	Irregular fluctuations in baseline FHR of two or more cycles per minute with peak to trough amplitude as follows:
	Absent variability = undetectable amplitude range
	Minimal variability = amplitude greater than undetectable but ≤5 beats/min
	Possible cause of absent or minimal variability: uteroplacental insufficiency or cord compression
	Hypoxic causes:
	Cord prolapse/compression
	Maternal hypotension
	Uterine hyperstimulation
	Abruptio placenta
	Uterine rupture
	Tachycardia
	Dysrhythmia
	Nonhypoxic causes:
	Prematurity
	Fetal sleep

	Medications
	Fetal anomaly
	Tachycardia, dysrhythmia
	Moderate variability = amplitude 6-25 beats/min
	Marked variability = amplitude >25 beats/min
	Possible cause of marked variability:
	Hypoxic causes:
	Cord prolapse/compression
	Maternal hypotension
	Uterine hyperstimulation
	Abruptio placenta
	Nonhypoxic causes:
	Fetal activity, fetal stimulation
Sinusoidal baseline:	Sinusoidal baseline is a smooth, wavelike pattern of regular frequency and amplitude, to be differentiated from baseline variability.
	May be seen in fetal anemia or hypoxia
Acceleration	Acceleration is an abrupt increase above the baseline with a peak above baseline of >15 beats/min and a duration of >15 seconds but <2 minutes from onset to return to baseline. Before 32 weeks of gestation, use >10 beats/min for peak above baseline and >10 seconds for duration.
Prolonged acceleration	This denotes an acceleration with a duration of >2 minutes but <10 minutes.
Decelerations	Decelerations of the FHR may be either periodic (occurring associated with contractions) or episodic (occurring without an association to contractions). Periodic decelerations may be described as recurrent if they occur with >50% of the contractions in a given 20-minute period.

Qualification of deceleration waveform may be defined as either abrupt (onset to nadir <30 seconds) or gradual (onset to nadir ≥30 seconds). Waveform qualification is key to differentiating between periodic decelerations that are defined as early or late versus those that are defined as variable.

Variable and prolonged decelerations may be quantified by the depth of the deceleration (nadir) in beats per minute. In addition, when describing prolonged decelerations, it may be helpful to include duration from onset to offset.

Early decelerations	Early deceleration is a gradual decrease and return to baseline associated with a contraction; the onset, nadir, and offset occur coincidentally with the contraction, with the nadir of the deceleration occurring at the peak of the contraction.
	Possible cause: head compression and vagal stimulation
	Clinical significance: a benign pattern in the setting of normal FHR and variability
Late decelerations	Late deceleration is a gradual decrease and return to baseline associated with a contraction; onset is delayed, with the nadir of deceleration always occurring after the peak of the contraction.
	Possible cause: uteroplacental insufficiency
	Related to maternal conditions:
	Hypertension/vascular disease
	Cardiac disease
	Hypotension
	Anemia
	Diabetes
	Smoking
	Uterine hyperstimulation
	Related to fetal/placental conditions:
	Postterm
	Intrauterine growth restriction
	Abruptio placenta

Continued

TABLE 16-1 Nomenclature for Fetal Heart Rate Interpretation—cont'd

	Chorioamnionitis
	Placenta previa/hemorrhage
Variable decelerations	Variable deceleration is an abrupt decrease in FHR of >15 beats/min lasting >15 seconds but <2 minutes. May be periodic or episodic. When associated with uterine contractions (periodic), variable decelerations may vary in onset, depth, and duration from contraction to contraction.
	Possible causes: Cord compression or vagal stimulation
	Related to maternal/fetal conditions:
	Positioning
	Second-stage labor
	Copious fluid loss with rupture of the membranes
	Monoamniotic multiple gestation
	Related to intrauterine conditions:
	Oligohydramnios
	Meconium
	Cord entanglement
	Short or knotted cord
	Nuchal or prolapsed cord
	Pure variable decelerations may have "shoulders" as a normal physiologic response.
	Overshoot and other variations are less reassuring.
Prolonged deceleration	Prolonged deceleration is a gradual or abrupt decrease of >15 beats/min lasting >2 minutes but <10 minutes. May be periodic or episodic.

FHR, Fetal heart rate.

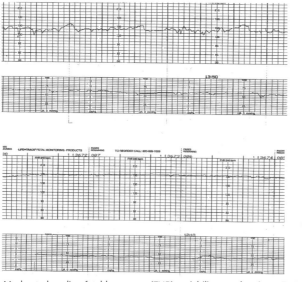

A, Moderate baseline
FHR variability

B, Baseline tachycardia
minimal FHR variability

FIGURE 16-1. A, Moderate baseline fetal heart rate (FHR) variability, accelerations. **B,** Baseline tachycardia, minimal FHR variability.

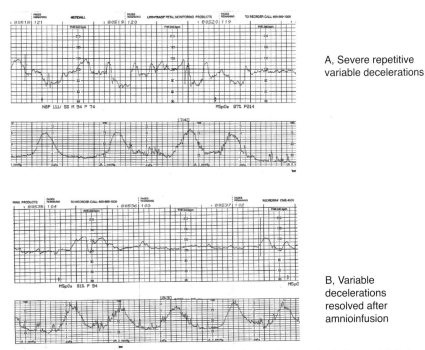

A, Severe repetitive variable decelerations

B, Variable decelerations resolved after amnioinfusion

FIGURE 16-2. A, Severe repetitive variable decelerations. **B,** Variable decelerations resolved after amnioinfusion.

II. MANAGEMENT OF NONREASSURING FETAL HEART RATE PATTERNS

A. Assess and Manage Cause of Nonreassuring Fetal Heart Rate Pattern

It is important for the birth attendant to look for a specific cause of the nonreassuring pattern and attempt to correct it. Table 16-1 describes physiologic causes of various FHR patterns. If a cause is found, measures may be instituted to correct underlying causes of abnormal FHR patterns and unnecessary interventions may be avoided.

B. Perform Intrauterine Fetal Resuscitation

General measures to improve fetal oxygenation and increase placental perfusion should be instituted. These include:

1. Administering maternal oxygen by face mask @ 8 to 10 L/min

2. Changing maternal position to improve uterine blood flow: lateral recumbent or knee-chest position
3. Reducing or discontinuing oxytocin infusion
4. Administering IV fluids to restore maternal intravascular volume and relieve maternal hypotension; for epidural-related hypotension, 2.5 to 10 mg ephedrine intravenously may be administered

C. Tocolytic Treatment of Nonreassuring Fetal Heart Rate Tracings

Tocolytic treatment will decrease or abolish uterine activity, which will remove the ischemic effect of uterine contractions and thereby improve the metabolic condition of the fetus before delivery.

1. Indication for tocolytic treatment
   a. Treatment of urgent nonreassuring FHR patterns: These would include bradycardia, persistent late or severe variable decelerations, lack of FHR variability, or fetal acidosis (scalp pH <7.20) for which immediate operative

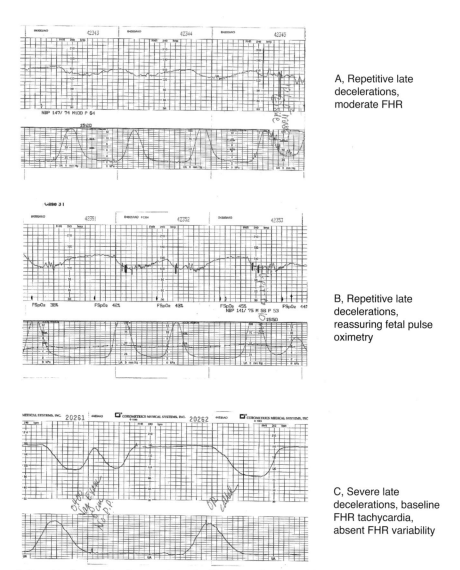

A, Repetitive late decelerations, moderate FHR

B, Repetitive late decelerations, reassuring fetal pulse oximetry

C, Severe late decelerations, baseline FHR tachycardia, absent FHR variability

FIGURE 16-3. A, Repetitive late decelerations, moderate fetal heart rate (FHR) variability. **B,** Repetitive late decelerations, reassuring fetal pulse oximetry. **C,** Severe late decelerations, baseline FHR tachycardia, absent FHR variability.

delivery would otherwise be indicated. Preparations should be made for potential cesarean delivery when the tocolytic is administered.

b. Treatment for less severe FHR patterns requiring operative delivery: Because of anticipated delay before delivery, it is thought further fetal decompensation might occur.

2. Posttocolytic treatment
After administration of the tocolytic, labor may be allowed to continue/resume if the FHR pattern resolves with a return of normal FHR variability. Personnel should be available for immediate cesarean delivery if the nonreassuring FHR pattern returns. A normal fetal scalp pH, fetal scalp

TABLE 16-2 Reassuring versus Nonreassuring Fetal Heart Rate Patterns

Reassuring Patterns	Nonreassuring Patterns
"Baseline"	
Normal rate	Bradycardia or tachycardia
Normal variability	Minimal or absent variability
Sinusoidal patterns	
"Periodic Changes"	
Accelerations	Late decelerations
	Variable decelerations
	Prolonged decelerations

oximetry, or fetal electrocardiogram (ECG) may also help reassure the birth attendant that continued labor is safe.

3. Methods of tocolytic treatment

  a. Terbutaline

    i. Administer subcutaneously (SQ) at a dose of 0.25 to 0.50 mg. This may be repeated every 10 to 15 minutes up to 4 doses.

    ii. Administer intravenously at a dose of 0.25 mg in 20 ml saline. This may be repeated once in 15 minutes.

    iii. Contraindications include maternal cardiovascular disease, preexisting maternal tachycardia, fluid overload, maternal thyrotoxicosis, and possibly abruptio placenta.

    iv. Possible side effects include maternal and fetal tachycardia, cardiac arrhythmia and ischemia, increased systolic and decreased diastolic blood pressure, tremor, pulmonary edema, nausea, vomiting, and headache.

  b. Magnesium sulfate ($MgSO_4$)

    i. Two to four grams $MgSO_4$ in 10% solution given as an initial 20 to 40 ml IV bolus over 15 to 20 minutes. An infusion of 1 to 4 g/hr may be started after the initial bolus.

    ii. A bolus is contraindicated if a $MgSO_4$ infusion is already running with a known therapeutic magnesium level.

    iii. Potential side effects include hyporeflexia and hypoventilation.

4. Outcomes and utilization

Two Cochrane metaanalyses[8,9] draw the following conclusions:

  a. Terbutaline tocolysis results in resolution of nonreassuring FHR patterns and decreased uterine activity.

  b. Terbutaline (and presumably other β-mimetics) is slightly more effective than $MgSO_4$.

  c. Terbutaline tocolysis is effective in "buying time" while preparing for vaginal or cesarean delivery.

  d. Administration of β-mimetics in second-stage labor has not been associated with improved outcomes. It has been associated with increased use of forceps.

D. Saline Amnioinfusion

Amnioinfusion is a technique of replacing amniotic fluid during labor via a transcervical intrauterine catheter (see Chapter 18, Section C). Infusion of fluid expands the amniotic cavity space and relieves cord compression.

1. Indication for saline amnioinfusion

Fetal heart abnormalities indicating umbilical cord compression (severe or repetitive variable decelerations) are effectively treated with a saline amnioinfusion.

2. Contraindications

  a. Overt, nonreassuring fetal surveillance for which delay in delivery could further compromise the fetus; examples include late decelerations with absent variability, scalp pH <7.20

  b. Active maternal infection, such as chorioamnionitis or genital herpes

  c. Known or suspected placenta previa or abruption

  d. Malpresentations

3. Technique of amnioinfusion

  a. A multiple lumen intrauterine pressure catheter is inserted. This will allow simultaneous measurement of contraction strength to detect uterine hypertonus.

  b. Normal saline or lactated Ringer's solution is infused at room temperature at a rate of 10 to 20 ml/min, to a maximum of 800 ml. A maintenance infusion of 1 to 3 ml/min may be continued thereafter.

  c. If bedside ultrasound is available, amniotic fluid index may be monitored and maintained at 10 cm or greater.

d. A rapid release of amniotic fluid with maternal position change may be replaced by a repeat bolus of 250 ml.

4. Complications of amnioinfusion
   a. Uterine hypertonus and overdistention, or polyhydramnios
   b. Uterine perforation, which is more common with a prior lower uterine segment scar
   c. Cord prolapse, which may result from too rapid of an infusion
   d. Infection

5. Outcomes of amnioinfusion
   a. A metaanalysis[10] of amnioinfusion for treatment of severe or repetitive variable decelerations had the following results:
      i. Reduced variable decelerations and bradycardia
      ii. Reduced cesarean and forceps delivery
      iii. Less meconium-stained amniotic fluid
      iv. Improved Apgar scores and cord pH
      v. Decreased rates of postpartum endometritis
   b. A Cochrane metaanalysis[11] of amnioinfusion for treatment of thick meconium had the following results:
      i. Decreased rates of heavy meconium staining and meconium aspiration syndrome
      ii. Reduced variable FHR decelerations
      iii. Reduced rates of cesarean delivery
      iv. Reduced neonatal intensive care unit admissions, neonatal ventilator use, and neonatal hypoxic ischemic encephalopathy
   c. A recent international, multicenter randomized controlled trial (RCT), however, demonstrated that amnioinfusion for the treatment of moderate-to-thick meconium did *not* reduce the incidence of meconium aspiration, neonatal morbidity, or cesarean delivery.[12] These authors concluded that amnioinfusion should *not* be recommended for reduction of meconium aspiration syndrome.

III. OTHER INTRAPARTUM FETAL SURVEILLANCE TECHNIQUES

A. Fetal Scalp pH Sampling
1. Indications for fetal scalp pH sampling
   a. Absent FHR variability without a clear cause
   b. Nonreassuring FHR patterns, unresponsive to oxygen, IV fluids, position change, or amnioinfusion

   c. Any other puzzling or worsening FHR patterns
2. Contraindications for scalp pH testing
   a. Known or suspected fetal blood dyscrasias
   b. Maternal human immunodeficiency virus (HIV)–positive status
   c. Active maternal genital infection (herpes simplex virus, group B streptococcus [GBS], gonorrhea [GC], chlamydia)
3. Actions based on results of scalp pH
   a. pH >7.25: allow labor to continue and resample as indicated
   b. pH 7.20 to 7.25: resample in 10 to 15 minutes
   c. pH <7.20: immediate resampling and delivery if confirmed
4. Is fetal scalp pH testing practical or necessary? Scalp pH testing can be technically difficult and is used relatively infrequently in the United States. The latest Cochrane review comparing continuous EFM versus IA demonstrated an increased relative risk (RR) of cesarean delivery with EFM (RR, 1.72; confidence interval [CI], 1.38-2.15). Continuous EFM plus scalp sampling reduced the RR to 1.24 (CI, 1.05-1.48). The use of scalp sampling appears to decrease the incidence of false-positive tracings that lead to unnecessary cesarean deliveries.[13]

B. Fetal Scalp Stimulation Testing
Fetal scalp stimulation is a reliable clinical alternative to scalp pH testing in fetuses with nonreassuring FHR tracings. A FHR acceleration of 15 beats/min over 15 seconds in response to firm digital pressure or the pinch of an Allis clamp consistently correlates with a scalp pH of greater than 7.20.[14]

C. Vibroacoustic Stimulation
A vibrating and sound-producing stimulus (artificial larynx) is applied to the maternal abdomen. An FHR acceleration of 15 beats/min over 15 seconds is associated with a normal fetal acid-base balance. Long-lasting (up to 2 hours) disturbances of the FHR have been reported after vibroacoustic stimulation. More RCTs need to be performed before the procedure can be recommended.[15]

D. Continuous Intrapartum Fetal Pulse Oximetry
In May 2000, the Federal Drug Administration (FDA) approved the first fetal pulse oximeter (OxiFirst by Nellcor, Inc.) A small probe is placed next to the fetal cheek or temple to measure continuous oxygen saturation.

1. Advantages
   a. Less invasive than scalp pH
   b. Continuous reading available
2. Disadvantages
   a. Placement of sensor difficult and easily dislodged
   b. Interference from hair, caput, and meconium
   c. Membranes must be ruptured
   d. Costs are high
3. Interpretation of fetal oxygen saturation ($FSPo_2$) results
   a. Normal $FSPo_2$ = 30 to 60%
   b. Continuous $FSPo_2$ >30% = reassuring
   c. $FSPo_2$ <30% during contractions but returning to >30% between contractions = observe and intervene
   d. $FSPo_2$ remaining <30% between contractions = deliver
   e. Observational trials continue to define these ranges
4. Initial multicenter trials[16,17]
   Cesarean delivery rate for "nonreassuring" FHR tracings decreased from 10% to 5% with use of fetal pulse oximetry. Cesarean delivery rate for "dystocia" more than doubled from 9% to 19%. There were no differences in fetal or neonatal outcomes, prompting lead authors to write, "we should proceed cautiously with any new technology."[17]
   ACOG's Committee Opinion from September 2001 states: "The American College of Obstetricians and Gynecologists Committee on Obstetric Practice currently cannot endorse the adoption of this device in clinical practice. The committee is particularly concerned that the introduction of this technology to clinical practice could further escalate the cost of medical care without necessarily improving clinical outcome."[18]
   With lack of widespread endorsement, Nellcor stopped production of their OxiFirst probes in January 2006. In a letter to users, the company states, "While the OxiFirst system has been a valuable assessment tool for the limited number of physicians who utilized the system, a lack of widespread acceptance, along with ongoing component obsolescence challenges, has prompted Nellcor to discontinue the system."[19]

E. Fetal Electrocardiography Monitoring

Animal and human studies have shown that fetal hypoxemia can alter the shape of the fetal electrocardiogram waveform, particularly ST-segment elevation or depression.[20] A Cochrane review supports the use of fetal ST waveform analysis via internal fetal scalp electrode as an adjunct to EFM when nonreassuring FHR patterns are present.

The FDA approved the STAN S31 (Neoventa Medical, Mölndal, Sweden) fetal heart monitoring system in 2006. This computer-enhanced fetal monitor records an "ST Event Flag" on the monitor tracing when fetal ECG changes are detected. ACOG will not endorse the system until further evidence is available that it is efficacious.

IV. EVIDENCE TO SUPPORT USE OF INTRAPARTUM FETAL STIMULATION TECHNIQUES

A metaanalysis of studies of scalp pH stimulation, Allis clamp stimulation, vibroacoustic stimulation, and digital scalp stimulation (N = 1297) revealed that an acceleration caused by any of the four techniques was reassuring of normal fetal status at the time of the test.[21]

V. USE OF INTRAPARTUM RESUSCITATION TECHNIQUES

A review of one tertiary care center revealed that adjuncts to EFM and intrapartum resuscitation maneuvers were underutilized compared with recommendations. They reviewed 134 cesarean deliveries for persistent nonreassuring FHR tracings. In only 37% of cases were either scalp stimulation or scalp pH attempted. Tocolytics were used in 25% of cases, and in those with persistent variable decelerations, only 40% received amnioinfusion.[22] Birth attendants should consider use of these techniques more frequently. Figure 16-4 is an algorithm suggesting an approach to fetal surveillance in labor for optimum diagnosis and treatment of fetal intolerance of labor.

VI. SOR A RECOMMENDATIONS

RECOMMENDATIONS	REFERENCES
Terbutaline tocolysis as intrauterine resuscitation results in resolution of nonreassuring FHR patterns and decreased uterine activity.	9

Continued

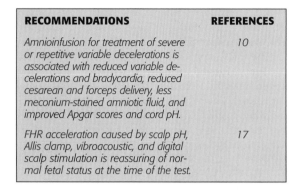

RECOMMENDATIONS	REFERENCES
Amnioinfusion for treatment of severe or repetitive variable decelerations is associated with reduced variable decelerations and bradycardia, reduced cesarean and forceps delivery, less meconium-stained amniotic fluid, and improved Apgar scores and cord pH.	10
FHR acceleration caused by scalp pH, Allis clamp, vibroacoustic, and digital scalp stimulation is reassuring of normal fetal status at the time of the test.	17

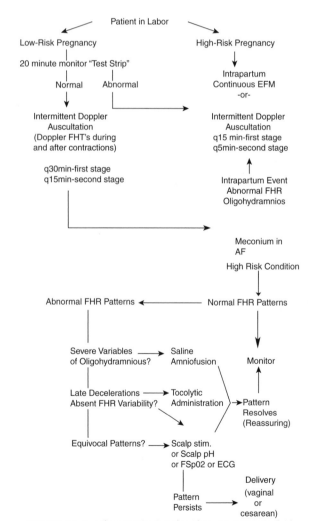

FIGURE 16-4. Labor monitoring algorithm. AF, Amniotic fluid; EFM, electronic fetal monitoring; ECG, electrocardiogram; FHR, fetal heart rate; FHT, fetal heart tracing.

REFERENCES

1. Freeman R: Intrapartum fetal monitoring—a disappointing story, N Engl J Med 322(9):624-626, 1990.
2. Mires G, William F, Howie P: Randomized controlled trial of cardiotocography versus Doppler auscultation of fetal heart at admission in labour in low risk obstetric population, BMJ 322:1457-1462, 2001.
3. ACOG technical bulletin: Fetal heart rate patterns: monitoring, interpretation, and management. Number 207—July 1995 (replaces No. 132, September 1989), Int J Gynaecol Obstet 51(1):65-74, 1995.
4. SOGC clinical practice guideline: Fetal health surveillance in labor. No. 112, March 2002, Society of Obstetricians and Gynaecologists of Canada, Vancouver, BC.
5. Electronic fetal heart rate monitoring: research guidelines for interpretation. National institute of Child Health and Human Development Research Planning Workshop, Am J Obstet Gynecol 177:1385-1390, 1997.
6. ACOG Committee on Obstetric Practice: Committee opinion: inappropriate use of the terms fetal distress and birth asphyxia, Committee Opinion #303, October 2004, American College of Obstetricians and Gynecologists (ACOG), Washington, DC.
7. ALSO Mnemonic Reference Cards. Available at: www.aafp.org/also. Accessed 2007.
8. Hofmeyr GJ, Kulier R: Tocolysis for preventing fetal distress in second stage of labour, Cochrane Database Syst Rev (1):CD000037, 1996.
9. Kulier R, Hofmeyr GJ: Tocolytics for suspected intrapartum fetal distress, Cochrane Database Syst Rev (1):CD000035, 1998.
10. Hofmeyr GJ: Amnioinfusion for potential or suspected umbilical cord compression in labour, Cochrane Database Syst Rev (1):CD000013, 1998.
11. Hofmeyr GJ: Amnioinfusion for meconium-stained liquor in labour, Cochrane Database Syst Rev (1):CD000014, 2002.
12. Fraser WE, Hofmeyr UJ, Lede R et al: Amnioinfusion for the prevention of the meconium aspiration syndrome, N Engl J Med 353:946-948, 2005.
13. Thacker SB, Stroup D, Chang M: Continuous electronic heart rate monitoring for fetal assessment during labor, Cochrane Database Syst Rev (2):CD000063, 2001.
14. Clark SL, Gimovsky ML, Miller FC: The scalp stimulation test: a clinical alternative to fetal scalp blood sampling, Am J Obstet Gynecol 148:274-282, 1984.
15. East CE, Smyth R, Leader LR et al: Vibroacoustic stimulation for fetal assessment in labour in the presence of a nonreassuring fetal heart rate trace, Cochrane Database Syst Rev (2):CD004664, 2005.
16. Garite TJ, Dilde GA, McNamara H et al: A multicenter controlled trial of fetal pulse oximetry in the intrapartum management of nonreassuring fetal heart rate patterns, Am J Obstet Gynecol 183(5):1049-1058, 2000.
17. East CE, Chan FY, Colditz PB: Fetal pulse oximetry for fetal assessment in labour, Cochrane Database Syst Rev (2):CD004075, 2004.
18. ACOG Committee on Obstetric Practice: committee opinion: fetal pulse oximetry. Committee Opinion #258, Obstet Gynecol 98:523-524, 2001.
19. Tyco Healthcare/Nellcor. Private letter to customers, Pleasanton, CA, November 1, 2005.
20. Neilson JP: Fetal electrocardiogram (ECG) for fetal monitoring during labour, Cochrane Database Syst Rev (2):CD000116, 2003.

21. Skupski DW, Rosenberg DR, Eglinton GS: Intrapartum fetal stimulation tests: a meta-analysis, *Obstet Gynecol* 99:129-134, 2002.
22. Hendrix NW, Chauhan SP, Scardo JA et al: Managing nonreassuring fetal heart rate patterns before cesarean delivery. Compliance with ACOG recommendations, *J Reprod Med* 45:995-999, 2000.

SECTION B Shoulder Dystocia

Osman N. Sanyer, MD

The complication of a shoulder dystocia during a cephalic vaginal delivery is one of the more feared occurrences in maternity care. The experience of managing a shoulder dystocia often proves to be memorable and emotionally traumatic for both the parents and caregivers. If efforts to reduce the dystocia are unsuccessful, fetal asphyxia may result. Even successful delivery of an infant from a shoulder dystocia can result in harm to the infant, the laboring mother, or both.

Though there are some characteristics of prenatal history and labor course that may raise concern for the occurrence of a shoulder dystocia, most occur in uncomplicated pregnancies absent these risk factors. The use of early induction of labor, or cesarean delivery, to prevent shoulder dystocia has not been supported by the literature.

Given the potentially disastrous outcomes of a labor complicated by a shoulder dystocia, it is encouraging to know that there are specific, rapid response techniques that have been shown to be effective in safely delivering the entrapped infant.

I. EPIDEMIOLOGY

A. Definition

Shoulder dystocia has been defined as the inability to deliver either of the infant's shoulders through the maternal pelvis using the usual manner of cephalic traction.[1] Usually the anterior fetal shoulder is trapped against the maternal pubic symphysis, though dystocia can occur in the face of entrapment of the posterior shoulder as well.

B. Incidence

The incidence of shoulder dystocia is greater in deliveries of infants weighing more than 4000 g (8 lb, 13 oz). However, it is essential to realize that more than 50% of dystocia cases occur in infants weighing less than 4000 g.[2]

Shoulder dystocia occurs in 0.5% to 2% of infants weighing less than 4000 g, with the incidence rate increasing to 5% to 10% in deliveries of infants weighing between 4000 and 4500 g (9 lb, 14 oz). In infants more than 4500 g, the incidence rate of shoulder dystocia has been found to be between 10% and 35%.[3,4]

II. RISK FACTORS

A. Antepartum Risk Factors

Infants weighing greater than 3000 g, who are being delivered of women with gestational diabetes, are at the greatest risk for being affected by a shoulder dystocia.[3,4] Antepartum risk factors for dystocia are listed in Table 16-3.[3-9]

B. Intrapartum Risk Factors

The most significant intrapartum risk factor for shoulder dystocia is the use of vacuum or forceps in assisting delivery. Additional risk factors are summarized in Table 16-4.[5,10,11]

Notably, fewer than 25% of deliveries complicated by shoulder dystocia are associated with any of the risk factors delineated.[12] These risk factors are therefore of limited clinical usefulness.[2]

TABLE 16-3 Antepartum Risk Factors for Shoulder Dystocia

Previous history of shoulder dystocia
Gestational diabetes
Previous history of delivering a large-for-gestational-age infant
Postdates pregnancy
Suspected fetal macrosomia
Maternal short stature
Abnormal maternal pelvic anatomy

TABLE 16-4 Intrapartum Risk Factors for Shoulder Dystocia

Protracted active phase of first-stage labor
Protracted second-stage labor
Assisted vaginal delivery (forceps or vacuum)

III. COMPLICATIONS ASSOCIATED WITH SHOULDER DYSTOCIA

The outcomes associated with shoulder dystocia include the range of possibilities from no complications or injury to the mother and fetus to severe trauma to each and even loss of life.

A. Maternal Complications

Maternal complications encountered during a delivery complicated by shoulder dystocia include lacerations of the perineum, vagina, rectum, and adjacent soft tissues. Hemorrhage can occur as a result of these lacerations or because of uterine atony.

B. Neonatal Complications

Neonatal complications associated with shoulder dystocia include:

1. Brachial plexus injury
   The most frequent brachial plexus injury is Erb's palsy. The infant will present with a flaccid arm, adducted at the shoulder, with internal rotation of that joint. The injury is a result of bruising and stretching of the brachial plexus on the affected side of the infant's neck. The symptoms resolve spontaneously in the majority of infants in the first few days after delivery, and recovery can continue for up to 12 months after birth. An exclusive association between shoulder dystocia and Erb's palsy is not clearly established. Erb's palsy has been diagnosed in infants delivered by cesarean delivery, as well as in the posterior arm of vaginally delivered infants.[13,14] A number of studies evaluating the outcomes of deliveries of macrosomic infants show a relatively high incidence of shoulder dystocia encountered during these deliveries (5.3-35%), but a very low incidence of permanent neurologic sequelae (<1%).[7,15-18]

2. Cervical spine injury
   Cervical spine injuries can occur as the result of excessive lateral stretching and rotational traction forces applied to the infant's neck.

3. Fractures
   Fractures of the clavicle and humerus are seen as the result of efforts to deliver the infant in a labor complicated by shoulder dystocia. Generally, these injuries heal spontaneously with minimal sequelae.

4. Neonatal asphyxia
   As a result of the entrapment of the fetal torso in the birth canal, the umbilical cord may be compressed. In such instances, severe fetal acidosis can occur in 7 minutes or less. The fetal pH declines approximately 0.04 each minute the head is trapped on the perineum. If uteroplacental insufficiency has been present before the cord compression, the fetal acidosis may develop much more quickly. It is this potential occurrence that adds the sense of urgency to delivery of an infant complicated by a shoulder dystocia.

IV. DIAGNOSIS

The diagnosis of a shoulder dystocia is made based on the clinical definition given earlier in this chapter. If the delivering physician is unable to deliver the infant's shoulders using the usual manner of cephalic traction, a shoulder dystocia has occurred. The infant's head will often retract against the maternal pelvis, pinning cheeks and forehead tightly against the perineum, making it difficult for the delivery assistant to pass fingers around and behind the infant's head.

V. PREVENTION OF SHOULDER DYSTOCIA

A. Prophylactic Cesarean or Elective Induction Not Indicated

Efforts have been made to prevent the occurrence of shoulder dystocia through antenatal intervention. Studies have shown that early induction and prophylactic cesarean delivery do not reduce the incidence of dystocia in women suspected of having fetal macrosomia.[16,19] A Cochrane analysis supports this conclusion as well.[20] An additional Cochrane review suggests that elective induction of women with diabetes may reduce the risk for fetal macrosomia but does not appear to reduce the risk for fetal or maternal morbidity.[21]

Efforts to identify fetal macrosomia by antenatal ultrasound have shown this technique to be unreliable. One study showed a predictive value of as high as 93% when the fetal abdominal circumference is used as the indicator of macrosomia.[17] However, other large studies show the positive predictive value of sonographic studies to be less than 50%.[11,22] Given that fetal macrosomia has been shown to be associated with a low incidence of neurologic sequelae in infants,[11,15-18] one would have to perform many cesarean deliveries in order to prevent one fetal brachial plexus injury due to shoulder dystocia.[23-25] Analytic decision models have estimated that 2345 cesarean deliveries, at a cost of nearly $5 million annually, would be needed to prevent one permanent brachial plexus injury in a patient without diabetes who had a fetus suspected of weighing more than 4000 g.[25]

In pregnant women with diabetes, more convincing evidence supports the use of prophylactic cesarean to prevent brachial plexus injury. The number needed to treat has been shown to be as low as 5 cesarean deliveries to prevent 1 brachial plexus injury in fetuses estimated to weigh greater than 5000 g, and 48 cesarean deliveries to prevent 1 such injury in infants estimated to be greater than 4000 g.[26] In a study that included 2000 women with diabetes, there was a reduction in shoulder dystocia from 2.4% to 1% with prophylactic cesarean for infants estimated to weigh greater than 4250 g by ultrasound. A concomitant increase in cesarean section rate, from 21.7% to 25.1% ($p < 0.04$), was reported. In the subgroup of women with diabetes, the frequency of shoulder dystocia, brachial plexus palsy, and cesarean delivery is greater, leading to the conclusion that a policy of elective cesarean delivery in this group potentially may have greater merit.[25]

Given the limited benefit of cesarean delivery in preventing shoulder dystocia, it is worthwhile to shift the focus to prevention of maternal and fetal injury when dystocia does occur. The development of a response algorithm, incorporating specific sequential maneuvers, when a dystocia has occurred has been shown to be effective in reducing the likelihood of fetal and maternal injury from dystocia.[10]

VI. MANAGEMENT OF DELIVERY

A. Prompt Recognition and Response

Earlier it was noted that the fetal pH will decline by 0.04 during every minute that the head is trapped on the perineum. It is therefore ideal to deliver the infant as promptly as possible once the diagnosis of dystocia is made. Quick recognition of the problem is essential. Each hospital and birthing center can set up an organized response to a birth attendant's call for help with a shoulder dystocia.

The protocol established to respond to a shoulder dystocia will vary based on the resources available to the labor and delivery unit. This protocol may include a request for the immediate presence of additional nursing personnel, a newborn resuscitation team, and an additional physician. One of the roles for a delivery team member is to record the timing and sequence of the maneuvers used to relieve the shoulder dystocia, not unlike the documentation of a cardiac resuscitation effort. In a delivery in which the concern for a potential shoulder dystocia is raised to a greater level by the presence of risk factors, the response team would ideally be notified in advance of the delivery.

It is important to include the laboring woman and her support persons as part of the team that is assembled to respond to a shoulder dystocia. Understanding of the maneuvers necessary to relieve the dystocia will enhance the ability of the woman to cooperate with those interventions, improving the chances for a successful and atraumatic delivery. After calling the response team, a brief explanation of the concerns and response related to the shoulder dystocia should be given to the woman in labor.

B. Consider Episiotomy

If an episiotomy has not been cut before delivery of the fetal head, the attendant should evaluate whether release of tension on the soft tissue of the perineum would provide more room for manipulation of the fetal shoulders or arms that may be required to relieve dystocia. Because McRoberts maneuver and suprapubic pressure relieve a large percentage of cases of shoulder dystocia, episiotomy can generally be done later in the sequence of treatment of dystocia.

C. McRoberts Maneuver

The McRoberts maneuver alone has been found to relieve more than 40% of all shoulder dystocias and, when combined with suprapubic pressure, may result in the resolution of more than 50% of shoulder dystocias.[27,28] It an ideal first step in the management of shoulder dystocia.

Two assistants hyperflex the mother's thighs back onto, or alongside, her abdomen. This position produces a rotation of the symphysis pubis and a flattening of the sacral promontory.[29] As a result of these positional changes in the maternal pelvis, the posterior shoulder moves over the sacral promontory, allowing it to fall into the hollow of the sacrum. The anterior shoulder is then able to more easily rotate from beneath the symphysis pubis. After this has occurred, the infant can generally be delivered with normal sacral traction.

D. Suprapubic Pressure

The suprapubic pressure maneuver can be done concurrently with, or subsequent to, the McRoberts maneuver. An assistant positioned at the patient's side, often standing on a stool or kneeling on the delivery bed, applies pressure to the maternal suprapubic region, rocking the infant's anterior shoulder forward, and thus under the maternal pubic symphysis. The birth attendant needs to guide the assistant in regard to the infant's presentation, to ensure that the anterior shoulder is being pushed in a forward rotation, to adduct the infant's shoulder, rather than backward, which would abduct the shoulder and increase the diameter of the shoulders, thus worsening the dystocia. The pressure is applied with the heel of the assistant's hand and can be continuous, or if delivery is not accomplished, a rocking motion may be used to dislodge the shoulder from behind the pubic symphysis. Fundal pressure may worsen the impaction, potentially injuring the fetus or mother, and should not be used in this situation.[30]

E. Shoulder Rotation

If the preceding efforts are unsuccessful at relieving the dystocia, the next maneuver involves reaching the fetal shoulders through the vagina and rotating them so that they traverse the pelvis in an oblique fashion. In the Rubin II maneuver, the delivery attendant applies two to three fingers to the posterior aspect of the infant's anterior shoulder (Figure 16-5), usually on the scapula, and then applies firm pressure to affect the forward rotation of that shoulder out from underneath the maternal symphysis pubis. If additional forces are needed, the attendant may use two to three fingers on the other hand to apply pressure to the anterior aspect of the posterior shoulder in what is known as the Woods corkscrew maneuver. This adds to the rotational forces being created by the hand on the anterior fetal shoulder. If the Woods

screw maneuver is not effective, the attendant can switch the direction of attempted rotation, applying pressure to the front of the fetal anterior shoulder, and the back of the fetal posterior shoulder, in what is known as the reverse Woods corkscrew maneuver (Figure 16-6). Continuous downward traction should be applied while conducting these maneuvers so that successful rotation will be recognized and delivery can be completed.

Regardless of which of these maneuvers proves to be the most successful, relief of the dystocia occurs when the anterior fetal shoulder rotates out from underneath the maternal symphysis pubis.

F. Delivery of Posterior Arm

The posterior arm may be delivered to relieve the shoulder dystocia. For the birth attendant to introduce a hand into the patient's vagina, an episiotomy will often be required. The attendant passes a hand in front of the baby's face, sliding two fingers along the fetal chest into the antecubital fossa of the posterior fetal arm. Pressure applied in this location flexes the fetal elbow, allowing the fetal forearm and hand to be grasped, drawn outward across the trunk and face, and then delivered. The posterior shoulder tends to follow the posterior arm. When the shoulder is delivered, the forces causing impaction of the anterior shoulder against the maternal symphysis are relieved.

G. All-Fours Position

In the event that the McRoberts maneuver is unsuccessful, assisting the mother to the "all-fours" position has been shown to quickly and atraumatically reduce most dystocias. Also known as the Gaskin maneuver, this is a safe, rapid, and effective tech-

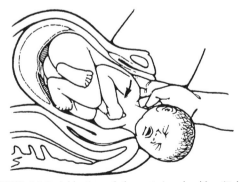

FIGURE 16-5. Adduction of the anterior shoulder (Rubin's maneuver).

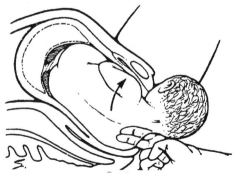

FIGURE 16-6. Abduction of the posterior shoulder (Woods screw maneuver).

TABLE 16-5 Delivery in the "All-Fours" Position

The posterior shoulder (now uppermost) can often be delivered from this position, using a midline episiotomy if necessary. If delivery of the posterior shoulder is still not possible, posterior arm extraction may be accomplished more readily in this position by passage of the attendant's hand in front of the fetal face and splinting along the uppermost humerus with the fingers passing along the sacral curve. The attendant should attempt to flex the elbow, grasp the fetal hand or wrist, and sweep the arm across the fetal chest. If the posterior (uppermost) shoulder is still entrapped in the sacral hollow, traction of the arm may convert both shoulders to an oblique lie and relieve the anterior shoulder impaction from behind the symphysis.

This maneuver has been used effectively in a series of more than 80 deliveries with shoulder dystocia.[19] The mean diagnosis-to-delivery interval in this series was 2.3 ± 1.0 (± standard deviation; range, 1-6) minutes. Rotation to this position is probably enhanced by having the mother change position during labor, avoidance of internal monitoring equipment and intravenous lines, and having at least two assistants present at the birth. It may be used prophylactically as a delivery position in anticipation of the delivery of a macrosomic infant.

From Bruner JP, Drummond SB, Meenan AL, Gaskin IM: All-fours maneuver for reducing shoulder dystocia during labor, *J Reprod Med* 43:439-443, 1998.

nique for the reduction of shoulder dystocia.[19] It has been widely practiced by midwives, and it may be instituted earlier than performing the Rubin or Woods screw maneuvers, or attempting to deliver a posterior arm.

This maneuver consists of assisting the delivering patient to the hands-and-knees position. This position straightens the angle of the sacral promontory and may disimpact the anterior shoulder simply by the change in position. It has been reported that the maneuver increases the true diagonal conjugate by as much as 10 mm and increases the sagittal dimension of the maternal pelvis by as much as 20 mm.[31] The maneuver is described in Table 16-5.

VII. SEVERE SHOULDER DYSTOCIA

If none of the preceding maneuvers is successful in relieving the dystocia, several other interventions may be attempted. These are regarded, to some degree, as measures of last resort. These methods are more likely to result in maternal or fetal injury, although

these injuries are considered acceptable when weighed against the risk for fetal asphyxia that will inevitably occur if the dystocia is not relieved.

A. Clavicle Fracture

The clavicle of the anterior fetal shoulder is deliberately fractured by applying direct outward pressure along the midpoint. As a result of this fracture, the clavicle collapses and the anterior shoulder is able to rotate out from beneath the maternal symphysis pubis.

B. Symphysiotomy

Symphysiotomy has been used infrequently in the United States but has been used with regularity in developing countries. The cartilage of the maternal symphysis pubis is sharply divided, causing the pubis to arch upward, and thus allowing the fetal anterior shoulder to slip beneath it.

A Foley catheter is used to displace the maternal urethra to one side and the incision is made under local anesthesia.[32] Patients may require 2 to 3 days of bedrest after the procedure, but morbidity is usually limited to short periods of discomfort while walking. Symphysiotomy provides an opportunity for safer delivery of severe shoulder dystocia in smaller hospitals that lack the presence of full-time anesthesia or timely obstetric consultation.

C. Zavanelli Maneuver

The Zavanelli maneuver involves cephalic replacement followed by cesarean delivery. The fetal head is rotated into a direct occiput anterior position, then flexed, and the vertex is pushed upward into the vagina. Pressure is then held on the fetal head until cesarean delivery can be achieved.[33] Tocolysis via terbutaline or inhaled anesthesia may be required to accomplish this procedure, although it has not been proved to enhance success over cases in which it was not used. This maneuver cannot be done if a nuchal cord has been cut and clamped. The birthing unit must have the personnel present to perform an immediate cesarean delivery. The ease with which the fetal head can be returned to the maternal vagina is unpredictable, making this an intervention of "last resort."[34]

VIII. PITFALLS AND CONTROVERSIES

The occurrence and outcome of a shoulder dystocia are unpredictable. Because of the risk for maternal and fetal injury or death, there is some risk for litigation, even if best practices are followed. Appropriate documentation of the events and interventions associated with a shoulder dystocia can be important to any response to a claim of negligence on the part of the care team. The delivery note should include the sequence and timing of the maneuvers used to relieve the dystocia. A description of the position the fetus, the condition of the infant at the time of delivery, and any subsequent resuscitation efforts should be included in the delivery note.

Just as communication with the laboring woman and her family before attempting to relieve the shoulder dystocia is important, communication with the patient and family after a difficult delivery is equally important. The anxiety and tension experienced by the woman and her family can be aided by a thorough explanation of this difficult obstetric problem. A review of the efforts made to relieve the dystocia, as well a discussion of the current status of the mother and infant, may provide reassurance to the family in the face of a frightening situation. A similar discussion with the delivering care team members can provide an opportunity to review the team's efforts, effectiveness, and emotional state.

VIII. SOR A RECOMMENDATIONS

RECOMMENDATIONS	REFERENCES
Labor induction for suspected fetal macrosomia results in an increased cesarean delivery rate without improving perinatal outcomes.	20
Induction of women with diabetes may reduce the risk for fetal macrosomia but does not reduce the risk for fetal and maternal morbidity.	21

REFERENCES

1. Resnick R: Management of shoulder dystocia girdle, *Clin Obstet Gynecol* 23:559-564, 1980.
2. Geary M, McParland P, Johnson H et al: Shoulder dystocia: is it predictable? *Eur J Obstet Gynecol Reprod Biol* 62:15-18, 1995.
3. Acker DB, Sachs BP, Friedman EA: Risk factor for shoulder dystocia, *Obstet Gynecol* 66:762-768, 1985.
4. Nocon JJ, McKenzie DK, Thomas LJ et al: Shoulder dystocia: an analysis of risks and obstetric maneuvers, *Am J Obstet Gynecol* 168:1732-1737, 1993.
5. Acker DB, Sachs BP, Friedman EA: Risk factor for shoulder dystocia in the average weight infant, *Obstet Gynecol* 67:614-618, 1986.
6. Benedetti TJ, Gabbe SC: Shoulder dystocia: a complication of fetal macrosomia and prolonged second stage of labor with mid-pelvic delivery, *Obstet Gynecol* 52:526-529, 1978.
7. Gonen R, Spiegel D, Abend M: Is macrosomia predictable and are shoulder dystocia and birth trauma preventable? *Obstet Gynecol* 88:526-529, 1996.
8. Lewis DF, Raymond RC, Perkins MB et al: Recurrence rate of shoulder dystocia, *Am J Obstet Gynecol* 172:1369-1371, 1995.
9. Morrison JC, Sanders JR, Magann EF et al: The diagnosis and management of dystocia of the shoulder, *Surg Gynecol Obstet* 175:515-522, 1992.
10. Baskett TF, Allen AC: Perinatal implications of shoulder dystocia, *Obstet Gynecol* 86:14-17, 1995.
11. Nesbitt TS, Gilbert WN, Herrchen B: Shoulder dystocia: an analysis of risk factors with macrosomic infants born in California, *Am J Obstet Gynecol* 179:476-480, 1998.
12. Lewis DF, Edwards MS, Asrat T et al: Can shoulder dystocia be predicted? Preconceptive and prenatal factors, *J Reprod Med* 43:654-658, 1998.
13. Gherman RB, Goodwin TM, Ouzounian JG et al: Brachial plexus associated with cesarean section: an in utero injury? *Am J Obstet Gynecol* 177:1162-1164, 1997.
14. Gherman RB, Ouzounian JG, Miller DA et al: Spontaneous vaginal delivery: a risk factor for Erb's palsy? *Am J Obstet Gynecol* 178:423-427, 1998.
15. Blickstein I, Ben-Arie A, Hagay ZJ: Antepartum risks of shoulder dystocia and brachial plexus injury for infants weighing 4200 g or more, *Gynecol Obstet Invest* 45:77-80, 1998.
16. Diani F, Venanzi S, Zanconato G et al: Fetal macrosomia and management of delivery, *Clin Exp Obstet Gynecol* 24:212-214, 1997.
17. Jayazeri A, Heffron JA, Phillips R et al: Macrosomia prediction using ultrasound fetal abdominal circumference of 35 centimeters or more, *Obstet Gynecol* 93:523-526, 1999.
18. Lipscomb KR, Gregory K, Shaw K: The outcome of macrosomic infants weighing at least 4500 grams, *Obstet Gynecol* 85:558-564, 1995.
19. Bruner JP, Drummond SB, Meenan AL, Gaskin IM: All-fours maneuver for reducing shoulder dystocia during labor, *J Reprod Med* 43:439-443, 1998.
20. Irion O, Boulvain M: Induction of labor for suspected fetal macrosomia, *Cochrane Database Syst Rev* (2):CD000938, 1998.
21. Boulvain M, Stan C, Irion O: Elective delivery in diabetic pregnant women, *Cochrane Database Syst Rev* (2):CD001997, 2001.
22. Smith GC, Smith MF, McNay MB et al: The relation between fetal abdominal circumference and birthweight: findings in 3512 pregnancies, *Br J Obstet Gynaecol* 104:186-190, 1997.
23. Bryant DR, Leonardi MR, Landwehr JB et al: Limited usefulness of fetal weight in predicting neonatal brachial plexus injury, *Am J Obstet Gynecol* 179:686-689, 1998.
24. Kolderup LB, Laros RK Jr, Musci TJ: Incidence of persistent birth injury in macrosomic infants: association with mode of delivery, *Am J Obstet Gynecol* 177:37-41, 1997.
25. Rouse DJ, Owen J, Goldenberg RL et al: The effectiveness and costs of elective cesarean delivery for fetal macrosomia diagnosed by ultrasound, *JAMA* 276:1480-1486, 1996.
26. Ecker JL, Greenberg JA, Norwitz ER et al: Birth weight as a predictor of brachial plexus injury, *Obstet Gynecol* 889:643-647, 1997.

27. Geary M, McParland P, Johnson H et al: Shoulder dystocia: is it predictable? *Eur J Obstet Gynecol Reprod Biol* 62:15-18, 1995.
28. Gherman RB, Goodwin, TM, Souter I et al: The McRoberts' maneuver for the alleviation of shoulder dystocia: how successful is it? *Am J Obstet Gynecol* 176:656-661, 1997.
29. Gobbo R, Baxley EG: Shoulder dystocia. *ALSO: advanced life support in obstetrics provider course syllabus,* Leawood, KS, 2000, American Academy of Family Physicians.
30. Gross SJ, Shime J, Farine D. Shoulder dystocia: predictors and outcome. A five-year review, *Am J Obstet Gynecol* 156:334-336, 1987.
31. Borell U, Fernstrom I: The mechanism of labor, *Radiol Clin North Am* 5:73-85, 1967.
32. White S, Thorpe R, Main D: Emergency obstetric surgery performed by nurses in Zaire, *Lancet* 2:612-613, 1987.
33. Sandberg EC: The Zavanelli maneuver: a potentially revolutionary method for the resolution of shoulder dystocia, *Am J Obstet Gynecol* 152:479-484, 1985.
34. Graham JM, Blanco JD, Wen T et al: The Zavenelli maneuver: a different perspective, *Obstet Gynecol* 79:882-884, 1992.

S E C T I O N   C
Chorioamnionitis

Stephen D. Ratcliffe, MD, MSPH

Chorioamnionitis, or infection of the amniotic membrane and space, is a common intrapartum complication. Its relation to preterm labor (PTL) is discussed in Chapter 12. This section addresses the recognition and management of chorioamnionitis in preterm and term pregnancies.

I. EPIDEMIOLOGY

A. Preterm Labor
Chorioamnionitis is commonly seen in patients experiencing PTL with intact membranes. Approximately 13% of such patients have a positive amniotic fluid culture, although only 1 of 8 women with a positive culture has clinically apparent chorioamnionitis. Thus, the clinician should maintain a high index of suspicion for this infection in patients presenting with PTL. Very-low-birth-weight infants whose labors have been complicated by chorioamnionitis are at increased risk for serious neurologic compromise.[1]

B. Term Pregnancy
Chorioamnionitis occurs in up to 12% of all term pregnancies.[1] Table 16-6 identifies factors that are associated with an increased risk for this intrapartum infection. Table 16-7 identifies intrapartum factors that have the greatest association with chorioamnionitis. In the setting of premature rupture of the membranes, the risk for chorioamnionitis increases with increasing numbers of vaginal examinations.[2] No association

TABLE 16-6 Risk Factors for Acute Chorioamnionitis

Presence of bacterial vaginosis	Meconium-stained fluid
Numerous vaginal examinations	Previous history of spontaneous or iatrogenic abortion
Prolonged labor	Colonization with group B streptococcus or gonorrhea
Prolonged spontaneous rupture of membranes	
Premature labor	Internal fetal monitoring

From Casey B, Cox S: Chorioamnionitis and endometritis, *Infect Dis Clin North Am* 11:203-222, 1997.

TABLE 16-7 Predictors of Chorioamnionitis

Risk Factor	Odds Ratio
>8 digital vaginal examinations (compared with 0-2 examinations)	5.07
7-8 digital vaginal examinations	3.80
5-6 digital vaginal examinations	2.62
3-4 digital vaginal examinations	2.06
Labor > 12 hours (compared with <3 hours)	4.12
Labor 9-12 hours	2.94
Labor 6-9 hours	1.97
Meconium-stained fluid	2.28
Time from ROM to active labor: >48 hours	1.76
Time from ROM to active labor: 24-48 hours	1.77
GBS colonization	1.71
Primipara	1.80

From Seaward P, Hannah M, Myhr T et al: International multicentre term PROM study: evaluation of predictors of neonatal infection in infants born to patients with premature rupture of membranes at term, *Am J Obstet Gynecol* 179:635-639, 1998.
GBS, Group B streptococcus; ROM, rupture of the membranes.

exists between water baths in labor and the development of chorioamnionitis.[3]

II. PATHOPHYSIOLOGY

A. Microbiology

Most cases of chorioamnionitis are polymicrobial and are derived from vaginal flora, predominantly anaerobes and genital mycoplasmas.[4]

1. Aerobes
   These include agents such as GBS, *Enterococcus faecalis, Streptococcus agalactiae,* and *Escherichia coli.*
2. Anaerobes
   These include bacteria such as *Peptostreptococcus, Clostridium, Bacteroides, Gardnerella,* and *Fusobacterium* species. Gardnerella, the causative agent of bacterial vaginosis, may increase the risk by a factor of 6.8.
3. Other infectious agents
   These include *Mycoplasma hominis, Ureaplasma urealyticum, Chlamydia,* herpes, and rarely *Candida. Ureaplasma* and *Mycoplasma* are associated with the pathogenesis of chorioamnionitis because they are isolated from infected amniotic fluid 30% to 45% of the time.[5]

B. Perinatal Effects

1. Maternal
   Chorioamnionitis is associated with greater rates of maternal blood transfusion, uterine atony, septic pelvic thrombophlebitis, and pelvic abscess.[1] Maternal mortality, although rare, does occur. Sepsis accounts for approximately 8% of maternity-related deaths.[5] The risk for endometritis is increased if cesarean delivery is required. Chorioamnionitis is associated with an increased incidence of labor dystocia (adjusted odds ratio [OR] of 2.3 for first-stage labor and 1.8 for second-stage labor) and cesarean delivery (adjusted OR of 1.8).[6]
   A multicenter study of 16,650 pregnancies studied the relation between time of diagnosis of chorioamnionitis to delivery with maternal and infant outcomes.[1] The only maternal complication associated with an increased duration of chorioamnionitis was uterine atony.
2. Neonatal
   Neonatal sepsis and mortality are increased when chorioamnionitis occurs in the preterm period. This is, in part, due to the increased vertical transmission of GBS in pregnancies lasting less than 35 weeks.[7] As a result, the Centers for Disease Control and Prevention recommends intrapartum chemoprophylaxis with penicillin or ampicillin for patients experiencing PTL or preterm premature rupture of the membranes (PPROM).[7] With this recommendation the incidence of early-onset group B streptococcal infections has decreased from 1.5 in 1000 in 1990 to 0.5 in 1000 in 1999. The discovery of *Ureaplasma* cultured from the amniotic cavity in the setting of preterm premature rupture of membranes is associated with a twentyfold increase in the risk for chronic lung disease in the premature infant.[8]
   Chorioamnionitis in the term pregnancy is associated with increased perinatal morbidity including:
   a. Incidence of 5-minute Apgar $\leq$ 3
   b. Neonatal sepsis
   c. Seizure[1]
   d. Maternal transfusion
   e. Septic pelvic thrombophlebitis
   f. Pelvic abscess
   An increased duration between diagnosis and delivery is associated with an increase in depressed 5-minute Apgar score and need for mechanical ventilation in the first 24 hours of life.
   A metaanalysis demonstrated an association between chorioamnionitis and an increased risk for cerebral palsy (RR, 1.9; 95% CI, 1.5-2.5) and cystic periventricular leukomalacia (RR, 2.6; 95% CI, 1.7-3.9).[8]

III. DIAGNOSIS

A. Clinical Presentation

Chorioamnionitis often occurs in the preterm pregnancy without any of the classic symptoms of infection. In the term pregnancy, the clinician should strongly suspect this diagnosis when one or more of the following signs or symptoms are present:

1. Maternal fever ($>100.5°F$)
2. Uterine tenderness
3. Fetal tachycardia
4. Foul-smelling amniotic fluid
5. Maternal tachycardia, chills, or rigor

Of these factors, maternal fever is one of the important predictors of infection. One of the potential confounding factors in making this diagnosis is the association between epidural anesthesia and low-grade intrapartum maternal fevers. In an analysis of 1235 nulliparous patients who had been randomized to receive active management of labor versus usual care, there was a nearly threefold increase in the diagnosis and treatment of suspected chorioamnionitis among women with epidurals (28%) compared with those without (10.8%).[9] Clinicians should carefully monitor for other signs and symptoms of chorioamnionitis in patients with epidural anesthesia. If the only sign is a low-grade fever (<100.5°F), it may be prudent to withhold antibiotic therapy.

B. Laboratory Findings

Leukocytosis, defined as a total white blood count greater than 12,000 cells/mm[3], is commonly encountered with chorioamnionitis, although it may occur during normal labor as well.[10] This degree of leukocytosis in labor has a sensitivity of 67% and a specificity of 86%. A leukocytosis accompanied by a left shift or bandemia greater than 3% bands is a more sensitive marker for chorioamnionitis. When the clinical diagnosis is in question, C-reactive protein (CRP) and erythrocyte sedimentation rates have been used as early markers of infection. However, these tests have a low specificity, generating a high rate of false-positive results.

C. Differential Diagnosis

Other entities can mimic chorioamnionitis, for example:
1. Genitourinary infections, including bladder and kidney infections
2. Intraabdominal processes, such as appendicitis and diverticulitis
3. Upper or lower respiratory tract infections

D. Amniotic Fluid Analysis

Amniocentesis is seldom used for diagnostic purposes in the term pregnancy; however, it is a useful tool in diagnosing chorioamnionitis in the preterm pregnancy when an adequate fluid pocket can be found. Gram stain of amniotic fluid has high positive and negative predictive values of 80% to 85% when confirmation of chorioamnionitis is based on a positive amniotic fluid culture.[4]

IV. MANAGEMENT

A. Timing of Antibiotic Therapy
1. PTL
   The clinician must always remain vigilant for signs of clinical chorioamnionitis and allow labor to progress if they occur. Prompt introduction of antibiotic therapy is indicated if chorioamnionitis is suspected. A Cochrane review indicates that the prophylactic use of antibiotics in women with PPROM results in a significant prolongation in the interval from rupture to delivery, a decrease in the incidence of neonatal sepsis, respiratory distress syndrome, and prolonged ventilation.[11] However, the use of antibiotics in the management of PPROM is not associated with an improvement in neonatal mortality.

2. Term pregnancy
   Unless vaginal delivery is imminent, use of antibiotic therapy is indicated when a clinical diagnosis of chorioamnionitis is made. Two RCTs demonstrated decreased neonatal infection rates when antibiotics are instituted during labor as opposed to after delivery.[12,13] Similarly, if the patient is known to be colonized with GBS, neonatal infectious morbidity is decreased when intrapartum antibiotic therapy is initiated during labor and the duration between this therapy and delivery is greater than 4 hours.[7]

B. Choice of Antibiotic Agents

Despite the presence of anaerobic bacteria in up to 50% of amniotic space infections, these infections can usually be adequately treated with antibiotics that have broad-spectrum aerobic coverage. Ampicillin, 2 g intravenously every 6 hours, or penicillin, 5 million units every 4 hours, have been shown to be effective in the treatment of women who are carriers of GBS. Ampicillin has the additional advantage of covering enterococcal infections. Expanded gram-negative coverage can be provided with the addition of an aminoglycoside, usually gentamicin. Gentamicin is given with a loading dose of 120 to 140 mg intravenously, followed by 1 to 1.5 mg/kg intravenously every 8 hours. If gentamicin is used on a prolonged basis, serum peak and trough levels should be followed to avoid potential fetal ototoxicity or maternal renal toxicity. Other acceptable single-agent antibiotic regimens are listed below. With the exception of patients allergic to penicillin, the combination of ampicillin and gentamicin is most commonly recommended. In situations in which anaerobic coverage is desirable, clindamycin, 500 to 750 mg every 6 hours, can be added to the following regimens. This coverage is usually added to treat postpartum endometritis when there is a lack of response to conventional aerobic antibiotic coverage.

1. Dosing of other antibiotics
   a. Piperacillin: 3 to 4 g intravenously every 4 hours
   b. Mezlocillin: 3 to 4 g intravenously every 4 hours
   c. Ticarcillin/clavulanic acid: 3 g intravenously every 6 hours
   d. Cefoxitin: 1 to 2 g intravenously every 6 hours
   e. Ampicillin/sulbactam: 1.5 to 3 g intravenously every 6 hours
2. Chorioamnionitis, cesarean delivery, and use of antibiotics
   An RCT by Turnquest and colleagues[14] provides evidence that patients with chorioamnionitis who require a cesarean delivery benefit from a single preoperative dose of IV clindamycin in addition to ampicillin and gentamicin. The patients in this trial did not benefit from additional postoperative antibiotics.

   Some experts recommend that patients undergoing cesarean section with chorioamnionitis be treated with antibiotic therapy after delivery until they are afebrile for at least 24 hours.[15] An adequately powered RCT demonstrated that administration of a single postpartum 900-mg dose of clindamycin given after cord clamping in conjunction with intrapartum treatment of chorioamnionitis with ampicillin and gentamicin was as effective in preventing infectious morbidity and was associated with shorter hospital stays when compared with conventional treatment.[15]

C. Monitoring the Maternal Condition

Most women with chorioamnionitis remain clinically stable and can be managed in an expectant manner. Providers should remain vigilant for the occasional patient who develops signs of hypotension and poor peripheral perfusion, indicating potential septic shock. This life-threatening complication requires an intensive-care level of treatment and monitoring.

D. Neonatal Management

The Centers for Disease Control and Prevention recommends that infants whose mothers have received intrapartum antibiotics for suspected chorioamnionitis undergo laboratory investigation for sepsis and receive antibiotic coverage pending those results of these studies.[7] This coverage consists of ampicillin (150-200 mg/kg/day intravenously or intramuscularly every 12 hours) and gentamicin (5 mg/kg/day intravenously or intramuscularly

every 12 hours) (see Chapter 19, Section E). Laboratory evaluation may include the following:

1. Complete blood cell count with differential
   Attention must be paid to the ratio of immature (bands)-to-total polymorphonuclear leukocytes (bands plus neutrophils). This immature (I)-to-total neutrophil series (T) ratio is considered increased if it is greater than 0.20.
2. Blood culture
3. C-reactive protein (CRP)
   Serial tests for CRP, an acute-phase reactant, may be helpful in evaluating the newborn. Two successive normal CRPs have a negative predictive value of greater than 97%. The sensitivity of CRP to diagnose sepsis at 24 hours of age is 78% and the specificity is 94%.[16]
4. Lumbar puncture
   Lumbar puncture should be performed when there is high index of suspicion for neonatal sepsis. Infants who have evidence of systemic infection should receive parenteral antibiotics for 7 to 10 days.

V. PREVENTION OF CHORIOAMNIONITIS

A series of more than 20,000 women who fell into one of three management strategies that was designed to decrease the incidence of invasive early-onset GBS infections in newborns showed that the strategy that incorporated GBS cultures between 35 and 37 weeks of gestation identified the maternal carriers of this infection.[17] Treatment of these carriers in labor to prevent early-onset disease resulted in a reduction in the incidence of chorioamnionitis in labor (RR, 0.7; 95% CI 0.6-0.8). The prevention of 1 case of chorioamnionitis required 23 prenatal cultures for GBS and administration of antibiotic prophylaxis to 4 women in labor.

The identification and intrapartum treatment of GBS carriers has also resulted in a 21% decrease of maternally invasive GBS infections from a baseline rate of 0.29 in 1000 in 1990 to 0.23 in 1000 in 1999.[7]

Other strategies to decrease the incidence of chorioamnionitis include:

1. Use of induction versus expectant management of labor with term premature rupture of membranes results in a reduction of chorioamnionitis of more than 50%.[18]
2. Avoid unnecessary or excessive number of vaginal examinations.[2]

3. Avoid the routine use of internal monitoring such as intrauterine pressure catheters.

4. Use of vaginal chlorhexidine during labor to prevent chorioamnionitis has been proposed as a preventive maneuver, but a Cochrane review of three studies did not demonstrate a decrease in maternal infection.[19]

VI. SOR A RECOMMENDATIONS

RECOMMENDATIONS	REFERENCES
The prophylactic use of antibiotics in women with PPROM results in a significant prolongation in the interval from rupture to delivery, a decrease in the incidence of neonatal sepsis, respiratory distress syndrome, and prolonged ventilation.	*12*
The use of induction versus expectant management of term premature rupture of membranes results in a decrease in the RR of chorioamnionitis of greater then 50%.	*19*
The treatment of GBS-positive carriers in labor results in a 30% decrease in the RR of chorioamnionitis.	*18*

REFERENCES

1. Rouse D, Landon M, Leveno K et al: The Maternal-Fetal Medicine Units cesarean registry: chorioamnionitis at term and its duration-relationship to outcomes, *Am J Obstet Gynecol* 191:211-216, 2004.
2. Schutte M, Treffers P, Kloostermen G et al: Management of premature rupture of membranes: the risk of vaginal examination to the infant, *Am J Obstet Gynecol* 146:395-400, 1983.
3. Robertson P, Huang L, Croughan-Minihane M et al: Is there an association between water baths during labor and the development of chorioamnionitis or endometritis? *Am J Obstet Gynecol* 178:1215-1221, 1998.
4. Gibbs R, Blanco J, St. Clair P et al: Quantitative bacteriology of amniotic fluid from patients with clinical intraamniotic infection at term, *J Infect Dis* 145:1-7, 1983.
5. Simpson KR: Sepsis during pregnancy, *J Obstet Gynecol Neonatal Nurs* 24:550-556, 1995.
6. Mark S, Croughan-Minihane M, Kilpatrick S: Chorioamnionitis and uterine function, *Obstet Gynecol* 95:909-1012, 2000.
7. Centers for Disease Control and Prevention: Prevention of perinatal group B streptococcal disease: revised guidelines from CDC, *MMWR Recomm Rep* 51(RR-11):1-22, 2002.
8. Wu Y, Escobar G, Grether J et al: Chorioamnionitis and cerebral palsy in term and near-term infants, *JAMA* 290: 2677-2684, 2003.
9. Goetzl L, Cohen A, Frigoletto F et al: Maternal epidural analgesia and rates of maternal antibiotic treatment in a low-risk nulliparous population, *J Perinatol* 23:457-461, 2003.
10. Casey B, Cox S: Chorioamnionitis and endometritis, *Infect Dis Clin North Am* 11:203-222, 1997.
11. Kenyon W, Boulvain M, Neilson J: Antibiotics for preterm rupture of membranes, *Cochrane Database Syst Rev* (2): CD001058, 2003.
12. Sperling RS, Ramamurthy RS, Gibbs RS: A comparison of intrapartum versus immediate postpartum treatment of intra-amniotic infection, *Obstet Gynecol* 70:861-865, 1987.
13. Gibbs RS, Dinsmoor MJ, Newton GR et al: A randomized trial of intrapartum versus immediate postpartum treatment of women with intraamniotic infection, *Obstet Gynecol* 72:823-828, 1988.
14. Turnquest M, How H, Cook C et al: Chorioamnionitis: is continuation of antibiotic therapy necessary after cesarean section? *Am J Obstet Gynecol* 179:1261-1266, 1998.
15. Edwards R, Duff P: Single additional dose postpartum therapy for women with chorioamnionitis, *Obstet Gynecol* 102:957-961, 2003.
16. Laborada G, Rego M, Jain A et al: Diagnostic value of cytokines and C-reactive protein in the first 24 hours of neonatal sepsis, *Am J Perinatol* 20:491-501, 2003.
17. Locksmith G, Clark P, Duff P: Maternal and neonatal infection rates with three different protocols for prevention of group B streptococcal disease, *Am J Obstet Gynecol* 180:416-422, 1999.
18. Hannah M, Ohlsson A, Farine D et al: Induction of labor compared to expectant management for prelabor rupture of the membranes at term. TERMPROM Study Group, *N Engl J Med* 334:1005-1010, 1996.
19. Lumbiganon P, Thinkhamrop J, Thinkhamrop B et al: Vaginal chlorhexidine during labour for preventing maternal and neonatal infections (excluding group B Streptococcal and HIV), *Cochrane Database Syst Rev* (4):CD004070, 2004.

SECTION D Intrapartum Bleeding

John C. Houchins, MD

This section covers specific intrapartum diagnostic and management strategies for placenta previa, placental abruption, and vasa previa. A more general perspective is included in Chapter 7, Section C.

I. INITIAL EVALUATION

A. History

On arrival, the patient should be questioned regarding the amount of bleeding she has experienced (e.g., "spotting" versus "as much as a period" or "enough to soak a pad"). Initial inquiries by nursing staff may also document perceived pain, the presence of contractions, or evidence of "show," or leakage of fluid.

Patients may not be accurate in their description of the quantity of blood, but overestimation is preferable until medical evaluation can take place.

B. Maternal Stabilization

Initial assessment of maternal and fetal stability is of primary importance and is directed at reviewing maternal vital signs, conducting a brief physical assessment, and FHR monitoring. This assessment is made more complex by the cardiovascular changes associated with pregnancy because a woman may not demonstrate any signs of shock until she has lost up to 35% of her blood volume. Normal blood pressures in pregnancy tend to be lower and the maternal heart rate is slightly greater than those seen in nonpregnant women. Alterations in blood pressure may be most difficult to assess in the patient with pregnancy-induced hypertension, in whom a "normal" blood pressure may actually reflect substantial volume depletion.

C. Initial Management

If bleeding is determined to be anything other than trivial, IV fluids should be started through a large-bore IV and oxygen should be applied. Nursing protocols should specify no vaginal examinations until seen by a physician. No digital examination should be performed unless the placental location is known to be distant to the cervical os. Reports of previous ultrasound scans should be obtained, and if not known from a previous examination, an ultrasound for placental location should be performed. Initial blood workup should include a complete blood cell count with platelets, type and crossmatch, prothrombin time/international normalized ratio (INR), and fibrinogen.

D. Indications for Immediate Cesarean Delivery

Indications for immediate cesarean delivery include a persistent nonreassuring FHR tracing and severe maternal hemorrhage. Otherwise, the evaluation may proceed in a more deliberate manner.

II. DIFFERENTIAL DIAGNOSIS OF VAGINAL BLEEDING

If the patient is in labor, bleeding may simply represent exuberant bloody "show," or may be caused by more concerning causes, such as vasa previa, abruption, or placenta previa. If the onset of bleeding coincides with rupture of membranes, vasa previa is more likely. Most patients with placenta previa present with bleeding before the onset of labor. Both of these serious causes of bleeding are also characterized by being painless (apart from contraction pain), unlike the associated pain of placental abruption.

A. Vasa Previa

Vasa previa is a fetal hemorrhage caused by the rupture of fetal vessels in a velamentous insertion of the umbilical cord (type I vasa previa) or of vessels traversing the membranes between two lobes of the placenta (type II vasa previa).[1] Although this condition is rare, rapid diagnosis is crucial because fetal mortality is greater than 50%. If initial FHR tracings are nonreassuring, an immediate cesarean delivery should be performed with neonatal resuscitation immediately available. If FHR tracings are stable and the diagnosis is in doubt, a rapid test should be performed to determine the presence of fetal blood. Kleihauer-Betke stains and hemoglobin electrophoresis are prohibitively time-consuming, making the following two methods more suitable:

1. Ogita test (approximately 4 minutes)
   Five drops of 0.1 M potassium hydroxide (KOH) is added to one drop of blood specimen and shaken vigorously for 2 minutes. Ten drops of precipitating solution, made from 400 ml of 50% saturated ammonium sulfate and 1 ml of 10 M hydrochloric acid, is then added to this and the mix dropped onto a filter paper to make a ring 20 mm in diameter. Denatured adult hemoglobin remains in the center, and fetal hemoglobin forms a colored ring at the periphery.

2. Modified Apt test (about 7 minutes)
   Pooled blood is collected with a syringe from the vaginal vault. The hemoglobin is lysed by the addition of an equal amount of tap water, and the mixture is centrifuged for several minutes. One milliliter of 1% NaOH is mixed with 5 ml of supernatant. In 2 minutes, the colorimetric reaction is read. A pink reaction indicates fetal hemoglobin; adult hemoglobin is yellow-brown.

   Although it should be emphasized that this diagnosis is primarily a clinical one that rarely requires laboratory confirmation, finding fetal hemoglobin in the setting of painless bleeding that commences with rupture of membranes confirms the diagnosis of vasa previa. The Ogita test is three times more sensitive than Apt and is quicker, but it requires more advanced preparation.[1,2]

B. Placental Abruption

1. Associated symptoms

    If intrapartum bleeding is associated with pain, abruption should be considered. Pain may be mild (similar to menstrual cramping), comparable with normal labor, or excruciating. It may be accompanied with uterine tenderness, or may be expressed solely as back pain in the patient with a posterior placenta.

2. Bleeding characteristics

    Hemorrhage may be externalized, either completely or partially, or may be concealed. The amount of bleeding is often underestimated clinically. Bleeding may also present as bloody amniotic fluid. Clinical presentation and grading of abruptions is discussed further in Chapter 7, Section C.

3. Ultrasound examination

    Ultrasound may demonstrate retroplacental or intraplacental hemorrhage, a separated placental edge, or no pathologic findings. Lack of sonographic findings should *not* be used to rule out a diagnosis of abruption.

C. Placenta Previa

1. Clinical evaluation

    Patients with spotting or minor amounts of vaginal bleeding can be evaluated by speculum examination to evaluate for cervical and vaginal causes of bleeding. It is prudent to visually inspect the cervix to rule out advanced cervical dilatation before vaginal probe examination.

2. Abdominal ultrasound

    This assessment can be made with a moderately full maternal bladder, but an empty bladder helps to avoid false-positive diagnoses.

3. Transperineal or transvaginal ultrasound

    This provides the most accurate means of assessing the relation of the cervical os to the placental edge. These scanning techniques are discussed in Chapter 18, Section A and Chapter 3, Section J. Transperineal scanning may be used to image a posterior placenta previa or to differentiate a marginal from a complete placenta previa. Transvaginal ultrasound may not be available in labor and delivery but may be used in the stable patient for evaluation of placenta previa.[3] The introduction of a vaginal probe into the vagina is at right angles to the cervical canal. The vaginal probe is covered with a sterile cover or condom and inserted only partially into the vaginal canal to image the lower uterine segment and cervix.

III. MANAGEMENT OF VAGINAL BLEEDING

Several general principles apply to treatment of all of the causes of severe vaginal bleeding in labor[4]:

- Antenatal RhoGAM (300 mg) should be given to all Rh-negative women with intrapartum bleeding for prophylaxis in the instance of possible fetomaternal hemorrhage. If a larger fetomaternal bleed is suspected, a Kleihauer-Betke test may be performed to determine the number of units of RhoGAM needed.
- The hematocrit should be maintained at 30% or greater with packed red cells or whole blood.
- Blood pressure is an insensitive estimate of blood volume in pregnancy. Fluid replacement with colloid or blood products should be guided by urine output, with a minimum goal of 30 ml/hr.

The overall strategy in managing the patient must take into account the amount of bleeding and the gestational age of the fetus. Diagnosis-specific management strategies are discussed in the following sections.

A. Placenta Previa

1. Effects of prematurity

    Because the greatest morbidity and mortality associated with placenta previa are due to prematurity, attempts should be made to continue a pregnancy that is less than 33 weeks of gestation. Tocolysis does not appear to be contraindicated to prolong the very preterm pregnancy, as long as the fetus is not compromised and hemorrhage is not massive.[5] Magnesium sulfate ($MgSO_4$) is the preferred agent. In many circumstances, the patient should be transferred as soon as stable to a perinatal center because the risk for rebleeding is substantial in the preterm gestation with placenta previa.

2. The double setup examination

    This is a treatment modality to determine whether a patient with equivocal findings of a marginal placenta previa may be permitted a trial of labor. Its utility is the prevention of unnecessary cesarean delivery in cases in which the bleeding edge of the placenta may be effectively tamponaded by the fetal head during labor. Palpation of the placental edge should not take place unless the patient is prepared and ready for immediate operative delivery, including having anesthesia in attendance and blood products ready. The patient may then be examined with digital vaginal examination with palpation of the placental edge. The advent of highly accurate transvaginal and transperineal ultrasound examinations has made this type of examination rarely necessary, however. Chances for a vaginal delivery increase dramatically (60% vs. 10%) when the placenta is 2.0 cm from the internal os, as determined by these scans.[6]

3. Operative delivery
   Cesarean delivery is indicated if bleeding is excessive, or if the fetus is mature and vaginal delivery is deemed unsafe or unlikely. An increased risk for placenta accreta exists for patients with placenta previa, especially multiparas and those with previous lower uterine incisions. The overall risk for this serious complication is 10% in patients with a low anterior placenta or placenta previa and previous cesarean operative delivery, and it increases with each successive cesarean delivery.[7,8] Because treatment might result in a cesarean hysterectomy, it is advisable for the physician and patient to be prepared for this possibility. These issues should be kept in mind when proceeding toward operative delivery, and transfer to a facility with more extensive blood-bank resources may need to be considered.

B. Placental Abruption

The management of placental abruption depends on the presence or absence of fetal life. In general, the risk for stillbirth in abruption is proportionate to the degree of placental separation.[9] Coagulopathy is rare in acute abruption with a surviving fetus (7%), but 28% of patients with abruption resulting in fetal demise experience development of a consumptive coagulopathy and disseminated intravascular coagulation (DIC) from the release of thromboplastin.[10] Although partial abruption may be stabilized such that a severely preterm gestation may continue, the following are guidelines for intrapartum management[4]:

1. Viable fetus in labor
   If the fetus is alive at the time of presentation, a fetal scalp electrode should be placed. Emergency cesarean delivery should be performed if a persistently nonreassuring FHR tracing is observed, unless vaginal delivery is imminent. In the setting of a more reassuring tracing, time can be allowed for stabilizing hemodynamic and coagulation parameters before cesarean delivery because this will

improve overall outcome.[4] Tocolysis is appropriate only in the case of severe prematurity, when the likelihood of extrauterine fetal survival is low.[11] In these cases, $MgSO_4$ is the tocolytic of choice. An individual experienced in neonatal resuscitation should be available for any delivery, vaginal or operative, when abruption is suspected.

   a. Monitoring patients with suspected abruption: The patient with abruption should be observed closely with serial complete blood cell counts and urine output as noted earlier. Fibrinogen levels and INR should also be evaluated. Normal pregnancy values for fibrinogen are increased (350-650 mg/dl). A fibrinogen value less than 150 mg/dl is indicative of significant coagulopathy and should be treated with fresh frozen plasma or whole blood. The blood bank should plan to stay at least three units ahead in cases of severe abruption.

   b. Bedside test for coagulopathy—the clot test: A red-top tube is drawn and taped beside the bed. Clot formation at 6 minutes is highly predictive of a fibrinogen level greater than 150 mg/dl. Absence of a clot or a fragile clot is evidence of coagulopathy.

   c. Monitoring contractions: Contractions should be monitored closely in abruption. The onset of tetanic contractions may precede appearance of abnormal FHR tracing. Placement of an intrauterine pressure catheter may help make the diagnosis. What feels like a tetanic contraction to palpation is manifested as frequent, small contractions superimposed on an elevated resting baseline.

2. The nonviable fetus and abruption
   If the fetus is nonviable, management is directed toward the safest means of delivering the patient. Vaginal delivery is preferable, if at all possible, with no absolute time limits as long as labor is progressing. Labor is often augmented to accomplish a vaginal delivery. Episiotomy and other measures that increase blood loss should be avoided. Cesarean delivery is performed only for severe maternal hematologic, hemodynamic, or other medical instability.

3. Postoperative management
   This includes continued monitoring of hemodynamic and hematologic parameters as described earlier. The incidence of all complications, including hemorrhage, DIC, acute tubular necrosis, and acute respiratory distress syndrome (ARDS) is

greater in abruption presenting with nonviable fetus than viable fetus (68% vs. 11%).[9] All of these are highly preventable with careful monitoring, which may require intensive care unit (ICU) admission and central line pressure monitoring.

REFERENCES

1. Oyelese Y, Lewis KM, Collea JV et al: Vasa previa: are most perinatal deaths preventable? *Contemp Obstet Gynecol* 48:43-56, 2003.
2. Odunsi K, Bullough CHW, Henzel J et al: Evaluation of chemical tests for fetal bleeding from vasa previa, *Int J Gynaecol Obstet* 55(3):207-212, 1996.
3. Timor-Tritsch IE, Yunis R: Confirming the safety of transvaginal sonography in patients suspected of placenta previa, *Obstet Gynecol* 81:742-744, 1993.
4. Gabbe SG: *Obstetrics: normal and problem pregnancies,* ed 4, New York, 2002, Churchill Livingstone.
5. Sharma A, Suri V, Gupta I: Tocolytic therapy in conservative management of symptomatic placenta previa, *Int J Gynaecol Obstet* 84(2):109-113, 2004.
6. Bhide A, Prefumo F, Moore J et al: Placental edge to internal os distance in the late third trimester and mode of delivery in placenta praevia, *BJOG* 110(9):860-864, 2003.
7. Miller DA, Chollet JA, Goodwin TM: Clinical risk factors for placenta previa-placenta accreta, *Am J Obstet Gynecol* 177:210-214, 1997.
8. Zaki ZM, Bahar AM, Ali ME et al: Risk factors and morbidity in patients with placenta previa compared to placenta previa non-accreta, *Acta Obstet Gynaecol Scand* 77:391-394, 1998.
9. Ananth CV, Berkowitz GS, Savitz DA et al: Placenta abruption and adverse perinatal outcomes, *JAMA* 282:1646-1651, 1999.
10. Witlin AG, Sibai BM: Perinatal and maternal outcome following abruptio placentae, *Hypertens Pregnancy* 20(2):195-203, 2001.
11. Combs CA, Nyberg DA, Mack LA et al: Expectant management after sonographic diagnosis of placental abruption, *Am J Perinatol* 9:170-174, 1992.

SECTION E Postpartum Hemorrhage

Janice M. Anderson, MD, FAAFP, and Narayana Rao V. Pula, MD

Postpartum hemorrhage (PPH) is an important cause of maternal morbidity in developed countries and a major cause of mortality internationally.[1] Prevention strategies exist, including active management of the third stage, but are underutilized.[2] Although there are known risk factors, not all cases are expected,[3] and even with the best care not all hemorrhages are avoidable.[4,5] Every maternity care service must be prepared to deal with severe hemorrhage.

This chapter discusses the importance of early recognition and systematic evaluation and treatment, as well as the use of preventive strategies, which can minimize the serious morbidity and mortality associated with PPH.

I. EPIDEMIOLOGY AND RISK FACTORS: GENERAL

PPH has been defined as more than 500 ml of blood loss in the first 24 hours after vaginal delivery, with more after cesarean delivery. A loss of 1000 ml, often described as severe, is recognized as clinically relevant. Definitions of PPH useful for research include a 10% decline in hematocrit, change in vital signs, or need for transfusion, though these all reflect recognition after the fact.[6] Estimating blood loss has been shown to be inaccurate, especially when there is a high-volume loss.[7] Depending on the definition used and the population studied, the incidence of PPH ranges from 3% to 18%.[8] According to expert consensus from the World Health Organization, PPH occurs in 10.5% of live births globally, with a case fatality rate of 1%.[1] The incidence of severe blood loss in developed nations remains at 3%, even with most effective management strategies.[4,5] Risk factors for PPH include, but are not limited to, prolonged third stage, prior PPH, multiple pregnancy, episiotomies, and fetal macrosomia.[9-11] It is important to remember that this is not always a predictable event, so one must be prepared to treat it at every delivery.[3]

II. EPIDEMIOLOGY, RISK FACTORS, AND PATHOGENESIS: CAUSE-SPECIFIC FEATURES

A. Uterine Atony

Uterine atony is responsible for the majority of PPH cases. Failure of the uterine smooth muscle to contract and constrict to create "living ligatures" around the spiral blood vessels in the placental bed[12] can lead to rapid blood loss. This blood loss can be significant because there is approximately 700 ml of blood per minute flowing through the term uterus.[13] Predisposing factors for uterine atony include overdistension of the uterus, chorioamnionitis, dysfunctional labor (e.g., protracted active phase, secondary arrest of labor, or prolonged second stage) or prolonged use of oxytocin, grand multiparity, and administration of $MgSO_4$.[13,14]

B. Genital Tract Trauma

Genital tract trauma, specifically lacerations/episiotomies, hematomas, uterine rupture, and uterine inversion, can each cause significant blood loss. The risk for lower genital tract trauma is increased if there has been a prolonged second stage, use of forceps or vacuum, episiotomy, or vulvar varicosities. Episiotomy is the most common risk factor for hematoma, but other risks include primiparity, preeclampsia, multiple gestation, vulvar varicosities, and coagulopathy.[15]

Clinically significant uterine rupture complicates 0.6% to 0.7% of pregnancies in patients undergoing a trial of labor after cesarean delivery (number needed to treat [NNT] = 370 elective cesarean deliveries to prevent 1 symptomatic rupture; 7142 to prevent 1 rupture-related hysterectomy).[16-18] Although this rate is increased compared with elective repeat cesarean delivery, the absolute risk remains low.[18] The risk for rupture increases primarily with previous classical uterine incision, and to a lesser extent with more than one prior cesarean delivery, puerperal fever, and augmentation or induction, particularly if prostaglandins and oxytocin are used sequentially.[17,19-21] Misoprostol should be avoided.[21] Ongoing studies are needed to confirm the suspected increased risk associated with single-layer closures, infection with prior cesarean delivery, or shortened interpregnancy interval.[17,19,20] Spontaneous rupture in an *unscarred* uterus is rare, reported to be 1 in 15,000. It occurs more often in women of high parity and is increased with the use of uterotonics.[22] Uterine inversion is rare, occurring in 0.05% of deliveries.[14] Active management of the third stage may reduce the incidence.[23] Classic risk factors for inversion are undue cord traction and excessive fundal pressure[24]; however, this has not been confirmed by recent studies.[25] Other predisposing factors are a fundally implanted placenta, delivery of a macrosomic fetus, use of oxytocin, and prior history of inversion.[26]

C. Retained Placenta, Invasive Placenta, or Both

The mean time from delivery until placental expulsion is 8 to 9 minutes.[5] As the length of the third stage increases, so does the risk for PPH, with a significant increase in the risk for PPH after 18 minutes.[5] Retained placenta, classically defined as the failure of the placenta to deliver by 30 minutes, occurs in less than 3% of vaginal deliveries,[27] but it is associated with a significantly greater risk for PPH compared with placental delivery in less than 30 minutes (OR, 6.2; 95% CI, 4.6-8.2; $p < 0.001$).[5] It is responsible for approximately 10% of all PPH.

If untreated, retained placenta has a high risk for maternal morbidity and even death.[28] Treatment often involves manual removal, which is associated with its own risks, including trauma, infection, or hemorrhage.[28] Retained placental fragments is the most common cause of delayed hemorrhage and can be responsible for persistent uterine atony that does not respond to uterotonics.[14]

Invasive placenta results from a defect in the decidual basalis, leading to an invasive implantation. Classification is based on the depth of invasion. Placenta accreta adheres, increta invades, and percreta penetrates the myometrium to, or beyond, the serosa.[29] The incidence of abnormal placentation has increased more than tenfold, from 0.003% in the 1950s to 0.04% in the 1990s, likely related to the increase in cesarean delivery rates.[30] The most important risk factors are previous cesarean delivery and placenta previa, particularly in combination. Additional risk factors include prior invasive placenta, history of uterine curettage or infection, fibroids or uterine anomalies, advanced maternal age, and high parity.[13,30]

D. Coagulopathies

Coagulation disorders, which are responsible for only a small percentage of PPH, are generally known before delivery, allowing advanced planning to prevent PPH. If not previously identified, they should be suspected if usual measures have failed to control hemorrhage and lack of clotting is noted. Thrombocytopenia, von Willebrand disease, and hemophilia are some of the disorders to consider. Patients can also experience development of a coagulopathy from HELLP (hemolysis, elevated liver enzymes, and low platelets) syndrome or DIC. Conditions that predispose to DIC include severe preeclampsia, amniotic fluid embolism (AFE), sepsis, placental abruption, and prolonged retention of fetal demise.[14,31] Abruption is associated with cocaine use and hypertensive disorders.[14] Excessive bleeding from any cause can deplete coagulation factors and lead to consumptive coagulation, which promotes further bleeding.

E. Late Postpartum Hemorrhage

Significant bleeding after 24 hours is termed delayed or late PPH. This may be caused by abnormal involution, sloughing of the eschar, or retained placental fragments.

III. DIAGNOSIS/CLINICAL FEATURES

In practice, the diagnosis of PPH is usually based on early recognition of excessive bleeding. Even though estimating blood volume has been shown to be inaccurate,[7] it is important to attempt to estimate ongoing blood loss. Changes in vital signs occur late and can be confusing in the puerperal period. For example, the increased blood volume that accompanies healthy pregnancy may delay the usual signs of volume loss, such as tachycardia and hypotension. Conversely, a decline of the blood pressure after delivery in a patient with preeclampsia cannot be assumed normal. In addition, the diagnosis may be delayed because of underestimation of blood loss or bleeding that develops while the patient is not being observed. Providers must be vigilant for less dramatic, but steady, bleeding and concealed hemorrhage.

In addition to recognizing PPH, a careful examination for its cause is essential to determine the best management plan. Usually, this is simply based on the clinical presentation, but occasionally, uterine exploration, ultrasound, or blood work is necessary. Clinical features that accompany several causes of PPH are detailed in the following sections.

A. Uterine Atony

A soft or boggy uterus on palpation typically suggests uterine atony. It may respond to uterine massage or uterotonics, if only briefly, by becoming firm, usually with an associated decrease in bleeding.

B. Trauma

Bleeding observed from vaginal or cervical lacerations and a uterus that is firm suggests genital tract trauma as a cause of the bleeding. Hematomas can cause pain and hemodynamic effects out of proportion with the estimated blood loss.

C. Inverted Uterus

The inverted uterus usually appears as a bluish gray mass protruding from the vagina and can be associated with vasovagal shock out of proportion with the amount of bleeding noted. Uterine exploration is often necessary to detect low-grade inversion.

D. Uterine Rupture

Uterine rupture usually occurs before delivery and presents with FHR abnormalities, most commonly bradycardia.

E. Retained Placenta

Excessive bleeding and a prolonged third stage, with or without atony, suggests retained placenta. This is especially true in the face of manual removal or incomplete placenta. Invasive placenta is likely if manual removal is difficult. If this is suspected and the patient is stable, ultrasound can help diagnose or determine the extent of invasion.

F. Coagulopathy

A noticeable lack of clotting and/or oozing from puncture sites is the main diagnostic feature of coagulopathy. Coagulation defects can be diagnosed by observing clot stability in a serum "red-top" tube of blood after 10 minutes. If no clot forms or it is easily disrupted, the fibrinogen level is likely less than 100 mg/dl and a clinically significant coagulopathy exists.[32] Confirmatory laboratory tests include platelet count, prothrombin time (INR), partial thromboplastin time, fibrinogen level, and fibrin split products (D-dimer).[14]

IV. PREVENTION

A. General Measures

It is prudent to minimize blood loss whenever possible to prevent the morbidity and mortality associated with PPH. This can be accomplished by identifying and correcting anemia or coagulopathies. Predelivery counseling of Jehovah's Witnesses, who are at a forty-four-fold increased risk for maternal death, will allow medically and ethically sound management.[33] Women at particularly high risk for abnormal placentation, such as a woman with a prior cesarean delivery who has an anterior low-lying placenta or previa, may benefit from an antenatal ultrasound to look for invasive placenta (especially percreta).[29,34,35] These patients, in addition to women with placenta previa, coagulopathy, or cervical pregnancy, can be offered delivery at a center with blood-banking facilities and anesthesia and surgery capabilities. Placing prophylactic catheters for angiographic embolization can be considered before cesarean delivery or labor in these patients.[14] Episiotomy should be avoided unless urgent delivery is necessary and the perineum is believed to be a limiting factor.[36] After delivery, continued observation for symptoms of slow or delayed postpartum bleeding is also important.

B. Active Management of the Third Stage

The most effective strategy for prevention of blood loss is *active management of the third stage of labor* (AMTSL).[37,38] This includes giving oxytocin with the anterior shoulder or immediately after delivery of the baby, controlled cord traction, and uterine massage after delivery of the placenta. As originally described AMTSL included early cord clamping, but recent trials have shown that a delay in cord clamping for about 60 seconds has benefits to the newborn. These benefits include increased iron stores and decreased anemia in term and preterm infants, and reduced incidence of intraventricular hemorrhage and sepsis in very preterm infants.[18,39-42] The delay has not been shown to increase neonatal morbidity or maternal blood loss.[39,40,42] When AMTSL is compared with expectant management, where the placenta is allowed to separate spontaneously, aided only by gravity or nipple stimulation, it has been shown to decrease blood loss, shorten the length of third stage, and decrease the incidence of PPH without an increase in manual removal of placenta or retained products.[8,37,43] The NNT is 12 to prevent 1 case of PPH and 67 to prevent 1 postpartum transfusion.[37] Despite this evidence, the application of AMTSL is underutilized.[2] Hospital guidelines encouraging use of active management result in significant reduction in the incidence of massive PPH.[44]

Oxytocin remains the drug of choice for prevention of hemorrhage, providing protection even if it is given after the placenta is delivered.[8,43] It is effective, has fewer side effects than ergot alkaloids or prostaglandins, and has no contraindications.[4,8,45]

Misoprostol has an important role in prevention of PPH because it is more effective than placebo (NNT is 18 to prevent 1 case of PPH) and has the following advantages over conventional uterotonics: It is inexpensive, heat and light stable, and requires no syringes.[46-48] These are important considerations for nonhospital and resource poor settings. Ongoing investigation is needed to determine the best dosage and route of administration to maximize effectiveness and minimize the common side effects of

shivering and pyrexia.[49] Misoprostol is not FDA approved for use in preventing PPH, but the U.S. Pharmacopeia considers this to be an acceptable off-label indication. The U.S. Pharmacopeia recommends it as an alternative agent when other uterotonic drugs are not available, suggesting a single dose of 400 to 600 μg orally or rectally immediately after delivery.[18]

V. TREATMENT

A. General Approach to Treatment

Once excessive blood loss is suspected, treatment must be initiated quickly. Many of the steps in the diagnosis and management must be carried out simultaneously (Figure 16-7). For brisk bleeding from any cause, a large-bore IV line should be started. Oxygen may be given and vital signs monitored. If bleeding occurs before placental delivery, attention is directed to removal of placenta. If atony is suspected, massage and uterotonics are started and blood loss and uterine tone are reevaluated frequently. During this time, the lower genital tract can be explored and lacerations repaired if needed. If uterine atony has been treated and no birth trauma or inversion recognized, it is useful to inspect the placenta and membranes, as well as explore the uterus, to determine whether retained placental fragments are responsible for continued bleeding. Uterine exploration will also allow detection of partial uterine inversion or rupture. Throughout the third stage, blood should be observed for appropriate clotting.

If not already present, help should be summoned if initial attempts to stop blood loss are unsuccessful. Blood loss greater than 1000 ml is considered severe and requires quick action using an interdisciplinary team approach, including anesthesia and surgery. Type and crossmatch should be obtained if this information was not previously ascertained. In addition to rapid infusion of crystalloid, type-specific blood may be needed. A Foley catheter can be placed to empty the bladder and monitor urine output. Intractable hemorrhage may require uterine packing or other tamponade procedures, such as a Foley catheter bulb. Hemostatic drugs, such as recombinant factor VIIa, may be administered.[14,50] Manual removal or uterine curettage can be considered if retained placenta is suspected. Compression of the aorta can be a temporizing measure.[51] Angiographic embolization, surgical ligation of the uterine arteries, and/or hysterectomy may be required.

Management of Postpartum Hemorrhage

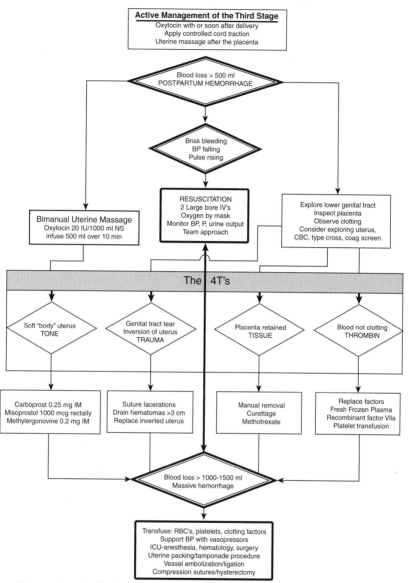

FIGURE 16-7. Many of the steps involved in diagnosing and treating postpartum hemorrhage (PPH) must be undertaken simultaneously. Although the steps in maternal resuscitation are consistent (center, bold), other actions taken may differ based on the actual cause. The causes are separated based on the Advanced Life Support and Obstetrics (ALSO) 4 Ts mnemonic: Tone Tissue Trauma Thrombin. Team Approach: Many hospitals run team drills to help standardize the approach to maternal resuscitation. Team approach requires all members of the medical team to be aware and involved (residents, attending staff, nursing, anesthesia, obstetric backup and/or critical care staff may be included). Coagulation screen includes platelet count, prothrombin time (international normalized ratio), partial thromboplastin time, fibrinogen level, and fibrin split products (D-dimer). BP, Blood pressure; CBC, complete blood cell count; Coag, coagulation; ICU, intensive care unit; IM, intramuscularly; NS, normal saline; P, pulse; RBCs, red blood cells. (Original figure courtesy Janice Anderson, MD, and Duncan Etches, MD)

B. Diagnosis-Specific Approach to Treatment

1. Uterine atony

Uterine atony may respond to uterine compression massage or uterotonics by becoming firm, usually with an associated decrease in bleeding. Bimanual uterine massage is the first, and sometimes only, action required to treat uterine atony. It is performed by placing one hand in the vagina and compressing the body of the uterus, whereas the other hand massages the fundus from above through the abdominal wall.

If bleeding persists, massage should be followed by drugs that promote contraction of the uterus (Table 16-8). If not already infusing, oxytocin (Pitocin), which rarely has side effects, can be given. If bleeding continues and there is no hypertension, methylergonovine (Methergine) may be given intramuscularly. The generalized smooth muscle stimulation affects the gastrointestinal and vascular systems in addition to the uterus, causing the side effects nausea, vomiting, and increased BP.[12] Carboprost (Hemabate) is an alternative uterotonic that has been shown to decrease blood loss when other means have failed.[60] It can be given intramuscularly or intramyometrially through the abdominal wall by elevating the uterus with an intravaginal hand. Carboprost has been shown to control hemorrhage in up to 87 % of cases.[60] In cases where carboprost was ineffective, chorioamnionitis was often present.[52,61] Side effects include nausea, vomiting, and diarrhea. Misoprostol (Cytotec) is effective in the treatment of PPH, although it is not FDA approved for this use. Side effects (nausea, vomiting, diarrhea, pyrexia, and shivering) may limit its usefullness.[36,59] Greater levels and larger doses are associated with more side effects.[59,62]

TABLE 16-8 Medications Used for Postpartum Hemorrhage

Medication	Dose	Contraindications/Cautions	Mechanism of Action
Oxytocin (Pitocin, Syntocinon)	10 IU IM 20-40 IU/L NS infusion 500 ml over 10 minutes, then 250 ml/hr[25] Alternate routes: IMM[53] IV bolus*	Contraindication: none	Stimulates the upper segment of the myometrium to contract rhythmically, constricting spiral arteries decreasing blood flow through the uterus[54]
Methylergonovine (Methergine)	0.2 mg IM repeat every 2-4 hours Alternative route: IMM[53]	Contraindication: hypertension/toxemia Caution: sepsis; vascular, hepatic, or renal disease	Vasoconstriction and contracts smooth muscles upper and lower segments of the uterus tetanically[12]
Carboprost (Hemabate) Prostaglandin F$_2\alpha$ analog	0.25 mg, IM or intramyometrially, repeated every 15-90 minutes for a total dose of 2 mg	Contraindication: active pulmonary, renal, hepatic, or cardiac disease Caution: history of asthma; hypertension; hypotension; cardiovascular, renal, or hepatic disease; anemia; jaundice; diabetes; or seizure disorder	Improves uterine contractility by increasing the number of oxytocin receptors and causes vasoconstriction[55]
Misoprostol† (Cytotec) Prostaglandin E$_1$ analog	200-600 μg PO or 400-1000 μg PR Best dose and route has yet to be determined‡	Contraindication: none Caution: cardiovascular disease	Generalized smooth muscle contraction [56]

Adapted from *Mosby's drug consult,* St. Louis, 2005, Mosby.
IM, Intramuscular; IMM, intramyometrially; IV, intravenous; NS, normal saline; PO, orally; PR, per rectum; prostaglandin F$_2\alpha$, 15-methyl prostaglandin F$_2\alpha$.
*A recent randomized controlled trial found that a 10-unit intravenous bolus did not cause significant hypotension.[57] This contradicts the long-held view that direct intravenous administration increases the risk for transient hypotension.[58]
†Despite widespread use, there is no Federal Drug Administration indication for misoprostol use in postpartum hemorrhage.
‡Dosages range from 200-1000 μg via oral, sublingual, rectal, and vaginal routes, sometimes in combination.[36,49,59]

2. Genital tract trauma

Bleeding lacerations should be repaired immediately. Small hematomas can be managed with close observation.[63] However, if the patient has signs of volume loss despite fluid replacement, or large or enlarging hematomas, then incision and evacuation of the clot is required.[63] The involved area should be irrigated and the bleeding vessels ligated. Where there is diffuse oozing, a layered closure will help to secure hemostasis and eliminate dead space. Broad-spectrum antibiotics are useful and drains are often necessary. Adequate anesthesia/analgesia is essential for exploration and repair.[15]

3. Uterine inversion

Every attempt should be made to replace the uterus quickly to its normal position. Concurrent intravascular support/maternal resuscitation are often needed. In approximately 50% of cases, the placenta is still attached and it can be left in place until after reduction to minimize blood loss.[23] The Johnson method of manual reduction begins with grasping the protruding fundus with palm of the hand, fingers directed toward the posterior fornix. The uterus is returned to position by lifting it up through the pelvis and into the abdomen with steady pressure toward the umbilicus.[64] Hydrostatic methods, which consist of infusing warm saline into vagina while occluding the introitus, have been successful as well. Various methods of occlusion have been reported, including the forearm and a vacuum extractor silastic cup.[50] Once the uterus is reverted, oxytocic agents can be given to promote uterine tone and prevent recurrence. If initial attempts to replace the uterus have failed or a cervical contraction ring develops, magnesium sulfate ($MgSO_4$), terbutaline, nitroglycerin, or general anesthesia may allow sufficient uterine relaxation for manipulation.[50] Failing this, the uterus will need to be replaced surgically.[23]

4. Uterine rupture

When found postpartum, a small asymptomatic lower uterine segment defect or bloodless dehiscence can be treated expectantly.[20] Symptomatic uterine rupture will require immediate fluid resuscitation and surgical repair of the defect, with probable hysterectomy. Temporary measures used while preparing for surgery include direct aortic compression and anteflexion, elevation, and compression of the uterus.[51]

5. Retained and invasive placenta

Firm traction on the umbilical cord with one hand, while applying suprapubic counterpressure with the opposite hand (Brandt maneuver), typically achieves placental delivery.[30] If retained, one management option is to inject the umbilical vein with 20 ml of a 0.9 % saline containing 10 to 20 units of oxytocin. This significantly reduces the need for manual removal of the placenta as compared with injecting saline alone.[28] Alternatively, one may proceed directly to manual removal of the placenta using appropriate analgesia. If retained fragments are suspected, they may be removed manually with a gauze sponge over the fingers or by curetting with a large loop.

The risk for PPH increases significantly if the placenta remains in place for more than 18 to 30 minutes.[5,10] If the tissue plane between uterine wall and placenta cannot be developed through blunt dissection with the edge of the gloved hand, invasive placenta should be considered (see Section F in this chapter).

The usual treatment for invasive placenta is intravascular volume support and hysterectomy. Dissection of tissue planes in placenta percreta involving pelvic organs can cause profuse, uncontrolled bleeding. Multiple case reports support conservative management of hemodynamically stable patients in this situation.[34] This includes leaving the placenta in place with or without weekly oral methotrexate[65] until beta human chorionic gonadotropin levels are zero.[34] Women treated for a retained placenta must be observed for late sequelae, including infection and secondary PPH.[34,65]

6. Coagulation disorders

In addition to maternal resuscitation measures, management of a coagulation disorder consists of treating the underlying disease process, serially evaluating the coagulation status, and replacing appropriate blood components.[14] Many smaller hospitals do not have platelets or fresh frozen plasma available, and emergency transportation systems may need to be activated.[66]

a. Maintain fibrinogen levels at more than 100 mg/ml with fresh frozen plasma. Each unit increases the fibrinogen 10 mg/100 ml. Cryoprecipitate can be used if the fibrinogen level is less than 50 mg/ml (expected increase is 2-5 mg/100 ml per bag of cryoprecipitate).

b. Maintain platelet count greater than 50,000. Each pack increases the platelet count by 5,000 to 10,000. Eight packs of random, pooled-donor platelets or one single-donor apheresis pack should be administered for every six units of packed red blood cells.

c. Maintain the hematocrit at or greater than 30% with packed red blood cells. Each unit increases the hematocrit by 3% and the hemoglobin by 1.5 g/ml.

d. Correct a prolonged prothrombin (INR) time with fresh frozen plasma. One unit is usually given for every four to five units of packed red blood cells or stored whole blood.

VI. CLINICAL COURSE

Women who have had PPH may experience postpartum dizziness from orthostatic hypotension or anemia with fatigue, which may make care of the newborn more difficult.[8] Postpartum anemia increases the risk for postpartum depression.[67] Transfusion may be necessary, which carries risks for transfusion reaction, HIV, hepatitis C, hepatitis B, cytomegalovirus, and syphilis.[68] In addition to mortality, severe cases of hemorrhage can lead to hypovolemic shock, renal or hepatic failure, DIC, myocardial ischemia, or ARDS.[59,69] Anterior pituitary ischemia (Sheehan syndrome) may delay or result in failure of lactation.[70,71] Though rare, severe PPH can be catastrophic; it is therefore important to practice prevention and aim for early recognition and treatment.

VII. SOR A RECOMMENDATIONS

RECOMMENDATIONS	REFERENCES

AMTSL decreases postpartum blood loss, length of third stage, and the incidence of PPH.
    Blood loss—weighted mean difference −80 ml (95% CI, −95 to −65)
    Length of third stage—NNT = 4 for >20 minutes; NNT = 10 for >40 minutes
    Incidence of PPH—NNT = 12 for >500 ml blood loss; NNT = 57 for >1000 ml blood loss
	37

There is no significant increase in the occurrence of retained placenta with AMTSL.	8, 37, 43
Oxytocin remains the first choice for prevention because it is as or more effective[8] than prostaglandins or ergot alkaloids and has fewer side effects.[4,45]	4, 8, 45

Elbourne[8]: *loss > 500 ml oxytocin vs. ergotamine: RR, 1.03 (95% CI, 0.73-1.47); loss > 1000 ml oxytocin vs. ergotamine: RR, 1.09 (95% CI, 0.45-2.66)*
    McDonald[45]: *oxytocin-ergotamine versus oxytocin alone: NNH = 6 for nausea and vomiting; NNH = 95 for increased diastolic blood pressure*
    Gulmezoglu[4]: *misoprostol versus oxytocin (or oxytocin-ergotamine): NNH = 7 for any negative side effects*	

Umbilical vein injection (20 units oxytocin in 20 ml saline) as treatment for retained placenta decreases need for manual removal of placenta (NNT = 8 for manual removal).	8
Misoprostol is effective for treatment of PPH but has more side effects than conventional uterotonic drugs:	36, 59
Mousa[59]: *NNT = 4 for persistent hemorrhage* Hofmeyr[36]: *NNT = 14 for blood loss > 500 ml; NNT = 101 for blood loss > 1000 ml (NS); NNH = 4 for any side effect*	
Misoprostol is effective for prevention of PPH and has advantages in resource-poor settings because it is inexpensive, heat stable, and simple to administer (NNT = 18 for any PPH[48]).	47, 48

Acknowledgments

Special thanks to Duncan Etches, MD, Marcy Brown, Linda Shab, and Janey Geier.

REFERENCES

1. AbouZahr C: Global burden of maternal death and disability, *Br Med Bull* 67:1-11, 2003.
2. Chong YS, Su LL, Arulkumaran S: Current strategies for the prevention of postpartum haemorrhage in the third stage of labour, *Curr Opin Obstet Gynecol* 16(2):143-150, 2004.
3. Bais JM, Eskes M, Pel M et al: Postpartum haemorrhage in nulliparous women: incidence and risk factors in low and high risk women. A Dutch population-based cohort study on standard (> or = 500 ml) and severe (> or = 1000 ml) postpartum haemorrhage, *Eur J Obstet Gynecol Reprod Biol* 115(2):166-172, 2004.
4. Gulmezoglu AM, Forna F, Villar J et al: Prostaglandins for prevention of postpartum haemorrhage, *Cochrane Database Syst Rev* (1):CD000494, 2004.

5. Magann EF, Evans S, Chauhan SP et al: The length of the third stage of labor and the risk of postpartum hemorrhage, *Obstet Gynecol* 105(2):290-293, 2005.

6. ACOG educational bulletin. Hemorrhagic shock. Number 235, April 1997 (replaces No. 82, December 1984). American College of Obstetricians and Gynecologists, *Int J Gynaecol Obstet* 57(2):219-226, 1997.

7. Razvi K, Chua S, Arulkumaran S et al: A comparison between visual estimation and laboratory determination of blood loss during the third stage of labour, *Aust N Z J Obstet Gynaecol* 36(2):152-154, 1996.

8. Elbourne DR, Prendiville WJ, Carroli G et al: Prophylactic use of oxytocin in the third stage of labour, *Cochrane Database Syst Rev* (4):CD001808, 2001.

9. Magann EF, Evans S, Hutchinson M et al: Postpartum hemorrhage after vaginal birth: an analysis of risk factors, *South Med J* 98(4):419-422, 2005.

10. Combs CA, Murphy EL, Laros RK Jr: Factors associated with postpartum hemorrhage with vaginal birth, *Obstet Gynecol* 77(1):69-76, 1991.

11. Stones RW, Paterson CM, Saunders NJ: Risk factors for major obstetric haemorrhage, *Eur J Obstet Gynecol Reprod Biol* 48(1):15-18, 1993.

12. De Costa C: St Anthony's fire and living ligatures: a short history of ergometrine, *Lancet* 359(9319):1768-1770, 2002.

13. Magann EF, Lanneau GS: Third stage of labor, *Obstet Gynecol Clin North Am* 32(2):323-332, 2005.

14. Alamia V Jr, Meyer BA: Peripartum hemorrhage, *Obstet Gynecol Clin North Am* 26(2):385-398, 1999.

15. Zahn CM, Yeomans ER: Postpartum hemorrhage: placenta accreta, uterine inversion, and puerperal hematomas, *Clin Obstet Gynecol* 33(3):422-431, 1990.

16. Chauhan SP, Martin JN Jr, Henrichs CE et al: Maternal and perinatal complications with uterine rupture in 142,075 patients who attempted vaginal birth after cesarean delivery: a review of the literature, *Am J Obstet Gynecol* 189(2):408-417, 2003.

17. Guise JM, McDonagh MS, Osterweil P et al: Systematic review of the incidence and consequences of uterine rupture in women with previous caesarean section, *BMJ* 329(7456):19-25, 2004.

18. Landon MB, Hauth JC, Leveno KJ et al: Maternal and perinatal outcomes associated with a trial of labor after prior cesarean delivery, *N Engl J Med* 351(25):2581-2589, 2004.

19. American Academy of Family Physicians (AAFP): Trial of labor after cesarean (TOLAC), formerly trial of labor versus elective repeat cesarean section for the woman with a previous cesarean section. AAFP Policy Action, March 2005.

20. ACOG practice bulletin #54: vaginal birth after previous cesarean, *Obstet Gynecol* 104(1):203-212, 2004.

21. ACOG Committee Opinion No. 342: induction of labor for vaginal birth after cesarean delivery, *Obstet Gynecol* 108(2):465-468, 2006.

22. Siddiqui M, Ranasinghe JS: Spontaneous rupture of uterus, *J Clin Anesth* 14(5):368-370, 2002.

23. Baskett TF: Acute uterine inversion: a review of 40 cases, *J Obstet Gynaecol Can* 24(12):953-956, 2002.

24. Kitchin JD 3rd, Thiagarajah S, May HV Jr et al: Puerperal inversion of the uterus, *Am J Obstet Gynecol* 123(1):51-58, 1975.

25. Gabbe SG: *Obstetrics: normal and problem pregnancies,* ed 4, New York, 2002, Churchill Livingston.

26. Brar HS, Greenspoon JS, Platt LD et al: Acute puerperal uterine inversion. New approaches to management, *J Reprod Med* 34(2):173-177, 1989.

27. Weeks AD, Mirembe FM: The retained placenta-new insights into an old problem, *Eur J Obstet Gynecol Reprod Biol* 102(2):109-110, 2002.

28. Carroli G, Bergel E: Umbilical vein injection for management of retained placenta, *Cochrane Database Syst Rev* (4):CD001337, 2001.

29. Miller DA, Chollet JA, Goodwin TM: Clinical risk factors for placenta previa-placenta accreta, *Am J Obstet Gynecol* 177(1):210-214, 1997.

30. Wu S, Kocherginsky M, Hibbard JU: Abnormal placentation: twenty-year analysis, *Am J Obstet Gynecol* 192(5):1458-1461, 2005.

31. Pritchard JA: Fetal death in utero, *Obstet Gynecol* 14:573-580, 1959.

32. The prevention and management of postpartum haemorrhage. In *WHO report of technical working group,* Geneva, 1990, World Health Organization.

33. Singla AK, Lapinski RH, Berkowitz RL et al: Are women who are Jehovah's Witnesses at risk of maternal death? *Am J Obstet Gynecol* 185(4):893-895, 2001.

34. O'Brien JM, Barton JR, Donaldson ES: The management of placenta percreta: conservative and operative strategies, *Am J Obstet Gynecol* 175(6):1632-1638, 1996.

35. ACOG committee opinion. Placenta accreta. Number 266, January 2002. American College of Obstetricians and Gynecologists, *Int J Gynaecol Obstet* 77(1):77-78, 2002.

36. Hofmeyr GJ, Walraven G, Gulmezoglu AM et al: Misoprostol to treat postpartum haemorrhage: a systematic review, *Br J Obstet Gynaecol* 112(5):547-553, 2005.

37. Prendiville WJ, Elbourne D, McDonald S: Active versus expectant management in the third stage of labour, *Cochrane Database Syst Rev* (2):CD000007, 2000.

38. Lalonde A, Daviss BA, Acosta A et al: Postpartum hemorrhage today: ICM/FIGO initiative 2004-2006, *Int J Gynaecol Obstet* 94(3):243-253, 2006.

39. Ceriani Cernadas JM, Carroli G, Pellegrini L et al: The effect of timing of cord clamping on neonatal venous hematocrit values and clinical outcome at term: a randomized, controlled trial, *Pediatrics* 117(4):e779-e786, 2006.

40. Chaparro CM, Neufeld LM, Tena Alavez G et al: Effect of timing of umbilical cord clamping on iron status in Mexican infants: a randomised controlled trial, *Lancet* 367(9527):1997-2004, 2006.

41. Rabe H, Reynolds G, Diaz-Rossello J: Early versus delayed umbilical cord clamping in preterm infants, *Cochrane Database Syst Rev* (4):CD003248, 2004.

42. van Rheenen P, Brabin BJ: Late umbilical cord-clamping as an intervention for reducing iron deficiency anaemia in term infants in developing and industrialised countries: a systematic review, *Ann Trop Paediatr* 24(1):3-16, 2004.

43. Jackson KW Jr, Allbert JR, Schemmer GK et al: A randomized controlled trial comparing oxytocin administration before and after placental delivery in the prevention of postpartum hemorrhage, *Am J Obstet Gynecol* 185(4):873-877, 2001.

44. Rizvi F, Mackey R, Barrett T et al: Successful reduction of massive postpartum haemorrhage by use of guidelines and staff education, *Br J Obstet Gynaecol* 111(5):495-498, 2004.

45. McDonald S, Abbott JM, Higgins SP: Prophylactic ergometrine-oxytocin versus oxytocin for the third stage of labour, *Cochrane Database Syst Rev* (1):CD000201, 2004.

46. McCormick ML, Sanghvi HC, Kinzie B et al: Preventing postpartum hemorrhage in low-resource settings, *Int J Gynaecol Obstet* 77(3):267-275, 2002.

47. Oboro VO, Tabowei TO: A randomised controlled trial of misoprostol versus oxytocin in the active management of the third stage of labour, *J Obstet Gynaecol* 23(1):13-16, 2003.

48. Derman RJ, Kodkany BS, Goudar SS et al: Oral misoprostol in preventing postpartum haemorrhage in resource-poor communities: a randomised controlled trial, *Lancet* 368(9543): 1248-1253, 2006.

49. Chong YS, Chua S, Shen L et al: Does the route of administration of misoprostol make a difference? The uterotonic effect and side effects of misoprostol given by different routes after vaginal delivery, *Eur J Obstet Gynecol Reprod Biol* 113(2):191-198, 2004.

50. Thomson AJ, Greer IA: Non-haemorrhagic obstetric shock, *Baillieres Best Pract Res Clin Obstet Gynaecol* 14(1):19-41, 2000.

51. Riley DP, Burgess RW: External abdominal aortic compression: a study of a resuscitation manoeuvre for postpartum haemorrhage, *Anaesth Intensive Care* 22(5):571-575, 1994.

52. *Mosby's drug consult*, St. Louis, 2005, Mosby.

53. Dildy GA 3rd: Postpartum hemorrhage: new management options, *Clin Obstet Gynecol* 45(2):330-344, 2002.

54. Blanks AM, Thornton S: The role of oxytocin in parturition, *Br J Obstet Gynaecol* 110(suppl 20):46-51, 2003.

55. Lamont RF, Morgan DJ, Logue M et al: A prospective randomised trial to compare the efficacy and safety of hemabate and syntometrine for the prevention of primary postpartum haemorrhage, *Prostaglandins Other Lipid Mediat* 66(3):203-210, 2001.

56. Magann EF, Lanneau GS: Third stage of labor, *Obstet Gynecol Clin North Am* 32(2):323-332, 2005.

57. Davies GA, Tessier JL, Woodman MC et al: Maternal hemodynamics after oxytocin bolus compared with infusion in the third stage of labor: a randomized controlled trial, *Obstet Gynecol* 105(2):294-299, 2005.

58. Hendricks CH, Brenner WE: Cardiovascular effects of oxytocic drugs used post partum, *Am J Obstet Gynecol* 108(5):751-760, 1970.

59. Mousa HA, Alfirevic Z: Treatment for primary postpartum haemorrhage, *Cochrane Database Syst Rev* (1):CD003249, 2003.

60. Oleen MA, Mariano JP: Controlling refractory atonic postpartum hemorrhage with Hemabate sterile solution, *Am J Obstet Gynecol* 162(1):205-208, 1990.

61. Duff P, Sanders R, Gibbs RS: The course of labor in term patients with chorioamnionitis, *Am J Obstet Gynecol* 147(4):391-395, 1983.

62. Lumbiganon P, Villar J, Piaggio G et al: Side effects of oral misoprostol during the first 24 hours after administration in the third stage of labour, *Br J Obstet Gynaecol* 109(11):1222-1226, 2002.

63. Benrubi G, Neuman C, Nuss RC et al: Vulvar and vaginal hematomas: a retrospective study of conservative versus operative management, *South Med J* 80(8):991-994, 1987.

64. Watson P, Besch N, Bowes WA Jr: Management of acute and subacute puerperal inversion of the uterus, *Obstet Gynecol* 55(1):12-16, 1980.

65. Mussalli GM, Shah J, Berck DJ et al: Placenta accreta and methotrexate therapy: three case reports, *J Perinatol* 20(5):331-334, 2000.

66. Skye DV: Management of peripartum hemorrhage, *WMJ* 97(11):43-46, 1998.

67. Corwin EJ, Murray-Kolb LE, Beard JL: Low hemoglobin level is a risk factor for postpartum depression, *J Nutr* 133(12):4139-4142, 2003.

68. Ekeroma AJ, Ansari A, Stirrat GM: Blood transfusion in obstetrics and gynaecology, *Br J Obstet Gynaecol* 104(3):278-284, 1997.

69. Karpati PC, Rossignol M, Pirot M et al: High incidence of myocardial ischemia during postpartum hemorrhage, *Anesthesiology* 100(1):30-36, discussion 5A, 2004.

70. Willis CE, Livingstone V: Infant insufficient milk syndrome associated with maternal postpartum hemorrhage, *J Hum Lact* 11(2):123-126, 1995.

71. Sert M, Tetiker T, Kirim S et al: Clinical report of 28 patients with Sheehan's syndrome, *Endocr J* 50(3):297-301, 2003.

SECTION F Retained Placenta

Jose Matthew Mata, MD, MS, and David Turok, MD, MPH

One of the more amazing aspects of childbirth is the routine release of the placenta minutes after delivery of the baby. When the third stage of labor exceeds 30 minutes, the diagnosis of retained placenta can be made. This condition may be complicated by PPH and, on rare occasion, may be a harbinger of a potentially catastrophic hemorrhage in the setting of the morbidly adherent placenta.

I. EPIDEMIOLOGY

Retained placenta occurs in 3% of vaginal deliveries,[1] with placenta accreta being a rare cause (1/2000).[2] Retained placenta is the cause of 6% of all PPHs[3] and is the second most common indication for blood transfusion in the third stage of labor, after uterine atony.[4] Risk factors for retained placenta include multiparity (≥5 prior deliveries), induced labor, excessive blood loss (≥500 ml), previous history of retained placenta, PTL, small placental weight (<500 g), history of dilation and curettage, and history of cesarean delivery.[5]

II. PATHOGENESIS AND CLINICAL FEATURES

A. Insufficient Uterine Contractions

Uterine contractions may not be sufficient to induce detachment of the placenta.

B. Entrapped Placenta

Detachment of the placenta may occur, but it may become trapped by contraction of the lower uterine segment.

C. Insufficient Decidual Tissue

The placenta may be abnormally adherent to the placenta because of scant or absent decidual layer, leading to an aberration of the normal cleavage plane. This situation creates a morbidly adherent placenta, classified by depth of invasion:

1. Placenta accreta (Table 16-9)
   The placenta is adherent to the myometrium.
2. Placenta increta
   The placenta invades the myometrium.
3. Placenta percreta
   The placenta penetrates the myometrium and the serosal surface.

The spectrum of adherent placenta can lead to considerable morbidity, or even mortality, through severe hemorrhage, uterine perforation, and in the case of percreta, placental invasion of surrounding structures.

III. DIAGNOSIS AND TREATMENT

A. Umbilical Cord Traction

Controlled traction on the umbilical cord may affect delivery of the trapped placenta. However, when applying controlled traction on the umbilical cord, suprapubic counter pressure should be applied to prevent uterine inversion.

B. Use of Intraumbilical Vein Injection of Oxytocin

Manual removal of the placenta is an option for the treatment of retained placenta, but it carries the risks for hemorrhage, infection, and genital tract trauma. In an attempt to avoid manual removal of the placenta, intraumbilical vein injection of oxytocin (10-20 units oxytocin in 20 ml of saline solution) has been proposed as an alternative to the management of retained placenta. A Cochrane review[6] of the use of intraumbilical vein oxytocin injection found that saline solution plus oxytocin compared with expectant management was associated with lower rates of manual removal of the placenta, but the differences were not statistically significant. No difference was found in blood loss, hemoglobin level, need for blood transfusion, need for curettage, infection, or length of hospital stay.[6] However, when saline solution and oxytocin were compared with saline alone, there was a significant reduction in the need for manual removal of the placenta (RR, 0.79; 95% CI, 0.69-0.91; NNT = 8).

TABLE 16-9 Identified Risk Factors for Placenta Accreta

Placenta previa

Prior cesarean delivery

Postpregnancy curettage

Prior myomectomy

Submucous leiomyomata

Prior retained placenta

Uterine infection

Maternal age >35 years

Adapted from Zahn CM, Yeomans ER: Postpartum hemorrhage: placenta accreta, uterine inversion, and puerperal hematomas, *Clin Obstet Gynecol* 3:422-431, 1990; and Bullarbo M, Tjuqum J, Ekerhovd E: Sublingual nitroglycerin for management of retained placenta, *Int J Gynaecol Obstet* 91:228-232, 2005.

Intraumbilical vein administration of oxytocin appears to have no significant side effects. Given its apparent safety and a possible reduction in the need for manual removal, intraumbilical vein injection of oxytocin can be considered for the management of retained placenta. To further clarify the efficacy of this treatment, a study is currently under way to randomize 572 women with retained placenta in the United Kingdom and Uganda.[7]

C. Sulprostone

A recent RCT from the Netherlands compared IV sulprostone, a synthetic prostaglandin E_2 derivative, with placebo in patients with retained placenta who had already received 60 minutes of AMTSL. Among the 50 randomized patients, 51.8% of those who received sulprostone expelled their placentas versus 17.6% of those receiving placebo ($p = 0.034$; NNT = 3).[8] Although this medication is not currently available in the United States, it may become an option in the future. Of note, the authors cite several case reports of adverse cardiac events in patients exposed to this medication, although none occurred in the study.

D. Uterine Relaxation for Entrapped Placenta

General anesthesia with halothane and tocolytics may allow delivery of a retained placenta by relaxing the uterus. Alternatively, general anesthesia may be used to assist in manual removal of the placenta.[9] However, this approach deserves caution because it may lead to excessive blood loss, which would require rapid reversal of uterine relaxation.

The use of IV or sublingual nitroglycerin has been proposed as an alternative to general anesthesia in the management of retained placenta. In a prospective study, a range of 50 to 200 μg IV nitroglycerin was adequate to cause uterine relaxation sufficient for manual removal of the placenta without any significant complications.[10] In an RCT, all 12 patients with retained placenta who received 1 mg sublingual nitroglycerin had successful delivery of the placenta versus 1 of 12 similar patients randomized to placebo.[11]

E. Manual Removal of the Placenta

If noninvasive measures fail to deliver the placenta, manual removal of the placenta can be performed. This is accomplished by attempting to identify the cleavage plane with a sterile, gloved hand placed inside the uterus. Before attempting manual removal, at least one, and preferably two, large-bore IV lines should be in place. Blood products, anesthesia, and surgical backup should be readily available because a complete placenta accreta may not bleed initially, but blood loss may be profuse once separation is attempted.

If a cleavage plane can be identified, the hand should be advanced between the placenta and uterus, attempting to deliver the placenta intact. When parts of the placenta are adherent, uterine curettage may be used to remove any fragments. After the placenta has been removed, uterotonic agents may be used to promote uterine contractility. If there is a resulting hemorrhage, an emergency hysterectomy may be required. Manual removal of the placenta places the patient at risk for late PPH, infection, and genital tract trauma. Prophylactic antibiotics, such as 1 g IV cefazolin administered at the time of the procedure, may be considered when performing manual removal of the placenta, though a Cochrane review failed to show any additional benefit from this procedure.[12]

F. Suspected Placenta Accreta

Risk factors for placenta accreta are listed in Table 16-9. There is a synergistic effect of placenta previa and prior cesarean delivery on the risk for placenta accreta. The risk for accreta with a placenta previa alone is 4% to 5%. If that same patient has a history of one prior cesarean delivery, the risk increases to 10% to 24%. If the patient has had two or more previous cesarean deliveries, the risk is 30% to 48%.[13-15] If there is a strong suspicion for placenta accreta

before delivery, the patient should be counseled about the likelihood of hysterectomy and blood transfusion. Cell saver should be considered and delivery should occur in a location with adequate available surgical support.[16]

IV. PREVENTION

A Cochrane review of the AMTSL (see Section E) with oxytocin at the time of delivery, early cord clamping, and cord traction was associated with a decreased incidence of retained placenta.[17] One study of 477 women has also shown that drainage of the umbilical cord reduced the incidence of retained placenta (RR, 0.28; 95% CI, 0.10-0.73).[18] A recent Cochrane review of drainage of the umbilical cord, which included the above study, found an overall significant reduction in the length of the third stage of labor.[19] However, this Cochrane review was performed with only two studies, and the authors state that it is difficult to draw conclusions from these studies because the use of oxytocics was not standardized and data for other outcome variables were not readily available. However, drainage of the umbilical cord is a simple procedure, has no known adverse effects, and can be considered as a preventative measure for retained placenta.

V. SOR A RECOMMENDATIONS

RECOMMENDATIONS	REFERENCES
AMTSL can reduce the incidence of retained placenta.	17
Oxytocin and saline solution given via the umbilical vein reduces the need for manual removal of the placenta (NNT = 8).	6

REFERENCES

1. Combs CA, Laros RK Jr: Prolonged third stage of labor: morbidity and risk factors, *Obstet Gynecol* 77(6):863-867, 1991.
2. Zahn CM, Yeomans ER: Postpartum hemorrhage: placenta accreta, uterine inversion, and puerperal hematomas, *Clin Obstet Gynecol* 3:422-431, 1990.
3. Weeks LR, O'Toole DM: Postpartum hemorrhage: a five year study at Queen of Angeles Hospital, *Am J Obstet Gynecol* 71:45-50, 1956.
4. Kamani AA, McMorland GA, Wadsworth LD: Utilization of red blood cell transfusion in an obstetric setting, *Am J Obstet Gynecol* 159:1177-1181, 1988.

5. Adelusi B, Soltan MH, Chowdhury N, Kangave D: Risk of re-tained placenta: multivariate approach, *Acta Obstet Gynecol Scand* 76:414-418, 1997.

6. Carroli G, Bergel E: Umbilical vein injection for management of retained placenta, *Cochrane Database Syst Rev* (4):CD001337, 2001.

7. Weeks A, Mirembe F, Alfirevic Z: The Release Trial: a ran-domized controlled trial of umbilical vein oxytocin versus placebo for the treatment of retained placenta, *BJOG* 112:1458, 2005.

8. Van Beekhuizen HJ, de Groot AN, De Boo T et al: Sulprostone reduces the need for the manual removal of the placenta in patients with retained placenta: a randomized controlled trial, *Am J Obstet Gynecol* 194(2):446-450, 2006.

9. Hood DD: Anesthetic techniques in obstetric emergencies, *Acta Anaesth Scand* 111:172-173, 1997.

10. Chedraui PA, Insuasti DF: Intravenous nitroglycerin in the management of retained placenta, *Gynecol Obstet Invest* 56:61-64, 2003.

11. Bullarbo M, Tjuqum J, Ekerhovd E: Sublingual nitroglycerin for management of retained placenta, *Int J Gynaecol Obstet* 91:228-232, 2005.

12. Chongsomchai C, Lumbiganon P, Laopaiboon M: Prophylactic antibiotics for manual removal of retained placenta in vaginal birth, *Cochrane Database Syst Rev* (2):CD004904, 2006.

13. Clark SL, Koonings PP, Phelan JP: Placenta previa/accreta and prior cesarean section, *Obstet Gynecol* 66:89-92, 1985.

14. Gesteland K, Oshiro B, Henry E et al: Rates of placenta previa and placental abruption in women delivered only vaginally or only by cesarean section. Abstract No. 403, *J Soc Gynecol Ivestig* 11:208A, 2004.

15. Miller DA, Chollet JA, Goodwin TM: Clinical risk factors for placenta previa-placenta accrete, *Am J Obstet Gynecol* 177: 210-214, 1997.

16. Placenta accreta. ACOG Committee Opinion No. 266. American College of Obstetricians and Gynecologists, *Obstet Gynecol* 99: 169-170, 2002.

17. Prendville WJ, Elbourne D, McDonald S: Active versus expectant management in the third stage of labour, *Cochrane Database Syst Rev* (3):CD000007, 2000.

18. Giacalone PL, Vignal J, Daures JP et al: A randomized evalua-tion of two techniques of management of the third stage of labour in women at low risk of postpartum hemorrhage, *BJOG* 107:396-400, 2000.

19. Soltani H, Dickinson F, Symonds I: Placental cord drainage after spontaneous vaginal delivery as part of the management of the third stage of labour, *Cochrane Database Syst Rev* (4): CD004665, 2005.

Section G **Preeclampsia and Eclampsia**

Lawrence Leeman, MD, MPH

Preeclampsia is a common complication of preg-nancy that affects approximately 2% to 8% of all preg-nancies.[1,2] It is the third leading cause of maternal mortality in the United States.[3] Neonatal morbidity and mortality result from the need for preterm deliv-ery for maternal reasons and directly from IUGR and placental abruption.

I. EPIDEMIOLOGY AND PATHOGENESIS

A. Associated Risk Factors

Factors that are strongly associated with an increased risk for preeclampsia include nulliparity, maternal age older than 40, multiple gestation, preeclampsia in a prior pregnancy (particularly when it was severe, be-fore 32 weeks, or both), chronic hypertension, chronic renal disease, antiphospholipid syndrome, elevated body mass index, and diabetes.[4]

B. Causative Factors

The cause of preeclampsia remains unknown; how-ever, abnormal placental implantation, endothelial cell abnormalities, altered levels of placental growth factor, and genetics all appear to be involved.[5]

Defective placental implantation and endothelial cell damage appear to underlie the development of preeclampsia. Pregnancies in which preeclampsia will develop demonstrate abnormal cytotrophoblas-tic invasion and incomplete transformation of uter-ine spiral arterioles during early pregnancy that leads to reduced placental perfusion.[6,7]

An increase of the serum level of soluble fms-like tyrosine kinase 1 (sFLT1) and a decrease in serum level of placental growth factor in the first half of pregnancy recently have been shown to be predictive of the later onset of preeclampsia.[8] Genetic factors are suggested by the familial incidence of preeclam-psia, although specific genes have not been identi-fied. The increased incidence of preeclampsia in first pregnancies may be caused by paternal genetic factors.[9,10]

II. DIAGNOSIS

Preeclampsia is a multiorgan disease process charac-terized by a classic triad of hypertension, proteinuria, and edema. The diagnostic criteria are based on the presence of hypertension and proteinuria without regard to the presence of edema because of the fre-quent occurrence of benign gestational edema.

1. Hypertension criteria
   Hypertension is defined as a sustained elevation of blood pressure to levels of 140 mmHg systolic

or 90 mmHg diastolic or greater.[1,11,12] Elevated blood pressure must be present on at least 2 occasions, 6 hours or more apart, with onset after 20 weeks of pregnancy.[11,12] A change in blood pressure of 30 mmHg systolic or 15 mmHg diastolic is no longer included in the definition of preeclampsia.[1] Blood pressure should be measured using an appropriately sized cuff with the patient in an upright position. If the initial blood pressure is elevated, then a repeat blood pressure should be checked after the patient has had at least a 10-minute rest period. Fair evidence exists to recommend universal blood pressure screening for preeclampsia at regular prenatal visits.[11,12]

2. Proteinuria

The presence of proteinuria distinguishes preeclampsia from gestational hypertension. Women with elevated blood pressure or random urinalysis with one plus protein or greater need quantitative evaluation. The gold standard is a 24-hour urine protein determination with more than 300 mg protein. A spot urine protein/creatinine ratio may help to rule out clinically significant proteinuria if the ratio is less than 0.19.[13] Women with the development of elevated blood pressure (140/90 mmHg) after 20 weeks of pregnancy without proteinuria have gestational hypertension. These patients may ultimately experience development of proteinuria and be diagnosed with preeclampsia, or they may be diagnosed after delivery as having had either chronic hypertension (if hypertensive 6 weeks after delivery) or transient hypertension of pregnancy (if blood pressure normalizes after delivery).

3. Mild versus severe preeclampsia

The prognosis and management of preeclampsia are dependent on whether the disease is mild or severe. The criteria for severe preeclampsia include the presence of any of the following signs, symptoms, or laboratory findings: systolic blood pressure greater than 160 mmHg, diastolic blood pressure greater than 110 mmHg, more than 5 g protein on a 24-hour urine protein determination, platelet counts less than 100,000/mm³, increased transaminases or lactate dehydrogenase level, persistent headache, right upper quadrant or epigastric pain, visual changes, oliguria (<500 ml in 24 hours), or a fetus with IUGR.[1]

III. TREATMENT

A. Timing of Delivery

Preeclampsia usually resolves rapidly after delivery, and delivery at any gestational age is of benefit to maternal health but must be weighed against neonatal morbidity and mortality due to prematurity.

B. Mild Preeclampsia

Expectant management is recommended until term (>37 weeks of gestation) unless the patient develops severe preeclampsia or nonreassuring fetal surveillance occurs.[14,15]

C. Severe Preeclampsia

Expectant management remains controversial and is usually recommended only in a tertiary care center as an inpatient until 32 to 34 weeks.[16-18] There are specific contraindications to expectant management beyond the time needed to administer corticosteroids. These include thrombocytopenia, uncontrollable hypertension, oliguria, headache, right upper quadrant pain, and pulmonary edema.

D. Antepartum Surveillance

A nonstress test should be performed as part of the initial evaluation when preeclampsia is diagnosed. An ultrasound is recommended to assess fetal growth and amniotic fluid volume as preeclampsia is associated with uteroplacental insufficiency and IUGR. During expectant management of mild preeclampsia, twice weekly nonstress testing with weekly amniotic fluid assessment is commonly recommended.[15] When severe preeclampsia is managed expectantly, more intensive surveillance is indicated that may include daily nonstress tests. Umbilical cord Doppler assessment of systolic-to-diastolic ratio or other indicators of increased placental resistance to flow have been demonstrated to be of benefit in women with preeclampsia undergoing expectant management.[19,20]

E. Treatment of Hypertension

No fetal benefits to treating elevated blood pressure in preeclampsia have been demonstrated, and the potential exists to worsen fetal condition (growth restriction or nonreassuring fetal surveillance) because of uteroplacental insufficiency. Severe hypertension (systolic blood pressure > 160 mmHg or diastolic blood pressure > 110 mmHg) does need to be treated to prevent maternal end-organ damage including cerebrovascular accident. IV medicines are recommended in labor with either labetalol (initial dose 10-20 mg IV) or hydralazine (initial dose 5-10 mg IV) as first-line agents.[14] Women with severe preeclampsia undergoing expectant management remote from term may be treated with oral labetalol or methyldopa (Aldomet).

F. Seizure Prophylaxis

Magnesium sulfate ($MgSO_4$) is the most effective drug for the prevention and treatment of eclamptic seizure. Because the risk for seizure in woman with severe preeclampsia is about 3%, all women with severe preeclampsia should receive $MgSO_4$ during labor.[21] $MgSO_4$ may be started before labor or induction depending on the severity of the disease. Controversy exists regarding the risks and benefits of treating women with mild preeclampsia as their risk for development of eclampsia is only 1 in 200 women.[22] In settings where it is difficult to monitor the presence of urine output and presence of deep tendon reflexes, such as in some developing countries, it may be safer to defer use of $MgSO_4$.

1. Dosing

   The recommended loading dose for $MgSO_4$ is 4 to 6 g over 15 to 20 minutes, followed by an infusion of 2 g/hr. A lower infusion rate is indicated (e.g., 1 g/hr) for women with altered renal function or oliguria. Therapeutic magnesium blood levels are in the range of 4 to 7 mEq/L; however, they do not need to be routinely checked in women with normal renal function and deep tendon reflexes. Magnesium toxicity proceeds in a stepwise fashion as the level increases above the therapeutic range with loss of patellar reflexes in the 8 to 10 mEq/L range and respiratory arrest at a level of 13 mEq/L.[23]

2. Duration of therapy

   $MgSO_4$ is usually continued for 12 to 24 hours, with the longer duration recommended for women with severe preeclampsia or worsening postpartum preeclampsia. An alternative approach is to base the length of postpartum magnesium therapy on the pace of disease resolution as determined by diuresis and blood pressure measurements.

G. Eclampsia

Eclamptic seizures are generalized tonic-clonic seizures, which are usually self-limited and last less than 60 seconds. $MgSO_4$ is the first-line therapeutic agent.

Women who are not receiving $MgSO_4$ when they develop eclampsia should receive a 6-g loading dose over 15 to 20 minutes, followed by an infusion of 2 g/hr. Women who experience development of eclampsia while receiving $MgSO_4$ should be given an additional 2-g IV bolus unless they are demonstrating signs or symptoms of magnesium toxicity. Polypharmacy in which benzodiazepines or barbiturates are given to women with eclampsia should generally be avoided, although an IV barbiturate drip may occasionally be needed in women with status eclamptic seizures.

H. HELLP Syndrome

A severe variant of preeclampsia is the syndrome of Hemolysis, Elevated Liver enzymes, and Lowered Platelets, known as HELLP syndrome, which was first described in 1982.[24] HELLP syndrome may require transfer to a tertiary care hospital; however, all maternity care providers must be prepared to care for women with HELLP syndrome, which may develop in active labor when transfer is difficult. As with preeclampsia, delivery is the cure. Because of the increased maternal risk, expectant management beyond the time to administer corticosteroids is rarely recommended even in the setting of severe prematurity, and some women may need to be delivered before completing the course of corticosteroids.

Severe thrombocytopenia and spontaneous rupture of a subcapsular liver hematoma are two potentially life-threatening complications of HELLP. Spontaneous bleeding or PPHs caused by coagulopathy are unlikely if the platelet count is more than 50,000/mm^3. Platelet transfusion should be considered if the platelet count is less than 20,000/mm^3 or with hemorrhage in the setting of thrombocytopenia. Unfortunately, transfused platelets have a short life span and are primarily of benefit when given before anticipated delivery or for management of spontaneous bleeding. High-dose corticosteroids have been recommended to transiently stabilize or increase platelet count; however, there is no evidence that maternal outcomes or fetal outcomes are improved other than the known fetal benefits of corticosteroids for fetuses less than 34 weeks of gestation.[25,26] Regional anesthesia may be safely administered to women with preeclampsia and/or HELLP as long as the platelet count remains greater than 100,000/mm^3 and is generally contraindicated if the platelet count is less than 50,000/mm^3. In the range of 50,000 to 100,000/mm^3, the use of regional anesthesia is controversial and will be dependent on the anesthesiologist. Right upper quadrant pain may occur secondary to liver inflammation in HELLP syndrome, and a dreaded complication is rupture of a hematoma of the liver capsule, which can rapidly result in shock, ascites, and death. An abdominal ultrasound or computed tomography (CT) scan should be obtained to evaluate for a hematoma in the setting of severe persistent right upper quadrant, epigastric, or shoulder pain. If a liver hematoma ruptures, emergent laparotomy and massive blood transfusions are potentially life-saving, although the mortality rate remains quite high.

I. Postpartum Care

Maternal status may worsen for several days after delivery. Preeclampsia or HELLP syndrome may be initially diagnosed after delivery, usually within the first week. Blood pressure medication is recommended if the postpartum blood pressure remains persistently elevated above 150 mmHg systolic or 100 mmHg diastolic. Magnesium is usually continued for 12 to 24 hours postpartum; however, occasionally a worsening clinical picture or de novo onset of severe preeclampsia or HELLP will require continuation of magnesium beyond 24 hours or initiation during the postpartum time period.

IV. PREVENTION

Calcium supplementation (1 g/day) in women at increased risk for preeclampsia (NNT = 7.4) and/or low dietary calcium (NNT = 67) is beneficial in preventing preeclampsia and its sequelae.[27,28] Low-dose aspirin similarly appears of modest benefit in specific groups of women at increased risk, including those with previous severe preeclampsia, diabetes, chronic hypertension, or renal or autoimmune disease (NNT = 18).[29]

A recent World Health Organization RCT examined the role of calcium supplementation among 8325 nulliparous women with low calcium intake.[28] The women randomized to the supplementation arm of the study received 1.5 g/day of calcium. This treatment was not associated with a decrease in the incidence of preeclampsia but was associated with decreases in severe preeclampsia, eclampsia, and neonatal mortality. A need exists to conduct additional studies to measure the impact of calcium supplementation in women at increased risk for preeclampsia and those with low baseline calcium intake.

V. SOR A RECOMMENDATIONS

RECOMMENDATIONS	REFERENCES
$MgSO_4$ is the treatment of choice for women with preeclampsia to prevent eclamptic seizures (NNT = 100) and placental abruption (NNT = 100).	30
$MgSO_4$ is more effective in preventing recurrent eclamptic seizures than diazepam or phenytoin.	31-33
Low-dose aspirin has small-to-moderate benefits for prevention of preeclampsia (NNT = 69), preterm delivery (NNT = 83), and perinatal mortality (NNT = 227) in women at greater risk for development of preeclampsia.	29
Calcium supplementation decreases the risk for development of hypertension and preeclampsia, particularly among women with low baseline calcium supplementation (NNT = 67) and those at high risk for development of hypertension (NNT = 7.4).	27, 28
Use of umbilical artery Doppler velocitometry for women with severe hypertension or IUGR decreased the need for labor induction or cesarean delivery compared with nonstress testing.	19, 20

REFERENCES

1. American College of Obstetricians and Gynecologists. ACOG Practice Bulletin No. 33: diagnosis and management of preeclampsia and eclampsia, *Obstet Gynecol* 99:159-167, 2002.
2. Duley L: Pre-eclampsia and the hypertensive disorders of pregnancy, *Br Med Bull* 67:161-176, 2003.
3. Berg CJ, Chang J, Callaghan WM et al: Pregnancy-related mortality in the United States, 1991-1997, *Obstet Gynecol* 101:289-296, 2003.
4. Milne F, Redman C, Walker J et al: The pre-eclampsia community guideline (PRECOG): how to screen for and detect onset of pre-eclampsia in the community, *BMJ* 330:576-580, 2005.
5. Davison JM, Homuth V, Jeyabalan A et al: New aspects in the pathophysiology of preeclampsia, *J Am Soc Nephrol* 15:2440-2448, 2004.
6. McMaster MT, Zhou Y, Fisher SJ: Abnormal placentation and the syndrome of preeclampsia, *Semin Nephrol* 24:540-547, 2004.
7. Merviel P, Carbillon L, Challier JC et al: Pathophysiology of preeclampsia: links with implantation disorders, *Eur J Obstet Gynecol Reprod Biol* 115:134-147, 2004.
8. Levine RJ, Thadhani R, Qian C et al: Urinary placental growth factor and the risk of preeclampsia, *JAMA* 293:77-85, 2005.

9. Esplin MS, Fausett MB, Fraser A et al: Paternal and maternal components of the predisposition to preeclampsia, *N Engl J Med* 344:867-872, 2001.

10. Morgan T, Ward K: New insights into the genetics of pre-eclampsia, *Semin Perinatol* 23:14-23, 1999.

11. Beaulieu MD: Prevention of preeclampsia. In Canadian Task Force on the Periodic Health Examination: *Canadian guide to clinical preventive health care,* Ottawa, 1994, Health Canada, pp 136-143.

12. U.S. Preventative Services Task Force: *Guide to clinical preventative services,* ed 2, Baltimore, 1996, Williams & Wilkins.

13. Rodriguez-Thompson D, Lieberman ES: Use of a random urinary protein-to-creatinine ratio for the diagnosis of significant proteinuria during pregnancy, *Am J Obstet Gynecol* 185:808-811, 2001.

14. National High Blood Pressure Education Program Working Group on High Blood Pressure in Pregnancy. Report of the National High Blood Pressure Education Program Working Group on High Blood Pressure in Pregnancy, *Am J Obstet Gynecol* 183:S1-S22, 2000.

15. Sibai BM: Diagnosis and management of gestational hypertension and preeclampsia, *Obstet Gynecol* 102:181-192, 2003.

16. Churchill D, Duley L: Interventionist versus expectant care for severe pre-eclampsia before term, *Cochrane Database Syst Rev* (3):CD003106, 2002.

17. Odendaal HJ, Pattinson RC, Bam R et al: Aggressive or expectant management of patients with severe pre-eclampsia between 28-34 weeks' gestation: a randomized controlled trial, *Obstet Gynecol* 76:1070-1075, 1990.

18. Sibai BM, Mercer BM, Schiff E et al: Aggressive versus expectant management of severe preeclampsia at 28 to 32 weeks' gestation: a randomized controlled trial, *Am J Obstet Gynecol* 171:818-822, 1994.

19. Neilson JP, Alfirevic Z: Doppler ultrasound for fetal assessment in high risk pregnancies, *Cochrane Database Syst Rev* (2):CD000073, 2000.

20. Williams KP, Farquharson DF, Bebbington M et al: Screening for fetal well-being in a high-risk pregnant population comparing the nonstress test with umbilical artery Doppler velocimetry: a randomized controlled clinical trial, *Am J Obstet Gynecol* 188: 1366-1371, 2003.

21. The Magpie Trial Collaboratve Group: Do women with pre-eclampsia, and their babies, benefit from magnesium sulphate? The Magpie Trial: a randomized placebo-controlled trial, *Lancet* 359:1877-1890, 2002.

22. Sibai B: Magnesium sulfate prophylaxis in preeclampsia: evidence from randomized trails, *Clin Obstet Gynecol* 48:478-488, 2005.

23. Dildy III GA: Complications of preeclampsia. In: Dildy III GA, Belfort MA, Saade GR et al, editors: *Critical care obstetrics,* ed 4, Malden, MA, 2004, Blackwell Science.

24. Weinstein L: Syndrome of hemolysis, elevated liver enzymes and low platelet count: a severe consequence of hypertension in pregnancy, *Am J Obstet Gynecol* 142:159-167, 1982.

25. Matchaba P, Moodley J: Corticosteroids for HELLP syndrome in pregnancy. *Cochrane Database of Systematic Reviews* 2004, Issue 1. Art. No.: CD002076. DOI: 10.1002/14651858. CD002076.pub2.

26. Sibai BM: Diagnosis, controversies, and management of the syndrome of hemolysis, elevated liver enzymes, and low platelet count, *Obstet Gynecol* 103:981-991, 2004.

27. Atallah AN, Hofmeyr GJ, Duley L: Calcium supplementation during pregnancy for preventing hypertensive disorders and related problems, *Cochrane Database Syst Rev* (3):CD001059, 2006.

28. Villar J, Abdel-Aleem H, Merialdi M et al: World Health Organization randomized trial of calcium supplementation among low calcium intake pregnant women, *Am J Obstet Gynecol* 194:639-649, 2006.

29. Knight M, Duley L, Henderson-Smart DJ, King JF: Antiplatelet agents for preventing and treating pre-eclampsia, *Cochrane Database Syst Rev* (2):CD000492, 2000.

30. Duley L, Gülmezoglu AM, Henderson-Smart DJ: Magnesium sulphate and other anticonvulsants for women with pre-eclampsia, *Cochrane Database of Systematic Reviews* (2): CD000025, 2003.

31. Duley L, Henderson-Smart DJ: Magnesium sulphate versus phenytoin for eclampsia, *Cochrane Database Syst Rev* (4): CD000128, 2003.

32. Duley L, Henderson-Smart DJ: Magnesium sulphate versus diazepam for eclampsia, *Cochrane Database Syst Rev* (4): CD000127, 2003.

33. Eclampsia trial collaborative group: Which anti-convulsant for women with eclampsia? Evidence from the collaborative trial, *Lancet* 345:1455-1463, 1995.

S E C T I O N   H   Medical Emergencies in Pregnancy

Lee T. Dresang, MD

Venous thromboembolism is the leading cause of maternal mortality in the United States and most developed countries.[1] Amniotic fluid embolism (AFE) accounts for approximately 10% of U.S. maternal deaths.[2] Although septic shock has decreased dramatically in developed countries because of factors including aseptic technique and antibiotics, it is still the second leading cause of maternal death worldwide.[3,4]

I. VENOUS THROMBOEMBOLISM

A. Epidemiology

Venous thromboembolism complicates 1.3 per 1000 pregnancies.[1] Untreated deep venous thrombosis (DVT) results in pulmonary embolism (PE) in 25% of cases, and undiagnosed PE has a 30% mortality rate.[5]

B. Pathophysiology

Antenatal thromboembolic disease is addressed in Chapter 8, Section D. The factors leading to antenatal venous thromboembolism can also cause intrapartum venous thromboembolism. All pregnancies involve some degree of predisposing hypercoagulation, venous stasis, and vascular damage.[6] Risk factors include multiparity (more than four deliveries), age older than 35, weight more than 80 kg, severe varicose veins, hyperemesis, preeclampsia, prolonged bed rest, immobility, infection/sepsis, dehydration, major medical problems (mechanical heart valve, inflammatory bowel disease, nephrotic syndrome, sickle cell disease, myeloproliferative disorders), and thrombophilic disorders.[6,7] Thrombophilic disorders include factor V Leiden, prothrombin G20210A and methylene tetrahydrofolate reductase mutations, antithrombin, protein C and protein S deficiencies, and antiphospholipid syndrome.[6,7] Additional venous thromboembolism risk factors unique to labor include instrumental delivery, cesarean delivery (especially if emergent), and PPH.[6,7]

C. Diagnosis

Unilateral leg pain, swelling and increased calf circumference, or a palpable cord should prompt an investigation for DVT. During pregnancy, 90% of DVTs occur in the left leg and 72% in the ileofemoral vein, compared with 55% and 9%, respectively, in nonpregnant patients.[7] Doppler is the test of choice for diagnosing DVT.[8]

PE has a wide variety of presentations from mild tachypnea and dyspnea to hemoptysis, respiratory distress, and cardiovascular collapse. When available, multidetector-row CT is the test of choice for diagnosing PE in pregnancy, with 99% sensitivity and specificity.[9] When CT is unavailable, ventilation perfusion (V/Q) scans remain the test of choice. However, even a high-probability V/Q scan is only 41% sensitive.[10]

D-dimer has a high negative predictive value for venous thromboembolism in pregnancy, but it is of little use when positive (elevated).[8] Arterial blood gas, chest radiograph, and ECG, although of lesser value, may suggest PE or other conditions.

D. Management

Evidence is lacking for the best intrapartum management of venous thromboembolism.[8] The best evidence regarding anticoagulation for venous thromboembolism is from studies of nonpregnant patients[11-13] with only case reports and expert opinion[14-16] to directly address management during pregnancy. Management of venous thromboembolism during labor can involve management of a woman receiving thromboprophylaxis because of risk factors for venous

thromboembolism, a woman receiving therapeutic anticoagulation because of a thromboembolic event earlier in pregnancy, and management of DVT and/or PE occurring during labor.

Women receiving prophylactic or therapeutic doses of heparin antenatally may be instructed to discontinue the heparin at the onset of labor or given 5000 units subcutaneous unfractionated heparin (UFH) every 12 hours until delivery.[8] For scheduled cesareans, heparin should be omitted the day of the procedure.[8] Protamine sulfate may be indicated before at least some cesarean deliveries, especially if a woman receiving antenatal anticoagulation is at high risk for perioperative bleeding (e.g., with possible placenta accreta) or at low risk for PE (e.g., >3 months after a DVT).[17] Discontinuing low-molecular-weight heparin (LMWH) 24 hours before elective inductions or epidural analgesia is recommended.[18] A woman's usual prophylactic dose of LMWH can be given 3 hours after epidural removal.[8] Therapeutic treatment regimens can be resumed the day after delivery.[8]

With acute venous thromboembolism during labor, the benefits of full therapeutic anticoagulation to prevent clot extension outweigh the risks for PPH.[17] When clinical suspicion of venous thromboembolism is greater, diagnostic and therapeutic actions may be initiated simultaneously.[8] Stabilization is the first priority; airway, breathing, and circulation (ABCs) should be addressed immediately. Anticoagulation may be started empirically and discontinued if venous thromboembolism is excluded. With significant PPH, the effects of heparin can be reversed using protamine sulfate; this is usually not necessary after a vaginal delivery.[17]

During pregnancy, anticoagulation options include LMWH and UFH, which can be given intravenously or SQ. The dose of the most commonly used LMWH in the United States is enoxaparin (100 units/mg) 1 mg/kg SQ every 12 hours.[6] With IV UFH, a loading dose of 5000 International Units (IU) or 80 IU/kg is followed by a continuous infusion of 1300 IU/hr or 18 IU/kg/hr.[19] With IV followed by subcutaneous UFH, an IV bolus of 5000 IU is followed by 15,000 to 20,000 IU SQ twice daily.[20] With UFH, unlike LMWH, the activated partial thromboplastin time (aPTT) must be monitored and the dosage adjusted to achieve an aPTT in the therapeutic range of 1.5 to 2.5 times the mean laboratory control value.[19,20] Expert opinion recommends IV UFH if venous thromboembolism occurs during labor.[17]

If anticoagulation is contraindicated or repeat PE occurs despite adequate anticoagulation, inserting a filter in the inferior vena cava may be necessary.[8] In the case of life-threatening massive PE, thrombolytic therapy, percutaneous catheter thrombus fragmentation, or surgical embolectomy may be used, depending on local expertise.[8,21]

E. Prevention

Identification of factors predisposing to venous thromboembolism and thromboprophylaxis are key elements for preventing intrapartum venous thromboembolism. Women with a personal or family history of thrombosis or thrombophilia should undergo a thrombophilia screen.[7] With thrombophilias and other high-risk conditions, LMWH throughout pregnancy can greatly reduce the likelihood of venous thromboembolism in labor and otherwise.[11-13]

Routine postpartum thromboprophylaxis is not indicated.[1] However, pharmacologic and mechanical prophylaxis may be indicated because of preexisting risk factors or new delivery-related risk factors including prolonged labor, mid-forceps, and immobility after delivery.[6] Graduated compression stockings (GCS) or pneumatic compression stockings (PCS) may be considered. A decision analysis concluded that the optimal postcesarean thromboprophylaxis strategy is routine use of PCS.[22] A Cochrane review showed that, in nonpregnant patients, GCS are effective in diminishing postoperative DVT risk, and that GCS combined with another method of prophylaxis is more effective than GCS alone.[23]

II. AMNIOTIC FLUID EMBOLISM

A. Epidemiology

Incidence and mortality figures vary widely because of the lack of sensitive and specific tests to definitively identify cases of AFE.[24] A decline in mortality rates from 86% in 1979 to 16% from 1997-2000 is probably due to improved ICU care and recognition of milder cases.[2]

B. Pathophysiology

The exact pathophysiology of AFE remains uncertain. One theory is that amniotic fluid enters maternal circulation, pulmonary vasculature constricts after exposure to immunologically active amniotic fluid, inflammatory material in the lungs depresses the myocardium and causes DIC and ARDS, and hypoxia leads to altered mental status and seizures.[24]

C. Diagnosis

The presentation of AFE is variable but often includes respiratory distress, hypotension, coagulopathy, hemorrhage, seizures, altered mental status, fetal distress, fevers, nausea, and vomitting.[24,25] It usually presents acutely during labor and delivery or immediately after delivery.[24] AFE is a diagnosis of exclusion: venous thromboembolism, preeclampsia/eclampsia, and peripartum cardiomyopathy are in the differential.

D. Management

AFE is life-threatening, but potentially reversible. Treatment involves oxygenation, circulatory support, and correction of coagulopathies.[25] An ICU is usually the best setting for managing AFE.[2]

E. Prevention

Currently, AFE cannot be predicted or prevented.[25]

III. SEPTIC SHOCK

A. Epidemiology

With approximately 5,768,000 cases annually, sepsis is the second most frequent cause of maternal death and is the leading cause of late postpartum death.[4] When women survive, morbidity is high: sepsis causes tubal scarring and infertility in approximately 450,000 women per year.[4]

B. Pathophysiology

Sepsis is the systemic response to infection; septic shock is sepsis with hypotension refractory to fluid resuscitation.[26] Pyelonephritis, pneumonia, septic abortion, and chorioamnionitis are common antepartum infections that increase the risk for sepsis.[26] In pregnant patients, it appears that the most common bacteria causing sepsis are gram-negative rods, followed by gram-positive bacteria and mixed or fungal infections.[26]

C. Diagnosis

Diagnosis of puerperal sepsis is challenging because, even with hospital deliveries, signs and symptoms are often not present until after a woman is discharged home.[3] The World Health Organization has defined puerperal sepsis as "infection of the genital tract occurring at any time between the rupture of membranes or labor, and the 42nd day postpartum in which two or more of the following are present: pelvic pain, fever (i.e. oral temperature 38.5 or higher on any occasion), abnormal vaginal discharge (e.g. presence of pus), abnormal smell/foul odor of discharge, delay in the rate of reduction of the size of the uterus (< 2cm/day during the first 8 days)."[3] Diagnostic criteria include general variables (fever, hypothermia, tachycardia, tachypnea, altered mental status, edema, positive fluid balance, hyperglycemia), inflammatory variables (leukocytosis, leukopenia, left shift, elevated CRP level, elevated procalcitonin level), hemodynamic variables (hypotension, Svo_2 >70%, cardiac index >3.5), organ dysfunction variables (hypoxemia, oliguria, increased creatinine, coagulation abnormalities, ileus, thrombocytopenia, and hyperbilirubinemia), and tissue perfusion variables (hyperlactatemia, decreased capillary refill, mottling).[26] Documentation of bacteremia is not sufficient to diagnose sepsis.[26]

D. Management

Management of septic shock is directed at stabilization, supportive care, and treatment of the underlying infection. Treatment may include fluids, vasopressors, transfusion of red blood cells and other blood products, mechanical ventilation, and broad-spectrum antibiotics.[26] At least in nonpregnant patients with sepsis, DVT prophylaxis with heparin and/or intermittent compression devices, H2 blockers or proton pump inhibitors, and tight glycemic control are beneficial.[26] A Cochrane review of intravenous immunoglobulin (IVIG) for treating sepsis and septic shock in nonpregnant patients found that polyclonal IVIG significantly reduced mortality.[27] Fetal monitoring may help assess the effectiveness of maternal resuscitation efforts and may indicate early delivery.[26]

E. Prevention

Aseptic technique and early diagnosis and treatment of various infections in pregnancy can help prevent the development of sepsis. According to a Cochrane review, antibiotic prophylaxis was associated with a RR of 0.44 (0.29-0.68) for a serious infectious outcome after cesarean delivery.[28]

Early recognition and treatment of sepsis is paramount to improved outcomes; an RCT of nonpregnant patients demonstrated improved survival with aggressive fluid, medicine, and blood administration to maintain and restore perfusion within the first 6 hours of resuscitation.[29]

IV. SOR A RECOMMENDATIONS

RECOMMENDATIONS	REFERENCES
In nonpregnant patients, LMWH has equivalent or better efficacy than UFH and is safe to use for the treatment of acute DVT.	11, 13
In nonpregnant patients, GCS are effective in diminishing the risk for postoperative DVT, and GCS combined with another method of prophylaxis is more effective than GCS alone.	19
Prophylactic antibiotics decrease the risk for endometritis, wound infection, and serious infection in women undergoing elective or nonelective cesarean section.	24

REFERENCES

1. Gates S, Brocklehurst P, Davis L: Prophylaxis for venous thromboembolic disease in pregnancy and the early postnatal period, *Cochrane Database Syst Rev* (2):CD001689, 2002.
2. Tuffnell D: Amniotic fluid embolism, *Curr Opin Obstet Gynecol* 15:119-122, 2003.
3. Dolea C, Stein C: Global burden of maternal sepsis in the year 2000. Geneva, 2003, World Health Organization.
4. World Health Organization. *World health report 2005; make every mother and child count*. Available at: http://www.who.int/whr/2005/whr2005_en.pdf. Accessed September 12, 2007.
5. Doyle N, Ramirez M, Mastrobattista J et al: Diagnosis of pulmonary embolism: a cost-effectiveness analysis, *Am J Obstet Gynecol* 191:1019-1023, 2004.
6. Nelson-Piercy C: Thromboprophylaxis during pregnancy, labour and after vaginal delivery. Royal College of Obstetricians and Gynaecologists guideline, 37, 2004, Royal College of Obstetricians and Gynaecologists.
7. Zotz R, Gerhardt A, Scharf R: Prediction, prevention and treatment of venous thromboembolic disease in pregnancy, *Semin Thromb Hemost* 29:143-153, 2003.
8. Greer I, Thomson A: Thromboembolic disease in pregnancy and the puerperium. Guidelines and Audit Committee of the Royal College of Obstetricians and Gynaecologists, 2007, Royal College of Obstetricians and Gynaecologists.
9. Quiroz R, Kucher N, Zou K et al: Clinical validity of a negative computed tomography scan in patients with suspected pulmonary embolism: a systematic review, *JAMA* 293:2012-2017, 2005.
10. The PIOPED investigators: Value of the ventilation/perfusion scan in acute pulmonary embolism: results of the Prospective Investigation of Pulmonary Embolism Diagnosis (PIOPED), *JAMA* 263:2753-2759, 1990.
11. Gould M, Dembitzer A, Doyle R et al: Low molecular weight heparins compared with unfractionated heparin for treatment

of acute venous thrombosis. A meta-analysis of randomized, controlled trails, *Ann Intern Med* 130:800-809, 1999.

12. Martinelli I, de Stefano V, Taiolo E et al: Inherited thrombophilia and first venous thromboembolism during pregnancy and the puerperium, *Thromb Haemost* 87:791-795, 2002.

13. Van Dongen C, Van den Belt A, Prins M et al: Fixed dose subcutaneous low molecular weight heparins versus adjusted dose unfractionated heparin for venous thromboembolism, *Cochrane Database Syst Rev* (4):CD001100, 2004.

14. Rodie V, Thomson A, Stewart F et al: Low molecular weight heparin for the treatment of venous thromboembolism in pregnancy: a case series, *BJOG* 109:1020-1024, 2002.

15. Kaaja R, Ulander V: Treatment of acute pulmonary embolism during pregnancy with low molecular weight heparin: three case reports, *Blood Coagul Fibrinolysis* 13:637-640, 2002.

16. Bates S, Greer I, Hirsh J et al: Use of antithrombotic agents during pregnancy: the seventh ACCP conference on antithrombotic and thrombolytic therapy, *Chest* 126:627S-644S, 2004.

17. Dildy G, Saade G, Phelan J et al: *Critical care obstetrics,* ed 4, New Orleans, 2003, Blackwell Publishing.

18. Thromboembolism in pregnancy. ACOG Practice Bulletin No. 19. American College of Obstetricians and Gynecologists, 2000.

19. Hyers T, Hull R, Weg J: Antithrombotic therapy for venous thromboembolic disease, *Chest* 108:335S-351S, 1995.

20. Prandoni P, Carnovali M, Marchori A: Subcutaneous adjusted-dose unfractionated heparin vs fixed-dose low-molecular-weight heparin in the initial treatment of venous thromboembolism, *Arch Intern Med* 164:1077-1083, 2004.

21. Pillny M, Sandmann W, Luther B et al: Deep venous thrombosis during pregnancy and after delivery: indications for and results of thrombectomy, *J Vasc Surg* 37:528-532, 2003.

22. Quinones J, James D, Stamilio D et al: Thromboprophylaxis after cesarean delivery, *Obstet Gynecol* 106:733-740, 2005.

23. Amaragiri S, Lees T: Elastic compression stockings for prevention of deep vein thrombosis, *Cochrane Database Syst Rev* (3): CD001484, 2000.

24. Moore J, Baldisseri M: Amniotic fluid embolism, *Crit Care Med* 33:S279-S285, 2005.

25. Davies S: Amniotic fluid embolus: a review of the literature, *Can J Anaesth* 48:88-98, 2001.

26. Fernandez-Perez E, Salman S, Pendem S et al: Sepsis during pregnancy, *Crit Care Med* 33:S286-S293, 2005.

27. Alejandria M, Lansang M, Dans L et al: Intravenous immunoglobulin for treating sepsis and septic shock, *Cochrane Database Syst Rev* (1):CD001090, 2002.

28. Smaill F, Hofmeyer G: Antibiotic prophylaxis for cesarean section, *Cochrane Database Syst Rev* (3):CD000933, 2002.

29. Rivers E, Nguyen B, Gavstad S et al: Early goal-directed therapy in the treatment of severe sepsis and septic shock, *N Engl J Med* 345:1368-1377, 2001.

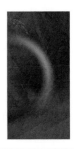

Malpresentation and Malpositions

S E C T I O N   A   Diagnosis

*Jamee H. Lucas MD, AAFP,
and Elizabeth G. Baxley, MD*

The term *lie* describes the relation of the long axis of the fetus to the mother. Longitudinal lies are present in more than 99% of pregnancies. The presenting part is the portion of the body of the fetus that is closest to the birth canal; it is the presenting part that determines the presentation. In the longitudinal lie, the presenting part is either breech or vertex. When the long axis is transverse, the shoulder is most often the presenting part.

In 96% of pregnancies near term, the fetus assumes a longitudinal lie with the vertex directed at the maternal pelvis, the back convex, and the head sharply flexed on the neck such that the chin is nearly in contact with the chest. In the remaining 4% of cases, a deviation occurs from this normal lie, constituting a malpresentation. Common factors associated with malpresentations include grand multiparity with lax maternal abdominal support, high fundal or lower uterine segment implantation of the placenta, prematurity, macrosomia, hydramnios, uterine malformations, fetal anomalies, and a contracted maternal pelvis. The literature also suggests that malpositions are more often seen with the use of epidural anesthesia.[1-3] It is not clear, however, if the relation is causal. It may be that by excessive relaxation of the pelvic musculature epidural anesthesia prevents appropriate rotation of the vertex, leading to occiput posterior (OP), persistent transverse, or asynclitic presentations.

Careful attention to prenatal diagnosis of a fetal malpresentation is essential to maximize fetal outcomes. Greater rates of maternal and perinatal mortality have been reported with fetal malpresentation.

In unstable or transverse lie, perinatal mortality rates from 3.9% to 24% have been reported, with up to 10% maternal mortality in some series.[4] Cord prolapse occurs 20 times as often in cases of transverse lie compared with vertex presentations.

I. INCIDENCE

The incidence of various malpresentations at or near term is detailed in the following sections.

A. Face Presentation

Face presentation is where the fetal neck is extended, with the occiput touching the back with the face toward the birth canal. The reported incidence of face presentation varies widely, from 0.1% to 2.0%; the majority of reports place the average incidence of this particular malpresentation at 0.2% to 0.3%, or 1 in 500 to 600 deliveries.[4-8]

B. Brow Presentation

Brow presentation is where the fetal neck is extended but not as much as the face presentation. Brow presentation is less common than face presentation, most likely because this is a transitional state that often converts to face or vertex presentation. Brow presentation has a reported incidence ranging from 1 in 468 to 3543 deliveries; most reports give an average incidence of 0.007%, or 1 in 1400 deliveres.[4,5,7-9]

C. Transverse Lie

The transverse lie malpresentation complicates 0.3% to 0.4% of all births, or 1 in 300 births.[4,5,7,8]

D. Breech Presentation

The incidence of breech presentation (see Section G) is highly dependent on gestational age, decreasing in frequency as the pregnancy progresses. Incidence rates at various gestational ages are as follows:

1. Incidence at 28 weeks: 22% to 25%
2. Incidence at 32 weeks: 7% to 13%
3. Incidence at 36 weeks: 5% to 7%
4. Incidence at 40 weeks: 2.5% to 6%

II. DIAGNOSIS

Several diagnostic measures can be used to determine the lie and presentation of a fetus, including abdominal palpation, vaginal examination, auscultation, and ultrasonography or, rarely, radiographically.

A. Abdominal Palpation

Abdominal palpation can be performed throughout the latter weeks of gestation, and between contractions in early labor, to gain information about the presentation and position of the fetus. A systematic set of four maneuvers, called *Leopold maneuvers,* is used to examine the gravid abdomen (Figure 17-1).[7]

1. First maneuver
   After outlining the contour of the uterus, the examiner gently palpates the fundus to determine which fetal pole is present.
2. Second maneuver
   This portion of the maneuver involves placing the palms of the examiner's hands on either side of the abdomen with gentle but deep pressure. This indicates the side on which the fetal back is located (hard, resistant structure) versus where the fetal limbs are located (numerous nodulations).
3. Third maneuver
   Using the thumb and fingers of one hand and grasping the lower portion of the maternal abdomen above the pubic symphysis, the examiner can differentiate between the head and breech.
4. Fourth maneuver
   Facing the mother's feet and using the fingertips of each hand, the examiner palpates above and to the sides of the symphysis pubis to determine the degree of head flexion in a cephalic presentation.

B. Vaginal Examination

Vaginal examination may be helpful in palpating the presenting part, although it can be inconclusive if the presenting part is very high or when palpating through a closed cervix and thick lower uterine segment. If the cervix is dilated enough to admit the examiner's gloved finger, the head versus breech usually can be readily distinguished from one another by differentiation of the sutures and fontanels from the sacrum and ischial tuberosities.

C. Auscultation

Auscultation by itself does not determine the fetal position, but it may reinforce what the examiner suspects from palpation. In the vertex and breech positions, fetal heart tones are best heard through the fetal back, whereas in a face presentation, they are heard through the fetal thorax. In vertex presentations, heart tones are heard with maximal intensity between the umbilicus and the anterior superior iliac spine of the mother. In breech presentations, this point of maximal intensity is closer to the level of the umbilicus. In the more common occipitoanterior position, fetal heart tones are heard best near the midline, whereas in transverse presentations, they are more lateral; in posterior presentations, the point of maximal intensity is back toward the mother's flank.

D. Diagnostic Ultrasonography

Bedside ultrasound in labor and delivery can be used to determine fetal presentation when abdominal and vaginal examinations are not confirmatory. Visualization of the fetal head versus breech in the lower uterine segment is definitive. When the presenting part is high, cord presentation may be discovered, although the absence of cord preceding the head does not guarantee safety of artificial rupture of membranes. Ultrasound also allows identification of placental location and may indicate fetal malformations associated with an abnormal lie.

E. X-Ray Examination

A single x-ray film may be used to aid in the diagnosis of fetal presentation. Information received in these cases far exceeds the minimal risk from plain film exposure. This type of examination may be more helpful in obtaining specific types of information, including type of breech presentation, extent of fetal neck extension, and gross maternal pelvic deformity.

REFERENCES

1. Saunders NJ Sr, Spiby H, Gilbert L et al: Oxytocin infusion during second stage of labour in primiparous women using epidural analgesia: a randomized double-blind placebo-controlled trial, *BMJ* 299:1423-1426, 1989.
2. Thorp JA, Hu DH, Albin RM et al: The effect of intrapartum epidural analgesia on nulliparous labor: a randomized, controlled prospective trial, *Am J Obstet Gynecol* 169:851-858, 1993.
3. Wittels B: Does epidural anesthesia affect the course of labor and delivery? *Semin Perinatol* 15:358-367, 1991.

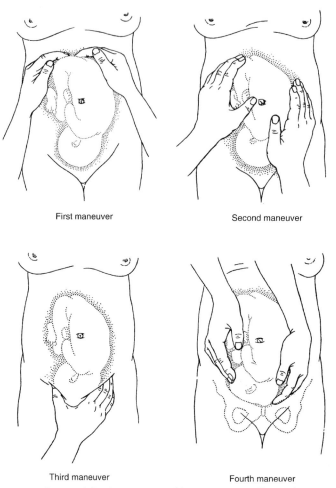

First maneuver

Second maneuver

Third maneuver

Fourth maneuver

FIGURE 17-1. Leopold maneuvers. (From Pritchard JA, Mac Donald PC, Gant NF: *Williams obstetrics,* ed 17, Norwalk, CT, 1985, Appleton-Century-Crofts.)

4. Seeds JW: Malpresentations. In Gabbe SG, Niebyl JR, Simpson JL, editors: *Obstetrics: normal and problem pregnancies,* ed 2, New York, 1991, Churchill Livingstone.

5. Cruickshank DP: Malpresentations and umbilical cord complications. In Scott JR, DiSaia PJ, Hammond CB, Spellacy WN, editors: *Danforth's obstetrics and gynecology,* ed 6, Philadelphia, 1990, JB Lippincott.

6. Duff P: Diagnosis and management of face presentation, *Obstet Gynecol* 57:105-112, 1981.

7. Pritchard JA, MacDonald PC, Gant NF: Dystocia caused by abnormalities in presentation, position, or development of the fetus and presentation, position, attitude and lie of the fetus. In Pritchard JA, MacDonald PC, Gant NF, editors: *Williams' obstetrics,* ed 21, Norwalk, CT, 2001, McGraw-Hill.

8. Shields JR, Medearis AL: Fetal malformations. In Hacker NF, Moore JG, editors: *Essentials of obstetrics and gynecology,* ed 2, Philadelphia, 1992, WB Saunders.

9. Levy DL: Persistent brow presentation: a new approach to management, *South Med J* 69:191-192, 1976.

SECTION B   Face Presentation

Elizabeth G. Baxley, MD, and Jamee H. Lucas, MD, AAFP

Face presentation occurs when the fetal head hyperextends such that the fetal face is the presenting part. The face as the presenting part occurs in

1 in 600 to 800 deliveries. Although the exact cause is unknown, factors that allow extension of the neck and restrict flexion, such as high maternal parity, contracted pelvis, and/or fetal macrosomia, are associated.[1] Anencephalic fetuses almost always present by the face because of lack of cranium development; this malformation has been reported to be seen in one third of cases of face presentation.[2]

I. DIAGNOSIS

The diagnosis of face presentation is usually not made until late in labor.[1] Only 3% of face presentations are diagnosed before labor, with 35% being diagnosed in the first stage, 27% in the second stage, and 35% at the time of delivery.

A. Abdominal Palpation

On Leopold maneuvers, face presentation is suspected when the cephalic prominence is on the same side as the fetal spine, occasionally with a palpable groove between them (Figure 17-2). Fetal heart tones are usually heard on the side of the small parts, below the umbilicus.[1]

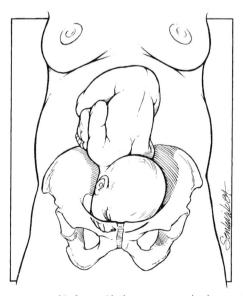

FIGURE 17-2. This fetus with the vertex completely extended on the neck enters the maternal pelvis in a face presentation. The cephalic prominence would be palpable on the same side of the maternal abdomen as the fetal spine.

B. Vaginal Examination

Face presentation is more often diagnosed by palpation of fetal mouth, nose, malar bones, and orbital ridges during vaginal examination. It is possible to confuse a face presentation with a breech presentation. In face presentations, the fetal mouth and malar prominences form the corners of a triangle, whereas in the breech presentation, the fetal anus is always on a line with the ischial tuberosities.

C. Radiologic Examination

Bedside ultrasound quickly reveals whether the breech or head is presenting and may demonstrate that the fetal neck is hyperextended. If ultrasound is not available or the diagnosis is uncertain, a conventional x-ray film of the abdomen also may demonstrate hyperextension of the fetal head.[1]

II. MANAGEMENT

The delivery position of the face is categorized according to the position of the fetal chin, or mentum. The majority (60-80%) of face presentations are in the mentum anterior position, whereas 10% to 12% are mentum transverse and 20% to 25% are mentum posterior.[2-4] This is an important clinical distinction because the mentum anterior position delivers by spontaneous vaginal delivery (SVD) 75% of the time, with the delivery of the head occurring by flexion rather than extension. The chin and mouth appear at the vulva initially followed by the nose, mouth, and brow. This is represented in an old obstetric adage "if a face is progressing, leave it alone."[3]

Protracted labor is not uncommon in face presentations and can be an ominous sign because it has been associated with an increased number of intrapartum deaths.[2] An increased incidence of fetal heart rate abnormalities also has been reported in labors with face presentations (predominantly variable decelerations), and continuous electronic fetal monitoring is recommended in these cases.[5,6] Internal fetal monitors must be applied carefully, avoiding ocular and cosmetic damage, and preferentially placing the electrode over the fetal chin.[7]

Almost all mentum transverse and a third to half of mentum posterior presentations spontaneously rotate to a mentum anterior position. However, a persistent mentum posterior position cannot deliver vaginally because the additional extension required to negotiate the pelvic curvature during descent is not possible. Cesarean section is indicated for persistent mentum posterior or when there is an arrest of dilatation or descent in any face presentation.[8] Maneuvers to convert a face presentation to a vertex result in increased perinatal morbidity and mortality, and should not be attempted. Face presentation is not a contraindication to use of oxytocin or forceps, although vacuum extraction should not be applied to the fetal face.

Close observation of the neonate must occur after delivery of a face presentation because laryngeal and tracheal edema are possible sequelae of the birth process and may require nasotracheal intubation if severe.[2] There is almost always severe facial edema in the newborn, causing transient distortion, about which parents need reassurance.

REFERENCES

1. Duff P: Diagnosis and management of face presentation, *Obstet Gynecol* 57:105-112, 1981.
2. Seeds JW: Malpresentations. In Gabbe SG, Niebyl JR, Simpson JL, editors: *Obstetrics: normal and problem pregnancies,* ed 2, New York, 1991, Churchill Livingstone.
3. Cruickshank DP: Malpresentations and umbilical cord complications. In Scott JR, DiSaia PJ, Hammond CB, Spellacy WN, editors: *Danforth's obstetrics and gynecology,* ed 6, Philadelphia, 1990, JB Lippincott.
4. Shields JR, Medearis AL: Fetal malformations. In Hacker NF, Moore JG, editors: *Essentials of obstetrics and gynecology,* ed 2, Philadelphia, 1992, WB Saunders.
5. Benedetti TJ, Lowensohn RI, Truscott AM: Face presentation at term, *Obstet Gynecol* 55:199-202, 1980.
6. Schwartz Z, Dgani R, Lancet M et al: Face presentation, *Aust N Z J Obstet Gynaecol* 26:172-176, 1986.
7. Miyashiro MJ, Mintz-Hittner HA: Penetrating ocular injury with a fetal scalp monitoring spiral electrode, *Am J Opthalmol* 128:526, 1999.
8. Danforth DN: Dystocia due to abnormal fetopelvic relations. In Danforth DN, Scott JR, editors: *Obstetrics and gynecology,* ed 5, Philadelphia, 1986, JB Lippincott.

SECTION C Brow Presentation

Elizabeth G. Baxley, MD,
and Jamee H. Lucas, MD, AAFP

A brow presentation occurs as a result of extension of the fetal head midway between the vertex and the face. The presenting part of the fetus visualized is between the orbits and the anterior fontanelle. The frontal bones form the point of designation (e.g., right frontal transverse), with frontum anterior as the most common position. Brow presentations are usually unstable, occurring when the head is in the process of converting from a vertex to a face or vice versa, and thus are seen in only 1 in 1400 deliveries.

The cause of brow presentation is similar to that of a face presentation. Any condition that causes abnormal neck extension and limits flexion of the fetal head can predispose to brow presentation. Fetal neck masses should be considered (e.g., cystic hygroma or teratoma) and ruled out by ultrasonography.

I. DIAGNOSIS

A. Abdominal Palpation
Rarely, by Leopold maneuvers, a brow presentation may be diagnosed when the examiner is able to palpate both the fetal chin and occiput.

B. Vaginal Examination
Brow presentation is more commonly diagnosed by palpating orbital ridges, eyes, frontal sutures, or the anterior fontanelle during vaginal examination (Figure 17-3). Like with a face presentation, this diagnosis is made before the second stage of labor in fewer than half of cases.[1,2]

C. Ultrasound versus X-Ray Diagnosis
Plain-film abdominal radiographs can demonstrate the degree of neck flexion better than ultrasonography and should not be avoided because of concerns about ionizing radiation, particularly in cases where labor is prolonged or has a secondary arrest.

II. MANAGEMENT

The prognosis of a brow presentation depends on the final presentation of the fetal vertex. It is an unstable lie, converting to a face or an occiput presentation in two thirds of cases. As with face presentations, management is expectant as long as labor is progressing normally. However, prolonged labors have been observed in 33% to 50% of brow presentations, and secondary arrest is common.[2,4] Persistent brow presentations are unable to deliver vaginally unless the fetus is very small or the pelvis very large, because of the large presenting diameter. Methods to convert

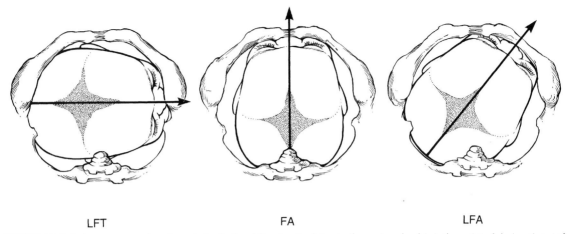

LFT   FA   LFA

FIGURE 17-3. In brow presentation, the anterior fontanel (frontum) relative to the maternal pelvis is the point of designation. *Left,* Fetus in left frontum transverse (LFT). *Middle,* Frontum anterior (FA). *Right,* Left frontum anterior (LFA).

the brow presentation are contraindicated. Cesarean section is the safest delivery method for a persistent brow presentation.[3]

REFERENCES

1. Cruickshank DP: Malpresentations and umbilical cord complications. In Scott JR, DiSaia PJ, Hammond CB, Spellacy WN, editors: *Danforth's obstetrics and gynecology,* ed 6, Philadelphia, 1990, JB Lippincott.
2. Seeds JW: Malpresentations. In Gabbe SG, Niebyl JR, Simpson JL, editors: *Obstetrics: normal and problem pregnancies,* ed 2, New York, 1991, Churchill Livingstone.
3. Danforth DN: Dystocia due to abnormal fetopelvic relations. In Danforth DN, Scott JR, editors: *Obstetrics and gynecology,* ed 5, Philadelphia, 1986, J.B. Lippincott.
4. Shields JR, Medearis AL: Fetal malformations. In Hacker NF, Moore JG, editors: *Essentials of obstetrics and gynecology,* ed 2, Philadelphia, 1992, WB Saunders.

S E C T I O N   D   Transverse Lie

Elizabeth G. Baxley, MD,
and Jamee H. Lucas MD, AAFP

In a transverse lie, the long axis of the fetus is perpendicular to that of the mother. Persistence of a transverse lie beyond 36 to 38 weeks of gestation is a significant clinical problem that must be managed carefully and systematically. In a transverse lie, the fetal head is in one iliac fossa and the buttock in the opposite. The fetal shoulder is typically the presenting part, and this condition is called a *shoulder presentation.*

The incidence of transverse lie is 10 times greater in grand multiparous patients (parity of 4 or more) than in nulliparous women. In addition, any condition that obstructs the lower uterine segment predisposes to transverse lie, including placenta previa or low-lying placenta, lower uterine segment uterine myomas, uterine anomalies, and fetal masses.

I. DIAGNOSIS
A. Abdominal Palpation
Even before abdominal palpation, a transverse lie is often recognizable by inspection alone, when the maternal abdomen is observed to be wider from side to side and the fundus does not extend very far beyond the umbilicus. In the case of a transverse lie, the fetal spine is either positioned up toward the maternal head or down toward the maternal cervix. With the first Leopold maneuver, neither the head nor the breech is found in the fundus, and on the second maneuver, the fetal head and buttocks are palpable in opposite iliac fossas. With abdominal palpation, the location of the fetal back (up or down) is readily identified.

B. Vaginal Examination
Neither the fetal head nor breech is found to be presenting on vaginal examination.

C. Radiologic Examination

Ultrasonography can rapidly confirm the diagnosis of transverse lie and can indicate the position of the fetal spine, the placental implantation site, and any fetal abnormalities that predispose to the transverse lie.

II. MANAGEMENT

A. External Version

Before the onset of labor, attempts at external cephalic version (ECV) are worthwhile if membranes are intact and if placenta previa and pelvic masses have been excluded as a cause. Emergency cesarean section and neonatal resuscitation capabilities must be immediately available if external version is attempted. Internal cephalic version is contraindicated because of the high rate of fetal and maternal complications. If the attempted version fails, or if rupture of membranes has occurred, vaginal delivery is impossible and cesarean section should be performed.[1]

B. Labor and Delivery Management

Spontaneous delivery of a term infant is impossible in cases of a persistent transverse lie. All of these women should be managed with elective cesarean section, often with a vertical uterine incision necessitated by the difficulty encountered in extraction of the fetus.

Unexpected spontaneous rupture of membranes (SROM) or artificial rupture of membranes (AROM) without a fetal part filling the pelvic inlet results in cord prolapse 20 times more often than in a vertex presentation, particularly for a "back up" transverse lie. AROM should be avoided when a shoulder presentation is present. Even with appropriate care, rates of maternal and fetal morbidity and death are greater with transverse lie because of the frequent association of this malpresentation with placenta previa, the greater risk for cord accidents, and the inevitability of abdominal delivery.

In cases of neglected transverse lie, the fetal shoulder is forced into the pelvis by the strength of the uterine contractions. After rupture of membranes, the corresponding arm often prolapses into the vagina. The shoulder arrests in the margins of the pelvic inlet after some descent but becomes impacted there as labor continues. This is an obstetric emergency. If not recognized and managed promptly, the uterus eventually ruptures as it contracts and tries to overcome the obstruction. The mother and fetus usually die if no treatment is given.

REFERENCE

1. Danforth DN: Dystocia due to abnormal fetopelvic relations. In Danforth DN, Scott JR, editors: *Obstetrics and gynecology,* ed 5, Philadelphia, 1986, JB Lippincott.

SECTION E   Transverse Arrest

Stephen D. Ratcliffe, MD, MSPH

I. DEFINITIONS AND CAUSES

The classic definition of transverse arrest is arrest of descent of the fetal head with the sagittal suture in a transverse position at the level of the midpelvis without the normal rotation of the head into the anteroposterior plane for 30 minutes.[1] This condition is caused by the shape of the maternal pelvis (flattened in the anteroposterior plane, the so-called platypelloid or android pelvis) or by ineffective uterine contractions.[1]

II. MANAGEMENT

A. Change in Maternal Position

A change in maternal position may encourage the fetus to rotate spontaneously.

B. Digital Rotation

Digital rotation is done by placing the index and middle fingers along the lambdoidal sutures. If the fetal head is in the left occiput transverse (OT) position, a counterclockwise rotation is accomplished using the clinician's right hand. If the fetal head is in the right OT position, the clinician applies left digital pressure along the lambdoidal sutures in a clockwise rotational manner.[1]

C. Attempted Manual Rotation from Occiput Transverse to Occiput Anterior

Once complete dilatation has occurred, the clinician can attempt a manual rotation from the OT position to occiput anterior (OA) position using the maneuver described in Section F. Maintaining flexion of the fetal head and using an abdominal hand to gently sweep the fetal shoulder out of the anterior-posterior plane are important aids to successfully complete this maneuver.[1]

D. Use of Oxytocin

If the cause of transverse arrest is believed to be ineffective uterine contractions, oxytocin augmentation is indicated (see Chapter 15, Section A). It is difficult to make a diagnosis of cephalopelvic disproportion (CPD) until this step has been carried out.

E. Vacuum-Assisted Delivery

If the fetal head has descended to a +2 or lower station, the vacuum can be applied to the point of maximum flexion approximately 2 to 3 cm anterior to the posterior fontanelle. Rotatory force should not be applied but rather allow the fetal head to "auto-rotate."[1]

F. Forceps-Assisted Delivery

If the above maneuvers have not been successful and the cause of the transverse arrest is believed to be an abnormally flattened maternal pelvis, cesarean section is indicated unless the operator is skilled in midforceps rotation with Kielland or Barton forceps. Midforceps rotations or applications at a station of 0 to +2 carry greater maternal and infant morbidity than cesarean section.[2,3] Midforceps application or rotation should be attempted by clinicians with advanced training in performing vaginally assisted deliveries.

REFERENCES

1. Stitely ML, Gherman RB: Labor with abnormal presentation and position, *Obstet Gynecol Clin N Am* 32:165-179, 2005.
2. Danforth DN: Dystocia due to abnormal fetopelvic relations. In Danforth DN, Scott JR, editors: *Obstetrics and gynecology,* ed 7, Philadelphia, 1998, J.B. Lippincott.
3. Plauche WC: Operative vaginal delivery and abnormal vertex presentation. In Plauche WE, Morrison JC, O'Sullivan MJ, editors: *Surgical obstetrics,* Philadelphia, 1992, W.B. Saunders.

SECTION F Occiput Posterior Position

Stephen D. Ratcliffe, MD, MSPH

I. DEFINITION, CAUSES, AND EFFECTS

The OP position occurs when the occipital portion of the fetal head presents in the posterior portion of the birth canal. This malposition is a common challenge for the clinician to recognize and manage.

A. Epidemiology

At the onset of labor, 10% to 20% of fetuses are in the OP position. Ultimately, about 5% of labors result in a persistent OP position. There is an increase in the incidence of the persistent OP position in women receiving epidural anesthesia (number needed to harm = 10).[1]

B. Natural History

Gardberg and colleagues[2] conducted a prospective study of 408 women in labor to track fetal positions throughout labor using bedside ultrasounds. Sixty-eight percent of the persistent OP positions began labor in the OA position. Eighty-seven percent of the fetuses that began labor in the OP position rotated spontaneously to OA before delivery. Women in labor whose fetuses are in the OP position tend to have "back labor" and may experience slower cervical dilatation and fetal descent. The duration of stage two is increased with persistent OP positions.

C. Effects on Perinatal Outcome

Effects on perinatal outcome of occiput posterior position include:
1. Maternal morbidity
   Laboring women with persistent OP position experience an increase in the following complications[3]:
   a. Episiotomy
   b. Third- and fourth-degree extensions
   c. Operative deliveries
   d. Cesarean deliveries
   e. Maternal blood loss
   f. Length of stay
2. Neonatal morbidity
   Neonatal morbidity is associated with the use of forceps or vacuum-assisted deliveries. An increased

incidence of Erb's and facial nerve palsies occurs with the use of forceps-assisted deliveries of newborns in the persistent OP position.[4]

II. DIAGNOSIS

The practitioner should be alerted to the possibility of an OP position when labor pains are primarily felt in the back. The clinician can make a diagnosis of OP position when the anterior fontanel (diamond-shaped, with four sutures emanating from the fontanel) is palpated in the anterior portion of the vagina and the posterior fontanel is palpated in the posterior portion of the birth canal. Occasionally, the fetal ears can be felt to assist in making the diagnosis. Use of a bedside ultrasound can confirm a diagnosis that is in doubt.

III. MANAGEMENT

A. Maneuvers to Correct an Occiput Posterior Position

1. Change of maternal position
   Although change of maternal position by putting the laboring mother in a hands-and-knees position during labor is widely used to promote the rotation from an OP to OA, a Cochrane review found insufficient evidence to support this practice.[5] Other recommended changes of positions include pelvic rocking and placing women into exaggerated lateral Sims' positioning.[6]

2. Manual rotation
   Rotation of the persistent OP to an OA position during stage two can avoid prolongation of this stage and many of the maternal/infant complications listed earlier. Factors that are associated with successful manual rotation include multiparity and maternal age younger than 35.[7] In this retrospective cohort study, successful manual rotation was associated with a 2% cesarean rate, whereas unsuccessful attempts were associated with a 34% cesarean rate.[7]
   The following steps to rotate a fetus from the OP to OA position are the methods used by the author:
   a. Inform the patient that effective pushing on her part is essential to help guide the rotation of her baby's head.
   b. If the fetus is in a left occiput posterior (LOP) position, the clinician should use the right hand to rotate the head in a counterclockwise direction about 90 degrees to a left occiput

anterior (LOA) position. Likewise, if the fetal head is in an ROP position, the clinician should use the left hand to rotate the head in a clockwise direction (also about 90 degrees) to the ROA position.

   c. Use of an assistant's hand to assist the rotation of the fetal shoulder can be a valuable addition to this procedure. The assistant's hand is applied in a lateral-to-medial "kneading" fashion to the patient's left lower abdomen when making a LOP-to-LOA rotation to help rotate the right fetal shoulder in a counterclockwise direction (from the vantage point of the clinician). This allows the fetus to make a rotation of its entire body and not merely its head. Likewise, the assistant's hand should apply gentle pressure to the right lower abdomen to move the left fetal shoulder in a clockwise direction when making a ROP-to-ROA rotation.

   d. The clinician's first maneuver is to locate the fetal posterior fontanel with the examiner's middle finger. Attempt to flex the fetal head by flexing the middle finger. *Do not elevate the fetal head.* During the ensuing manual rotation, maintain the fetal head in a flexed position.

   e. During a contraction the mother is asked to push and the assistant is asked to begin a "kneading" motion over the appropriate side of the lower maternal abdomen. The clinician will have already flexed the fetal head and now places the middle finger along the upper lambdoidal suture to move the head in a rotary motion from LOP to LOA or from ROP to ROA. Try to maintain flexion of the fetal head during the rotation maneuver.

3. Prevention of OP position
   A recent Australian randomized controlled trial (RCT) examined the question whether doing hands-and-knees exercises during the last 2 to 4 weeks of pregnancy would reduce the incidence of persistent OP at term. This study did not show any beneficial effect of this intervention.[8]

B. Delivery from an Occiput Posterior Position

1. Spontaneous vaginal delivery (SVD)
   Persistent OP position is associated with a lower incidence of SVDs than an OA position. Fitzpatrick and colleagues[3] conducted a prospective observational study of 246 women with a persistent OP position over a 2-year period. Fifty-five percent of

multiparous and 29% of nulliparous women achieved SVDs in this study. These women experienced a sevenfold increase in third-degree extensions. This increased incidence of posterior trauma is related to the increased biparietal diameter of the nonflexed fetal head. In this study, the women with persistent OP positions experienced 12% of the cesarean sections of the due to labor dystocia, although they represented 1.1% of the total study population. As the fetal head "crowns" just before delivery, some OP position fetuses will spontaneously rotate to an OA position.

2. Vacuum-assisted vaginal delivery

The vacuum device should be applied over the apex (point of maximum flexion) of the head 2 to 3 cm from the posterior fontanel. This may be difficult to do with the persistent OP position. Attempts should be made to avoid paramedian placement of the vacuum cup because of its association with an increased risk for neonatal cephalhematomas.[9] RCT evidence has been reported that the use of softer vacuum cups versus rigid ones is associated with a decreased number of successful vaginal deliveries, particularly with delivery of the fetus in the OP position (NNH = 20), but the use of the soft cups is associated with a decrease in significant scalp trauma (NNT = 14).[10]

3. Forceps-assisted vaginal delivery

Forceps may be applied to deliver an infant in the OP position. All of the prerequisites discussed in Chapter 18, Section D should be met. The handles of the forceps should not be elevated to deliver the baby's face in the OP position. As a result, third- and fourth-degree extensions are common. In Pearl and co-workers' series,[4] the percentage of infants experiencing Erb's palsy was 1% and facial nerve palsy was 3% when forceps were used to deliver babies in the OP position. Family physicians must be prepared to abandon this procedure and proceed to cesarean section if excessive traction is required to effect a vaginal delivery.

4. Cesarean section

When managing the woman with a persistent OP position, the clinician should make plans for the possibility of the diagnosis of CPD that will necessitate a cesarean intervention. This is especially true for the nulliparous patient. The diagnosis of CPD is usually made with failure to descend with adequate uterine contractions with complete cervical dilatation or when there is an unsuccessful attempt at a vacuum- or forceps-assisted delivery.

IV. SOR A RECOMMENDATION

RECOMMENDATION	REFERENCE
An increased incidence of persistent OP position occurs in women who receive epidural anesthesia (NNH = 10).	*1*

REFERENCES

1. Anim-Somuah M, Smyth R, Howell CJ: Epidural versus non-epidural analgesia in labour, *Cochrane Database Syst Rev* (4): CD000331, 2005.
2. Gardberg M, Laakkonen E, Salevaara M: Intrapartum sonography and persistent occiput posterior position: a study of 408 deliveries, *Obstet Gynecol* 91:746-749, 1998.
3. Fitzpatrick M, McQuillan K, O'Herlihy C: Influence of persistent occiput posterior position on delivery outcome, *Obstet Gynecol* 98:1027-1031, 2001.
4. Pearl M, Roberts J, Laros R et al: Vaginal delivery from the persistent occiput posterior position: influence on maternal and neonatal morbidity, *J Reprod Med* 38:955-961, 1993.
5. Hofmeyr G, Kulier R: Hands and knees posture in late pregnancy or labour for fetal malposition, *Cochrane Database Syst Rev* (2):CD001063, 2005.
6. Fenwick L, Simkin P: Maternal positioning to prevent or alleviate dystocia in labor, *Clin Obstet Gynecol* 30:83-89, 1987.
7. Shaffer BL, Cheng YW, Vargas JE et al: Manual rotation of the fetal occiput: predictors of success and delivery, *Am J Obstet Gynecol* 194:e7-e9, 2006.
8. Kariminia A, Chamberlain M, Keogh J et al: Randomised controlled trial of effect of hands and knees posture on the incidence of occiput posterior position at birth, *BMJ* 328: 490-496, 2004.
9. Teng FY, Sayre JW: Vacuum extraction: does duration predict scalp injury? *Obstet Gynecol* 89:281-285, 1997.
10. Johanson R, Menon V: Soft versus rigid vacuum extractor cups for assisted vaginal delivery, *Cochrane Database Syst Rev* (2):CD000446, 2000.

SECTION G **Breech Presentation**

Stephen D. Ratcliffe, MD, MSPH

I. EPIDEMIOLOGY

A. Incidence
Breech deliveries occur in 3% to 4% of all deliveries but occur in 15% of infants weighing less than 2500 g.[1]

B. Predisposing Factors
Predisposing factors for breech presentation include[2]:
1. Fetal anomalies
   These include major structural abnormalities such as hydrocephaly and anencephaly, and the major chromosomal anomalies.
2. Uterine overdistention
   Major causes of overdistention include polyhydramnios and multiple gestation.
3. Uterine abnormalities/pelvic obstruction
   Conditions include septate and bicornuate uterus. Pelvic obstructions include uterine fibroids, placenta previa, and low-lying placenta.

II. NATURAL HISTORY

A. Spontaneous Conversion from Breech to Vertex
Of all fetuses that are breech at 32 weeks of gestation, about 60% spontaneously convert to vertex.[2] Factors that reduce the conversion to vertex include nulliparity, previous breech, and extended fetal legs.[3]

B. Associated Fetal/Neonatal Conditions
Central nervous system malformations occur in 1.5% to 2.0% of infants with a breech presentation. The incidence of trisomy 21 is 0.5%. Overall, 9% of all infants with breech presentations have some type of congenital malformation.

C. Effect on Perinatal Morbidity/Mortality
There is a fourfold increase in perinatal mortality among term infants and a threefold increase among preterm infants.[4,5] Two thirds of these deaths are a result of congenital malformations or infections. Thus, only one third of the increased risk for perinatal mortality is attributed to preventable factors, such as trauma and asphyxia.[6] The Term Breech Trial demonstrated that the increase in perinatal morbidity and mortality occurred both during labor and the vaginal delivery.[7,8]

III. DIAGNOSIS

When the clinician performs the Leopold maneuvers during an antenatal exam, the fetal head is palpated in the fundus and the softer breech is felt over the lower abdomen. A vaginal examination may be done to reveal soft fetal buttocks, genitalia, an anus or small parts. When the examination is in doubt, an ultrasound examination will resolve any questions as to the presenting fetal part.[2] The types of breech presentations at term are shown in Figure 17-4.

A. Frank Breech
Frank breech occurs when the fetal hips are flexed and the knees are extended; this accounts for about 60% of breeches.

B. Incomplete or Footling Breech
In the incomplete or footling breech presentation, the fetus has one or both of its hips incompletely flexed so that some part of the lower extremity is the presenting part. This presentation occurs about 25% to 35% of the time and is more common among premature fetuses.

C. Complete Breech
In the complete breech presentation, the fetus has its hips and knees flexed. This accounts for 5% of breech presentations.

IV. MANAGEMENT

The family physician should have a strategy to recognize and manage the breech presentation during the third trimester and in labor.

A. Antenatal Management
1. Recognition
   It is important to begin to assess the fetal lie beginning at 32 to 34 weeks of gestation using the techniques as described earlier.
2. Maneuvers to convert the breech to the vertex position
   a. External version: This maneuver can be carried out safely by a qualified operator beginning at

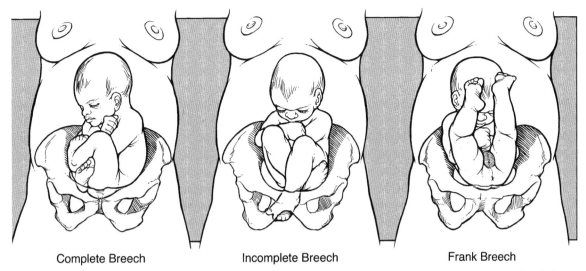

Complete Breech   Incomplete Breech   Frank Breech

FIGURE 17-4. The complete breech is flexed at the hips and flexed at the knees. The incomplete breech shows incomplete deflexion of one or both knees or hips. The frank breech is flexed at the hips and extended at the knees.

36 weeks of gestation for the nullipara and 38 weeks of gestation for the multipara. (See Section H for a complete description of the procedure.)

b. Use of moxibustion: This is a type of traditional Chinese medicine that uses moxibustion (burning herbs to stimulate acupuncture points) of acupoint BL 67 (located beside the outer corner of the fifth toenail). An RCT reported that the application of moxibustion for nullipara breech presentations beginning at 33 weeks of gestation resulted in increased fetal activity during the treatment period and an increased spontaneous conversion to the vertex presentation (relative risk, 1.58; 95% confidence interval [CI], 1.29-1.94) although this cephalic version did not lead to a decrease in cesarean section rates.[9] This author replicated this study in Italy among nulliparous women at 33 weeks of gestation and did not find an increase in spontaneous conversion to the vertex presentation. There was a much greater nonadherence to the moxibustion treatment group in this study, which may have confounded the treatment effect.[10]

c. Postural management: The Cochrane meta-analysis of three RCTs involving a total number of 192 women showed that the use of postural management (elevation of the maternal pelvis) was associated with a nonsignificant trend toward fewer noncephalic births. The author of this review states, "There is not enough evidence to evaluate the use of postural management for breech presentation."[11]

B. Intrapartum Management

Since the landmark Term Breech Trial was published, the debate about the management of the term breech presentation has been, for the most part, resolved in favor of offering an elective cesarean delivery.

1. Term Breech Trial

   The Term Breech Trial was a landmark study involving 2088 women with singleton breech presentations at term that randomized them into planned vaginal breech deliveries versus cesarean sections. This study was conducted in 121 centers in 26 countries spanning developed and developing countries with different baseline perinatal mortality rates.[7] This study demonstrated that elective vaginal breech deliveries by experienced obstetricians was associated with a threefold increase in perinatal serious morbidity and mortality. Overall, 5% of the vaginal breech deliveries versus 1.6% of the elective cesarean deliveries experienced this morbidity and mortality. The number of elective cesarean sections needed to prevent 1 infant with serious morbidity or mortality was 14. Maternal outcomes were comparable in the control and treatment groups both in the immediate period after childbirth and at 3 months after delivery.[12] This study resulted in an ACOG Committee opinion that "planned vaginal delivery of a term singleton breech may no longer be appropriate."[13]

2. Follow-up Term Breech Trials
   a. Maternal outcomes at 2 years[14]
      No significant differences in maternal outcomes 2 years after delivery were found with respect to sexual function, family relationships, urinary incontinence, depression, or distressing memories of the birth experience. Women in the planned cesarean group did have an increased incidence of constipation.
   b. Pediatric outcomes at 2 years[15]
      Using an intention-to-treat analysis, researchers found that the risk for death or neurodevelopmental delay was not increased in the planned vaginal birth group compared with the planned cesarean section group.
   c. Economic analysis[16]
      Overall costs were approximately $877 less in the planned cesarean versus vaginal delivery group. This occurred largely because of increased physician charges and increased use of the neonatal intensive care unit in the planned vaginal delivery group.
   d. Mothers' views of childbirth experience
      Patients had variable feelings about their childbirth that were associated with allocation to either planned cesarean or vaginal birth. Women allocated to the planned cesarean section group were more likely to appreciate being able to schedule the delivery, feel reassured about their infants' health, and perceive less pain with childbirth. Women allocated to the vaginal birth group were more likely to perceive that the birth was more natural and liked being more of a participant in the birth process. These views, however, did not affect the evaluations of the quality of intrapartum care, support from their clinicians, or amount of involvement in decision making.[17]

3. New evidence demonstrating safety with vaginal breech delivery: The PREMODA Study[18]
   A nonrandomized, observational, prospective study with intent-to-treat analysis involving 8105 French and Belgium women demonstrated a low rate of perinatal mortality or serious neonatal morbidity (1.59% overall and 1.60% in the planned vaginal delivery group). Other than the difference in study design between this study and the Term Breech Trial, this study applied rigorous management criteria for the management of the vaginal breech patient in labor including routine use of pelvimetry, use of intrapartum ultrasound to exclude fetuses with hyperextended heads, continuous electronic fetal surveillance, and stage two practices designed to aim for delivery within 1 hour of pushing. This study provides evidence to support offering women the option for elective vaginal breech delivery in systems that provide the safeguards and physician expertise found in this study.

C. Factors Favorable for Vaginal Breech Delivery

Factors favorable for vaginal breech delivery include[2]:
1. Frank breech
2. Gestational age between 36 and 38 weeks
3. Multiparous patient with previous vaginal breech delivery of infant more than 3200 g or cephalic delivery of infant more than 3600 g
4. Estimated fetal weight between 2700 and 3200 g (6 and 7 pounds)
5. Favorable (soft, effaced) cervix dilated 3 cm or more
6. Presenting part at or below 0 station at labor's onset
7. Adequate pelvimetry (particularly in the anteroposterior diameter): anteroposterior dimension of the inlet, 11 cm or greater; transverse diameter of the inlet and anteroposterior diameter of the midpelvis, 12 cm or greater; interspinous distance of the midpelvis, 9.5 cm or greater
8. Flexed fetal neck
9. Experienced operator

D. Factors Unfavorable for Vaginal Breech Delivery

Factors unfavorable for vaginal breech delivery include:
1. Footling or complete breech presentation
2. Gestational age less than 36 or more than 38 weeks
3. Estimated fetal weight of less than 2700 g or more than 3800 g
4. No previous vaginal deliveries or difficult previous vaginal delivery
5. Unfavorable cervix
6. High presenting part at onset of labor

7. Maternal pelvis flattened in the anteroposterior diameter
8. Hyperextended fetal neck
9. Inexperienced operator

E. Special Precautions for Estimating Fetal Weight in Labor

A sonographic estimate of fetal weight can be helpful in deciding whether to attempt a vaginal breech delivery. It is important to note, however, that even skilled sonographers can estimate plus or minus 15% of the actual fetal weight.

F. Techniques to Assess Maternal Pelvimetry

Once a determination of estimated fetal weight has occurred, a number of methods are available to assess maternal pelvimetry. The initial test of choice is a radiograph or bedside ultrasound of the maternal abdomen to ensure that the fetal head is not extended and to look for other congenital anomalies. X-ray pelvimetry can produce the pelvic measurements as detailed earlier. Computed tomography pelvimetry has the advantage of using radiation that is 80% less than conventional x-rays. An RCT that compared the use of magnetic resonance imaging (MRI) versus clinical pelvimetry showed that the use of the latter technology did not significantly reduce the overall cesarean rate. MRI pelvimetry was associated with a lower emergency cesarean rate.[19]

G. Technique of Vaginal Breech Delivery

The following is the procedure for delivering a vaginal breech presentation in an advanced state of labor.[2,20] The family physician may encounter this malpresentation when there is insufficient time to proceed with a cesarean section.

1. Expect spontaneous dilatation and descent at a normal rate
   If the progress of labor is abnormal, consider abandoning vaginal delivery in favor of cesarean section if time allows. Avoid early amniotomy because it may increase the risk for cord prolapse.
2. Use of anesthesia
   If used, anesthesia that permits full maternal cooperation is best (i.e., local, pudendal, low spinal, or epidural rather than general). Epidural anesthesia is associated with a prolonged stage two but not with an increase in breech extraction or cesarean

sections.[21] Anesthesia personnel should be available on standby for the second stage of labor in case general anesthesia is required.

3. Delivery of the breech
   The operator needs to have patience during this process and should monitor for fetal well-being throughout the delivery. Await descent of the breech until the perineum is distended. Delivery of the infant up to the umbilicus should occur by spontaneous contractions and maternal pushing. Once the fetal umbilicus has passed the perineum, the fetal head will have entered the maternal pelvis and vaginal breech delivery becomes the only available route of delivery.
4. Ensure that the fetal back is anterior
   Grasp the hips to ensure that the fetal back is anterior (Figure 17-5). If the back rotates posteriorly, the head will be OP and the chin is likely to extend against the symphysis pubis with potentially disastrous results.
5. Freeing the umbilical cord
   After the umbilicus is delivered, pull out a few inches of the umbilical cord if it appears to have excessive traction on it; otherwise, do not manipulate the umbilical cord.
6. Delivery of the body
   Maternal pushing should be the major force to help deliver the fetal body. The operator can use a towel placed around the fetal pelvis with thumbs applied over the sacroiliac joints and fingers over the anterior thigh to apply gentle downward traction. *The operator must not apply pressure to the fetal abdomen; this could result in significant visceral injuries.*
7. Delivery of the shoulders and arms
   If the shoulders and arms do not deliver spontaneously, sweep the posterior arm across the chest and out. If this is ineffective, rotate the trunk to place the other shoulder posterior and sweep that arm out if it does not deliver spontaneously (Figure 17-6). It is often helpful to have an assistant elevate the fetal trunk and legs by cradling it in a towel sling.
8. Delivery of the fetal head
   An assistant maintains suprapubic pressure to keep the head flexed. An episiotomy may be necessary to provide the exposure to accomplish the following maneuvers.
   a. Apply digital pressure on the malar eminence with the same hand supporting the chest and the opposite hand pulling downward on the

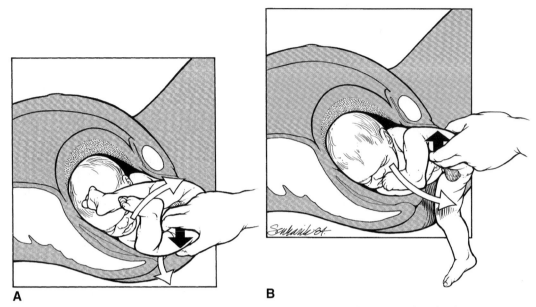

FIGURE 17-5. After spontaneous expulsion to the umbilicus, external rotation of each thigh **(A)** combined with opposite rotation of the fetal pelvis results in flexion of the knee and delivery of each leg **(B).**

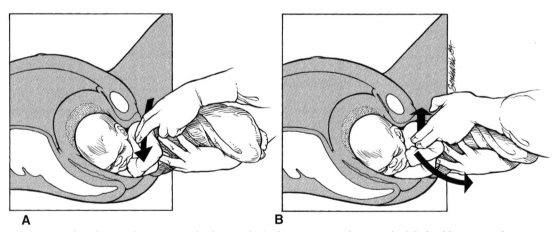

FIGURE 17-6. When the scapulae appear under the symphysis, the operator reaches over the left shoulder, sweeps the arm across the chest **(A),** and delivers the arm **(B)**.

shoulders (Mauriceau-Smellie-Veit maneuver) (Figure 17-7).

b. Apply digital pressure on the malar eminence as above with the opposite hand applying suprapubic pressure to maintain head flexion (Wigand-Martin maneuver).

c. Use Piper forceps (Figure 17-8).

The fetal body should not be elevated any more than being parallel to the floor to avoid hyperextension injuries. The operator may need to kneel on the floor to deliver the fetal head, particularly if forceps are applied.

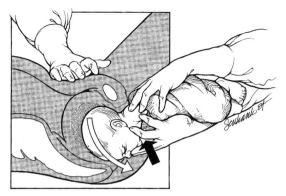

FIGURE 17-7. Cephalic flexion is maintained by pressure *(black arrow)* on the fetal maxilla (not mandible). Often, delivery of the head is easily accomplished with continued expulsive forces from above and gentle downward traction.

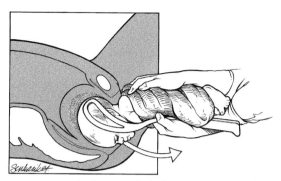

FIGURE 17-8. The fetus may be laid on the forceps and delivered with gentle downward traction as illustrated here.

V. SOR A RECOMMENDATIONS

RECOMMENDATIONS	REFERENCES
Use of elective cesarean delivery versus vaginal delivery to manage the term breech presentation results in a significant decrease in perinatal mortality and serious neonatal morbidity.	7, 12
Use of elective cesarean deliver versus vaginal delivery to manage the term breech presentation does not result in any significant maternal outcomes 2 years after the delivery except for an increase in constipation in the cesarean group.	14
Use of elective cesarean delivery versus vaginal delivery to manage the term breech presentation does not decrease mortality or neurodevelopmental delay by the age of 2 years.	15

REFERENCES

1. Weiner CP: Vaginal breech delivery in the 1990s, *Clin Obstet Gynecol* 35:559-569, 1992.
2. Cruickshank DP: Malpresentations and umbilical cord complications. In Danforth DN, Scott JR, editors: *Obstetrics and gynecology*, ed 7, Philadelphia, 1998, JB Lippincott.
3. Westgren M, Edvall H, Nordstrom L et al: Spontaneous cephalic version of breech presentation in the last trimester, *Br J Obstet Gynaecol* 92:19-24, 1985.
4. Croughan-Minihane MS, Petitti DB, Gordis L, Golditch I: Morbidity among breech infants according to method of delivery, *Obstet Gynecol* 75:821-825, 1990.
5. Thorpe-Beeston JG, Banfield PJ, Saunders NJ Sr: Outcomes of breech delivery at term, *BMJ* 305:746-747, 1992.
6. Cheng M, Hannah M: Breech delivery at term: a critical review of the literature, *Obstet Gynecol* 82:605-610, 1993.
7. Hannah ME, Hannah WJ, Hewson SA et al: Planned caesarean section versus planned vaginal birth for breech presentation at term: a randomized multicentre trial. Term Breech Trial Collaborative Group, *Lancet* 356:1375-1383, 2000.
8. Su M, Hannah WJ, Willan A et al: Planned caesarean section decreases the risk of adverse perinatal outcome due to both labour and delivery complications in the Term Breech Trial, *BJOG* 111:1065-1074, 2004.
9. Cardini F, Weixin H: Moxibustion for correction of breech presentation, *JAMA* 280:1580-1584, 1998.
10. Cardini F, Lombardo P, Regalia AL et al: A randomized controlled trial of moxibustion for breech presentation, *BJOG* 112:743-747, 2005.
11. Hofmeyr GJ: Cephalic version by postural management (Cochrane review). *The Cochrane Library,* Oxford, 2006, Wiley Publishing.
12. Hannah ME, Hannah WJ, Hodnett ED et al: Outcomes at 3 months after planned cesarean vs planned vaginal delivery for breech presentation at term: the international randomized Term Breech Trial, *JAMA* 287:1822-1831, 2002.
13. ACOG Committee Opinion. Mode of term singleton breech delivery. Number 265, December 2001. American College of Obstetricians and Gynecologist, *Int J Gynaecol Obstet* 77:65-66, 2002.
14. Hannah ME, Whyte H, Hannah WJ et al: Maternal outcomes at 2 years after planned cesarean section versus planned vaginal birth for breech presentation at term: the international randomized Term Breech Trial, *Am J Obstet Gynecol* 191:917-927, 2004.
15. Whyte H, Hannah ME, Saigal S et al: Outcomes of children at 2 years after planned cesarean birth versus planned vaginal birth for breech presentation at term: the International Randomized Term Breech Trial, *Am J Obstet Gynecol* 191:864-871, 2004.
16. Palencia R, Gafni A, Hannah ME et al: The costs of planned cesarean versus planned vaginal birth in the Term Breech Trial, *CMAJ* 174:1109-1113, 2006.
17. Hodnett ED, Hannah ME, Hewson S et al: Mothers' views of their childbirth experiences 2 years after planned Caesarean

versus planned vaginal birth for breech presentation at term, in the international randomized Term Breech Trial, *J Obstet Gynaecol Can* 27:224-231, 2005.

18. Goffinet F, Carayol M, Foidart J et al: Is planned vaginal delivery for breech presentation at term still an option? Results of an observational prospective survey in France and Belgium, *Am J Obstet Gynecol* 194:1002-1011, 2006.

19. Van Loon AJ, Mantingh A, Serlier D et al: Randomised controlled trial of magnetic-resonance pelvimetry in breech presentation at term, *Lancet* 350:1799-1804, 1997.

20. Yasin S, O'Sullivan MJ: Assisted breech extraction. In Plauche WC, Morrison JC, O'Sullivan MJ, editors: *Surgical obstetrics,* Philadelphia, 1992, WB Saunders.

21. Chadha YG, Mahmoud TA, Dick MJ et al: Breech delivery and epidural analgesia, *Br J Obstet Gynaecol* 99:96-100, 1992.

SECTION H **External Cephalic Version**

Kent Petrie, MD

External cephalic version (ECV) is a procedure to manually guide a fetus from a breech to a vertex presentation. It is performed to reduce the incidence of breech presentation at delivery. Fetuses found to be in the breech presentation at 36 weeks of gestation or later are candidates for ECV.

I. INCIDENCE OF BREECH

There is a natural tendency toward spontaneous version from breech to cephalic presentation as pregnancy progresses. Twenty-five percent of fetuses are breech at 28 weeks of gestation. This percentage declines to 13% by 32 weeks. Nine percent of fetuses are breech at 36 weeks of gestation, and half of these will turn spontaneously to cephalic presentation in the last month of pregnancy.[1]

Smaller fetuses are more likely to be breech at 40 weeks. Eight percent of 2000-g fetuses are breech, whereas only 3% of 3000-g fetuses are breech.

II. NATURAL HISTORY

A. Conditions Associated with Breech Presentation

Multiple gestation, multiparity, uterine relaxation, both polyhydramnios and oligohydramnios, pelvic tumors, uterine fibroids and septa, and a history of breech all are factors increasing the incidence of breech presentation.

B. Congenital Anomalies

Congenital anomalies are seen more frequently in breech fetuses. These include hydrocephaly and anencephaly, and disorders of the gastrointestinal, genitourinary, cardiovascular, and musculoskeletal systems. Fetuses with Down syndrome are also more commonly found in the breech presentation; this is thought to be due to relative hypotonia, which reduces spontaneous version.

III. EFFECT ON PERINATAL OUTCOMES

A. Morbidity Associated with Breech Presentation

Breech presentation is a common problem that can cause hazards to both mother and fetus. Perinatal morbidity and mortality for vaginal breech delivery at term are significantly greater than for vertex delivery.

B. Maternal Morbidity and Mortality with Cesarean Delivery

Twelve percent of cesarean deliveries in the United States are now performed for breech presentation, ranking as the third most frequent indication, after repeat cesarean and labor dystocia.[2] This modern trend toward cesarean for breech presentation at term has been accompanied by increased postsurgical maternal morbidity compared with vaginal delivery. Potential injury to the infant in breech, however, still exists at cesarean delivery.

C. Cost-Effectiveness of External Cephalic Version versus Cesarean Delivery

Two studies have reviewed the cost-effectiveness of ECV. The first study, a decision analysis, found that routine use of ECV would decrease the number of cesarean deliveries and would cost significantly less than either a scheduled cesarean or a trial of labor without ECV.[3] The second study, a retrospective cohort study, found that ECV reduced both maternal and fetal morbidity associated with cesarean delivery and saved, on average, $2462 per patient.[4]

IV. DIAGNOSIS

Ultrasound is useful for confirmation of breech presentation and to "rule out" certain birth defects and uterine anomalies that predispose to breech presentation.

V. ALTERNATIVE TREATMENTS FOR THE VERSION OF THE BREECH PRESENTATION

Alternative treatments for the version of the breech presentation are discussed in the following sections.[5]

A. Prenatal Exercises

Studies in which patients assumed the knee-chest position with chest and head against the floor or bed and hips elevated, accompanied by gentle pelvic rocking for 20 minutes three times a day, demonstrate version rates greater than control patients.[6,7] This posture allows the fetus to "fall forward" out of the pelvis and promotes turning. If the knee-chest position is uncomfortable, the patient may achieve the same effect by lying supine with her hips supported on several firm pillows. A Cochrane metaanalysis, however, has demonstrated an overall nonsignificant trend toward reduction in breech presentation with these exercises.[8]

B. Hypnosis

Mehl[9] studied 100 volunteer patients whose fetuses were found to be breech at 37 to 40 weeks of gestation. The patients received weekly office hypnosis sessions with suggestions for general relaxation and release of fear and anxiety. Relaxation audiotapes were provided for each patient to use daily at home. Mehl reports 81% of the fetuses in the intervention group turned compared with 48% in a matched control group.

C. Traditional Chinese Medicine

Moxibustion has been studied, applied at acupuncture point UB 67 on the lateral aspect of the fifth toe. When performed bilaterally for 15 minutes each day beginning at 33 weeks of gestation, Cardini and Weixin[10] demonstrated a 75% version rate by 35 weeks compared with 47% in matched control subjects. It is postulated that this stimulation causes increased maternal adrenocortical activity, increasing uterine tone and fetal activity that stimulates spontaneous version.

VI. PREDICTING SUCCESS OF EXTERNAL CEPHALIC VERSION

A. Success Rates

The overall success rate of ECV has been variably reported in the literature from 35% to 86%.[11-17] Many authors have identified prognostic factors for ECV success. ECV is most successful in multiparous patients, with placental location lateral or fundal, with normal or increased amniotic fluid, and with the fetus in a nonfrank breech presentation with the fetal spine to the mother's side and crossing the maternal midline.

B. Scoring System for External Cephalic Version

Newman and associates[18] developed a scoring system that can help predict success of ECV (Table 17-1). The scoring system is most helpful at the extremes, with rare successful versions with a score of 2 or less and a high likelihood of success with scores of 9 or 10.[18]

C. Tocolysis

Most available evidence supports the use of a tocolytic agent during ECV, especially in nulliparous patients.[15,16,19-21] A recent metaanalysis using terbutaline reported a 50% increase in successful ECV regardless of parity.[22]

D. Use of Anesthesia with External Cephalic Version

Available evidence does not support the routine use of anesthesia for ECV. Concern exists that the loss of patients' pain perception could result in the clinician applying excessive force during ECV. Studies using epidural anesthesia report increased success rates, but dural puncture and marginal placental abruption were noted in the epidural groups.[23,24] Epidural use also negated the overall cost savings of vaginal birth over cesarean delivery. An RCT evaluating the effect of spinal anesthesia on ECV found no significant differences.[25]

TABLE 17-1 **Newman Score**

	0	1	2
Parity	0	1	≥2
Dilation	≥3 cm	1-2 cm	0 cm
Estimated fetal weight	<2500 g	2500-3500 g	>3500 g
Placenta	Anterior	Posterior	Lateral/fundal
Station	≥−1	−2	≤−3

From Newman RB, Peacock BS, Van Dorsten JP et al: Predicting success of external cephalic version, *Am J Obstet Gynecol* 169:245-249, 1993.

VII. CONTRAINDICATIONS TO EXTERNAL CEPHALIC VERSION

Contraindications to ECV include:

1. Multiple pregnancy (except version of the second twin after delivering the first)
2. Oligohydramnios
3. Uterine malformation
4. Placenta previa
5. Fetal anomaly
6. Previous placental abruption during this pregnancy
7. Suspected fetal distress or IUGR
8. Ruptured membranes (because of the risk for cord prolapse)
9. Nonreassuring fetal heart rate tracings
10. Preeclampsia (relative contraindication because of increased risk for abruption)
11. Previous uterine surgery: Little information is available on the effects of a previous uterine scar on the success and safety of ECV. One small study indicates that it is comparable with patients without a prior cesarean section.[26]
12. Patient in labor (not considered a contraindication in some institutions): A small number of studies report successful ECV when patients are in labor.[20,22]

VIII. PERFORMING AN EXTERNAL CEPHALIC VERSION

A. Informed Consent

Written informed consent for ECV should be signed after careful discussion of the procedure, alternatives, and risks.[2,27,28]

B. Preparation for the Procedure

1. The procedure should be performed in a labor room with the operating room notified (and consultant privileged to do cesarean notified, if the doctor attempting version is not) in the event of complications requiring emergency cesarean delivery. A nonstress test should be performed while an IV is started and blood sent for possible type and crossmatch.
2. The patient should empty her bladder, be placed in a hospital gown, and assume a supine position in bed with a slight left lateral tilt in mild Trendelenburg position, with knees slightly bent.
3. If tocolysis is chosen, it may be administered as terbutaline 5 to 10 mg orally 30 minutes before the procedure or 0.25 mg subcutaneously or intravenously 10 minutes before the procedure.
4. Two operators are helpful because the procedure can be strenuous.
5. Operators should have well-trimmed fingernails.
6. Ultrasound gel or mineral oil applied to the abdomen will reduce friction on the skin as the infant is moved.

C. Performing the Procedure

1. Elevate the breech with a hand placed in the suprapubic area below the breech.
2. With slow, steady pressure, push the breech into the iliac fossa with the lower hand, in the direction to begin a forward roll movement of the fetus.
3. Keeping the fetal head flexed, manipulate the fetus into the oblique and then transverse diameter. Avoid rapid, sharp movements. Firm pressure will allow the progress to occur in stages. Pause occasionally to allow the infant to "squirm" a bit. Typically, about two thirds of the force needs to be applied to the breech, whereas one third is applied to the head, mainly to keep the head flexed.
4. When the technique is applied using two operators, the second operator may monitor the progress with frequent ultrasound observations of fetal position and heart rate, as well as assist the first operator with manual pressure on one of the fetal poles.
5. When the baby is just past transverse, it will usually rotate the rest of the way with little effort on the part of the operators.
6. Set the fetal head into the pelvis by manual manipulation and fundal pressure. Move the patient out of the Trendelenburg position.
7. If a forward roll fails, try a backward flip, particularly if the head and breech lie on the same side of the midline.
8. If ultrasound reveals that the fetal spine is directly anterior, it may be difficult to perform these maneuvers. One randomized trial found that fetal acoustic stimulation produced fetal motion resulting in a shift of the fetal spine to the maternal right or left, dramatically increasing the success of ECV (86% vs. 8%).[29]
9. If the procedure is unsuccessful in 15 to 20 minutes, discontinue the procedure.
10. If bradycardia occurs during the procedure, stop. If it persists, revert to the original breech position. If bradycardia further persists despite oxygen administration and maternal position change, prepare for emergency cesarean delivery.

11. Perform a nonstress test when the procedure is completed, regardless of whether the version is successful.

12. Discharge patient when the nonstress test is reactive, the patient feels well, and there is no evidence of active labor.

IX. COMPLICATIONS OF EXTERNAL CEPHALIC VERSION

A. Fetal and Maternal Complications

1. Incidence/Type

   Rare complications of ECV have been reported (overall incidence of 1-2%), and include fetal bradycardia and fetal distress caused by knotted or entangled cords, placental abruption, fetal hemorrhage, maternal hemorrhage, preterm labor, and premature rupture of the membranes. By far the most common complication is fetal heart rate changes. One series found an incidence rate of fetal heart rate changes of 39%, but they were transient and had no relation to the final outcome of the pregnancy.[30]

2. Fetal mortality

   Fetal mortality is extremely rare and is reported only in cases of attempted ECV under general anesthesia or in settings without electronic monitoring and ultrasound. A follow-up study in the same institution, after a change in protocol, did not find the same adverse outcomes.[14] When attempting an ECV, facilities and personnel must be available for performing an emergency cesarean section to prevent this rare complication.

3. Impact on cesarean rates

   A lower cesarean delivery rate has been reported in women who have had a successful ECV compared with women who have not attempted ECV.[11-14] After successful version, however, the intrapartum cesarean section rate has been reported to be twice that of a control group of vertex vaginal deliveries.[31]

4. Fetal-maternal transfusions

   Fetal-maternal transfusions have been reported to occur in up to 6% of patients undergoing external version. A dose of RhoGAM is recommended in the Rh-negative patient.

B. Reversion to Breech

Reversion to breech after successful ECV is more common when version is attempted before 36 weeks of gestation. Reports of spontaneous reversion up to 40% if version is done before 36 weeks emphasize that fetal lie is generally unstable until the last month of pregnancy. Most reports of ECV after 36 weeks show a stable vertex presentation at labor in 90% to 100% of cases.[32,33]

ECV before term is no longer recommended because of this greater rate of reversion, the risk for premature birth, and the potential need to perform an emergency cesarean delivery of a premature infant because of fetal distress. Most protocols now recommend a first attempt after 36 weeks of gestation.

X. MANAGEMENT AFTER ATTEMPTED EXTERNAL CEPHALIC VERSION

A. Unsuccessful External Cephalic Version

If ECV is unsuccessful, the following steps may be taken:

1. Version may be attempted again in several days to one week.

2. Version may be attempted again with spinal or epidural anesthesia before a scheduled cesarean section delivery.

3. Cesarean delivery may be scheduled without an additional attempt.

4. Cesarean delivery may be performed when patient presents in labor if spontaneous version has not occurred in the interim.

B. Successful External Cephalic Version

If ECV is successful, the following steps may be taken:

1. Patient may resume routine prenatal care until onset of labor with close surveillance by examination, ultrasound, or both to assure maintenance of vertex presentation.

2. If the cervix is favorable and the patient is term, induction of labor may be considered immediately after ECV.

XI. MULTIPLE PREGNANCY

A. Version of the Second Twin

Although multiple pregnancy is listed as a contraindication to ECV, version of the second twin after the first twin has been delivered vaginally is acceptable. After delivery of the first twin and before rupture of the membranes surrounding the second twin, the head of the second twin can generally be guided into the pelvis for vertex delivery. The procedure is made easier if real-time ultrasound is available at the bedside in the delivery room. Some evidence suggests that breech extraction of the second twin is associated with fewer complications than cesarean delivery and may be the preferred choice if the birth attendant is skilled at breech extraction.[34]

XII. SOR A RECOMMENDATION

RECOMMENDATIONS	REFERENCES
Routine tocolysis increases the success rate of ECV at term (NNT = 4.1).	22
Caesarean section for the birth of a second twin not presenting cephalically is associated with increased maternal febrile morbidity with as yet no identified improvement in neonatal outcome.	34

REFERENCES

1. Westgren M, Edvall H, Nordstrom L et al: Spontaneous cephalic version of breech presentation in the last trimester, *Br J Obstet Gynaecol* 92:19-22, 1985.
2. Coco AS, Silverman SD: External cephalic version, *Am Fam Physician* 58:731-748, 1998.
3. Gifford DS, Keeler E, Kahn KL: Reductions in cost and cesarean rate by routine use of external cephalic version: a decision analysis, *Obstet Gynecol* 85:930-936, 1995.
4. Mauldin JG, Mauldin PD, Feng TI et al: Determining the clinical efficacy and cost savings of successful external cephalic version, *Am J Obstet Gynecol* 175:1639-1644, 1996.
5. Tiran D, Mack S: *Complementary therapies for pregnancy and childbirth*, ed 2, London, 2000, Bailliere Tindall.
6. Chenia F, Crowther CA: Does advice to assume the knee-chest position reduce the incidence of breech presentation at delivery? A randomized clinical trial, *Birth* 14:75-78, 1987.
7. Smith C, Crowther C, Wilkinson C et al: Knee-chest postural management for breech at term: a randomized controlled trial, *Birth* 26:71-75, 1999.
8. Hofmeyr GJ, Kulier R: Cephalic version by postural management for breech presentation, *Cochrane Database Syst Rev* (3): CD000051, 2000.
9. Mehl LE: Hypnosis and conversion of the breech to vertex presentation, *Arch Fam Med* 3:883-887, 1994.
10. Cardini F, Weixin H: Moxibustion for correction of breech presentation: a randomized controlled trial, *JAMA* 280:1580-1584, 1998.
11. Brocks V, Philipsen T, Secher NJ: A randomized trial of external cephalic version with tocolysis in late pregnancy, *Br J Obstet Gynecol* 91:653-656, 1984.
12. Dyson DC, Ferguson JE, Hensleigh P: Antepartum external cephalic version under tocolysis, *Obstet Gynecol* 67:63-68, 1986.
13. Marchick R: Antepartum external cephalic version with tocolysis: a study of term singleton breech presentations, *Am J Obstet Gynecol* 158:1339-1346, 1988.
14. Hofmeyr GJ, Gyte G: Interventions to help external cephalic version for breech presentation at term, *Cochrane Database Syst Rev* (1):CD000184, 2004.

15. Robertson AW, Kopelman JN, Read JA et al: External cephalic version at term: is a tocolytic necessary? *Obstet Gynecol* 70:896-899, 1987.
16. Van Veelen AJ, Van Capellen W, Flu PK et al: Effect of external cephalic version in late pregnancy on presentation art delivery: a randomized controlled trial, *Br J Obstet Gynecol* 96:916-921, 1989.
17. Zhang MJ, Bowes WA, Fortney JA: Efficacy of external cephalic version: a review, *Obstet Gynecol* 82:306-313, 1993.
18. Newman RB, Peacock BS, Van Dorsten JP et al: Predicting success of external cephalic version, *Am J Obstet Gynecol* 169:245-249, 1993.
19. Chung T, Neale E, Lau TK et al: A randomized double blind controlled trial of tocolysis to assist external cephalic version in late pregnancy, *Acta Obstet Gynecol Scand* 75:720-724, 1996.
20. Marquette GP, Boucher M, Theriault D et al: Does the use of a tocolytic agent affect the success rate of external cephalic version? *Am J Obstet Gynecol* 175:859-861, 1996.
21. Stock A, Chung T, Rogers M et al: Randomized double blind placebo controlled comparison of ritodrine and hexaprenaline for tocolysis prior to external cephalic version at term, *Aust N Z J Obstet Gynecol* 33:265-268, 1993.
22. Fernandez CO, Bloom SL, Smulian JC et al: A randomized, placebo controlled evaluation of terbutaline for external cephalic version, *Obstet Gynecol* 90:775-779, 1997.
23. Rozenburg P, Goffinet F, de Spirlet M et al: External cephalic version with epidural anesthesia after failure of a first trial with beta-mimetics, *Br J Obstet Gynecol* 107:406-410, 2000.
24. Schorr SJ, Speights SE, Ross EL et al: A randomized trial of epidural anesthesia to improve external cephalic version success, *Am J Obstet Gynecol* 177:1133-1137, 1997.
25. Dugoff L, Stamm CA, Jones OW et al: The effect of spinal anesthesia on the success rate of external cephalic version: a randomized trial, *Obstet Gynecol* 93:345-349, 1999.
26. Flamm BL, Fried MW, Lonky NM et al: External cephalic version after previous cesarean section, *Am J Obstet Gynecol* 165:370-372, 1991.
27. American College of Obstetricians and Gynecologists (ACOG): External cephalic version. ACOG Practice Bulletin No. 13, February 2000, Washington, DC, 2000, ACOG.
28. Eisinger SH: Malpresentations, malpositions and multiple gestations. *Advanced Life Support in Obstetrics (ALSO) course syllabus*, ed 4, Leawood, KS, 2000, American Academy of Family Physicians.
29. Johnson RL, Elliott JP: Fetal acoustic stimulation, an adjunct to external cephalic version: a blinded randomized crossover study, *Am J Obstet Gynecol* 173:1369-1372, 1995.
30. Phelan JP, Stine LE, Mueller E et al: Observations of fetal heart rate characteristics related to external cephalic version and tocolysis, *Am J Obstet Gynecol* 149:658-661, 1984.
31. Lau TK, Lo KW, Robers M: Pregnancy outcomes after successful external cephalic version for breech presentation at term, *Am J Obstet Gynecol* 176:218-223, 1997.
32. Kasule J, Chimbira TH, Brown IM: Controlled trial of external cephalic version, *Br J Obstet Gynecol* 92:14-18, 1985.
33. Kornman MT, Kimball KT, Reves KO: Preterm external cephalic version in an outpatient environment, *Am J Obstet Gynecol* 172:1734-1738, 1995.
34. Crowther CA: Caesarean delivery for the second twin, *Cochrane Database Syst Rev* (2):CD000047, 2000.

SECTION I Twin Gestation

Ellen L. Sakornbut, MD

I. PRESENTATION OF TWIN GESTATION

As term approaches, crowding of the uterus decreases the freedom of movement of the fetuses. Conventionally, the presenting twin in the intrapartum setting is often referred to as twin A and the after-coming twin as twin B. This may not be consistent with the designations provided during serial ultrasound examinations throughout pregnancy, and indeed, it may be difficult to predict early in pregnancy which twin will present in labor. Management of the delivery necessitates knowledge of the position of each twin. Approximately 43% of twins present as vertex, vertex; 38% as vertex, nonvertex (either breech or transverse); and 19% as breech with twin B any presentation.[1]

II. MANAGEMENT OF TWIN LABOR

A. Ultrasound

Intrapartum use of ultrasound is helpful both at presentation to the labor unit and during vaginal delivery for assessment of position, presentation, and heart rate of the fetuses. With practice, the clinician can determine degree of fetal head flexion and position of extremities in the nonvertex second twin (frank, complete, footling breech).

B. Use of Oxytocin

One study comparing oxytocin augmentation and induction of labor in twin and singleton pregnancies found use of oxytocin to be safe and effective. Patients with twin pregnancy were not more likely to encounter hyperstimulation or less likely to respond to oxytocin therapy than patients with singleton pregnancies.[2]

C. Timing of Delivery

Timing of delivery should be determined based on obstetric indications. These may include deterioration of fetal condition caused by twin-twin transfusion or maternal indication such as preeclampsia. The risks for delivery before 37 weeks are primarily those associated with prematurity. A 7-year study of uncomplicated twin gestations in one center found a thirteenfold increased risk for neonatal complications in pregnancies delivered before 38 weeks compared with pregnancies delivered at or after 38 weeks.[3] It is reassuring to note that infants born from multiple gestation pregnancies do not experience increased risk at the same gestational age. A large prospective study of multiple gestations provides evidence of similar neonatal outcomes at all viable premature weeks of gestation comparing twins and triplets with singletons.[4] A small RCT compared expectant management (spontaneous labor) versus induction of labor at 37 weeks. Birth weights did not differ significantly, but there was a lower incidence of infection in the expectant management group.[5] Evidence does not, therefore, support elective induction for twin gestation in the absence of specific fetal or maternal indication.

D. Fetal Heart Rate Monitoring

In twin pregnancies, it may be technically more difficult to obtain adequate documentation of fetal heart rates. A combination of methods may be needed to monitor the status of each twin.

E. Planning for the Newborns

Resuscitation planning for the newborns should include adequate equipment and personnel for both twins, whether delivery is vaginal or operative. Although it has been proposed that the after-coming twin is at greater risk than the presenting twin, the most experienced pediatric resuscitator should initiate activity with the presenting twin if that infant appears unstable at birth.

F. Vaginal Birth after Prior Cesarean Section

Two larger studies are available, both retrospective, addressing safety issues with trial of labor. A comparison of 186 women with twin gestation choosing trial of labor with 226 women choosing elective cesarean found a 64.5% success rate overall with no increase in maternal mortality or morbidity or uterine rupture and no difference in neonatal outcomes.[6] A cohort study of 535 women with twin gestation found a decreased likelihood of choice for trial of labor (adjusted odds ratio, 0.3; 95% CI, 0.2-0.4) but no more likelihood of failure of trial of labor, uterine rupture, endometritis, other maternal morbidity, or neonatal morbidity and mortality compared with more than 24,000 singleton pregnancies.[7] No RCTs are available.

G. Monoamniotic Twin Gestation

Monoamniotic twin gestation is seen infrequently. A recent longitudinal study from 1986 through 2002 showed a 60% survival rate for fetuses, with the cause of intrauterine death in 8 of 10 fetuses due to documented cord entanglement.[8] Patients who are documented with a monoamniotic gestation should be referred for perinatal high-risk services as soon as a diagnosis is made because of the need for intensive monitoring and the potential for benefit from interventions.

III. CHOICE OF ROUTE OF DELIVERY

A. Presenting Fetus Vertex

Route of delivery remains a controversial issue in which decision making is likely determined more by local practice and nonmedical factors than by evidence. The majority of studies are retrospective. A metaanalysis of 67 studies from 1980 through 2001 was performed to evaluate route of delivery. Sixty-three of 67 studies were discarded from analysis because of quality issues. The authors concluded that planned cesarean section may decrease the risk for a low 5-minute Apgar score, particularly if twin A is breech. Otherwise, there was no evidence to support planned cesarean section for twins.[9]

A Cochrane systematic review in 2000 found only one good-quality RCT comparing outcomes in vaginal versus cesarean delivery for after-coming twins in nonvertex presentations.[10] No improvement of neonatal outcome was reported for second twins born by cesarean compared with cesarean, but maternal febrile morbidity was increased with cesarean delivery.[11] As of publication of this textbook, a Medline search for RCTs occurring since publication of the 2000 Cochrane review shows no recent randomized trials addressing this issue.

B. Presenting Fetus Breech

Although most clinicians in the United States will choose cesarean delivery for breech-first twins, a retrospective study of more than 239 vaginal and 374 cesarean deliveries did not find increased neonatal morbidity or mortality in fetuses weighing more than 1500 g with vaginal delivery.[12] A major concern, however, for the delivery of breech-first twins is encountered if the second twin is vertex with the potential for interlocking heads.

C. Clinical Considerations

Decision making regarding route of delivery should include an informed consent discussion with the patient. Other obstetric risks may influence the decision for operative or vaginal delivery because some women plan for a tubal ligation after delivery. Individual and labor unit resources may additionally contribute to this process because fewer clinicians currently offer experience in breech extraction or even vaginal delivery of the frank breech. Even with the presumed lower risk for vaginal delivery for vertex, vertex, cord prolapse in the after-coming fetus or abruption may necessitate cesarean delivery. Breech delivery is covered separately in Section G.

REFERENCES

1. Adams PM, Chervenak FA: Intrapartum management of twin gestation, *Clin Obstet Gynecol* 33:52-60, 1990.
2. Fausett MB, Barth WH Jr, Yoder BA, Satin AJ: Oxytocin labor stimulation of twin gestations: effective and efficient, *Obstet Gynecol* 90:202-204, 1997.
3. Udom-Rice I, Singlis SR, Skupski D et al: Optimal gestation age for twin delivery, *J Perinatol* 20:231-234, 2000.
4. Garite TJ, Clark RH, Elliott JP et al: Twins and triplets: the effect of plurality and growth on neonatal outcome compared with singleton infants, *Am J Obstet Gynecol* 191(3):700-707, 2004.
5. Suzuki S, Otsubo Y, Sawa R et al: Clinical trial of induction of labor versus expectant management in twin pregnancy, *Gynecol Obstet Invest* 49(1):24-27, 2000.
6. Cahill A, Stamilio DM, Pare E et al: Vaginal birth after cesarean (VBAC) attempt in twin pregnancies: is it safe? *Am J Obstet Gynecol* 193(3 pt 2):1050-1055, 2005.
7. Varner MW, Leindecker S, Spong CY et al: The Maternal-Fetal Medicine Unit cesarean registry: trial of labor with a twin gestation, *Am J Obstet Gynecol* 193(1):135-140, 2005.
8. Ezra Y, Shveiky D, Ophir E et al: Intensive management and early delivery reduce antenatal mortality in monoamniotic twin pregnancies, *Acta Obstet Gynecol Scand* 84(5):432-435, 2005.
9. Hogle KL, Hutton EK, McBrien KA et al: Cesarean delivery for twins: a systematic review and meta-analysis, *Am J Obstet Gynecol* 188(1):220-227, 2003.
10. Crowther CA: Caesarean delivery for the second twin, *Cochrane Database Syst Rev* (2):CD000047, 2000.
11. Rabinovici J, Barkai G, Reichman B et al: Randomized management of the second nonvertex twin, *Am J Obstet Gynecol* 156(1):52-56, 1987.
12. Blickstein I, Goldman RD, Kupferminc M: Delivery of breech first twins: a multicenter retrospective study, *Obstet Gynecol* 95(1):37-42, 2000.

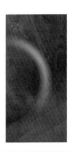

CHAPTER 18

Intrapartum Procedures

SECTION A Use of Ultrasound in Labor and Delivery

Ellen L. Sakornbut, MD

Many patients presenting to labor and delivery are in need of sonographic evaluation. Common indications for diagnostic use of ultrasound in labor and delivery include the evaluation of patients with unknown dates or size-dates discrepancy, determination of fetal position, evaluation of preterm labor or preterm premature rupture of membranes, evaluation of patients with vaginal bleeding, and investigation of possible fetal demise. This section addresses the use of ultrasound as it is applied in urgent or emergent intrapartum problems. Physicians who provide intrapartum care can become familiar with basic uses of ultrasound in this context. Some intrapartum applications require more advanced skills and extended amounts of training. The maternity care provider must recognize that intrapartum sonographic examinations are often difficult to perform because of fetal crowding, low station of the presenting part, oligohydramnios, and patient discomfort. Sonographic examinations in labor and delivery may be limited to specific information that is sought quickly because of clinical necessity and are not intended to supplant standard or basic obstetric examination as defined by the American Institute of Ultrasound in Medicine and the American College of Obstetricians and Gynecologists (ACOG).[1,2]

I. APPLICATIONS

Initially, the clinician should perform a general uterine survey with longitudinal and transverse sweeps of the maternal abdomen. The basic information revealed by the survey is detailed in the following sections.

A. Fetal Presentation

1. Breech

   If breech, it may be difficult to ascertain whether it is complete, frank, or footling. It is possible to identify extremity position, but a single plain film (fetogram) more completely defines position of extremities if one is considering vaginal delivery and sonographic findings are inconclusive.

2. Transverse lie

   If transverse lie is confirmed, the position of the spine (back up or down) is important to determine. Cord prolapse is much more likely with the back up, and the uterine incision may be modified for operative delivery.

B. Multiple Gestation

Multiple gestation is usually suspected when fetal size is greater than dates would indicate or if more than two fetal poles are palpated. Confirmation of twins is achieved by visualizing two separate fetal heads and heartbeats. Diagnosis of twin gestation should always be followed by a careful check to detect multiples of greater magnitude than twin gestation.

If twin gestation is diagnosed, the examiner should attempt to locate a separating membrane. The membrane may be difficult to visualize because of crowding, but a gentle tap on the side of the maternal abdomen may demonstrate the membrane fluttering in the fluid wave. Monoamniotic twins are rare; because of the danger of cord entanglement, delivery is usually operative. Position and presentation of each fetus should be determined for intrapartum management. Difficulties in the diagnosis of a twin gestation include the following:

1. Diagnosis of a "stuck" twin

   The "stuck" twin, either demised or living, may be contained within an oligohydramniotic sac. This fetus may be difficult to visualize depending on its position in the uterus.

2. Diagnosis of conjoined twins

   Although rare, this diagnosis may be suspected because of persistent face-to-face or chest-to-chest presentation.

C. Fetal Life

Locating fetal heart tones may be difficult in some patients on presentation to labor and delivery. Sonographic location of fetal cardiac activity is usually easy to determine. Diagnosis of fetal demise can be confirmed by the following findings:

1. No cardiac activity
2. Hydropic changes (pleural effusions, skin edema, and ascites)
3. Overriding of cranial bones, as with x-ray

D. Amniotic Fluid Assessment

1. Technique for amniotic fluid index (AFI)

   The maternal abdomen is divided into four quadrants using the midline and the umbilicus. Keeping the transducer perpendicular to the floor, the deepest pocket of amniotic fluid is located in each quadrant. A vertical measurement of this pocket is performed, avoiding any areas of the pocket that contain extremity or umbilical cord. The sum of these measurements, in centimeters, is the AFI. A sum of less than 5 cm is considered oligohydramnios, 5 to 8 cm is considered borderline, 8 to 20 cm is considered normal, and greater than 20 to 25 cm is considered polyhydramnios.[3]

2. Outcomes

   The impact of oligohydramnios on pregnancy outcomes is controversial. Although oligohydramnios has been considered a marker for placental insufficiency and increased risk, some outcome studies do not demonstrate any difference in outcomes comparing women with normal amniotic fluid and women with oligohydramnios as measured by either the AFI or largest vertical pocket, sometimes referred to as single deepest pocket.[4,5] Specifically, neither measurement of AFI nor single deepest pocket failed to prospectively identify pregnancies with fetal heart rate abnormalities resulting in amnioinfusion, variable or late decelerations, cesarean delivery for apparent fetal

compromise, or admission to a neonatal intensive care unit.[6] Furthermore, a prospective study comparing amniotic fluid distribution did not demonstrate any influence on outcome whether the greatest distribution of amniotic fluid was present in the upper quadrants or the lower quadrants, where cord compression might be expected because of fetal structures.[7]

E. Placental Evaluation

The placenta is generally easy to identify by its characteristic homogeneous appearance; some lobulation often appears in late pregnancy. Certain challenges and pitfalls can be encountered.

1. Placental grading

   Ultrasound is not reliable as a means of assessing fetal lung maturity. Less than 50% of patients will demonstrate a grade 3 placenta at term; therefore, lack of a "mature" placenta does not indicate inadequate lung maturation. Conversely, the presence of a grade 3 placenta is usually associated with fetal lung maturity.[8]

2. Placenta previa

   a. Anterior placenta previa: When this is suspected in a patient with a full bladder, the patient should empty her bladder with repeat scanning to eliminate the possibility of a false-positive result because of a low-lying anterior placenta.

   b. Posterior placenta previa: When this is suspected, the patient should be placed in the Trendelenburg position and attempts should be made to displace the fetal presenting part gently so that the lower uterine segment and cervical os may be visualized.

   c. Transvaginal or transperineal scanning (Figure 18-1): This can be used to define more completely the relation of the placenta to the cervical os when transabdominal scanning is inconclusive. Transvaginal ultrasound results in lower rates of false-positive and -negative findings than transabdominal ultrasound,[9] with a positive predictive value of 71% and a negative predictive value of 100%. Many labor and delivery units do not have transvaginal transducers, and transperineal scanning may be substituted. This technique produces a similar field of view, demonstrating the internal cervical os and placental relations. Transvaginal scanning of placenta previa can be performed safely because the probe is only partially inserted into the vagina for

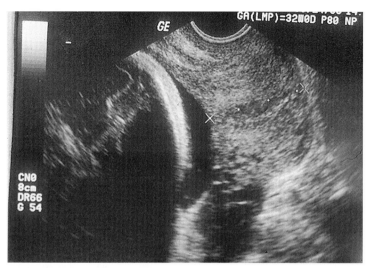

FIGURE 18-1. A transvaginal image of the cervix demonstrates the echogenic mucus of the endocervix and the internal cervical os. The fetal head is presenting. The calipers are placed to measure the cervical length.

optimal visualization of the cervix; the endocervical canal is approximately perpendicular to the vagina, making intracervical insertion unlikely.

3. Succenturiate lobes

A succenturiate lobe may be missed with ultrasound scanning. It should be suspected if echo patterns characteristic for placental tissue are noted to be discontinuous with the main body of the placenta. Because vascular connections are present between the succenturiate lobe and the rest of the placenta, disruption of these vascular structures at the time of rupture of membranes may result in vasa previa (see Chapter 16, Section D). Patients diagnosed with a succenturiate lobe should have color flow Doppler scanning to evaluate vascular structures with emergent cesarean delivery for patients at high risk for vasa previa.

4. False-positive diagnosis

Other structures that may be mistaken for placental tissue are as follows:

a. Segmental myometrial contractions: These may be seen throughout pregnancy and last 20 to 30 minutes. Usually there is a slight difference in echogenicity and a characteristic contour to the segmental contraction. No echogenic reflection is on the fetal side of the subsegmental contraction, as is noted with the chorionic plate of the placenta.

b. Blood clots: Blood clots may demonstrate similar echodensity and consistency as does placental tissue.

F. Assessment for Nuchal Cord

The presence of a nuchal cord is a common finding at the time of delivery and often is suspected before delivery because of variable decelerations. Nuchal cord has been associated in one prospective blinded study with a greater rate of operative delivery in nulligravidas and with lower 1- and 5-minute Apgar scores.[10] However, a large, retrospective study of more than 11,000 deliveries found no increase in 5-minute Apgar scores less than 7 or in admission to neonatal intensive care units.[11] Meconium staining was significantly increased only in the instance of multiple nuchal cords in a postterm pregnancy. The authors of that study conclude that evaluation for nuchal cord on presentation in labor is unnecessary and does not result in improved outcomes.

G. Assessment of Lower Uterine Segment in Managing Vaginal Birth after Cesarean

One small, prospective, observational study evaluated outcomes after examination of the lower uterine segment during trial of labor in women with previous cesarean delivery.[12] These authors suggest the critical cutoff value for safe management of labor (i.e., avoidance of uterine dehiscence) in this instance is 2.5 mm, but no other studies are currently available to support this finding.

H. Assessment of Cord Presentation

A retrospective study of cord prolapse and cord presentation examined whether cord prolapse was predictable from previous ultrasounds and whether identification of cord presentation could predict a need for surgical intervention. In the first series, cord prolapse was not reliably predicted by previous ultrasound. In a second retrospective series, when cord presentation was identified in the third trimester, approximately half of these patients had persistent cord presentation or cord presentation combined with malpresentation and/or cord prolapse requiring cesarean delivery.[13] The authors suggest close follow-up of women who have cord presentation identified with serial ultrasound to delineate management decisions if abnormal presentation persists.

II. ASSESSMENT OF PRETERM LABOR AND PRETERM RUPTURE OF MEMBRANES

Assessment of preterm labor and preterm rupture of membranes is discussed in the following sections (see also Chapter 12 for a more detailed discussion).

A. Gestational Age/Estimated Fetal Weight Assessment

Patients presenting in labor may have inadequate or no documentation of gestational age. Even when there is some estimate of gestational age from menstrual dating and antenatal visits, accuracy of dating may be limited. Because ultrasound dating in the third trimester is no more accurate than ±3 weeks, estimates made in labor and delivery may be erroneous. Nonetheless, an estimate of fetal size is of some management and prognostic value.

1. Fetal biometry
   Fetal biometry is a more advanced skill and beyond the scope of this chapter. This is most accurate when based on measurement of multiple parameters, preferably fetal head, abdomen, and femur measurements.
2. Estimation of fetal weight
   Fetal weight estimates in the third trimester commonly vary from actual weights by 10% to 15%.[14,15]

B. Assessment of the Lower Uterine Segment and Cervix

Assessment of the lower uterine segment and cervix can be facilitated by use of transperineal or transvaginal scanning (see Figure 18-1), avoiding the acoustic shadows created by the symphysis pubis and avoiding the risks of digital examination for patients with placenta previa.[16-18]

1. Technique for visualization of the cervix and lower uterine segment
   The curvilinear probe is placed on the perineum or the vaginal probe is partially inserted into the vagina. The image is oriented so that a symmetric image of the external cervical os is obtained with the internal os visualized as a "T" or an isosceles triangle or funnel.[19] Transperineal and transvaginal scanning demonstrate comparable results.[20] The use of transvaginal ultrasound does not increase the risk for infection in women with preterm premature rupture of membranes.[21]
2. Accuracy of the technique
   Cervical dilatation has been demonstrated with some accuracy up to four centimeters. Cervical effacement and lower uterine segment changes may antedate cervical dilatation.
   a. Funneling: "Funneling" of the lower uterine segment or development of a V-shaped or U-shaped segment can be seen in early preterm labor. When coupled with a short cervical length, it has been associated with poor neonatal outcome (i.e., preterm labor, chorioamnionitis, abruption, rupture of the membranes, and serious neonatal morbidity and mortality) compared with pregnancies with short cervical length but no funneling.[22]
   b. Cervical effacement: This has been determined with more accuracy than dilatation. The uneffaced cervix in the third trimester usually measures between 3.5 and 4.8 cm. Fifty percent effacement corresponds to a cervical length of 1.5 cm, and 75% effacement corresponds to 1.0 cm. A cervical length ≤2.0 cm has been associated with a short time interval between ruptured membranes and delivery in women presenting with preterm rupture of membranes.[23] In addition, a cervical length ≤2.0 cm has been strongly associated with premature delivery at less

than 27 weeks in women who were being evaluated for cervical incompetence.[10]

c. Cervical length: Cervical length measurements are addressed elsewhere in this textbook. Their utility in prevention of preterm birth remains controversial. An early study of cervical length measurement found a strong association between very preterm birth (<27 weeks) and short cervical length (<2.0 cm) in women who were being assessed for possible cervical incompetence.[24] A metaanalysis of well-designed randomized trials found cerclage to be effective in prolonging pregnancy in singleton pregnancies with a short cervical length measured between 16 and 24 weeks, especially in pregnancies with a previous preterm birth (relative risk [RR], 0.61) or second-trimester pregnancy loss (RR, 0.57).[25] Apparent cervical length is altered if the operator uses the transabdominal approach or with bladder filling. Accurate cervical length measurements should be conducted using transvaginal or transperineal approach. Cervical length measurement as a technique can be learned in approximately 25 supervised scans in learners not previously trained in transvaginal ultrasound and is learned even more rapidly by individuals who have previous training in transvaginal ultrasound.[26]

Although cervical length measurement may be used to predict the presence of an incompetent cervix with measurements conducted at less than 24 weeks gestational age, cervical length measurements may also be used for evaluation of patients with preterm contractions or preterm labor to predict which patients are at low risk for preterm delivery. A prospective study with measurements of cervical length in all patients presenting with premature contractions compared pregnancies where clinicians were blinded to cervical length measurement (controls) and pregnancies where clinicians used cervical length measurements, with a cutoff of 25 mm, as a basis for discharge from the hospital. The two groups did not differ in rates of delivery within 7 days, rates of delivery before 37 weeks, or use of tocolytics, but the number of hospital days was significantly shorter in the group managed using cervical length measurements.[27]

Another observational study of women with painful contractions and intact membranes between 24 and 35 weeks found a cutoff value of 15 mm predictive of increased risk for delivery within 7 days.[28]

III. ASSESSMENT FOR ABRUPTION

Abruption is a clinical diagnosis. It may be supported by sonographic findings, but lack of sonographic evidence does not rule out an abruption. The size of a bleed is often underestimated by ultrasound examination. Possible sonographic findings of abruption include the following:

1. Abnormal thickening of the placenta
   This may be caused by the presence of a recent retroplacental hemorrhage. Fresh hemorrhage is usually echogenic.
2. "Torn up" or abnormally rounded edge of the placenta
3. Increased area of sonolucency
   This may occur between the myometrium and the placenta, and may represent a retroplacental clot (Figure 18-2). Areas of sonolucency may occur within the substance of the placenta. These may be mimicked by placental lakes, which are normal in mature placentas.

IV. ASSESSMENT OF FETAL WELL-BEING

A. Amniotic Fluid Index
The use of the AFI to assess fetal well-being is discussed in Chapter 11, Section B.

B. Biophysical Profile
The use of the biophysical profile is discussed in Chapter 11, Section B. The technique as described by Manning and colleagues[29] is as follows:

1. Amniotic fluid pocket measuring 1×2 cm: 2 points
2. Fetal breathing movements, 3 periods of 30 seconds each in 30 minutes: 2 points
3. Fetal extremity movements, 3 in 30 minutes: 2 points
4. Fetal tone, 3 episodes of extension with return to flexion in 30 minutes: 2 points
5. Reactive NST: 2 points
   A perfect score on a biophysical profile is described as 10 of 10 with an NST of 8 of 8 without NST.

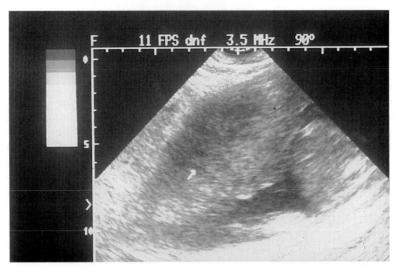

FIGURE 18-2. *Arrow* indicates a small abruption, which is demonstrated as an echolucent retroplacental clot. The patient presented after a motor vehicle accident and was tender to palpation over this aspect of the uterine fundus.

V. USE OF ULTRASOUND TO DETERMINE EXCESS FETAL WEIGHT

A systematic quantitative review of ultrasound biometry in detecting macrosomia concluded that use of standard biometric formulas for prediction of estimated fetal weight (EFW) and measurement of abdominal circumference were equivalent in accuracy of predicting macrosomia.[30] The likelihood of predicting a macrosomic fetus was 5.7 to 6.9 times more likely with a positive result and 0.37 to 0.48 times less likely with a negative result, using an EFW of 4000 g or an abdominal circumference of 36 cm. These authors suggest that either method for predicting macrosomia is more reliable in ruling in macrosomia than in ruling out macrosomia.

Ultrasound prediction of macrosomia appears to influence clinical behavior with increased rates of labor induction and cesarean delivery without reduction in shoulder dystocia or birth trauma.[31] Thus, although rates of shoulder dystocia are greater in macrosomic infants, ultrasound determination has not been demonstrated to be of benefit in preventing permanent neurologic sequelae in infants of women without diabetes who are suspected of macrosomia. Further discussion of this issue is included in other chapters of this textbook.

VI. USE OF ULTRASOUND FOR INTRAPARTUM PROCEDURES

Ultrasound is used as part of the following intrapartum procedures:
1. Amniocentesis (see Section F)
2. External version (see Chapter 17, Section H)
3. Twin delivery (see Chapter 17, Section I)
   Monitoring of position and cardiac activity of the second twin may be helpful while manually guiding the twin into cephalic position or to determine position of feet and spine if a breech extraction is to be performed.

VII. SUMMARY

Ultrasound is frequently useful in the intrapartum setting. Although some skills are easily learned, other skills, such as biometry and assessment of preterm labor, may take greater amounts of training and experience. The use of ultrasound in labor and delivery for limited examinations has been recognized as a valuable adjunct in patient management. Use of ultrasound for limited examinations is not intended to supplant diagnostic use of ultrasound for basic and targeted examinations as defined by the ACOG and the American Institute of Ultrasound in Medicine (which includes full biometry and organ survey). The physician performing the sonographic examination must be aware of the pitfalls in diagnosis and the limitations associated with the intrapartum setting.

REFERENCES

1. Ultrasound imaging in pregnancy. American College of Obstetricians and Gynecologists Committee Opinion, Number 96, August 1991, Washington, DC.
2. Antepartum Obstetrical Ultrasound Examination Guidelines: Official Guidelines and Statements on Obstetrical Ultrasound, Laurel, MD, October 1985, The American Institute of Ultrasound in Medicine.
3. Rutherford SE, Phelan JP, Smith CV et al: The four-quadrant assessment of amniotic fluid volume: an adjunct to antepartum fetal heart rate testing, *Obstet Gynecol* 70:353-356, 1987.
4. Verrotti C, Bedocchi L, Piantelli G et al: Amniotic fluid index versus largest vertical pocket in the prediction of perinatal outcome in post-term pregnancies, *Acta Biomed* 75(suppl 1):67-70, 2004.
5. Ott WJ: Reevaluation of the relationship between amniotic fluid volume and perinatal outcome, *Am J Obstet Gynecol* 192(6):1803-1809, 2005.
6. Moses J, Doherty DA, Magann EF et al: A randomized clinical trial of the intrapartum assessment of amniotic fluid volume: amniotic fluid index versus the single deepest pocket technique, *Am J Obstet Gynecol* 190(6):1564-1570, 2004.
7. Magann EF, Chauhan SP, Doherty DA et al: Predictability of intrapartum and neonatal outcomes with the amniotic fluid volume distribution: a reassessment using the amniotic fluid index, single deepest pocket, and a dye-determined amniotic fluid volume, *Am J Obstet Gynecol* 188(6):1523-1527, 2003.
8. Hopper KD, Komppa GH, Williams BP et al: A reevaluation of placental grading and its clinical significance, *J Ultrasound Med* 3:261-265, 1984.
9. Farine D, Peisner DB, Timor-Trisch IE: Placenta previa—is the traditional approach satisfactory? *J Clin Ultrasound* 18:328-330, 1990.
10. Assimakopoulos E, Zafrakas M, Garmiris P et al: Nuchal cord detected by ultrasound at term is associated with mode of delivery and perinatal outcome, *Eur J Obstet Gynecol Reprod Biol* Epub 123:188-192, 2005.
11. Schaffer L, Burkhardt T, Zimmermann R et al: Nuchal cords in term and postterm deliveries—do we need to know? *Obstet Gynecol* 106(1):23-28, 2005.
12. Sen S, Malik S, Salhan S: Ultrasonographic evaluation of lower uterine segment thickness in patients of previous cesarean section, *Int J Gynaecol Obstet* 87(3):215-219, 2004.
13. Ezra Y, Strasberg SR, Farine D: Does cord presentation on ultrasound predict cord prolapse? *Gynecol Obstet Invest* 56(1):6-9, 2003.
14. Ott WJ, Doyle S, Falmm S: Accurate ultrasonic estimation of weight, *Am J Perinatol* 2:178-182, 1985.
15. Sabbagha RE, Minogue J, Tamura RK: Estimation of birth weight by use of formulas targeted to large-, appropriate-, and small-for-gestational-age fetuses, *Am J Obstet Gynecol* 160:854-862, 1989.
16. Jeanty P, d'Alton M: Romero R et al: Perineal scanning, *Am J Perinatol* 3:289-295, 1986.
17. Mahony BS, Nyberg DA, Luthy DA et al: Translabial ultrasound of the third trimester cervix, *J Ultrasound Med* 9:717-723, 1990.
18. Zilianti M, Azuaga A, Calderon F et al: Transperineal sonography in second trimester to term pregnancy and early labor, *J Ultrasound Med* 10:481-485, 1991.
19. Burger M, Weber-Rossler T, Willmann M et al: Measurement of the pregnant cervix by transvaginal sonography: an interobserver study and new standards to improve interobserver variability, *Ultrasound Obstet Gynecol* 9:188-193, 1991.
20. Kurtzman JT, Goldsmith LJ, Gall SA et al: Transvaginal versus transperineal ultrasonography: a blinded comparison in the assessment of cervical measurement at midgestation, *Am J Obstet Gynecol* 179:852-857, 1998.
21. Carlan SJ, Richmond LB, O'Brien WF: Randomized trial of endovaginal ultrasound in preterm premature rupture of membranes, *Obstet Gynecol* 89:458-461, 1997.
22. Rust OA, Atlas RO, Kimmel S et al: Does the presence of a funnel increase the risk of adverse perinatal outcome in a patient with a short cervix? *Am J Obstet Gynecol* 192(4):1060-1066, 2005.
23. Rizzo G, Capponi A, Angelini E et al: The value of transvaginal ultrasonographic examination of the uterine cervix in predicting preterm delivery in patients with preterm rupture of membranes, *Ultrasound Obstet Gynecol* 11:23-29, 1998.
24. Guzman ER, Mellon R, Vintzileos AM et al: Relationship between endocervical canal length between 15–24 weeks and obstetric history, *J Matern Fetal Med* 7:269-272, 1998.
25. Berghella V, Odibo AO, To MS et al: Cerclage for short cervix on ultrasonography: meta-analysis of trials using individual patient-level data, *Obstet Gynecol* 106(1):181-189, 2005.
26. Vayssiere C, Moriniere C, Camus E et al: Measuring cervical length with ultrasound: evaluation of the procedures and duration of a learning method, *Ultrasound Obstet Gynecol* 20(6):575-579, 2002.
27. Sanin-Blair J, Palacio M, Delgado J et al: Impact of ultrasound cervical length assessment on duration of hospital stay in the clinical management of threatened preterm labor, *Obstet Gynecol Surv* 60(5):283-284, 2005.
28. Fuchs IB, Henrich W, Osthues K et al: Sonographic cervical length in singleton pregnancies with intact membranes presenting with threatened preterm labor, *Ultrasound Obstet Gynecol* 24(5):554-557, 2004.
29. Manning FA, Baskett TF, Millison I et al: Fetal biophysical profile scoring: a prospective study in 1,184 high-risk patients, *Am J Obstet Gynecol* 140:289-293, 1981.
30. Coomarasamy A, Connock M, Thornton J et al: Accuracy of ultrasound biometry in the prediction of macrosomia: a systematic quantitative review, *BJOG* 112(11):1461-1466, 2005.
31. Weeks JW, Pitman, T, Spinnato JA: Fetal macrosomia: does antenatal prediction affect delivery route and birth outcome? *Am J Obstet Gynecol* 173:1215-1219, 1995.

S E C T I O N   B   Pudendal and Paracervical Blocks

Rachel Elizabeth Hall, MD, FAAFP

A woman's satisfaction with the birth experience is less related to the absence of pain than to her control over the perception of pain.[1,2] A variety of pain relief methods, both pharmacologic and nonpharmacologic, should be discussed during prenatal visits to help the patient prepare to achieve acceptable pain relief. Some examples are alternative focus techniques such as Lamaze; labor room support persons such as doulas; sensory distractions such as acupressure or transcutaneous electrical nerve stimulation units[1]; intravenous, intrathecal,[2] or intraepidural narcotics; and local anesthetic options such as pudendal or paracervical blocks.

During the first stage of labor, pain results from uterine contractions; stretching, distention, and dilation of the cervix and lower uterine segment; and pressure on the pelvis. This pain is mediated by C-fibers, which produce visceral pain in the distribution of T10 through L1.[1-3] Pain during the second stage of labor is caused by stretching of the vagina and perineum, and is mediated by Aδ fibers causing a somatic pain in the S2-4 distribution.[1-3] Pain relief for the first two stages of labor can be reduced using a local anesthetic via paracervical and pudendal blocks. These are relatively simple and easily learned techniques, and the toxic effects of local anesthetic agents (seizures, hypotension, arrhythmias) are rare, especially with careful administration and frequent aspiration.[1]

I. PARACERVICAL BLOCK

A. Indications
The paracervical block can provide pain relief during the first stage of labor, typically lasting 30 to 90 minutes. Several randomized controlled trials (RCTs) demonstrate that paracervical block was 75% effective in achieving good or excellent pain relief.[4] A paracervical block may also alleviate the urge to push that some patients experience before complete dilatation, thus decreasing the risk for cervical laceration. A single, small, double-blinded study (n = 117) compared the intravenous opiate, pethidine, with paracervical blocks. The average pain relief in the paracervical block group was significantly greater than that in the pethidine group, and the labors were significantly shorter, with no difference in fetal heart rate abnormalities, instrumented or surgical delivery, or subsequent epidural requests.[5]

B. Contraindications
1. Allergy to local anesthetic agent
2. Evidence of fetal compromise
3. Pelvic infection

4. Coagulopathy
Informed consent should be obtained before performing the procedure.

C. Complications
1. Transient fetal bradycardia
   Episodes of fetal bradycardia have been strongly associated with paracervical blocks[3] and may last from 3 to 6 minutes, but they are not associated with adverse fetal outcome. With slow infusion of the anesthetic, use of newer anesthetics that appear to have lesser effects on fetal heart rate, and careful submucosal placement with frequent aspiration, this complication should be reduced.[1] However, the resultant patient and provider anxiety, as well as availability of other pain relief methods such as epidurals, has led to infrequent use of this technique.
2. Intravascular or intrafetal injection
   This may occur with improper technique.
3. Inhibition of labor
   If given before 4 cm dilation, labor may be inhibited.

D. Technique
When performing a paracervical block, the patient is placed in a modified lithotomy position with a pillow under her side to avoid inferior vena cava and aortic compression. The procedure is as follows:
1. Place fetal monitor.
2. Check cervical dilation.
3. Perform antibacterial perineal preparation.
4. Using a 10-ml syringe with a 20- or 22-gauge 6-inch needle and trumpet guide, draw up 10 ml of 1% lidocaine, 1% mepivacaine, or 1.5% chloroprocaine.
5. Using the index and middle fingers, guide the trumpet to the cervicovaginal junction (Figure 18-3) at the 3 to 4 o'clock position, depending on the cervical dilation. Earlier in labor, the nerves are located at 4 and 8 o'clock positions; later, they migrate to 3 and 9 o'clock positions.
6. Allowing no more than 3 mm of the needle tip to protrude, aspirate for blood and, if negative, inject 5 to 10 mm of anesthetic.
7. If no bradycardia occurs after 5 minutes, repeat at the 8 to 9 o'clock position.
8. Continue fetal monitoring for 30 minutes after the procedure.

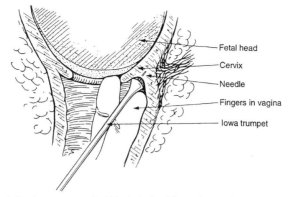

FIGURE 18-3. Technique of administering a paracervical block during labor using an Iowa trumpet. (From Pfenninger JL, Fowler GC, editors: *Procedures for primary care physicians,* St. Louis, 1994, Mosby.)

II. PUDENDAL BLOCK

A. Indications

Pudendal block provides pain relief during the second stage of labor, as well as for episiotomy and repair, but does not relieve contraction pain. It is most often used for vacuum or forceps deliveries. A successful procedure blocks all three branches of the pudendal nerve, which supplies sensory and motor innervation to the perineum.[2] However, bilateral relief is achieved only 50% of the time.[1] A study comparing intrathecal narcotics with epidural anesthesia found that intrathecal anesthesia, when combined with an adequately placed pudendal, was nearly as effective as epidural in accomplishing pain relief.[2]

B. Contraindications

Contraindications for pudendal block are the same as for paracervical block, with the exception of abnormal fetal heart rate patterns that do not occur as a result of pudendal block unless anesthetic is injected intravascularly or intrafetally.

C. Complications

1. Intravascular injection
2. Hematoma
3. Infection

D. Technique

The technique for administering a pudendal block is as follows[6]:

1. Place the patient in the modified dorsal lithotomy position as for a paracervical block.
2. Institute electronic fetal monitoring.
3. Perform a vaginal examination for dilatation and descent to avoid injection of the fetal scalp.
4. Perform a perineal preparation.
5. Using a 10-ml 20-gauge 6-inch needle, draw up 10 ml of 1% lidocaine.
6. Using the index and middle fingers, guide the tip to the ischial spine (Figure 18-4).
7. Allowing 7 to 10 mm of the tip to protrude, aspirate for blood. The vessels are lateral to the nerve, so if blood is aspirated, move the needle tip medially. If negative, inject 2 to 4 ml of 1% lidocaine at two to three sites: inferior to the tip of the ischial spine, medial to the tip of the spine, and into the ligament. Limit the total amount injected to 10 ml per site to avoid systemic reactions.

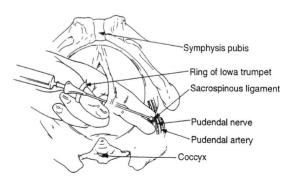

FIGURE 18-4. Left hand is directing a guide and needle toward the pudendal nerve. This illustration shows the hand directed more laterally to better show the anatomy. (From Pfenninger JL, Fowler GC, editors: *Procedures for primary care physicians,* St. Louis, 1994, Mosby.)

8. Repeat on the opposite side.
9. After 5 minutes, check anesthesia by gently drawing an Allis forceps over each side of the perineum and observing for the anal "wink" response. Additional local anesthesia may be required before performing other procedures.

III. SUMMARY

Both paracervical and pudendal block techniques can easily be learned by any level maternity care provider. Because the ACOG published a Committee Statement outlining that maternal request is a sufficient medical indication for pain relief during labor,[1] it is important to be able to discuss and offer as many types of pain relief options to women to allow a greater sense of control over pain and improvement in perception of the birth experience.

REFERENCES

1. Fields SA, Wall EM: Obstetrics analgesia and anesthesia, *Prim Care* 20:705-712, 1993.
2. Stephens MB, Ford RE: Intrathecal narcotics for labor analgesia, *Am Fam Physician* 56:463-470, 1997.
3. American College of Obstetricians and Gynecologists (ACOG). ACOG Practice Bulletin No. 36: obstetric analgesia and anesthesia, *Obstet Gynecol* 100:177-191, 2002.
4. Leeman L, Fontaine P, King V et al: The nature and management of labor pain: part II. Pharmacologic pain relief, *Am Fam Physician* 68:1115-1120, 2003.
5. Bricker L, Lavender T: Parenteral opioids for labor pain relief: a systematic review, *Am J Obstet Gynecol* 186:S94-S109, 2002.
6. Marquardt DN: Paracervical block. *Procedures for primary care physicians,* St. Louis, 1994, Mosby.

SECTION C Amnioinfusion and Use of Intrauterine Pressure Catheter

Stephen D. Ratcliffe, MD, MSPH

The clinical significance of oligohydramnios and its relation to placental insufficiency and umbilical cord compression is discussed in Chapter 7, Section G and Chapter 11, Section B. The scientific basis for the use of amnioinfusion is described in Chapter 16, Section A. This section describes the related procedures of placement of an intrauterine pressure catheter (IUPC) and administration of an amnioinfusion.

I. INTRAUTERINE PRESSURE CATHETER

A. Indications
IUPCs are used when clinicians need to document the intrauterine pressure and for the use of instilling and infusion of fluid into the intrauterine cavity. For example, in the setting of dystocia and suspected inadequate uterine contractions, placement of an IUPC yields objective measurements of intrauterine pressure.

B. Contraindications
The following are relative contraindications to the placement of an IUPC:
1. Chorioamnionitis
2. Malpresentation
3. Known or suspected placenta previa
4. Known or suspected placental abruption

C. Complications
Clinically significant complications are rare, but there are case reports of uterine perforation, umbilical cord prolapse,[1] and placental abruption.

D. Equipment
IUPCs have a sensing device to measure intrauterine pressure and a port through which to instill the infusion of normal saline (NS) or lactated Ringer's (LR) solution.

E. Intrauterine Pressure Catheter Placement Technique
The technique to place the IUPC is as follows:
1. The fetal presenting part is known; the cervix is usually dilated more than 1 cm.
2. Using sterile technique, the clinician introduces the tip of the plastic guide between the fetal head and posterior lip of the cervix.
3. The IUPC is then gently inserted to a depth of 30 cm. The clinician should encounter only mild resistance in placing the IUPC. Marked resistance should be an indication to abort the procedure.
4. The fetal monitor is then calibrated so that intrauterine pressures can be readily measured. Resting tone should be less than 15 mmHg.

II. AMNIOINFUSION

A. Indications

1. Evidence of umbilical cord compression
   A major indication for amnioinfusion is to provide an additional fluid cushion when there is evidence of umbilical cord compression during labor. Repetitive variable decelerations, particularly if they are severe or prolonged, are thought to be a result of umbilical cord compression.[2] Amnioinfusion is more effective in relieving variable decelerations in the presence of oligohydramnios (AFI < 5 cm). A summary of published RCTs indicates that there is evidence that use of amnioinfusion for the treatment of suspected cord compression results in a decreased rate of variable decelerations (number needed to treat [NNT] = 3), cesarean section (NNT = 8), cord pH less than 7.20 (NNT = 8), and postpartum endometritis (NNT = 17).[1] Prophylactic amnioinfusion in the presence of oligohydramnios has resulted in varied clinical outcomes. The Cochrane review[3] does not demonstrate improved outcomes, although another metaanalysis supports the use of this treatment strategy.[4]

2. Presence of thick meconium-stained fluid
   Until a recent major clinical trial indicated otherwise, another indication for amnioinfusion has been the presence of moderate-to-thick meconium-stained fluid. The Cochrane review of 12 small RCTs and another metaanalysis demonstrated that in settings with standard perinatal surveillance, amnioinfusion was associated with a decrease in heavy meconium staining, variable decelerations, and reduced cesarean sections.[5,6] Under limited perinatal surveillance, amnioinfusion was associated with a decrease in the incidence of meconium aspiration syndrome, neonatal hypoxic-ischemic encephalopathy and neonatal ventilation. The usefulness of this procedure in settings with limited perinatal surveillance was confirmed in a recent from India.[7] It is not known whether these beneficial effects are due to the dilution of the meconium or the primary alleviation of umbilical cord compression.
   A recent international multicenter RCT demonstrated that in settings with standard peripartum fetal surveillance, the use of amnioinfusion for the treatment of moderate-to-thick meconium did not reduce the incidence of perinatal morbidity or mortality.[8] This study was conducted in 56 centers in 13 countries and involved 1998 women. Amnioinfusion for this indication did not decrease the incidence of cesarean section or meconium aspiration syndrome. The authors conclude that "amnioinfusion should not be recommended for the prevention of the meconium aspiration syndrome in such settings."[8]

B. Contraindications

Amnioinfusion has the same contraindications noted previously with regard to placement of an IUPC. Amnioinfusions can be used safely with patients undergoing an attempt at vaginal birth after a previous cesarean section.[9,10]

C. Complications

1. Polyhydramnios
   In addition to the rare complications associated with placement of an IUPC, polyhydramnios may occur if the rate and duration of the amnioinfusion are not carefully monitored.

2. Uterine hypertonus
   A possible effect of polyhydramnios is uterine hypertonus. The incidence of cord prolapse is not increased with the use of amnioinfusion.

D. Equipment

1. IUPC
2. Intravenous tubing
3. NS or LR solution
4. Fetal monitor

E. Procedure

1. Indications are met for amnioinfusion
2. Informed consent is obtained
3. The IUPC is placed
4. Performing the amnioinfusion
   An initial bolus of 250 to 600 ml NS or LR solution is administered. The infusion may be administered using gravity drainage or a pump. The case reports of complications because of uterine overdistention have occurred with the use of an infusion pump; hence, some centers have opted to use the gravity drainage method. No evidence supports the original recommendation that the NS or LR solution be warmed before starting the amnioinfusion.[11]
5. Postamnioinfusion maintenance
   After the initial bolus, a maintenance infusion of 1 to 3 ml/min is used. If intrapartum ultrasound is used, the amnioinfusion can be adjusted to keep

the AFI between 8 and 12 cm. An infusion of 250 ml fluid results in an average increase of the AFI of 4 cm and often results in a small increase in the basal uterine tone.[12] Clinicians who can obtain an AFI during labor can easily determine when an adequate fluid cushion has been achieved (an AFI between 8 and 12 cm). When an AFI is not available, it is recommended that the total quantity infused not exceed 800 ml.

III. SOR A RECOMMENDATION

RECOMMENDATION	REFERENCE
Amnioinfusion is an effective treatment of suspected umbilical cord compression that occurs in the presence of recurrent variable decelerations. Use of amnioinfusion for this indication results in a decrease in the number of variable decelerations (NNT = 3), cesarean intervention (NNT = 8), and postpartum endometritis (NNT = 16).	*1*

REFERENCES

1. Hofmeyr GJ: Amnioinfusion in intrapartum umbilical cord compression (Cochrane review), *The Cochrane Library*, Oxford, 2006, Update Software.
2. Spong C, McKindsey F, Ross M: Amniotic fluid index predicts the relief of variable decelerations after amnioinfusion bolus, *Am J Obstet Gynecol* 175:1066-1070, 1996.
3. Hofmeyr GJ: Prophylactic versus therapeutic amnioinfusion for oligohydramnios in labour, *Cochrane Database Syst Rev* (2):CD000176, 2007.
4. Pitt C, Sanchez-Ramos L, Kaunitz AM et al: Prophylactic amnioinfusion for intrapartum oligohydramnios: a meta-analysis of randomized controlled trials, *Obstet Gynecol* 96:861-866, 2000.
5. Hofmeyr GJ: Amnioinfusion for meconium-stained liquor in labour, *Cochrane Database Syst Rev* (2):CD000014, 2002.
6. Pierce J, Gaudier FL, Sanchez-Ramos L: Intrapartum amnioinfusion for meconium-stained fluid: meta-analysis of prospective clinical trials, *Obstet Gynecol* 95:1051-1056, 2000.
7. Rathore AM, Singh R, Ramji S et al: Randomised trial of amnioinfusion during labour with meconium stained amniotic fluid, *BJOG* 109:17-20, 2002.
8. Fraser WE, Hofmeyr UJ, Lede R et al: Amnioinfusion for the prevention of the meconium aspiration syndrome, *N Engl J Med* 353:946-948, 2005.
9. Ouzounian J, Miller D, Paul R: Amnioinfusion in women with previous cesarean births: a preliminary report, *Am J Obstet Gynecol* 174:783-786, 1996.
10. Hicks P: Systematic review of the risk of uterine rupture with the use of amnioinfusion after previous cesarean delivery, *South Med J* 98:458-461, 2005.
11. Glantz J, Letteney D: Pumps and warmers during amnioinfusion: Is either necessary? *Obstet Gynecol* 87:150-155, 1996.
12. Strong TH, Hetzler G, Paul RH: Amniotic fluid volume increase after amnioinfusion of a fixed volume, *Am J Obstet Gynecol* 162:746-748, 1990.

Section D Assisted Deliveries

Stephen D. Ratcliffe, MD, MSPH, and James R. Damos, MD

The assisted vaginal delivery, either with forceps or vacuum extraction, is an important skill to acquire when managing the second stage of labor. This section discusses the indications and prerequisites for an assisted vaginal delivery using forceps and vacuum extraction. The evidence comparing forceps with vacuum extraction is examined.

I. INDICATIONS FOR ASSISTED VAGINAL DELIVERY

A. Maternal Exhaustion
Maternal exhaustion may occur when first- or second-stage labor is prolonged.

B. Anesthesia and Analgesia
The use of epidural anesthesia is strongly associated with an increased use of an assisted vaginal delivery.[1] For every 10 patients receiving epidural anesthesia, an additional forceps- or vacuum-assisted delivery occurs.

C. Prolonged Second Stage of Labor
The ACOG previously defined prolonged second-stage labor as greater than 1 hour for the multiparous patient and greater than 2 hours for the nulliparous patient. In recognizing that regional anesthesia has the effect of prolonging second-stage labor, ACOG amended these definitions for women with epidural anesthesia as follows[2]:

1. Prolonged second-stage labor for the multiparous patient lasting longer than 2 hours
2. Prolonged second-stage labor for the nulliparous patient lasting longer than 3 hours

D. Nonreassuring Fetal Heart Tones

If vaginal delivery can be accomplished expeditiously, the presence of a nonreassuring fetal heart tracing may be an indication for assisted delivery. Cesarean backup should always be anticipated.

E. Patients with Chronic Medical Conditions

Women with chronic conditions whose health will be adversely affected with repeated Valsalva maneuvers are candidates for an assisted delivery.

F. Malposition

Fetuses in a persistent occiput posterior (OP) position, or with transverse presentation or mild degrees of deflexion or asynclitism, may have their delivery assisted through use of forceps or vacuum devices. A persistent OP position increases the need for an assisted delivery.[3]

II. STRATEGIES TO DECREASE THE NEED FOR ASSISTED DELIVERY

A. Provide Continuous Labor Support

The use of continuous support during labor reduces the need for assisted deliveries (odds ratio [OR], 0.89; confidence interval [CI], 0.84-0.96; NNT = 59). The optimal support comes from the use of a trained labor support person, a doula.[4] One-on-one nursing support or the use of female family members or friends may serve as a helpful substitute when doula support is not available.

B. Delay the Onset of Maternal Pushing with Epidural Anesthesia

In women with epidural anesthesia, delaying the onset of pushing until they have a strong urge to push, up to a 2-hour period, results in lower rates of assisted delivery with comparable neonatal outcomes.[5]

C. Perform Manual Rotation from Occiput Posterior to Occiput Anterior

If the fetal head can be manually rotated from OP, which is a partially deflexed cephalic attitude, to OA with a partially flexed head, the resulting smaller diameters may prevent the need for an assisted delivery (see Chapter 17, Section F). When assisted delivery is used in the persistent OP position, greater rates of third- and fourth-degree perineal extensions and need for subsequent interventions, such as cesarean delivery, may occur.[3,6]

D. Use Oxytocin during Second-Stage Labor When Progressive Fetal Descent Fails to Occur

Second stage use of oxytocin in nulliparas with epidural anesthesia is associated with a decrease in the need for assisted delivery (NNT = 12) and cesarean delivery rates (NNT = 65).[7]

E. Encourage Position Change during Second-Stage Labor

Use of the upright and lateral pushing positions versus the "traditional" dorsal lithotomy position is associated with a decrease in assisted deliveries, a reduction in duration of second-stage labor, a reduction in episiotomy rates, and an increase in second-degree extensions.[8]

III. PREREQUISITES FOR ASSISTED VAGINAL DELIVERY

The prerequisites for assisted vaginal delivery are discussed in the following sections.[9]

A. Membranes Must Be Ruptured

The presence of membranes may interfere with application of either vacuum or forceps devices. Furthermore, knowledge of the presence or absence of meconium-stained fluid can affect early neonatal management.

B. Cervix Must Be Completely Dilated

To avoid maternal trauma, the clinician must be certain that there is no remaining cervical lip or rim before applying the forceps or vacuum.

C. Vertex Presentation Is Present and Position of the Fetal Head Is Known

As progression of cervical dilation occurs through first-stage labor, it is important to determine the fetal head position. It becomes increasingly difficult to make this determination during second-stage labor as the fetal caput develops. The anterior fontanelle is larger and forms a cross or a diamond with *four* sutures emanating from it. The posterior fontanelle is smaller and forms a Y with *three* sutures extending from it. The clinician can also feel for an ear and see which way it bends. When in doubt, bedside ultrasound may be used to determine position.

D. Fetal Head Must Be Deeply Engaged

If the cephalic prominence can still be palpated above the pubic symphysis on abdominal examination, the fetal head is not likely to be sufficiently engaged for assisted delivery. A vertex presentation with considerable molding may appear to be at a lower station of descent than is accurate. If much of the sacral hollow is empty, fetal descent is likely to be higher than a $+2$ station. This would involve a midforceps or vacuum application and should be avoided if possible.

E. Knowledge of Delivering Instruments

Clinicians performing assisted deliveries must know what types of forceps and vacuum devices are available at their institution and be familiar with them before attempting their use. In many hospitals, a mentoring program can be arranged to help a physician become familiar with a particular instrument.

F. Maternal-Fetal Size Relationship Should Be Assessed

Macrosomic babies with weights greater than 4000 to 4500 g have a greater incidence of shoulder dystocia, particularly if the mother has gestational diabetes.[10] The clinician should assess the maternal-fetal size relationship before attempting a vaginally assisted delivery. If fetal macrosomia is suspected, the clinician should prepare the team to respond appropriately should a shoulder dystocia occur.

G. Adequate Anesthesia

Regional anesthesia usually provides adequate pain relief for assisting a delivery. An effective pudendal block provides some relief that may be augmented with local infiltration of 1% lidocaine.

H. Empty Bladder

The patient's bladder should be empty before an instrumented delivery is attempted. Time permitting, a straight catheterization can be performed.

I. Abandoning the Procedure

If assisted delivery does not proceed easily or does not produce progress toward deliver, the clinician must be willing to abandon the procedure and be prepared to proceed to immediate cesarean delivery. During the transition time to cesarean, if the fetal condition is in jeopardy, an intrauterine fetal resuscitation can be done by administering subcutaneous terbutaline, 0.25 to 0.5 mg, and oxygen to the patient (see Chapter 16, Section A).[11] The ACOG recommends that multiple attempts at assisted vaginal delivery using different instruments (vacuum, different types of forceps) be avoided because of the greater potential for maternal and/or fetal injury.[2]

IV. CLASSIFICATION OF FORCEPS APPLICATION

A. Engagement

Engagement occurs when the biparietal diameter of the fetal head has passed the plane of the pelvic inlet (Figure 18-5). Clinically, one can determine engagement when the presenting part is palpated at the level of the ischial spine and determined to be at 0 station. After vigorous labor, the fetal skull may be elongated and molded with caput formation. There may also be asynclitism, in which the sagittal suture is not in the midline of the pelvis. These factors may create the erroneous impression that engagement has occurred when, in fact, the biparietal diameter has not passed through the inlet.

B. Forceps Definitions

Because of problems defining engagement and concern over the need for guidelines for midforceps application, the Maternal-Fetal Medicine Committee of ACOG reclassified forceps applications in 1988.[2]
1. Outlet forceps
   The fetal skull has reached the pelvic floor. The scalp is visible between contractions. The sagittal suture is in the anteroposterior diameter, or in the right or left occiput anterior or posterior position, but not more than 45 degrees from the midline.
2. Low forceps
   The leading edge of the fetal skull is at $+2$ station or lower. The head is not on the pelvic floor but fills the hollow of the sacral space. Rotations are divided into 45 degrees or less and more than 45 degrees.

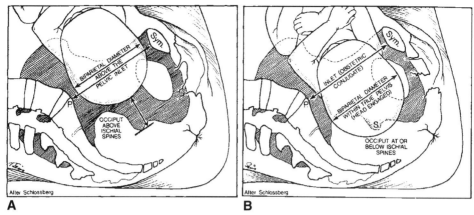

A   **B**

FIGURE 18-5. A, When the lowermost portion of the fetal head is above the ischial spines, the biparietal diameter of the head is not likely to have passed through the pelvic inlet and, therefore, is not engaged. **B,** When the lowermost portion of the fetal head is at or below the ischial spines, it is usually engaged. Exceptions occur when there is considerable molding, caput formation, or both. *P,* Sacral promontory; *S,* ischial spine; *Sym,* symphysis pubis. (From Cunningham FG, MacDonald P, Gant N et al, editors: *Williams obstetrics,* ed 19, East Norwalk, CT, 1993, Appleton & Lange.)

3. Midforceps
   The head is engaged, but the leading edge of skull is above +2 station.

V. PROCEDURE FOR FORCEPS

The procedures for forceps-assisted delivery is discussed in the following sections.[11,12]

A. Choice of Instrument
1. Simpson forceps (Figure 18-6)
   The Simpson forceps and its modifications (Simpson, Luikart-Simpson, and DeLee) have long, shallow, tapered blades and are most suitable to large and extensively molded fetal heads.

2. Elliot forceps
   The Elliot forceps and its modifications (Elliot, Tucker-McLane, Tucker-Luikart) have shorter blades and an accentuated cephalic curve that is more suitable for a rounded fetal head that has not undergone extensive molding. In addition, Elliot instruments, because of their overlapping shanks, do not distend the perineum in the same way as the separated shanks of the Simpson-type forceps.

B. Application
1. Forceps insertion
   After ensuring that indications and prerequisites for forceps application are present, the forceps blades can be coated with soapy lubricant for ease of

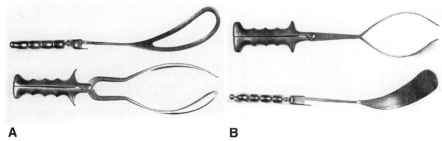

A   **B**

FIGURE 18-6. A, Simpson forceps. Note the ample pelvic curve in the single blade above and cephalic curve evident in the articulated blades below. The fenestrated blade and the wide shank in front of the English-style lock characterize the Simpson forceps. **B,** Tucker-McLane forceps. The blade is solid; the shank is overlapping. (From Cunningham FG, MacDonald P, Gant N et al, editors: *Williams obstetrics,* ed 19, East Norwalk, CT, 1993, Appleton & Lange.)

application. Some evidence has been reported that the application of foam pads to the forceps blades or coating the blades with a soft rubber coating may decrease neonatal facial trauma.[12,13] The left forceps handle, determined in relation to maternal position, is held in the operator's left hand during insertion using a "pencil grip." Insertion begins with the cephalic curve facing inward toward the vulva, with the shank perpendicular to the floor. The blade is applied to the left side of the fetal head, assuming an occiput anterior position, using the operator's right hand to protect the maternal left pelvic sidewall and guide the blade into position. The right thumb is placed on the heel of the forceps blade and is used as the inserting force as the handle is brought through a wide arc with the operator's left hand.

The right forceps handle is then held in the operator's right hand and is applied to the right side of the fetal head on the mother's right side. Similarly, the operator's left hand protects the mother's right pelvic sidewall and guides the blade into position. The left thumb is placed on the heel of the forceps blade, as the inserting force. The handles should fit together and lock if the blades are applied correctly.

2. Position for safety

The posterior fontanel should be midway between the shanks and 1 cm anterior to the plane of the shanks. This ensures proper flexion of the fetal head to present the narrowest diameter to the pelvis. If the posterior fontanelle is higher than 1 cm above the plane of the shanks, traction will cause extension of the head, thus presenting a larger fetal diameter to the pelvis and making delivery more difficult. If there is a fenestration in the forceps being used, it should be barely palpable. If more than a fingertip is able to be inserted, the forceps blades are not in far enough to be below the malar eminence. Finally, fetal sutures should be assessed. The sagittal suture should be in the midline between the blades to ensure proper forceps application. Some also check the lambdoidal sutures, which should be above and equidistant from the upper surface of each blade. In summary, to make sure the forceps are applied correctly, check **P**osition **F**or **S**afety—**P**osterior fontanel, **F**enestration, **S**utures.

C. Delivery

Traction is made with a gentle pulling motion that gradually increases and decreases to mimic the uterine contraction, unless circumstances dictate a more expedient approach. Using Pajot's maneuver, the pelvic curve will be followed. As the fetal head begins to descend under the pubic symphysis, the handle of the forceps should be elevated to lessen the pressure and distension of the perineum. It is at this junction that the clinician may need to perform an episiotomy that should be modest and extended into the vaginal mucosa and away from the anal sphincter. It is quite feasible to avoid making an episiotomy for the multiparous patient. The operator should closely observe the perineum as the head begins to crown. If the perineum begins to tear or an episiotomy begins to extend, one should slow down the procedure to avoid further trauma. Once the fetal head has "crowned," the forceps should be removed carefully to avoid causing a sulcus or vaginal sidewall laceration. A modified Ritgen maneuver may be necessary to help deliver the head at this point (Figure 18-7).

D. Follow-up Care

1. A thorough maternal cervical, vaginal, and rectal examination should be conducted to rule out lacerations.
2. The infant should be examined for evidence of birth trauma, looking specifically for fractured clavicle, cephalhematoma, lacerations or abrasions, or facial nerve palsy.

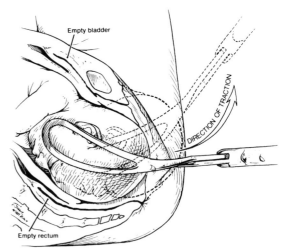

FIGURE 18-7. Occiput anterior. Delivery by outlet forceps (Simpson). The direction of gentle traction for delivery of the head is indicated. (From Cunningham FG, MacDonald P, Gant N et al, editors: *Williams obstetrics*, ed 19, East Norwalk, CT, 1993, Appleton & Lange.)

3. An operative note should be completed that includes the indications for the procedure and a detailed account of the operation. The ABCDEFGHIJ mnemonic taught in the Advanced Life Support and Obstetrics course provides a systematic method for documentation of the procedure.[11]

4. On the first postpartum day, the mother and any other significant family members should be questioned about their perceptions of the need for assisting the delivery and their experience regarding how the delivery went. Clarification of any misperceptions can be carried out with support and empathy.

5. Stool softeners should be ordered when third- or fourth-degree extensions of an episiotomy have occurred. Patients should be told to expect that the first bowel movement or two may be painful. Forceps-assisted deliveries are associated with an increased risk for anal sphincter injury, and dysfunction related to this injury has been noted to last over a 10-year period.[14]

VI. VACUUM EXTRACTION

The vacuum device rivals forceps in safety and efficacy. During a vacuum delivery, the operator assists by adding to the momentum of the maternal expulsive efforts, rather than simply pulling the baby out with the instrument alone.[11,15] Plastic cup extractors are safer and easier to assemble. Metal cups, no longer available in the United States, are more capable of solving rotational problems and can provide more traction.

A. Indications and Prerequisites

The same indications and prerequisites outlined for forceps application apply for use of the vacuum device.

B. Advantages of Vacuum Application

1. The vacuum instrument is easier than forceps to apply.
2. The vacuum-assisted delivery teaches the clinician to follow the pelvic curve.
3. The vacuum applies less force to the fetal head.
4. The vacuum requires less anesthesia and results in fewer vaginal and cervical lacerations.
5. Studies show a lower incidence of anal sphincter tears with vacuum application compared with forceps.[16]

C. Disadvantages of Vacuum Application

1. Traction can be applied only during contractions.
2. Proper traction is necessary to avoid losing vacuum.
3. Delivery may take longer than with forceps because vacuum pressure is applied only during contractions. This may not be as ideal when rapid delivery is necessary.
4. There may be difficulty in maintaining vacuum suction on the fetal head if molding is present.
5. There is an increase in the incidence of cephalhematomas and retinal hemorrhages with vacuum use compared with spontaneous delivery or forceps.[17] Predelivery factors found to predispose to neonatal cephalhematoma formation include increasing asynclitism, paramedian placement of the vacuum, and time from application to delivery exceeding 5 to 10 minutes.[17,18]
6. Potentially fatal subgaleal hemorrhages have been reported in recent years, resulting in an FDA advisory described in Section G.[19]

D. Contraindications to Vacuum Assistance

1. Prematurity at less than 37 weeks of gestation requires special caution
2. Breech, face, brow, or transverse presentation
3. Incomplete cervical dilatation
4. Cephalopelvic disproportion
5. Fetal vertex not engaged
6. If greater than 45 degrees rotation of the fetal head is necessary, special caution must be taken

E. When to Stop with Vacuum Efforts

1. Failure to achieve extraction after 10 minutes at maximal pressure
2. Failure to achieve extraction within 20 minutes of initiation of procedure
3. Disengagement of extractor cup three times
4. No significant progress in three consecutive pulls
5. Fetal scalp trauma inflicted by extractor cup

F. Procedure

To effect a vaginal delivery, the fetal head must rotate and flex at the neck to allow the passage of the widest diameter of the head through the pelvis (Figures 18-8 and 18-9). This pathway is simulated

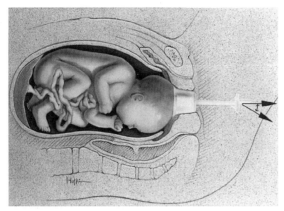

FIGURE 18-8. Correct position of the vacuum cup and the correct direction of traction before the vertex clears the symphysis pubis. (From Epperly T, Breitinger R: Vacuum extraction, *Am Fam Physician* 38:205-210, 1988.)

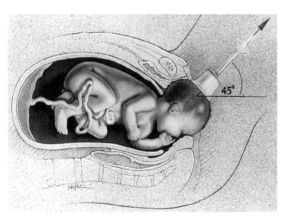

FIGURE 18-9. Change in the direction of traction as the vertex crowns. (From Epperly T, Breitinger R: Vacuum extraction, *Am Fam Physician* 38:205-210, 1988.)

when the mentovertical diameter points in the direction of the delivering pathway. The "flexion point" is the location on the fetal head where outward traction pulls the head to allow the mentovertical diameter to be oriented in the direction of the birth canal. The flexion point is located in the midline, over the sagittal suture, approximately 6 cm from the anterior fontanelle and 2 to 3 cm from the posterior fontanelle. The center of the vacuum cup should be applied in this location. Because most vacuum cups have diameters ranging

from 50 to 70 mm, when the center of the cup is placed over the flexion point, the edges of the cup should be approximately 3 cm from the anterior fontanelle and just at the edge of the posterior fontanelle.

The anterior fontanelle is a good reference point for checking cup application because access to the posterior fontanelle is partially blocked once the vacuum cup is in place. A finger is swept around the edge of the cup to make sure no maternal tissue is trapped beneath the cup. Negative pressure is then raised to the yellow area on the dial. The cup is then reexamined for position and presence of maternal tissue. With the next contraction, negative pressure is rapidly raised to the green area on the dial. Traction is applied while trying to avoid a rotary force that may break the seal. The J-shaped pelvic curve can be appreciated as the head descends through the pelvis.

G. Complications
On May 21, 1998, an FDA public advisory was published cautioning health-care providers about use of vacuum-assisted delivery devices.[19] One type of life-threatening complication noted with vacuum-assisted delivery is subgaleal hematoma. This occurs when emissary veins are damaged and blood accumulates in the potential space between the galea aponeurotica and the periosteum of the skull. Signs of subgaleal hematoma include diffuse swelling of the head that may shift dependently when the infant's head is repositioned. This swelling indents easily on palpation and may be significant enough to result in hypovolemic shock. Intracranial hemorrhage may also occur and be life-threatening. Signs of intracranial hemorrhage include convulsions, lethargy, obtundation, apnea, bulging fontanelle, poor feeding, increased irritability, bradycardia, and/or shock. Thus, this FDA advisory cautions physicians to use discretion and make sure that there are definite indications for vacuum-assisted delivery.

H. Follow-up Care after a Vacuum-Assisted Delivery
1. Documentation
   An operative report that describes the indication, procedure, and any complications of the procedure should be completed.
2. Patient communication
   Misunderstandings or misperceptions are common when quick decisions must be made toward the end

of a delivery. Every attempt should be made to understand the perceptions of the patient and her family as to why the assisted delivery occurred and to address any possible misunderstanding.

3. Fetal scalp trauma

   If fetal scalp emphysema or erythema occurred after the vacuum was applied, it will typically resolve within 1 week without complications. Examine for cephalhematomas, subgaleal hemorrhages, and subsequent jaundice. Parental reassurance plays an important role.

VII. DELIVERING AN OCCIPITOPOSTERIOR PRESENTATION BY FORCEPS OR VACUUM

The fetus in the OP position rotates spontaneously to an OA presentation in more than 90% of cases. If the OP presentation is persistent, delivery can occur in this position. Vacuum or forceps delivery with the fetus in an OP position, or cesarean delivery, is safer and, in most cases, preferable to forceps rotation.[11,15] The persistent OP presentation is a cause of relative cephalopelvic disproportion and is associated with an increased incidence of a failed assisted delivery. Therefore, preparations should be made for emergent cesarean delivery if the procedure fails or the fetal condition deteriorates.

A. Vacuum

The vacuum is the preferable instrument for delivering an OP presentation because autorotation may occur without trauma to maternal sidewalls. A built-in safety factor is disengagement of the cup three times.

B. Forceps

Forceps rotation should be done only by skilled and experienced operators. For less experienced clinicians, a vacuum or forceps delivery with the fetus in an OP position or a cesarean intervention is safer. Forceps delivery when the fetus is in an OP position occurs as follows:

1. Forceps are applied in the manner described earlier.
2. Traction initially is straight out, because flexion of the head is limited and extension of the head presents greater diameters to the pelvis and will not occur.

3. Traction is applied until the nose is visible beneath the symphysis; then upward motion brings the occiput into view. This is followed by downward pressure to deliver the rest of the face.

VIII. FORCEPS VERSUS VACUUM: WHICH IS BETTER?

The vacuum extractor rivals forceps in safety and efficacy, depending on the experience of the operator. Use of the vacuum extractor is associated with an increased risk for cephalhematoma (absolute risk increase of 5.5%; number needed to harm [NNH] = 18) and retinal hemorrhage (absolute risk increase of 15.4%; NNH = 6.5).[16] However, use of vacuum prevents significant maternal injury (absolute risk reduction = 11%; NNT = 9). Forceps is often preferred in emergent situations when time is a factor.

IX. PROPHYLACTIC ANTIBIOTICS AFTER ASSISTED VAGINAL DELIVERY

Women with cesarean or assisted vaginal delivery are at increased risk for rehospitalization, principally because of infectious morbidities.[20] A recent Cochrane review looked at all randomized trials comparing any prophylactic antibiotic regimen with placebo, or no treatment, in women undergoing vacuum or forceps deliveries.[21] The authors' conclusions were that the data were too few and of insufficient quality to make any recommendations for practice. Future research on antibiotic prophylaxis for operative vaginal delivery is needed to conclude whether it is useful for reducing postpartum morbidity.

X. DEVELOPMENTAL OUTCOMES OF ASSISTED VAGINAL DELIVERY

There are no apparent long-term cognitive or neurologic sequelae for infants delivered with forceps or vacuum. Evaluations comparing 3413 five-year-olds delivered by assisted versus spontaneous vaginal route found no difference in cognitive testing.[22] A cohort study of nearly 25,000 births did not find any association between forceps delivery and adult seizure disorder.[23]

XI. SOR A RECOMMENDATIONS

RECOMMENDATIONS	REFERENCES
Use of the vacuum extractor versus use of forceps is associated with an increased risk for cephalematoma (NNH = 18) and retinal hemorrhage (NNH = 6.5).	16
Use of the vacuum extractor versus use of forceps is associated with prevention of significant maternal injury (NNT = 9).	16
Use of epidural anesthesia is associated with increased use of a vaginally assisted delivery (NNH = 10).	1
The use of continuous support during labor reduces the need for assisted deliveries (NNT = 59).	4

REFERENCES

1. Howell CJ: Epidural vs. non-epidural analgesic for pain relief, *Cochrane Database Syst Rev* (4):CD000331, 2005.
2. American College of Obstetricians and Gynecologists Practice Bulletin: operative vaginal delivery. Number 17, June 2000, Washington, DC.
3. Benavides L, Wu JM, Hundley AF et al: The impact of occiput posterior fetal head position on the risk on anal sphincter injury in forceps-assisted vaginal deliveries, *Am J Obstet Gynecol* 192:1702-1706, 2005.
4. Hodnett ED, Gates S, Hofmeyr GJ et al: Continuous support for women during childbirth, *Cochrane Database Syst Rev* (3): CD000198, 2003.
5. Fraser WD, Marcoux S, Krauss I et al: Multicenter, randomized, controlled trial of delayed pushing for nulliparous women in the second stage of labor with continuous epidural analgesia. The PEOPLE (Pushing Early or Pushing Late with Epidural) Study Group, *Am J Obstet Gynecol* 182(5): 1165-1172, 2000.
6. Cargill YM, MacKinnon CJ: Guidelines for operative vaginal birth, *J Obstet Gynaecol Can* 26:747-753, 2004.
7. Saunders NJ, Spiby H, Gilbert L et al: Oxytocin infusion during second stage of labour in primiparous women using epidural analgesia: a randomized double-blind placebo-controlled trial, *BMJ* 299:1423-1426, 1989.
8. Gupta JK, Hofmeyr GJ: Position during second stage of labour, *Cochrane Database Syst Rev* 1:CD002006, 2004.
9. Cunningham FG, MacDonald P, Gant N et al: Forceps delivery and related techniques. In Cunningham FG, MacDonald P, Grant N, editors: *Williams obstetrics,* ed 19, East Norwalk, CT, 1993, Appleton & Lange.
10. Geary M, McParland P, Johnson H et al: Shoulder dystocia—is it predictable? *Eur J Obstet Gynecol Reprod Biol* 62:15-18, 1995.
11. Damos JR, Bassett R: Forceps and vacuum extraction: Advanced Life Support in Obstetrics. American Academy of Family Physicians Course Syllabus, 2003.
12. Roshan DF, Petrikovsky B, Sichinava L et al: Soft forceps, *Int J Gynaecol Obstet* 88:249-252, 2005.
13. Johanson RB: Obstetric forcep pad designed to reduce trauma. In Enkin MW, Keirse MHNC, Renfrew MH, Neilson JP, editors: Pregnancy and Childbirth Module, *Cochrane Database Syst Rev,* Review No. 07086. Cochrane Updates on Disk. Oxford, Update Software, 1994.
14. Fornell EU, Matthiesen L, Sjodahl R et al: Obstetric anal sphincter injury ten years after: subjective and objective long term effects, *BJOG* 12:312-316, 2005.
15. Vacca A: *Handbook of vacuum assisted delivery in obstetric practice,* ed 2, Brisbane, Australia, 2003, Vacca Research.
16. Johanson RB, Menon VJ: Vacuum extraction versus forceps delivery, *Cochrane Database Syst Rev* (2):CD000224, 2000.
17. Bofill JA, Rust OA, Devidas M et al: Neonatal cephalohematoma from vacuum extraction, *J Reprod Med* 42:565-569, 1997.
18. Teng FY, Sayre JW: Vacuum extraction: does duration predict scalp injury? *Obstet Gynecol* 89:281-285, 1997.
19. Burlington DB: FDA Public Health Advisory: need for CAUTION when using vacuum-assisted delivery devices, Rockvale, MD, May 21, 1998, Food and Drug Administration.
20. Lydon-Rochelle M, Holt VL, Martin DP et al: Association between method of delivery and maternal rehospitalization, *JAMA* 283:2411-2416, 2000.
21. Liabsuetrakul T, Choobun T, Peeyananjarassri K et al: Antibiotic prophylaxis for operative vaginal delivery, *Cochrane Database Syst Rev* (3):CD004455, 2004.
22. Wesley BD, Van Den Berg BJ, Reece EA: The effect of forceps delivery on cognitive development, *Am J Obstet Gynecol* 169:1091-1095, 1993.
23. Murphy DJ, Libby G, Chien P et al: Cohort study of forceps delivery and the risk of epilepsy in adulthood, *Am J Obstet Gynecol* 191:392-397, 2004.

S E C T I O N   E

Episiotomy and Repair of Perineal Lacerations and Episiotomies

Robert W. Gobbo, MD,
and Lawrence Leeman, MD, MPH

I. INTRODUCTION AND HISTORY

Concern for perineal trauma in childbirth dates back to the writings of Aristotle, yet it was not until 1742 that Ould described a technique for repairing the perineum.[1] For many years, it was believed that episiotomies prevented excessive pressure to the fetal scalp and laxity to the mother's pelvic floor, thus preventing uterine, bladder, and rectal prolapse later in the women's life. In 1920, DeLee[2] advocated for the routine use of forceps and episiotomy to protect the perineum and pelvic floor from future relaxation.

II. ROUTINE USE OF EPISIOTOMY

A. Lack of Benefit

Routine episiotomy has no demonstrated benefit other than a reduction in the incidence of anterior perineal lacerations, which are usually not clinically significant.[3]

B. Risk for Anal Sphincter Laceration

Episiotomy and operative vaginal delivery have been identified as the primary remediable risk factors for anal sphincter lacerations.[4-8] Episiotomy is also associated with increased perineal pain, dyspareunia, and anal sphincter lacerations.[9] Minimal information exists regarding long-term functional outcomes after episiotomy or perineal lacerations other than the association with anal incontinence symptoms.[9]

C. Episiotomy Rates

Episiotomy rates vary widely across practitioners and maternity care settings; however, the overall rate is gradually declining and was 29% in 2003.[10] A university center reported an episiotomy rate of 1% in a low-risk population served by nurse-midwives,[11] suggesting that many unnecessary episiotomies are being performed annually in the United States.

D. Epidemiology of Anal Sphincter Lacerations

Severe perineal tears that involve the anal sphincters and/or the rectal mucosa are identified in up to 6% of vaginal deliveries.[12-15] Studies demonstrate that 20% to 50% of women will develop anal incontinence symptoms despite appropriate repair.[16-18] Risk factors for third- and fourth-degree tears have been identified mainly in retrospective studies. Birth weight more than 4000 g, OP delivery, short perineal body, and nulliparity are nonpreventable risk factors,[19] and episiotomy[6,15] and operative vaginal delivery[20,21] are the primary preventable risk fasctors. One study found a 29% rate of third-degree lacerations with forceps and a 12% rate with vacuum-assisted vaginal delivery.[20] A metaanalysis of seven RCTs demonstrated that one anal sphincter laceration was avoided for every 18 women delivered with vacuum assist rather than forceps.[21] Since the introduction of endo-anal ultrasound, occult damage to the anal sphincter anatomy has been identified in up to 36% of women after vaginal delivery in a prospective study.[22] Occult damage may represent lacerated anal sphincters below intact perineal muscles or sphincter lacerations that were missed because of inadequate postpartum visual examination.[23]

III. PERINEAL AND PELVIC FLOOR ANATOMY

A. Perineal Body

The female perineal body is a mass of interlocking muscular, fascial, and fibrous components lying between the vagina and anus, and is an integral attachment point for the anal sphincter complex. Perineal anatomy and techniques for repair of injuries to the perineal body are often neglected in medical education.[24] The bulbocavernosus and the transverse perineal muscles form the perineal body (Figure 18-10) with additional muscle fibers added from the puborectalis and external anal sphincter (EAS) muscles.

B. Anal Sphincter Complex

The internal anal sphincter (IAS) and EAS and the rectal mucosa comprise the anal sphincter complex, which extends for a distance of 3 to 4 cm from the anal verge (Figure 18-11). The IAS is composed of smooth muscle, which provides most of the resting anal tone and is continuous with the smooth muscle of the colon.[25] The EAS is a circular striated muscle lying anterior to the rectal mucosa and IAS, and provides the squeeze tone.

IV. DEFINITIONS AND CLASSIFICATION OF EPISIOTOMIES AND LACERATIONS

All physicians and midwives offering maternity care will have the need to repair perineal lacerations and, on occasion, to perform an episiotomy. This section describes the classification and repair of these wounds.

A. Types of Episiotomy

1. Midline episiotomy

   This is a surgical incision in the median or midline raphe of the perineal body. Episiotomy, if necessary, is best done when the presenting head is crowning and the perineal tissues have thinned. Performing an episiotomy earlier than this will

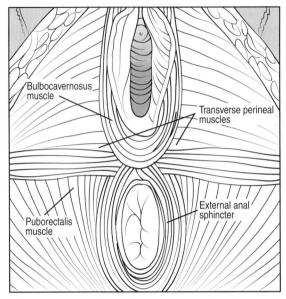

FIGURE 18-10. Muscles of the perineal body. (Copyright Brooks Hart. Ciné Med, Inc., Woodbury, CT.)

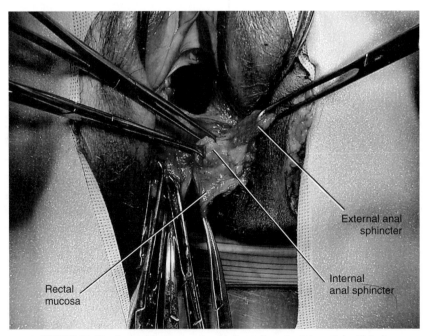

FIGURE 18-11. Anal sphincter complex (cadaver dissection) (see Color Plates).

usually not hasten delivery and will only lead to increased blood loss. A finger or tongue blade is placed between the neonatal scalp and the perineum to protect the fetal presenting part. Mayo or bandage scissors slide in into this space and cut directly downward toward the patient's rectum. Sometimes it is also necessary to cut slightly inward toward the hymen to provide for more room; this is especially true if the perineum has not thinned out before incision. The length required to cut will vary with the clinical situation and the individual patient's perineal anatomy. Inexperienced clinicians may cut a longer incision than is required and increase the likelihood of extension into the rectum. Some women have a short perineum and any incision downward will easily extend into the rectum.[26,27]

2. Mediolateral episiotomy

A surgical incision should be directed from the posterior fourchette to either the right or left at a 30- to 45-degree angle from the vertical. Although common in many European and Third World countries, this type of incision is not commonly used in the United States, perhaps because of lack of clinician experience or the belief that mediolateral episiotomies are more difficult to repair and result in increased postpartum pain, although little evidence exists to support these concerns.[28,29] This approach is associated with a decreased incidence of third- and fourth-degree extensions compared with midline episiotomy.[28,29]

B. Laceration Classification

For purposes of classification, perineal lacerations, episiotomies, and extensions of episiotomies are considered in the same manner and defined as first through fourth degree. Third-degree lacerations have been categorized based on the extent to which the EAS and IAS are involved.

1. First degree

This laceration is confined to the perineal skin or vaginal mucosa, or both, without involvement of the perineal muscles. These usually do not need repair unless they are bleeding.

2. Second degree

This laceration involves the perineal muscles (transverse perineal, bulbocavernosus, or both) but does not involve the anal sphincter complex (Figure 18-12).

3. Third degree

This laceration involves the anal sphincter but does not extend through the rectal mucosa. These may be subclassified[30] as:

a. Less than 50% of the EAS
b. More than 50% of EAS
c. Involves the IAS

4. Fourth degree

This laceration extends into the rectal mucosa (Figure 18-13). Uncommonly, a "buttonhole" injury may occur where the EAS is intact, yet an extension has entered the rectal lumen approximately 3 to 4 cm above the anorectal verge, where a very thin layer of tissue separates the vagina and the rectum.

V. INDICATIONS FOR EPISIOTOMY

Episiotomy use should be restricted to births in which there is a need to shorten the second stage because of nonreassuring fetal heart tones or in which additional room is needed to facilitate the performance of a maneuver or procedure.[9,28]

A. Nonreassuring Fetal Heart Tones

Episiotomy may be indicated to expedite vaginal delivery if a bradycardia or deep repetitive fetal heart decelerations occur in the second stage.

B. Shoulder Dystocia

Shoulder dystocia is a soft-tissue dystocia, and episiotomy does not relieve the dystocia. However, it may help provide room for the birth attendant's hands if internal rotational maneuvers are needed.

C. Breech Delivery

Occasionally, an episiotomy may be needed to assist in delivery of the after-coming head with the Mauriceau-Smellie-Veit maneuver or to apply Piper forceps.

D. Operative Vaginal Delivery

Episiotomy is not routinely indicated for operative vaginal delivery[31] but may be needed on occasion to facilitate adequate space for a safe forceps application.

VI. RELATIVE CONTRAINDICATIONS TO EPISIOTOMY

Episiotomy should be avoided in the setting of maternal coagulopathy, large perivulvar varicosities, or maternal infection with human immunodeficiency virus (HIV), hepatitis B, or hepatitis C.

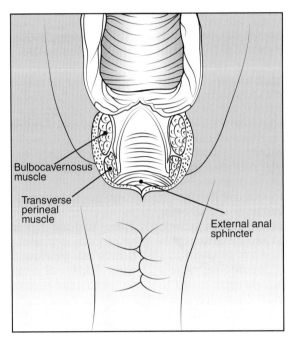

FIGURE 18-12. Second-degree laceration with preservation of the external anal sphincter and rectal mucosa. (Copyright Brooks Hart, Ciné Med, Inc., Woodbury, CT.)

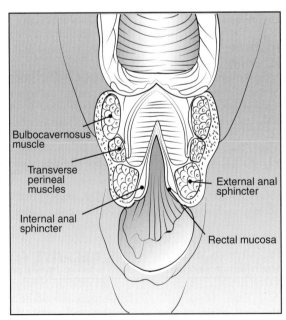

FIGURE 18-13. Fourth-degree laceration with extension through the external anal sphincter into the rectal mucosa. (Copyright Brooks Hart, Ciné Med, Inc., Woodbury, CT.)

VII. REPAIR OF PERINEAL LACERATION OR EPISIOTOMY[32]

A. Equipment

1. Sterile drapes
2. Irrigation solution
3. Needle holder
4. Metzenbaum scissors
5. Suture scissors
6. Forceps with teeth
7. Allis clamps (for anal sphincter lacerations)
8. Gelpi (Figure 18-14) or Deaver retractor (for use in visualizing anal sphincter complex or deep vaginal lacerations)
9. 10-ml syringe with 22-gauge needle
10. 1% lidocaine (Xylocaine)
11. 2-0 or 3-0 polyglactin 910 suture on a taper point CT-1 (Ethicon) or GS-21 (Syneture) needle (for vaginal mucosa)
12. 2-0 or 3-0 polyglactin 910 suture on a taper point CT-1 (Ethicon) or GS-21 (Syneture) needle (for perineal muscle sutures)
13. 4-0 polyglactin 910 suture on a taper point SH (Ethicon) or GS-22 (Syneture) needle (for perineal skin repair)
14. 4-0 chromic or polyglactin 910 on taper point SH (Ethicon) or GS-22 (Syneture) needle (for rectal mucosa)
15. 2-0 polyglactin taper point CT-1 (Ethicon) or GS-21 (Syneture) needle (for repair of IAS)
16. 2-0 polydioxanone sulfate (PDS-Ethicon), monofilament polyglyconate (Maxon-Syneture) or polyglactin 910 taper point CT-1 (Ethicon) or GS-21 (Syneture) needle (for the EAS)

B. Anesthesia

Local anesthesia can be administered before cutting an episiotomy or before the repair. Anesthetic choice is at the discretion of the provider, but commonly used anesthetic agents include lidocaine or bupivacaine. Additional anesthesia options include pudendal nerve block, intravenous analgesia, or "topping off" an existing epidural analgesia. Regional anesthesia by spinal or epidural may be of particular benefit to facilitate repairs in women with anal sphincter complex lacerations by relaxing the anal sphincters, which often are retracted laterally.[30,32]

C. Repair Techniques

First-degree lacerations or very small second-degree lacerations may not need to be repaired unless there is active bleeding. The SUNS trial found no differ-

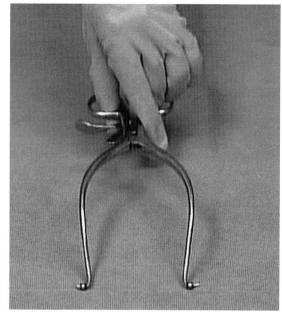

FIGURE 18-14. A Gelpi retractor (see Color Plates).

ence in pain in unsutured first- and second-degree lacerations, although the wounds were not as well approximated at 6 weeks.[33] A prospective cohort study showed no difference in postpartum pelvic floor outcomes in women with unsutured vs. sutured second degree lacerations except greater pain in the sutured group.[33a]

1. Repair of vaginal mucosa
   a. Repairing the apex: The vaginal mucosa is repaired by placing a suture approximately 1 cm above the apex of the laceration to incorporate any retracted blood vessels and prevent bleeding. If the apex is deep in the vagina, it may be difficult to visualize. The clinician can place a single interrupted suture as high in the defect as possible and then place a hemostat on the free end of the suture. The wound can then be retracted inferiorly, and subsequent interrupted sutures can be placed superiorly until the apex is exposed for repair.
   b. Closing the vaginal mucosa: Once the apex suture is secured, the vaginal mucosa is approximated by passing the needle through one side of the vagina mucosa and the underlying rectovaginal septum, and back out to the opposing side through the rectovaginal septum and vaginal mucosa. Locking each stitch

provides better hemostasis, but it is not necessary if the tissue is not bleeding. Care should be taken not to place the sutures too lateral to the midline incision. This may result in excessive imbrication of the vaginal epithelium that can lead to epidermal inclusion cysts as the wound heals. Incorporating the rectovaginal septum can potentially prevent future rectocele development, but care must be taken not to enter the rectal lumen.

   c. Suturing: The suture may be either tied proximal to the hymenal ring or brought under the hymenal ring and held for repair of the perineal muscles. Appropriate suture for the vaginal mucosa and perineal muscles repair is 2–0 or 3–0 polyglactin (Vicryl or Polysorb), an absorbable synthetic suture, which decreases the women's experience of short-term pain (OR, 0.53; 95% CI, 0.43-0.64; adjusted relative risk [ARR], 13%; NNT = 7.5), the need for analgesia (OR, 0.63; 95% CI, 0.49-0.80; ARR, 11%; NNT = 9), and suture dehiscence (OR, 0.41; 95% CI, 0.25-0.67; ARR, 10%; NNT = 10) compared with chromic suture.[34] Use of a rapidly absorbable polyglactin suture (Vicryl Rapide) has the additional advantage of a decrease likelihood of requiring postpartum suture removal.[35]

2. Repair of the perineal muscles

   a. Perineal muscles: The perineal muscles may be reapproximated using a series of interrupted sutures or by a continuation of the running suture from the vaginal mucosa. When using interrupted sutures, one or two sutures of 2–0 or 3–0 polyglactin are initially placed through the transverse perineal muscles (Figure 18-15). A large amount of muscle may be reapproximated by using a large CT-1 needle, which is initially directed through the muscles approximately 5 mm from the skin edge. The needle then exits through the deeper region of the transverse perineal muscles. The needle is carried across the midline, enters deep on the opposing side, and exits approximately 5 mm from the skin edge. Depending on the length of the perineal body laceration, a second interrupted suture is placed above the first suture in a similar fashion.

   b. Bulbocavernosus repair: The perineal body repair is completed with a single interrupted suture of 2–0 or 3–0 polyglactin to reunite the bulbocavernosus muscle. A large CT-1 needle

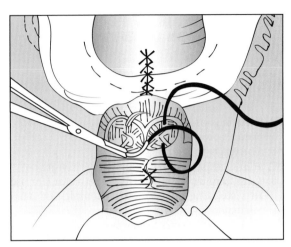

FIGURE 18-15. Repair of the bulbocavernosus muscle. (Copyright University of New Mexico Family Medicine, 2007.)

is directed superiorly and posteriorly to grasp the muscle and then exits in the inferior region of the bulbocavernosus muscle. The needle is then directed to the opposing side to enter the bulbocavernosus inferiorly and exit superiorly. A gentle downward tug after exiting the bulbocavernosus on each side should demonstrate movement of the labia majora as the muscle runs through the labia. A lack of downward movement of the labia suggests that the bulbocavernosus has not been successfully reached.

   c. Repairing perineal muscles using continuous suturing from the vaginal mucosal repair: Alternatively, the suture from the vaginal mucosa may be used to close the perineal body with a running suture.

   d. Repair of deep perineal laceration: Some patients may have too deep of a defect to repair the perineum with single bites of the remaining suture. In this situation, the deep layers of the perineum can be closed with interrupted stitches before using the running suture.

3. Repair of the perineal skin

The skin may be either left unsutured or repaired with a running subcuticular suture of 4–0 polyglactin starting at the deepest point of the skin laceration. Although skin repair has been traditional, recent evidence supports leaving the perineal skin unsutured. Placement of the interrupted sutures through the perineal body as described earlier usually results in excellent reapproximation without use of skin sutures.

a. Oboro and colleagues[36] compared a two-layer closure with a three-layer closure and found patients with a two-layer closure and the skin left unsutured had less perineal pain at 48 hours (57% vs. 65%; RR, 0.87; 95% CI, 0.78-0.97) and 14 days (22% vs. 28%; RR, 0.77; 95% CI, 0.61-0.98), less need for suture removal, and less dyspareunia at 3 months. Rates of wound healing were similar.

b. The Ipswich Childbirth Studies compared a two-layer closure (leaving the skin edges unsutured) with a three-layer closure. They found a trend toward decreased pain, decreased dyspareunia at 3 months, and less altered perineal sensation at 1 year in the two-layer group compared with the three-layer group.[37]

At the top of the subcuticular skin closure, the needle is passed into the vagina behind the hymenal ring and tied to itself. If skin sutures are placed, the subcuticular method is superior to interrupted sutures through the skin because of less pain for up to 10 days postpartum (OR, 0.68; 95% CI, 0.53-0.86; ARR, 7%; NNT = 14).[35] A small nonrandomized clinical trial demonstrated that the use of enbucrilate tissue adhesive results in less postoperative pain and similar cosmetic outcomes compared with subcuticular sutures.[38]

4. Repair of third- and fourth-degree lacerations
Limited data are available to recommend one method of repair over another for third- and fourth-degree lacerations; it is our opinion that careful attention to the visualization of anatomic structures, the principles of sterile technique, hemostasis, adequate exposure, and gentle handling of tissue will result in better patient outcomes.[39] Several retrospective studies have looked at the outcome of primary repair in terms of reported anal incontinence symptoms, anal manometry, and endoanal ultrasound, although the method of repair is rarely detailed.[40-43] Although anal sphincter defects on endoanal ultrasound in women with a history of a sphincter laceration are clearly associated with anal incontinence symptoms, most women with anatomic defect on endoanal ultrasound did not have symptoms.[42,44] A thorough inspection of the full extent of the wound is necessary. Identifying the apex of the rectal mucosal tear and the often-retracted ends of

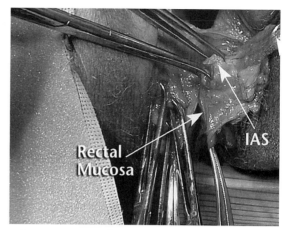

FIGURE 18-16. Rectal mucosa and internal anal sphincter (IAS) (see Color Plates).

the EAS and IAS (Figure 18-16) is essential to reapproximate the anatomy. A Gelpi retractor (see Figure 18-14) may be helpful in providing exposure, or additional assistance should be obtained to provide necessary exposure. Irrigation of the area with warm saline, redraping and regloving, and the use of antibiotics for surgical prophylaxis may potentially reduce the incidence of complications of tissue breakdown and secondary infection with accompanying breakdown of the repair.

a. Rectal mucosa repair: The rectal mucosa is repaired with continuous suture of 4–0 chromic, or polyglycolic acid on a tapered needle is started at the apex of the mucosal incision. The suture is placed in a manner that imbricates or inverts the rectal mucosa. The sutures should be placed to avoid passing the needle into the bowel lumen. Traditional recommendations have emphasized that sutures should not penetrate the complete thickness of the mucosa into the anal canal, to avoid promoting fistula formation.

Some operators find it helpful to place a double-gloved little finger of the nondominant hand into the rectum to assist in providing optimal exposure while performing this phase of the repair, although care must be used to avoid needlestick injury. The sutures are continued to the anal verge. Once at the anal verge, the clinician can place a suture back inside the repair and tie the suture off to itself to avoid tying the knot on the anal skin.

b. IAS repair
   i. After closing the rectal lumen the surgeon should reirrigate the wound.
   ii. The IAS is identified as a glistening, white fibrous structure between the rectal mucosa and EAS. This is a structure that often is not mentioned in obstetric textbooks. A postpartum defect in the IAS on endoanal ultrasound is associated with anal incontinence symptoms supporting the need to attempt to repair the IAS.[44] It is often retracted laterally, and placement of Allis clamps is useful because identification may be difficult.
   iii. Interrupted or running sutures of 2–0 polyglactin are used to reapproximate the IAS. This step previously was referred to as the second imbricating suture layer over the rectal mucosa.
   iv. Because of the association of a persistent postpartum defect in the IAS with anal incontinence, it is hoped that the identification and repair of the IAS will improve functional outcomes after anal sphincter complex repair; however, studies are needed to assess this.

c. EAS repair
   i. End to end versus overlap technique: The overlap technique of repair for third- and fourth-degree tears was initially described with a separate repair of the internal sphincter. In the original description, women whose tears were repaired using the end-to-end technique were compared with historical control patients, and there was a reduction in anal incontinence from 41% to 8% in the overlap group.[45]

   In an RCT comparing end-to-end and overlap technique, no significant differences in continence symptoms, anorectal manometry, or ultrasound appearance of the sphincter were identified at 3-month follow-up. In this RCT (N = 112), both groups were repaired with long-acting suture material.[17] However, the IAS was not repaired. A small study (n = 64) that included use of PDS suture and repair of the IAS demonstrated a greater incidence of anal incontinence (24% vs. 0%;

$p = .009$; RR, 0.07; 95% CI, 0.00-1.21) and fecal urgency (32% vs. 3.7%; $p = .02$; RR, 0.12; 95% CI, 0.02-0.86) in the end-to-end repair group than in the overlapping repair group. A Cochrane review of three studies concluded that the evidence was insufficient to recommend one type of repair without further research.[46,47] There are no completed Cochrane systematic reviews on the method of repair for external rectal sphincter. Studies of secondary sphincter repair for anal incontinence remote from delivery showed a significant increase in continence rate with overlap repair.[48,49] However, one study showed a deterioration of anal incontinence 5 years after secondary repair.[50]

   ii. Type of suture: No Cochrane reviews or RCTs to assess the best suture material for repair of the rectal sphincter were identified. However, monofilament suture material such as PDS or polyglyconate (Maxon) appears to be better than chromic catgut or braided polyglactin (Vicryl) in the repair of the anal sphincter because of a longer half-life and lower likelihood of infection.[30,45] Use of fine sutures (such as 3–0) may cause less irritation and discomfort.[30] Knot migration over time is a potential complication of using long-acting absorbable suture.[30]

   iii. End-to-end repair (Figure 18-17)
      (a) The ends of the EAS often retract laterally and must be clearly identified as facilitated by adequate lighting, visualization, and anesthesia. The muscle and its capsule can be grasped and brought anteriorly and medially using Allis clamps.
      (b) The EAS may be repaired in the end-to-end fashion that is traditional to obstetric repair or in the overlapping technique used by colorectal surgeons for sphincteroplasty.
      (c) The sphincter is reapproximated using four carefully placed 2–0 or 3–0 PDS sutures on a CT-1 needle. Figure-of-eight sutures are not recommended because of the theoretic risk for tissue strangulation with resultant devascularization and poor healing.[3]

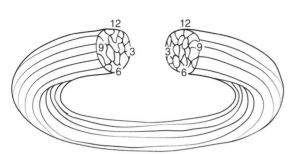

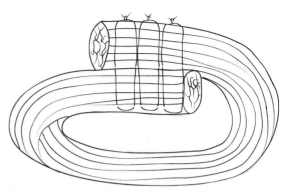

FIGURE 18-17. PISA (posterior, inferior, superior, and anterior poles) or "clock repair."

FIGURE 18-18. Overlapping repair of perineal laceration or episiotomy.

(d) For end-to-end repair, the severed ends of the sphincter muscle and its capsule should be oriented to identify the posterior, inferior, superior, and anterior poles (mnemonic: PISA). For the sake of description of this repair, these represent the position of these poles to the surgeon and are not the anatomic descriptions relative to the patient. The first suture should be placed at the quadrant most posterior (to the operator) portion of the sphincter (3 o'clock position), the second suture should be placed in the inferior quadrant (nearest to the rectal mucosa; 6 o'clock position), the third suture is then superior (closest to the hymen; 12 o'clock position), and the fourth suture is anterior (just underlying to the skin; 9 o'clock position). Follow the order of placement of these sutures to get all four positions approximated and not to close access for the repair by placing a suture in front of or superior to the other positions before these are completed, to prevent the surgeon from "painting herself or himself into anatomic corner."

iv. Overlapping repair (Figure 18-18)
   (a) The overlapping repair uses mattress suture to bring together the ends of the sphincter.
   (b) Dissection with Metzenbaum scissors may be required to have adequate length to overlap the muscles.
   (c) The suture is passed from top to bottom through the superior and inferior flaps and then bottom to top back through the inferior and superior flaps.
   (d) A straight (Keith) needle may make this repair easier for the surgeon.
   (e) Two additional sutures are placed in a similar fashion, and after all three are in place they are each tied with the knots on top of the overlapped sphincter ends.
   (f) The overlapping technique may potentially result in improved healing because of the larger surface area of tissue contact, although results from studies currently are mixed.[11,17,45,46]

v. Repair of skin overlying the anal sphincter complex: Once anal sphincter repair is complete it may be helpful to start the subcuticular skin repair slightly beyond the anopectineal line to the perineum before starting the second-degree or vaginal/perineal portion of the repair. This may help in preventing a buttonhole defect and make it easier to close the skin in this area rather than waiting until later in the repair.

5. Lacerations of the vulva and anterior vaginal wall
Anterior vaginal wall lacerations are more common with restrictive use of episiotomies.[3,6] The urethra, bladder, and clitoris can all be involved with resulting hemorrhage or fistula formation, or both. The

placement of a Foley catheter can aid in distinguishing the urethra from the surrounding structures. Suturing of periurethral, periclitoral, and labial laceration may only be required generally for deep wounds or for hemostasis, although bilateral labial lacerations do have the potential for labial fusion.[51]

VIII. POSTPARTUM CARE

A. Antibiotics
Perioperative broad-spectrum antibiotics are commonly recommended for surgical prophylaxis because of the contaminated nature of the repair. Development of infection increases the likelihood of dehiscence of the anal sphincter repair with increased risk for anal incontinence and fistula formation. A Cochrane review found inadequate evidence to recommend for or against the use of prophylactic antibiotic for anal sphincter complex obstetric repairs. If antibiotics are used, inclusion of drugs that cover anaerobic bacteria from fecal contamination is recommended.[30] A second-generation cephalosporin with anaerobic coverage (e.g., cefoxitin) and combining a first-generation cephalosporin with either clindamycin or metronidazole are potential options.

B. Comfort Measures
Ice packs are used initially in postpartum care, followed by local heat and anesthetic sprays. Ibuprofen, sitz baths, therapeutic ultrasound, and oral narcotics have demonstrated effectiveness in reducing postrepair pain and discomfort.[52,53]

Laxatives are recommended during the postoperative period to prevent disruption of the repair by straining or hard stool. Use of a stool softener such as lactulose and a bulking agent such as psyllium is recommended for 2 weeks.[30] No medications are administered rectally, including enemas, suppositories, and stool softeners.

IX. CHART DOCUMENTATION

Chart documentation is important, and it is highly recommended to dictate the repair of third- and fourth-degree lacerations as a formal operative report including the specific procedure and sutures used.[54] In a recent review of 50 cases, only 30% of the charts surveyed reported any method of external sphincter repair, and only 20% documented a rectal examination.[54]

X. CODING THE PROCEDURE

A. Procedure Codes (Current Procedural Terminology)
1. 59400 Vaginal delivery including repair
2. 59300 Laceration repair by provider other than attending

B. Diagnosis Codes (International Classification of Disease Ninth Revision)
1. 664.0_ First degree perineal laceration
2. 664.1_ Second degree perineal laceration
3. 664.2_ Third degree perineal laceration
4. 664.3_ Fourth degree perineal laceration
5. Add fifth digit: 0 = "unspecified," 1 = delivered without complication, 2= postpartum complication

The International Classification of Disease Ninth Revision requires all five digits for a complete code. These codes apply to the 2005 Current Procedural Terminology codes.

XI. POSTPARTUM FOLLOW-UP

Perineal infection is an uncommon complication. Superficial infection is characterized by local erythema, edema, exudate, and tenderness. Management includes opening the perineal wound and debridement of the infected tissue, which can then heal by secondary intention. Physicians need to consider necrotizing fasciitis and obtain surgical consultation for this life-threatening condition. The use of stool softeners is recommended to decrease the possibility for breakdown of the repair secondary to passage of hard stool and to decrease pain with defecation.[30,55]

A. Postpartum Anal Incontinence
Routine postpartum care must include careful assessment of all women with anal sphincter lacerations to determine the anatomic integrity of the repair and presence of anal incontinence symptoms. Decreased rectal tone, an attenuated perineal body, or a rectovaginal fistula may be found on examination. Patients with a third- or fourth-degree laceration repair initially may experience a sensation of tearing or pulling with bowel movements. About 20% to 50% of women will experience at least episodic incontinence of stool or flatus, which may be caused by disruption of the sphincters or their innrevation.[13,42]

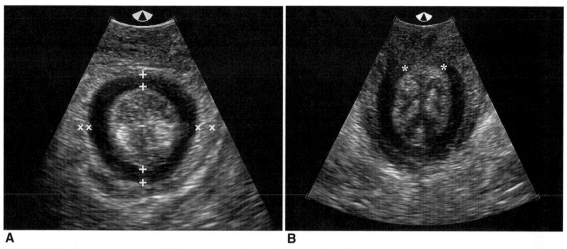

A   **B**

FIGURE 18-19. Endoanal ultrasound. **A,** Intact internal (+) and external (x) sphincters. **B,** Disruption of the internal anal sphincter at 12 o'clock position *(asterisk).*

1. Rectovaginal fistulas

   Rectovaginal fistulas are uncommon and may present with passage of stool or flatus per vagina, but some degree of decreased rectal tone may still occur with an appropriate repair of the sphincter.

2. Anal incontinence

   Patients with anal incontinence symptoms at 6 weeks should be offered the option of consultation with a urogynecologist or colorectal surgeon who may perform endoanal ultrasound to assess the IAS and EAS (Figure 18-19).

XII. SOR A RECOMMENDATIONS

RECOMMENDATIONS	REFERENCES
Vacuum-assisted vaginal delivery results in a lower incidence of anal sphincter laceration than forceps delivery.	*20, 21, 56*
Synthetic absorbable suture should be used for repair of vaginal mucosa and perineal muscles rather than chromic catgut because of a lower incidence of postpartum pain.	*34, 57*
Continuous subcuticular closure of the perineal skin results in less pain and need for suture removal compared with interrupted transcutaneous sutures and should be used when the perineal skin is sutured.	*35*

REFERENCES

1. Ould F: *A treatise of midwifery,* London, 1741, J. Buckland.
2. DeLee JB: The prophylactice forceps operation, *Am J Obstet Gynecol* 1:34-44, 1920.
3. Carroli G, Belizan J: Episiotomy for vaginal birth, *Cochrane Database Syst Rev* (2):CD000081, 200.
4. Bodner-Adler B, Bodner K, Kaider A et al: Risk factors for third-degree perineal tears in vaginal delivery, with an analysis of episiotomy types, *J Reprod Med* 46:752-756, 2001.
5. Donnelly V, Fynes M, Campbell D et al: Obstetric events leading to anal sphincter damage, *Obstet Gynecol* 92:955-961, 1998.
6. Klein MC, Gauthier RJ, Robbins JM et al: Relationship of episiotomy to perineal trauma and morbidity, sexual dysfunction, and pelvic floor relaxation, *Am J Obstet Gynecol* 171:591-598, 1994.
7. Renfrew MJ, Hannah W, Albers L et al: Practices that minimize trauma to the genital tract in childbirth: a systematic review of the literature, *Birth* 25:143-160, 1998.
8. Riskin-Mashiah S, O'Brian Smith E, Wilkins IA: Risk factors for severe perineal tear: can we do better? *Am J Perinatol* 19:225-234, 2002.
9. Hartmann K, Viswanathan M, Palmieri R et al: Outcomes of routine episiotomy: a systematic review, *JAMA* 293:2141-2148, 2005.
10. Kozak LJ, Owings MF, Hall MJ: National Hospital Discharge Survey: 2001 annual summary with detailed diagnosis and procedure data, *Vital Health Stat* 13:1-198, 2004.
11. Garcia V, Rogers RG, Kim SS et al: Primary repair of obstetric anal sphincter laceration: a randomized trial of two surgical techniques, *Am J Obstet Gynecol* 192:1697-1701, 2005.
12. Eason E, Labrecque M, Marcoux S et al: Anal incontinence after childbirth, *CMAJ* 166:326-330, 2002.
13. Handa VL, Danielsen BH, Gilbert WM: Obstetric anal sphincter lacerations, *Obstet Gynecol* 98:225-230, 2001.
14. Sultan AH, Kamm MA, Hudson CN et al: Anal-sphincter disruption during vaginal delivery, *N Engl J Med* 329:1905-1911, 1993.

15. Zetterstrom J, Lopez A, Anzen B et al: Anal sphincter tears at vaginal delivery: risk factors and clinical outcome of primary repair, *Obstet Gynecol* 94:21-28, 1999.

16. Fenner DE, Genberg B, Brahma P et al: Fecal and urinary incontinence after vaginal delivery with anal sphincter disruption in an obstetrics unit in the United States, *Am J Obstet Gynecol* 189:1543-1550, 2003.

17. Fitzpatrick M, Behan M, O'Connell PR et al: A randomized clinical trial comparing primary overlap with approximation repair of third-degree obstetric tears, *Am J Obstet Gynecol* 183:1220-1224, 2000.

18. Pollack J, Nordenstam J, Brismar S et al: Anal incontinence after vaginal delivery: a five-year prospective cohort study, *Obstet Gynecol* 104:1397-1402, 2004.

19. Power D, Fitzpatrick M, O'Herlihy C: Obstetric anal sphincter injury: how to avoid, how to repair: a literature review, *J Fam Pract* 55:193-200, 2006.

20. Bofill JA, Rust OA, Schorr SJ, et al. A randomized prospective trial of the obstetric forceps versus the M-cup vacuum extractor, *Am J Obstet Gynecol* 175:1325-1330, 1996.

21. Eason E, Labrecque M, Wells G et al: Preventing perineal trauma during childbirth: a systematic review, *Obstet Gynecol* 95:464-471, 2000.

22. Faltin DL, Boulvain M, Irion O et al: Diagnosis of anal sphincter tears by postpartum endosonography to predict fecal incontinence, *Obstet Gynecol* 95:643-647, 2000.

23. Andrews V, Sultan AH, Thakar R et al: Occult anal sphincter injuries: myth or reality? *BJOG* 113:195-200, 2006.

24. Sultan AH, Kamm MA, Hudson CH: Obstetric perineal trauma: an audit of training, *J Obstet Gynaecol* 15:19-23, 1995.

25. Woodman PJ, Graney DO: Anatomy and physiology of the female perineal body with relevance to obstetrical injury and repair, *Clin Anat* 15:321-334, 2002.

26. Deering SH, Carlson N, Stitely M et al: Perineal body length and lacerations at delivery, *J Reprod Med* 49:306-310, 2004.

27. Goldberg J, Hyslop T, Tolosa JE et al: Racial differences in severe perineal lacerations after vaginal delivery, *Am J Obstet Gynecol* 188:1063-1067, 2003.

28. American College of Obstetricians and Gynecologists. Episiotomy. ACOG Practice Bulletin No. 71, *Obstet Gynecol* 107:957-962, 2006.

29. Coats PM, Chan KK, Wilkins M et al: A comparison between midline and mediolateral episiotomies, *Br J Obstet Gynaecol* 87:408-412, 1980.

30. Royal College of Obstetricians and Gynaecologists: Management of third- and fourth-degree perineal tears following vaginal delivery. Available at: http://www.rcog.org.uk/resources/Public/pdf/green_top29_management_third.pdf. Accessed October 12, 2001.

31. Youssef R, Ramalingam U, Macleod M et al: Cohort study of maternal and neonatal morbidity in relation to use of episiotomy at instrumental vaginal delivery, *BJOG* 112:941-945, 2005.

32. Leeman L, Spearman M, Rogers R: Repair of obstetric perineal lacerations, *Am Fam Physician* 68:1585-1590, 2003.

33. Fleming VE, Hagen S, Niven C: Does perineal suturing make a difference? The SUNS trial, *BJOG* 110:684-689, 2003.

33a. Leeman LM, Roger RG, Greulich B et al: Do unsutured second-degree perineal lacerations affect postpartum functional outcomes? *J Am Board Fam Med* 20(5):451-457, 2007.

34. Kettle C, Johanson RB: Absorbable synthetic versus catgut suture material for perineal repair, *Cochrane Database Syst Rev* (2):CD000006, 2000.

35. Kettle C, Johanson RB: Continuous versus interrupted sutures for perineal repair, *Cochrane Database Syst Rev* (2):CD000947, 2000.

36. Oboro VO, Tabowei TO, Loto OM et al: A multicentre evaluation of the two-layered repair of postpartum perineal trauma, *J Obstet Gynaecol* 23:5-8, 2003.

37. Gordon B, Mackrodt C, Fern E et al: The Ipswich Childbirth Study: 1. A randomised evaluation of two stage postpartum perineal repair leaving the skin unsutured, *Br J Obstet Gynaecol* 105:435-440, 1998.

38. Bowen ML, Selinger M: Episiotomy closure comparing enbucrilate tissue adhesive with conventional sutures, *Int J Gynaecol Obstet* 78:201-205, 2002.

39. McLennan MT, Melick CF, Clancy SL et al: Episiotomy and perineal repair. An evaluation of resident education and experience, *J Reprod Med* 47:1025-1030, 2002.

40. Gjessing H, Backe B, Sahlin Y: Third degree obstetric tears; outcome after primary repair, *Acta Obstet Gynecol Scand* 77:736-740, 1998.

41. Poen AC, Felt-Bersma RJ, Strijers RL et al: Third-degree obstetric perineal tear: long-term clinical and functional results after primary repair, *Br J Surg* 85:1433-1438, 1998.

42. Sultan AH, Kamm MA, Hudson CN et al: Third degree obstetric anal sphincter tears: risk factors and outcome of primary repair, *BMJ* 308:887-891, 1994.

43. Wood J, Amos L, Rieger N: Third degree anal sphincter tears: risk factors and outcome, *Aust N Z J Obstet Gynaecol* 38: 414-417, 1998.

44. Kammerer-Doak DN, Wesol AB, Rogers RG et al: A prospective cohort study of women after primary repair of obstetric anal sphincter laceration, *Am J Obstet Gynecol* 181:1317-1323, 1999.

45. Sultan AH, Monga AK, Kumar D et al: Primary repair of obstetric anal sphincter rupture using the overlap technique, *Br J Obstet Gynaecol* 106:318-323, 1999.

46. Fernando RJ, Sultan AH, Kettle C et al: Repair techniques for obstetric anal sphincter injuries, *Obstet Gynecol* 107:1261-1268, 2006.

47. Fernando R, Sultan AH, Kettle C et al: Methods of repair for obstetric anal sphincter injury. *Cochrane Database of Systematic Reviews* (3). Art. No.: CD002866. DOI: 10.1002/14651858. CD002866.pub2, 2006.

48. Londono-Schimmer EE, Garcia-Duperly R, Nicholls RJ et al: Overlapping anal sphincter repair for faecal incontinence due to sphincter trauma: five year follow-up functional results, *Int J Colorectal Dis* 9:110-113, 1994.

49. Norderval S, Oian P, Revhaug A et al: Anal incontinence after obstetric sphincter tears: outcome of anatomic primary repairs, *Dis Colon Rectum* 48:1055-1061, 2005.

50. Malouf AJ, Norton CS, Engel AF et al: Long-tern results of overlapping anterior anal-sphincter repair for obstetric trauma, *Lancet* 355:260-265, 2000.

51. Arkin AE, Chern-Hughes B: Case report: labial fusion postpartum and clinical management of labial lacerations, *J Midwifery Womens Health* 47:290-292, 2002.

52. Kymplova J, Navratil L, Knizek J: Contribution of phototherapy to the treatment of episiotomies, *J Clin Laser Med Surg* 21:35-39, 2003.

53. Peter EA, Janssen PA, Grange CS et al: Ibuprofen versus acetaminophen with codeine for the relief of perineal pain after childbirth: a randomized controlled trial, *CMAJ* 165:1203-1209, 2001.

54. Nichols CM, Lahaye L, Hullfish K: Chart documentation of surgical methods for severe perineal laceration repair, *J Pelvic Med Surg* 11:39-43, 2005.
55. Mahony R, Behan M, O'Herlihy C et al: Randomized, clinical trial of bowel confinement vs. laxative use after primary repair of a third-degree obstetric anal sphincter tear, *Dis Colon Rectum* 47:12-17, 2004.
56. Johanson RB, Menon BK: Vacuum extraction versus forceps for assisted vaginal delivery, *Cochrane Database Syst Rev* (2): CD000224, 2000.
57. Kettle C, Hills RK, Jones P et al: Continuous versus interrupted perineal repair with standard or rapidly absorbed sutures after spontaneous vaginal birth: a randomised controlled trial, *Lancet* 359:2217-2223, 2002.

S E C T I O N   F   Amniocentesis during the Third Trimester of Pregnancy

Mark Deutchman, MD

Amniocentesis is an important procedure in the third trimester of pregnancy when amniotic fluid sampling is necessary to determine fetal lung maturity, diagnose chorioamnionitis, or follow the course of pregnancies affected by Rh isoimmunization. This section includes a discussion of the indications for amniocentesis, technique for performing this procedure, and interpretation of results of amniotic fluid analysis. The indications and interpretation of genetic amniocentesis are not included in this section because this testing is performed in the first or second trimester, although the technique is substantially the same.

I. INDICATIONS FOR THIRD-TRIMESTER AMNIOCENTESIS

A. Assessing Fetal Lung Maturity

Amniocentesis is done to obtain amniotic fluid for lung maturity testing in any of the following situations:

1. Before repeat cesarean delivery, if fetal lung maturity is in doubt
2. In the case of preterm labor, to aid in the decision of whether to initiate tocolysis
3. For patients in labor with unresolved gestational age by history, physical examination, and ultrasound fetal biometry

4. As an aid to deciding when to stop tocolysis in women being treated for premature labor

B. Suspected Chorioamnionitis

Amniocentesis may be performed to obtain amniotic fluid for white blood cell count, Gram's stain and culture, or rapid tests for infection described later in Section IV. The clinical setting in which this testing is most common is preterm premature rupture of membranes. In preterm labor without ruptured membranes, routine amniocentesis to assess for infection has not been shown to improve perinatal outcomes.[1]

C. Rh Isoimmunization

In Rh-isoimmunized pregnancies, serial amniocentesis procedures may be performed to diagnose and evaluate the degree of fetal hemolysis, as represented by increasing amniotic fluid bilirubin levels.

II. LUNG MATURITY TESTING METHODS AND INTERPRETATION

Several tests may be performed on amniotic fluid samples to assess fetal lung maturity. All of the tests described are much better at predicting the absence of respiratory distress than predicting that the infant will have respiratory distress syndrome.[2] Each of these tests measures either phospholipid pulmonary surfactants or the effects of surfactants. The choice of test will often be based on which is available in a particular clinical setting.

A. Lecithin/Sphingomyelin Ratio

The lecithin/sphingomyelin (L:S) ratio is the traditional standard for fetal lung maturity testing. A ratio of greater than 2:1 is 98% predictive of fetal lung maturity. Falsely mature values can be obtained in mothers with diabetes (classes A through C), asphyxiated infants, or in cases of Rh isoimmunization.[3] Because this test is performed by thin-layer chromatography, it is cumbersome and time-consuming. It is therefore commonly replaced by one of the tests described in the following sections.

B. Phosphatidyl Glycerol

The presence of phosphatidyl glycerol in excess of 3% (i.e., a positive test) indicates functional lung maturity and is a more reliable predictor of lung maturity than the L:S ratio in clinical situations in which the L:S may be falsely mature, such as maternal diabetes. The appearance of phosphatidyl glycerol is also accelerated in clinical situations associated with fetal stress, such as maternal hypertension and premature rupture of the membranes.[3] Testing for phosphatidyl glycerol is performed by thin-layer chromatography or by a slide agglutination test using antisera. This test is not affected by blood, meconium, or vaginal secretions.

C. Fetal Lung Maturity

Fetal lung maturity (Abbott Laboratories, Irving, TX) is a test for total surfactant relative to albumin in amniotic fluid using fluorescent polarization technology. A value of 70 or greater is considered mature.

D. Foam Stability Index

Foam stability index (Beckman Instruments, Fullerton, CA) is a test kit that measures the effects of total surfactants. Amniotic fluid is added to wells in a cassette that contains varying preloaded volumes and concentrations of ethanol. The entire cassette is shaken vigorously for 30 seconds and observed after an additional 60 seconds. The end point is the observation of stable bubbles in the wells of varying ethanol/amniotic fluid concentrations. Stable bubbles in the well labeled "47" or greater indicate lung maturity. The presence of blood or meconium interferes with this test. Silicone from collection tubes causes a falsely mature result.

E. The Tap Test

The tap test is a bedside test in which 1 ml amniotic fluid is mixed with 1 drop of 6 N hydrochloric acid and 1.5 ml diethyl ether. The tube containing this mixture is tapped 3 or 4 times, creating 200 to 300 bubbles in the ether layer. Fluid from a mature fetus causes the bubbles to break down rapidly. If no more than five bubbles persist in the ether layer after 10 minutes, the result is considered mature.[4] More rapid disappearance of bubbles provides more assurance of lung maturity.[5]

F. Turbidity of Amniotic Fluid

Turbidity of amniotic fluid is a potent indicator of fetal lung maturity. If a tube of amniotic fluid is turbid enough to prevent the reading of newsprint through it, fetal lung maturity is predicted with 97% certainty.[5] This test is fast, simple, and inexpensive, and should be considered the primary rapid screening test.

G. Optical Density

The optical density of amniotic fluid at 650 nm is a useful test for amniotic fluid that is contaminated by blood, but not by meconium. Optical density values 0.15 or more predict maturity and agree well with L:S ratio testing.[5]

H. Lamellar Body Counts

Surfactant extruded from fetal pneumocytes is present in "packages" about the same size as platelets. The presence of these structures in quantities of at least $32,000/\mu l$ is 99% predictive of fetal lung maturity, with a negative predictive value of 63%.[6] The advantage of this test is that it can be performed rapidly on uncentrifuged amniotic fluid with a standard hematology analyzer. Bloody fluid will reduce the density of lamellar bodies.

I. Causes of False-Positive Results

Both blood and meconium can cause falsely mature results for the fetal lung maturity test, foam stability index, and tap test.[7] An assay for phosphatidyl glycerol should be reliable even in the face of meconium and bloody fluid.[2,8]

J. Testing from Vaginal Pool Specimens

Testing on an amniotic fluid sample obtained from the vaginal pool after spontaneous rupture of membranes must be interpreted with caution. Some studies have found testing for phosphatidyl glycerol testing to be more reliable than L:S testing, but others have found that certain vaginal bacteria can create false-positive results.[5] Because they are surfactants, soaps and detergents should be carefully excluded from any amniotic fluid sample being tested for fetal lung maturity.

K. Use of Multiple Tests

Commonly available tests are so strongly predictive of lung maturity that testing by multiple methods is not recommended if the result of a first test is "positive."[2]

III. DIAGNOSIS OF CHORIOAMNIONITIS IN PRETERM PREMATURE RUPTURE OF MEMBRANES

Only 1% to 2% of women who present with preterm premature rupture of membranes have traditional clinical signs of chorioamnionitis, but 25% to 40% will have a positive culture when amniocentesis is performed on initial presentation.[9] Because a positive amniotic fluid culture may take several days, a more rapid test is desirable. Table 18-1 shows the amniotic fluid tests used to help diagnose chorioamnionitis

TABLE 18-1 **Amniotic Fluid Tests Correlation with Positive Amniotic Fluid Culture**

Test	Sensitivity (%)	Specificity (%)	PPV (%)	NPV (%)
Gram's stain	24	99	91	68
Amniotic fluid WBC (>30/mm³)	57	78	—	—
Leukocyte esterase	19	87	42	68
Glucose (<10 mg/dl)	57	74	57	74
Interleukin-6	81	75	67	86
Glucose, amniotic fluid WBC, and Gram's stain	76	60	61	80

Adapted from Strassner HT Jr, Golde SH, Mosley GH et al: Effect of blood in amniotic fluid on the detection of phosphatidylglycerol, *Am J Obstet Gynecol* 138:697-701, 1980.
PPV, Positive predictive value; NPV, negative predictive value; WBC, white blood cell count.

and their sensitivities, specificities, and positive and negative predictive values. A combination of Gram's stain, white blood cell count, and glucose offers the greatest clinical value.

A. Gram's Stain

The presence of any organisms seen on a Gram's stain of unspun amniotic fluid obtained by amniocentesis indicates an abnormal finding.[10] If fluid is obtained by aspiration through an IUPC, the first 10 ml of this fluid should be discarded to avoid contamination.[11]

B. Amniotic Fluid White Blood Cell Count

The abnormal threshold of the amniotic fluid white blood cell count test is 30/mm³.

C. Rapid Test for Leukocyte Esterase

A positive rapid test for leukocyte esterase suggests infection.

D. Amniotic Fluid Glucose

The abnormal threshold for the amniotic fluid glucose test is 10 mg/dl.

IV. AMNIOTIC FLUID BILIRUBIN IN THE Rh-ISOIMMUNIZED PREGNANCY

Bilirubin levels are indirectly assessed by measuring the optical density of amniotic fluid at 450 nm. The value obtained is plotted against gestational age on a Liley graph or a Queenan graph; these are available in standard obstetric textbooks. The absolute value and trend over time determines management, which may include continued surveillance, intrauterine transfusion, or delivery.

V. ULTRASOUND EXAMINATION BEFORE THE PROCEDURE

Before a patient undergoes an amniocentesis, she should have an ultrasound evaluation with particular attention paid to assessment of fluid volume, location of fluid pockets, fetal presentation, and placental location. It is desirable, but not absolutely essential, to avoid the placenta. The main contraindication to amniocentesis is severe oligohydramnios. Unless a prior ultrasound has been performed to rule out fetal anomalies and establish accurate dating, an ultrasound should be obtained before amniocentesis because the finding of anomalies or readjustment of dating may alter the clinical diagnosis and management plan.

VI. THE AMNIOCENTESIS PROCEDURE

The amniocentesis procedure is detailed in the following sections.[12,13]

A. Informed Consent

Written informed consent should be obtained, making sure that the patient understands the reason for the procedure, diagnostic alternatives, and risks.

B. Identifying a Fluid Pocket

Ultrasound is used to locate an accessible pocket of fluid. Ideally, a pocket away from the fetal face and free of umbilical cord should be chosen. In cases of oligohydramnios or a large anterior placenta, the examiner may lift the fetal head, creating a pocket of fluid in the lower uterine segment appropriate for amniocentesis. The maternal bladder should be empty. This suprapubic technique carries an increased risk for rupture of the membranes. The transplacental route for amniocentesis is less desirable but not absolutely contraindicated if no other appropriate site is available.

C. Use of Anesthesia/ Local Preparation

Local anesthesia with 1% lidocaine may be used to anesthetize the skin. Some operators believe that because this is a "one-stick" procedure, local anesthesia is not necessary. This option should be discussed with the patient. After an appropriate site is selected, the skin is prepped in a sterile fashion. Making a "dent" in the skin with the hub of a needle or other round object can help keep the operator from losing the operative site during the prep.

D. Preparation for the Amniocentesis

The anticipated depth of insertion of the needle is measured sonographically. A 3.5-inch, 21-gauge spinal needle is commonly used, but a 1.5-inch needle may be sufficient in thin patients. Needles, syringes, and collection tubes are assembled on a sterile drape, and the operator should wear sterile gloves. The ultrasound transducer may be covered with a sterile glove or drape. If ultrasound coupling gel is used, it should be sterile. However, antiseptic soaps, such as povidone iodine and chlorhexidine, work well as ultrasound conductive media during the procedure.

E. Steps of the Amniocentesis Procedure

1. Technique

   The operator holds the needle in one hand and the ultrasound transducer in the other hand, continuously observing the progress of the needle through the maternal tissues into the target pocket of amniotic fluid (Figure 18-20). The transducer is held a few centimeters away from the tap site, often under the sterile drape. Alternatively, an experienced assistant may hold the ultrasound transducer. If the transducer is not covered by a sterile drape or glove, it should not contact the needle.

2. Aspiration of amniotic fluid

   The stylet is removed from the needle, and if amniotic fluid is seen to appear in the hub, a short piece of flexible tubing is attached and a 20- to 30-ml syringe is used to aspirate fluid. If the operator

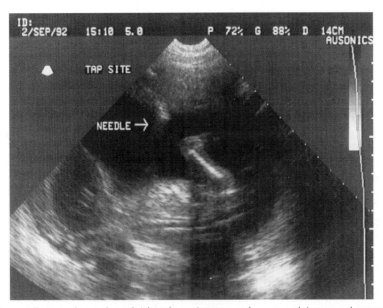

FIGURE 18-20. The needle tip is observed as a bright echo as it traverses the maternal tissues and enters the amniotic fluid.

is holding both the needle and the transducer, an assistant can connect the tubing and aspirate the fluid. If no fluid comes back, the needle is repositioned, usually slightly deeper. If the needle tip is seen to be within fluid but there is no fluid return, the membranes may be tented over the tip. This can be alleviated either by rotating the needle, which causes the bevel of the needle to tear through the membranes, or by further advancing the needle under sonographic guidance. If blood-tinged fluid is obtained, the first few milliliters are discarded until clear fluid is obtained.

3. Postamniocentesis care

After an adequate sample is obtained, usually 10 to 30 ml, the needle is withdrawn. It is not unusual for the baby to "bump" the needle during the procedure, often resulting in a withdrawal response by the fetus.[14] If a large amount of fetal movement is noted while the preparation is being done, the patient should be rescanned before needle insertion to confirm the presence of the target pocket. Another site should be chosen if the pocket has disappeared. The amniotic fluid is placed in a sterile container and taken directly to the laboratory for analysis. It is strongly recommended that the laboratory be warned before the procedure that a sample is on the way. If a kit test is being used, the results can be available in a few minutes.

After amniocentesis, the tap site is inspected sonographically. "Streaming" of blood into the amniotic fluid is sometimes seen and usually stops promptly. If this continues, the pregnancy should be monitored closely. A period of maternal observation for uterine contractions is necessary, and nonstress testing should be considered.

4. Special considerations

If optical density testing is to be performed for assessment of bilirubin in Rh isoimmunization, the fluid should be shielded from light. Mothers who are Rh-negative, and who are not already sensitized, should receive $Rh_o(D)$ immunoglobulin after amniocentesis.

VII. RISKS OF AMNIOCENTESIS

Amniocentesis risks can be minimized by using simultaneous real-time sonographic guidance to avoid injury to maternal and fetal structures.[15] Most studies of amniocentesis risks deal with early second-trimester procedures performed for genetic testing, not the third-trimester applications discussed here. Many reports of fetal injury were made before sonographic monitoring was available. All risks listed below, for both mother and fetus, are rare in occurrence.

A. Maternal Risks

1. Perforation of intraabdominal organs with infection or bleeding
2. Amniotic fluid embolism
3. Rh isoimmunization

B. Fetal Risks

1. Initiation of labor
2. Amnionitis
3. Rupture of the membranes
4. Puncture of fetus or umbilical cord
5. Placental abruption

VIII. SOR A RECOMMENDATION

RECOMMENDATION	REFERENCE
Commonly available amniotic fluid tests of fetal lung maturity are so strongly predictive that testing by multiple methods is not recommended if the result of a first test is "positive."	2

REFERENCES

1. Agency for Healthcare Research and Quality (AHRQ): Management of preterm labor. Evidence Report/Technology Assessment No 18. AHRQ Publication No. 01-E021, Rockville, MD, 2000, AHRQ.
2. American College of Obstetricians and Gynecologists (ACOG): Assessment of fetal lung maturity. ACOG Educational Bulletin No. 230, November 1996, Washington, DC, 1996, American College of Obstetricians and Gynecologists.
3. Jobe A: Evaluation of fetal lung maturity. In Creasy R, Resnik R, editors: Maternal-fetal medicine: principles and practice, Philadelphia, 1989, WB Saunders.
4. Socol M: The tap test: confirmation of a simple, rapid, inexpensive, and reliable indicator of fetal pulmonary maturity, Am J Obstet Gynecol 162:218-222, 1990.
5. Field NT, Gilbert WM: Current status of amniotic fluid tests of fetal maturity, Clin Obstet Gynecol 40:366-386, 1997.
6. Lewis, PS, Lauria MR, Dzieczkowski J et al: Amniotic fluid lamellar body count: cost-effective screening for fetal lung maturity, Obstet Gynecol 93:387-391, 1999.
7. Keniston RC, Noland GL, Pernoll ML: The effect of blood, meconium and temperature on the rapid surfactant test, Obstet Gynecol 48:442-445, 1976.
8. Strassner HT Jr, Golde SH, Mosley GH et al: Effect of blood in amniotic fluid on the detection of phosphatidylglycerol, Am J Obstet Gynecol 138:697-701, 1980.

9. Canavan TP, Hyagriv NS, Caritis S: An evidence-based approach to the evaluation and treatment of premature rupture of membranes: part I, *Obstet Gynecol Surv* 59(8):669-677, 2004.

10. Gibbs RS, Blanco JD, St Clair PJ et al: Quantitative bacteriology of amniotic fluid from patients with clinic intra-amniotic infection at term, *J Infect Dis* 145:1-8, 1982.

11. Listwa HM, Sobel AS, Carpenter J, Gibbs RS: The predictability of intrauterine infection by analysis of amniotic fluid, *Obstet Gynecol* 48:31-33, 1976.

12. Bowman J: Technique of amniocentesis. In Creasy R, Resnik R, editors: *Maternal-fetal medicine: principles and practice*, Philadelphia, 1989, WB Saunders.

13. Goldberg JD, Norton ME: Genetics and prenatal diagnosis. In Callen PW, editor: *Ultrasonography in obstetrics and gynecology*, ed 4, Philadelphia, 2000, WB Saunders.

14. Petrikovsky MB, Kaplan GP: Fetal responses to inadvertent contact with the needle during amniocentesis, *Fetal Diagn Ther* 10:83-85, 1995.

15. Jeanty P, Rodesch F, Romero R et al: How to improve your amniocentesis technique, *Am J Obstet Gynecol* 146:593-596, 1983.

SECTION G   Cesarean Delivery

Mark Deutchman, MD, and Neil J. Murphy, MD

This section covers indications for cesarean delivery, perioperative patient care, and an overview of surgical technique. The actual techniques of cesarean delivery must be learned by practical, supervised experience. The ability to perform cesarean delivery as primary surgeon is part of the surgical skills of many family physicians, particularly those in rural areas. Every family physician should be able to function as a first assistant at surgery and should be prepared to perform perimortem cesarean delivery.

I. OVERVIEW AND INCIDENCE

The total cesarean delivery rate in the United States has been steadily increasing from 21% in 1996 to more than 29% in 2004.[1] The primary cesarean rate has increased from 15% to 20.6% during that same time period. Much of this change is due to the precipitous drop in vaginal delivery after previous cesarean from 28% to 9%, after a 1999 ACOG Practice Bulletin expressed concern about the possibility of catastrophic uterine rupture.[2] The bulletin stated that vaginal delivery after previous cesarean should be attempted only when surgical intervention is "immediately" available.[2] A discussion of the merits and dangers of VBAC is beyond the scope of this section but can be found in a report by the Agency for Healthcare Research and Quality[3] and a Cochrane review.[4]

A. Role of the Family Physician

Family physicians and midwives have established a positive record of lower than average cesarean delivery rates in several published outcome studies.[5-7] Family physicians who perform their own cesarean deliveries have reported excellent patient outcomes.[8,9] Clinicians can help assure their patients a reasonable chance of vagial delivery by using the following approaches[5,10-12]:

1. Encourage a trial of vaginal birth after previous cesarean section for properly selected patients in appropriate settings.
2. Adhere to the definition of active labor before admitting low-risk mothers to the hospital (see Chapter 14, Section A).
3. Interpret fetal heart rate tracings properly to avoid overdiagnosis of nonreassuring fetal heart rate patterns (see Chapter 16, Section A).
4. Use intrapartum amnioinfusion in appropriate situations (see Section C in this chapter).
5. Use epidural anesthesia judiciously.
6. Use oxytocin to judiciously augment labor but avoid hyperstimulation and resultant fetal intolerance of labor (see Chapter 15, Sections A and B).
7. Encourage patients to be informed about, and prepared for, their childbirth experience.
8. Establish "second opinion" or preoperative consultation guidelines within the hospital.

II. INDICATIONS FOR CESAREAN DELIVERY

A. Maternal Indications

1. Hemorrhage caused by placenta previa or placental abruption
2. Inability of mother to tolerate labor because of cardiac, pulmonary, or other medical disease
3. Contracted pelvis because of congenital deformity or old fracture
4. Previous reconstructive vaginal surgery, particularly vesicovaginal fistula
5. Pelvic tumors
6. Previous placement of a cerclage by the abdominal route

7. When previous surgery involved the active segment of the uterus as in cases of classical cesarean or myomectomy

8. Maternal desire to forgo a trial of labor after prior cesarean delivery

9. Perimortem, as a possible aid to maternal resuscitation when cardiopulmonary resuscitation has been in progress for more than 5 minutes[13]

10. Some mothers may simply request cesarean delivery.

A discussion of this topic is beyond the scope of this section but can be found in a National Institutes of Health report[14] and in a Cochrane review.[15]

B. Fetal Indications

1. Transverse lie, including shoulder presentation
2. Transverse arrest
3. Brow presentation
4. Face presentation with mentum posterior
5. Failed forceps delivery
6. Failed vacuum extraction if head too high for forceps
7. Truly arrested labor after trial of augmentation
8. Breech presentation of single pregnancy[16] or for breech second twin[17]
9. Nonreassuring fetal heart rate pattern, usually after intrauterine resuscitation efforts
10. Umbilical cord prolapse
11. Infant with very low birth weight (<1500 g)
12. Macrosomic infant, with consideration of the inaccuracy of sonographic estimation of fetal weight (see Section A)
13. Conjoined twins
14. Active maternal genital herpes simplex virus infection
15. Maternal thrombocytopenia
16. Uterine rupture, including abdominal trauma or rupture of previous cesarean delivery scar
17. Delivery of infant of an HIV-positive mother to decrease likelihood of transmission to the infant[18]
18. Perimortem for fetal salvage in case of mother undergoing cardiopulmonary resuscitation for more than 5 minutes[13]

III. TECHNIQUE AND OTHER SURGICAL ISSUES AND CHOICES

A. Preoperative Preparation

1. Make sure patient's prenatal record, including laboratory data, is available. Review preoperative hematocrit levels. Assess the patient's risk for complications and consider whether appropriate facilities and personnel are available.

2. If time permits, it is desirable to check mother's blood type and check for antibodies in case blood is required for transfusion. It is usually not necessary to crossmatch blood unless the likelihood of transfusion is high.

3. Volume-load normotensive patients who will receive epidural or spinal anesthesia with 1000 ml of LR solution or NS.

4. Administer nonparticulate antacid and/or H_2 blocker/metoclopramide in case of vomiting to minimize risk for pulmonary damage if aspiration occurs.

5. Establish whether the father or other support person will be present.

6. Identify family members who will be in the waiting area and, if possible, have them designate a spokesperson for communications.

7. Document in the chart the indications for the procedure and the discussion with the patient providing the basis for her informed consent. Risks to document include bleeding, infection, damage to maternal organs, hysterectomy, and death.

8. For mothers with low-to-moderate risk for bacterial endocarditis, antibiotic prophylaxis for subacute bacterial endocarditis is not recommended.[19]

B. Choice of Anesthesia

The types of anesthesia that can be used during cesarean delivery are[20,21]:

1. General anesthesia is typically used in life-threatening emergent cases such as cord prolapse, severe hemorrhage, or severe fetal distress.

2. Spinal or epidural anesthesia is used if time is not critical. This permits the mother to be awake and avoids passage of anesthetic agents to the infant across the placenta. Spinal anesthesia is easier to perform and has faster onset than epidural anesthesia but carries increased risk for hypotension because of peripheral vasodilatation. In either case, the patient should receive a fluid bolus (500-1000 ml of NS or LR solution) before anesthesia, and ephedrine should be available in case hypotension occurs (25-50 mg intramuscularly or 10 mg intravenously [IV]).

3. Technique of spinal anesthesia

    a. Perform a lumbar puncture at L4-5 or L3-4 interspace with mother in sitting or lateral decubitus position. A 21-gauge or smaller needle should be used to avoid a spinal headache caused by a leak from the tap site. Insert the needle with the bevel parallel to the long axis of the spine to make smaller hole in dura, along its fibers, rather than create a flap in the dura. A smaller needle (25-gauge) can be used through a larger, shorter needle inserted through the skin.

b. Mix 0.8 mg tetracaine, 0.2 ml of 1:1000 epinephrine, and 1 ml of 10% dextrose in a syringe. When cerebrospinal fluid flows from the needle hub, attach the syringe containing anesthetic mixture and draw a few drops of cerebrospinal fluid into it to demonstrate free flow. Inject over a period of a few seconds and immediately withdraw needle and place mother supine with uterus displaced to one side. While testing abdominal skin sensation, roll operating table to right, left, head up or down to control level of block.

c. An alternative medication for spinal anesthesia is bupivacaine 0.75% in 8% dextrose. Use 1.5 ml for women shorter than 5 feet 4 inches and 1.75 ml for those taller than 5 feet 4 inches tall.

d. Narcotics can be added to the spinal anesthetic for both short- and long-lasting postoperative analgesia. Useful agents are fentanyl 25 µg plus morphine injection (Duramorph) 0.2 to 0.3 ml. Some institutional protocols require continuous postoperative monitoring using pulse oximetry when intraspinal narcotics are used because of the possibility of maternal respiratory depression. The period of monitoring ranges from the duration of the spinal anesthesia to 24 hours.

4. Local anesthesia may be used as a primary technique or to augment an incomplete spinal or epidural block. After the infant has been delivered, general anesthesia can be induced or sedation can be added.

C. Instruments Used during Cesarean Delivery

1. Scalpel to open skin and deeper layers
2. Electrocautery pencil, set to "coagulation" current to control bleeding
3. Electrocautery pencil, set to "cutting" current to open subcutaneous tissue and fascia
4. Scissors (curved Mayo or Metzenbaum) to open fascia and peritoneum
5. Hemostats to clamp bleeding vessels before electrocoagulation or ligature
6. Kocher or Ochsner clamps to hold fascia

7. Bladder retractor
8. Richardson retractors for abdominal wall
9. Thumb forceps (Russian or Bonney) to elevate peritoneum and bladder reflection as these tissues are handled
10. Smooth thumb forceps to handle peritoneum on entering the abdomen
11. Ring forceps to help remove membranes and placental fragments
12. Allis or Pennington clamps to hold the cut edges of the uterus and limit blood loss
13. Suction tips: pool or Yankauer depending on stage of operation
14. The choice of suture is entirely optional; absorbable suture is appropriate for all layers; a long-lasting suture should be chosen for the fascia if absorbable suture is used

D. Essential Steps in the Operation

1. Prepare the patient as described earlier
2. Administer anesthesia
3. Scrub the skin and position patient
   a. A variety of skin scrub regimens are suitable, including but not limited to povidone iodine and chlorhexidine, as for any other abdominal surgery.
   b. Consider clipping pubic hair that interferes with the incision area.
   c. The patient should be positioned with a lateral tilt to decrease hypotension caused by vena cava compression by the uterus.[22]
4. Decompress the urinary bladder with an indwelling Foley bladder catheter.
5. Perform the skin incision.
   a. A Pfannenstiel incision is cosmetically preferable but may take longer depending on experience of the surgeon. Its repair is stronger because there is less strain on the underlying transversely incised fascia than when fascia is incised vertically. This incision is made transversely about two fingerbreadths above the symphysis pubis. Incisions at least 15 cm long provide greater ease of infant delivery than shorter incisions.
   b. A midline vertical incision from the symphysis to the umbilicus can offer more room, particularly if difficulty is expected delivering the infant because of abnormal lie, hydrocephalus, or other unusual conditions.

c. In either case, the rectal muscles may also be divided to obtain more room.

d. If a previous skin scar is present, it may be excised as the incision is made or closed, although this is not usually necessary in cases of Pfannenstiel incision.

6. Divide subcutaneous tissues and secure hemostasis. The assistant should be ready with sponges, a hemostat, and electrocautery or ligation material depending on operator's preference.

7. Divide the fascia in the same direction as the skin incision. When making a low transverse abdominal entry, the assistant should be ready with Kocher clamps to grasp the fascia upper and lower edges.

8. Free the fascia from underlying rectus muscles in the case of Pfannenstiel incision. This is usually done bluntly with fingers; if adhesions are present, sharp dissection may be necessary. This is a critical step in obtaining good exposure and must be done both above and below the incision. Be prepared to identify and clamp the inferior epigastric arteries, which are exposed during this step.

9. Separate the rectus muscles by placing fingers between the rectus muscles and pulling laterally.

10. Open the peritoneum: using a hemostat or smooth thumb forceps, grasp the peritoneum high in the incision to avoid injury to the bladder. Regrasp the peritoneum close to the original spot and drop the original site to allow bowel to fall away, then carefully open the peritoneum with Metzenbaum scissors.

11. Palpate the uterus and presenting part.

12. Develop the bladder flap: Grasp the peritoneum where it reflects off the bladder onto the uterus and open the plane with scissors. Extend the flap to both sides as the assistant rotates the bladder and abdominal wall retractors to the side the operator is working on.

13. Open the uterus[23]

a. A low transverse incision is most commonly used. The initial uterine incision is made with a knife. Lateral extension is made with blunt pressure or with bandage scissors. The assistant should maintain exposure using suction and retractors.

i. In most cases, the lower uterine segment is thin and therefore less vascular.

ii. This incision heals well, reducing the risk for dehiscence in later pregnancies, thus permitting subsequent trial of labor.

iii. The main risk associated with transverse incision is lateral extension into the uterine vessels.

b. The classical incision reaches into the "active" upper uterine segment or the fundus. Vertical extension is made with a knife or bandage scissors. It is associated with increased blood loss and uterine rupture during subsequent pregnancies but is appropriate in the following situations:

i. The lower uterine segment is very thick, underdeveloped, or occupied by fibroids or an anterior placenta previa

ii. When delivering a very-low-birth-weight infant

iii. The infant is in a transverse lie with its back down

iv. Fetal anomalies are present requiring a large incision (e.g., hydrocephalus)

c. The low vertical incision may also be used but often extends upward into the active uterine segment making it similar to the classical incision

14. Deliver the infant

a. If the infant is in a cephalic presentation, scoop the head out of the pelvis and deliver the body in the usual fashion.

b. If the infant is in a breech presentation, grasp the pelvis or feet and then follow the same steps described for assisted breech delivery (see Chapter 17, Section G). Be prepared with a larger incision and maneuvers to maintain neck flexion, including availability of Piper forceps.

c. During this time, the assistant should be prepared to perform these functions at the operator's request:

i. Suction amniotic fluid and blood from the surgical field.

ii. Remove the bladder retractor to give the operator room to grasp the presenting part.

iii. Suction the infant's nose and mouth.

iv. Apply fundal pressure.

v. Reinsert retractors after infant is delivered.

15. Deliver the placenta and membranes. Massaging the uterus and allowing the placenta to expel spontaneously through the incision rather than manually removing it results in decreased maternal blood loss and decreased incidence in postpartum endometritis.[24] Ring forceps are used to retrieve fragments.

16. Request oxytocin and antibiotic administration.
    a. Request the addition of 20 units oxytocin to the intravenous drip or administer 10 units as an intravenous bolus.
    b. Prophylactic antibiotics: Cesarean deliveries are by definition "contaminated cases," particularly if the membranes were ruptured before surgery. Prophylactic antibiotic use has been shown to reduce postpartum morbidity, wound infection, and other serious infections.[25]
    c. There appears to be no advantage to multiple doses over a single perioperative dose.[26]
    d. Ampicillin or a first-generation cephalosporin (such as cefazolin, 1 g IV, after delivery of the infant) are inexpensive and effective.[26]
    e. Irrigation with antibiotic is less effective than systemic antibiotic administration.[26]
17. Place ring, Allis clamps, or Pennington clamps on the cut edges of the uterus to aid closure and limit blood loss.
18. Evacuate the uterus of remaining fluids and tissues using a laparotomy sponge.
19. Close the uterus.
    a. The assistant should maintain exposure and be ready to remove clamps before sutures are placed to avoid sutures being placed through the opening in the clamps.
    b. Some operators bring the uterus out of the abdomen while it is being closed.[27] This may make the uterine incision more accessible if exposure is difficult but often causes an awake patient to become nauseated because of vagal stimulation when traction is applied to the peritoneum.
    c. The uterus may be closed in one or two layers.[28] Additional or imbricating layers can be added if required for hemostasis.
20. Evacuate blood and amniotic fluid from the pelvis using a pool suction tip or gauze wrapped over a Yankauer suction tip. Many clinicians choose to irrigate the peritoneal cavity with NS to assist in the evacuation of blood clots. Laparotomy sponges may be used.
21. Bladder flap and peritoneal closure is not necessary.[29]
22. Close the fascia. Grasp the fascia in the midline with Kocher clamps. The assistant should demonstrate the corner of the fascial incision with a small Richardson retractor at the start of the repair.
23. Irrigate the subcutaneous tissues. Closure of the subcutaneous tissue (Camper fascia closure) has been shown to decrease the incidence of wound infection, separation, seromas, and hematomas, independent of all factors except obesity and four or more vaginal examinations.[30] Drains are normally not necessary in a cesarean delivery[31] but may be indicated if there is concern about incomplete hemostasis, a hematoma, or possible infection.
24. Close the skin with suture or staples. Subcuticular closure of Pfannenstiel incisions results in less pain and better cosmetic appearance.[32]
25. Apply a sterile dressing.
26. To ensure uterine drainage, compress the uterus with the palm of a hand on the abdomen to squeeze out blood and clots. If necessary, palpate the cervical os from below to make sure it is open for drainage, particularly for patients whose membranes were not ruptured before surgery.

E. The Simplified "Misgav Ladach" Cesarean Section Technique

The simplified "Misgav Ladach" cesarean section technique is a modification of the Joel-Cohen method of cesarean delivery; it is faster and produces less blood loss. This technique involves the following main features[33]:

1. The skin incision is made just through the skin, and not the subcutaneous tissue. Incision placement is higher than a Pfannenstiel incision, about 1 inch below a line connecting the anterior superior iliac spines.
2. The subcutaneous fat is opened sharply only in the midline to expose the fascia, which is opened in the midline with a knife.
3. The fascia is "zipped" open with slightly opened scissor tips beneath the fat.
4. The fascia is pulled off the midline cranially and caudally.
5. The muscles, fascia, and subcutaneous fat are slowly pulled laterally seeking to open the incision bloodlessly.
6. The peritoneum is opened bluntly by stretching with fingers.
7. The uterus is closed in a single layer.
8. The bladder flap and peritoneum are not closed.
9. The fascia is closed with one running layer of 1–0 Vicryl with the operator working away from himself or herself.
10. The skin is closed loosely with widely spaced mattress sutures.

F. The "Bloodless" Cesarean Delivery

The "bloodless" cesarean delivery technique has been described for use on mothers infected with human immunodeficiency virus. The main features of this technique are as follows[34]:

1. The wound is irrigated and redraped before the uterus is opened.
2. The surgeon cleans or changes gloves before the uterus is opened.
3. The uterus is opened without rupturing membranes, and a surgical stapling device is used to enlarge the uterine incision.
4. The infant is delivered, leaving membranes intact over the presenting part if possible.
5. The infant is initially bathed on the operating table before being handed off.

G. Writing an Operative Note

1. Specify type of skin and uterine incision, and note if tubal ligation has been done; when the uterine incision is vertical, note whether it extended into the active segment.
2. Indication, preoperative and postoperative diagnoses
3. Age of mother, G__P__ at ____ weeks
4. Sex, cord vessel number, weight, Apgar scores, and cord pH of newborn, if obtained
5. Anesthesia type
6. Estimated blood loss; the average blood loss at cesarean delivery is 1000 ml[35]
7. Tubes/drains
8. Complications
9. Surgeons

IV. COMPLICATIONS

A. Difficult Cesarean Delivery/ Abdominal Dystocia

1. If the abdominal incision is too tight, both skin and fascia may be extended, or the rectus muscles may be divided.
2. If the head is deeply engaged, it can be lifted from below (vaginally) by an assistant or grasped with forceps or a vacuum extractor. A vacuum extractor should not be applied over the infant's face.
3. Low transverse or low vertical incisions may be extended vertically to obtain extra room. Low transverse incisions may be extended in either a "T" (central) or "L" (lateral) fashion. If the vertical extension reaches into the active segment of the uterus, the patient should not attempt a trial of labor in a subsequent pregnancy because of the risk for uterine rupture.

B. Cesarean Delivery omplicated by Chorioamnionitis

Cesarean delivery complicated by chorioamnionitis (see Chapter 16, Section C) has the following features:

1. Chorioamnionitis affects up to 10% of pregnancies.
2. Infectious complications are increased when patients with chorioamnionitis undergo cesarean delivery.
3. An RCT of chorioamnionitis patients undergoing cesarean delivery found that continuing antibiotics after surgery did not show any benefit in reducing endometritis over treatment with ampicillin during labor and a single dose of clindamycin and gentamicin before surgery.[36]

C. Uterine Hemorrhage

Uterine hemorrhage may be treated with a variety of techniques. Significant intraoperative blood loss should be treated in a timely fashion with blood products and/or autotransfusion by cell saver, if available.

1. Administer oxytocin, 5 to 20 units IV, intramuscularly, or directly into the uterus for atony.
2. Administer methylergonovine (Methergine®), 0.2 mg intramuscularly, for atony.
3. Prostaglandin $F_2\alpha$ (Hemabate) may be given intramuscularly or into the myometrium, in doses of 0.25 mg every 30 to 60 minutes to a maximum dose of 2 mg, for atony.
4. Administer misoprostol, 400 to 800 mg rectally. This is an off-label use of this drug.
5. A tourniquet may be applied to the lower uterine segment by tying a latex or rubber urinary-type catheter around it. This can provide time for uterine artery ligation or hysterectomy, or while help is being summoned.
6. Directly suture bleeding points.
7. Perform the B-Lynch suture procedure, which strangulates the arterial blood supply to the myometrium.[37]
8. Ligate the uterine artery by placing sutures in the lateral aspect of the uterus.
9. Ligate the uterine arteries medial to the ovaries.
10. Place interrupted, circular sutures parallel to the uterine incision anteriorly and completely through the wall of the uterus posteriorly.[38]

11. Proceed with hypogastric artery ligation.
12. Inflate a Foley catheter balloon (30 ml) in the lower uterine segment with the rest of the catheter protruding out the vagina and apply moderate traction.
13. Selective arterial embolization may be used but is often not timely or feasible.
14. Hysterectomy is often the procedure of last resort.

D. Bladder Injury

Bladder injury usually occurs during repeat cesarean delivery and is often due to adhesions.[35]

1. Superficial or partial-thickness injuries can be repaired with a single layer of 3–0 absorbable suture.
2. Larger injuries should be repaired in two layers with 2–0 or 3–0 absorbable suture.
3. Bladder repair integrity can be tested by inflating the bladder with sterile milk (infant formula), which, unlike methylene blue or indigo carmine, does not stain tissues.
4. Bladder drainage with a Foley catheter for 1 to 5 days is indicated for larger injuries.

E. Bowel Injury

Bowel injury is rare. Previous surgery and pelvic infection with adhesion formation are predisposing factors.[35] Bowel injury repair techniques are as follows:

1. Simple serosal tears can be oversewn with 3–0 or 4–0 absorbable suture.
2. Enterotomy should be repaired in two layers.
3. The suture line should be placed at a right angle to the bowel long axis to avoid narrowing the bowel lumen and creating stenosis.
4. Extensive bowel injury should be repaired by end-to-end anastomosis.
5. Any defects in the mesentery should be closed to avoid internal hernias.
6. After bowel repair, patients must be observed for return of bowel motility and for infection.

F. Criteria for Postoperative Blood Replacement

Young, stable, otherwise healthy patients can tolerate a low hematocrit level if blood volume is maintained with crystalloid. Blood replacement should be based on symptoms rather than laboratory data.

G. Postoperative Fever

1. The differential diagnosis of postoperative fever[39] includes the following:
   a. Endomyometritis
   b. Urinary tract infection
   c. Respiratory infection
   d. Pulmonary atelectasis
   e. Wound infection
   f. Septic pelvic thrombophlebitis
2. The workup includes the following:
   a. Perform a general physical examination with particular attention to the wound; the uterus and lochia; and the lungs, particularly in smokers.
   b. Obtain a complete blood cell count, urinalysis, urine culture, and culture of wound drainage.
   c. Order a chest radiograph if there are abnormal lung findings on physical examination.
   d. Open the wound if signs of wound infection are present.
   e. Consider blood cultures.
3. Treatment includes broad-spectrum antibiotic therapy to cover both aerobic and anaerobic organisms while cultures are pending. A synthetic penicillin and an aminoglycoside or a second- or third-generation cephalosporin are acceptable initial choices. Lack of defervescence after initiation of antibiotics should prompt suspicion of septic pelvic thrombophlebitis. Treatment of this condition consists of a trial of anticoagulation with heparin, which usually produces defervescence in 48 to 72 hours. Anticoagulation is not usually necessary beyond 7 to 10 days.

H. Pulmonary Embolus

Pulmonary embolus should be considered, as in any other postoperative patient with chest pain, respiratory distress, or other suggestive symptoms.

I. Spinal Headaches

Headaches after spinal anesthesia, or a "wet" epidural anesthetic in which the dura was punctured, can typically be alleviated by an epidural blood patch, which involves injecting 10 ml of the patient's own blood into the epidural space close to the original puncture site.

V. POSTOPERATIVE CARE AND PATIENT COUNSELING

A. General Principles of Postoperative Care and Order Writing

1. As with all orders, strive for clarity and simplicity.
2. Avoid nonstandard abbreviations.

3. Specify start and stop times for medications, particularly antibiotics.
4. Each patient's postoperative course is unique; there is no substitute for frequent hands-on patient reevaluation by a consistent observer.

B. Typical Initial Postoperative Orders

Always record date and time of postoperative orders.

1. Vital signs are obtained every 15 minutes until stable, every 30 minutes until anesthesia wears off, and then every 4 hours after the patient is returned to her room.
2. Nothing by mouth (NPO) is ordered until anesthesia has worn off and the patient is not nauseated; then offer clear liquids.[40]
3. The patient should sit up at bedside and dangle legs as soon as anesthesia has worn off.
4. Intravenous fluids should be ordered as D5/0.45 NS to run at 125 ml/hr continuously.
5. Ten units of oxytocin should be added to first 1000 ml of intravenous fluids and the need for continuation reassessed before the second liter of fluids is started.
6. A hematocrit is ordered on the morning of the first postoperative day.
7. Foley catheter is left to closed drainage.
8. Dressing is reinforced with dry gauze as needed. The physician should be called if dressing becomes saturated or wound becomes swollen.
9. The physician should also be called if patient develops a fever more than 100.4°F, increasing uterine tenderness, or foul-smelling lochia.
10. Antibiotics should be ordered, if needed, beyond the perioperative dose.
11. If the patient is a smoker, consider incentive inspirometer and nicotine patch.
12. Record the number and degree of saturation of perineal pads.
13. If vaginal flow is excessive, the uterus can be massaged through the abdominal wall, and 5 units oxytocin given by intravenous push while calling the physician.
14. Pain medication options include:
    a. If patient had intraspinal narcotics administered at the time of surgery, there may be no need for additional pain medication during the first 24 hours after surgery.
    b. Patient-controlled analgesia pump may be ordered, specified by institutional protocol.
    c. Oral pain medication may be given, when the patient can tolerate them, on subsequent postoperative days. This may include nonsteroidal agents.[41]
15. Antiemetic options include:
    a. Promethazine, 12.5 to 25 mg IV, every 4 hours as needed
    b. Prochlorperazine, 2.5 to 10 mg IV, every 4 hours as needed
    c. Trimethobenzamide, 250 mg intramuscularly or 200 mg rectally, every 6 hours as needed
    d. Ondansetron, 4 mg IV or intramuscularly every 4 hours
16. Indicate if workup for $Rh_o(D)$ immunoglobulin is to be done.
17. Review prenatal laboratory data to determine whether hepatitis prophylaxis is needed for the newborn.
18. Review prenatal laboratory data to determine whether rubella immunization is needed for the patient.
19. Specify the phone number to be called if there are questions or problems.

C. Immediate Postoperative Patient Counseling

1. Explain the condition of the patient and her infant.
2. Inform the patient of where her infant and family are located, and when she will be able to see them.
3. Explain that the usual postoperative length of hospital stay is approximately 3 days, assuming no complications.
4. Explain to the patient how to get pain medication using the call button or patient-controlled analgesia pump.
5. Tell the patient that her uterus will cramp and that nurses will be massaging her uterine fundus.
6. Offer to try to answer any additional questions, particularly a review of the circumstances leading to the cesarean delivery, if it was not planned.

D. Considerations on First Postoperative Day

1. Review the nurse's notes and graphic chart.
2. Ask the patient how she feels; acknowledge her incisional pain and uterine cramps.
3. Ask if her pain medication is adequate.
4. Review the items listed previously as "immediate postoperative counseling."

5. Listen to patient's chest and abdomen, and remove dressing to inspect the incision. If necessary, reapply only a light dressing.
6. Review results of postpartum hematocrit, if available, and compare with preoperative value.
7. Encourage patient to ambulate and warn her of possibility for postural hypotension.
8. Typical orders include the following:
   a. Discontinue Foley catheter.
   b. Ambulate at least once during each day and evening shift.
   c. May shower and wash hair, with assistance on first attempt.
   d. Advance diet if patient is hungry.
   e. If gastrointestinal motility has returned, stop parenteral medications and change to oral route.
   f. Decrease rate of intravenous fluids, or convert to a heparin lock if the patient has been taking oral fluids well.
   g. Follow up to see whether $Rh_o(D)$ immunoglobulin was administered, if indicated.
9. If patient is nursing, ask how this is progressing and order lactation consultation, if needed.
10. Instruct patient in how to hug a pillow to splint abdomen during coughing.
11. Consider performing a newborn examination in the presence of parents; if necessary, arrange to return to do that when father can be present.
12. Assess the progress of maternal-infant bonding.
13. Assess if social services will be needed, particularly for single mothers or if the patient seems vague about where she will live, lacks support people, or does not have baby clothes, car seat, and other accessories already assembled.
14. Remind the new parents that an infant car seat is needed before discharge.

E. Considerations on Second Postoperative Day

1. Repeat items 1 through 6 as on the first day.
2. Assess progress in advancing diet.
3. Change to oral pain medication, if not done the previous day.
4. For constipation, consider 30 ml Milk of Magnesia.
5. For "gas pains," consider ambulation or a return flow enema.
6. Repeat items 9 through 14 from previous section on first postoperative day.
7. Discuss infant care and feeding.
8. Restart prenatal vitamins for nursing mothers.

F. Considerations before Discharge

1. The mother should be able to eat, ambulate, urinate, and have her pain controlled by oral medications before discharge.
2. Infant care and self-care teaching should be completed.
3. Birth control and timing of resumption of intercourse should be discussed.
4. Discuss expectations for vaginal bleeding.
5. Write instructions or prescriptions for pain medication, iron, and vitamins if applicable.
6. If patient has a stapled transverse wound, consider removing staples and applying tape reinforcing strips. If the wound was closed using subcuticular sutures, consider applying fresh tape. In either case, tell patient what bathing is permitted; that powder can help itching and ingrown hairs; that a light dressing is helpful to prevent rubbing on clothes; and that a thick scar will normally develop as healing progresses, then smooth out over subsequent months.
7. Answer questions about lifting and exercise. Patients with Pfannenstiel incisions should have their exercise dictated by their comfort. For vertical skin incisions, they should avoid lifting anything heavier than the infant until the 6-week follow-up visit. Kegel exercises, single leg lifts, and pelvic tilt back exercise can start as soon as comfort permits.
8. Consider a dietary consult for overweight or underweight patients and those who are nursing for the first time.
9. Make specific appointments in writing for both the baby and mother at 1 to 2 weeks and 6 to 8 weeks after delivery, respectively. Mothers who go home very soon (second or third postoperative day) should be seen sooner than 6 weeks after delivery. A wound check, or removal of staples from vertical incisions, at 5 to 7 days after surgery can also include answering questions about self-care and infant care. Telephone follow-up may suffice in some situations.
10. Discuss the importance of well-child visits and immunizations.
11. Direct mother to community services, including Women, Infants and Children (WIC), for assistance with nutritional services, if indicated.
12. Infant car seat is needed.

G. Considerations at the First Outpatient Visit

1. Review the indications for the cesarean delivery and inquire as to how mother feels about having had a surgical, rather than a vaginal, delivery.
2. Answer specific questions.
3. Discuss the possibility of a future trial of labor.
4. Examine incision. Confirm that the thickening under the incision is a normal process that indicates healing and that it will smooth out over a few months.
5. Discuss normal postpartum vaginal bleeding.
6. Discuss resumption of intercourse and need for extra lubrication because of the relative estrogen deficiency normally present postpartum, particularly during lactation.
7. Discuss birth control.
8. Discuss physical activity.
9. Discuss diet.
10. Always allow time for questions about the infant and an examination of the infant with the parents present.
11. Discuss medications (e.g., for pain, vitamins, iron, bowel care).
12. Set specific date for next visit.

VI. SOR A RECOMMENDATIONS

This table is based on individual Cochrane reviews. In addition, Dodd and colleagues[4] provide a summary of evidence-based cesarean delivery.

RECOMMENDATIONS	REFERENCES
Planned caesarean for term breech delivery compared with planned vaginal birth reduces perinatal or neonatal death or serious neonatal morbidity, at the expense of somewhat increased maternal morbidity.	16
Caesarean delivery for the birth of a second twin not presenting cephalically is associated with increased maternal febrile morbidity, with no identified improvement in neonatal outcome.	17
Zidovudine, nevirapine, and delivery by elective caesarean delivery appear to be effective in decreasing the risk for mother-to-child transmission of HIV infection.	18

RECOMMENDATIONS	REFERENCES
Both spinal and epidural techniques are shown to provide effective anesthesia for caesarean delivery.	21
When lateral tilt is used during caesarean delivery, there are fewer low Apgar scores and improved cord blood pH measurements and oxygen saturation.	22
Manual removal of the placenta at caesarean delivery may do more harm than good, by increasing maternal blood loss and increasing the risk for infection.	24
Prophylactic antibiotics reduce endometritis by two thirds to three fourths and decrease wound infections in women undergoing cesarean delivery.	25
Both ampicillin and first-generation cephalosporins have similar efficacy in reducing postoperative endometritis. There does not appear to be added benefit in utilizing a more broad-spectrum agent or a multidose regimen.	26
There appear to be no advantages or disadvantages for routine use of single-layer uterine closure compared with two-layer closure, except perhaps a shorter operation time.	28
No evidence has been reported to justify the time taken for peritoneal closure.	29
The risk for hematoma or seroma is reduced with fat closure compared with nonclosure, as is the risk for wound complications such as hematoma, seroma, wound infection, or wound separation.	30
Routine use of wound drains at caesarean delivery confers no benefit.	31
When closing the skin at cesarean delivery, the use of absorbable subcuticular suture results in less postoperative pain and yields a better cosmetic result at the postoperative visit.	32
No evidence has been reported to justify a policy of withholding oral fluids after uncomplicated caesarean delivery.	40
Naproxen sodium 550 mg, naproxen 400 mg, and naproxen sodium 440 mg administered orally are effective analgesics for the treatment of acute postoperative pain in adults.	41

REFERENCES

1. Centers for Disease Control and Prevention National Center for Health Statistics: *Preliminary births for 2004: infant and maternal health.* Available at: http://www.cdc.gov/nchs/products/pubs/pubd/hestats/prelimbirths04/prelimbirths04health.htm. Accessed August 20, 2006.

2. ACOG practice bulletin. Vaginal birth after cesarean delivery. Number 5, July 1999 (replaces practice bulletin number 2, October 1998). American College of Obstetricians and Gynecologists, *Int J Gynaecol Obstet* 66:197-204, 1999.

3. Centers for Disease Control and Prevention Agency for Healthcare Research and Quality: Vaginal birth after cesarean (VBAC). Summary, evidence report/technology assessment: Number 71. AHRQ Publication Number 03-E017, March 2003. Rockville, MD, 2003, Agency for Healthcare Research and Quality. Available at: http://www.ahrq.gov/clinic/epcsums/vbacsum.htm. Accessed August 20, 2006.

4. Dodd JM, Crowther CA, Huertas E et al: Planned elective repeat caesarean section versus planned vaginal birth for women with a previous caesarean birth, *Cochrane Database Syst Rev* (4):CD004224, 3, 2007.

5. Applegate JA, Walhout MF: Cesarean section rate: a comparison between family physicians and obstetricians, *Fam Pract Res J* 12:255-262, 1992.

6. Deutchman ME, Sills D, Connor PD: Perinatal outcomes: a comparison between family physicians and obstetricians, *J Am Board Fam Pract* 8:440-447, 1995.

7. Hueston WJ: Specialty differences in primary cesarean section rates in a rural hospital, *Fam Pract Res J* 12:245-253, 1992.

8. Deutchman M, Connor P, Gobbo R et al: Outcomes of cesarean sections performed by family physicians and the training they received: a 15-year retrospective study, *J Am Board Fam Pract* 8:81-90, 1995.

9. Deutchman ME, Connor PD: Cesarean section by family physicians: a national multi-site study of surgical outcomes and training. Presented at the 25th Annual Meeting of the North American Primary Care Research Group, Orlando, FL, 1997.

10. Iglesias S, Burn R, Saunders LD: Reducing the cesarean section rate in a rural hospital, *CMAJ* 145:1459-1463, 1991.

11. Meyers SA, Gliecher N: A successful program to lower cesarean section rate, *N Engl J Med* 319:1511-1516, 1988.

12. Sanchez-Ramos L, Peterson HB, Martinex-Schnell B et al: Reducing cesarean sections at a teaching hospital, *Am J Obstet Gynecol* 163:1081-1088, 1990.

13. American Heart Association: 2005 guidelines for cardiopulmonary resuscitation and emergency cardiovascular care part 10.8: cardiac arrest associated with pregnancy, *Circulation* 112:150-153, 2005.

14. National Institutes of Health: *NIH State-of-the-Science Conference: cesarean delivery on maternal request.* Available at: http://consensus.nih.gov/2006/2006cesareanSOS027main.htm. Accessed September 16, 2007.

15. Lavender T, Hofmeyr GJ, Neilson JP et al: Caesarean section for non-medical reasons at term, *Cochrane Database Syst Rev* (3):CD004660, 3, 2007.

16. Hofmeyr GJ; Hannah ME: Planned caesarean section for term breech delivery, *Cochrane Database Syst Rev* (3):CD000166, 3, 2007.

17. Crowther CA: Caesarean delivery for the second twin, *Cochrane Database Syst Rev* (2):CD000047, 3, 2007.

18. Brocklehurst P: Interventions for reducing the risk of mother-to-child transmission of HIV infection, *Cochrane Database Syst Rev* (1):CD000102, 3, 2007.

19. Dajani A, Bolger A, Taubert K et al: Prevention of bacterial endocarditis: American Heart Association recommendations, *JAMA* 277:1794-1801, 1997.

20. Spielman FJ, Cefalo RC: Anesthesia for obstetrics. In Plauche WC, Morrison JC, Sullivan MJ, editors: *Surgical obstetrics,* Philadelphia, 1992, WB Saunders.

21. Ng K, Parsons J, Cyna AM et al: Spinal versus epidural anaesthesia for caesarean section, *Cochrane Database Syst Rev* (2): CD003765, 3, 2007.

22. Wilkinson C, Enkin MW: Lateral tilt for caesarean section, *Cochrane Database Syst Rev* (2):CD000120, 3, 2007.

23. Rodriguez AI, Porter KB, O'Brien WF: Blunt versus sharp expansion of the uterine incision in low-segment transverse cesarean section, *Am J Obstet Gynecol* 171:1022-1025, 1994.

24. Wilkinson C, Enkin MW: Manual removal of placenta at caesarean section, *Cochrane Database Syst Rev* (2):CD000130, 3, 2007.

25. Smaill F, Hofmeyr GJ: Antibiotic prophylaxis for cesarean section, *Cochrane Database Syst Rev* (3):CD0933, 3, 2007.

26. Hopkins L, Smaill F: Antibiotic prophylaxis regimens and drugs for cesarean section, *Cochrane Database Syst Rev* (2): CD001136, 3, 2007.

27. Jacobs-Jokhan D, Hofmeyr GJ: Extra-abdominal versus intra-abdominal repair of the uterine incision at caesarean section, *Cochrane Database Syst Rev* (4):CD000085, 3, 2007.

28. Enkin MW, Wilkinson C: Single versus two layer suturing for closing the uterine incision at Caesarean section, *Cochrane Database Syst Rev* (2):CD000192, 3, 2007.

29. Bamigboye AA, Hofmeyr GJ: Closure versus non-closure of the peritoneum at caesarean section, *Cochrane Database Syst Rev* (4):CD000163, 3, 2007.

30. Anderson ER, Gates S: Techniques and materials for closure of the abdominal wall in caesarean section, *Cochrane Database Syst Rev* (4):CD004663, 3, 2007.

31. Gates S, Anderson ER: Wound drainage for caesarean section, *Cochrane Database Syst Rev* (1):CD004549, 3, 2007.

32. Alderdice F, McKenna D, Dornan J: Techniques and materials for skin closure in caesarean section, *Cochrane Database Syst Rev* (2):CD003577, 3, 2007.

33. Chez RA: The Misgav Ladach method of cesarean section, *Contemp Ob/Gyn* 81-88, 1998.

34. Towers CV, Deveikis AA, Asrat T et al: A "bloodless cesarean section" and perinatal transmission of the human immunodeficiency virus, *Am J Obstet Gynecol* 179:708-714, 1998.

35. Yasin SY, Walton DL, O'Sullivan MJ: Problems encountered during cesarean delivery. In Plauche WC, Morrison JC, Sullivan MJ, editors: *Surgical obstetrics,* Philadelphia, 1992, W.B. Saunders.

36. Turnquest MA, How HY, Cook CR et al: Chorioamnionitis: is continuation of antibiotic therapy necessary after cesarean section? *Am J Obstet Gynecol* 179:1261-1266, 1998.

37. B-Lynch C, Coker A, Lawal AH et al: The B-Lynch surgical technique for the control of massive post partum hemorrhage: an alternative to hysterectomy? Five cases reported, *Br J Obstet Gynaecol* 104:372-375, 1997.

38. Cho JY, Kim SJ, Cha KY et al: Interrupted circular suture: bleeding control during cesarean delivery in placenta previa accreta, *Obstet Gynecol* 78:876-879, 1991.
39. Gabert HA: Complications common to obstetric operative procedures. In Plauche WC, Morrison JC, Sullivan MJ, editors: *Surgical obstetrics*, Philadelphia, 1992, WB Saunders.
40. Mangesi L; Hofmeyr GJ: Early compared with delayed oral fluids and food after caesarean section, *Cochrane Database Syst Rev* (3):CD003516, 3, 2007.
41. Mason L, Edwards JE, Moore RA et al: Single dose oral naproxen and naproxen sodium for acute postoperative pain, *Cochrane Database Syst Rev* (4):CD004234, 3, 2007.

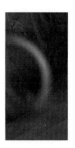

CHAPTER **19**

The First Month of Life

SECTION A Initial Management of the Normal Newborn

Patricia Fontaine, MD, MS

Family physicians have a unique advantage in providing care for infants they deliver. Having already established a relationship with one or both parents, and being well acquainted with maternal prenatal factors that can have significant impact on the newborn's condition, family physicians can provide high-quality medical care for infants while promoting bonding and family adjustment.

I. CARE OF THE HEALTHY TERM INFANT AT BIRTH

A. Initial Steps
1. The infant is delivered into a warm environment and quickly dried.[1]
2. When necessary, the nose and mouth are suctioned with a bulb syringe.[1]
3. Further stimulation may be provided by vigorously rubbing the infant's back with a dry towel, or slapping or flicking the infant's feet.[1]
4. Every attempt should be made to respect parents' expressed preferences for their involvement in the delivery, such as having the father cut the umbilical cord or having the baby placed immediately in skin-to-skin contact with the mother. Early breastfeeding should be encouraged. As long as the infant appears stable and hypothermia is avoided, these activities may be encouraged for their value in family bonding. Early skin-to-skin contact has been associated with less infant crying and positive effects on breastfeeding.[2]

B. Apgar Scoring
1. The Apgar score provides a systematic appraisal of the infant's adaptation to extrauterine life. Five characteristics (heart rate, respiratory effort, tone, reflex response, and color) are scored at 1 minute and 5 minutes of life (Table 19-1).[3]
2. Infants with Apgar scores of 7 to 10 are considered normal; a score of 4 to 6 indicates mild-to-moderate depression; and a score of 0 to 3 indicates severe depression.
3. If the 5-minute score is less than 7, additional scores are noted every 5 minutes, up to 20 minutes.
4. Although the Apgar score has little value in predicting long-term outcomes, it is a systematic way of reflecting the extent of neonatal depression and the effectiveness of resuscitation[3] (see Section B, Neonatal Resuscitation).

C. Initial Assessment
The newborn assessment in the delivery room should be brief, to minimize stress on the infant and unnecessary disruption of the family. It should include an assessment of temperature, heart rate, breathing, color, and activity; auscultation of the heart and lungs; and a visual inspection for physical anomalies or birth injury.[3,4]
1. Assessment of heart rate, breathing, and color
   a. Heart rate: The heart rate should always be more than 100 beats/min and generally stabilizes in the 120 to 160 range. Irregularities in cardiac rhythm are occasionally present, most often because of premature atrial contractions that are benign and self-limited.[3]
   b. Respiratory rate: The normal respiratory rate is 30 to 60 breaths/min. Moist rales may be present during the first several minutes of life. Rales are not concerning as long as the infant is well suctioned, is not cyanotic, and is not

TABLE 19-1 Determination of Infant Apgar Score

Sign	0	1	2
Color (Appearance)	Blue, pale	Body pink, extremities blue	Completely pink
Heart rate (Pulse)	Absent	<100	≥100
Reflex response (Grimace)	No response	Grimace	Cough, sneeze, cry
Muscle tone (Activity)	Limp	Slow flexion of extremities	Well flexed
Respiratory effort	Absent	Weak cry, hypoventilation	Strong cry

showing signs of respiratory distress such as grunting or retractions.[3]

c. Acrocyanosis: This is a blue coloration of the hands and feet that is common in healthy newborns, especially in response to a cool environment. Generalized cyanosis and pallor are two signs reflecting inadequate oxygenation or poor peripheral circulation. Generalized cyanosis requires immediate evaluation for significant cardiac or lung abnormalities.[3]

2. Inspection for physical anomalies and evidence of birth injury

a. Congenital anomalies or birth defects: These occur in 1 of every 33 live births in the United States.[5] Major anomalies are ideally detected during prenatal care, by ultrasound, or by other studies, so that an appropriate management plan is in place for the delivery.

b. Minor anomalies: Common minor deviations from normal may be noted on initial physical examination. The features, significance, and management of selected abnormalities are described in Table 19-2.

c. Birth injuries: A birth injury may result from unavoidable pressure as the infant passes through the birth canal, or from medical interventions such as use of the vacuum extractor.

d. Scalp edema (caput succedaneum)/bruising: This occurs commonly over the presenting part.

e. Subperiosteal hemorrhage (cephalhematoma): This occurs over the fetal parietal bones often after passage through a tight maternal pelvis.[6]

f. Clavicular/shoulder injuries: When shoulder dystocia occurs, the infant should be examined for a fractured clavicle or brachial plexus palsy.[6]

D. Disposition

The initial assessment, combined with history of exposure to maternal risk factors, determines whether the infant will require extended observation or may be treated as a healthy newborn. For the healthy newborn, the optimal family-centered program is rooming in, where mother and infant spend time together with attention from an understanding and helpful nurse, and with essentially unrestricted visits from the father, siblings, and other key support persons.[4] Rooming in offers advantages for breastfeeding instruction, as well as potential protective effects against hospital-acquired infections, as the infant becomes colonized with maternal microorganisms.

II. CARE IN THE HEALTHY NEWBORN NURSERY

A. Physical Examination

When the initial delivery room assessment is normal, the first complete newborn examination takes place sometime during the first 24 hours of life, after admission routines have been accomplished and the infant's general condition and temperature have stabilized.

1. Estimation of gestational age

The maternal due date may provide a reliable estimate of the infant's gestation, particularly when derived from ultrasound measurements in the first trimester. When maternal dates are uncertain, the infant's physical and neurologic maturity can be assessed using the instrument shown in Figure 19-1. The infant's weight, length, and head circumference are plotted against the estimated gestational age on a standard growth curve, ideally one that has been standardized for the infant's population of origin. Infants may be classified as small (SGA) or large for gestational age (LGA) at the extremes of

TABLE 19-2 Common and Uncommon Deviations from Normal on Newborn Physical Examinations

Condition	Description	Causes	Evaluation/Treatment
HEENT (head, ears, eyes, nose, and throat)			
Cephalhematoma	Subperiosteal hemorrhage causing localized swelling, usually over parietal bone	Pressure against fetal skull as it passes through birth canal	Observation; if severe, rule out underlying fracture
Subconjunctival hemorrhage	Red patch in sclera, adjacent to iris	Rupture of small conjunctival capillaries during birth process	Observation; resolves in 7-10 days
Abnormal red reflex; "white pupil"	Ophthalmoscope examination: lack of typical red-yellow reflection from retina	Cataract; neuroblastoma (rare)	Ophthalmologic referral for complete evaluation
Congenital glaucoma	Cornea cloudy, large (>11 mm)	Congenital	Early recognition and referral for treatment
Nasolacrimal duct obstruction	Eye watering; conjunctivitis may develop secondarily	Developmental; may manifest during first few days to weeks of life	Warm pack, massage, treat conjunctivitis with topical antibiotic; refer for probing if not resolved by 9-12 months
Low-set external ear	Upper attachment of ear (not pinna) falls below a horizontal line determined by the inner and outer canthus of the eye	Renal anomalies (Potter syndrome); trisomies; other congenital anomalies	Investigate for trisomy, renal anomalies as indicated
Preauricular skin tags	Unilateral or bilateral; broad vs. pedunculated base; mainly cosmetic concern	Familial/embryogenic anomaly	Pedunculated tag: ligate tightly at base; sloughs in 1-2 weeks Broad-based tag, or one containing cartilage: refer to surgeon, consider Goldenhar syndrome
Cleft lip or palate	Incomplete closure of lip's vermilion border; may also involve nasolabial fold, palate	Multifactorial: genetic, chromosomal, and nongenetic; cleft lip or palate occurs in 1/1000 births; cleft palate alone occurs in 1/2500 births	Multidisciplinary team approach; surgical correction (lip) as early as 1-3 months; feeding assessment important
Gingival retention cysts (epithelial pearls)	"Ricelike" white nodules on gingiva (may be mistaken for teeth)	Keratin-containing cysts lined with squamous epithelium	Observation; anticipate spontaneous resolution
Neck mass	Branchial cleft cyst/sinus; thyroglossal duct cyst; cystic hygroma	Developmental/embryogenic anomalies	Surgical referral
Chest			
Heart murmur	Characterize quality, intensity, and timing in cardiac cycle	1. Transitional—changeover from fetal to infant circulatory system 2. Functional 3. Pathologic—congenital anomalies	Evaluate infant's overall status; cyanosis or respiratory distress in the presence of murmur needs urgent evaluation
Abdomen mass	Palpable mass	50% are of genitourinary origin	Ultrasound examination

Condition	Description	Causes	Evaluation/Treatment
Chest—Cont'd			
Two umbilical vessels (check freshly cut cord section at birth)	Only one umbilical artery present in cord stump	More common in twins; other congenital defects possible (cerebrovascular, gastrointestinal, genitourinary), but low incidence	Perform additional diagnostic tests if other findings also suggest abnormality
Genitalia			
Vaginal tags/discharge	Mucosal skin tags protrude from vagina; mucus or blood-tinged discharge in first days of life	Tags: common variant Discharge: probably normal response to maternal hormone withdrawal	Tags: observe; surgical removal rarely required for unacceptable tags not resolving in childhood
Undescended testes	Location of testes: intraabdominal, in inguinal canal, high scrotal, or ectopic	Cause unclear Incidence: 3-5% term births, higher for preterm If bilateral cryptorchidism, consider ambiguous genitalia	Observe for spontaneous descent between 3 and 6 months; refer for surgical exploration/orchiopexy at 6-12 months; long-term risk for testicular malignancy, infertility
Hypospadias	Urethral meatus located proximal to tip of glans (base of glans, penile shaft, scrotum)	Developmental anomaly Incidence: 1/500 male births	Avoid circumcision; surgical referral, repair at 6-9 months
Hernia, inguinal	Inguinal swelling or mass; may extend into scrotum; does not transilluminate; may be reducible	Less common in newborn than hydrocele	Prompt surgical referral because of risk for incarceration
Hydrocele	Scrotal swelling that transilluminates	Patent processus vaginalis allows fluid accumulation around testes	Observe for resolution over 4-6 months; refer for surgical repair if persists beyond 6-12 months
Extremities, back			
Clavicle fracture	Infant cries when affected side is examined; decreased movement of arm on that side	Large-for-gestational-age infant, shoulder dystocia; break often occurs as anterior shoulder is delivered from under maternal pubic symphysis	Heals spontaneously
Hip dislocation	Head of femur lies outside or is easily displaced from acetabulum; leg lengths may be unequal, and hip abduction may be limited, with palpable "click"	Multifactorial: genetic predisposition to acetabular dysplasia and joint laxity; environmental (breech position) Incidence: 1/1000 births	Early detection important; orthopedic referral
Pilonidal dimple/tract	Pinpoint invagination of skin over caudal portion of spinal column	May be associated with spina bifida occulta, nonfusion of posterior arches of spine Patch of abnormal hair, lipoma or hemangioma may also mark spina bifida occulta	Perform neurologic examination; neurosurgical referral if deficits present
Skin			
Salmon patch or "Stork's beak mark"	Light red, irregularly shaped macule found on the upper eyelids, glabella, or occiput	Superficial capillary malformation, extremely common among light-skinned newborns	Facial lesions fade over months; occipital lesions may persist into adulthood

Continued

TABLE 19-2 Common and Uncommon Deviations from Normal on Newborn Physical Examinations—cont'd

Condition	Description	Causes	Evaluation/Treatment
Skin—Cont'd			
Port wine stain or "nevus flammeus"	Dark red or purplish macule that does not blanch to pressure	Capillary malformation; on the face, suggests Sturge-Weber syndrome; on extremity, Klippel-Trenaunay syndrome	Refer to dermatologist for pulsed dye laser treatment; evaluate for underlying syndromes as appropriate
Hemangioma	Red, rough-surfaced nodule	Benign tumor of capillary endothelial cells	Expect lesion to enlarge initially, then involute; 50% are gone by age 5, 70% by age 7, 90% by age 9
Milia	Pinpoint-sized white papules scattered over the nose, cheeks, and forehead	Sebaceous retention cysts; present in up to 40% of newborns	Expect spontaneous rupture and disappearance within a few weeks
Erythema toxicum	Blotchy erythematous macules; may develop urticarial centers. Size varies from a few millimeters to 2-3 cm; appears on trunk or extremities during the first days of life	Cause unknown. Smears of lesions show eosinophils. More common in term infants; in preterm, seek other causes for rash	Expect spontaneous resolution within 7-10 days

expected weight for the gestational week. Traditionally, SGA was defined as weight below the 10th percentile; however, a cutoff at the 3rd percentile is more highly associated with morbidity and mortality among term infants.[7]

2. Physical examination by organ system

The physician reviews the infant's measurements and vital signs (temperature, pulse, respiratory rate) and then examines the infant in the following order:

a. Auscultate heart and lungs. These are the initial maneuvers because they are best accomplished while the infant is quiet.

b. Perform general examination. Examine the head, eyes, ears, nose, throat (HEENT), neck, chest, abdomen, genitalia, back, and extremities in head-to-toe order.

c. Perform neurologic examination. This includes assessing resting posture, muscle tone, and reflexes. Check for the rooting, suck, and grasp reflexes. Evaluate the traction response (head lag) as the infant is pulled to sitting position and observe the Moro reflex.

Table 19-2 summarizes the typical physical findings and minor deviations from normal that can be observed on newborn physical examinations.[6]

B. Preventive Health Measures for Newborns

Routine screening tests and preventive measures in the newborn nursery are designed to prevent short- and long-term morbidity. The American Academy of Pediatrics (AAP) and the American College of Obstetricians and Gynecologists have developed clinical guidelines describing the recommended measures.[4]

1. Vitamin K prophylaxis

Vitamin K is used to prevent vitamin K deficiency bleeding (VKDB) in neonates. VKDB, also known as hemorrhagic disease of the newborn, is due to the deficiency of vitamin K–dependent clotting factors II, VII, IX, and X, which results from the limited stores of vitamin K available to the infant at birth.[8]

a. Types of VKDB

VKDB is characterized as "early" when bleeding occurs within the first 24 hours of life, "classic" if it occurs during the remainder of the first week, and "late" if it occurs during weeks 2 through 12.[8]

b. Incidence

VKDB occurs in approximately 5 to 7 cases per 100,000 live births.[8]

c. Risk factors

Exclusive breastfeeding is associated with VKDB because vitamin K is not present in appreciable

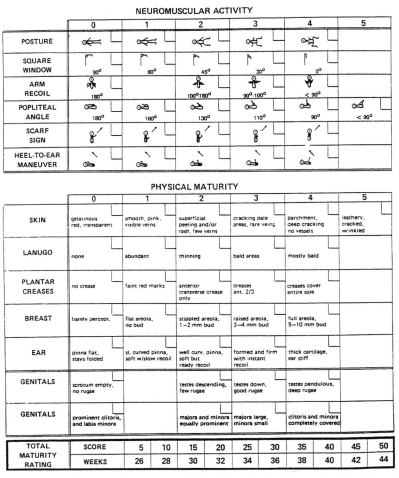

NEUROMUSCULAR ACTIVITY

	0	1	2	3	4	5
POSTURE						
SQUARE WINDOW	90°	60°	45°	30°	0°	
ARM RECOIL	180°		100°-180°	90°-100°	< 90°	
POPLITEAL ANGLE	180°	160°	130°	110°	90°	< 90°
SCARF SIGN						
HEEL-TO-EAR MANEUVER						

PHYSICAL MATURITY

	0	1	2	3	4	5
SKIN	gelatinous red, transparent	smooth, pink, visible veins	superficial peeling and/or rash, few veins	cracking pale areas, rare veins	parchment, deep cracking no vessels	leathery, cracked, wrinkled
LANUGO	none	abundant	thinning	bald areas	mostly bald	
PLANTAR CREASES	no crease	faint red marks	anterior transverse crease only	creases ant. 2/3	creases cover entire sole	
BREAST	barely percept.	flat areola, no bud	stippled areola, 1–2 mm bud	raised areola, 3–4 mm bud	full areola, 5–10 mm bud	
EAR	pinna flat, stays folded	sl. curved pinna, soft w/slow recoil	well curv. pinna, soft but ready recoil	formed and firm with instant recoil	thick cartilage, ear stiff	
GENITALS	scrotum empty, no rugae		testes descending, few rugae	testes down, good rugae	testes pendulous, deep rugae	
GENITALS	prominent clitoris, and labia minora		majora and minora equally prominent	majora large, minora small	clitoris and minora completely covered	

TOTAL MATURITY RATING	SCORE	5	10	15	20	25	30	35	40	45	50
	WEEKS	26	28	30	32	34	36	38	40	42	44

FIGURE 19-1. To assess gestational age, rate the Neuromuscular Activity and Physical Maturity of the infant; then combine these ratings to derive Total Maturity Rating at the bottom of the form. (From Klaus MH, Fanaroff AA: *Care of the high-risk infant,* Philadelphia, 1977, WB Saunders.)

amounts in breast milk, and the newborn is unable to synthesize the vitamin.[8,9] Liver disease and cholestasis are also associated with VKDB because bile salts are needed for the absorption of fat-soluble vitamin K from the intestine.[9,10]

d. Clinical presentation

  i. Classic VKDB: This usually presents with spontaneous bleeding from the skin, nose, circumcision site, umbilical cord, or gastrointestinal tract.[8]

  ii. Late VKDB: This most commonly presents as intracranial, cutaneous, or gastrointestinal bleeding.[8] Intracranial

hemorrhage may cause seizures, altered sensorium, and death.[11]

e. Laboratory findings in VKDB include a prolonged international normalized ratio (or prothrombin time) coupled with a normal platelet count and fibrinogen level.[8]

f. Treatment

  i. One dose of intramuscular (IM) vitamin K given shortly after birth has been shown to reduce the incidence of classic VKDB.[8] In the United States, the standard is to administer 0.5 to 1 mg vitamin K by the IM route within 1 hour of birth.[12]

    ii. Oral vitamin K

Currently, no oral preparations of vitamin K are licensed for use in newborns in the United States. In other countries, concerns over high vitamin K levels after IM injection and a controversial association with childhood leukemia (subsequently substantially refuted) have prompted investigation into more physiologic oral dosage schedules. Oral vitamin K has been evaluated using varying dosage schedules: a single oral dose on the first day of life, a series of three doses, or weekly doses until age 3 months for exclusively breastfed infants.[13] Each regimen improves laboratory measures of clotting function in the first week. Extended daily or weekly dose schedules have shown promise in suppressing clinical VKDB[13] but have not been tested in randomized trials.[8]

2. Conjunctivitis of the newborn

Conjunctivitis of the newborn, or *ophthalmia neonatorum,* refers to the presence of conjunctival inflammation and discharge in an infant younger than 1 month.

  a. Causes and incidence

In the United States, the most common cause of newborn conjunctivitis is *Chlamydia trachomatis,* with an incidence of 8 per 1000 live births. Gonococcal ophthalmia neonatorum is less common (0.3/1000 live births), but it is significant because of its potential to result in corneal scarring and blindness if left untreated.[14] Without prophylaxis, conjunctivitis develops in approximately one third of infants exposed to chlamydia and 30% to 50% exposed to gonococci.[15]

  b. Prophylaxis

In the United States, prophylaxis against neonatal conjunctivitis is required by federal law. Agents used for prophylaxis include 0.5% erythromycin ointment, 1% tetracycline ointment (single-dose tubes), and 1% silver nitrate solution (single-dose wax ampules).[14] All three treatments are effective in preventing gonococcal ophthalmia,[16] but they do not reliably protect against conjunctivitis caused by chlamydia.[17] The solution or ointment is instilled into the infant's inferior conjunctival sacs and is most effective when administered as soon as possible after birth. However, a delay of 1 hour may be acceptable to facilitate maternal-infant bonding.[17]

  c. Treatment for infants exposed to active maternal infections

    i. Gonorrhea

In addition to receiving topical ocular prophylaxis, infants born to mothers with active gonococcal disease should receive a single IM or intravenous dose of ceftriaxone, 25 to 50 mg/kg, with a maximum dose of 125 mg.[3]

    ii. Chlamydia

Because no topical agent has been shown to prevent exposed infants from development of nasopharyngeal colonization with chlamydia, infants born to mothers with untreated chlamydial infections should be treated with oral erythromycin, 30 mg/kg/day in divided doses every 8 to 12 hours for 14 days.[3]

3. Hepatitis B immunization

Reducing perinatal hepatitis B virus (HBV) transmission by immunizing newborns is part of a comprehensive strategy to prevent HBV infection in the United States. Because acute and chronic HBV infections result in major health problems, and because strategies that rely on vaccinating only high-risk groups are unsuccessful, universal HBV immunization is recommended for all infants.[4,18]

Ninety percent of infants infected with HBV go on to become chronic carriers, and up to 25% die in adulthood of HBV-associated liver disease, including cirrhosis and hepatocellular carcinoma.[18,19]

Appropriate immunization has been shown to decrease perinatal transmission and to reduce the number of chronic carriers. The number of new infections per year has declined from an average of 260,000 in the 1980s to 60,000 in 2004.[20]

  a. Hepatitis B immunoglobulin (HBIG): HBIG is administered to infants of HBsAg-positive mothers to provide passive immunity while the hepatitis B vaccine series is completed. HBIG is prepared from human plasma known to contain a high titer of antibody against HbsAgs.[19]

  b. Hepatitis B vaccine (Hep B): Hep B is produced by recombinant DNA technology using common yeast. It is available as a monovalent vaccine and as part of multicomponent vaccines. All hepatitis B vaccines are available without mercury (previously a component of the preservative thimerosal), eliminating the potential for mercury toxicity with repeated doses.[19]

c. Administration and dosage schedule[21]: According to the U.S. Advisory Committee on Immunization Practices, all infants should receive monovalent (single antigen) Hep B before hospital discharge. The dose should be omitted only if there is a specific order from the physician and the mother's immunity status (HBsAg test report) is documented in the medical record.

d. Infants born to HBsAg-positive mothers: These infants should also receive 0.5 ml HBIG. HBIG and Hep B are injected at different sites, within 12 hours of birth.

e. Mother's hepatitis B status is unknown: The infant should receive Hep B within 12 hours of birth. Maternal HBsAg status should be checked as soon as possible. If the mother tests positive for HBsAg, the infant should receive HBIG as soon as results are available and no later than the first week of life.

The Hep B vaccine series should be completed with either monovalent or combination vaccine, as outlined in Table 19-3.

f. Adverse effects of hepatitis B vaccine: These appear to be minimal. A serious allergic reaction to a prior dose of hepatitis B vaccine (or to yeast) is a contraindication to further doses. Research to investigate a possible link between multiple childhood vaccines and autoimmune conditions has been reassuring.[19]

C. Screening Tests

1. Hospitals may be governed by state laws requiring newborn screening for inborn errors of metabolism and other medical conditions. Examples include phenylketonuria, galactosemia, hypothyroidism, and hemoglobinopathies.

TABLE 19-3 Hepatitis B Vaccine Schedules for Newborn Infants, by Maternal Hepatitis B Surface Antigen (HBsAg) Status

Maternal HBsAg Status	Single-Antigen Vaccine		Single Antigen + Combination Vaccine	
	Dose	Age	Dose	Age
Positive	1[†]	Birth (≤12 hrs)	1[†]	Birth (≤12 hrs)
	HBIG[§]	Birth (≤12 hrs)	HBIG	Birth (≤12 hrs)
	2	1-2 mos	2	2 mos
	3[¶]	6 mos	3	4 mos
			4[¶]	6 mos (Pediarix) or 12-15 mos (Comvax)
Unknown**	1[†]	Birth (≤12 hrs)	1[†]	Birth (≤12 hrs)
	2	1-2 mos	2	2 mos
	3[¶]	6 mos	3	4 mos
			4[¶]	6 mos (Pediarix) or 12-15 mos (Comvax)
Negative	1[†,††]	Birth (before discharge)	1[†,††]	Birth (before discharge)
	2	1-2 mos	2	2 mos
	3[¶]	6-18 mos	3	4 mos
			4[¶]	6 mos (Pediarix) or 12-15 mos (Comvax)

From Centers for Disease Control and Prevention: A comprehensive immunization strategy to eliminate transmission of hepatitis B virus infection in the United States: recommendations of the Advisory Committee on Immunization Practices (ACIP); Part 1: Immunization of Infants, Children, and Adolescents, *MMWR* 54(RR-16):1-12, 2005.
†Recombivax HB or Engerix-B should be used for the birth dose. Comvax and Pediarix cannot be administered at birth or before age 6 weeks.
§Hepatitis B immune globulin (0.5 mL) administered intramuscularly in a separate site from vaccine.
¶The final dose in the vaccine series should not be administered before age 24 weeks (164 days).
**Mothers should have blood drawn and tested for HBsAg as soon as possible after admission for delivery; if the mother is found to be HBsAg positive, the infant should receive HBIG as soon as possible but no later than age 7 days.
††On a case-by-case basis and only in rare circumstances, the first dose may be delayed until after hospital discharge for an infant who weighs ≥2000 g and whose mother is HBsAg negative, but only if a physician's order to withhold the birth dose and a copy of the mother's original HBsAg-negative laboratory report are documented in the infant's medical record.

2. Hearing screening

The prevalence of congenital hearing loss is 2 to 3 per 1000 live births.[22] The rationale for early identification of hearing loss is to allow interventions that will optimize the infant's development and acquisition of language skills.[4,22]

Risk factors for hearing loss include[4]:

a. Family history of hereditary sensorineural hearing loss

b. History of cytomegalovirus, rubella, syphilis, herpes, or toxoplasmosis infection in utero

c. Craniofacial anomalies, including morphologic abnormalities of the pinnae and ear canals

d. Ototoxic medications, including aminoglycosides used in multiple courses or in combination with loop diuretics

e. Birth weight less than 1500 g, mechanical ventilation lasting 5 days or longer, and bacterial meningitis

A national public health goal outlined in *Healthy People 2010* is to "increase the proportion of newborns who are screened for hearing loss by age 1 month, have audiologic evaluation by age 3 months, and are enrolled in appropriate intervention by age 6 months."[22]

It is important for results of all screening tests performed in the newborn nursery to be documented on the infant's outpatient medical record after discharge, and to arrange appropriate follow-up for any abnormal results.

REFERENCES

1. 2005 American Heart Association guidelines for cardiopulmonary resuscitation and emergency cardiovascular care. Part 13: neonatal resuscitation guidelines, *Circulation* 112(suppl 1):188-195, 2005.

2. Anderson GC, Moore E, Hepworth J, Bergman N: Early skin-to-skin contact for mothers and their healthy newborn infants, *Cochrane Database Syst Rev* (2):CD003519, 2003.

3. Thilo EH, Rosenberg AA: The newborn infant. In Hay WW, Levin MJ, Sondheimer JM, Deterding RR, editors: *Current pediatric diagnosis and treatment,* ed 17, Norwalk, CT, 2005, Appleton & Lange.

4. American Academy of Pediatrics (and) the American College of Obstetricians and Gynecologists: Care of the neonate. *Guidelines for perinatal care,* ed 5, Elk Grove Village, IL and Washington, DC, 2002.

5. Centers for Disease Control and Prevention: *Birth defects.* Available at http://www.cdc.gov/node.do/id/0900f3ec8000dffe. Accessed January 13, 2007.

6. Lewan RB, Wood CR, Ambuel B: Problems of the newborn and infant. In Taylor RB, editor: *Family medicine principles and practice,* ed 6, New York, 2003, Springer-Verlag.

7. McIntire DD, Bloom SL, Casey BM et al: Birth weight in relation to morbidity and mortality among newborn infants, *N Engl J Med* 340:1234-1238, 1999.

8. Puckett RM, Offringa M: Prophylactic vitamin K for vitamin K deficiency bleeding in neonates, *Cochrane Database Syst Rev* (4):CD002776, 2000.

9. Souter AH: New aspects of vitamin K prophylaxis, *Semin Thromb Hemost* 29:373-376, 2003.

10. Hey E: Vitamin K—what, why, and when, *Arch Dis Child Fetal Neonatal Ed* 88:80-83, 2003.

11. D'Souza IE, Rao SD: Late hemorrhagic disease of newborn, *Indian Pediatr* 40:226-229, 2003.

12. Nock ML, Blumer JL: Therapeutic agents. *Fanaroll and Martin's neonatal-perinatal medicine: diseases of the fetus and infant,* ed 8, St. Louis, 2006, Mosby.

13. Hansen KN, Minousis M, Ebbesen F: Weekly oral vitamin K prophylaxis in Denmark, *Acta Paediatrica* 92:802-805, 2003.

14. O'Hara MA: Ophthalmia neonatorum, *Pediatr Rev* 40:715-725, 1993.

15. Foster A, Klauss V: Ophthalmia neonatorum in developing countries, *N Engl J Med* 332:600-601, 1995.

16. Chen JY: Prophylaxis of ophthalmia neonatorum: comparison of silver nitrate, tetracycline, erythromycin and no prophylaxis, *Pediatr Infect Dis J* 11:1026-1030, 1992.

17. Bausch LC: Newborn eye prophylaxis—where are we now? *Nebraska Med J* 78:383-384, 1993.

18. Centers for Disease Control and Prevention: A comprehensive immunization strategy to eliminate transmission of hepatitis B virus infection in the United States: recommendations of the Advisory Committee on Immunization Practices (ACIP); Part 1: Immunization of Infants, Children, and Adolescents, *MMWR* 54(RR-16):1-12, 2005.

19. Centers for Disease Control and Prevention: *Hepatitis B fact sheet, December 2006.* Available at: http://www.cdc.gov/ncidod/diseases/hepatitis/b/vaxfact.pdf. Accessed February 3, 2007.

20. Centers for Disease Control and Prevention, National Center for HIV/AIDS, Viral Hepatitis, STD, and TB Prevention: *Viral hepatitis B fact sheet.* Available at: http://www.cdc.gov/ncidod/diseases/hepatitis/b/fact.htm. Accessed February 3, 2007.

21. Centers for Disease Control and Prevention: *Recommended childhood and adolescent immunization schedule, U.S. 2007.* Published January 25, 2007. Available at: http://www.cdc.gov/vaccines/recs/schedules/downloads/child/2007/child-schedule-bw-print.pdf. Accessed February 7, 2007.

22. U.S. Department of Health and Human Services: *Healthy People* 2010, focus area 28, vision and hearing. Available at: http://www.healthypeople.gov/Document/HTML/Volume2/28Vision.htm#_Toc489325915. Accessed February 7, 2007.

S E C T I O N   B   Neonatal Resuscitation

Patricia Adam, MD, MSPH, and Patricia Fontaine, MD, MS

I. PREPARATION FOR RESUSCITATION

Overall, approximately 10% of all newborns will require resuscitation.[1] Even under the best of circumstances, instruments for scoring antepartum and intrapartum risk will not identify all infants at risk for adverse outcomes.[2] Family physicians who practice obstetrics should acquire and maintain skills in neonatal resuscitation so they can respond with confidence when called on to attend to an infant in unanticipated distress.

A. Anticipation

Anticipate the need for resuscitation in high-risk situations. See Chapter 12 for obstetric events associated with adverse newborn outcomes.

B. Assemble Team

Have one to two additional people present whose sole responsibility is the newborn. These individuals should be skilled or certified in neonatal resuscitation. The first person should be trained in all aspects of resuscitation, including endotracheal intubation and administration of medications. The second person is needed if the resuscitation becomes complicated; he or she should be able to assist with tactile stimulation, suctioning, bag and mask ventilation, or chest compressions.[1,3]

C. Equipment

Assemble and check necessary equipment (Table 19-4).

II. RESUSCITATION OF THE DEPRESSED INFANT

The AAP in collaboration with the American Heart Association has established the Neonatal Resuscitation Program (NRP).[1,4] The NRP consists of a series of well-ordered steps in which evaluation of the infant's respiratory effort, heart rate, and peripheral perfusion leads to decisions regarding appropriate actions. The impact of the NRP on neonatal health was evaluated using statewide data from Illinois; after widespread implementation of NRP training, the percentage of high-risk neonates with 1- and 5-minute Apgar scores greater than 7 increased by 1 to 2 percentage points.[5] The following is a summary based on the NRP recommendations.[1,4]

A. Initial Steps

1. Warm, dry, suction, and stimulate the infant during the first 30 seconds after delivery. For healthy newborns, this can be accomplished at the foot of the bed.
2. If necessary, place the infant, head toward you, under a preheated radiant warmer. If the neonate is born to a febrile mother, care should be taken to minimize persistent hyperthermia.[4]

TABLE 19-4 Preparation of Delivery Room Equipment

Procedure	Equipment	Preparation
Thermal protection	Radiant warmer Towel/blanket	Preheat warmer Warm towel/blanket
Clearing airway	Bulb syringe Mechanical suction Suction catheters: 5 or 6, 8, and 10 French	Set pressure to 100 mmHg
	For meconium infants: Laryngoscope (#0 and 1 straight blade) Endotracheal tubes (2.5, 3.0, 3.5, 4.0 mm) Stylet Endotracheal tube suction adapter	Attach appropriate size blade and check light
Positive-pressure ventilation	Oxygen tubing/flowmeter Resuscitation bag Mask Feeding tube, 8 French 20-ml syringe Endotracheal tube Stethoscope	Attach to bag; set at 5-L flow Check for function Select appropriate size On hand for gastric suction
Medications	Epinephrine 1:10,000 Sodium bicarbonate 0.5 mEq/ml Naloxone Volume expander Syringes and needles	Prepare medications in syringe Anticipate needing
Universal precautions	Gloves	

3. Position the infant's head so the airway is open. Suction the mouth and then the nose with a bulb syringe, removing mucus and amniotic fluid. A suction catheter attached to mechanical suction set at 100 mmHg may also be used.
4. Dry the infant with a warm towel, stimulating with vigorous strokes over the back. Remove the wet towel. Newborns lose body heat rapidly from wet skin, particularly given their large surface area-to-body mass ratio. Cold stress must be

avoided because it causes peripheral vasoconstriction and exacerbates metabolic acidosis.[1]

B. Rapid Assessment

Follow each assessment with the appropriate resuscitation steps outlined in Figure 19-2. Each intervention should last no more than 30 seconds, after which the newborn should be assessed again. If there is no improvement in respiratory effort, color, or heart rate, then move to the next level of resuscitation.[1]

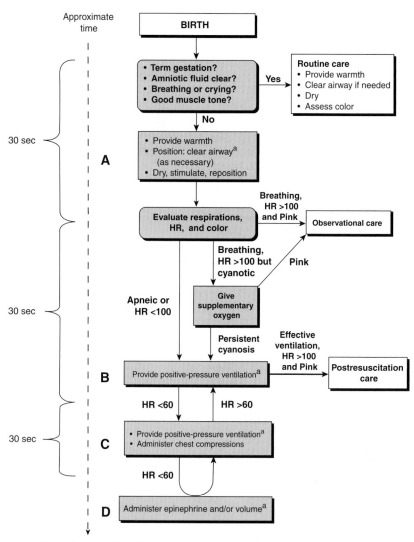

FIGURE 19-2. Overview of resuscitation in the delivery room. HR, Heart rate. (From Goldsmith JP: *Textbook of neonatal resuscitation,* ed 5, Elk Grove, IL, 2006, American Academy of Pediatrics.)

C. Bag and Mask Ventilation

Bag and mask ventilation is a simple and effective means of delivering positive-pressure ventilation with 100% oxygen that restores respiration in most moderately depressed newborns. Positive-pressure ventilation should be instituted immediately for the indications below. The longer it takes to restore spontaneous heart rate and breathing, the greater the likelihood of anoxic cerebral insult.[1]

1. Indications
   a. Heart rate less than 100 beats/min
   b. Absent or gasping respirations
2. Equipment
   a. Self-inflating bags: Bags such as neonatal Laerdal or Hope II are most commonly used. Check for connection to oxygen supply, oxygen reservoir (needed to deliver 100% oxygen to patient), and pressure relief or pop-off valve. The pop-off valve prevents pressures greater than 30 to 40 cm H_2O from being delivered to the infant, a precaution against pneumothorax.
   b. Masks: These should have cushioned rims for adapting to the contours of the face. Sizes are available for infants weighing 500 to 4500 g. Proper fit is achieved when the infant's nose and mouth, but not eyes, are covered by the mask.
   c. Oxygen: A metaanalysis of five studies comparing resuscitation with 100% O_2 to room air (RA) found that positive-pressure ventilation with RA is as good as 100% O_2. In term infants, the use of RA appears to shorten resuscitation time and decrease mortality from 9.8% to 5.9% (odds ratio [OR], 0.59; 95% confidence interval [CI], 0.40-0.87).[6] The 2006 revised NRP recommendations consider the pertinent evidence insufficient to recommend for the use of positive-pressure ventilation with RA and continue to recommend resuscitation with 100% O_2. If O_2 is not available, resuscitation should proceed with RA.[4]
3. Technique
   a. Position the infant with the neck slightly extended to open the airway in the "sniffing" position.
   b. Place the mask on the face to obtain a seal whereas avoiding pressure over the eyes or larynx.
   c. Ventilate by compressing the bag enough to achieve a visible, easy rise of the infant's chest. Remember that the first breath requires more

pressure than subsequent breaths. If there is difficulty getting the infant's chest to rise, check for the following problems:
   i. Presence of an air leak around the mask from improper size or positioning
   ii. Excessive secretions blocking the airway
   iii. An equipment malfunction, such as a pop-off valve stuck in the open position
   d. Continue to ventilate 40 to 60 times per minute. Effective ventilation is best confirmed by an increasing heart rate; after 30 seconds of positive-pressure ventilation, an assistant should report the heart rate.
   e. If bag and mask ventilation is needed for more than a few minutes, insert an orogastric tube to evacuate air that accumulates in the stomach, which could potentially compromise diaphragmatic excursion. Tape the tube in place and leave it open for continued air release.
   f. Discontinue ventilation when the heart rate is greater than 100 beats/min, spontaneous respirations have returned, and central cyanosis is improving.

D. Chest Compressions

Chest compressions are required for severe depression. This step should be instituted only after ventilation has been established, because chest compression in the absence of ventilation is of little, if any, value.[1,4]

1. Indications: heart rate less than 60 beats/min, despite 30 seconds of positive-pressure ventilation
2. Technique
   a. Hand position: The preferred method is to encircle the infant's chest with both hands, placing the two thumbs over the sternum below the nipple line and above the xiphoid process. If access to the umbilical vein is needed, the resuscitator can perform cardiopulmonary resuscitation with the index and middle fingers of one hand compressing the sternum in the same location.[1,4]
   b. Technique: The sternum should be depressed one third the anteroposterior diameter of the chest at a rate of 90 compressions per minute. For the thumb technique, pressure should be exerted vertically by flexing both thumbs at the proximal interphalangeal joint.
   c. Use of bag and mask: Bag and mask ventilation at 30 breaths/min (the addition of chest compressions decreases the amount of time available for ventilations) should accompany the compressions in a 1:3 ratio.

d. Chest compressions: After 30 seconds of chest compressions and ventilations, assess the pulse. Chest compressions may be discontinued when the heart rate is more than 60 beats/min.

E. Endotracheal Intubation

Endotracheal intubation offers more control over ventilation and eliminates the concern that air will enter the infant's stomach but requires more skill than bag and mask ventilation.[1,7] A study of neonatal resuscitation teams composed of residents, neonatal fellows, and neonatologists in a tertiary care hospital found that, on average, the team successfully intubated the neonate 50% of the time.[7] As a result, the Cochrane Collaboration has designed a protocol to review the literature comparing endotracheal intubation and bag and mask ventilation.[8] Other preliminary data suggest that laryngeal mask airways may be a reasonable alternative for failed intubations; the NRP currently does not support the routine use of laryngeal mask airways.[4]

1. Indications
   a. Ineffective or prolonged bag and mask ventilation
   b. Tracheal suctioning for the depressed infant born through meconium-stained amniotic fluid (MSAF)
   c. Anticipated need for longer-term ventilation (e.g., birth weight <1000 g)
   d. Possible access route for administering medications during resuscitation
   e. An infant with a known diaphragmatic hernia
2. Personnel and equipment
   a. Two people are needed—one to intubate and ventilate, and one to assist in managing equipment and confirming proper tube placement by listening to the infant's lungs.
   b. A laryngoscope with a straight blade, size 1 (term) or 0 (preterm), should be tested and in good working order. A spare lightbulb should always be available.
   c. Endotracheal tubes (2.5-4.0 mm in internal diameter) should be available. A 3.5- or 4.0-mm tube works well for most infants more than 38 gestational weeks or 3000 g. Stylets are often used to stiffen the tube. The stylet must be secured so that its tip does not extend beyond the tube itself.
   d. A suction catheter of appropriate caliber for the endotracheal tube should be available. The catheter is connected to mechanical suction set at a maximum of 100 mmHg.

3. Technique
   a. Regarding timing, data from videotaped intubations found that mean time to intubate ranged from 23.6 to 31.9 seconds. No infant decompensated between 20 and 30 seconds, suggesting that 30 seconds is a realistic and also a safe goal.[7]
   b. Preoxygenate with 100% O_2 and maintain a source of 100% free-flow O_2 near the neonate's mouth while intubating.
   c. Position the infant with the head slightly extended to open the airway. A small towel roll behind the infant's shoulders may be helpful. Hyperextension moves the trachea forward and makes landmarks difficult to visualize.
   d. With the laryngoscope in the left hand (for both left- and right-handed individuals), advance the blade carefully over the infant's tongue until the glottis is visualized. Use a lifting motion in the direction of the scope handle rather than a lever-like motion, which places undue pressure on the infant's maxilla. Have an assistant put gentle pressure over the larynx, which may help bring the glottis into view in difficult circumstances.
   e. When properly positioned, the tip of the blade will be either in the vallecula behind the epiglottis, or over the epiglottis, with the vocal cords clearly in view.
   f. Insert the endotracheal tube by advancing it gently from the right side of the infant's mouth. A common mistake is to advance the tube through the center of the laryngoscope blade, preventing direct visualization of the intubation. The clinician should be able to see the endotracheal tube pass directly through the vocal cords.
   g. The depth of insertion should be midway between the vocal cords and carina. To assist in proper placement, most endotracheal tubes now have a dark line marked near the tip (vocal cord guide) that should be positioned at the level of the cords.
   h. Shorten the endotracheal tube so that less than 4 cm extends from the lips and tape it into place.
   i. Attach a ventilation bag to the endotracheal tube and deliver positive-pressure ventilations (but not if meconium is present). Look for a rise in the infant's chest and listen for bilateral breath sounds in the axilla to ensure proper endotracheal tube position. A CO_2 detector can be helpful in confirming proper position as well.[1,4,9]

F. Drugs and Volume Expansion

Drugs for neonatal resuscitation are given for the following indications. The dosages and routes of administration are summarized in Table 19-5.[1,4]

1. Bradycardia or cardiac arrest
   Epinephrine is indicated when the heart rate is less than 60 beats/min and does not respond to oxygen, positive-pressure ventilation, and 30 seconds of chest compressions.
   Epinephrine, 1:10,000 solution in doses of 0.01 to 0.03 mg/kg, is administered rapidly intravenously via umbilical vein catheter. Delivery via the endotracheal tube used to be an option, but has never been studied and may likely be ineffective. The 2006 NRP no longer recommends endotracheal administration, although one may consider administering epinephrine endotracheally at a greater dose (0.1 mg/kg) while establishing intravenous access.[4]

2. Hypovolemia
   The neonate may develop low intravascular volume as a result of sepsis, hemorrhage, placental abruption, or maternal shock.
   Treatment consists of volume expansion with normal saline or lactated Ringer's solution, given through an umbilical catheter. The initial bolus of 10 ml/kg over 5 to 10 minutes can be repeated if necessary. Whole blood may be used for volume replacement in situations where fetal blood loss is suspected.[1,4]

3. Acidosis
   Acidosis is the ultimate outcome of ineffective cardiopulmonary function in the depressed neonate. Current standards are to treat acidosis as a last resort, after prolonged resuscitation.
   Sodium bicarbonate should be used only after ventilation, chest compressions, epinephrine, and possibly fluids have been administered. In these rare instances, sodium bicarbonate, 4.2% solution, can be given (1 mEq/kg/min intravenously).[1]

4. Narcotic-induced respiratory depression
   Narcotic analgesics administered to the mother before delivery can result in poor respiratory effort and decreased tone in the newborn.
   NRP no longer recommends administration of naloxone during the initial steps of resuscitation.[4] Naloxone may be indicated if resuscitation using positive-pressure ventilation has failed to reverse respiratory depression in a neonate whose mother was treated within the last 4 hours with a narcotic. Treatment consists of naloxone hydrochloride (1 mg/ml solution) given intravenously or intramuscularly. Endotracheal administration is no longer recommended because of lack of data.[4] If effective, the infant must be observed for rebound narcotic-induced respiratory depression because the effect of the narcotic typically outlasts that of the naloxone.[1,4]

G. Unsuccessful Resuscitation Attempts

Consider the following causes if the infant does not respond to resuscitation:

1. Airway obstruction caused by a plug of meconium or mucus
2. Choanal atresia—congenital obstruction of the posterior nasopharynx
3. Robin syndrome—micrognathia with the tongue obstructing the posterior pharynx
4. Pneumothorax, tension pneumothorax, or pleural effusion
5. Diaphragmatic hernia

Resuscitation is rarely successful after 10 minutes of asystole and should be discontinued if there are no signs of life.[4]

III. MANAGEMENT OF MECONIUM-STAINED AMNIOTIC FLUID

A. Background and Epidemiology

1. Meconium-stained amniotic fluid (MSAF)
   MSAF traditionally has been regarded as a sign of fetal distress because the passage of meconium can result from hypoxia and subsequent parasympathetic stimulation of the fetal gut and anal sphincter.[10] Passage of meconium is not always a sign of fetal distress, however. In mature fetuses, physiologic activation of the vagal system may be responsible for meconium passage in the absence of distress. MSAF is present in 10% to 15% of pregnancies at 40 weeks, compared with 25% to 30% at 41 weeks.[11]

2. Meconium aspiration syndrome (MAS)
   About 2% to 36% of infants born through MSAF go on to experience development of MAS.[12] MAS is defined as respiratory distress in a neonate born through MSAF with symptoms that have no alternative explanation[12] and is often associated with characteristic radiologic findings.[13] Fortunately, the incidence and mortality of MAS has declined since the mid-1970s, with some of the reduction attributable to the decrease in deliveries beyond 41 weeks.[3,14]

TABLE 19-5 Medications for Neonatal Resuscitation

Medication	Concentration to Administer	Preparation	Dosage/Route	Weight	Total Dose	Total Dose/ Infant	Rate/Precautions
Epinephrine	1:10,000	1 ml	0.1-0.3 ml/kg IV	1 kg 2 kg 3 kg 4 kg		0.1-0.3 ml 0.2-0.6 ml 0.3-0.9 ml 0.4-1.2 ml	Give rapidly If give via ET, then use 0.3-1 ml/kg in 3- to 5-ml syringe
Volume expanders	Normal saline Whole blood	40 ml	10 ml/kg IV	1 kg 2 kg 3 kg 4 kg		10 ml 20 ml 30 ml 40 ml	Give over 5-10 minutes
Sodium bicarbonate	0.5 mEq/ml (4.2% solution)	20-ml or two 10-ml prefilled syringes	2 mEq/kg IV	1 kg 2 kg 3 kg 4 kg	2 mEq 4 mEq 6 mEq 8 mEq	4 ml 8 ml 12 ml 16 ml	Give slowly, no faster than 1 mEq/kg/min Give only if infant is being effectively ventilated
Naloxone hydrochloride	1 mg/ml	1 ml	0.1 mg/kg IV, IM	1 kg 2 kg 3 kg 4 kg	0.1 mg 0.2 mg 0.3 mg 0.4 mg	0.1 ml 0.2 ml 0.3 ml 0.4 ml	Give only in rare cases Give rapidly IV preferred IM acceptable

Modified from Bloom RS, Cropley C: *Textbook of neonatal resuscitation*, Dallas, TX, 1996, American Heart Association.
ET, Endotracheal; IM, intramuscularly; IV, intravenously.

B. Recognition and Characterization of Meconium in Amniotic Fluid

1. At-risk pregnancies

   MAS is not caused exclusively by the aspiration of meconium in the intrapartum period, but rather by a combination of peripartum or chronic in utero stressors on the fetus. The literature is conflicting, and the exact cause for MAS has yet to be determined.[3,13,15-18] Multiple observational studies have documented associations/risk factors for MAS that include thick meconium,[13,18] intrapartum fetal heart rate abnormalities,[13,16-18] low pH,[16] and the need for resuscitation.[17]

   To prepare for possible MAS, consider amniotomy during labor in at-risk pregnancies, such as postdates, intrauterine growth restriction, and fetal heart rate abnormalities.

2. Consistency of the meconium-stained fluid

   a. Thin meconium: This results when relatively small amounts of meconium are well dispersed throughout the amniotic fluid. The fluid is slightly discolored, but no solid particles are visible.

   b. Thick meconium: Moderately thick meconium is opaque fluid without particles. Thick meconium is both opaque and particulate, often likened to "pea soup." The thicker the meconium, the greater the risk for development of MAS. In a study of 2094 infants born through MSAF, the odds of developing MAS with thick meconium were nearly 10 times that with thin meconium (OR, 9.85; 95% CI, 4.4-22.1).[13]

C. Management

1. Intrapartum management for MSAF

   a. Fetal monitoring: Continuous fetal monitoring is the preferred method for monitoring labors with thick meconium (see Chapter 14, Section E).

   b. Amnioinfusion: Evidence regarding the effectiveness of amnioinfusion is conflicting, and outcomes vary depending on the population studied.[19-21] (See Chapter 18, Section C regarding amnioinfusions for significant variable decelerations.)

      i. A 2002 Cochrane review recommended amnioinfusion for labors complicated by thick MSAF based on a meta-analysis of 12 trials that showed a decrease in MAS by at least 50% (N = 1877; RR, 0.24; 95% CI, 0.12-0.48).[20]

      ii. A 2005 randomized controlled trial (RCT) by Fraser and colleagues[21] contradicted these results, finding no difference in MAS among 1998 women with labors complicated by thick meconium who were randomized to amnioinfusion versus usual care (RR of MAS, 1.39; 95% CI, 0.88-2.19). The discrepancy in findings may be explained by different risk levels for MAS. In the RCT, neonates were at lower risk for stressors associated with MAS, fetal monitoring was universal, and the cesarean section rate was approximately 30%.

      iii. In U.S. settings where labors are monitored closely and cesarean deliveries are common, amnioinfusion offers little benefit to the neonate and should no longer be recommended.

2. Neonatal management according to NRP

   a. Perineal suctioning: Based on the negative findings of an RCT comparing oropharyngeal suctioning at the perineum with no suctioning in 2514 neonates born through MSAF, perineal suctioning is no longer recommended.[4,22]

   b. Vigorous infant: This is defined as having a heart rate of more than 100 beats/min, spontaneous respiration, and some movement including extremity flexion—the 1-minute Apgar score will be 8 or greater, and routine assessment and care are the only steps needed. Intubation and endotracheal suction are not necessary unless subsequent respiratory distress develops.

   c. Signs of distress at delivery: If there are any signs of distress, the newborn should be intubated and endotracheal suction performed.

   d. Endotracheal suctioning: The procedure is repeated with reintubation and suctioning until the returns from the trachea are free of meconium. If at any point the infant develops profound bradycardia and central cyanosis, the resuscitator may need to give positive-pressure ventilation, despite the fact that not all the meconium has been cleared.

IV. SOR A RECOMMENDATION

RECOMMENDATION	REFERENCE
Neonates born through MSAF who are not vigorous should be intubated and suctioned (if meconium is present below the cords) to decrease the risk for MAS.	23

REFERENCES

1. Katwinkel J: *Textbook of neonatal resuscitation,* ed 4, Dallas, TX, 2000, American Heart Association/American Academy of Pediatrics.
2. Leeman L, Leeman R: Do all hospitals need cesarean delivery capacity? An outcomes study of maternity care in a rural hospital without on-site cesarean capability, *J Fam Pract* 51(2): 129-134, 1992.
3. Hermansen MC, Hermansen MG: Pitfalls in neonatal resuscitation, *Clin Perinatol* 32:77-95, 2005.
4. 2005 American Heart Association guidelines for cardiopulmonary resuscitation and emergency cardiovascular care. Part 13: neonatal resuscitation guidelines, *Circulation* 112(suppl 1): 188-195, 2005.
5. Patel D, Piotrowski ZH, Nelson MR et al: Effect of a statewide neonatal resuscitation training program on Apgar scores among high-risk neonates in Illinois, *Pediatrics* 107(4): 648-655, 2001.
6. Saugstad OD, Ramji S, Vento M: Resuscitation of depressed newborn infants with ambient air or pure oxygen: a meta-analysis, *Biol Neonate* 87(1):27-34, 2005.
7. Lane B, Finer N, Rich W: Duration of intubation attempts during neonatal resuscitation, *Pediatrics* 145(1):67-70, 2004.
8. O'Donnell CPF, Davis PG, Morley CJ: Endotracheal intubation versus face mask for newborns resuscitated with positive pressure ventilation at birth. (Protocol), *Cochrane Database Syst Rev* (4). Art. No.: CD004948. DOI: 10.1002/14651858. CD004948, 2004.
9. Finer NN, Rich WD: Neonatal resuscitation: raising the bar, *Curr Opin Pediatr* 16:157-162, 2004.
10. Gabbe SG, Niebyl JR, Simpson JL, editors: *Obstetrics: normal and problem pregnancies,* ed 4, New York, 2002, Churchill Livingstone.
11. Sedaghatian MR, Othman L, Hossain MM et al: Risk of meconium-stained amniotic fluid in different ethnic groups, *J Perinatol* 4:275-261, 2000.
12. Cleary GM, Wiswell TE: Meconium-stained amniotic fluid and the meconium aspiration syndrome: an update, *Pediatr Clin North Am* 45:511-529, 1998.
13. Wiswell TE, Gannon CM, Jacob J et al: Delivery room management of the apparently vigorous meconium-stained neonate: results of the multicenter, international collaborative trial, *Pediatrics* 105:1-7, 2000.
14. Yoder BA, Kirsch EA, Barth WH et al: Changing obstetric practices associated with decreasing incidence of meconium aspiration syndrome, *Obstet Gynecol* 99:731-739, 2002.
15. Blackwell SC, Moldenhauer J, Hassan AA et al: Meconium aspiration syndrome in term neonates with normal acid-base status at delivery: is it different? *Am J Obstet Gynecol* 184: 1422-1426, 2001.
16. Paz Y, Solt I, Zimmer EZ: Variables associated with meconium aspiration syndrome in labors with thick meconium, *Eur J Obstet Gynecol Reprod Biol* 94:27-30, 2001.
17. Meydanli MM, Dilbaz B, Caliskan E et al: Risk factors for meconium aspiration syndrome in infants born through thick meconium, *Int J Gynecol Obstet* 72:9-15, 2001.
18. Liu WF, Harrington T: Delivery room risk factors for meconium aspiration syndrome, *Am J Perinatol* 19(7):367-377, 2002.
19. Institute for Clinical Systems Improvement (ICSI): *Intrapartum fetal heart rate management,* Bloomington, MN, 2004, ICSI.
20. Hofmeyer GJ: Amnioinfusion for meconium-stained liquor in labour, *Cochrane Database Syst Rev* (1):CD000014, 2002.
21. Fraser WD, Hofmeyr J, Lede R et al: Amnioinfusion for the prevention of the meconium aspiration syndrome, *N Engl J Med* 353(9):909-917, 2005.
22. Vain NE, Szyld EG, Prudent LM et al: Oropharyngeal and nasopharyngeal suctioning of meconium-stained neonates before delivery of their shoulders: multicentre, randomised controlled trial, *Lancet* 364:597-602, 2004.
23. Halliday HL, Sweet D: Endotracheal intubation at birth for preventing morbidity and mortality in vigorous, meconium-stained infants born at term, *Cochrane Database Syst Rev* (1). Art. No.: CD000500. DOI: 10.1002/14651858. CD000500, 2001.

S ECTION C Neonatal Circumcision

Patricia Fontaine, MD, MS

Newborn circumcision is surgical removal of the foreskin (prepuce) from the penis. It is a common procedure in the United States, performed largely for cultural and religious reasons. The question whether circumcision conveys medical benefits sufficient to outweigh risks and costs has sparked decades of debate.[1]

In 1999, the AAP issued a policy statement concluding that existing scientific evidence is not sufficient to recommend routine neonatal circumcision, that the procedure is not essential to an infant's well-being, and that parents should be the ones to decide in their son's best interest.[2]

International observational studies and clinical trials, mostly in Africa, have shown that circumcised men acquire human immunodeficiency virus (HIV) infection at lower rates than uncircumcised, demonstrating a substantial public health benefit in those settings, where HIV prevalence is high and heterosexual acquisition is common.[3-7] Studies are under way to evaluate the potential value and risk-benefit profile of circumcision as an HIV prevention strategy in the United States.[3]

I. EPIDEMIOLOGY

A. U.S. Circumcisions during the Mid-Twentieth Century

At the peak of its acceptance between the late 1940s and the early 1970s, up to 1.5 million newborn circumcisions were performed annually, and in some U.S. hospitals, 85% to 90% of male infants were circumcised.[8]

B. Trends during the Late Twentieth Century

Circumcision rates remained relatively stable from 1979 to 1999, with approximately two thirds of male newborns being circumcised before hospital discharge (65% in 1999).[9]

C. Variation by Geography, Race, and Religion

1. Geographic variation
   Circumcision rates in the United States are greater in the Midwest (81%) than in the Northeast (66%), South (64%), or West (37%).[9]
2. Ethnic differences
   In 1999, because of decreases in circumcisions for white Americans and an increase among African Americans, the rates were approximately 65% for both races.[9] For Hispanic Americans, the circumcision rate has been reported to be 54%.[10]
3. Religious practices
   Jewish and Muslim religious teachings stipulate newborn circumcision.[1]

II. RISKS, BENEFITS, AND INFORMED CONSENT

Ideally, the family physician should discuss the potential risks and benefits of circumcision with one or both parents before the birth. Prenatal visits are an opportune time for this discussion.

A. Physician's Role

The physician's role regarding circumcision is to:
1. Provide accurate and unbiased information for parents' decisions
2. Support the decision once it is made
3. Perform the circumcision with skill, utilizing appropriate analgesia

B. Risks versus Benefits

A comprehensive review of hospital-based neonatal circumcisions in Washington State evaluated the complication rate in relation to potential benefits and concluded that six urinary tract infections can be prevented for every complication that occurs; almost two complications can be expected for every case of penile cancer prevented.[11] Table 19-6 summarizes the indications, contraindications, benefits, and risks of routine neonatal circumcision, together with the supporting evidence.

III. ANALGESIA

A. Rationale

Effective analgesia decreases the physiologic stress responses newborns would otherwise experience during circumcision, including crying, changes in heart rate and blood pressure, decreased oxygen saturation, and increased serum cortisol levels.[1]

The importance of pain control for newborn circumcision is highlighted by the AAP's 1999 Circumcision Policy Statement, which states, "Analgesia is safe and effective in reducing the procedural pain… and should be provided if neonatal circumcision is performed."[2]

B. Options for Pain Management

Several options are available for managing procedural and postoperative pain from newborn circumcision. Methods may be used in combination, for example, oral sucrose plus dorsal penile nerve block (DPNB).

1. DPNB (with 1% lidocaine)
   DPNB blocks the dorsal penile nerves as they exit from beneath the symphysis pubis, providing anesthesia of the foreskin, glans, and distal penile shaft. The DPNB technique is presented in the next section. Risks and benefits are presented in Table 19-7.
   DPNB is the most thoroughly studied method for managing the pain of neonatal circumcision. Several small RCTs have confirmed the effectiveness of DPNB in achieving decreased crying, smaller increases in heart rate, smaller decreases in oxygen saturation, and lower serum cortisol levels than placebo injections or no analgesia.[1,12]
   DPNB carries a low risk for minor side effects, the most common being ecchymosis or brief bleeding at the injection site.[13]
2. Ring block
   "Ring block" is the term for local infiltration of 1% lidocaine (Xylocaine) in a circumferential ring around the penis, either at the base or midshaft. One RCT (N = 52 infants) found ring block to be equivalent to DPNB and eutectic mixture of local

TABLE 19-6 Newborn Circumcision: Risks and Benefits

	Comments
Indications for Circumcision	
Religious belief	Jewish and Muslim religions have stipulations regarding circumcision.
Strong parental preference	
Contraindications to Circumcision	
Medically unstable infant	Delay circumcision until the infant is stable.
Preterm infant	Delay circumcision until infant is ready for discharge.
Genital anomalies—hypospadias, webbed penis, congenital megalourethra	With hypospadias, the foreskin may be needed for later surgical correction.
Abnormal bleeding or family history of bleeding disorder	Check appropriate coagulation studies before circumcision.
Potential Risks*	
Pain and behavioral changes	The central nervous system pain pathways are well developed in newborns. Heart rate, blood pressure, cortisol levels, and crying all increase during circumcision; use of local anesthesia can blunt these effects.
Hemorrhage	Bleeding requiring treatment occurs in approximately 0.1% of circumcisions.[13] Typical management includes direct pressure and use of hemostatic agents (silver nitrate, absorbable gelatin or cellulose products). If bleeding skin edges are widely separated, circumferential sutures may be needed.
Infection	The true incidence of infection is unknown. Minor erythema or yellowish crusting occurs not uncommonly during healing.
Removal of too much or too little skin	A poor cosmetic result can be avoided with careful attention to technique. Identify the coronal sulcus and aim to remove skin 1-2 mm distal to that landmark. Avoid excessive traction on the foreskin, which can pull skin from the penile shaft into the cone or bell.
Foreskin adhesions, skin bridges	Make sure the tissue plane between foreskin and glans is completely developed before removing the foreskin.
Retained plastic bell apparatus	The plastic bell should be removed after 7 days if it has not dropped off spontaneously. Rarely, prolonged attachment may result in urosepsis or formation of a permanent sulcus.
Potential Benefits	
Reduced risk for penile cancer	Penile cancer is rare, 9-10 cases per year per 1 million U.S. men.[1] Invasive penile cancer is associated with being uncircumcised (relative risk, >3), with phimosis, and with human papillomavirus infection.
Reduced incidence of urinary tract infection	The risk for uncircumcised infants is 4 to 10 times greater than circumcised infants.[1,22] Most of the excess risk occurs in infants <12 months old. The absolute risk rate of urinary tract infection in an uncircumcised infant is 1%.
Reduced risk for STDs/HIV infection	Behavioral factors are more important than circumcision status in acquiring STDs. Conclusions from studies are conflicting and vary by disease; however, noncircumcised status appears to be a risk factor for syphilis and HIV.[5]
Avoiding circumcision later in life	Conditions requiring circumcision later in life are uncommon: Phimosis (nonretractable foreskin)—90% of uncircumcised male infants will have a fully retractable foreskin by age 5 years. Paraphimosis (retracted foreskin trapped behind the glans) may occur in elderly men requiring bladder catheterization. Balanitis (infection of the glans and foreskin) is more common in uncircumcised boys and men.[6]

*Most complications are minor. Overall incidence rate of complications is approximately 0.2% to 0.6%.[1]
HIV, Human immunodeficiency virus; STD, sexually transmitted disease.

TABLE 19-7 Risks and Benefits of Anesthesia for Newborn Circumcision

	Comments
Risks	
Bleeding from injection site: ecchymosis or hematoma at injection site	Bleeding and ecchymosis are usually of minor degree; incidence rate of small ecchymosis is 10% in a series of dorsal penile nerve blocks
Methemoglobinemia	Rare; may be induced by a variety of local anesthetics; presents with cyanosis and decreased oxygen saturation
Transient penile ischemia	Theoretic; not reported in newborn circumcision with local anesthesia
Lidocaine toxicity: cardiac arrhythmias, seizures	Theoretic; should not occur if dosage is kept within guidelines and intravascular injection is avoided
Benefits	
During circumcision procedure: 1. Less crying 2. Better transcutaneous oxygen levels 3. Smaller increases in heart rate, blood pressure	Overall, local anesthesia has been shown to reduce pain and stress of newborn circumcision (most studies have involved the dorsal penile nerve block)
After surgery: 1. Cortisol levels less indicative of stress 2. Less interference in infant's behavioral state and sleep patterns 3. Less interference in maternal-infant interaction	Behavioral changes are transient; have not been documented beyond 24 hours after the procedure

anesthetics (EMLA) cream in reducing infant crying and more effective than either in minimizing heart rate changes during lysis of foreskin adhesions.[14]

3. Distal branch block

Injecting lidocaine at the junction the glans and the penile shaft is termed "distal branch block" or simply "local anesthesia." Distal block has been tested against DPNB in one randomized trial (N = 30 infants) and found to be associated with significantly smaller increases in heart rate, less time crying, and lower serum cortisol levels.[15]

Caution is warranted because distal injections can distort anatomic landmarks, making the circumcision procedure more difficult and, in some cases, leading to unsatisfactory cosmetic results.[16]

4. Topical anesthesia

A mixture of 2.5% lidocaine and 2.5% prilocaine, known as EMLA cream (AstraZeneca, Wilmington, DE), has been shown to be effective in reducing overall infant crying and heart rate changes when compared with placebo.[17] EMLA cream is not as effective as DPNB in reducing pain responses.[18] Approximately 1 to 2 g EMLA cream is applied to the distal half of the penis and secured with an occlusive dressing 60 to 90 minutes before the procedure.[17,18]

5. Sucrose solution on a pacifier

This has been shown to reduce signs of pain during circumcision with the Gomco clamp.[19]

6. Acetaminophen

This can be given after the circumcision to decrease pain responses such as crying during diaper changes.[20,21]

C. Technique of Dorsal Penile Nerve Block

The DPNB technique is as follows[22]:

1. Assemble the necessary equipment: a 1-ml tuberculin syringe, a 31- to 33-gauge needle, and 1% lidocaine without epinephrine.

2. Prepare the penis and the prepubic skin with a topical surgical scrub.

3. Draw 0.8 ml of 1% lidocaine into the tuberculin syringe; 3 to 4 mg/kg may be used for more precise dosing.

4. Stabilize the penis by gentle traction with one hand.

5. Identify the two injection sites at the base of the penis. They will be at the 10 and 2 o'clock

positions, 0.5 to 1.0 cm distal to the point where the penile root passes under the pubic symphysis.

6. Pierce the skin with the needle at an acute angle, directed slightly downward. A depth of 1 to 3 mm is required to reach the appropriate fascial layer superficial to the corpora cavernosa.
7. Check that the tip of the needle is freely mobile (i.e., not embedded in the corpus cavernosum).
8. Aspirate to ensure against intravascular injection.
9. Inject 0.4 ml lidocaine, or half the total calculated dose of lidocaine.
10. Repeat the injection at the second site.
11. Allow 3 to 5 minutes for the block to take effect.

IV. CIRCUMCISION TECHNIQUES

Clamp techniques (e.g., Gomco or Mogen) and Plastibell device (Hollister, Libertyville, IL) all achieve good results with appropriate patient selection,

attention to asepsis, and careful surgical technique.[23] The Gomco technique may take nearly twice as long as the Mogen technique.[19]

A. Steps for Circumcision with the Gomco Clamp

Steps for circumcision with the Gomco clamp (Figure 19-3) are as follows[23]:

1. Set up the sterile circumcision tray; check all equipment.
2. Identify anatomic landmarks; consider marking the coronal sulcus with sterile pen.
3. Grasp the rim of the foreskin at 10 and 2 o'clock positions with curved mosquito hemostats.
4. Insert a blunt-tipped probe or straight hemostat under the foreskin to the coronal sulcus. Sweep the probe or hemostat over the glans penis, freeing the foreskin from the glans.
5. Make the crush line for the dorsal slit by inserting one blade of a straight hemostat under the

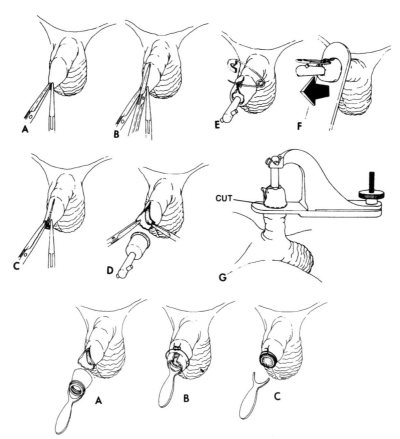

FIGURE 19-3. Two common techniques for newborn circumcision. *Top,* Using the Gomco clamp. *Bottom,* Using the plastic bell.

foreskin at the 12 o'clock position, to within a few millimeters of the corona. One technique is to slide the hemostat blade all the way to the corona and then withdraw it by one third of the total distance. Close the hemostat and remove after a few seconds.

6. Cut the dorsal slit along the crush line with scissors.
7. Retract the foreskin to expose the entire glans and coronal sulcus. Break down any remaining adhesions with the probe or a 4 × 4 gauze pad.
8. Insert a properly sized cone over the glans. Cones of 1.1 or 1.3 cm are usually appropriate for term infants.
9. Draw the foreskin back over the cone, bring the two edges of the dorsal slit together, and secure with a sterile safety pin.
10. Bring the safety pin up parallel with the shaft of the cone. Use the pin to draw the foreskin through the hole in the Gomco base plate. (An alternative technique is to use a curved mosquito hemostat to approximate the edges of the dorsal slit and guide the foreskin through the base plate.)
11. Hook the Gomco top plate under the arms of the cone and position it properly over the base plate.
12. Check landmarks.
    a. Is there a symmetric cuff of foreskin above the base plate?
    b. Is the entire length of the dorsal slit visible above the base plate?
13. Attach the nut to the bolt on the base plate and fasten firmly. Many authorities recommend waiting 5 minutes to ensure hemostasis.
14. Excise the foreskin just above the base plate, holding the scalpel nearly parallel to the plate.
15. Unfasten the nut and remove the upper and lower plates.
16. Gently brush the crushed skin line off the cone with gauze and remove the cone.
17. Cover the glans with petroleum jelly or precut petrolatum gauze.

B. Steps for Circumcision with the Plastibell Device

Steps for circumcision with the Plastibell device are as follows[23]:

1. Free adhesions and make a dorsal slit as in preceding steps 1 through 6.
2. Place the plastic cone inside the foreskin. It should fit snugly but without pressure on the glans. The

groove in the cone should lie beyond the apex of the dorsal slit.

3. If the cone catches on the frenulum, use scissors to shape the lower edge of the cone to fit.
4. Hold the foreskin firmly over the cone and tie a suture around the cone to compress the foreskin into the groove.
5. Trim off the foreskin distal to the ligature with tissue scissors.
6. Break off the disposable cone handle.

C. Steps for Circumcision with the Mogen Clamp

Steps for circumcision with the Mogen clamp are as follows[23]:

1. Identify anatomic landmarks.
2. Free adhesions with probe or straight forceps.
3. Pull an appropriate length of foreskin beyond the tip of the glans.
4. Apply Mogen clamp distal to the tip of the glans and tighten.
5. Excise foreskin with scalpel.
6. Use gentle pressure to expose the tip of the glans.

V. POSTCIRCUMCISION CARE

A. Circumcisions Performed with Gomco or Mogen Clamps

1. Observe carefully for 1 to 2 hours for any signs of excessive bleeding.
2. Apply petroleum jelly to the glans and reapply with each diaper change.
3. The infant will usually urinate normally within 6 to 8 hours after the procedure; it is not necessary to delay hospital discharge to document voiding.
4. Parents should expect the tip of the penis to appear red and have slight yellowish coating initially, but to report frank bleeding or signs of infection. The healing process will take 7 to 10 days.

B. Circumcisions Performed with the Plastibell Device

1. The cone and ligature should not be disturbed; they will fall off spontaneously in 5 to 8 days. The cone should be removed if it remains in place beyond that time.
2. Parents should report any persistent bleeding or signs of infection.

VI. SOR A RECOMMENDATIONS

RECOMMENDATIONS	REFERENCES
In populations where HIV prevalence is great and heterosexual acquisition is common, circumcision is associated with a decreased risk for acquiring HIV infection.	4-6
An effective method for local analgesia should be used for neonatal circumcision to decrease stress responses and alleviate pain.	12, 14-18

REFERENCES

1. Alanis MC, Lucidi RS: Neonatal circumcision: a review of the world's oldest and most controversial operation, *Obstet Gynecol Surv* 59:379-395, 2004.
2. American Academy of Pediatrics, Task Force on Circumcision: Circumcision Policy Statement, *Pediatrics* 103:686-693, 1999.
3. Department of Health and Human Services, Center for Disease Control and Prevention: *Male circumcision and risk for HIV transmission: implications for the United States, December 2006.* Available at: http://www.cdc.gov/hiv/resources/factsheets/circumcision.htm. Accessed January 7, 2007.
4. Weiss HA, Quigley MA, Hayes R: Male circumcision and risk of HIV infection in sub-Saharan Arica: a systematic review and meta-analysis, *AIDS* 14:2361-2370, 2000.
5. Siegfried N, Muller M, Volmink J et al: Male circumcision for prevention of heterosexual acquisition of HIV in men, *Cochrane Database Syst Rev* (3):CD003362, 2003.
6. Auvert B, Taljaard D, Lagarde E et al: Randomized, controlled intervention trial of male circumcision for reduction of HIV infection risk: the ANRS 1265 Trial, *PLoS Med* 2:e298, 2005.
7. National Institutes of Health, National Institute of Allergy and Infectious Diseases: *Adult male circumcision significantly reduces risk of acquiring HIV, December 13, 2006.* Available at: http://www3.niaid.nih.gov/news/newsreleases/2006/AMC12_06.htm. Accessed January 7, 2007.
8. Schoen EJ, Fischell AA: Pain in neonatal circumcision, *Clin Pediatr* 30:429-432, 1991.
9. National Center for Health Statistics: *Trends in circumcisions among newborns.* Available at: http://www.cdc.gov/nchs/products/pubs/pubd/hestats/circumcisions/circumcisions.htm. Accessed January 7, 2007.
10. Laumann EO, Masi CM, Zuckerman EW: Circumcision in the United States: prevalence, prophylactic effects, and sexual practice, *JAMA* 277:1052-1057, 1997.
11. Christakis DA, Harvey E, Zerr DM et al: A trade-off analysis of routine newborn circumcision, *Pediatrics* 2000;105(1 pt 3): 246-249, 2000.
12. Stang HJ, Gunnar MR, Snellman L et al: Local anesthesia for neonatal circumcision: effects on distress and cortisol response, *JAMA* 259:1507-1511, 1988.
13. Fontaine P, Dittberner D, Scheltema K: The safety of dorsal penile nerve block for anesthesia in circumcision, *J Fam Pract* 39:243-248, 1994.
14. Lander J, Brady-Fryer B, Metcalfe JB et al: Comparison of ring block, dorsal penile nerve block, and topical anesthesia for neonatal circumcision: a randomized clinical trial, *JAMA* 78:2157-2162, 1997.
15. Masciello AL: Anesthesia for neonatal circumcision: local anesthesia is better than dorsal penile nerve block, *Obstet Gynecol* 75:834-838, 1990.
16. Lenhart JG, Lenhart NM, Reid MA et al: Local anesthesia for circumcision: which technique is most effective? *J Am Board Fam Pract* 10:13-19, 1997.
17. Taddio A, Ohlsson K, Ohlsson A: Lidocaine-prilocaine cream for analgesia during circumcision in newborn boys, *Cochrane Database Syst Rev* (2):CD000496, 2000.
18. Choi WY, Irwin MG, Hui TWC et al: EMLA cream versus dorsal penile nerve block for postcircumcision analgesia in children, *Anesth Analg* 96:396-399, 2003.
19. Kaufman GE, Cimo S, Miller LW et al: An evaluation of the effects of sucrose on neonatal pain with 2 commonly used circumcision methods, *Am J Obstet Gynecol* 186:564-568, 2002.
20. Howard CR, Howard FM, Weitzman ML: Acetaminophen analgesia in neonatal circumcision: the effect on pain, *Pediatrics* 93:641-649, 1994.
21. Macke JK: Analgesia for circumcision: effects on newborn behavior and mother/infant interaction, *J Obstet Gynecol Neonatal Nurs* 30:507-514, 2001.
22. Fontaine P, Toffler W: Dorsal penile nerve block for neonatal circumcision, *Am Fam Physician* 43:1327-1333, 1991.
23. Holman JR, Lewis EL, Ringler RL: Neonatal circumcision techniques, *Am Fam Physician* 52:511-518, 1995.

SECTION D Neonatal Jaundice

Karen Jankowski Fruechte, MD, and Patricia Fontaine, MD, MS

Neonatal jaundice is a yellow discoloration of the skin, sclera, and deeper tissue resulting from deposition of bilirubin. Jaundice is common in newborns and is usually due to benign physiologic processes requiring no intervention. Infants with significant jaundice, as determined by risk factors and total serum bilirubin (TSB) levels, should undergo evaluation for pathologic causes and will sometimes require treatment with phototherapy. In rare instances, severe jaundice can lead to kernicterus, causing permanent central nervous system (CNS) damage. This complication can be prevented by a policy of routine risk assessment and screening, monitoring TSB levels, and initiating therapy in a timely manner.

I. EPIDEMIOLOGY

Approximately 60% of newborns appear clinically jaundiced during the first days of life, most often because of benign physiologic processes.[1] Excessive hyperbilirubinemia, defined as a TSB level greater than the 95th percentile for age in hours, occurs in 5% to 6% of healthy newborns.[2] It may be due to physiologic or pathologic causes.

II. RISK FACTORS

The conditions associated with excessive hyperbilirubinemia are listed in Table 19-8. Factors most commonly associated include breastfeeding, prematurity, significant jaundice in a sibling, and jaundice noted before discharge.[3]

A. Gestational Age

Infants born at greater than 38 weeks are at low risk for development of excessive hyperbilirubinemia. Infants between 35 and 37 6/7 weeks of gestation are at intermediate risk. Premature newborns less than 35 weeks of gestation are at high risk.[3]

B. Ethnicity

Infants of Asian, African, and Mediterranean decent have increased risk for glucose-6-phosphate dehydrogenase deficiency. Gilbert syndrome is present in 10% to 19% of the Eastern Scottish population.[4] The black race has been associated with a decreased risk for excessive hyperbilirubinemia.[3]

III. PATHOGENESIS

A. Physiologic Jaundice

Several aspects of bilirubin metabolism contribute to physiologic neonatal jaundice.

1. Increased bilirubin production
   Newborns have high levels of circulating erythrocytes that are broken down into heme, then into iron, carbon monoxide, biliverdin, and eventually bilirubin.[5]
2. Decreased bilirubin uptake and conjugation
   Serum albumin binds bilirubin and carries it to the liver, where the newborn's transient deficiency of the enzyme glucuronyl transferase leads to reduced bilirubin conjugation. In addition, newborns have a reduced amount of ligandin (a bilirubin binding protein), which assists with uptake of bilirubin into the liver cell.[5]

TABLE 19-8 Risk Factors for Development of Severe Hyperbilirubinemia in Infants of 35 or More Weeks of Gestation (in approximate order of importance)

Major Risk Factors

Predischarge TSB or TcB level in the high-risk zone (see Figure 19-4)

Jaundice observed in the first 24 hours

Blood group incompatibility

Gestational age <37 weeks

Previous sibling received phototherapy

Cephalohematoma or significant bruising

Exclusive breastfeeding, especially if poor latch and excessive weight loss (>10%)

East Asian race

Minor Risk Factors

Predischarge TSB or TcB level in the high intermediate-risk zone

Gestational age 37-38 weeks

Jaundice observed before discharge

Previous sibling with jaundice

Macrosomic infant of a mother with diabetes

Adapted from American Academy of Pediatrics, Subcommittee on Hyperbilirubinemia: Management of hyperbilirubinemia in the newborn infant 35 or more weeks of gestation, *Pediatrics* 114:297, 2004.
TcB, Transcutaneous bilirubin; TSB, total serum bilirubin.

3. Increased enterohepatic circulation
   Conjugated bilirubin is excreted through the bile into the intestine, where it is deconjugated by a mucosal enzyme, β-glucuronidase, and reabsorbed into the enterohepatic circulation before it can be excreted with the stool. Newborns have slow intestinal motility because of a paucity of gut flora and relative caloric deprivation in the first days of life, both of which promote physiologic hyperbilirubinemia through increased enterohepatic circulation.[5]

B. Breastfeeding-Associated Jaundice

Jaundice associated with breastfeeding may represent a prolonged or exaggerated physiologic jaundice caused by decreased caloric intake and increased enterohepatic circulation of bilirubin.[6] Among infants with identical amounts of weight loss, there are equivalent TSB levels in breastfed and formula-fed newborns.[5]

C. True Breast Milk Jaundice

An unknown factor in human milk prolongs increased enterohepatic circulation by promoting the intestinal absorption of unconjugated bilirubin. This may occur in association with a genetic mutation identical to Gilbert syndrome that causes prolonged unconjugated hyperbilirubinemia in breastfed newborns.[5]

D. Pathologic Jaundice

Table 19-9 lists the causes of pathologic jaundice, grouped into three main categories: overproduction of bilirubin, decreased conjugation of bilirubin, and decreased bilirubin excretion.[1,6]

IV. DIAGNOSIS

History, physical examination, and serum bilirubin level are the first steps in diagnosing clinically significant jaundice.

A. History

1. Ascertain the type of nutrition—breast milk, formula, or combination.
2. Assess latch and suck reflex.
3. Voiding/stooling pattern also indicate adequacy of intake. A well-hydrated newborn will have 4 to 6 wet diapers in 24 hours and 3 to 4 stools per day by the fourth day of life.

B. Physical Examination

Perform a visual estimation of jaundice in a well-lit room or preferably in natural light.

1. Technique
   Blanch the skin with digital pressure to reveal the underlying color of the subcutaneous tissue.
2. Assessment
   Jaundice progresses in a cephalocaudal direction. Jaundice above the nipple line can generally predict a TSB level less than 12.0 mg/dl, but predicting levels greater than 12 mg/dl is difficult and often inaccurate.[7]

TABLE 19-9 Causes of Pathologic Jaundice

Overproduction of Bilirubin

1. Immune-mediated hemolysis (positive Coombs' test)

ABO incompatibility (the type A or type B infant of a type O mother)

Rh incompatibility (the Rh-positive infant of an Rh-negative mother)

Other blood group incompatibilities (e.g., Kell, Duffy)

2. Coombs'-negative hemolysis

RBC membrane defects (spherocytosis and other abnormally shaped RBCs)

RBC enzyme abnormalities (G6PD, pyruvate kinase, and hexokinase deficiencies)

3. Nonhemolytic causes of increased bilirubin load

Extravascular hemorrhage (skin, scalp, central nervous system, adrenal glands)

Polycythemia

Decreased Rate of Bilirubin Conjugation

1. Gilbert syndrome (an autosomal-dominant deficiency of BGT; affects 3-6% of the population)

2. Crigler-Najjar syndrome, types I and II (rare genetic deficiencies of BGT)

Decreased Excretion of Bilirubin

1. Cholestatic syndromes

2. Obstruction of the biliary tree

3. Congenital cirrhosis, hepatitis

4. Exaggerated enterohepatic circulation (gastrointestinal obstruction, ileus)

BGT, Bilirubin glucuronosyltransferase; G6PD, glucose-6-phosphate dehydrogenase; RBC, red blood cell.

3. Assess weight loss
   A loss of greater than 10% of birth weight during the first week of life is a sign of feeding problems and inadequate caloric intake.[8]
4. Verify the gestational age
   Preterm infants are at increased risk for jaundice.
5. Check for excessive bruising or cephalohematoma
   Increased red blood cell breakdown causes increased TSB level.
6. Assess for signs of sepsis
   Lethargy, irritability, hepatosplenomegaly, temperature instability, and poor feeding are serious indicators of underlying disease and deserve aggressive workup.

C. Total Serum Bilirubin

The capillary TSB level should be measured if the newborn appears jaundiced within the first 24 hours of life, jaundice is excessive for the infant's age, or there is any doubt about the degree of jaundice.[3]

D. Transcutaneous Bilirubin

Several devices provide noninvasive transcutaneous bilirubin (TcB) measurements that correlate well with TSB. TcB meters can correct for varying levels of melanin and hemoglobin. Measurements are within 2 to 3 mg/dl of TSB level, particularly for TSB level less than 15 mg/dl, but accuracy between racial groups is yet to be determined.[3,9]

E. Predischarge Bilirubin Assessment

The American Academy of Pediatrics (AAP) recommends that all infants receive a predischarge bilirubin test, either TSB or TcB. The bilirubin level is then plotted on an age-in-hours–specific nomogram to assess an infant's risk for subsequent hyperbilirubinemia (Figure 19-4). Infants who have hour-specific values more than 95% are at increased risk for development of severe hyperbilirubinemia.[3]

V. CLINICAL COURSE

A. Physiologic Jaundice

Clinical jaundice appears *after* 24 hours of age and in term newborns resolves within 7 to 10 days.[6] Peak TSB level occurs between 3 and 5 days of age with an average peak of 5 to 6 mg/dl. Unconjugated serum bilirubin increases by less than 5 mg/dl per day.

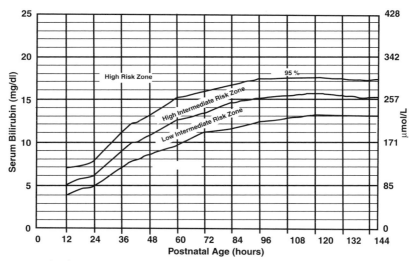

FIGURE 19-4. Nomogram for designation of risk in 2840 healthy newborns at 36 or more weeks of gestational age with birth weight of 2000 g or more or 35 or more weeks of gestational age and birth weight of 2500 g or more based on the hour-specific serum bilirubin values. The serum bilirubin level was obtained before discharge, and the zone in which the value fell predicted the likelihood of a subsequent bilirubin level exceeding the 95th percentile (high-risk zone). This nomogram should not be used to represent the natural history of neonatal hyperbilirubinemia. (From American Academy of Pediatrics, Subcommittee on Hyperbilirubinemia: Management of hyperbilirubinemia in the newborn infant 35 or more weeks of gestation, *Pediatrics* 114:297, 2004. Copyright American Academy of Pediatrics.)

B. Breastfeeding-Associated Jaundice

Most breastfed infants experience only mild unconjugated hyperbilirubinemia; however, 9% to 13% have levels exceeding 12 mg/dl during the first 5 days of life.[5] Resolution may extend beyond the typical 7 to 10 days.

C. True Breast Milk Jaundice

TSB levels start to increase by 3 to 5 days of age. Most do not exceed 10 to 12 mg/dl, but the levels may reach as high as 22 to 24 mg/dl in rare cases.[5] Half of newborns with breast milk jaundice continue to have TSB levels greater than 5 mg/dl by week 3 of life and are clinically jaundiced. Increased levels decline gradually and may not return to normal for 2 to 3 months.[5]

VI. ADDITIONAL TESTING

A. Rapidly Increasing Total Serum Bilirubin Levels

Infants with rapidly increasing TSB levels or levels requiring phototherapy require the following additional laboratory tests, particularly if the cause of jaundice is not evident from history and physical examination[3]:
1. Blood type and Coombs' test
2. Complete blood cell count and smear
3. Direct or conjugated bilirubin

B. Total Serum Bilirubin Level Approaching Exchange Transfusion Level

When the TSB level approaches exchange transfusion level, the clinician should obtain[3]:
1. Reticulocyte count
   If elevated, this may indicate hemolysis.
2. Glucose-6-phosphate dehydrogenase level
   Consider this in jaundiced newborns from an at-risk ethnic background.
3. Albumin
   The bilirubin/albumin ratio is an approximate measurement of the unbound bilirubin level. Increases of unbound bilirubin have been associated with kernicterus in sick, preterm infants.[3]
4. End-tidal carbon monoxide
   Infants with hemolysis have increased levels of exhaled carbon monoxide, and this can be measured by the end-tidal carbon monoxide.[10]

C. Evaluating an Increased Direct or Conjugated Bilirubin Level

The following steps are necessary to evaluate an increased direct or conjugated bilirubin level[3]:
1. Obtain a urinalysis and urine culture to assess for risk for sepsis.
2. Initiate further evaluation for sepsis if indicated by clinical examination (see Section IV.B).

D. Jaundice after Three Weeks of Age

Distinguishing direct versus indirect bilirubin levels may be useful in evaluating jaundice in an infant beyond 3 weeks of age.
1. Direct (conjugated) bilirubin level
   If increased, consider disorders such as cholestasis, biliary atresia, or sepsis.
2. Indirect (unconjugated) bilirubin level
   If increased, consider Gilbert syndrome, Crigler-Najjar syndrome, or true breast milk jaundice. Check the results of the newborn thyroid and galactosemia screen.

VII. TREATMENT

A. Physiologic Jaundice

No treatment is needed for strictly physiologic jaundice. Parents generally appreciate reassurance and education about how jaundice develops.

B. Jaundice Associated with Breastfeeding

Management of breastfeeding-associated jaundice is based on the assumption that breast milk is the optimal infant nutrition, and that health-care providers should support a mother's decision to breastfeed during treatment for hyperbilirubinemia.
1. Encourage mothers to begin breastfeeding as soon as possible. Feedings should be on demand or at least every 3 hours.
2. Request a certified lactation consultant if the mother has difficulty establishing nursing or there are signs of excessive infant weight loss.
3. If a woman chooses to interrupt breastfeeding, assure her that there is nothing wrong with her milk, and she can resume nursing once the hyperbilirubinemia has resolved. An electric breast pump can be used to maintain her milk supply during the temporary interruption.

4. Unless there is evidence of dehydration, supplementation with intravenous fluids or dextrose water is not necessary because it has been associated with decreased breast milk intake and increased bilirubin levels in the first week of life.[3]
5. Substitution with formula
   a. AAP recommendation: Consider substitution only if the infant is dehydrated, has more than 10% weight loss, or has inadequate intake.[3]
   b. Effect on TSB levels in infants receiving phototherapy: Formula-fed infants have a quicker decline in TSB levels than strictly breastfed infants, but no significant reduction in the overall duration of phototherapy has been seen.[11]

C. Phototherapy

1. Overview
   Phototherapy is the standard treatment for significant hyperbilirubinemia because it is effective, safe, and relatively noninvasive.[12] The most demonstrated value of phototherapy lies in its ability to reduce the risk that the TSB will increase to a level at which exchange transfusion is indicated.[13]
2. Mechanism
   Light converts bilirubin into isomeric forms that are less toxic and more easily excreted in urine and bile than native bilirubin itself.
3. Indications
   For infants more than 35 weeks of gestation, the AAP has issued clinical practice guidelines for initiation of phototherapy (Figure 19-5). The guidelines recognize three risk categories based on TSB and take into account gestational age and other risk factors. The guidelines refer to the TSB level at which intensive phototherapy should be initiated based on hour-specific TSB.[3]
4. Types of phototherapy
   a. Conventional: Fluorescent white light is placed 15 to 20 cm above the infant with a usual dose of 6 to 12 $\mu W/cm^2$.[14]

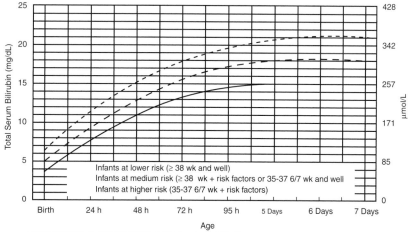

FIGURE 19-5. Guidelines for phototherapy in hospitalized infants of 35 or more weeks of gestation. *Note:* These guidelines are based on limited evidence and the levels shown are approximations. The guidelines refer to the use of intensive phototherapy, which should be used when the total serum bilirubin (TSB) exceeds the line indicated for each category. Infants are designated as "higher risk" because of the potential negative effects of the conditions listed on albumin binding of bilirubin, the blood–brain barrier, and the susceptibility of the brain cells to damage by bilirubin. G6PD, Glucose-6-phosphate dehydrogenase. (From American Academy of Pediatrics, Subcommittee on Hyperbilirubinemia: Management of hyperbilirubinemia in the newborn infant 35 or more weeks of gestation, *Pediatrics* 114:297, 2004. Copyright American Academy of Pediatrics.)

b. Intensive: A dose of 30 $\mu W/cm^2$ per nanometer of blue-green light is placed 10 to 12 cm from above the infant. A fiberoptic pad or special fluorescent tubes are placed beneath the infant.[14]

c. Fiberoptic blankets: Placing these blankets next to the infant's body rather than using overhead lights allows time for parent-child bonding and may increase parent satisfaction. This method, however, is generally less effective at lowering the TSB level than conventional therapy alone.[15]

d. Home phototherapy: Consider this for infants without risk factors when the TSB level is 2 to 3 mg/dl less than those shown in Figure 19-5 for each risk category.[3]

5. Side effects

a. Overheating and increased insensible water loss

b. Retinal damage is a hypothetical concern for which an infant's eyes are shielded

c. Bronze infant syndrome: a gray-brown discoloration of the skin that can occur in infants with cholestatic jaundice; this rare side effect often resolves within a few weeks after phototherapy and has few deleterious consequences[3]

D. Intravenous immunoglobulin

Intravenous immunoglobulin is used in infants with isoimmune hemolytic disease (ABO or Rh incompatibility) with increasing TSB levels despite intensive phototherapy or infants who are approaching the need for exchange transfusion.[16]

E. Exchange Transfusion

1. Indications
Exchange transfusion is needed for the rare infant with extreme hyperbilirubinemia that is unresponsive to intensive phototherapy.[14] The goal of exchange transfusion is to keep the TSB levels less than that at which kernicterus has been reported (see Section VIII.B).

2. Technique
The transfusion removes approximately 25% of the infant's total body bilirubin by replacing twice the infant's blood volume with donor red cells and plasma. An exchange transfusion will also remove the majority of abnormal red blood cells in cases of hemolysis.[6]

3 Risks
These include electrolyte disturbances, hypoglycemia, thrombocytopenia, necrotizing enterocolitis, graft-versus-host disease, and cardiac arrest. The mortality rate for exchange transfusion is estimated at 3 per 1000 procedures.[17]

VIII. COMPLICATIONS OF HYPERBILIRUBINEMIA

A. Acute Bilirubin Encephalopathy

Acute bilirubin encephalopathy can manifest in different phases: early, intermediate, and advanced.[18]

1. Early phase
This occurs in the first few days of a severely jaundiced infant and is characterized by lethargy, poor sucking, hypotonia, and a slightly high-pitched cry.

2. Intermediate phase
This evolves by the end of the first week and consists of moderate stupor, irritability, fever, and hypertonia with backward arching of the neck (retrocollis) and trunk (opisthotonos). Anecdotal evidence indicates a possible reversal of the CNS changes with exchange transfusion at this stage.

3. Advanced stage
This results in pronounced retrocollis-opisthotonos, shrill cry, no feeding, apnea, fever, deep stupor to coma, and sometimes seizures or even death. Permanent CNS damage likely occurs at this stage.

B. Kernicterus

Kernicterus is the chronic form of bilirubin encephalopathy that develops over months to years in infants who survive the acute stages. These infants may experience severe neurologic abnormalities including cerebral palsy, sensorineural hearing loss, dental enamel hypoplasia, and paralysis of upward gaze.[18] Kernicterus has been reported at TSB levels ranging from 23.6 to 41.5 mg/dl, but most cases occur at levels greater than 30 mg/dl.[19,20]

The true incidence of kernicterus is difficult to determine; currently, only case reports exist. Kernicterus has been reported in apparently healthy, full-term, breastfed infants. Forty-one cases of kernicterus have occurred since the late-1970s, and 31 of these have been reported since 1990.[19]

C. Less Severe Bilirubin Toxicity

Discussion continues whether a less severe form of bilirubin encephalopathy can occur, one that is asymptomatic in the newborn period but associated with subtle deficits in hearing, neurodevelopment, or motor function later in life.[1,3]

IX. PREVENTION

A. Hospital Protocols

The 2004 AAP guidelines stress the importance of hospital protocols for the early detection and treatment of significant jaundice. The following components are recommended[3]:

1. Systematic risk assessment
   This is done by the physician on all infants before discharge.
2. Reminders or checklists
   These should be centered on risk factor assessment or laboratory interpretation and provided by the hospital as guidance for appropriate follow-up.
3. Nursing protocols
   A protocol in place to give a Registered Nurse the ability to obtain a TcB or TSB level.

B. Parent Education

Hospital stays have become shorter, and infants who are discharged early are at risk for having undetected jaundice. At the time of discharge, the hospital should provide written and verbal information for parents explaining jaundice and how to monitor for it in their newborn.

C. Postdischarge Follow-up

Follow-up within 3 to 5 days of discharge is important for identifying an emerging problem with significant jaundice.

1. Infants discharged before 24 hours of age should be seen for follow-up by 72 hours of age; those discharged between 24 and 48 hours by 96 hours; and those between 48 and 72 hours by 120 hours.
2. The history and physical examination should include the infant's feeding, voiding, and stooling patterns; weight and percentage weight loss; and evaluation for the presence of jaundice.

X. PITFALLS AND CONTROVERSIES

A. Clinical Factors

Researchers continue to question how clinical factors such as the level and duration of hyperbilirubinemia, gestational age, hemolysis, or acidosis affect the likelihood of development of kernicterus or chronic bilirubin encephalopathy.

B. Continuation versus Discontinuation of Breastfeeding

Advantages and disadvantages are associated with discontinuing breastfeeding and starting formula feeding in jaundiced newborns, and this should be a conversation between parents and clinician.

C. Cost-effectiveness

Risks, cost, and benefits of different strategies to prevent and treat hyperbilirubinemia are currently unknown.

D. Evidence to Guide Treatment

There is a paucity of experimental evidence to inform the management of neonatal jaundice and particularly the prevention of kernicterus. The existing evidence is mostly based on observational studies or expert opinion.

REFERENCES

1. American Academy of Pediatrics, Provisional Committee for the Quality Improvement and Subcommittee on Hyperbilirubinemia: Practice parameter: management of hyperbilirubinemia in the healthy term newborn, *Pediatrics* 94:558-565, 1994.
2. Bhutani V, Gourley GR, Adler S et al: Noninvasive measurement of the total serum bilirubin in a multiracial predischarge newborn population to assess the risk of severe hyperbilirubinemia, *Pediatrics* 106:1-9, 2000.
3. American Academy of Pediatrics, Subcommittee on Hyperbilirubinemia: Management of hyperbilirubinemia in the newborn infant 35 or more weeks of gestation, *Pediatrics* 114:297-316, 2004.
4. Monaghan G, Mclellan A, McGeehan A et al: Gilbert's syndrome is a contributory factor in prolonged unconjugated hyperbilirubinemia of the newborn, *J Pediatr* 134:441-446, 1999.
5. Gartner LM, Herschel M: Jaundice and breastfeeding, *Pediatr Clin North Am* 48:389-399, 2001.
6. Thilo EH, Rosenberg AA: The newborn infant. In Hay WW, Hayward AR, Levin MJ et al, editors: *Current pediatric diagnosis and treatment*, ed 17, Norwalk, CT, 2005, Appleton & Lange.
7. Moyer VA, Ahn C, Sneed S: Accuracy of clinical judgement in neonatal jaundice, *Arch Pediatr Adolesc Med* 154:391-394, 2000.
8. Laing IA, Wong CM: Hypernatraemia in the first few days: is the incidence rising? *Arch Dis Child Fetal Neonatal Ed* 87: F158-F162, 2002.
9. Rubaltelli FF, Gourley GR, Loskamp N et al: Trancutaneous bilirubin measurement: a multicenter evaluation of a new device, *Pediatrics* 107:1264-1271, 2001.
10. Herschel M, Karrison T, Wen M et al: Evaluation of the direct antiglobulin (Coombs') test for identifying newborns at risk

for hemolysis as determined by end-tidal carbon monoxide concentration (ETCO$_2$); and comparison of the Coombs' test with ETCO$_2$ for detecting significant jaundice, *J Perinatol* 22:341-347, 2002.

11. Tan KL: Decreased response to phototherapy for neonatal jaundice in breastfed infants, *Arch Pediatr Adolesc Med* 152:1187-1190, 1998.

12. Scheidt PC, Bryla DA, Nelson KB et al: Phototherapy for neonatal hyperbilirubinemia: six-year follow-up of the National Institute of Child Health and Human Development Clinical Trail, *Pediatrics* 85:455-463, 1990.

13. Maisels MJ: Phototherapy—traditional and nontraditional, *J Perinatol* 21(suppl 1):S93-S97, 2001.

14. Dennery PA, Seidman DS, Stevenson DK: Neonatal hyperbilirubinemia, *N Engl J Med* 344:581-590, 2001.

15. Mills JF, Tudehope D: Fibreoptic phototherapy for neonatal jaundice, *Cochrane Database Syst Rev* (1):CD002060, 2001.

16. Gottstein R, Cooke R: Systematic review of intravenous immunoglobulin in haemolytic disease of the newborn, *Arch Dis Child Fetal Neonatal Ed* 88:F6-F10, 2003.

17. Keenan WJ, Novak KK, Sutherland JM et al: Morbidity and mortality associated with exchange transfusion, *Pediatrics* 75(suppl):417-421, 1985.

18. Ip S, Chung M, Kulig J et al: An evidence-based review of important issues concerning neonatal hyperbilirubinemia, *Pediatrics* 114:130-153, 2004.

19. Brown AK, Johnson L: Loss of concern about jaundice and the reemergence of kernicterus in full-term infants in the era of managed care. In Fanaroff AA, Klaus MH, editors: *Yearbook of neonatal and perinatal medicine,* St. Louis, 1996, Mosby-Yearbook.

20. Centers for Disease Control and Prevention (CDC): Kernicterus in full-term infants—United States, 1994-1998, *MMWR Morb Mortal Wkly Rep* 50:491-494, 2001.

SECTION E Evaluation and Management of Infection in the Newborn

Laura Chambers-Kersh, MD, and Patricia Fontaine, MD, MS

Infections are an important cause of morbidity and mortality during the newborn period. They can be caused by a wide variety of agents including bacteria, viruses, fungi, protozoa, and mycoplasma. This section focuses primarily on bacterial sepsis and includes a discussion about neonatal herpes. Diagnosing infection in the newborn can be challenging because the symptoms are nonspecific and initially may be subtle. Management strategies may include preventive actions taken at the time of delivery (e.g., cesarean section for active maternal genital herpes, antibiotic prophylaxis for group B streptococcus [GBS]), careful monitoring in the newborn nursery for infants at high risk, and transfer to an intensive care unit for evaluation and treatment in cases when clinical signs of infection develop.

I. EPIDEMIOLOGY AND RISK FACTORS

A. Definitions

Bacterial sepsis, the leading infectious cause of mortality, ranked fifth among all causes of neonatal death.[1] In newborns, it is characterized as either early or late onset.

1. Early-onset infection
   This occurs during the first week of life and has an incidence of 4 to 5 cases per 1000 live births. Early-onset infections are generally due to organisms acquired from the mother.

2. Late-onset infections
   These infections begin after the first week of life, although some studies extend this definition to positive blood cultures after 72 hours of life.

B. Risk Factors

1. Maternal colonization with GBS
   a. GBS colonization is a significant risk factor. Women with prenatal GBS colonization are more than 25 times more likely than GBS-negative women to have early-onset GBS infections in their infants.[2]
   b. Prenatal screening with vaginal/rectal cultures and intrapartum antibiotic prophylaxis (IAP) for women colonized with GBS have resulted in a significant decrease in GBS infections in newborns.[3,4] Early-onset infections declined by 70% between 1993 and 2002.[2]
   c. The incidence of late-onset GBS disease has remained stable, indicating that IAP has less impact there.[2]
   d. The incidence of non-GBS pathogens including *Escherichia coli* has been stable during the era of IAP.[2] Several studies have been done since recommendations were first published in 1996 to look for the emergence of antibiotic-resistant strains of GBS, and an increased incidence in neonatal infections caused by organisms other than GBS has occurred. Increases in the frequency of non-GBS early-onset sepsis have been limited to preterm, low-birth-weight, or very-low-birth-weight neonates.[5]

2. Prolonged rupture of the membranes and chorioamnionitis

   Rupture of the amniotic membranes for over 24 hours increases the rate of neonatal infection to 1 in 100 live births. If chorioamnionitis is present, the rate increases to 1 in 10 live births.[6]

3. Prematurity

   Preterm infants are five times more likely to develop sepsis than term infants.[6]

   a. Preterm infants have increased exposure to infectious agents during birth because of the association of infection and preterm labor.[7] Histologic chorioamnionitis has been found in 70% of preterm deliveries versus 15% of term deliveries[8] and carries a strong association with increased risk for sepsis.[9]

   b. Interventions required for neonatal intensive care, such as placement of indwelling vascular catheters and endotracheal tubes, increase the premature infant's risk for infection.[10]

4. Epidural analgesia

   Epidural anesthesia has not been shown to be a risk factor for neonatal sepsis. However, the increase in maternal temperature that occurs in association with epidural analgesia can suggest the possibility of chorioamnionitis. As a result, infants of women who received epidurals are more likely to be evaluated for sepsis and treated with antibiotics.[11]

II. PATHOGENESIS

A. Modes of Transmission

The three main modes of transmission for neonatal infections are as follows[6]:

1. Transplacental or blood-borne
2. Ascending infection from the maternal genital tract after disruption of the amniotic membranes
3. Direct contact with an infected birth canal or infected blood during delivery

B. Bacterial Causes

1. Early onset

   GBS, *Staphylococcus aureus, Klebsiella pneumoniae,* and *E. coli* are the most frequent causes of early-onset infections.[6,12] Other pathogens such as *Haemophilus influenzae* and *Listeria monocytogenes* are occasionally responsible.

2. Late onset

   In addition to the organisms that cause early-onset sepsis, nosocomial organisms such as coagulase-negative staphylococci, enterococcus, pseudomonas, and other gram-negative organisms begin to play a more prominent role in late-onset infections.[6]

C. Viral Causes

Neonatal viral infections may be acquired either in utero (congenital infection) or at the time of delivery. Congenital infections include cytomegalovirus, rubella, varicella, and syphilis. Acquired infections include herpes simplex virus (HSV), hepatitis, and HIV. Perinatal aspects of these infections are discussed in Chapter 9, Section A.

III. CLINICAL FEATURES

A. Signs and Symptoms

Clinical signs of neonatal sepsis may be present at birth or develop rapidly during the first 24 hours of life. Symptoms at birth include unanticipated low Apgar scores, poor perfusion, and hypotension.[6] Symptoms within first 24 hours include the following:

1. Respiratory distress

   This is the most common sign, with a typical clinical picture of persistent tachypnea exceeding 60 breaths/min, substernal and intercostal retractions, and failure to maintain adequate oxygenation.

2. Temperature instability

   Temperature instability raises concern if measurements are outside the expected range, less than 36.5°C or exceeding 37.5°C. Only about 50% of infants with sepsis will have a temperature greater than 37.8°C axillary.[7]

3. Other warning signs

   These include sustained tachycardia (heart rate > 160 beats/min), lethargy, hypotonia, poor feeding, vomiting, abdominal distention, unexplained jaundice, petechiae, purpura, and bleeding.[13]

B. Clinical Course

Infants at risk for sepsis should be reassessed frequently. If not recognized and properly treated, sepsis may progress to respiratory failure, cardiac failure, pulmonary hypertension, shock, renal failure, liver dysfunction, cerebral edema or thrombosis, adrenal hemorrhage and/or insufficiency, neutropenia, anemia, thrombocytopenia, and disseminated intravascular coagulopathy.[14]

Mortality rates from neonatal sepsis have been reported to be as low as 10% when all bacteremic infections are included; if limited to full sepsis syndrome, the rate probably approaches 50%.[14] Fatality rate is greatest for gram-negative and fungal sepsis (36.2% and 31.8%, respectively), compared with 11.2% for gram-positive sepsis.[15]

IV. DIAGNOSIS

A. Indications for Testing

A full diagnostic evaluation is required for infants with signs of sepsis, or those whose mothers received intrapartum for suspected chorioamnionitis.

B. Recommended Tests

Recommended tests to diagnose sepsis include[16]:
1. Complete blood cell count and differential
2. Blood culture
3. Chest radiograph (if respiratory abnormalities are present)
4. Lumbar puncture (if feasible).

C. Culture Sources and Follow-up

Blood, cerebrospinal fluid, or another normally sterile source are considered standard culture sources for documenting neonatal infection.[13] Blood culture should be obtained from an umbilical catheter only at the time of initial insertion.[14] Surface cultures and cultures of gastric aspirates are not sufficiently accurate to be clinically helpful.[17]

The standard of care is generally to give antibiotics until cultures have been negative for 48 hours.[6] However, in a retrospective trial of 416 blood cultures, 36 hours was considered sufficient to rule out sepsis in an asymptomatic neonate.[18]

D. Chest Radiograph

Chest radiograph is useful for ruling out other causes of respiratory distress, such as a pneumothorax or congenital anomalies of the heart or lungs. The presence of infiltrates on the chest radiograph is a nonspecific finding, seen with pneumonia, atelectasis, or excessive interstitial fluid.

E. Lumbar Puncture

Lumbar puncture continues to have a role in evaluating asymptomatic newborns at risk for sepsis, albeit a controversial one.[13] Lumbar puncture may be unnecessary for the term infant with risk factors but no clinical signs of sepsis because meningitis occurs in at most 4 per 1000 infants in that situation.[19] However, a retrospective study demonstrated that 37% of in-fants with culture-proven meningitis (16/43) would have escaped diagnosis if lumbar puncture had not been performed routinely.[20] When signs of sepsis are present, the AAP states that a lumbar puncture, if feasible, should be performed.[16]

F. Serum Markers

Many markers have been evaluated for predictive value, including the white blood cell count, absolute neutrophil count, immature/total neutrophil ratio (I:T ratio), C-reactive protein (CRP), and erythrocyte sedimentation rate.[21] The range of values used to predict infection are shown in Table 19-10. In general, negative tests are better at excluding infection than positive tests are in predicting infections subsequently confirmed with blood cultures.

A combination of two tests, interleukin-8 (IL-8) and CRP, shows promise for reducing the use of empiric antibiotics without increasing the risk for missing diagnoses of infants with infection. A trial of 1291 infants randomized to receive standard empiric antibiotic therapy versus therapy when only IL-8 and CRP were elevated found that only seven infants with suspected infection would have to be evaluated with IL-8 and CRP to avoid one course of unnecessary antibiotic therapy (number needed to treat = 7; 95% CI, 5-12).[22]

G. Other Laboratory Abnormalities

Thrombocytopenia, hypoglycemia, and hyperbilirubinemia have also been independently associated with neonatal bacterial sepsis.

H. Urine Antigen Testing

Urine antigen testing with latex agglutination is not recommended as a screening test because of its insufficient sensitivity and specificity (28.6% and 86.7%, respectively) and its lack of demonstrable clinical impact.[23]

V. TREATMENT

A. Management of Infants with Symptoms of Sepsis

Any infant with a clinical picture suggesting sepsis, pneumonia, or meningitis should receive care in a setting where full diagnostic evaluation and treatment are available, generally in a special care nursery or neonatal intensive care unit. A full diagnostic evaluation should be performed (see earlier). Empiric treatment with antibiotics should be initiated.

TABLE 19-10 Presumptive Tests for Predicting Neonatal Infection

Test	Cutoff Values for Predicting Infection	Positive Predictive Value (%)	Negative Predictive Value (%)
WBC	<5000/mm³	27	92
ANC	<1500-1750 mm³	NA	NA
I:T ratio	>20%	11	100
ESR	>10 mm/hr days 0-3; >15 mm/hr thereafter	24	95
CRP	>10 mg/L	NA	86
IL-8 and/or CRP	≥70 pg/ml >10 mg/L	68	93

Data from Allen SR: Management of asymptomatic term neonates whose mothers received intrapartum antibiotics—part 2: diagnostic tests and management strategies, *Clin Pediatr* 36:617-624, 1997; and Gerdes JS, Polin RA: Sepsis screen in neonates with evaluation of plasma fibronectin, *Pediatr Infect Dis J* 6:443-446, 1987.
ANC, Absolute neutrophil count; CRP, C-reactive protein; ESR, erythrocyte sedimentation rate; IL-8, interleukin-8; I:T, immature/total neutrophil ratio; NA, data not available from the referenced studies; WBC, white blood cell count.

B. Antibiotic Treatment

No evidence has been reported from randomized trials to guide the treatment of presumed early-onset neonatal sepsis. A retrospective review of 67,260 infants found 25 cases of early-onset group B sepsis, none with isolates resistant to ampicillin, penicillin, cephalosporins, or vancomycin.[24]
1. First choice of antibiotic coverage
   This is a combination of ampicillin and gentamicin, which gives broad-spectrum coverage for the common pathogens transmitted from the mother, that is, GBS and enteric gram-negative organisms.[25]
   a. Ampicillin 100-150 mg/kg/day divided every 12 hours
   b. Gentamicin 2.5 mg/kg every 12 to 24 hours depending on gestational age
2. Cefotaxime
   An alternative regimen is cefotaxime 100 mg/kg/day divided every 12 hours.
3. Treatment based on culture results
   The antibiotic choice can be adjusted based on results of cultures and sensitivities.[16] Resistant organisms are of greater concern in late-onset sepsis, in which organisms are usually nosocomial. In these organisms there is an increasing trend toward antibiotic resistance, and in the hospital setting, it is not uncommon to use vancomycin as first-line empiric therapy.

4. Duration of treatment[6]
   Sepsis is treated for 10 to 14 days. Meningitis requires 21 days of treatment.

C. Other Treatments

If sepsis progresses, further treatment measures may be necessary, such as extracorporeal membrane oxygenation in respiratory failure, fluid resuscitation and inotropic agents in shock, corticosteroids in adrenal insufficiency, phototherapy or exchange transfusion for hyperbilirubinemia, and parenteral feeding when unable to sustain enteral feeding.[14]

D. Management of Infants Born to Mothers Colonized with Group B Streptococcus

Management of infants born to mothers with GBS depends on whether adequate IAP was given, the infant's gestational age, and whether signs of sepsis are present (Figure 19-6).
1. Term infants with adequate maternal IAP
   Term infants with no symptoms, whose mothers were GBS positive but received penicillin or ampicillin more than 4 hours before delivery, can be regarded as healthy, low-risk newborn requiring nothing more than an appropriate period of hospital observation. Because more than 90% of early-onset infections will manifest symptoms by 24 hours of life, 24 hours is the minimum

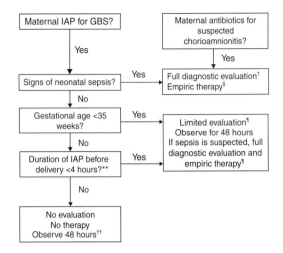

* If no maternal intrapartum prophylaxis for GBS was administered despite an indication being present, data are insufficient on which to recommend a single management strategy.

† Includes complete blood cell count and differential, blood culture, and chest radiograph if respiratory abnormalities are present. When signs of sepsis are present, a lumbar puncture, if feasible, should be performed.

§ Duration of therapy varies depending on results of blood culture, cerebrospinal fluid findings, if obtained, and the clinical course of the infant. If laboratory results and clinical course do not indicate bacterial infection, duration may be as short as 48 hours.

¶ CBC with differential and blood culture.

** Applies only to penicillin, ampicillin, or cefazolin and assumes recommended dosing regimens.

†† A healthy-appearing infant who was 38 weeks of gestation at delivery and whose mother received >4 hours of intrapartum propylaxis before delivery may be discharged home after 24 hours if other discharge criteria have been met and a person able to comply fully with instructions for home observation will be present. If any of these conditions is not met, the infant should be observed in the hospital for at least 48 hours and until criteria for discharge are achieved.

FIGURE 19-6. Sample algorithm for management of a newborn whose mother received intrapartum antimicrobial agents for prevention of early-onset group B streptococcal disease (GBS) or suspected chorioamnionitis. This algorithm is not an exclusive course of management. Variations that incorporate individual circumstances or institutional preferences may be appropriate. (From Schrag S, Gorwitz R, Fultz-Butts K, Schuchat A: Prevention of perinatal group B streptococcal disease. Revised guidelines from CDC, *MMWR Recomm Rep* 51:1-22, 2002.)

recommended hospital stay.[2,16] Monitoring should include regular vital signs and observation for the signs of sepsis described earlier.

2. Term infants with inadequate maternal IAP
If the mother is GBS positive or had another indication for IAP but did not receive dose of antibiotic at least 4 hours before delivery, there is insufficient

evidence to recommend one definitive management strategy for the newborn.[2,26]

One practice is to administer IM penicillin to the infant within 1 hour of birth, based on observational studies showing a decline in early-onset GBS sepsis with universal administration of penicillin to newborns.[27] A limited laboratory evaluation should be performed, including a complete blood cell count with differential and blood culture.[2] Clinical monitoring should take place in the hospital for at least 48 hours.[2]

E. Management of Infants of Gestational Age Less than 35 Weeks

Infants less than 35 weeks of gestation who are at high risk for GBS by virtue of maternal history require, at a minimum, a 48-hour in-hospital observation period and a limited laboratory evaluation with blood culture and a complete blood cell count with differential. There is a low threshold for obtaining full diagnostic evaluation and beginning empiric antibiotic therapy if sepsis is suspected.[2,16]

VI. PREVENTION

A. Intrapartum Antibiotic Prophylaxis

IAP is effective in decreasing early-onset GBS infection in newborns.[4] Maternal indications for IAP for GBS and recommended drugs and doses are described in Chapter 9, Section A.

B. Breastfeeding

Exclusive breastfeeding has been shown to reduce the incidence of early-onset sepsis in a case–control study (OR, 0.33; 95% CI, 0.1-0.8).[12]

C. Hand Hygiene

The most common source of postnatal infections in hospitalized newborns is from contact with the contaminated hands of health-care personnel. An observational study found that, on average, physicians comply with Centers for Disease Control and Prevention (CDC) hand hygiene guidelines less than 60% of the time.[28] After instituting a problem-based and task-oriented education program to increase hand hygiene in the neonatal intensive care unit, health-care–associated infection rate decreased from 17.2 per 100 patient admissions to 9.1 per 100 patient admissions.[29]

D. Other Interventions

Interventions such as vaginal chlorhexidine during labor have not been shown to be effective in changing infant outcomes.[30]

VII. HERPES SIMPLEX VIRUS

Before the availability of antiviral drugs, most babies with neonatal herpes died.[31] With antiviral treatment, most notably acyclovir, the mortality rate has decreased to less than 1 in 3 with disseminated disease, and less than 1 in 20 with CNS disease. However, two of three infants with CNS infection suffer sequelae, approximately the same rate as before antiviral treatment.[32] Data generated over 20 years suggest that there has been no improvement in time of initiation of antiviral therapy, a delay often longer than 1 week.[33] Better knowledge and earlier consideration of neonatal herpes could improve outcomes, decreasing the time between onset of infection and initiation of therapy. Chapter 9, Section IX.A details maternal HSV infections and perinatal management.

A. Epidemiology

1. Incidence
   The incidence of neonatal herpes varies by population, but has been found to be 11 to 31 in 100,000 births.[34,35]
2. Role of HSV-1
   HSV-2 traditionally has been considered the cause of genital ulcerations, and continues to be in the developing world, but the incidence of genital HSV-1 has now come to surpass HSV-2 in some developed nations.[36] A 2003 U.S. study showed of 18 infants with neonatal herpes, 8 had HSV-1 and 10 had HSV-2.[34] No differences in diagnosis and treatment between the two strains are reported in the literature.
3. Seasonal variation
   In the United States, neonatal CNS herpes is more common in winter in spring, as enterovirus predominates in summer and fall.

B. Risk Factors

1. Exposure to maternal HSV through vaginal delivery
   a. First episode, primary infection: A previously seronegative women with new vesicular HSV lesions has a 57% likelihood of transmission to the infant.
   b. First episode, nonprimary infection: A first episode of lesions in a woman who has previously seroconverted without an outbreak gives a 25% transmission rate.
   c. Recurrent clinical infections: These are associated with only a 2% transmission rate.[37]
   d. Asymptomatic transmission: It is important to remember that as many as 80% of infants with neonatal HSV are born to mothers without any symptoms during the peripartum period.
2. Social and ethnic factors
   Black, Mexican American, and women living in poverty have an overall greater rate of seropositivity.[38] Therefore, they are less likely to have a primary infection during pregnancy and their infants are at lower risk.
3. Fetal monitoring
   Invasive monitoring, such as fetal scalp electrode, has been repeatedly found to be a risk factor for neonatal HSV infection.[34]

C. Clinical Features

Neonatal herpes is classified into three subgroups:
1. Local skin, eye, and/or mouth
   Infants should be checked on a daily basis for the typical skin lesions, grouped vesicles on an erythematous base. These may appear on the scalp and face, buttocks, and oral mucosa at any point in the disease process.
2. CNS
   Manifestations of local CNS disease are usually noted 10 days to 4 weeks after birth. Nonspecific findings include lethargy, irritability, or poor feeding; herpes is more likely if convulsions occur.
3. Disseminated disease
   If left untreated, about 70% of localized infection in the neonate will progress to CNS or disseminated disease. Disseminated disease is more common in premature infants and most often affects the liver.

D. Diagnosis

1. HSV should be considered in any newborn with negative bacterial blood or CSF cultures and a progressively worsening clinical condition.
2. Viral blood and CSF cultures should be done, as well as skin and eye cultures in the presence of suspicious lesions. If adequately obtained, viral cultures are usually positive within 2 days and infrequently are positive after 4 days. CSF abnormalities tend to increase over the first few days, as

opposed to improving (such as seen with entero-viral meningitis).

3. Complete blood cell counts, DIC panel, and trans-aminases should be obtained.
4. Low CRP levels are more consistent with viral than bacterial/fungal infections.
5. Magnetic resonance imaging or computerized tomography evaluation of the brain may be useful in CNS neonatal herpes, though such studies often are negative initially.

E. Treatment

Suspicious findings and risk factors should prompt isolation precautions and consideration of antiviral therapy.

1. Recommended dosage
   Intravenous acyclovir 20 mg/kg every 8 hours (60 mg/kg/day) should be administered.
2. Duration
   The duration of treatment is 14 days for disease that is limited to the skin, eyes, or mouth (i.e., normal CSF), and 21 days for other forms of neonatal HSV infection.[39]
3. Acyclovir resistance
   Be alert for the possibility of acyclovir-resistant HSV strains in neonates born to mothers with HIV.[40]
4. Ophthalmic consultation
   This should be obtained to monitor for ocular findings. Ocular disease can be unilateral or bilateral, progressive, and cause cortical blindness.
5. Dermatology consultation
   This can be helpful in differential diagnosis of skin lesions.[40]

F. Prevention

1. Primary HSV infection
   After vaginal delivery to a woman with active lesions thought to be an initial genital HSV infection, there is a 30% to 50% risk for neonatal herpes, and prophylactic acyclovir therapy is generally recommended. For a proven primary first episode, guidelines recommend continuing prophylaxis for a 14-day course.[39]
2. Recurrent HSV infection
   Because of low transmission rate, empiric treatment is not recommended for neonates born to mothers with recurrent genital HSV infections at time of delivery. There is still a 1% to 4% chance of transmission in recurrent active infections, so these infants should be monitored closely with

weekly practitioner examinations and parent instruction.[40]

VIII. SOR A RECOMMENDATIONS

RECOMMENDATIONS	REFERENCES
IAP for GBS is effective in reducing the incidence of early-onset GBS disease in newborns.	27
High-dose acyclovir is effective in reducing infant mortality in cases of neonatal HSV infections.	34, 35, 40

REFERENCES

1. Anderson RN, Smith BL: Death: leading causes for 2002, *Natl Vital Stat Rep* 53:1-89, 2005.
2. Schrag, S, Gorwitz R, Fultz-Butts K et al: Prevention of perinatal group B streptococcal disease. Revised guidelines from CDC, *MMWR Recomm Rep* 51:1-22, 2002.
3. Schrag SJ, Zywicki S, Farley M et al: Group B streptococcal disease in the era of intrapartum antibiotic prophylaxis, *N Engl J Med* 342:15-20, 2000.
4. Smaill F. Intrapartum antibiotics for Group B streptococcal colonisation, *Cochrane Database Syst Rev* (1):CD000115, 1996.
5. Moore MR, Schrag SJ, Schuchat A: Effects of intrapartum antimicrobial prophylaxis for prevention of group-B-streptococcal disease on the incidence and ecology of early-onset neonatal sepsis, *Lancet Infect Dis* 3:201-213, 2003.
6. Thilo EH, Rosenberg AA: The newborn infant. In Hay WW, Levin MJ, Sondheimer JM, Deterding RR, editors: *Current pediatric diagnosis and treatment*, ed 17, Norwalk, CT, 2004, Appleton & Lange.
7. Goldenberg RL, Hauth JC, Andrews WW: Intrauterine infection and preterm delivery, *N Engl J Med* 342:1500-1507, 2000.
8. Mueller-Heubach E, Rubinstein DN, Schwarz SS: Histologic chorioamnionitis and preterm delivery in different patient populations, *Obstet Gynecol* 75:622-626, 1990.
9. Mehta R, Nanjundaswamy S, Shen-Schwarz S et al: Neonatal morbidity and placental pathology, *Indian J Pediatr* 73:2-28, 2006.
10. Brady MT: Health care-associated infections in the neonatal intensive care unit, *Am J Infect Control* 33:268-275, 2005.
11. Lieberman E, O'Donoghue C: Unintended effects of epidural analgesia during labor: a systematic review, *Am J Obstet Gynecol* 186:S31-S68, 2002.
12. Bhutta ZA, Yusuf K: Early-onset neonatal sepsis in Pakistan: a case-control study of risk factors in a birth cohort, *Am J Perinatol* 14:577-581, 1997.
13. Allen SR: Management of asymptomatic term neonates whose mothers received intrapartum antibiotics—part 2: diagnostic tests and management strategies, *Clin Pediatr* 36:617-624, 1997.
14. Stoll BJ: Infections of the neonatal infant, pathogenesis and epidemiology. In Behrman RE, editor: *Nelson textbook of pediatrics*, ed 17, Philadelphia, 2004, WB Saunders.

15. Stoll BJ, Hansen N, Fanaroff AA et al: Late-onset sepsis in very low birthweight neonates: the experience of the NICHD Neonatal Research Network, *Pediatrics* 110:285-291, 2002.

16. American Academy of Pediatrics Committee on Infectious: *The Red Book,* ed 26, Elk Grove Village, IL, 2003, American Academy of Pediatrics.

17. Dobson SRM, Isaacs D, Wilkinson AR et al: Reduced use of surface cultures for suspected neonatal sepsis and surveillance, *Arch Dis Child* 67:44-47, 1992.

18. Kumar Y, Qunibi M, Neal TJ et al: Time to positivity of neonatal blood cultures, *Arch Dis Child Fetal Neonatal Ed* 85:182-186, 2001.

19. Fielkow S, Reuter S, Gotoff SP: Cerebrospinal fluid examination in symptom-free infants with risk factors for infection, *J Pediatr* 119:971-973, 1991.

20. Wiswell TE, Baumgart S, Gannon CM et al: No lumbar puncture in the evaluation for early neonatal sepsis: will meningitis be missed? *Pediatrics* 95:803-806, 1995.

21. Gerdes JS, Polin RA: Sepsis screen in neonates with evaluation of plasma fibronectin, *Pediatr Infect Dis J* 6:443-446, 1987.

22. Franz AR, Bauer K, Schalk A et al: Measurement of interleukin 8 in combination with C-reactive protein reduced unnecessary antibiotic therapy in newborn infants: a multicenter, randomized, controlled trial, *Pediatrics* 114:1-8, 2004.

23. Hayden RT, Frenkel LD: More laboratory testing: greater cost but not necessarily better, *Pediatr Infect Dis J* 19:290-292, 2005.

24. Puopolo KM, Madoff LC, Eichenwald EC: Early-onset group B streptococcal disease in the era of maternal screening, *Pediatrics* 115:1240-1246, 2005.

25. Mtitimila EI, Cooke RW: Antibiotic regimens for suspected early neonatal sepsis, *Cochrane Database Syst Rev* (4):CD004495, 2004.

26. Siegel JD, Cushion NB: Prevention of early-onset group B streptococcal disease: another look at single-dose penicillin at birth, *Obstet Gynecol* 87:692-698, 1996.

27. Ungerer RL, Lincetto O, Mcguire W et al: Prophylactic versus selective antibiotics for term newborn infants of mothers with risk factors for neonatal infection, *Cochrane Database Syst Rev* (4):CD003957, 2004.

28. Pittet D, Simon A, Hugonnet S et al: Hand hygiene among physicians: performance, beliefs, and perceptions, *Ann Intern Med* 141:1-8, 2004.

29. Lam BC, Lee J, Lau YL: Hand hygiene practices in a neonatal intensive care unit: a multimodal intervention and impact on nosocomial infection, *Pediatrics* 114:e565-e571, 2004.

30. Stade B, Shah V, Ohlsson A: Vaginal chlorhexidine during labour to prevent early-onset neonatal group B streptococcal infection, *Cochrane Database Syst Rev* (3):CD003957, 2004.

31. Whitley RJ, Nahmias AJ, Soong SJ et al: Vidarabine therapy of neonatal herpes simplex virus infection, *Pediatrics* 66:495-501, 1980.

32. Kimberlin DW, Lin CY, Jacobs RF et al: Safety and efficacy of high-dose intravenous acyclovir in the management of neonatal herpes simplex virus infections, *Pediatrics* 108:230-238, 2001.

33. Kimberlin DW, Lin CY, Jacobs RF et al: Natural history of neonatal herpes simplex virus infections in the acyclovir era, *Pediatrics* 108:223-229, 2001.

34. Brown ZA, Wald A, Morrow RA et al: Effect of serologic status and cesarean delivery on transmission rates of herpes simplex virus from mother to infant, *JAMA* 289:203-209, 2003.

35. Gutierrez KM, Flakovitz H, Maldonado Y et al: The epidemiology of neonatal herpes simplex virus infections in California from 1985 to 1995, *J Infect Dis* 180:199-202, 1999.

36. Nilsen A, Myrmel H: Changing trends in genital herpes simplex virus infection in Bergen, Norway, *Acta Obstet Scand* 79:693-696, 2000.

37. Brown ZA, Benedetti J, Ashley R et al: Neonatal herpes simplex virus infection in relation to asymptomatic maternal infection at the time of labor, *N Engl J Med* 324:1247-1252, 1991.

38. Nahmias AJ, Neonatal HSV infection part II: obstetric considerations—a tale of hospitals in two cities (Seattle and Atlanta, USA), *Herpes* 11:41-44, 2004.

39. Pass R, Weber T, Whitley RJ, editors: *Herpesvirus infections in pregnancy. Recommendations from the IHMF Management Strategies Workshop. International Herpes Management Forum, 1999.* Available at: http://www.ihmf.org/guidelines/summary9.asp. Accessed March 15, 2006.

40. Nahmias AJ: Neonatal HSV infection part i: continuing challenges, *Herpes* 11:33-37, 2004.

SECTION F Infant Feeding and Nutrition

Patricia Fontaine, MD, MS

Family physicians play important roles in providing parents information about infant nutritional requirements and optimal feeding practices. The physician may also help by supporting the mother's decision to bottle-feed or breastfeed. Qualified nursing personnel and trained lactation consultants can enhance the physician's efforts by working closely with mothers and infants in the immediate postpartum period.

I. BREASTFEEDING

A. Advantages for Infants

Human breast milk is widely recognized as the optimal source of infant nutrition for the first 6 months of life.[1,2] It provides adequate calories for optimal growth and development, appropriately distributed among protein, fats, and carbohydrates. In addition, colostrum and breast milk together contain many immunologic factors that are not present in commercial formulas, including secretory IgA, lysozyme, lactoferrin, bifidus factor, and macrophages.[3] Infants fed human milk have been shown in epidemiologic studies to have decreased incidences of diarrhea, lower respiratory tract infection, otitis media, bacterial meningitis, urinary tract infection, and necrotizing enterocolitis. In addition, an infant diet of human milk appears to confer a measure of protection against certain chronic illnesses, including insulin-dependent diabetes mellitus, Crohn's disease, ulcerative colitis, lymphoma, and allergic conditions.[4] A detailed discussion of the advantages of breastfeeding appears in Chapter 4, Section D.

B. Prevalence

In 2002, 70% of mothers breastfed their infants in the early postpartum period and 33% continued for 6 months. National goals as outlined in *Healthy People 2010* are to increase the percentage of women who breastfeed to 75% in the early postpartum period, 50% at 6 months and 25% at 1 year.[5] Factors that influence breastfeeding rates are discussed in Chapter 20, Section C.

C. Breastfeeding Routines

Some breastfeeding routines (see Chapter 4, Section D) are as follows[4]:

1. Breastfeeding should be initiated as soon as possible after delivery. Many mother-infant pairs are able to begin nursing within the first hour of life.
2. Rooming in is desirable because it enhances the full-time, exclusive nature of the early breastfeeding experience.
3. An on-demand feeding schedule is optimal. Infant signs of hunger include increased alertness and activity, mouthing, and rooting. Crying is a late sign of hunger.
4. Breastfed infants require frequent feedings. (The gastric emptying time for breast milk is 1.5 hours, compared with nearly 4 hours for formula.) Mothers should be prepared initially to nurse their infants every 2 to 2.5 hours, or approximately 8 to 12 times in 24 hours.
5. No supplements such as formula, water, or dextrose solutions should be given to breastfeeding newborns, unless there is a specific medical indication.
6. The AAP recommends that when a breastfeeding infant is discharged less than 48 hours after birth, there should be follow-up at 2 to 4 days of age for evaluation of successful breastfeeding behavior.[4]

D. Pumping and Storing Breast Milk

Women may experience difficulty in pumping a significant volume of breast milk before letdown is well established. Hospital-style electronic pumps can be helpful, particularly in the early postpartum period.

Pumped breast milk can be safely stored at room temperature for 8 hours or kept in the refrigerator at 0° to 4°C for 72 hours with no degradation of its many beneficial constituents.[6] Freezing allows the milk to be stored for up to 6 months, although cellular activity and concentrations of vitamins B_6 and C are decreased.[6] A clean plastic or glass container may be used, although glass has the potential to break with freezing. Milk may be thawed in the refrigerator or under running water. Once thawed, any milk not used within 24 hours should be discarded.[7]

E. Precautions

Mothers who are positive for HBsAg may breastfeed, provided the infant receives HBIG and hepatitis B vaccine according to immunization guidelines.[8]

1. Maternal contraindications to breastfeeding
   Mothers who are unable to discontinue illicit drug use, those taking certain medications (e.g., radioactive isotopes, antimetabolites, cancer chemotherapy agents),[9] and those with active infectious tuberculosis should not breastfeed. Women who are positive for HIV have a small chance of transmitting infection to their infants through breast milk and, in the United States, are generally counseled not to breastfeed.[4]
2. Infant contraindications to breastfeeding
   Galactosemia in the infant is one widely recognized contraindication to breastfeeding; otherwise, infant contraindications are rare. Human milk is the preferred feeding for preterm infants and infants with most medical conditions. When direct breastfeeding is not possible, pumped breast milk should be considered the first alternative.[4]

F. Vitamin and Mineral Supplements for the Breastfed Infant

1. Vitamin K
   Low levels of vitamin K in breast milk make it advisable for the infant to receive the standard dose of parenteral vitamin K in the newborn nursery.[10]
2. Vitamin D
   Vitamin D may be given as a supplement to infants at high risk for deficiency, such as those not exposed to adequate sunlight or those whose mothers are vitamin D deficient.[4]
3. Thiamine (B_1), cobalamin (B_{12}) and folate
   Deficiencies of B_1, B_{12}, and folate develop uncommonly in breastfed infants, usually associated with

problems in the mother's dietary intake or absorption of these vitamins.[3]

   a. Thiamine deficiency may develop if the mother is an alcoholic or has a poor diet.

   b. B_{12} deficiency may occur in infants of mothers with untreated pernicious anemia or an unsupplemented vegetarian diet.

   c. Maternal folate deficiency can result in a similar deficiency in the infant, particularly in preterm infants.

4. Iron

Iron is well absorbed by breastfed infants, who acquire 0.06 mg/kg/day of iron from breast milk. This daily intake, combined with iron stores accumulated in utero, gives the healthy breastfed infant enough iron to meet ongoing requirements without supplementation for the first 6 months of life.[11] Certain infants at high risk, or those with documented anemia, are candidates for iron supplementation. For example, infants of mothers with poorly controlled diabetes and small-for-gestational-age and preterm infants are born with reduced iron stores and may be at risk.[11]

5. Fluoride

Although the addition of fluoride to municipal water supplies has been an important public health measure for reducing dental caries among U.S. children, excessive supplementation can lead to dental fluorosis (cosmetic dental changes ranging from white striations to brownish gray strains). Fluoride supplements are not recommended for infants younger than 6 months. This applies to both bottle-fed and breastfed infants, regardless of the amount of fluoride in the municipal water supply.[4]

II. BOTTLE-FEEDING

Bottle-feeding with commercial infant formula is an alternative to consider when breastfeeding is not possible.[12] This may occur when breastfeeding is unacceptable to the mother, has failed despite best attempts at management of common minor difficulties, or when maternal illness or employment dictate. Commercial infant formulas are manufactured either from cow's milk or soy-based protein. Soy-based formulas have no advantage over cow's milk formulas for most infants, but they are safe for use in special circumstances (e.g., infants with galactosemia or hereditary lactose deficiency, infants of vegetarian parents).[13]

Formulas are patterned as closely as possible after human breast milk and are fortified with selected vitamins, minerals, fatty acids, and nucleotides.[12]

A. Preparation and Storage of Infant Formula

Infant formula comes in three types: ready to feed, liquid concentrate, and powder. Ready-to-feed formula is conveniently prediluted and is the most expensive. Concentrated formula must be mixed 1:1 with water. Powdered formula is the most economical choice, prepared as one scoop to 2 ounces of water. Boiling the water is not necessary when sanitized city water is used.[7]

1. Preventing lead contamination

To alleviate concerns of lead contamination from water pipes, parents may let tap water run for 2 minutes before mixing it with formula.

2. Warming formula

Once prepared, formulas may be heated by warm running water, in a bottle warmer, or on the stove. Microwave heating is sometimes discouraged because it may cause "hot spots" in formula; at a minimum, thorough mixing is required after heating.

3. Storing formula

Once opened, cans of liquid formula or concentrate should be refrigerated and used within 48 hours. Diluted formula should be used within 24 hours.

B. Bottle-Feeding Routines

During the first days of life, formula-fed newborns will take 1/2 to 1 ounce every 3 to 5 hours. By the end of the first week, amounts have increased to 1 to 3 ounces per feeding. By the end of the first month, a typical feeding schedule will be 2 to 4 ounces, 7 to 8 times a day.

C. Vitamins and Minerals

1. Iron

Infant formulas are classified as "low-iron" or "iron fortified." Iron-fortified formulas range in concentration from 10 to 12 mg/L, which are adequate amounts to meet requirements for the first 12 months of life (assuming the addition of appropriate solid foods in the second 6 months). "Low-iron" formulas contain 1.1 to 4.5 mg/L, a range that fails to meet minimum iron requirements for infants and results in unacceptably high rates of iron deficiency by age 9 months.[11]

Controlled studies have found no difference between low-iron and iron-fortified formulas in the occurrence of infant infections or gastrointestinal disturbances such as diarrhea and constipation.[14,15] Iron-fortified formulas are therefore the recommended option.

2. Fluoride
Ready-to-feed formulas have fluoride concentrations less than 0.3 ppm, the minimum standard beyond which supplementation is recommended. Infants older than 6 months, who are maintained exclusively on ready-to-feed formulas with no additional fluoride intake from fluoridated municipal water or other sources, will therefore require fluoride supplementation. The concentration of fluoride in bottled waters is variable; parents should be discouraged from using bottled water for preparing powdered or concentrated formula.[7]

REFERENCES

1. American Dietetic Association: Position of the American Dietetic Association: promoting and supporting breastfeeding, *J Am Diet Assoc* 105:810-818, 2005.
2. Kramer MS, Kakuma R: The optimal duration of exclusive breastfeeding: a systematic review, *Adv Exp Med Biol* 554: 63-77, 2004.
3. Howard CR, Weitzman M: Breast or bottle: practical aspects of infant nutrition in the first 6 months, *Pediatr Ann* 21:619-621, 1992.
4. American Academy of Pediatrics Work Group on Breastfeeding: Breastfeeding and the use of human milk (RE9727), *Pediatrics* 100:1035-1039, 1997.
5. U.S. Department of Health and Human Services: *Healthy People* 2010. Healthy People 2010 midcourse review. Available at: http://www.healthypeople.gov/Data/2010prog/focus16. Accessed February 28, 2007.
6. Lawrence RA: Storage of human milk and the influence of procedures on immunological components of human milk, *Acta Paediatr* 88:14-18, 1999.
7. Krebs NF, Primak LE: Normal childhood nutrition and its disorders. In Hay WW, Levin MJ, Sondheimer JM, Deterding RR, editors: *Current pediatric diagnosis and treatment,* ed 18, New York, 2007, Lange Medical Books/McGraw-Hill.
8. Hill JB, Sheffield JS, Kim MJ et al: Risk of hepatitis B transmission in breastfed infants of chronic hepatitis B carriers, *Obstet Gynecol* 99:1049-1052, 2002.
9. American Academy of Pediatrics Committee on Drugs: The transfer of drugs and other chemicals into human milk, *Pediatrics* 108:776-789, 2001.
10. Greer FR: Vitamin K status of lactating mothers and their infants, *Acta Paediatr Suppl* 430:95-103, 1999.
11. American Academy of Pediatrics Committee on Nutrition: Iron fortification of infant formulas, *Pediatrics* 104:119-123, 1999.
12. Motil KJ: Infant feeding: a critical look at infant formulas, *Curr Opin Pediatr* 12:469-476, 2000.
13. American Academy of Pediatrics Committee on Nutrition: Soy protein-based formulas: recommendations for use in infant feeding, *Pediatrics* 101:148-153, 1998.
14. Singhal A, Morley R, Abbott R et al: Clinical safety of iron-fortified formulas, *Pediatrics* 105:E38, 2000.
15. Scariati PD, Grummer-Strawn LM, Fein SB et al: Risk of diarrhea related to iron content of infant formula: lack of evidence to support the use of low-iron formula as a supplement for breastfed infants, *Pediatrics* 99:E2, 1997.

SECTION G   Bonding and Family Adaptation

Patricia Fontaine, MD, MS

I. BACKGROUND

A. Definition
Bonding is a positive, emotionally based relationship between infant and parent that is long term, reciprocal, and includes the concept of attachment. Secure infant attachment develops over time as a mother or other primary caretaker who is sensitive to infant behavioral cues meets the infant's needs appropriately and consistently.[1]

B. Infant Attachment Style
The importance of attachment cannot be overstated. By age 12 to 18 months, infants develop a characteristic attachment style that can be objectively judged to be either secure or insecure. Investigations have repeatedly shown that infants with secure attachment exhibit more competent behavior as toddlers and preschoolers. Some authorities consider security of attachment to be of paramount importance to mental health across the life span.[2,3]

C. Bonding Theory
Early studies of bonding indicated that maternal-infant contact within the first 3 hours of birth, combined with extended contact in a rooming-in arrangement, could lead to significant positive effects on subsequent maternal behavior.[4] Additional research since the late 1980s, however, has been unable to substantiate whether there is a "sensitive period" after birth during which bonding must take place, how long the sensitive period may last, and how much and what type of maternal-infant contact is optimal for bonding.[5] Nevertheless, it is highly

consistent with the philosophy of family-centered perinatal care to provide opportunities for appropriate physical contact and to educate parents regarding the physiologic and emotional responses of infants and parents throughout pregnancy, birth, and postpartum. Family physicians may find themselves in a position to review and modify existing hospital routines that arbitrarily interrupt the bonding process.

II. PRENATAL BONDING

A. Maternal Attachment

Maternal attachment to the infant may begin to develop during the prenatal period.[5,6] The level of emotional attachment can be assessed by talking with the mother about her emotional acceptance of the pregnancy, the amount of social support she has for child-rearing, what fantasies she has for her child's future, and what physical preparations she has made for the infant's arrival. In addition, formal assessment tools have been created to rate mother-infant bonding.[7,8] Failure to exhibit expected responses may be a clue to a high-risk situation that would benefit from additional social services or support.

B. Paternal Attachment

The father can be encouraged to participate in a broad range of activities that promote attachment. During prenatal visits, both parents appear to be emotionally affected by experiences such as hearing the fetal heartbeat or viewing the infant via ultrasound. However, the outcomes of such experiences on paternal attachment have not been well studied.

III. BONDING AFTER BIRTH

A. Sensory Components

1. Tactile sensation
   Tactile sensation plays a key role in the bonding process. Parents tend to touch their newborns in a specific pattern, fondling the hands and feet before touching the body, implying an innate process. Tactile stimulation enhances the parent-child relationship from the beginning, providing relaxation, comfort, and positive effects on breastfeeding. Direct skin-to-skin contact has been recommended.[4,5,9] In a trial designed to test the

hypothesis that increased physical contact would promote secure infant attachment, mothers of newborns were randomized to receive either a soft infant carrier or a plastic car seat when discharged from the hospital. Infants whose mothers kept them in close body contact with the soft carrier were significantly more likely to be securely attached at 1 year of age.[10]

2. Mother's voice
   The mother's voice is familiar to the infant from many months of in utero perception. Tone, pitch, cadence, and accent all contribute to familiarity and comfort. Newborns show a significant preference for voices speaking the language they heard in utero.[11] Parents may be encouraged to talk, hum, or sing to the newborn.

3. Eye contact
   This plays an important role in initial parent-infant bonding. Mothers and their infants exhibit a preference for viewing one another at close range with eyes aligned. Parents should be informed that the baby focuses best at a distance of several inches, roughly from the crook of the parent's arm to the face. Drops or ointments used to prevent newborn conjunctivitis can cause irritation and tearing. Instillation may be postponed for 1 hour, until after the initial bonding experiences with mother and father.[5]

4. Nursing and the mother's milk
   These are among the strongest stimuli for attachment, having psychobiologic effects beyond their nutritive value. Although breastfeeding is a powerful bonding influence, it is not strictly essential. Mothers who choose to bottle-feed should be particularly encouraged to engage in other bonding behaviors.[12]

B. Emotional Components

Most mothers, though certainly not all, will develop maternal feelings toward their infants the first time they hold the baby for more than a few minutes.[12] There is typically an outpouring of affection followed by a feeling that the baby belongs to her.[6]

However, the emotional bonding response may be delayed because of medical emergencies, maternal addiction, or depression. For example, women who score higher on the Edinburgh Postnatal Depression Scale after delivery have been shown to have lower bonding scores during the first weeks of life.[8] Parents should be reassured that a satisfying bonding experience can occur after the adverse conditions have stabilized. In cases of cesarean section delivery under regional anesthesia, the mother should be given the opportunity to view and touch her infant while still in the operating room.

C. Rooming In

Rooming in should be encouraged for the extended opportunities it allows for parent-infant contact.[13]

IV. BONDING AND ATTACHMENT ISSUES FOR THE FATHER AND OTHER FAMILY MEMBERS

A. Paternal Bonding

No conclusive statements can be made about the effects of paternal birth attendance, early contact, and extended contact on the father's subsequent involvement with the infant.[14] However, many of the factors involved in maternal bonding may also be experienced by the father. Physical contact and the father's involvement in routine infant care can be encouraged.[15]

B. Sibling Bonding

Sibling visits can be encouraged in the immediate postpartum period, although the effects of visits on sibling attachment to the new baby are largely unstudied.[13] It is prudent for a child with a fever or symptoms of an acute illness, such as upper respiratory infection or gastroenteritis, to be excluded from early visits.[13] Healthy siblings may be taught how to touch, stroke, and speak to the baby within the first days of birth. Allowing a brother or sister of appropriate age to participate in infant care such as feeding or dressing may facilitate positive attachment. Possible sibling jealousy should be anticipated, and clear limits should be set against hitting or rough handling. Sibling classes, analogous to birth preparation classes for parents, are available in some communities. They have not definitively been shown to decrease sibling rivalry or alter reactions to the newborn.[16]

C. Extended Family

The grandmother may be a key support person, particularly for adolescent mothers. One observational study found that infants who were insecurely attached to adolescent mothers were securely attached to the maternal grandmothers who had a significant care-taking role.[17]

V. MARITAL ADAPTATION

The first month of the infant's life is a redefining period in the parents' relationship, characterized by vulnerability and the potential for growth (see Chapter 21, Section C). Lack of sleep, continuing constraints on the sexual relationship, and new physical, emotional, and financial responsibilities may weigh on both father and mother. Family physicians may explore issues of marital adjustment during both postpartum and well-infant visits. Satisfactions inherent in the bonding process and adequate support from an extended social network may serve to counteract the frustrations inherent in new parenting roles.[18,19]

REFERENCES

1. Bowlby J: *Attachment and loss,* vol 1, *Attachment,* New York, 1982, Basic Books.
2. Van Jzendoorn MH, Juffer F, Duyvesteyn MGC: Breaking the intergenerational cycle of insecure attachment; a review of the effects of attachment-based interventions on maternal sensitivity and infant security, *J Child Psychol Psychiatry* 36: 225-247, 1994.
3. Wright JC, Binney V, Smith PK: Security of attachment in 8-12 year-olds: a revised version of the separation anxiety test, its psychometric properties and clinical interpretation, *J Child Psychol Psychiatry* 36:757-774, 1995.
4. Klaus MH, Jerauld R, Kreger NC et al: Maternal attachment: importance of the first post-partum days, *N Engl J Med* 286:460-463, 1972.
5. Symanski ME: Maternal-infant bonding: practice issues for the 1990s, *J Nurse Midwifery* 37:67S-73S, 1992.
6. U.S. Department of Health and Human Services: *Mental health: a report of the Surgeon General.* Chapter 3. *Children and mental health, 1999.* Available at: http://www.surgeongeneral.gov/library/mentalhealth/chapter3/sec1.html. Accessed March 5, 2007.
7. Brockington IF, Oates J, George S et al: A screening questionnaire for mother-infant bonding disorders, *Arch Women's Mental Health* 3:133-140, 2001.
8. Taylor A, Atkins R, Kumar R et al: A new mother-to-infant bonding scale: links with early maternal mood, *Arch Womens Ment Health* 8:45-51, 2005.
9. Anderson GC, Moore E, Hepworth J et al: Early skin-to-skin contact for mothers and their healthy newborn infants, *Cochrane Database Syst Rev* (2):CD003519, 2003.
10. Anisfeld E, Casper V, Nozyce M et al: Does infant carrying promote attachment? An experimental study of the effects of increased physical contact on the development of attachment, *Child Dev* 61:1617-1627, 1990.
11. Fifer WP, Moon CM: The role of mother's voice in the organization of brain function in the newborn, *Acta Paediatr Suppl* 397:86-93, 1994.
12. Troy NW: Early contact and maternal attachment among women using public health care facilities, *Appl Nurs Res* 6: 161-166, 1993.

13. American Academy of Pediatrics (and) the American College of Obstetricians and Gynecologists: Care of the neonate. *Guidelines for perinatal care*, ed 5, Elk Grove, IL and Washington, DC, 2002.
14. Palkovitz R: Changes in father-infant bonding beliefs across couples' first transition to parenthood, *Matern Child Nurs J* 20:141-154, 1992.
15. American Academy of Pediatrics: Becoming a father. In Shelov SP, Hannemann RE, editors: *Caring for your baby and young child: birth to age 5*, ed 4, New York, 1999, Bantam. Excerpt available at: http://www.aap.org/healthtopics/parenting.cfm. Accessed March 6, 2007.
16. Anderberg GJ: Initial acquaintance and attachment behavior of siblings with the newborn, *J Obstet Gynecol Neonatal Nurs* 17:49-54, 1988.
17. Patterson DL: Adolescent mothering: child-grandmother attachment, *J Pediatr Nurs* 12:228-237, 1997.
18. Gjerdingen DK, Froberg DG, Fontaine P: The effects of social support on women's health during pregnancy, labor and delivery, and the postpartum period, *Fam Med* 23:370-375, 1991.
19. Gjerdingen DK, Chaloner KM: The relationship of women's postpartum mental health to employment, childbirth, and social support, *J Fam Pract* 38:465-472, 1994.

SECTION H   General Care of the Neonate

Patricia Fontaine, MD, MS, and Sherri Fong, BS

Parents of healthy babies should leave the hospital with basic written information on home care and feeding. The predischarge interview should include reviewing the instructions with the mother or both parents. In addition, reputable websites can provide resources for new parents.[1-3]

I. CORD CARE

The umbilical cord will dry up and fall off in 1 to 3 weeks. A slight bloody discharge is normal, both before and after the cord falls off. Pyogenic granuloma, a firm, pink nodule developing in the umbilicus after the cord falls off, may be treated with silver nitrate cautery.

II. PENIS/CIRCUMCISION CARE

A. Circumcision Healing

A circumcised penis should heal within a week to 10 days. During healing, the glans oozes small amounts of blood or yellowish serum. Petroleum jelly should be applied to the tip of the penis at each diaper change until it heals to prevent sticking to the diaper.

B. Care of the Uncircumcised Penis

No special care is necessary for the uncircumcised penis during the first month of life. Parents should be instructed not to retract the foreskin forcibly.[4]

III. BATHING

A. Bathing in the First Weeks of Life

The newborn requires only sponge bathing two to three times a week until the cord falls off. After that, the baby may be bathed in a small tub, using mild soap if necessary. Overzealous washing with soap can lead to drying of the skin.

B. Use of Powder, Oil, and Lotions

Powder, oil, and lotion are generally unnecessary and are not recommended because they can clog pores and theoretically increase the risk for contact dermatitis from perfumes, dyes, and other chemicals.

C. Treatment of "Cradle Cap"

Baby shampoo and a soft scalp brush are helpful for dislodging the scales of seborrhea or "cradle cap."

IV. SLEEPING

A. Newborn Sleeping Patterns

Newborns sleep 10 to 12 hours out of 24, waking every 2 to 4 hours for feeding. They will gradually sleep less often for longer periods and be awake longer. At 12 to 13 pounds, they may sleep 8 to 9 hours at a time, or through the night.

B. Sleeping Position

Healthy term newborns should be placed on their backs to sleep to decrease the risk for sudden infant death syndrome (SIDS).[5] Preterm infants are at greater risk for SIDS than term infants.[5,6] Although direct studies are lacking, the consensus is that preterm infants should also be placed on their backs to sleep.[7]

Soft thick bedding, pillows, and compressible mattresses are associated with SIDS and should be avoided. Side sleeping is less desirable because infants may roll onto their stomachs from their sides.[7]

The "Back to Sleep" campaign initiated in 1994 by the National Institute of Child Health and Human Development and the AAP has improved public awareness of the link between SIDS and prone (stomach) sleeping.[8] Between 1992 and 1998 the frequency of prone sleeping among U.S. infants decreased from more than 70% to approximately 20%, and the deaths from SIDS declined by more than 40%.[7]

V. CRYING

A. Possible Causes

A crying infant may be hungry, overfed, hot, cold, wet, tired, or just want to be held. When the problem is corrected, the infant usually stops crying and goes to sleep.

B. Colic

When crying is more persistent, it may be classified as colic. The most widely used definition of colic describes the infant as being unexplainably irritable, fussy, or crying.[9,10] Colic may be frightening to new parents because the infant appears to be in physical distress, with flushed face, clenched fists, and legs pulled up to the abdomen.

Colic develops as early as 2 weeks of life and usually subsides by age 4 months.[10] It typically occurs late in the day and may last for several days.[9] Although the cause of colic remains unknown, common explanations point to gastrointestinal, psychosocial, and neurodevelopmental causes.[10]

When an otherwise healthy infant cries for a prolonged period, parents should be advised to take the infant to the doctor to exclude physiologic causes. Many treatments have been proposed for infant colic, but there is no conclusive evidence of their effectiveness. The best recommendation is to support parents and reassure them that colicky symptoms will resolve in a matter of time.[10]

VI. CAR SEATS

Laws in all 50 states require children to be restrained in car seats when traveling. Infants less than 20 pounds should be in rear-facing infant seats. Proper use of infant safety seats can reduce hospitalizations and fatalities by approximately 70%.[11]

VII. PACIFIERS

During the early months, pacifiers can provide the baby sucking comfort after a full stomach or for short periods of fussiness at sleep time. They are handy, harmless, and often effective. Pacifiers are preferable to thumb sucking because they can be eliminated after 6 to 12 months, and the habit broken.

VIII. BURPING AND VOMITING

A. Burping

Burping expels air swallowed during feeding. Parents typically "burp the baby" after feeding about 5 minutes, holding the baby upright against the shoulder or prone across the knees, and gently patting or rubbing its back. If the baby has not burped within 3 to 5 minutes, continue feeding and try again.

B. "Spitting Up"

"Spitting up" is normal and can be reduced by gentle handling, feeding smaller amounts, and by placing the baby in an upright position after feeding. Projectile vomiting should be reported to the doctor if it occurs repeatedly.

C. Hiccups

Hiccups are caused by a full stomach pressing on the diaphragm, causing it to contract rhythmically and involuntarily. Hiccups may continue for an hour, but are harmless. Burping the baby or offering additional sips of warm water, milk, or formula may interrupt the hiccups.

IX. BOWEL AND BLADDER FUNCTION

A. Normal Infant Bowel Movements

Bowel movements may occur after every feeding or as infrequently as every few days. The typical breast-fed infant's stools will be yellow, soft, and "seedy" in appearance. Stools of formula-fed infants are more formed and brown. Parents should understand that variation in color is common and rarely signifies pathology.

B. Constipation

If the stools are small, hard pellets, the infant is constipated. Fluid intake may be supplemented by giving the infant a little warm water. Parents should not use enemas or bowel stimulants without physician supervision.

C. Frequency of Urination

The baby should urinate every 2 to 4 hours.

X. FEVER

A. Significance of Fever in Infancy

Fever may be a sign of serious illness during the first month of life. The rate of bacterial infection has been found to be roughly 4% when the temperature is 38.1° to 39°C, 8% for 39.1° to 39.9°C. and 18% for 40°C or more.[12] Parents should report to the physician a rectal temperature more than 38.8°C.

B. Thermometers

Every household with an infant should be equipped with a thermometer. Glass thermometers with mercury, digital thermometers, and tympanic thermometers all give accurate measurements.[13] Liquid crystal strips applied to the forehead are inaccurate in infants younger than 1 month.[14] Mercury and digital thermometers can be used by the oral, rectal, or axillary routes. The rectal measurements may be up to 1°C more than a simultaneous axillary determination.[14]

C. Antipyretics

Liquid formulations of acetaminophen or ibuprofen can be used for managing fever in infants older than 2 months.[13]

REFERENCES

1. *American Academy of Pediatrics parenting corner.* Available at: http://www.aap.org/parents.html. Accessed March 7, 2007.
2. *KidsHealth from the health experts of Nemours.* Available at: http://www.kidshealth.org/index.html. Accessed March 7, 2007.
3. *Zero to three.* Available at: http://www.zerotothree.org. Accessed March 7, 2007.
4. American Academy of Pediatrics: *Newborns: care of the uncircumcised penis,* Elk Grove, IL, 2007, AAP Professional Publication.
5. Oyen N, Markestad T, Skaerven R et al: Combined effects of sleeping position and prenatal risk factors in sudden infant death syndrome: the Nordic epidemiologic SIDS study, *Pediatrics* 100:613-621, 1997.
6. Malloy MH, Hoffman HJ: Prematurity, sudden infant death syndrome, and age of death, *Pediatrics* 96:464-471, 1995.
7. American Academy of Pediatrics Task Force on Infant Sleep Position and Sudden Infant Death Syndrome: Changing concepts of sudden infant death syndrome: implications for infant sleeping environment and sleep position, *Pediatrics* 105:650-656, 2000.
8. Willinger M, Hoffman HJ, Wu KT et al: Factors associated with the transition to nonprone sleep positions of infants in the United States: the National Infant Sleep Position Study, *JAMA* 280:329-335, 1998.
9. Wessel MA, Cobb JC, Jackson EB et al: Paroxysmal fussing in infancy, sometimes called "colic," *Pediatrics* 14:421-435, 1954.
10. Roberts DM: Infantile colic, *Am Fam Physician* 70:735-740, 2004.
11. American Academy of Pediatrics Policy Statement: Safe transportation of newborns at hospital discharge, *Pediatrics* 104: 986-987, 1999.
12. Bonadio WA, Romine K, Gyuro J: Relationship of fever magnitude to rate of serious bacterial infection, *J Pediatr* 116:733, 1990.
13. Brayden RM, Daley MF, Brown JM: Ambulatory & community pediatrics. In Hay WW, Levin MJ, Sondheimer JM, Deterding RR, editors: *Current pediatric diagnosis and treatment,* ed 18, New York, 2007, Lange Medical Books/McGraw-Hill.
14. Shann F, Mackenzie A: Comparison of rectal, axillary, and forehead temperatures, *Arch Pediatr Adolesc Med* 150:74-78, 1996.

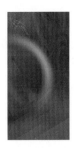

Postpartum Biomedical Concerns: Breastfeeding

SECTION A **Delayed Postpartum Hemorrhage**

Charles Carter, MD,
and Elizabeth G. Baxley, MD

I. DEFINITION

Late postpartum bleeding (secondary postpartum hemorrhage) is defined as abnormal or excessive vaginal bleeding occurring anywhere from 24 hours until 12 weeks after delivery.[1] This postpartum complication occurs most commonly as a result of uterine subinvolution, that is, failure of vessels at the former placental site to return to normal size or obliterate, or both.[2] This may result from partial retention of placental tissue or blood clots or infection. Retained placental fragments that do not cause immediate postpartum hemorrhage undergo necrosis and fibrin deposition, leading to formation of a placental polyp. As the polyp eschar detaches from the myometrium, a brisk late postpartum hemorrhage may occur. Other less common causes include a ruptured varix, submucosal leiomyomata, genital tract hematomas, and clotting disorders.[3]

II. DIAGNOSIS

The diagnosis is made when heavier bleeding, in excess of normal lochia, develops after the first postpartum day. Once hemorrhage is noted, a source must be identified. The perineum and vagina should be explored for a bleeding source or hematoma. Uterine size should be assessed by bimanual examination.

Clinical assessment for retained placental tissue has a 67% positive predictive value (PPV) and a 94% negative predictive value (NPV).[4]

If examination does not reveal a cause, or if the patient does not respond to initial treatment, laboratory tests should be ordered, including hematocrit and hemoglobin, platelet count, prothrombin time, partial thromboplastin time, fibrinogen, and fibrin split products.

When bleeding is moderate, but not severe enough to require immediate surgical intervention, ultrasound may be a helpful diagnostic tool because it can potentially exclude retained placental fragments as the cause. However, it should be used with a measure of caution, because there is poor correlation between clinical assessment and ultrasound findings. Although quite sensitive (93-94%), its use is limited by a poor specificity (16-62%), with a PPV of 46% and a NPV of 96%.[5,6] This is due, in part, to the finding that 51% of women with normal postpartum bleeding at 7 days will have intrauterine echogenic foci seen on ultrasound.[7] Thus, a negative ultrasound is considered reassuring, whereas a positive study may lead to unnecessary curettage.

III. TREATMENT

Initial therapy is directed at controlling the bleeding. However, a paucity of quality evidence exists regarding treatment, with a Cochrane review finding no randomized controlled trials (RCTs) available to guide therapy.[1] Oxytocin, in concentrations of 20 to 24 units per liter of fluid, given intravenously at a rate of 250 ml/hr, or methylergonovine, at a dose of 0.2 mg given intramuscularly, are commonly used drug regimens for postpartum hemorrhage. Prostaglandin E_2

vaginal suppositories, or intramuscular or intramyo-metrial injection of 0.25 mg prostaglandin F_2, have been shown to work in refractory cases of bleeding.[1,3] Misoprostol is another potentially effective treatment for delayed postpartum hemorrhage. However, current evidence supports its use only in primary postpartum hemorrhage, and further quality trials are needed to decide the best dose and route of administration.[8] Its use in delayed postpartum hemorrhage is limited to a case report, albeit with positive results.[9]

Adequate blood replacement, appropriate anesthesia, and surgical assistance should be obtained as needed. Curettage is usually effective in stopping immediate hemorrhage and may be helpful in identifying the cause of bleeding if placental fragments or large blot clots are retrieved. Selective arterial embolization via interventional radiology is effective when curettage has failed and has the potential to preserve fertility.[10] In severe cases of hemorrhage, uterine packing, surgical intervention, or both are necessary, often with ligation of the uterine or hypogastric artery, or both. Occasionally, subtotal or total hysterectomy must be performed.

REFERENCES

1. Alexander J, Thomas P, Sanghera J: Treatments for secondary postpartum haemorrhage, *Cochrane Database Syst Rev* (1): CD002867, 2002.
2. Neill AC, Nixon RM, Thornton S: A comparison of clinical assessment with ultrasound in the management of secondary postpartum haemorrhage, *Eur J Obstet Gynecol Reprod Biol* 104:113-115, 2002.
3. James AH: More than menorrhagia: a review of the obstetric and gynaecological manifestations of bleeding disorders, *Haemophilia* 11:295-307, 2005.
4. Neill AC, Nixon RM, Thornton S: A comparison of clinical assessment with ultrasound in the management of secondary postpartum haemorrhage, *Eur J Obstet Gynecol Reprod Biol* 104:113-115, 2002.
5. Pather S, Ford M, Reid R et al: Postpartum curettage: an audit of 200 cases, *Aust N Z J Obstet Gynaecol* 45:368-371, 2005.
6. Neill AC, Nixon RM, Thornton S: A comparison of clinical assessment with ultrasound in the management of secondary postpartum haemorrhage, *Eur J Obstet Gynecol Reprod Biol* 104:113-115, 2002.
7. Edwards A, Ellwood DA: Ultrasonographic evaluation of the postpartum uterus, *Ultrasound Obstet Gynecol* 16:640-643, 2000.
8. Mousa HA, Alfirevic Z: Treatment for primary postpartum haemorrhage, *Cochrane Database Syst Rev* (1):CD003249, 2007.
9. Adenkanmi OA, Purmessur S, Edwards G et al: Intrauterine misoprostol for the treatment of severe recurrent atonic secondary postpartum haemorrhage, *BJOG* 108:541-542, 2001.
10. Pelage J, Soyer P, Repiquet D et al: Secondary postpartum hemorrhage: treatment with selective arterial embolization, *Radiology* 212:385-389, 1999.

SECTION B Postpartum Endometritis

Elizabeth G. Baxley, MD, and Charles Carter, MD

I. DEFINITION AND EPIDEMIOLOGY

Postpartum endometritis is the most common puerperal infection, occurring in 1.6% to 2.5% of women after vaginal delivery, and in 6% to 18% of women who undergo cesarean delivery, depending on the risk factors that led to operative delivery.[1-3] It refers to a spectrum of infections.[3]

A. Endometritis
Endometritis represents the initial stage of infection involving the endometrium and superficial myometrium.

B. Endomyometritis
Endomyometritis indicates a moderate stage of infection involving the endometrium and the full thickness of the myometrium.

C. Endomyoparametritis
Endomyoparametritis indicates a severe infection, in which infection has progressed through the myometrium and has extended into the broad ligaments. Endometritis should be suspected when a woman experiences development of persistent fever in the postpartum period and another source of infection is not found.

II. CAUSES OF POSTPARTUM ENDOMETRITIS

A. Causative Agents
Endometritis occurs as an ascending infection of normal vaginal organisms. The majority of cases are polymicrobial in origin (Table 20-1).

Gram-positive aerobic cocci, predominantly streptococci, are most common. Other less common aerobic organisms include *Escherichia coli* and *Enterococcus*. *Enterococcus* has been isolated in up to one fourth of women who receive cephalosporin prophylaxis before delivery.[4]

Anaerobic gram-negative bacilli make up approximately one third of isolates, with *Bacteroides* being the most common. These women are more likely to

TABLE 20-1 Commonly Isolated Organisms in Women with Endometritis

Aerobes	*Anaerobes*
Gram-positive cocci	Gram-positive cocci
Group B streptococcus	*Peptococcus* sp.
Group A streptococcus	*Peptostreptococcus* sp.
Enterococcus	Gram-positive bacilli
Streptococcus sp. (other)	*Clostridium* sp.
Staphylococcus sp.	Gram-negative bacilli
Gram-negative cocci	*Bacteroides bivius*
Escherichia coli	*Bacteroides fragilis*
Klebsiella pneumoniae	*Bacteroides sp (other)*
Proteus mirabilis	

Adapted from Cox S, Gilstrap L: Postpartum endometritis, *Obstet Gynecol Clin North Am* 16(2):363-371, 1989.

have severe endometritis or acquire a wound infection.[2,5] *Gardnerella vaginalis* and other anaerobes that are typically associated with bacterial vaginosis (BV) also should be considered likely pathogens.

III. RISK FACTORS

A. Route of Delivery
The dominant predictor of postpartum endometritis is cesarean delivery.[1,4,5] A retrospective review of 32,834 women that included 22,270 spontaneous vaginal deliveries, 4908 assisted vaginal deliveries, and 5656 cesarean deliveries demonstrated this risk as shown in Table 20-2.[1]

TABLE 20-2 Influence of Cesarean Section on Endometritis

Primary cesarean delivery with a trial of labor	21.2 RR increase	95% CI: 15.4-29.1
Primary cesarean delivery without a trial of labor	10.3 RR increase	95% CI: 5.9-17.9
Repeat cesarean delivery after a trial of labor	14.6 RR increase	95% CI: 9.2-23.1

Adapted from Burrows LJ, Meyn LA, Weber AM: Maternal morbidity associated with vaginal versus cesarean delivery, *Obstet Gynecol* 103:907-912, 2004.
RR, Relative risk; CI, confidence interval.

Wide variation exists in reported rates of endometritis after abdominal delivery. In low-risk situations, such as elective repeat cesarean, the incidence rate may be as low as 2.7%. However, when operative delivery follows prolonged labor and rupture of membranes, and in women who have undergone a large number of vaginal examinations, endometritis rates increase to 9.4%.[1,4] Furthermore, duration of surgery in patients undergoing cesarean delivery is directly proportional to endometritis rates.

It is not uncommon for women who have postpartum endometritis after a cesarean delivery to also experience development of an abdominal incision infection. The causative organism is typically derived from the patient's skin flora. *Staphylococcus aureus* is most common, and community-acquired, methicillin-resistant strains are also possible pathogens.[2]

B. Length of Labor
Increased labor length correlates positively with the risk for endometritis because of increased colonization of the lower uterine segment from the greater number of cervical examinations performed.

C. Prolonged Rupture of Membranes
Prolonged rupture of the membranes confers a two-fold increased risk for postpartum endometritis.[1] Positive amniotic fluid cultures have been reported in women with membrane rupture longer than 24 hours, although this appears to relate more to corresponding long labor length. When the effect of labor length has been removed, rupture of membranes alone has not been confirmed as an independent risk factor for endometritis.[4]

D. Internal Fetal Monitoring
Little evidence has been reported to support greater endometritis rates as a result of internal fetal monitoring. Studies that have reported an association between these practices and endometritis have selected women who have had longer labors, more vaginal examinations, and a protracted period of ruptured membranes.[4]

E. Manual Placental Removal
Manual removal of the placenta and uterine exploration after placental delivery have both been implicated as contributing risk factors in the development of postpartum endometritis.[6] Manual placental removal at the time of cesarean delivery also increases rates of postpartum endometritis, with a relative risk of 1.7.[7,8]

F. Maternal Obesity

Cesarean delivery in a woman with a body mass index greater than 25 or weighing more than 200 pounds increases the likelihood of development of endometritis by 30%.[1,2]

G. Chorioamnionitis

Pregnancies complicated by chorioamnionitis are 3.2 times more likely to also be complicated by postpartum endometritis.[1] However, women with chorioamnionitis who receive appropriate antibiotic therapy after delivery are unlikely to experience development of postpartum endometritis.[2]

H. Anal Sphincter Lacerations

Women who experience anal sphincter lacerations are 2.9 to 4.5 times more likely to experience development of postpartum endometritis compared with those who did not have a laceration.[1]

IV. DIAGNOSIS

A. History and Clinical Examination

Postpartum endometritis is a clinical diagnosis, suggested primarily by fever and the exclusion of extrapelvic sources of infection. Postpartum fever less than 101°F in the first 24 hours after delivery often resolves spontaneously. However, maternal temperatures of $\geq$100.4°F (38°C) on 2 or more occasions, at least 6 hours apart, after the first 24 hours postpartum, or fever of more than 101.0°F at any time, when accompanied by lower abdominal pain and uterine tenderness, heralds the diagnosis of endometritis.

Maternal tachycardia commonly parallels the fever. The patient may have foul-smelling lochia, although this is not a consistent finding. Associated findings may include dynamic ileus, pelvic peritonitis, or pelvic abscess. It is rare to find a palpable mass distinct from the tender uterus on initial examination.

B. Differential Diagnosis

Other causes of postpartum fever should be excluded as the cause of the fever, including urinary tract infection, pneumonia or atelectasis, wound infection, intravenous site phlebitis, viral syndrome, and mastitis. The clinical examination should be comprehensive in nature, including auscultation of the lungs and palpation of the breasts, back, and extremities. Examination of abdominal or perineal wounds also should include looking for abscess or cellulitis. Septic pelvic thrombophlebitis is a rare cause of postpartum fever and should be considered when a woman fails to respond to conventional therapy for endometritis (see Chapter 20, Section F).

C. Laboratory Studies

Leukocytosis in the range of 15,000 cells/mcL to 30,000 cells/mcL is typical for women with postpartum endometritis. However, this leukocytosis is difficult to differentiate from the physiologic leukocytosis of pregnancy; thus, serial changes in white blood cell count may be more helpful in aiding in the diagnosis and treatment response. Urine cultures should be collected routinely in postpartum patients with fever to rule out a urinary tract infection. Genital cultures are frequently contaminated and rarely provide clinically useful information. Blood cultures should be obtained from women experiencing shaking chills or rigors,[2] though they are positive in only 5% to 10% of patients and rarely implicate a single causative agent.[4] Culture findings are not available at the time treatment is initiated, which further limits their usefulness.

D. Imaging Studies

In women with puerperal fever refractory to antimicrobial therapy, contrast-enhanced computed tomography (CT) is the initial study of choice. Magnetic resonance imaging is an alternative, whereas sonography is unreliable.[9]

V. PREVENTION OF ENDOMETRITIS

A. Antenatal Prevention

Altered vaginal microflora before the onset of labor (e.g., BV; heavy vaginal colonization by *Streptococcus agalactiae, Streptococcus pyogenes,* or *E. coli*) has been associated with greater rates of endometritis.[2] In one cohort study with 924 patients enrolled, the risk for postpartum endometritis was tripled among women with BV in early pregnancy (RR, 3.26).[10] However, no trials to date have demonstrated that screening for and treating BV reduces infectious complications.[11]

A Cochrane analysis that examined 6 RCTs, involving 2184 women, concluded that in high-risk patients, defined as those with a previous preterm birth, antibiotic prophylaxis in the second and third trimester results in a reduced risk for postpartum endometritis (odds ratio [OR], 0.46; 95% confidence interval, 0.24-0.89).[12] These studies used various antibiotics and delivery units. Thus, the ideal prophylactic regimen remains uncertain.

B. Prevention at Time of Delivery

Studies of prophylactic antibiotic use at delivery are conflicting. Antibiotics often are used at the time of cord clamping to prevent postpartum endometritis in women undergoing cesarean delivery. A Cochrane review of 81 RCTs comparing antibiotic prophylaxis with no treatment in women undergoing elective and nonelective cesarean delivery showed that use of prophylactic antibiotics reduced the incidence of postpartum endometritis by two thirds.[13]

Single-dose antibiotic prophylaxis with ampicillin/ sulbactam, cefazolin, or cefotetan appears to be effective for uninfected, at-risk women undergoing cesarean delivery.[14] Single-dose ampicillin/sulbactam provides better prophylaxis than single-dose ampicillin in women undergoing cesarean section with rupture of membranes. In one small RCT, failure of prophylaxis and subsequent endometritis was documented in 8.8% of patients who received ampicillin and sulbactam and 35.3% of patients who received ampicillin alone ($p < 0.02$).[15]

VI. TREATMENT

A. Antibiotic Choices

Once endometritis is diagnosed, treatment should be initiated with parenteral antibiotics. Broad-spectrum coverage is necessary because of the polymicrobial nature of the disease, but there is no consensus on the safest and most efficacious regimen.[4] Systematic literature review supports the standard treatment of clindamycin for coverage of gram-positive and anaerobic organisms, but in combination with an aminoglycoside, typically gentamicin, for gram-negative coverage.[16] Once-daily dosing of gentamicin at 4.5 to 5 mg/kg has been shown to achieve therapeutic peak levels without drug accumulation and with substantial cost savings.[16-18] Fewer treatment failures have been demonstrated with once-daily dosing of gentamicin as compared with thrice-daily dosing.[16,17] In addition, once-daily dosing with clindamycin (2700 mg) has also been evaluated together with gentamicin (5 mg/kg) in women with postpartum endometritis, and it has demonstrated a similar success rate as the standard every 8 hours dosing schedule.[19]

B. Length of Treatment

Antibiotic therapy administered early in the infection will usually produce a positive response in more than 90% of patients within 48 hours of initiation.[2,20] Parenteral antibiotics should be continued until the patient has been afebrile and asymptomatic for 24 to 48 hours.[21] RCTs have shown no benefit from oral antibiotic therapy after successful parenteral treatment for endometritis, which has led to the conclusion that this common practice is unnecessary.[15,20]

C. Treatment Failure

Bacterial pathogen resistance is a rare cause of antibiotic treatment failure. Rather, inappropriate response parenteral antibiotic therapy should prompt a search for additional diagnoses. Other pelvic pathologies presenting similarly to endometritis include pelvic or surgical site abscess, abscess involving the episiotomy and deeper vaginal tissue, and septic pelvic thrombophlebitis. The patient should also be reevaluated for extrapelvic sources of infection, and her medication list should be reviewed for adequacy of antibiotic dosing and to assess for the possibility of drug fever.

VII. SUMMARY

Postpartum endometritis is the most common cause of puerperal infection. It occurs more frequently in women undergoing cesarean delivery. It is usually an anaerobe predominant, polymicrobial infection. Diagnosis is based predominantly on the clinical examination and the exclusion of other causes of postpartum fever. Most women respond to parenteral, single-daily dose therapy with clindamycin and an aminoglycoside. Oral antibiotics are not indicated after clinical improvement is achieved with intravenous therapy.

VIII. SOR A RECOMMENDATIONS

RECOMMENDATIONS	REFERENCES
Gentamicin and clindamycin, in combination, are the drugs of choice when treating endometritis. Once-daily dosing of gentamicin is associated with fewer treatment failures than thrice-daily dosing.	*16*
Oral therapy is not needed once uncomplicated endometritis has clinically improved with intravenous therapy.	*16*
Prophylactic antibiotics should be given to women undergoing elective or nonelective cesarean delivery.	*13*

REFERENCES

1. Burrows LJ, Meyn LA, Weber AM: Maternal morbidity associated with vaginal versus cesarean delivery, *Obstet Gynecol* 103:907-912, 2004.
2. Faro S: Postpartum endometritis, *Clin Perinatol* 32:803-814, 2005.
3. Morales WJ, Collins EM, Angel JL et al: Short course of antibiotic therapy in treatment of postpartum endomyometritis, *Am J Obstet Gynecol* 161:568-572, 1989.
4. Cox SM, Gilstrap LC: Postpartum endometritis, *Obstet Gynecol* 16(2):363-371, 1989.
5. Newton ER, Prihoda TJ, Gibbs RS: A clinical and microbiologic analysis of risk factors for puerperal endometritis, *Obstet Gynecol* 75:402-406, 1990.
6. Ely JW, Rijshinghani A, Bowdler NC et al: The association between manual removal of the placenta and postpartum endometritis following vaginal delivery, *Obstet Gynecol* 86:1002-1006, 1995.
7. Dehbashi S, Honarvar M, Fardi FH: Manual removal or spontaneous delivery and postcesarean endometritis and bleeding, *Int J Gynecol Obstet* 86:12-15, 2004.
8. Wendy Atkinson M, Owen J, Wren A et al: The effect of manual removal of the placenta on postcesarean endometritis, *Obstet Gynecol* 87(1):99-102, 1996.
9. Kubik-Huch RA, Huch R, Hilfiker P et al: Role of duplex color Doppler ultrasound, computed tomography, and MR angiography in the diagnosis of septic puerperal ovarian vein thrombosis, *Abdom Imaging* 24:85-91, 1999.
10. Jacobsson B, Pernevi P, Chidekel L et al: Bacterial vaginosis in early pregnancy may predispose for preterm birth and postpartum endometritis, *Acta Obstet Gynecol Scand* 81(11):1006-1010, 2002.
11. Kekki M, Kurki T, Pelkonen J et al: Vaginal clindamycin in preventing preterm birth and periparital infections in asymptomatic women with bacterial vaginosis: a randomized, controlled trial, *Obstet Gynecol* 97:643-648, 2001.
12. Thinkhamrop J, Hofmeyr GJ, Adetoro O et al: Prophylactic antibiotic administration in pregnancy to prevent infectious morbidity and mortality, *Cochrane Database Syst Rev* (4):CD002250, 2002.
13. Smaill F, Hofmeyr GJ: Antibiotic prophylaxis for cesarean section, *Cochrane Database Syst Rev* (3):CD00093, 2002.
14. Noyes N, Berkeley AS, Freedman K et al: Incidence of postpartum endomyometritis following single-dose antibiotic prophylaxis with either ampicillin/sulbactam, cefazolin, or cefotetan in high-risk cesarean section patients, *Infect Dis Obstet Gynecol* 6:220-223, 1998.
15. Rijshinghani A, Savopoulos SE, Walters JK et al: Ampicillin/sulbactam versus ampicillin alone for cesarean section prophylaxis: a randomized double-blind trial, *Am J Perinatol* 12:322-324, 1995.
16. French LM, Smaill FM: Antibiotic regimens for endometritis after delivery, *Cochrane Database Syst Rev* (4):CD001067, 2004.
17. Mitra AG, Whitten MK, Laurent SL et al: A randomized, prospective study comparing once-daily gentamicin versus thrice-daily gentamicin in the treatment of puerperal infection, *Am J Obstet Gynecol* 177:786-792, 1997.
18. Sunyecz JA, Wiesenfeld HC, Heine RP: The pharmacokinetics of once-daily dosing with gentamicin in women with postpartum endometritis, *Infect Dis Obstet Gynecol* 6:160-162, 1998.
19. Livingston JC, Llata E, Rinehart E et al: Gentamicin and clindamycin therapy in postpartum endometritis: the efficacy of daily dosing versus dosing every 8 hours, *Am J Obstet Gynecol* 188:149-152, 2003.
20. Dinsmoor MJ, Newton ER, Gibbs RS: A randomized, double-blind, placebo-controlled trial of oral antibiotic therapy following intravenous antibiotic therapy for postpartum endometritis, *Obstet Gynecol* 77:60-62, 1991.
21. Larsen JW, Hager WD, Livengood CH et al: Guidelines for the diagnosis, treatment and prevention of postoperative infections, *Infect Dis Obstet Gynecol* 11:65-70, 2003.

SECTION C Breastfeeding

Mary Rose Tully, MPH, IBCLC,
and Patricia Ann Payne, BSN, CNM, MPH

Family practitioners are in an ideal position to both promote and manage breastfeeding. Breastfeeding is natural, but not automatic; therefore, it is important for physicians to be familiar with common feeding problems that may lead to premature weaning. Breastfeeding is not always trouble free; therefore, knowledgeable physician support can be important to breastfeeding outcomes.[1]

I. INFLUENCE OF THE HEALTH-CARE SYSTEM

A. Provider Behavior

Physicians can have enormous impact on breastfeeding duration by working from the premise that breastfeeding is the standard for infant feeding, guiding mothers to effective resources, and being available to breastfeeding patients.[2] By bringing their practice settings into compliance with the *International Code of Marketing of Breast-milk Substitutes*[3] and subsequent resolutions, family practice physicians can assure that women benefit from continuity of care in a breastfeeding-friendly environment.

Raisler[4] used focus groups to examine qualitatively the experience of low-income women around breastfeeding within the existing health-care system. The women identified helpful providers as those who had accurate information, established a caring relationship, had a repertoire of effective interventions/suggestions, were enthusiastic, and made referrals to other professionals for problems they themselves could not manage. The women identified provider behaviors that were not helpful as being difficult to reach to ask questions, giving misinformation, encouraging formula supplementation as an answer to breastfeeding problems, and using a routine and impersonal approach.

B. Prenatal and Postpartum Practices

Routine procedures that may seem innocuous have been shown to negatively impact breastfeeding initiation and duration. A number of studies have evaluated the deleterious effects of hospitals dispensing formula sample packs on breastfeeding duration.[1,5] Researchers have begun to look at the influence of prenatal exposure to formula advertising and free samples on breastfeeding initiation and continuation rates. Howard and colleagues[6] report on the effects of formula advertising materials distributed prenatally in an office setting on breastfeeding practices. The study involving 547 women found that, although breastfeeding initiation was not affected, exposure to formula promotion materials significantly increased breastfeeding cessation in the first 2 weeks. Among women with uncertain goals for breastfeeding or goals of 12 weeks or less, exclusive, full, and overall breastfeeding durations was shortened. Although this study lacks socioeconomic and racial diversity, similar studies bear out the general results. The distribution of formula samples by health-care providers, even when specifically designated as "breastfeeding kits," decreases breastfeeding duration.[6]

II. BENEFITS OF BREASTFEEDING

A. Breastfeeding as the Infant Feeding Paradigm

When thinking about infant feeding or talking with parents, consider breastfeeding as the paradigm, rather than a way to give the infant some "advantages." This is critical both as the physician weighs intervention options when there are feeding problems and in conveying the significance of breastfeeding for infant health in the short and long term.[7] For example, explaining that the child who is formula-fed has an increased risk for respiratory infections, just as the infant who lives with secondhand smoke does, may be more honest and effective than saying that the child who is breastfed has the advantage of fewer ear infections.

B. The Costs of Not Breastfeeding

Ball and Wright reviewed the health-care costs for a cohort of infants who were formula-fed in the late 1990s.[8] They found it cost an additional $331 to $475 to provide health care for an infant *never* breastfed in the first year of life. These data do not include loss of income or productivity while caring for the infants or the loss of revenue to the employers when employees are out with sick children.

C. Benefits of Breastfeeding to the Mother

1. Immediate postpartum benefits
   Breastfeeding in the immediate postpartum period promotes uterine contractions and decreases blood loss. The stimulation of oxytocin production by the suckling infant has also been shown to increase the mother's engrossment with and attachment to her infant.[9]

2. Protection against breast cancer
   In a case–control study, Jernstom and colleagues found that among women who carry the *BRCA1* gene, cumulative lactation for at least a year is protective against breast cancer; however, it does not provide protection for those with *BRCA2*.[10] Although there appears to be a protective effect of breastfeeding against postmenopausal breast cancer, the research remains inconclusive.[10,11] Breastfeeding has also been found to be protective against ovarian cancer.[12]

3. Bone density status
   A review by Karlsson and co-workers[13] found that, although there is bone density loss during pregnancy and lactation, there is at least a return to prepregnancy status, if not an improved bone density status, among women who breastfeed. The authors also found that risk for fracture was slightly less than, or equal to, that for nulliparous women in all studies. Additional studies are necessary, and calcium supplementation still appears to be important for women during childbearing years.

4. Family planning
   Optimal child spacing of 3 to 5 years allows a woman to recover from pregnancy and childbearing. The lactational amenorrhea method (LAM) has been shown to be an effective method of child spacing.[14,15] Essentially, as long as the interval between breastfeedings during the day does not exceed 4 hours and there is no more than one 6-hour interval at night, ovulation is suppressed, even if menses returns.[14] Even though it is not commonly used in the United States, LAM can be an effective approach to pregnancy prevention during the first 6 months after delivery if a woman is exclusively breastfeeding. The woman must be

instructed carefully about the implications of supplementing the infant, and that once the number of breastfeedings per day decreases she will need another form of contraception. Trained personnel should instruct women in the other parameters of natural family planning (NFP) such as keeping a basal body temperature chart and evaluating cervical mucus, especially if they are interested in using this method long term.

D. Contraindications

True contraindications to breastfeeding are extremely rare and include mothers taking chemotherapy drugs and mothers who are human immunodeficiency virus (HIV)–positive with access to safe feeding alternatives.[16] Mothers who are human T-cell lymphotrophic virus–positive can pump and freeze their milk to destroy the virus, but they should not breastfeed.[17] Infants with galactosemia cannot breastfeed, and those with some rare metabolic disorders, such as phenylketonuria disease, may need to combine breastfeeding with a specially developed formula to meet their nutritional needs.[16] Occasionally, a mother may need to temporarily stop breastfeeding while she is taking a medication, but she can pump and discard her milk until the medication has cleared her system.[18]

III. BREAST ASSESSMENT

A. Breast Examination

Breast examination is a part of routine care. This is a good time to introduce the discussion of breastfeeding.[19] A careful history of breast problems and surgeries is important.

B. Breast Surgeries

If milk ducts have been cut during a surgical procedure, they may be blocked by scar tissue or no longer be connected to allow milk to flow. With reduction mammoplasty, the milk ducts and nerves in the areolar area may be severed or scarred. Breast implants are rarely a problem when breastfeeding because they are placed under the muscle, and placement does not interfere with either nerves or ducts. However, if the implants were placed to change the appearance of tuber-shaped (long, narrow), hypoplastic, or asymmetric breasts, rather than just as size enhancement, there may be a problem with inadequate glandular tissue for milk production. Radiation treatment that includes the breasts can also affect milk production.

The infant of a woman who has had breast surgery should be followed closely to assess milk transfer until weight gain is well established (Tables 20-3 and 20-4). Careful monitoring of milk transfer can guide the clinician in determining whether there is a need to supplement and the volume the infant will require. Nipple piercing does not prevent successful breastfeeding, although the jewelry must be removed before breastfeeding.

TABLE 20-3 Signs That Feeding Is Progressing Successfully

Infant
- At least 3 stools every 24 hours (changing from meconium to breast milk stools by day 4)
- At least 6 wet diapers with pale urine every 24 hours by day 4
- Infant is content between feedings
- Infant rouses easily or wakes for feedings about every third hour

Mother
- Breasts soften or lighten as the baby feeds
- Breast changes signaling lactogenesis stage II around 72 hours
- Nipples may be tender but are not abraded or cracked, and pain eases as milk flows during feeding
- Signs of oxytocin and prolactin release: uterine contractions/increased lochia flow from oxytocin (in the first 3-4 days), and drowsy and thirsty from prolactin

---

TABLE 20-4 Signs of Correct Latch/Milk Transfer

- Sustained, rhythmic suck/swallows with short pauses
- Audible swallows (mother may not recognize this at first)
- Infant's arms and hands relaxed during feeding
- Infant's mouth moist after feeding
- Mother feels a strong tug, but not pain, on the nipple after initial latch
- Mother experiences signs of hormone release (see Table 20-3)
- Breasts soften or lighten during feeding
- Nipples are elongated at end of feeding but not pinched or abraded

C. Anatomic Variants

Neifert found that women who experience little or no prenatal breast enlargement were at greater risk for insufficient milk production.[20] Although breast size has no influence on milk production, some variations in anatomy are associated with insufficient milk production.[21] Tuber-shaped breasts, hypoplastic breasts, breasts that are set wide enough to allow placement of the palm of a hand between them, and markedly asymmetric breasts are all associated with increased risk for insufficient milk production. However, not all women with these breast variations have problems. Again, careful monitoring of milk transfer and infant weight gain can guide the clinician's management.

D. Inverted Nipples

About 10% of women have truly inverted nipples that retract when stimulated.[22] Although wearing plastic breast shells is often suggested in the prenatal period, Neifert found their use was not predictive of breastfeeding success at 6 weeks.[22] Although some interventions such as Hoffman's exercises have been described in the literature for encouraging the nipple to evert prenatally, no evidence exists that they make a difference. Nipple shields can be used for infants that have difficulty latching on to an inverted nipple (see Box 20-1).

IV. IMMEDIATE POSTPARTUM MANAGEMENT ISSUES

A. Optimal Feeding Practices

Clinical management in the first 48 hours after birth can significantly affect breastfeeding duration.[1,19] Early initiation of breastfeeding, typically in the first hour, is associated with establishment of effective feeding, as well as enhanced maternal-infant interaction. Unrestricted breastfeeding, at least every third hour, is associated with less pathologic engorgement, earlier onset of mature milk production, lower infant bilirubin levels, more stable infant blood glucose levels, decreased initial infant weight loss, and greater weight gain.[1]

B. Assessment of the Newborn

Healthy term infants do not typically experience development of symptomatic hypoglycemia as a consequence of poor or infrequent feedings, but they may experience development of transient hypoglycemia in the immediate newborn period. Exclusive breastfeeding is adequate to meet the needs of these healthy

---

BOX 20-1   NIPPLE SHIELDS

Some infants have no difficulty latching on to an inverted nipple, and their sucking draws the nipple into the mouth effectively. If the infant is having difficulty, a silicone nipple shield (Figure 20-1) can be used to facilitate latch-on. Nipple shields are available in three sizes. To work effectively, the base of the shield should fit the base of the nipple, not the size of the infant's mouth. Again, the infant needs to be monitored for effective milk transfer until a weight gain pattern is established. The mother needs to use a hospital-grade electric breast pump if her breasts are not softer or lighter after feeding with a nipple shield, and the infant will need to be assessed for adequate milk intake and supplemented as appropriate.

A nipple shield may also be useful if a mother has flat nipples. However, frequent feedings immediately after birth while the breast tissue is fairly soft can help some infants to learn to draw the nipple into the mouth without need of a shield. For the infant whose mother does not have protruding nipples, it is important to avoid sticking a finger in the infant's mouth to assess the suck, and to avoid pacifiers and bottles at least until breastfeeding is well established and the infant can latch on easily and effectively feed at the breast.

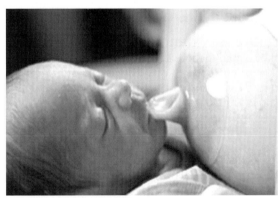

FIGURE 20-1. Nipple shield.

---

term infants.[23] Infants at risk for development of hypoglycemia include small- and large-for-gestational-age infants, infants of mothers with diabetes, those who weigh less than 2500 g, and those with certain medical problems. However, even among the at-risk infants, monitoring blood glucose does not preclude breastfeeding immediately after birth, and breastfeeding can often minimize hypoglycemia.[23] If there is a concern about glucose levels, early and frequent assessment of latch and milk transfer is more important than ever (see Tables 20-3 and 20-4). Likewise, a weight loss of greater than 5% within the first 2 days after birth is more likely to signal an inaccurate recording of birth weight than a lack of caloric intake. In rare instances, it may signal dehydration and should always be evaluated.[24]

Since frequent breast emptying is critical for the establishment of prolactin receptors for adequate milk production, use of pacifiers and bottles before breastfeeding can shorten breastfeeding duration. Furthermore, introducing foreign protein, including infant formulas, into the infant's gut increases risk for atopic disease, infection,[25] and diabetes,[26,27] and should be done with caution.

There is a tendency to assume that feeding is taking place whenever the infant is at the breast. However, evaluation of effective milk transfer is an important part of postpartum care and early infant assessment. The infant who is feeding more frequently than about every third hour (8-12 times per 24 hours) may need assistance to latch on more effectively. The mother may need to be encouraged to breastfeed longer to ensure a complete feeding has occurred. The easy digestibility of human milk, which allows for rapid gastric emptying[28] and causes less stress on the infant's digestive system, does not necessitate feeding more frequently than if the infant were being fed formula (the composition and caloric value of formula is based on human milk). Digestion only begins in the stomach; thus, if the infant is taking sufficient volume at a feeding, he or she will be satisfied and grow well feeding every 2 to 3 hours.

Assessment of breastfeeding should include information about the feeding pattern throughout a 24-hour period and a report of signs of correct latch-on and milk transfer during each feeding (see Tables 20-3 and 20-4).[1]

A systematic review of the literature on the introduction of complementary feeding by the World Health Organization (WHO)[29] supports the American Academy of Pediatrics recommendation of exclusive breastfeeding for approximately 6 months before introduction of any complementary feedings.[30]

V. SELECTED MANAGEMENT ISSUES

A. Maternal Medications

Few medications are contraindicated for the breastfeeding mother.[18] For most medical conditions that require medication, a risk/benefit analysis, including the amount of drug that potentially might reach the infant and the effect it might have on the infant, will suggest that breastfeeding be continued. Medication that a mother can safely take while pregnant can generally be continued while breastfeeding, unless there is a potential effect on milk production.[31] When considering the safety of a drug, some issues to consider include whether the drug is absorbed in the gastrointestinal tract, the molecular weight, the lipid solubility, the protein binding, the half-life, and the maternal plasma level of the drug, as well as the age and size of the infant.[31]

Clinical practice libraries should include copies of *Medications and Mothers' Milk*,[31] *Clinical Therapy in Breastfeeding Patients*,[32] and *Drugs in Pregnancy and Lactation*,[33] either in hard copy or CD-ROM with a subscription for periodic updates. There are also several on-line databases, including Perinatology.com (www.Perinatology.com) and Drugs and Lactation Database (LactMed; http://toxnet.nlm.nih.gov/cgi-bin/sis/htmlgen?LACT). These resources include the most recent literature references and American Academy of Pediatrics recommendations, and they serve as excellent guides for both pharmacologic agents and herbal preparations.

B. Sore Nipples

Sore nipples is one of the leading concerns for mothers and a common cause of untimely weaning. Nipple pain is usually a normal adjustment to breastfeeding, but it can be caused by incorrect latch. Sore nipples can also be caused by a yeast infection or a dermatitis.[1,19] Frequency and duration of feedings are not correlated with degree of soreness. Both clinical experience and a study of the physiology of infant suck show that careful positioning of the infant on the breast with the nipple in the intraoral space at the back of the mouth not only promotes optimal milk transfer (the nipple is not pinched and milk can flow freely) but also minimizes nipple trauma and increases comfort during feedings even after trauma has occurred.[1,19]

It is important to teach the mother to position her infant at her breast with good support to keep the infant's hips in the same plane as the head through the entire feeding (Figure 20-2). She should then grasp the infant by the shoulders with her thumb and forefinger supporting the head below the ears, separate the infant's arms to hug the breast, and as the infant roots with a wide-open mouth, pull the infant quickly to her breast.[34] It is important to continue supporting the breast as the infant latches on, or the nipple may not go deeply enough into the infant's mouth.

FOUR COMMON BREASTFEEDING POSITIONS

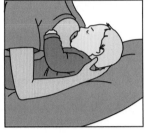

Football

- Hold the baby's back and shoulders in the palm of your hand.

- Tuck the baby under your arm, keeping the baby's ear, shoulder, and hip in a straight line.

- Support the breast. Touch baby's lips. Once the baby's mouth is open wide, pull the baby quickly to you.

- Continue to hold your breast until the baby feeds easily.

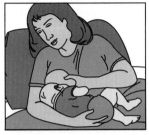

Lying Down

- Lie on your side with a pillow at your back and lay the baby so you are facing each other.

- To start, prop yourself up on your elbow and support your breast with the hand.

- Pull the baby close to you, bring up the baby's mouth with your nipple.

- Once the baby is feeding well, lie back down. Hold your breast with the opposite hand.

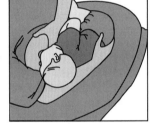

Cradling

- Cradle the baby in the arm closes to the breast, with the baby's head in the crook of your arm.

- Have the baby's body facing you tummy to tummy.

- Use your opposite hand to support the breast.

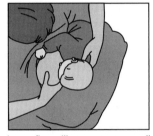

Across The Lap

- Lay your baby on firm pillows across your lip.

- Turn the baby facing you.

- Reach across your lap to support the baby's back and shoulders with the palm of your hand.

- Support your breast from underneath. Once the baby's mouth is open wide, pull your baby quickly onto your breast.

FIGURE 20-2. Breastfeeding positions. (Copyright by Lactation Consultants of North Carolina, reprinted with permission.)

Several therapies for healing sore nipples have been tried over the years; however, using the principles of moist wound healing seems to be the most successful. Applying a hydrogel dressing (www. Hollister.com) until the next feeding is minimally invasive, offers the mother comfort, and when used in conjunction with correct latch-on techniques, fosters rapid nipple healing. Purified lanolin designed for use by breastfeeding mothers can also be applied, but it may irritate the skin or foster yeast growth, particularly in humid climates. Breast milk, which contains infection-fighting immunoglobulins and fat-soluble vitamins associated with healing including A and E, can be expressed and rubbed into the sore areas to promote healing and does not need to be washed off before the next feeding.[19]

C. Engorgement

Although breast engorgement is one of the most common difficulties encountered by breastfeeding women, not all women become engorged. If an infant is feeding well and the mother is not experiencing painful swelling, she may not recognize the transition from colostrum to mature milk as engorgement. However, adequate breast emptying during the first 2 weeks is critical to establishing the prolactin receptors that will regulate milk production the entire time the mother is lactating.[1] Swollen breast tissue can be effectively treated with cold compresses or cabbage leaves, or both.[35-37] As with any other swollen tissue, applying heat will draw more fluid to the affected area and is counterproductive. Engorgement inhibits milk flow because the swollen tissue is compressing the milk ducts, not because the mother is failing to experience the letdown or milk ejection reflex. Frequent, effective feedings and/or milk expression to treat engorgement are crucial for long-term milk supply.[1]

D. Mastitis

Mastitis is an infection of the breast tissue usually caused by either *S. aureus* or *Staphylococcus epidermis.* Symptoms may include a tender, swollen, red area on one breast; fever of more than 101°F; and flu-like symptoms of a systemic illness. The infection is not in the milk itself, and it is important for the mother to continue breastfeeding. Potential consequences of inflammation and breast infection are diminished milk supply, the risk for abscess, and untimely weaning. As with any systemic bacterial infection, mastitis should be treated with an antibiotic, analgesics for pain (ibuprofen can also reduce inflammation), frequent breast emptying, especially by breastfeeding, extra fluids, and bed rest.[25,38] Because most cases of mastitis are staphylococcal infections, they can be treated with dicloxacillin, nafcillin, or cephalexin. Women who are allergic to penicillin can be treated with erythromycin or clindamycin.[38] If the infant is younger than 1 month, sulfa drugs should be avoided. If the infant is not emptying the breasts adequately, the mother needs to use a hospital-grade electric pump to finish emptying the breast after each feeding. Women who wean while they have mastitis are a greater risk for abscess.[25] In rare cases where the mother has group B streptococcal mastitis, the infection can be transmitted to the infant.[39] Any case of early postpartum mastitis should be treated aggressively and the infant observed carefully.

VI. INFANT ISSUES

A. Weight

Normal infant weight loss after birth is 5% to 7% in the first 72 hours because of passage of meconium and excess fluid. By 72 hours, the infant's weight should stabilize and the infant should begin to gain an average of 30 g/day by the fifth day.[1] Continued weight loss, lack of transitional stools, lack of increased urine output, increased bilirubin, and infant lethargy or irritability are all signs of inadequate milk intake.[1]

Lack of intake is a feeding management issue that is amenable to early intervention. It may be related to infrequent feedings, lack of milk transfer because of poor latch, poor positioning, incorrect suck, shortened feedings because of infant sleepiness or maternal pain, or rarely, low milk production. With prefeeding and postfeeding weights as a guide, the source of poor intake can be assessed and an infant can be encouraged to take sufficient volume at each feeding to be satisfied and to grow well.[22,40] A scale accurate to 2 g (e.g., scales available from Tanita Scales [www.tanita.com] and Medela, Inc. [www.medela.com]) must be used to accurately determine prefeeding and postfeeding weights. One gram equals 1 ml milk.

B. Milk Composition

Colostrum is dense in calories, primarily protein, and consistent in composition throughout a feeding. However, the composition of mature milk changes from skim milk (fore milk) to whole milk to cream (hind milk) during each feeding on each breast. Occasionally, an infant or mother will end the feeding before the infant gets the higher fat hind milk. This may be because the mother has been told to feed for a certain number of minutes per side, because the mother takes the infant off as soon as he or she pauses, or because the infant stops sucking when the nipple slips forward in his or her mouth and is no longer stimulating the medial tongue. Although the typical infant will feed for about 15 minutes on each breast to get sufficient hind milk, this is only an average.[1] If an infant is gaining less than an average of 30 g/day, it may be that keeping the infant on the first breast for a few additional minutes at each feeding will increase caloric intake sufficiently to increase rate of weight gain and also allow the infant to go a little longer between feedings.

C. Hyperbilirubinemia

Elevated bilirubin levels in the first 24 hours is a sign of illness and is not associated with feeding. Breastfeeding does not exacerbate the problem, and because the infant is ill, the more of his or her mother's milk the infant can be fed, the better.

Elevated unconjugated bilirubin levels after 24 hours is usually associated with inadequate caloric intake.[41] Meconium contains a significant amount of bilirubin. Delayed passage of meconium is associated with increased bilirubin levels and inadequate calorie intake and dehydration. The newborn lacks intestinal bacteria and, consequently, unconjugated bilirubin is reabsorbed into the hepatic circulation, contributing to increased serum bilirubin levels.[41] Establishing adequate breastfeeding frequency with effective milk transfer is key to preventing hyperbilirubinemia in the otherwise healthy breastfed infant. Supplementation of breastfed infants with water does not lead to decreased bilirubin levels.[41]

A rare, late-onset (after day 5), prolonged increase of unconjugated bilirubin occurs when the infant is gaining weight well, stooling appropriately, and otherwise thriving. This late-onset form of jaundice is associated with a yet undefined component in some mother's milk. This is called *breast milk jaundice*[19] and can last for several weeks. If the bilirubin level is of concern, a differential diagnosis can be made by interrupting breastfeeding for 24 hours. If feeding the infant donor human milk or formula causes a decrease in bilirubin level, the infant can safely return to breastfeeding and the bilirubin level will gradually decline.

Regardless of the cause of hyperbilirubinemia, feeding is a significant component of the treatment. Continued breastfeeding with or without supplementation and phototherapy is appropriate. Evaluation of milk transfer and frequency of feedings can guide the treatment plan. If the infant is not emptying the breasts well, the mother can use a hospital-grade pump to keep her breasts well stimulated and emptied. Using a nursing supplement at the breast to deliver extra pumped milk, donor milk, or formula to increase caloric intake at the breast is optimal.[1]

D. Short Frenulum

Occasionally, an infant has difficulty achieving a good enough latch to transfer sufficient milk or breastfeed without causing nipple damage because of a short frenulum. Clipping the frenulum is the rea-sonable option if the short frenulum is interfering with breastfeeding.[42,43]

E. Use of Donor Milk

Donor human milk is available on physician's order through donor human milk banks. The milk banks operate similarly to donor blood banks, but with more thorough screening of the donors and their breastfeeding infants. All donors are serum screened for HIV-1 and -2, human T-cell lymphotrophic virus, hepatitis C, hepatitis B, and syphilis. The milk is stored frozen, heat treated (Holder pasteurization, 62.5°C for 30 minutes), and refrozen for storage until it is needed.[44] A current list of active donor milk banks that follow the Human Milk Banking Association of North America (HMBANA) guidelines can be found via the Internet (www.hmbana.org).

F. Nutritional Supplementation for the Breastfed Infant

Women who are strict vegan vegetarians or who have had a gastric bypass are at risk for vitamin B_{12} deficiency and their infants will require supplemental vitamins.[45]

G. Rickets

All infants and children need sufficient sunlight exposure cumulative each week to produce vitamin D. The minimum is 30 minutes per week with only a diaper or 2 hours per week fully clothed without a hat for a light-skinned infant. Darker skinned infants require longer exposure. Maternal consumption of vitamin D does not influence the level in the mother's milk.[46] Infants at risk for development of rickets (primarily preterm infants and very dark-skinned infants who have minimal sun exposure) do need to be supplemented with vitamin D after about 2 months.[47]

H. Fussy Infants

Until an infant is gaining weight adequately and is not jaundiced, pacifiers should be avoided.[1] A fussy infant who is signaling that he or she is hungry, regardless of how long ago a feeding occurred, should be fed again. If an infant constantly needs to suck, it is important to evaluate latch, effectiveness of milk transfer, and length of feeding for volume of milk transfer.[1]

Occasionally, a mother will have such overproduction of milk that she changes the infant from the first side to the second side just to ease her fullness before the infant has gotten to the higher fat hind milk. If her infant is having explosive stools, acting "constantly" hungry, but gaining well, it may be that by changing the feeding pattern to thoroughly soften one breast before going to the second side, the infant will get the more satisfying hind milk on the first side and not take so much of the higher lactose fore milk on the second side.[48]

I. Appetite Spurts

Typically babies go through "appetite spurts" or "growth spurts" at around 1 week, 6 weeks, 3 months, 6 months, and 9 months. More frequent feedings for about 48 hours will increase the mother's milk production (the more milk is removed, the more will be made); then the infant will spread out the feedings again. At the 6-month appetite spurt, the infant will probably be ready to begin intake of some solid food. Solids should be fed *after* breastfeeding until about 9 months because the infant's primary source of calories should still be milk.

VII. SUPPORT FOR EVIDENCE-BASED PRACTICE

Breastfeeding and human lactation management is a dynamic field of practice that requires attention to the literature for best practice. Many resources are available for health-care professionals who are working to change their practice from management by anecdote to an evidence-based approach. The American Academy of Family Physicians (www.aafp.org) has a breastfeeding policy statement, the International Lactation Consultant Association (ILCA; www.ilca.org) has published *Clinical Guidelines for the Establishment of Exclusive Breastfeeding* and several other related documents, the Academy of Breastfeeding Medicine (www.bfmed.org) offers several breastfeeding protocols on its website, and the American Academy of Pediatrics (www.aap.org) has a statement on breastfeeding and the use of human milk to mention a few.

VIII. LACTATION CONSULTANTS

A new allied health profession focusing exclusively on appropriate clinical management and support of breastfeeding began in 1985 with the first certification examination for breastfeeding/human lactation specialists offered by the International Board of Lactation Consultant Examiners (IBLCE). The International Board Certified Lactation Consultant (IBCLC) has met the extensive academic and clinical experience prerequisites of IBLCE and passed a rigorous 6-hour examination including both didactic and clinical portions. To maintain the IBCLC credential, one must recertify by continuing education or examination every 5 years (the examination recertification is required at least every 10 years). Lactation consultants come from a variety of academic backgrounds; however, the majority of consultants are registered nurses (RNs). A few IBCLCs are physicians, midwives, or advanced practice nurses. Most IBCLCs in the United States are not licensed primary care providers but rather work collaboratively with primary care providers. (For more information about the examination or a list of IBCLCs in your area, contact IBLCE at iblce@erols.org.)

Because the IBCLC is not licensed, there is no regulation of the use of the title "lactation consultant" in the United States, and there are some breastfeeding management courses that provide a certification. However, none of these certifications requires the same prerequisites, scrutiny of preparation, recertification, or adherence to a code of ethics that are required by the IBLCE. Several programs also train paraprofessionals to provide breastfeeding support (with varying degrees of hands-on assistance), usually to WIC recipients. These paraprofessionals are typically supervised by an IBCLC or other health-care professional and can be a great resource for breastfeeding mothers.

IX. CONCLUSION

Family physicians can be key players in women's decisions to breastfeed and to continue to breastfeed. The evidence that human milk is the species-specific food for the human infant is not new. There is increasing research evidence to support the effectiveness of promotion and encouragement of breastfeeding is increasing. The majority of breastfeeding problems can be resolved with appropriate clinical information and support. In addition, IBCLCs or Registered Lactation Consultants (R-LCs) have the extensive training and education to provide evidence-based clinical support to assess and solve breastfeeding problems. Several strategies are presented that family physicians will want to routinely incorporate into their clinical practice to promote optimal health for mothers and infants, solutions specific to more common issues/concerns of the breastfeeding mother, and resources for referral.

X. RECOMMENDATIONS

Breastfeeding management is an area of health care that does not lend itself to randomized clinical trials. It would not be ethical to assign mothers not to breastfeed or to practice less than optimal feeding patterns to provide a randomized control group for a study on the effects of not breastfeeding. Likewise, it would not be possible to blind a woman to the interventions that are used to assist her with breastfeeding difficulties. However, from clinical observations, retrospective studies, observational studies, case–control studies, and basic bench research, it has been well established that there are health consequences for both the mother and the infant of not breastfeeding and not breastfeeding exclusively.[1,26,27,30,49-53,57] Strong evidence links regular use of pacifiers with shortened breastfeeding duration,[54] but conclusive evidence does not exist regarding whether regular pacifier use is a marker for breastfeeding difficulties or is the causative agent. In either case, pacifier use is something to be noted and addressed by the physician as part of a breastfeeding assessment. Exclusive breastfeeding for 6 months with appropriate introduction of iron-rich solids beginning at 6 months is recommended based on extensive clinical observation.[29,55] Clear evidence exists that clinical support from health-care providers is linked to improved initiation and duration.[56]

REFERENCES

1. International Lactation Consultant Association (ILCA): *Clinical guidelines for the establishment of exclusive breastfeeding,* Raleigh, NC, 2005, ILCA.
2. Taveras EM, Li R, Grummer-Strawn L, Richardson M et al: Opinions and practices of clinicians associated with continuation of exclusive breastfeeding, *Pediatrics* 113(4):e283-e290, 2004.
3. World Health Assembly: *International code of marketing of breast-milk substitutes,* 1981.
4. Raisler J: Against the odds: breastfeeding experiences of low income mothers, *J Midwifery Womens Health* 45(3):253-263, 2000.
5. Donnelly A, Snowden HM, Renfrew MJ et al: Commercial hospital discharge packs for breastfeeding women, *Cochrane Database Syst Rev* (2):CD002075, 2000.
6. Howard C, Howard F, Lawrence R et al: Office prenatal formula advertising and its effect on breast-feeding patterns, *Obstet Gynecol* 95(2):296-303, 2000.
7. Wiessinger D: Watch your language! *J Hum Lact* 12(1):1-4, 1996.
8. Ball T, Wright A: Health care costs of formula-feeding in the first year of life, *Pediatrics* 103(suppl):870-876, 1999.
9. Kennell JH, Klaus MH: Bonding: recent observations that alter perinatal care, *Pediatr Rev* 19(1):4-12, 1998.
10. Jernstrom H, Lubinski J, Lynch HT et al: Breast-feeding and the risk of breast cancer in BRCA1 and BRCA2 mutation carriers, *J Natl Cancer Inst* 96(14):1094-1098, 2004.
11. European Society on Human Reproduction and Embryology Capri Workshop Group: Hormones and breast cancer, *Hum Reprod Update* 10(4):281-293, 2004.
12. Tung KH, Wilkens LR, Wu AH et al: Effect of anovulation factors on pre- and postmenopausal ovarian cancer risk: revisiting the incessant ovulation hypothesis, *Am J Epidemiol* 161(4):321-329, 2005.
13. Karlsson MK, Ahlborg HG, Karlsson C: Maternity and bone mineral density, *Acta Orthop* 76(1):2-13, 2005.
14. Labbok MH, Hight V, Peterson AE et al: Multicenter study of the lactational amenorrhea method (LAM): I. efficacy, duration, and implications for clinical application, *Contraception* 55:327-336, 1997.
15. Tommaselli GA, Guida M, Palomba S et al: Using complete breastfeeding and lactational amenorrhoea as birth spacing methods, *Contraception* 61(4):253-257, 2000.
16. Lawrence RA: *Maternal and child health technical information bulletin: a review of medical benefits and contraindications to breastfeeding in the United States,* Washington, DC, 1997, U.S. Government Printing Office.
17. Ando Y, Ekuni Y, Matsumoto Y et al: Long-term serological outcome of infants who received frozen-thawed milk from human T-lymphotropic virus type-I positive mothers, *J Obstet Gynaecol Res* 30(6):436-438, 2004.
18. American Academy of Pediatrics Committee on Drugs: Transfer of drugs and other chemicals into human milk, *Pediatrics* 108:776-789, 2001.
19. Smith JW, Tully MR: Midwifery management of breastfeeding: using the evidence, *J Midwifery Womens Health* 46(6): 423-438, 2001.
20. Neifert M, DeMarzo S, Seacat J et al: The influence of breast surgery, breast appearance, and pregnancy-induced breast changes on lactation sufficiency as measured by infant weight gain, *Birth* 17(1):31-38, 1990.
21. Neifert MR, Seacat JM, Jobe WE: Lactation failure due to insufficient glandular development of the breast, *Pediatrics* 76(5):823-828, 1985.
22. Neifert M: Clinical aspects of lactation, *Clin Perinatol* 26(2):281-306, 1999.
23. Williams AF: *Hypoglycemia of the newborn: review of the literature,* Geneva, 1997, WHO.
24. Yaseen H, Salem M, Darwich M: Clinical presentation of hypernatremic dehydration in exclusively breast-fed neonates, *Indian J Pediatr* 71(12):1059-1062, 2004.
25. Lawrence RA, Lawrence RM: *Breastfeeding: a guide for the medical profession,* ed 6, Philadelphia, 2005, Mosby.
26. Sadauskaite-Kuehne V, Ludvigsson J, Padaiga Z et al: Longer breastfeeding is an independent protective factor against development of type 1 diabetes mellitus in childhood, *Diabetes Metab Res Rev* 20(2):150-157, 2004.
27. Taylor JS, Kacmar JE, Nothnagle M et al: A systematic review of the literature associating breastfeeding with type 2 diabetes and gestational diabetes, *J Am Coll Nutr* 24(5):320-326, 2005.
28. Broussard DL: Gastrointestinal motility in the neonate, *Clin Perinatol* 22(1):37-59, 1995.

29. World Health Organization (WHO): *Expert consultation on the optimal duration of exclusive breastfeeding,* Geneva, 2001, WHO.

30. Gartner LM, Morton J, Lawrence RA et al: Breastfeeding and the use of human milk, *Pediatrics* 115(2):496-506, 2005.

31. Hale T: *Medications and mothers' milk,* ed 10, Amarillo, TX, 2006, Pharmasoft Publishing.

32. Hale T: *Clinical therapy in breastfeeding patients,* Amarillo, TX, 1999, Pharmasoft Medical Publishing.

33. Briggs GG, Freeman RK, Yaffe SJ: *Drugs in pregnancy and lactation,* ed 5, Baltimore, MD, 1998, Williams & Wilkins.

34. Tully MR, Overfield ML: *Breastfeeding counseling guide,* ed 2, Raleigh, NC, 1989, Lactation Consultants of North Carolina.

35. Nikodem VC, Danziger D, Gebka N et al: Do cabbage leaves prevent breast engorgement? A randomized, controlled study, *Birth* 20(2):61-64, 1993.

36. Roberts KL: A comparison of chilled cabbage leaves and chilled gel packs in reducing breast engorgement, *J Hum Lact* 11:17-20, 1995.

37. Snowden HM, Renfrew MJ, Woolridge MW et al: Treatments for breast engorgement during lactation, *Cochrane Database Syst Rev* (2):CD000046, 2001.

38. Mass S: Breast pain: engorgement, nipple pain and mastitis, *Clin Obstet Gynecol* 47(3):676-682, 2004.

39. Kotiw M, Zhang GW, Daggard G et al: Late-onset and recurrent neonatal group B streptococcal disease associated with breast-milk transmission, *Pediatr Dev Pathol* 6(3):251-256, 2003.

40. Neifert MR, Seacat JM, DeMarzo SM et al: The association between infant weight gain and breast milk intake measured by office test weights, *Am J Dis Child* 144(4):420-421, 1990 (abstract).

41. Gartner LM, Herschel M: Jaundice and breastfeeding, *Pediatr Clin North Am* 48(1):389-400, 2001.

42. Ballard JL, Auer CE, Khoury JC: Ankyloglossia: assessment, incidence, and effect of frenuloplasty on the breastfeeding dyad, *Pediatrics* 110(5):e63, 2002.

43. Ricke LA, Baker NJ, Madlon-Kay DJ et al: Newborn tongue-tie: prevalence and effect on breast-feeding, *J Am Board Fam Pract* 18(1):1-7, 2005.

44. Human Milk Banking Association of North America (HMBANA): *Guidelines for the establishment and operation of a donor human milk bank,* ed 13, Raleigh, NC, 2006, HMBANA.

45. Graham SM, Arvela OM, Wise GA: Long-term neurologic consequences of nutritional vitamin B_{12} deficiency in infants, *J Pediatr* 121:710-714, 1992.

46. Specker BL, Valanis B, Hertzberg V et al: Sunshine exposure and serum 25-hydroxyvitamin D concentrations in exclusively breast-fed infants, *J Pediatr* 107(3):372-376, 1985.

47. Kreiter SR, Schwartz RP, Kirkman HN et al: Nutritional rickets in African American breast-fed infants, *J Pediatr* 137(8): 153-157, 2000.

48. Woolridge MW, Fisher C: Colic, "overfeeding," and symptoms of lactose malabsorption in the breastfed baby: a possible artifact of feeding management? *Lancet* 2(8607):382-384, 1988.

49. Arenz S, Ruckerl R, Koletzko B et al: Breast-feeding and childhood obesity—a systematic review, *Int J Obes Relat Metab Disord* 28(10):1247-1256, 2004.

50. Bullen CL, Tearle PV, Stewart MG: The effect of "humanised" milk and supplemented breastfeeding on the faecal flora of infants, *J Med Microbiol* 10(4):403-413, 1977.

51. Labbok M: Effects of breastfeeding on the mother, *Pediatr Clin North Am* 48(2):143-158, 2001.

52. Mimouni Bloch A, Mimouni D, Mimouni M et al: Does breastfeeding protect against allergic rhinitis during childhood? A meta-analysis of prospective studies, *Acta Paediatr* 91(3):275-279, 2002.

53. Uhari M, Mantysaari K, Niemela M: A meta-analytic review of the risk factors for acute otitis media, *Clin Infect Dis* 22(6):1079-1083, 1996.

54. Ullah S, Griffiths P: Does the use of pacifiers shorten breast-feeding duration in infants? *Br J Community Nurs* 8(10): 458-463, 2003.

55. Kramer MS, Kakuma R: The optimal duration of exclusive breastfeeding: a systematic review, *Adv Exp Med Biol* 554: 63-77, 2004.

56. Sikorski J, Renfrew MJ, Pindoria S et al: Support for breast-feeding mothers: a systematic review, *Paediatr Perinat Epidemiol* 17(4):407-417, 2003.

57. Ip S, Chung M, Raman G et al: Breastfeeding and maternal and infant health outcomes in developed countries. Evidence Report/Technology Assessment No. 153 (Prepared by Tufts-New England Medical Center Evidence-based under Contract No. 290-02-0022). AHRQ Publication No. 07-E007. Rockville, MD: Agency for Healthcare Research and Quality, April 2007.

S E C T I O N   D   Mastitis

Charles Carter, MD,
and Elizabeth G. Baxley, MD

I. DEFINITION AND INCIDENCE

Lactation mastitis is an acute mammary cellulitis involving the interlobular connective tissue of the breast.[1-3] This breastfeeding complication occurs in approximately 2% to 33% of nursing mothers, depending on the population studied.[2,4] Risk factors include improper nursing techniques; nipple cracking and soreness (OR, 3.4); use of antifungal cream (OR, 3.4); manual breast pump use (OR, 3.3); breast trauma; blocked ducts; engorgement/stasis; maternal fatigue or high levels of stress; poor diet; and professional, technical, or managerial occupations for both parents.[1,2,4-7] Women with a history of mastitis have a greater rate of recurrence in both current and subsequent nursing periods with other children (OR, 4.0).[1,2,6] Feeding duration is not associated with mastitis.[2] Mastitis during the first 3 weeks postpartum is associated with breastfeeding cessation, indicating a need for physician counseling should it occur.[8]

A. Pathophysiology

Milk stasis and engorgement often precede mastitis by promoting milk leakage into surrounding breast tissue, resulting in an inflammatory response and offering a favorable substrate for bacterial growth.[1,9] Prevention, therefore, is aimed at preventing and treating milk stasis and noninfectious inflammation by frequent feedings, nipple care, and a gradual increase in the duration of nursing at each breast. The most commonly isolated organisms are *S. aureus* and coagulase-negative staphylococci. Other isolates include group A and B β-hemolytic streptococci, *E. coli,* and *Bacteroides* species.[1] Based on a series of case reports and one retrospective review, community-acquired, methicillin-resistant *S. aureus* is emerging as an important pathogen in cases of mastitis and breast abscess.[10-13]

B. Clinical Presentation

Mastitis typically presents 2 to 7 weeks after breast-feeding initiation, and it begins with the abrupt onset of fever, chills, and flu-like symptoms. It is usually unilateral, with breast erythema, induration, and pain.[1,2,9] These systemic manifestations help differentiate it from other causes of breast pain such as duct blockage or engorgement.[9] Clinical examination reveals a well-demarcated, V-shaped area of warmth and inflammation. Most women will be ill enough to restrict their activities or resort to bed rest.[2]

II. TREATMENT

The aim of treatment is to prevent complications, control pain, and allow lactation to continue.[1,15] Standard practice antibiotic therapy is directed at *S. aureus* with either a penicillinase-resistant penicillin or a first- or second-generation cephalosporin.[1] Cultures are typically unnecessary, unless needed to direct treatment should empiric coverage fail. First-line options are dicloxacillin or cephalexin for 10 days.[9] Mothers of infants younger than 1 month should avoid use of sulfonamides. A few limited quality RCTs examining antibiotic treatment suggest improved outcomes with antibiotics; however, studies defining ideal treatment duration or coverage spectra are unavailable.[1]

Adjunctive treatments should include regular breast emptying, massage, and warm compresses for symptomatic pain relief. Analgesics, including codeine-containing preparations, can be used when discomfort is severe; however, nonsteroidal antiinflammatory medications such as ibuprofen are typically adequate.

Mastitis need not halt breastfeeding or lactation because maintaining lactation may enhance the resolution of inflammation by reducing congestion, thereby shortening the duration of symptoms and improving outcomes.[1,9] Furthermore, breast engorgement may contribute to abscess formation.[1,3] Maternal mastitis does not harm the newborn, with the exception of women with HIV who breastfeed because mastitis increases the vertical transmission risk.[1,16] Thus, continued breastfeeding support is important during episodes of mastitis.

III. BREAST ABSCESS

Breast abscess develops in approximately 5% to 11% of women with lactation mastitis. Milk stasis, as well as delayed, inappropriate, or lack of treatment for mastitis, increases the risk.[1,17] Clinically, a breast abscess presents similarly to mastitis, but exquisite tenderness is present in the region of the abscess. Fluctuation may be present but should not be expected. Ultrasound examination of the breast when persistent induration, swelling, or tenderness is present aids in the diagnosis of breast abscess.[17,18] Breast abscess should also be suspected when initial antibiotic therapy for mastitis fails.[9]

No studies of mastitis-associated breast abscess treatment have been published. Current treatment includes either incision and drainage or repeated needle aspirations. Antibiotic coverage should include *S. aureus* and anaerobes. Women may resume breastfeeding once pain and adequate wound healing allow.[1,9] A wound culture may help direct therapy. Furthermore, community-acquired, methicillin-resistant *S. aureus* can cause mastitis, and these infections may be more prone to abscess formation.[1,13,14]

REFERENCES

1. Barbosa-Cesnik C, Schwartz K, Foxman B: Lactation mastitis, *JAMA* 289:1609-1612, 2003.
2. Foxman B, D'Arcy H, Gillespie B et al: Lactation mastitis: occurrence and medical management among 946 breastfeeding women in the United States, *Am J Epidemiol* 155:103-116, 2002.
3. Niebyl JR, Spence MR, Parmley TH: Sporadic (nonepidemic) puerperal mastitis, *J Reprod Med* 20:97-100, 1978.
4. Kaufmann R, Foxman B: Mastitis among lactating women: occurrence and risk factors, *Soc Sci Med* 33:701-705, 1991.
5. Fetherston C: Risk factors for lactation mastitis, *J Hum Lact* 14:101-109, 1998.
6. Foxman B, Schwartz K, Looman SJ: Breastfeeding practices and lactation mastitis, *Soc Sci Med* 38:755-761, 1994.
7. Riordan JM, Nichols FH: A descriptive study of lactation mastitis in long-term breastfeeding women, *J Hum Lact* 6:53-58, 1990.

8. Schwartz K, D'Arcy HJS, Gillespie B et al: Factors associated with weaning in the first 3 months postpartum, *J Fam Pract* 51:439-444, 2002.

9. Prachniak GK: Common breastfeeding problems, *Obstet Gynecol Clin North Am* 29:77-88, 2002.

10. Gastelum DT, Dassey D, Mascola L et al: Transmission of community-associated methicillin-resistant *Staphylococcus aureus* from breast milk in the neonatal intensive care unit, *Pediatr Infect Dis J* 24(12):1122-1124, 2005.

11. Laibl VR, Sheffield JS, Roberts S et al: Atypical presentation of community-acquired methicillin-resistant *Staphylococcus aureus* in pregnancy, *Obstet Gynecol* 106(3):461-465, 2005.

12. Behari P, Englund J, Alcasid G et al: Transmission of methicillin-resistant *Staphylococcus aureus* to preterm infants through breast milk, *Infect Control Hosp Epidemiol* 25(9):778-780, 2004.

13. Amir L: Breastfeeding and *Staphylococcus aureus:* three case reports, *Breastfeed Rev* 10(1):15-18, 2002.

14. Saiman L, O'Keefe M, Graham PL 3rd et al: Hospital transmission of community-acquired methicillin-resistant *Staphylococcus aureus* among postpartum women, *Clin Infect Dis* 37(10):1313-1319, 2003.

15. Thomsen AC, Espersen T, Maigaard S: Course and treatment of milk stasis, noninfectious inflammation of the breast, and infectious mastitis in nursing women, *Am J Obstet Gynecol* 149:492-495, 1984.

16. Michie C, Lockie F, Lynn W: The challenge of mastitis, *Arch Dis Child* 88:818-821, 2003.

17. Dener C, Inan A: Breast abscesses in lactating women, *World J Surg* 27:130-133, 2003.

18. Hayes R, Michell M, Nunnerley HB: Acute inflammation of the breast—the role of breast ultrasound in diagnosis and management, *Clin Radiol* 44:253-256, 1991.

SECTION E Postpartum Thyroiditis

Charles Carter, MD, and Elizabeth G. Baxley, MD

Postpartum thyroiditis is the most common postpartum thyroid syndrome, with a prevalence of 5% to 7% in the first year after delivery.[1] It manifests as transient hyperthyroidism between 1 and 3 months after delivery and hypothyroidism between 3 and 6 months after delivery.[2] Although postpartum thyroiditis is most common, there are other causes, notably a syndrome of postpartum reactivation of Graves' disease in women who have previously been treated for it.[3,4]

I. EPIDEMIOLOGY/RISK FACTORS

The incidence of postpartum thyroiditis is greatest in Hispanic women, less common in white women, and uncommon among black women.[5] Rates of thyroid dysfunction are not dependent on age, parity, or breastfeeding, but a family history of thyroid disorders is common.

II. PATHOGENESIS

Postpartum thyroiditis is an autoimmune thyroiditis characterized by a destructive lymphocytic infiltration of the thyroid gland.[1,2] The syndrome is strongly associated with the presence of thyroid peroxidase antibodies (TPOAb) in maternal serum.[1,6-9]

III. CLINICAL FEATURES

The majority of women have a brief, often asymptomatic, thyrotoxic phase, followed by a more long-lasting symptomatic hypothyroid phase.[1,8] The onset of the hyperthyroid phase is typically around the fourth postpartum week, with symptoms peaking at 8 to 12 weeks. The hypothyroid phase begins at 4 to 8 months postpartum and lasts 4 to 6 months.[1] Symptoms are initially subtle and insidious, making it difficult to distinguish between postpartum thyroiditis and other frequently encountered postpartum complaints such as fatigue, weight gain, dry skin, constipation, loss of initiative, memory impairment, depression, anxiety, and emotional lability. Thus, although it can be associated with significant morbidity, postpartum thyroiditis is underdiagnosed.

Women with lethargy persisting beyond several weeks should have their thyroid function evaluated. Thyroid enlargement may be found on physical examination, although a persistent goiter is uncommon. Patients with a symptomatic thyrotoxic phase during the early stages of postpartum thyroiditis often experience an abrupt onset of neck pain and tenderness, fatigue, and palpitations. Occasionally, this mimics panic attacks or postpartum psychosis.[10]

IV. DIAGNOSIS

The diagnosis of postpartum thyroiditis is based on the presence of abnormal thyroid function tests in a postpartum woman who has increased TPOAb.[6] During the hypothyroid phase, thyroid-stimulating hormone (TSH) levels are increased, peaking at 4 to 6 months. The severity of symptoms usually follows the trend of TSH variation. Patients who do have increased TSH levels should be followed expectantly by repeating TSH and thyroid antibody levels every 8 to 12 weeks until these values return to normal.[5,11]

Ultrasound reveals diffuse or multifocal hypoechogenicity of the thyroid, correlating with lymphocytic infiltration.[1,6,12] If Graves' disease needs to be ruled out, it may be distinguished from the thyrotoxic phase of postpartum thyroiditis by the finding of TSH receptor antibodies and low, rather than high, radioactive iodine or technetium uptake.[1,8] For breastfeeding women who require an uptake scan, radioactive iodine is contraindicated. Breastfeeding should be interrupted for 3 days for an iodine-123 scan or 24 hours for a technetium scan, although women may continue to pump and discard the breastmilk.[1]

V. TREATMENT

Women with mild-to-moderate thyroid dysfunction may have minimal symptoms and may not even present for care. Furthermore, of women who do seek medical attention, not all require treatment. Treatment should be reserved for symptomatic women with laboratory evidence of thyroid dysfunction and is not indicated for patients with increased thyroid antibody titers alone.[3]

Treatment consists of β-blockers for moderate-to-severe symptoms in the hyperthyroid phase and levothyroxine for the hypothyroid phase.[8,13] Antithyroid drugs are unnecessary because there is no increased hormone production.[1] Thyroid hormone replacement improves symptoms but does not alter the illness course and is continued for 12 to 18 months after diagnosis.[14]

In most cases, normal thyroid function returns within 1 year. High thyroid antibody titers and low radioactive iodine uptake herald a more severe hypothyroid phase and greater likelihood of persistent hypothyroidism. In addition, permanent hypothyroidism develops in many women.[1,12,13,15,16] As many as 50% of women who have experienced development of postpartum thyroiditis will have hypothyroidism 7 to 9 years later, with women who are euthyroid during the first postpartum year carrying a thirteenfold relative risk for thyroid dysfunction.[6,12] Factors predictive of long-term thyroid dysfunction include a hypothyroid form of postpartum thyroid dysfunction, TSH level more than 20 mU/L, and greater TPOAb levels during the postpartum period (relative risk, 32).[6]

Relapse with subsequent pregnancies occurs in up to 70% of women. Peak antibody levels and duration of illness are similar in each relapse for individual patients.[12-14]

VI. PITFALLS AND CONTROVERSIES

A. Screening

Some authors view postpartum thyroiditis as an exacerbation of ongoing, subclinical autoimmune thyroid disease because it is consistent with the typical behavior of other autoimmune thyroid diseases, and because immunologic abnormalities can be observed before thyroid dysfunction occurs.[1] Half of TPOAb-positive pregnant women go on to experience development of postpartum thyroid dysfunction, suggesting TPOAb screening could be valuable as part of routine prenatal care.[7,17] These antibodies occur in 10% of pregnant women at 14 weeks of gestation,[17] and the test is readily available, relatively inexpensive, and sensitive.[7,13] However, the specificity in early pregnancy is 62% and the PPV for postpartum thyroiditis is only 48%.[7] Most women with postpartum thyroiditis do not require treatment and would not have otherwise been identified.[16] Furthermore, limited evidence currently exists that subclinical hypothyroidism is associated with adverse outcomes.[18]

Thus, the benefit of screening remains controversial. A joint statement from three endocrinology associations advocates for routine thyroid disease screening in pregnancy but makes no comment on TPOAb screening.[19] Guidelines by the American College of Obstetricians and Gynecologists recommend against routine TPOAb screening.[16] Screening with TSH prenatally and at 3 and 6 months after delivery may be valuable in women with other autoimmune disorders such a history of postpartum thyroiditis (69% prevalence of recurrence) or type 1 diabetes mellitus (25-25% prevalence of postpartum thyroiditis).[8,13,17,18] Because of the symptom overlap, all women with postpartum depression are candidates for thyroid dysfunction testing.[13] However, depressive symptoms do not appear to be predictive of postpartum thyroiditis or vice versa.[9,20]

Gaps in knowledge about postpartum thyroiditis include the impact on maternal and child outcomes, and a prospective trial is under way to address this.[17] At this juncture, remaining alert for signs and symptoms that suggest thyroid dysfunction and having a low threshold for evaluating thyroid status in high-risk patients is likely the most effective approach for a clinician to take until more evidence becomes available.

REFERENCES

1. Muller AF, Drexhage HM, Berghout A: Postpartum thyroiditis and autoimmune thyroiditis in women of childbearing age: recent insights and consequences for antenatal and postnatal care, *Endocr Rev* 22:605-630, 2001.
2. Lucas A, Pizarro E, Granada ML et al: Postpartum thyroiditis: epidemiology and clinical evolution in a non-selected population, *Thyroid* 10:71-77, 2000.
3. Jansson R, Dahlberg PA, Karlsson FA: Postpartum thyroiditis, *Baillieres Clin Endocrinol Metab* 2:619-635, 1988.
4. Jansson R, Dahlberg PA, Winsa B et al: The postpartum period constitutes an important risk for the development of clinical Graves' disease in young women, *Acta Endocrinol* 116:321-325, 1987.
5. Hayslip GC, Fein HG, O'Donnell VM et al: The value of serum antimicrosomal antibody testing in screening for symptomatic postpartum thyroid dysfunction, *Am J Obstet Gynecol* 159:203-209, 1988.
6. Premawardhana LDKE, Parkes AB, Ammari F et al: Postpartum thyroiditis and long-term thyroid status: prognostic influence of thyroid peroxidase antibodies and ultrasound echogenicity, *J Clin Endocrinol Metab* 85(1):71-75, 2000.
7. Premawardhana LDKE, Parkes AB, John R et al: Thyroid peroxidase antibodies in early pregnancy: utility for prediction of postpartum thyroid dysfunction and implications for screening, *Thyroid* 14:610-615, 2004.
8. Terry AJ, Hague WM: Postpartum thyroiditis, *Semin Perinatol* 22:497-502, 1998.
9. Lucas A, Pizarro E, Granada ML et al: Postpartum thyroid dysfunction and postpartum depression: are they two linked disorders? *Clin Endocrinol* 55:809-814, 2001.
10. Bokhari R, Bhatara VS, Bandettini F et al: Postpartum psychosis and postpartum thyroiditis, *Psychoneuroendocrinology* 23:643-650, 1998.
11. Vargas MT, Briones-Urbina R, Gladman D et al: Antithyroid microsomal autoantibodies and HLADRS are associated with postpartum thyroid dysfunction: evidence supporting an autoimmune pathogenesis, *J Clin Endocrinol Metab* 67:327-333, 1988.
12. Lazarus JH: Clinical manifestations of postpartum thyroid disease, *Thyroid* 9:685-689, 1999.
13. Amino N, Tada H, Hidaka Y et al: Therapeutic controversy: screening for postpartum thyroiditis, *J Clin Endocrinol Metab* 84:1813-1821, 1999.
14. Kampe O, Jansson R, Karlsson FA: Effects of l-thyroxine and iodide on the development of autoimmune postpartum thyroiditis, *J Clin Endocrinol Metab* 70:1014-1018, 1990.
15. Lazarus JH, Ammari F, Oretti R et al: Clinical aspects of recurrent postpartum thyroiditis, *Br J Gen Pract* 418:305-308, 1997.
16. American College of Obstetricians and Gynecologists: ACOG Practice Bulletin. Clinical management guidelines for obstetrician-gynecologists. Number 37, August 2002. (Replaces Practice Bulletin Number 32, November 2001). Thyroid disease in pregnancy, *Obstet Gynecol* 100:387-396, 2002.
17. Lazarus JH, Premawardhana LDKE: Screening for thyroid disease in pregnancy, *J Clin Pathol* 58:449-452, 2005.
18. Surks MI, Ortiz E, Daniels GH et al: Subclinical thyroid disease: scientific review and guidelines for diagnosis and management, *JAMA* 291:228-238, 2004.
19. Gharib H, Tuttle RM, Baskin HJ et al: Subclinical thyroid dysfunction: a joint statement on management from the American Association of Clinical Endocrinologists, the American Thyroid Association, and The Endocrine Society, *Thyroid* 15:24-28, 2005.
20. Kent GN, Stuckey BGA, Allen JR et al: Postpartum thyroid dysfunction: clinical assessment and relationship to psychiatric affective morbidity, *Clin Endocrinol* 51:429-438, 1999.

SECTION F   Septic Pelvic Thrombophlebitis

Charles Carter, MD

Septic pelvic thrombophlebitis is a rare postpartum complication of endometritis or postsurgical infection.[1,2] It occurs in less than 1% of patients with postpartum endometritis.[1] There is a lack of high-quality evidence regarding its evaluation and treatment, with most literature in the form of case reports and retrospective series.

I. EPIDEMIOLOGY AND RISK FACTORS

A. Incidence

The reported incidence of septic pelvic thrombophlebitis varies depending on the population studied, although 1 in 2000 deliveries is most often reported.[1-3] The incidence after vaginal delivery is 1 in 9000 to 13,500 compared with 1 in 400 to 800 for cesarean delivery.[2,4]

B. Risk Factors

The principle risk factors of septic pelvic thrombophlebitis are endometritis or surgical infection.[2] It is more common after cesarean deliveries.[2,4] Though unlikely now, older case series report "criminally induced abortion" as a risk factor.[5] Chorioamnionitis in patients undergoing cesarean section increased the absolute risk 0.4% (relative risk increase of 2.74).[6] One study suggests preeclampsia as a risk factor, though this is not mentioned in other literature.[7]

II. PATHOGENESIS

Pathogenic factors of septic pelvic thrombophlebitis include inherent factors of pregnancy (venous stasis, hypercoagulable state) and bacterial injury to the pelvic venous intima.[3,5,8] Although sharing some features, this is a different process than is encountered in typical venous thrombosis.[5]

III. CLINICAL FEATURES

In cases of postpartum endometritis or wound infection, or both, the expected course is defervescence and clinical improvement after initiation of antibiotics and, if necessary, wound drainage. However, in cases where fever persists, clinicians must reassess the patient to ensure appropriate antibiotic coverage and reevaluate for other possible diagnoses (e.g., infected hematoma).

If fever persists despite addressing these factors, septic pelvic thrombophlebitis should be considered. Thus, prolonged fever ($\geq$38°C) despite adequate antibiotic coverage is the principle defining symptom. Patients typically have an undulating temperature pattern and tachycardia.[8]

Current understanding divides septic pelvic thrombophlebitis into two distinct clinical syndromes: ovarian vein thrombophlebitis and "enigmatic fever."[1,3,8] These syndromes have distinct characteristics (Table 20-5) and differential diagnoses.

IV. DIAGNOSIS

Clinicians should consider a diagnosis of septic pelvic thrombophlebitis in women with endometritis or postoperative infections who have persistent fever after 72 hours of appropriate parenteral antibiotic treatment.[9] Definitive diagnosis is problematic because there is no confirmatory test barring surgery. Thus, positive tests are helpful, whereas negative imaging does not necessarily rule out the diagnosis.

A. Diagnostic Modalities

Contrast-enhanced CT scan is the initial imaging modality of choice, and magnetic resonance angiography is an acceptable alternative/adjunct. Patients with thrombophlebitis of the smaller pelvic veins may not have findings despite having the clinical syndrome. Doppler ultrasonography is unreliable.[9-11]

B. Blood Cultures

Although septic thrombosis is assumed, blood cultures are positive in only a minority of cases.[2,12]

C. Acute Ovarian Vein Thrombosis

In patients with symptoms characteristic of the acute ovarian vein thrombosis syndrome (see Table 20-5), the differential includes abscess, appendicitis, adnexal hematoma, ovarian torsion, pyelonephritis, and renal calculi. The differential for enigmatic fever includes abscess, collagen-vascular disease, drug fever, and viral syndrome.[1,3]

TABLE 20-5 Clinical Comparison of Ovarian Vein Thrombophlebitis and Enigmatic Fever

Clinical Features	Acute Ovarian Vein Thrombophlebitis	"Enigmatic Fever"
Postpartum onset	48-96 hours	Varies
General appearance	Acutely ill	Nontoxic
Fever, chills	Yes	Yes
Tachycardia	Yes	Yes
Symptoms	Abdominal, flank pain; possible nausea, vomiting	May initially have abdominal pain
Physical examination	Lower quadrant pain, guarding; palpable mass on bimanual, most often on right side	Unrevealing
Imaging	Typically reveals thrombus	May be unrevealing
Other	Ileus may occur	Endometritis symptoms may improve after antibiotics, but fever and tachycardia persist

Data from Duff P: Serious sequelae of puerperal infection. In Gabbe SG: *Obstetrics: normal and problem pregnancies,* ed 4, New York, 2002 Churchill Livingstone; Gibbs RS: Severe infections in pregnancy, *Med Clin North Am* 73:713-721, 1989; Dunnihoo DR, Gallaspy JW, Wise RB et al: Postpartum ovarian vein thrombophlebitis: a review, *Obstet Gynecol Surv* 46;415-427, 1991; and Larsen JW, Hager WD, Livengood CH et al: Guidelines for the diagnosis, treatment and prevention of postoperative infections, *Infect Dis Obstet Gynecol* 11:65-70, 2003.

V. TREATMENT

A. Medical Treatment

Historical cornerstones of treatment include broad-spectrum antibiotics for endometritis and heparin anticoagulation. Most authors recommend therapeutic heparin as treatment. Many reports remark on defervescence after heparin treatment and suggest a "heparin challenge" to confirm an uncertain diagnosis.[1,3,8,13,14] However, these recommendations are not based on prospective, randomized trials. Only one randomized trial has been performed and its findings call into question the importance of heparin treatment, finding no difference in outcomes between the heparin and nonheparin groups.[4] Given the lack of prospective evidence, current guidelines acknowledge that some patients will improve without heparin and present two options:

1. Broad-spectrum antibiotics for endometritis alone
2. Broad-spectrum antibiotics for endometritis plus therapeutic heparin until the patient is afebrile 24 to 48 hours[9]

B. Surgery

Surgery is reserved for nonresponsive patients.[1]

C. Prolonged Anticoagulation

Prolonged anticoagulation is unnecessary unless complications such as pulmonary embolism arise.[1,9] Septic pulmonary embolism is a potential complication, and patients with signs suggesting this should be evaluated. However, although not common, the current incidence of this complication is unknown. Brown and colleagues[4] did not find this complication in their clinical trial. However, this trial was not large enough to preclude that heparin protects from embolization.

VI. SUMMARY: PITFALLS AND CONTROVERSIES

The principle controversy surrounding septic pelvic thrombophlebitis treatment regards heparin therapy. Appropriately designed RCTs are needed to address whether heparin improves outcomes. As mentioned earlier, treatment may involve either broad-spectrum antibiotics alone or antibiotics with heparin anticoagulation.

REFERENCES

1. Duff P: Serious sequelae of puerperal infection. In Gabbe SG, editor: *Obstetrics: normal and problem pregnancies,* ed 4, New York, 2002, Churchill Livingstone.
2. Witlin AG, Mercer BM, Sibai BM: Septic pelvic thrombophlebitis or refractory postpartum fever of undetermined etiology, *J Matern Fetal Med* 5:355-358, 1996.
3. Gibbs RS: Severe infections in pregnancy, *Med Clin North Am* 73:713-721, 1989.
4. Brown CE, Stettler RW, Twickler D et al: Puerperal septic pelvic thrombophlebitis: incidence and response to heparin therapy, *Am J Obstet Gynecol* 181(1):143-148, 1999.
5. Collins CG, MacCallum EA, Nelson EW et al: Suppurative pelvic thrombophlebitis: incidence, pathology, and etiology, *Surgery* 30:298-310, 1951.
6. Rouse DJ, Landon M, Leveno KJ et al: The maternal-fetal medicine units cesarean registry: chorioamnionitis at term and its duration-relationship to outcomes, *Am J Obstet Gynecol* 191:211-216, 2004.
7. Isler CM, Rinehart BK, Terrone DA et al: Septic pelvic thrombophlebitis and preeclampsia are related disorders, *Hypertens Pregnancy* 23(1):121-127, 2004.
8. Dunnihoo DR, Gallaspy JW, Wise RB et al: Postpartum ovarian vein thrombophlebitis: a review, *Obstet Gynecol Surv* 46:415-427, 1991.
9. Larsen JW, Hager WD, Livengood CH et al: Guidelines for the diagnosis, treatment and prevention of postoperative infections, *Infect Dis Obstet Gynecol* 11:65-70, 2003.
10. Twickler DM, Setiawan AT, Evans RS et al: Imaging of puerperal septic thrombophlebitis. Prospective comparison of MR imaging, CT, and sonography, *AJR Am J Roentgenol* 169:1039-1043, 1997.
11. Kubik-Huch RA, Huch R, Hilfiker P et al: Role of duplex color Doppler ultrasound, computed tomography, and MR angiography in the diagnosis of septic puerperal ovarian vein thrombosis, *Abdom Imaging* 24:85-91, 1999.
12. Cohen MB, Pernoll ML, Gevirtz CM et al: Septic pelvic thrombophlebitis: an update, *Obstet Gynecol* 62:83-89, 1983.
13. Dunn LJ, Van Voorhis LW: Enigmatic fever and pelvic thrombophlebitis. Response to anticoagulants, *N Engl J Med* 276(5):265-268, 1967.
14. Josey WE, Staggers SR: Heparin therapy in septic pelvic thrombophlebitis: a study of 46 cases, *Am J Obstet Gynecol* 120:228-233, 1974.

S E C T I O N G Postpartum Contraception

Christine Stabler, MD, FAAFP

Comprehensive prenatal care includes a careful discussion of postpartum family planning. The prenatal period will give the couple ample opportunity to explore all factors determining their choice for contraception after delivery. It is the responsibility of the clinician to elucidate the determining factors for the couple to consider and to provide supportive information. Unfortunately, much of the information available for couples is in written form only. Abike and colleagues[1] found that low literacy was directly related to nonuse of contraception before unplanned pregnancies and also was associated with failure to use contraception at 2 months postpartum. Information tailored to the patient and delivered in an understandable form is important for successful postpartum contraception.

I. FACTORS THAT DETERMINE CONTRACEPTIVE CHOICES

Factors that determine a couple's contraceptive choice include their age, number of living children, the need for temporary or permanent contraception, desire for spacing of children, existing medical conditions, personal attitudes, and the woman's lactation status. Recommendations for postpartum contraception should take these factors into consideration.

II. RETURN TO SEXUAL ACTIVITY

Perineal healing is usually sufficient to return to sexual activity by 4 weeks after delivery, although those with episiotomies or tears may experience discomfort for a more prolonged period. The vagina, which is dusky, engorged, spacious, and smooth after delivery, diminishes in size and regains its normal rugated, pink appearance by approximately 3 weeks after delivery. Activation of the pituitary-ovarian axis in the nonlactating woman begins as early as 25 days after delivery with a mean time until ovulation of 45 days. Resumption of sexual activity will be determined by comfort, return of libido, and fatigue. The couple should be prepared for contraception before resumption of sexual activity. Ideally, the couple will have chosen their method of contraception before leaving the hospital postpartum.

III. CONTRACEPTIVE CHOICES FOR BREASTFEEDING WOMEN

1. Lactational amenorrhea method (LAM)
   Breastfeeding delays the onset of ovulation in the postpartum period. The LAM requires that a mother must be fully, or exclusively breastfeeding, amenorrheic, and that it be used for no more than 6 months. With these provisions the LAM is more than 98% effective in preventing a pregnancy.[2] The patient choosing the LAM should begin breastfeeding immediately after delivery. Nipple stimulation

is essential for ovarian suppression; thus, breastfeeding must be continuous, including nighttime. The LAM is a flexible, well-tolerated method of contraception. It has been used in a variety of cultures and socioeconomic groups. It is ideal for the patient who prefers a natural method of family planning. Failure rates have been shown to be greater in working women, when the goal of 10 short or 6 long episodes of breastfeeding per day is more difficult to achieve.[2,3] Still, satisfaction rates with the LAM are quite high.

Once menses have resumed, or feedings are supplemented with solids or formula, it is important for the patient to have an available alternative or additional method to use for contraception. Natural family planning (NFP) can replace LAM when menstrual periods resume; however, cervical mucus consistency can be affected by continued breastfeeding, and basal body temperatures can be altered by nighttime awakenings for breastfeeding.

2. Hormonal contraception
   It has been demonstrated that the estrogen component of combined oral contraceptives (COCs) has a moderate inhibitory effect on breast milk supply.[4] WHO data suggest that at 1 year of age, breastfed infants exposed to COCs weighed, on average, 1 kg less than nonexposed infants. This difference disappeared at 2 years of age, when solids constituted a larger portion of the infant diet.[5] A variety of progestin-only contraceptives has been found acceptable for lactating women. They can be started as early as 3 days after delivery. The following summarizes the progestin-only contraceptives:

a. Progestin-only pills (POPs): POPs deliver small, continuous levels of progestin throughout the cycle but require a high degree of compliance. Under the influence of continuous progestin, cervical mucus becomes viscid and sticky, preventing passage of sperm. Ovulation is suppressed in 15% to 40% of cycles in nonlactating women, but this increases to more than 80% in breastfeeding mothers.[6] Although failure rates are greater than for COCs, POPs are effective when combined with lactation, with more than 99% efficacy. No inhibition of milk supply occurs, and no adverse effects have been found in infants exposed to POPs.[4] When women opt to supplement feedings or discontinue lactation, an alternative contraceptive must be offered as a backup to ensure contraceptive efficacy.

b. Depot medroxyprogesterone acetate (DMPA): DMPA does not suppress milk production and affords a high level of efficacy even as women supplement feedings or discontinue lactation. The irregular bleeding women experience when receiving DMPA appears to be acceptable, although prolonged but not excessive bleeding can occur when the contraceptive is administered immediately postpartum.[7] A dose of 150 mg is administered intramuscularly every 12 weeks. Women weighing less than 115 pounds should shorten the interval to 10 weeks. Efficacy is not reduced in overweight women. Common side effects include telogen effluvium (progestin-related hair loss) with the first injection, weight gain of 2 to 4 pounds per year of use, depression, acne, and irregular menses. At year 1, 60% of users are amenorrheic. By year 2, 70% are still amenorrheic. Median time of return to fertility is 10 months, but delays of up to 18 months may occur.

c. Etonogestrel (Implanon): Implanon is a single-rod subdermal system that delivers continuous levels of etonogestrel, a progestin, over a 3-year period similar to the Norplant system (Levonorgestrel implant). Levels of progestin slowly wane over the 3 years from 60 to 70 μg/day in the first year of use to 25 to 35 μg/day by the third year. Women more than 130% of ideal body weight may not achieve the 99% contraceptive efficacy at these levels as compared with women of ideal body weight, although postmarketing data have not shown this decreased efficacy in overweight women.[8] As a progestin-only method, it is compatible with breastfeeding. Implanon does not affect the amount of breast milk produced by the mother or the number of feedings needed by the infant. No difference exists in the composition of the breast milk in women using Implanon. In one study that observed the breastfed children of mothers using Implanon for contraception for 3 years, there was no difference in their growth rates or general health compared with breastfed children whose mothers were not using hormonal contraception.[8]

d. COCs: The effect of low-dose (≤35 μg ethinyl estradiol) COC on lactation is controversial. The amount of estrogen that is secreted in breast milk is not harmful to the infant. Small reductions in breast milk can be overcome with increased feedings when COCs are started after 1 month of lactation when good breastfeeding patterns have been achieved. If breastfeeding motivation is marginal, the reduction in supply may be sufficient to discourage continuation and other methods of contraception are recommended.

3. Barrier methods

Barrier methods are readily available, inexpensive, and well-accepted methods of contraception for postpartum woman. Condoms with spermicide, diaphragms, and sponges have the advantage of no effect on menses, breast milk, or weight gain. Efficacy is user dependent in that actual failure rates are greater than those quoted with perfect use of the method.

a. Condoms with spermicide via film, foam, or gel: These are useful in breastfeeding women alone or as an adjunct to POPs when the mother begins supplementation of feedings. Failure rates in breastfeeding mothers are lower than the 2 to 21 per 100 women-years quoted for nonlactating women. Latex condoms are recommended. Hepatitis B and HIV viruses may pass through natural skin condoms. Spermicide-containing nonoxynol-9 is also somewhat effective in protection against some infectious diseases. Polyethylene and polyurethane condoms are less available but afford equivalent protection to latex condoms.

b. Diaphragms: Diaphragms are a good choice of contraceptive method for lactating women. Spermicide used with the diaphragm can make insertion more feasible for lactating women who may have vaginal dryness. Diaphragms can be fitted after 6 weeks postpartum, but weight gain or loss of more than 15 pounds may necessitate refitting the device. Failure rates are variable from 2.4 to 19.6 per 100 women-years.[9] Careful instruction regarding voiding before and after intercourse can minimize the small increased risk for urinary tract infections seen in diaphragm users. Although the cervical cap failed to gain much favor with American women, the new Lea Barrier (distributed by Yama, Inc., New Jersey), a silicone barrier that covers the cervix, may provide more flexibility and acceptance.[9] The Lea comes in one size. It is placed over the cervix and uses suction to maintain its position over the cervix. It has a strap for easy removal, is used with a spermicide, and is available by prescription. Failure rates are similar to those for the diaphragm.

c. Vaginal sponges: These are polyurethane sponges that offer an immediate and continuous presence of spermicide (nonoxynol-9 or benzalkonium chloride) throughout a 24-hour period. The sponge needs no fitting and is available online and over the counter. Failure rates approximate other barrier methods of contraception. Initially available from 1983 through 1995, Today sponges were withdrawn from the market until manufacturing problems were solved. The Today Sponge was reintroduced in 2005. Other sponge-based contraceptive systems such as the Avert are also available with similar efficacy.

4. Intrauterine devices (IUDs)
Worldwide, the IUD is the most popular reversible method of contraception. U.S. acceptance is more limited (approximately 2% of contraceptive use vs. 33% in China), but newer devices and better information on the method has led to greater use of the IUD. Two IUDs are currently available in the United States, The Paragard CopperT and the Mirena levonorgestrel system. The Paragard is effective for 10 years of use. The Mirena has approval for 5 years of contraception. IUDs are 99.2% to 99.9% effective as birth control.[9] Multiple mechanisms of action contribute to the efficacy of the IUD, among them changes in cervical mucus, changes in the endometrium, and alteration in sperm and tubal motility. The degree to which prevention of implantation plays a role is unclear, but the CopperT works primarily by affecting motility. They do not protect against sexually transmitted infections, including HIV/AIDS. Women participating in high-risk behaviors for sexually transmitted infection should be counseled against the IUD for contraception, but in women at low risk, no increase in infections or tubal infertility has been demonstrated. Pregnancies that occur while using the IUD are at increased risk for complications including spontaneous abortion, preterm delivery, and ectopic implantation. The absolute risk for an ectopic pregnancy is 1 per 1000 woman-years, which is less than half the risk for women using no contraception. Neither IUD has significant effect on breastfeeding. Trivial amounts of levonorgestrel are secreted into breast milk in women using the Mirena system. Nursing and its associated oxytocin release has not been associated with increased expulsion rates for IUDs. Retention rates for the IUD are improved when the IUD is placed at least 6 weeks after delivery.

IUDs placed immediately after delivery were associated with increased pain and bleeding; however, a Cochrane review of the topic made no clear recommendation as timing of insertion was not randomized in the studies reviewed.[10]

5. Sterilization
The postpartum period is a logical time for tubal sterilization when women desire permanent contraception. Tubal ligations can be perfumed at the time of cesarean section or within 2 days after delivery, and they do not increase the length of stay in the hospital. Many women elect to delay the procedure to 6 to 8 weeks after delivery to ensure that the infant is healthy and to reflect on their decision. Failure rates range from 0.14% to 1%, with slightly greater rates in procedures performed postpartum.[11] Vasectomies are a safe alternative to tubal sterilization for women. This 30-minute ambulatory procedure is performed under local anesthesia and carries a failure rate of 0.1% to 0.3%. Most failures result from spontaneous recanalization, which can occur any time after vasectomy. The risk for recanalization appears to be related to the surgical techniques used during the procedure. Fascial interposition can reduce the risk for failure by about 50% when performed with ligation and excision. Using cautery instead of ligation and excision may further reduce the risk for failure, making vasectomy an even more effective contraceptive method. Another caveat of vasectomy is the mandatory use of alternative contraception for 8 to 12 weeks after the procedure until azoospermia can be achieved.

6. Contraception for nonlactating women
Although most nonbreastfeeding women will resume menstrual cycles within 4 to 6 weeks after delivery, only about one third of first cycles will be ovulatory and even fewer will result in pregnancy. If a couple wishes to avoid all risk for pregnancy, however, contraception should be started at the time of (barriers, spermicide, NFP) or before (hormonals, IUDs, or permanent contraception) the first postpartum sexual intercourse. All of the options available for breastfeeding mothers apply to nonlactating women. POPs alone are less effective (approximately 85% vs. 99% for COCs) and should be discouraged as a single method in nonlactating women.

a. When to initiate therapy: COCs are an acceptable choice and can be started within the second to third postpartum week. This delay reduces the procoagulant effects of estrogen on the postpartum woman as coagulation and fibrinolysis is close to normal by 2 weeks. Seven days of hormonal contraception should be sufficient to suppress any ovarian follicle in development; therefore, backup contraception such as a condom plus spermicide should be used if sexual activity begins less than 1 week after initiation of the COC.

b. NFP: NFP is a set of methods of family planning that help women to achieve or avoid pregnancy by identifying times of infertility and potential fertility. The Sympto-Thermal Method is based on daily fertility awareness; a couple charts the woman's common signs of fertility (cervical mucus, basal body temperature, and cervical position) and uses that information to determine her fertile and infertile times.[12] It can be used both to achieve and to avoid or postpone pregnancy. When used to avoid pregnancy, the couple abstains from intercourse during the fertile time. Alternately, couples can use NFP to reduce use of other contraceptives such as barrier devices by using them only during the fertile periods. Other methods make statistical estimates as to when a woman is fertile (Rhythm Method and the Standard Days Method). Education is essential for success, and on average, couples need 6 months of practice to achieve efficacy. The Rhythm Method, the most well-known method of NFP, has a perfect-use failure rate of 9% per year, whereas other types of NFP have lower perfect-use failure rates of 1% to 3% per year.[12]

REFERENCES

1. Abike J, Bennett I, Gadsden V et al: Maternal literacy and postpartum contraception, *Contraception* 73:613-617, 2006.
2. Nichols-Johnson V: The breastfeeding days and contraception, *Breastfeed Abstr* 21:11-12, 2001.
3. Labbok M, Cooney K, Coly S: *Guidelines: breastfeeding, family planning, and the lactational amenorrhea method—LAM*, Washington, DC, 1994 Institute for Reproductive Health.
4. Diaz S, Zepeda A, Maturana X et al: Fertility regulation in nursing women. IX. Contraceptive performance, duration of lactation, infant growth, and bleeding patterns during use of progesterone vaginal rings, progestin-only pills, Norplant implants, and Copper T 380-A intrauterine devices, *Contraception* 56(4):223-232, 1997.
5. WHO Task Force on Oral Contraceptives: Effects of hormonal contraceptives on milk volume and infant growth, *Contraception* 30(6):505-521, 1984.
6. Díaz SP, Miranda A, Brandeis H et al: Mechanism of action of progesterone as contraceptive for lactating women. In Seppala M, Hamberger L, editors: *Frontiers in human reproduction*, New York, June 1991, New York Academy of Sciences.
7. Curtis K, Peterson H: Long-acting methods of contraception, *N Engl J Med* 353:2169-2175, 2005.
8. Oloto E: Questions regarding implanon, *Mayo Clin Proc* 79:519-524, 2004. Available at: http://www.mayoclinic.com/health/implanon/DI00074.
9. Levitt C, Shaw E, Wong S et al: Systematic review of the literature on postpartum care, *Birth* 31:203-212, 2004.
10. Grimes DA, Schulz KF, Vliet H et al: Immediate post-partum insertion of intrauterine devices. In the *Cochrane Database of Systematic Reviews*, CD003036, 3, 2007.
11. Peterson HB, Xia Z, Hughes JM: Risk of pregnancy after tubal sterilization: findings from the U.S. Collaborative Review of sterilization, *Am J Obstet Gynecol* 1161-1168, 1996. Available at: http://www.contraception.net/resource_centre/barrier.asp
12. ACOG natural family planning pamphlet, Am College of OBGYN, Washington, DC, 2003. Available at: http://www.ccli.org

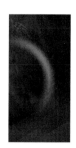

CHAPTER 21

Postpartum Psychosocial Concerns

Dwenda K. Gjerdingen, MD, MS, Elizabeth Ann Shaw, BSc, MD, FCFP, and Sharon S.-L. Wong, PhD, RD

SECTION A Maternal Adjustment

The postpartum period is a time of significant transition for a woman and her family. Aside from adjustment to physical changes in their bodies, women are also coping with fatigue and changes in both relationships and their parenting roles within the family. Women may also experience a variety of psychological and psychiatric disorders after childbirth, from the milder and more common transient "blues," to severe depression, posttraumatic stress, and psychosis. At least one trial indicates that in the first 5 postpartum weeks, women are three times more likely to experience an episode of major depression.[1] This condition often goes unrecognized because many of the symptoms of depression are also complaints in the normal postpartum period (fatigue, sleep disturbance, emotional lability), and the newborn is often the focus for both parents and caregivers. In addition to this impact on the mother, there is evidence of a significant association between mothers' mental health and their children's cognitive, behavioral, and physical development, up to 5 years of age.[2]

I. POSTPARTUM BLUES

Postpartum blues are commonly experienced by new mothers, with prevalence rates of 26% to 85% depending on the diagnostic criteria used.[3] Symptoms, which are usually short-lived, begin within the first week after birth, peak around day 5, and usually resolve by 12 days after delivery. These symptoms include dysphoria, mood lability, crying, anxiety, insomnia, poor appetite, and irritability.[3] Although the blues are considered to be a simple adjustment disorder of childbirth, they also are known to be a risk factor for subsequent postpartum depression.[4] The symptoms usually resolve spontaneously, and women often benefit from reassurance and support.

II. POSTPARTUM DEPRESSION

A. Epidemiology

Reported prevalence rates of postpartum depression are dependent on the definition and diagnostic criteria chosen. A metaanalysis of studies from the United Kingdom, United States, and Australia reports an overall prevalence rate of 13%.[5] A recent systematic review of studies using objective criteria for the diagnosis of major depression indicates a prevalence rate of 1.0% to 5.9% during the first postpartum year, and 6.5% to 12.9% for major and minor depression combined.[1] (Minor depression refers to the presence of two to four symptoms of major depressive disorder, as listed in Table 21-1, where the symptoms are not accounted for by another psychiatric disorder.[6]) Between 20% and 40% of women with a history of postpartum depression will suffer a recurrence with subsequent pregnancies.[5]

B. Risk Factors

Based on a systematic review of the literature, factors with the strongest statistical association with postpartum depression include poor marital adjustment, recent life stresses (bereavement, unemployment, illness), maternal prenatal depression, lack of social support, abuse of the mother, and a history of previous psychiatric disorder in the mother.[7]

TABLE 21-1 Criteria for Major Depressive Episode

Five or more of the symptoms listed below, together with these qualifications:

    Must include symptoms 1 or 2

    Symptoms are present nearly every day for the same 2-week period

    Symptoms represent a change from baseline

    Symptoms produce clinically significant distress or change in functioning

    Symptoms are not due to drugs, another medical condition, or bereavement (unless prolonged, i.e., >2 months)

    Symptoms do not meet criteria for a mixed episode

Symptoms

1. Depressed mood most of the day
2. Markedly diminished interest or pleasure in all or almost all activities most of the day
3. Marked decrease or increase in appetite, resulting in significant unintentional weight loss or weight gain (i.e., >5% body weight in 1 month)
4. Insomnia or hypersomnia
5. Psychomotor agitation or retardation
6. Fatigue or loss of energy
7. Feelings of worthlessness or inappropriate guilt
8. Decreased ability to think or concentrate
9. Recurrent thoughts of death or recurrent suicidal thoughts (with or without a plan)

Adapted from American Psychiatric Association: *Diagnostic and statistical manual of mental disorders,* ed 4, Washington, DC, 2000, American Psychiatric Association.

C. Pathogenesis

The fact that women are at increased risk for mood disorders in the postpartum period implies that gonadal steroids may play a role in the pathogenesis of depression in women. In women with postpartum depression, there is also a much stronger family history of psychiatric disorders or depression (71% and 48%, respectively) than in the population at large, which suggests a familial component.[3]

D. Clinical Features

Because postpartum depression is a type of major depressive disorder, with symptoms beginning sometime during the first 4 weeks after delivery, the clinical characteristics are those of major depression (see Table 21-1). The *postpartum onset* modifier can also be applied to manic or mixed episode in major depressive disorder, bipolar I disorder, bipolar II disorder, or brief psychotic disorder.[6] Although this definition specifies an onset within the first postpartum month, women remain at increased risk for depression for up to 1 year after delivery.[5] The duration of depressive symptoms in childbearing women is similar to that of non-childbearing women: 44% and

47%, respectively, continue to show symptoms at 6 month follow-up.[8]

1. Role of history and physical examination
   A careful history and physical examination should be done on all women presenting with postpartum mood symptoms. Important components of the history are the psychiatric history, including previous postpartum episodes, a family history of Axis I disorders, and stressful life events. Recording the woman's current symptoms enables the provider to rate these prospectively over the course of follow-up.

2. Exclusion of other common medical conditions
   Women who are thought to be depressed should be evaluated for thyroid dysfunction because depression is sometimes associated with the hypothyroid phase of postpartum thyroiditis.[9] Seen in 1.1% to 16.7% (mean, 7.5%) of postpartum women, postpartum thyroiditis is marked by an increased level of thyroid-stimulating hormone and anti-thyroid antibodies.[9] For these patients, treatment of postpartum thyroid dysfunction is important to the effective management of postpartum depression. Postpartum depression may

also be associated with anemia; a hemoglobin or hematocrit should be ordered, particularly when depressed patients specify fatigue as a primary complaint.

E. Diagnosis and Screening

Although many antenatal risk factors have been identified, the benefits of screening women at risk in the prenatal period and then intervening to prevent postpartum depression have yet to be clearly demonstrated. Currently, no antenatal screening tool is available with acceptable predictive validity that can be recommended for use. Several screening tools have been evaluated in the postpartum population, including the Beck Depression Inventory (BDI), the Postpartum Depression Screening Scale (PDSS), the Edinburgh Postnatal Depression Scale (EPDS), and the Center for Epidemiological Studies Depression Scale (CES-D). For major depression, a positive screen on any of these scales reliably predicts with good specificity women who have postpartum depression. Although the sensitivity for the EPDS and PDSS scales is quite high (75-100%), the sensitivity of the other scales tends to be lower. For minor depression, the sensitivity rates are even lower (43-71%), significantly increasing the risk for missing women with minor depression.[1]

The most widely used screening tool for postpartum depression in large populations is the EPDS. This scale, consisting of 10 mood-related statements (Table 21-2), has been validated, computerized, and used as a telephone screen.[10] Mothers who score above a threshold of 12 (of 30 total) are likely to be suffering from a major depressive illness (sensitivity, 100%; specificity, 79%).[1]

In view of the high risk for depression within the first 5 weeks, consideration should be given to scheduling visits before the traditional 6 weeks in women at risk for postpartum depression. Because most women do not seek professional help, home visits may be appropriate to assess the new mother's parenting skills and to screen for depressive symptoms.

The Patient Health Questionnaire-9 is a relatively new nine-item depression screen that is based on *Diagnostic and Statistical Manual of Mental Disorders,* Fourth Edition (DSM-IV) criteria (Table 21-3). It has been validated in more than 6000 patients in a primary care population and in a general obstetrics and gynecology clinic. In these settings, the sensitivity and specificity for depression compared with a structured mental health interview were both 88% at a cutoff

TABLE 21-2 Edinburgh Postnatal Depression Scale

In the past 7 days:
1. I have been able to laugh and see the funny side of things:
   As much as I always could
   Not quite so much now
   Definitely not so much now
   Not at all
2. I have looked forward with enjoyment to things:
   As much as I ever did
   Rather less than I used to
   Definitely less than I used to
   Hardly at all
*3. I have blamed myself unnecessarily when things went wrong:
   Yes, most of the time
   Yes, some of the time
   Not very often
   No, never
4. I have been anxious or worried for no good reason:
   No, not at all
   Hardly ever
   Yes, sometimes
   Yes, very often
*5. I have felt scared or panicky for no very good reason:
   Yes, quite a lot
   Yes, sometimes
   No, not much
   No, not at all
*6. Things have been getting on top of me:
   Yes, most of the time I haven't been able to cope at all
   Yes, sometimes I haven't been coping as well as usual
   No, most of the time I have coped quite well
   No, I have been coping as well as ever.
*7. I have been so unhappy that I have had difficulty sleeping:
   Yes, most of the time
   Yes, sometimes
   Not very often
   No, not at all
*8. I have felt sad or miserable:
   Yes, most of the time
   Yes, quite often
   Not very often
   No, not at all

Continued

TABLE 21-2 Edinburgh Postnatal Depression Scale—cont'd

---

*9. I have been so unhappy that I have been crying:

Yes, most of the time

Yes, quite often

Only occasionally

No, never

*10. The thought of harming myself has occurred to me:

Yes, quite often

Sometimes

Hardly ever

Never

score of 10 or more.[11] Although it has not been specifically validated for use in postpartum depression, it has a similar advantage to the EPDS in that it can be self-administered. An abbreviated two-question version of this questionnaire (the first two questions in the tool), is also being used as a quick screen for depressive disorders in general populations.

Women who screen positive for depression using any of the tools discussed earlier should ideally have the diagnosis confirmed using an interview to evaluate for the presence of DSM-IV criteria of depression (see Table 21-1).

F. Management Recommendations

1. Antidepressant drugs and psychotherapy
   Postpartum depression can generally be treated with antidepressant medications or psychotherapy; combined therapy has not shown additional benefit. Only two small randomized controlled trials (RCTs) have evaluated pharmacotherapy plus psychotherapy specifically in the treatment of postpartum depression.[12,13] In the first trial, fluoxetine was found to be as effective as a full course of cognitive behavioral therapy (CBT) in the treatment of postpartum depression at 12 weeks. No additional benefit was shown when psychotherapy was combined with pharmacotherapy.[12] Similarly, in the second trial, women with a DSM-IV diagnosis of depression with comorbid anxiety benefited from paroxetine but did not derive any additional benefit from the combination of a 1-hour weekly CBT session plus paroxetine. There was no placebo group in this trial.[13] Although a variety of other antidepressants may be used to treat postpartum depression, none of them has been studied in proper RCTs. Of three classes of antidepressants (selective serotonin reuptake inhibitors [SSRIs], tricyclic antidepressants [TCAs], and other antidepressants), the TCAs produce the most side effects and carry the greatest risk for toxicity when taken in overdose.

   A number of RCTs have examined the impact of different psychotherapy techniques alone in the treatment of postpartum depression. Supportive counseling, CBT, interpersonal psychotherapy, and psychodynamic therapy all reduced EPDS scores in the first 3 to 4 months after delivery.[14-17] Only one trial looked at longer term outcomes, and it found no difference between the control and intervention groups at 9 months after delivery, which likely reflects the timing of spontaneous remission of postpartum depression.[15]

2. Antidepressant therapy for breastfeeding women
   Although TCAs traditionally have been prescribed for breastfeeding women because of a lack of demonstrated harm in published case reports, SSRIs are becoming more popular because of their greater tolerability and relative safety when taken in overdose. Although there are no major RCTs of TCA treatment in breastfeeding women, a review of 45 small trials and case reports found that no adverse events had been reported for nursing infants exposed to nortriptyline, desipramine, and imipramine.[18] However, doxepin should be used with caution in breastfeeding women based on reports of neonatal sedation and high serum levels of this drug or its metabolites in nursing infants.[18]

TABLE 21-3 Patient Health Questionnaire-9 Nine-Symptom Checklist

Over the last 2 weeks, how often have you been bothered by any of the following problems?

	Not at all	Several days	More than half of the days	Nearly every day
1. Little interest or pleasure in doing things	0	1	2	3
2. Feeling down, depressed or hopeless	0	1	2	3
3. Trouble falling or staying asleep or sleeping too much	0	1	2	3
4. Feeling tired or having little energy	0	1	2	3
5. Poor appetite or overeating	0	1	2	3
6. Feeling bad about yourself—or that you are a failure or have let yourself or your family down	0	1		
7. Trouble concentrating on things, such as reading the newspaper or watching T.V.	0	1	2	3
8. Moving or speaking so slowly that other people could have noticed? Or the opposite—being so fidgety or restless that you have been moving around a lot more than usual	0	1	2	3
9. Thoughts that you would be better off dead or of hurting yourself in some way	0	1	2	3

(For office coding: Total score_____ = _____ + _____ + _____)

If you checked off *any* problems, how *difficult* have these problems made if for you to do your work, take care of things at home, or get along with other people?

Not difficult at all	Somewhat difficult	Very difficult	Extremely difficult
☐	☐	☐	☐

From the Primary Care Evaluation of Mental Disorders Patient Health Questionnaire (PRIME-MD-PHQ). The Patient Health Questionnaire was developed by Drs. Robert Spitzer, Janet B. W. Williams, Kurt Kroenke, and colleagues. PRIME-MD is a trademark of Pfizer Inc. Copyright 1999, Pfizer Inc. All rights reserved.

Several reviews of SSRIs in breastfeeding women have concluded that all SSRIs are excreted into breast milk in small quantities.[18-20] Serum levels in the infant appear to be the lowest with sertraline, fluvoxamine, and paroxetine and the highest with fluoxetine and citalopram.[20,21] Generally, the SSRIs have not been associated with significant short-term adverse effects. However, there have been reports of irritability and reduced postnatal growth in infants exposed to fluoxetine and lethargy in infants exposed to citalopram and paroxetine (one report each).[19,21] Limited data are available on escitalopram. Although there are some short-term safety concerns with paroxetine, sertraline, and fluoxetine, little research has examined the long-term neurodevelopmental implications of exposure to any of these medications during breastfeeding.

Although the data would not support switching a woman from one SSRI to another if the current medication is effective, it would make some sense when starting a new medication to choose one that is associated with lower neonatal serum concentrations. Currently, sertraline is the most frequently prescribed drug in nursing mothers and is approved by the U.S. Food and Drug Administration for this purpose.[18] There are fewer data available for other (non-TCA, non-SSRI) antidepressants. Safety reports on venlafaxine (a serotonin-norepinephrine reuptake inhibitor) showed detectable serum levels in 10 of 12 infant cases reported, but no adverse neurodevelopmental effects. Two infants were observed for 6 months.[19] Limited to no data exist on bupropion, mirtazapine, and reboxetine, thus these should not be used as first-line drugs to treat depression in breastfeeding women.[19]

The lack of long-term data on breastfeeding infants' exposures to maternal antidepressants must, however, be balanced with the known impact of depression on the infant, including impairments in bonding and the mother-child relationship, delayed motor development, and lower intelligence quotients.[2] Therapy should be instituted at the lowest effective dose, and the infant should be monitored carefully for growth and behavior. Particular caution may need to be taken with premature infants because their ability to metabolize these drugs is lower than for term infants.[18]

3. Estrogen therapy

One RCT evaluated the use of transdermal 17β-estradiol, 200 μg daily, in the treatment of women with postpartum depression. Although there were improvements in the group treated with estrogen, more women in the treatment group received conventional antidepressants, and the women in the control group had been depressed for a longer period.[22] These clinically significant differences between groups may negate the conclusions of the study. Estrogen therapy is not recommended for breastfeeding women because it is associated with decreased milk production.

4. Other recommendations

In women with postpartum depression who desire contraception, the physician must be aware of the potential negative impact of progesterone-containing contraceptives on mood. Although such contraceptives are not contraindicated for depressed patients, their impact on mental well-being should be monitored.

G. Prevention of Postpartum Depression

1. Postpartum support

Postpartum hospital stays in North America are often less than 48 hours for a vaginal birth; thus, most of the provision of postpartum care takes place in the community and in ambulatory settings. Psychosocial postpartum support programs have been developed to improve parenting, maternal mental and physical health, and maternal quality of life.

Several trials have evaluated the ability of various postpartum support programs (telephone calls, home visitation) to reduce the risk for postpartum depression in low-risk postpartum women.

A recent metaanalysis suggested that, taken as a whole, postpartum women who received a supportive psychological or psychosocial intervention were just as likely to experience postpartum depression as women who received standard postpartum care.[23] Programs that had only a postpartum component were more likely to be beneficial than those that had both an antepartum and a postpartum component.

In contrast, when women at high risk for postpartum depression or family dysfunction were enrolled, both less intensive peer counseling from trained volunteers and more intensive nurse home visitation and case conferencing reduced EPDS scores.[23,24] It also appears that postpartum depression rates are reduced when women are offered home support based on a needs assessment that also screens for depression.[25]

2. Pharmacotherapy

One small RCT showed that prophylactic use of sertraline, 50 to 75 mg daily, for 20 weeks led to a reduction in postpartum depression (7% vs. 50%) in women with a history of postpartum depression.[26] Thus, there is some evidence that screening for depressive symptoms in postpartum women, together with intervention (either pharmacotherapy or a peer- or health-professional–based support program) in those at greater risk, does improve mental health outcomes.

III. POSTPARTUM PSYCHOSIS

A. Epidemiology/Risk Factors

Psychotic mood disorders occur in approximately 1 to 2 in 1000 women who have recently given birth.[27] A history of bipolar illness increases the risk for postpartum psychosis to as much as 25%, and prior postpartum psychosis further increases the risk to 50% to 75%.[27]

B. Clinical Features

Early symptoms of psychosis consist of irritability, mood lability, and agitation, and these rapidly progress to confusion, mood changes similar to a mixed manic episode, and frank psychotic symptoms, such as hallucinations, disorganized thoughts, bizarre behavior, delusions, and loss of reality. The theme of the delusion often involves the newborn and may evolve into feeling a need to harm or kill the baby. These delusional thoughts do not produce distress in affected mothers.[28]

C. Treatment

Postpartum psychosis is a psychiatric emergency because these mothers are at increased risk for harming themselves and their children. Untreated, the disorder is associated with a 5% suicide rate and up to a 4% infanticide rate.[28] Therefore, these women should be hospitalized. There are no known trials to date on the treatment of psychosis during pregnancy and postpartum; however, experts recommend that active treatment include one or more of the following: mood stabilizers, neuroleptics, benzodiazepines, and electroconvulsive therapy.[27,29] Associated insomnia and bipolar disorder should also be treated; however, lithium should not be used in breastfeeding mothers.[29]

D. Clinical Course

Symptoms usually begin within the first 2 to 3 weeks after childbirth, sometimes as early as 2 to 3 days postpartum.[28] The prognosis of individual episodes is usually good; however, some women have a protracted course despite treatment. A majority of women will have future recurrences, whereas only a small minority (4%) has exclusively puerperal episodes.[29]

IV. OTHER MENTAL DISORDERS THAT OCCUR DURING THE POSTPARTUM PERIOD

Other more common mental disorders that may have their onset in the postpartum period or be exacerbated by childbirth-related factors include posttraumatic stress disorder (PTSD), panic disorder, obsessive-compulsive disorder (OCD), and eating disorders. Although these conditions have been well studied in general populations, there have been relatively few studies on their occurrence in the postpartum period. Therefore, in some cases, prevalence and treatment recommendations are based on studies from general populations. The DSM-IV does not currently include a postpartum modifier for these four conditions.[6]

A. Posttraumatic Stress Disorder

1. Epidemiology and risk factors
   Because of the potentially traumatizing effects of childbirth (e.g., due to pain, prolonged labor, emergency cesarean sections, and sense of loss of control), mothers may experience childbirth-related PTSD. However, even though childbirth-related trauma and stress are relatively common, only a small minority of women who experience such trauma will develop PTSD. In a community-based sample of 499 women, 33% of women identified a traumatic birthing event and the presence of at least three trauma symptoms, but only 5.6% of the group met criteria for acute PTSD.[30] A longitudinal study found the incidence rate of PTSD at 6 weeks after delivery to be 2.8%, which was greater than the 1.5% incidence rate at 6 months after delivery, suggesting that PTSD symptoms may indeed be provoked by adverse birthing events.[31] Factors that have been associated with acute trauma symptoms in the postpartum period include level of obstetric intervention and perception of inadequate care during labor.[30]

2. Clinical features/diagnosis
   Criteria for PTSD include:
   a. Exposure to a traumatic event that produced persistent symptoms of increased arousal (e.g., exaggerated startle response, difficulty sleeping, irritability, outbursts of anger, difficulty concentrating, hypervigilance)
   b. Persistent reexperiencing the traumatic event (e.g., through recurrent distressing recollections or dreams of the event, or psychological reactivity on exposure to cues that symbolize the event)
   c. Persistent avoidance of the event (e.g., efforts to avoid thoughts or conversations related to the event, inability to recall the trauma, feeling detached or estranged from others); in addition, these symptoms last more than 1 month and produce significant distress or functional impairment[6]

3. Treatment
   Research has primarily addressed the treatment of PTSD in general populations rather than in postpartum women. A metaanalysis of RCTs on PTSD treatment found that pharmacotherapy for this disorder appears to have positive effects, with odds ratios for treatment response with various agents ranging from 2.2 to 5.6. The SSRIs appear both safe and effective for this indication.[32] In addition, a Cochrane review showed that both individual and group trauma-focused CBT and stress management are effective in the treatment of PTSD.[33]

4. Prevention
   A recent Cochrane review found no beneficial effect of a single session of psychological debriefing

for the prevention of PTSD in (nonpostpartum) trauma-exposed individuals.[34] Neither has significant benefit from prophylactic debriefing seen in women with childbirth-related trauma.

B. Panic Disorder

1. Epidemiology
   Panic disorder affects 1% to 3% of people in the general population at some point in their lives.[35] The age at onset is most often between late adolescence and the mid-thirties—the childbearing years—and twice as many women as men suffer from panic disorder.[36]

2. Clinical features/diagnosis
   Panic disorder is defined as the presence of recurrent, unexpected panic attacks followed by at least 1 month of persistent concern about having another panic attack, worry about the possible implications or consequences of the panic attacks, or a significant behavioral change related to the attacks.[36] Panic attacks are characterized by symptoms such as shortness of breath, palpitations, chest pain, dizziness, nausea, sweating, fear of losing control or "going crazy," and a sense of impending doom.[36] Mothers may fear the infant, based on the awesome responsibility of care, or they may fear crib death, with the result that they become sleep deprived.[37] In a qualitative study based on interviews with six mothers who had experienced postpartum panic disorder, the following themes emerged: panic seriously complicated mothers' lives, cognitive function diminished during attacks, women struggled to maintain control during attacks and worked hard at preventing future attacks, negative lifestyle changes resulted, self-esteem dropped, and mothers were haunted by the prospect of negative residual effects on themselves and their families.[36]

3. Treatment
   Antidepressants improve panic symptoms and global functioning; two metaanalyses found that SSRIs and TCAs are equally effective in reducing panic severity and the number of attacks.[35] Benzodiazepines also help reduce panic severity but are most useful in improving depression and functioning when used in combination with other therapies.[35] Metaanalyses have also found CBT to be effective in reducing panic frequency and severity; however, many of the trials were conducted in select groups and, therefore, may not be applicable to general or postpartum populations.[35]

4. Clinical course
   Preexisting panic disorder may either worsen or improve with pregnancy, as noted in a review of eight noncontrolled studies regarding the effect of pregnancy on panic disorder. Of the 215 pregnancies described in these studies, 41% showed improvement in panic disorder symptoms during pregnancy, whereas 38% showed onset or exacerbation of symptoms in the postpartum period.[38]

C. Obsessive-Compulsive Disorder

1. Epidemiology and risk factors
   The lifetime prevalence rate of OCD in the general population is 2% to 3%, and the incidence of OCD in women is thought to be greatest during childbearing years.[28] In a case-controlled retrospective study of 68 patients with OCD, the birth of a live child was the only life event significantly more reported by OCD patients than by control patients.[39]

2. Clinical features/diagnosis
   OCD is an anxiety disorder with the following characteristics: (1) intrusive and inappropriate thoughts, ideas, or images (obsessions) that lead to increased anxiety or distress, and that are not simply excessive worries about real-life problems; or (2) repetitious, intentional rituals (compulsions) performed to neutralize the anxiety or distress. At some point, the individual recognizes that the obsessions or compulsions are excessive or unreasonable, to the degree that they often interfere with normal function.[6] When OCD occurs in the postpartum period, the content of obsessional thoughts is often related to the theme of harming the newborn; these thoughts are very distressing to mothers.[28]

3. Treatment
   Large RCTs have demonstrated the efficacy of SSRIs for the treatment of OCD in general populations.[28] In addition, a quantitative review of OCD treatments found that certain psychotherapeutic approaches, such as exposure with response prevention or cognitive therapy, are highly effective in reducing OCD symptoms.[40] However, similar studies have not been conducted on postpartum populations.

D. Eating Disorders

1. Epidemiology and risk factors
   After giving birth, mothers are also at risk for eating disorders—for example, bulimia nervosa,

anorexia nervosa, and eating disorders not otherwise specified—because of their concerns about residual weight gain after giving birth.[41] The lifetime prevalence rate in female individuals for bulimia nervosa is 1% to 3% and for anorexia nervosa is 0.5%.[6] Point prevalence estimates for eating disorders in young western women are 1% for bulimia and 2% to 5% for partial eating disorder syndromes or eating disorder not otherwise specified.[42]

2. Clinical features/diagnosis

Features of *bulimia nervosa* include:

a. Uncontrolled episodes of binge eating

b. Recurrent inappropriate compensation to prevent weight gain, such as self-induced vomiting, laxatives, diuretics, fasting, or excessive exercising, with criteria 1 and 2 occurring at least twice weekly for 3 months

c. Self-evaluation that is unduly influenced by body shape and weight

Anorexia nervosa is characterized by:

a. Disturbance of body image

b. Intense fear of becoming fat, even though underweight

c. Refusal to maintain body weight at or above a minimally normal weight for age and height (e.g., body weight 15% or more below expected weight)

d. In female individuals of childbearing age, absence of three consecutive menstrual cycles without other cause[6]

3. Treatment

In a systematic review of studies on the treatment of eating disorders in the general population, the combination of pharmacologic and psychological treatments was found to be superior to the single psychotherapeutic approach, which, in turn, was superior to single drug treatment (just superior to placebo). Among drug treatments, SSRIs are considered first line.[43] A Cochrane review on the use of psychotherapy for bulimia nervosa and binging found that there is a small body of evidence for the efficacy of CBT in bulimia nervosa and similar syndromes, but the quality of trials was variable and the sample sizes were often small.[42]

4. Clinical course

In a general population sample of 97 healthy primigravid women who were followed for several months after delivery, eating disorder symptoms increased markedly in the first 3 months after delivery and then plateaued over the next 6 months.[41]

REFERENCES

1. Gaynes BN, Gavin N, Meltzer-Brody S et al: Perinatal depression: prevalence, screening accuracy and screening outcomes. Evidence Report/Technology Assessment No. 119. AHRQ Publication No. 05-E006-2, Rockville, MD, February 2005, Agency for Healthcare Research and Quality.
2. Grace SL, Evindar A, Stewart DE: The effect of postpartum depression on child cognitive development and behavior: a review and critical analysis of the literature, *Arch Womens Ment Health* 6:263-274, 2003.
3. Steiner M: Perinatal mood disorders: position paper, *Psychopharmacol Bull* 34:301-306, 1998.
4. Stowe Z, Nemeroff CB: Women at risk for postpartum-onset major depression, *Am J Obstet Gynecol* 173:639-645, 1995.
5. Priest SR, Austin M, Sullivan E: Antenatal psychosocial screening for prevention of antenatal and postnatal anxiety and depression, *Cochrane Database Syst Rev* (1):CD005124, 2005.
6. American Psychiatric Association: *Diagnostic and statistical manual of mental disorders,* ed 4, Washington, DC, 2000, American Psychiatric Association.
7. Wilson LM, Reid AJ, Midmer DK et al: Antenatal psychosocial risk factors associated with adverse postpartum family outcomes, *CMAJ* 154(6):785-799, 1996.
8. Whiffen VE, Gotlib IH: Comparison of postpartum and non-postpartum depression: clinical presentation, psychiatric history and psychosocial functioning, *J Consult Clin Psychol* 61(3):485-494, 1993.
9. Stagnaro-Green A: Postpartum thyroiditis, *Best Pract Res Clin Endocrinol Metab* 18(2):303-316, 2004.
10. Cox JL, Holden JM, Sagovsky R: Detection of postnatal depression: development of the 10-item Edinburgh Postnatal Depression Scale, *Br J Psychiatry* 150:782-786, 1987.
11. Kroenke K, Spitzer RL, Williams JB: The PHQ-9: validity of a brief depression severity measure, *J Gen Intern Med* 16: 606-613, 2001.
12. Appleby L, Warner R, Whitton A et al: A controlled study of fluoxetine and cognitive-behavioural counselling in the treatment of postnatal depression, *BMJ* 314:932-936, 1997.
13. Misri S, Reebye P, Corral M et al: The use of paroxetine and cognitive-behavioral therapy in postpartum depression and anxiety: a randomized controlled trial, *J Clin Psychiatry* 65(9):1236-1241, 2004.
14. O-Hara MW, Stuart S, Gorman L et al: Efficacy of interpersonal psychotherapy for postpartum depression, *Arch Gen Psychiatry* 57:1039-1045, 2000.
15. Cooper PJ, Murray L, Wilson A et al: Controlled trial of the short and long-tern effect of psychological treatment of postpartum depression, *Br J Psychiatry* 182:412-419, 2003.
16. Wickberg B, Hwang CP: Counselling of postnatal depression: a controlled study on a population based Swedish sample, *J Affect Disord* 39:209-216, 1996.
17. Holden JM, Sagovsky R, Cox JL: Counselling in a general practice setting: controlled study of health visitor intervention in treatment of postnatal depression, *BMJ* 289:223-226, 1989.
18. Whitby DH, Smith KM: The use of tricyclic antidepressants and selective serotonin reuptake inhibitors in women who are breastfeeding, *Pharmacotherapy* 25(3):411-425, 2005.
19. Gentile, S: The safety of newer antidepressants in pregnancy and breastfeeding, *Drug Safety* 28(2):137-152, 2005.
20. Hallberg P, Sjöblom V: The use of selective serotonin reuptake inhibitors during pregnancy and breast-feeding: a review and clinical aspects, *J Clin Psychopharmacol* 25(1):59-73, 2005.

21. Weissman AM, Levy BT, Hartz AJ et al: Pooled analysis of antidepressant levels in lactating mothers, breast milk and nursing infants, *Am J Psychiatry* 161:1066-1078, 2004.
22. Lawrie TA, Herxheimer A, Dalton K: Oestrogens and progestogens for preventing and treating postnatal depression, *Cochrane Database Syst Rev* (2):CD001690, 2000.
23. Dennis CL: Psychosocial and psychological interventions for prevention of postnatal depression: systematic review, *BMJ* 331:15-22, 2005.
24. Armstrong KL, Fraser JA, Dadds MR et al: A randomized, controlled trial of nurse home visiting to vulnerable families with newborns, *J Paediatr Child Health* 35:237-244, 1999.
25. MacArthur C, Winter HR, Bick DE et al: Effects of redesigned community postnatal care on women's health 4 months after birth: a cluster randomized controlled trial, *Lancet* 359:378-385, 2002.
26. Wisner KL, Perel JM, Peindl KS et al: Prevention of postpartum depression: a pilot randomized clinical trial, *Am J Psychiatry* 161:1290-1292, 2004.
27. Pedersen CA: Postpartum mood and anxiety disorders: a guide for the nonpsychiatric clinician with an aside on thyroid associations with postpartum mood, *Thyroid* 9(7):691-697, 1999.
28. Brandes M, Soares CN, Cohen LS: Postpartum onset obsessive-compulsive disorder: diagnosis and management, *Arch Womens Ment Health* 7(2):99-110, 2004.
29. Sharma V: Pharmacotherapy of postpartum psychosis, *Exp Opin Pharmacother* 4(10):1651-1658, 2003.
30. Creedy DK, Schochet IM, Horsfall J: Childbirth and the development of acute trauma symptoms: incidence and contributing factors, *Birth* 27(2):104-111, 2000.
31. Ayers S, Pickering AD: Do women get posttraumatic stress disorder as a result of childbirth? A prospective study of incidence, *Birth* 28(2):111-118, 2001.
32. Stein DJ, Seedat S, Van der Linden GJ et al: Selective serotonin reuptake inhibitors in the treatment of post-traumatic stress disorder: a meta-analysis of randomized controlled trials, *Int Clin Psychopharmacol* 15(suppl 2):S31-S39, 2000.
33. Bisson J, Andrew M: Psychological treatment of post-traumatic stress disorder (PTSD), *Cochrane Database Syst Rev* (3):CD003388, 2005.
34. Rose S, Bisson J, Churchill R et al: Psychological debriefing for preventing post traumatic stress disorder (PTSD), *Cochrane Database Syst Rev* (3):CD000560, 2005.
35. Ham P, Waters DB, Oliver N: Treatment of panic disorder, *Am Fam Physician* 71:733-739, 2005.
36. Beck CT: Postpartum onset of panic disorder, *Image J Nurs Sch* 31(2):131-135, 1998.
37. Brockington I: Postpartum psychiatric disorders, *Lancet* 363:303-310, 2004.
38. Hertzberg T, Wahlbeck K: The impact of pregnancy and puerperium on panic disorder: a review, *J Psychosom Obstet Gynecol* 20:59-64, 1999.
39. Maina G, Albert U, Gobetto F et al: Recent life events and obsessive-compulsive disorder (OCD): the role of pregnancy/delivery, *Psychiatry* 89:49-58, 1999.
40. Abramowitz JS: Effectiveness of psychological and pharmacological treatments for obsessive-compulsive disorder: a quantitative review, *J Consult Clin Psychol* 65(1):44-52, 1997.
41. Stein A, Fairburn CG: Eating habits and attitudes in the postpartum period, *Psychosom Med* 58:321-325, 1996.
42. Hay PJ, Bacaltchuk J, Stefano S: Psychotherapy for bulimia nervosa and binging, *Cochrane Database Syst Rev* (3):CD000562, 2004.
43. Bellini M, Merli M: Current drug treatment of patients with bulimia nervosa and binge-eating disorder: selective serotonin reuptake inhibitors versus mood stabilizers, *Int J Psychiatry Clin Pract* 8(4):235-243, 2004.

SECTION B   Paternal Adjustment

I. EPIDEMIOLOGY/RISK FACTORS

Fathers may also experience emotional disturbances after the birth of an infant, though at a lower frequency than mothers. Studies on fathers' postdelivery adjustment have found that 10% or more of fathers experience psychological distress in the postpartum period.[1] Risk factors that contribute to psychological problems in fathers include having a depressed partner, having an unsupportive relationship, and being unemployed.[1]

II. CLINICAL FEATURES

Specific psychiatric conditions seen in new fathers include depression, anxiety disorders, neurotic disorders, sexual problems, and problem drinking.[1] In addition, fathers may experience declines in their general health, vitality, and quality of life after the birth of a first child.[2]

III. DIAGNOSIS

Fathers with depressed partners should be screened for depression because there is a 50% prevalence rate of psychiatric morbidity among fathers who have partners with psychiatric problems.[1] Like mothers, fathers may also be screened for depression with the EPDS, but a lower cutoff (e.g., positive screen: >5) is recommended to maintain the validity of this screen in fathers.[3]

IV. TREATMENT

Fathers with moderate-to-severe depression usually benefit from measures similar to those used in treating maternal depression, including antidepressant therapy, psychotherapy, social support, and exercise.

It is also important to encourage fathers' and mothers' mutual support, including emotional and practical support.

V. CLINICAL COURSE

Depression in new fathers generally follows a course similar to that seen in depressed mothers or other individuals.

REFERENCES

1. Ballard C, Davies R: Postnatal depression in fathers, *Int Rev Psychiatry* 8:65-71, 1996.
2. Gjerdingen DK, Center BA: First-time parents' prenatal to postpartum changes in health, and the relation of postpartum health to work and partner characteristics, *J Am Board Fam Pract* 16:304-311, 2003.
3. Matthey M, Barnett B, Kavanagh DJ et al: Validation of the Edinburgh Postnatal Depression Scale for men, and comparison of item endorsement with their partners, *J Affect Disord* 64:175-184, 2001.

S E C T I O N C Marital Adjustment

Not only is the arrival of a child often difficult for mothers and fathers as individuals, but it also tends to be stressful on the marriage, as documented by research showing general marital decline across the transition to parenthood.[1] This dynamic is also reflected in population-based studies, where individuals with young children (ages 0-13) in the household have been shown to have significantly less marital satisfaction than individuals with no children.[2] These postpartum marital declines are associated with, and likely exacerbated by, other marital changes, including changes in marital structure, sexual relationship, and work roles.

I. CHANGES IN WORK ROLES AND MARITAL STRUCTURE

The birth of a first child dramatically expands parents' work responsibilities, as noted in one study that reported that total work time increased 64% for mothers and 37% for fathers after delivery.[3] However, the nature of these work changes differs between fathers and mothers. Although both mothers and fathers experience increases in time devoted to childcare and total work, this change is greater for

mothers. To compensate, mothers decrease their participation in the workforce after the birth of a first child (by about 11 hours/week), whereas fathers' paid work time remains about the same.[3] Thus, when spouses or partners become parents, they tend to move to a more traditional division of labor, where mothers invest more of their work energies at home and fathers more in the paid workforce.[1]

These postpartum role changes may produce marital tension because wives' marital satisfaction is often related to their husbands' participation in household chores.[4] Some experts believe that imbalances in the division of labor are the greatest source of conflict in a marriage. Couples who have recently become parents are particularly susceptible to this source of conflict because work roles shift so dramatically at this time.

II. CHANGES IN SEXUAL RELATIONSHIP

The sexual relationship of a couple also changes after the birth of a child. In a systematic review of 59 studies on parental sexuality during pregnancy and the postpartum period, it was noted that most couples do not practice intercourse for about 2 months after delivery. Thereafter, sexual interest and activity tend to be reduced for several months, and sexual problems occur fairly often.[5] In one prospective study of more than 1000 postpartum women, less than 10% of women who reported sexual problems felt that they had received adequate help.[6] In the Wisconsin Maternity Leave and Health Study, 570 mothers and their husbands or partners completed a sex questionnaire four times, from the 5th month of pregnancy through 1 year after delivery. Results showed that sexual patterns were similar at the 4th month of pregnancy, 4 months after delivery, and 12 months after delivery, but that sexual expression (both intercourse and masturbation) was considerably reduced at 1 month after delivery. On average, couples resumed intercourse at 7.3 weeks after delivery.[7] Other studies have found that approximately 90% of couples have resumed sexual activity by 6 months after childbirth.[8] Importantly, for many women, return of sexual desire after delivery lags behind resumption of sexual activity.[6,7]

Several factors may negatively impact postpartum sexual relationships, including breastfeeding,[6,7] assisted vaginal delivery,[9] vaginal or perineal lacerations,[9,10] mediolateral episiotomy,[11] breakdown of the muscle or skin sutures in the early postpartum period,[9] fatigue and work demands, depression,[12] and vaginal atrophy secondary to estrogen withdrawal, which may be exacerbated by breastfeeding.[13] For women with spontaneous perineal/vaginal lacerations, the degree of injury is also important. Women with second-degree perineal trauma have been found to be 80% more likely and those with third- or fourth-degree perineal trauma 270% more likely to report dyspareunia at 3 months after delivery, compared with women without trauma.[10] However, postpartum dyspareunia is not always directly related to birthing trauma. In a prospective study of 62 women who had recently given birth, 45% of women developed entry dyspareunia, but only 6% had pain at the sites of vulvar repair. The median length of symptoms in the 39% with nonfocal introital dyspareunia was 5.5 months, and tenderness lasted up to 1 year. Such dyspareunia developed in women having a first (42%) or second (47%) infant, delivering vaginally (42%) or by cesarean section (29%), and lactating (41%) or not lactating (22%).[14]

Unlike mothers, fathers do not usually lose interest in sexual activity after delivery, but their sexual activity declines in response to their partners' disinterest.[15] This male/female discordance in sexual desire may contribute to marital distress and, for some men, extramarital sex.[16]

III. TREATMENT

It is important that the practitioner specifically inquire about sexual function and concerns in the postpartum period. In addition, providers should advise partners to:

1. Regularly affirm their care and support of one another.
2. Plan ways in which they will show tangible support to each other after delivery, particularly through the sharing of childcare and household responsibilities.
3. Be aware of anticipated postpartum changes in their sexual relationship. Anticipatory guidance may prevent the development of long-term problems.
4. Understand the hormonal effects of breastfeeding on sexual function, so they do not wrongly attribute such effects to a problem in their relationship or terminate breastfeeding prematurely.
5. Limit episiotomies.[17]
6. Consider the use of vaginal lubricants or short-term use (e.g., up to a few months) of estrogen cream or suppositories for postpartum dyspareunia caused by vaginal atrophy and dryness.

IV. CLINICAL COURSE

For parents with young children, the decline in marital satisfaction continues until children reach school age and then begins to improve as children grow into adolescence and early adulthood.[18]

REFERENCES

1. MacDermid SM, Huston TL, McHale SM: Changes in marriage associated with the transition to parenthood: individual differences as a function of sex-role attitudes and changes in the division of household labor, *J Marriage Fam* 52:475-486, 1990.
2. Orbuch TL, House JS, Mero RP et al: Marital quality over the life course, *Social Psychol Q* 59:162-171, 1996.
3. Gjerdingen DK, Center BA: First-time parents' postpartum changes in employment, childcare, and housework responsibilities, *Social Sci Res* 34:103-116, 2005.
4. Watson WJ, Watson L, Wetzel W et al: Transition to parenthood: what about fathers? *Can Fam Physician* 41:807-812, 1995.
5. Von Sydow K: Sexuality during pregnancy and after childbirth: a metacontent analysis of 59 studies, *J Psychosom Res* 47(1):27-49, 1999.
6. Glazener CMA: Sexual function after childbirth: women's experiences, persistent morbidity and lack of professional recognition, *Br J Obstet Gynaecol* 104:330-335, 1997.
7. Hyde JS, DeLamater J: Sexuality during pregnancy and the year postpartum. In Travis CB, White JW, editors: *Sexuality, society, and feminism. Psychology of women* 2000.
8. Connolly A, Thorp J, Pahel L: Effects of pregnancy and childbirth on postpartum sexual function: a longitudinal prospective study, *Int Urogynecol J Pelvic Floor Dysfunct* 192:1293-1296, 2005.
9. Abraham S, Child A, Ferry J et al: Recovery after childbirth: a preliminary prospective study, *Med J Australia* 152(1):9-12, 1990.
10. Signorello LB, Harlow BL, Chekos AK et al: Postpartum sexual functioning and its relationship to perineal trauma: a retrospective cohort study of primiparous women, *Am J Obstet Gynecol* 184(5):881-890, 2001.
11. Sartore A, De Seta F, Maso G et al: The effects of mediolateral episiotomy on pelvic floor function after vaginal delivery, *Obstet Gynecol* 103(4):669-673, 2004.
12. Morof D, Barrett G, Peacock J et al: Postnatal depression and sexual health after childbirth, *Obstet Gynecol* 102(6): 1318-1325, 2003.
13. Walbroehl GS: Sexuality during pregnancy, *Am Fam Physician* 29:273-275, 1984.
14. Goetsch MF: Postpartum dyspareunia. An unexplored problem, *J Reprod Med* 44(11):963-968, 1999.
15. Gielen AC, O'Campo PJ, Faden RR: Interpersonal conflict and physical violence during the childbearing year, *Soc Sci Med* 39:781-787, 1994.
16. Ali MM, Cleland JG: The link between postnatal abstinence and extramarital sex in Cot d'Ivoire, *Stud Fam Plann* 32(3):214-219, 2001.

17. Flynn P, Faniek J, Janssen P et al: How can second-stage management prevent perineal trauma? Critical review, *Can Fam Physician* 43:73-84, 1997.
18. Bigner JJ: *Parent-child relations: an introduction to parenting*, Columbus, OH, 1998, Merrill (Prentice Hall).

SECTION D   Sibling Adjustment

Sibling reactions to the birth of an infant vary by the sex of the infant and sibling, the length of time since the birth, and the age of the sibling. Same-sex sibling dyads have been reported to show more problematic behaviors. Problems tend to diminish as time progresses; siblings older than 6 years of age show fewer negative behaviors than do younger siblings.[1]

I. BIRTH IMPACT ON MOTHER'S RELATIONSHIP TO THE OLDER SIBLING

Direct observations of families before and after the birth of a second child reveal changes in mothers' interactions with the older siblings after the arrival of the infant. After childbirth, mothers tend to decrease the attention they give to older siblings and to increase their negative interactions with this child.[2] These changes may explain, at least partially, the negative behaviors of older children after the arrival of a new infant.

II. REACTIONS OF A SIBLING TO THE BIRTH

Children may react to the birth of a sibling in various ways, for example:
1. Attention-seeking behavior
2. Imitating behaviors
3. Direct aggression or confrontation (with the mother or infant)
4. Regression
5. Anxiety behaviors
6. Maturity and independence[1,3]

III. TREATMENT

Both parents should regularly give focused, positive attention to older children. Parents can be encouraged to find ways to include older children in providing care to the infant.

REFERENCES

1. Stewart RB, Mobley LA, Van Tuyl SS et al: The firstborn's adjustment to the birth of a sibling: a longitudinal assessment, *Child Dev* 58:341-355, 1987.
2. Dunn J, Kendrick C: The arrival of a sibling: changes in patterns of interaction between mother and first-born child, *J Child Psychol Psychiatry* 21:119-132, 1980.
3. Griffin EW, de la Torre C: Sibling jealousy: the family with a new baby, *Am Fam Physician* 28:143-146, 1983.

SECTION E   Specific Family Situations

I. SINGLE-PARENT FAMILIES

A. Epidemiology

Single-parent families are growing in number and are predominantly led by women. In the United States, almost 13 million families, or approximately 18% of all American families, are headed by women.[1] Almost half of these families live below the poverty line.[1] In Canada in 1991, about 1 million families, or approximately 13% of all Canadian families, were single-parent families, 80% of which were headed by women.[2] In recent reports on fertility trends, today's single mothers are not necessarily teenage girls, but rather women in their twenties and thirties who are bearing children on their own.[2]

B. Risks to the Single Parent and Child

The stresses felt by single-parent families are likely even greater than those felt by dual-parent families because the burdens of financial support, child care, household chores, and other work responsibilities generally rest on a single individual. The literature on single-parent families focuses primarily on single mothers and less so on single fathers; thus, this section draws from the literature on single mothers.

Female-headed families are particularly vulnerable to increased poverty, intergenerational family violence, high levels of everyday stressors, low self-esteem, lower educational levels, and high levels of depressive symptoms,[1,3,4] which place them at greater risk for poor physical and mental health and other adverse outcomes.[4]

Various single-parent subgroups may have especially high risks for adverse outcomes. A study of single mothers who were enrolled in an undergraduate university program reported that the mothers' major health concerns were chronic tiredness and overwhelming worries.[5] A study of low-income single mothers reported that more than 75% manifested some depressive symptoms.[6] Single mothers with a history of abuse or neglect have an increased risk for poor mental health.[7] Although the literature focusing on postpartum single mothers is scarce, it is anticipated that the many stressors faced by single mothers are only intensified in the postpartum period with the great demands of caring for an infant and adjusting to the many physical and psychosocial changes after childbirth.

Children in single-parent families often have fewer resources and are more likely to have behavioral problems and health vulnerability than children from dual-parent families.[1] Children in single-parent families have a reportedly 80% greater risk for suffering serious injury or harm from abuse or neglect.[8] In single-parents families where the parent experiences limited support and overwhelming responsibilities, abusive forms of punishment appear to be more prevalent and acceptable. Children in low-income families also have greater risks for sexual abuse, educational neglect, and serious injury from maltreatment and abuse than children from higher income families.[8]

C. Treatment

The postpartum period is an opportune time to provide interventions for families at high risk such as single-parent families that may otherwise be marginalized from traditional services. Screening for risk factors for mental disorders in postpartum single mothers may improve maternal and child outcomes. One study done in vulnerable families, about 60% of which were single-parent families, suggested that a home-visiting intervention in the immediate postnatal period aimed at identifying depression levels, stress levels, and coping has the potential to prevent cases of child abuse and neglect.[9] In another study, providing parental training to single mothers of school-aged children was associated with positive outcomes in both the mother (e.g., reduced coercive parenting, improved effective parenting practices) and child (e.g., improved adjustment).[10]

One study in postpartum mothers reported that low-income mothers have high levels of unmet learning and information needs.[3] This study highlights the importance of providing accessible and appropriate community-based information resources for low-income mothers. Because single mothers fall in the lowest income brackets,[1] appropriate referrals to potential resources, such as networks for assistance with childcare, household chores, or other responsibilities, may be of benefit. Further studies on parental training of single mothers in the postpartum period are warranted, and it is anticipated that some form of support or educational intervention, or both, would be of benefit to single mothers and their children in the postpartum period.

In conclusion, the postpartum period is a time of physical and psychosocial changes for single parents, many of whom have few social and financial resources. Limited evidence exists to support the use of educational and supportive interventions, and screening for mental disorders (e.g., depression and anxiety) in postpartum single mothers.

II. ADOLESCENT MOTHERS

A. Epidemiology

Since the 1990s, there has been an overall decline in teenage pregnancy rates in both the United States and Canada, which has led to associated declines in teenage birth rates.[11,12] Although teenage pregnancy rates tend to be greater in certain minority groups (e.g., black and Hispanic populations), declines in adolescent pregnancies have been seen in white, black, and Hispanic adolescent groups. In the United States in 2000, the teen pregnancy rate was 71 per 1000 for white adolescents (aged 15-19 years), 153 per 1000 for black adolescents, and 138 per 1000 for Hispanic adolescents.[11] These trends may be related to the increasingly wide availability of contraceptives and awareness of the risks of unprotected sex. In the United States in 2000, there were 468,990 births to teenagers 15 to 19 years of age, giving an all-time low birth rate of 48 births per 1000 teenagers.[11] In Canada in 1997, there were 19,724 births to teenagers 15 to 19 years of age, giving an all-time low teen birth rate of 20 births per 1000 teenagers.[12]

B. Risks to the Mother and Child

During the postpartum period, adolescent mothers face unique personal challenges, social challenges, and risks, such as social isolation, lack of maternal competence, poor mental health, subsequent pregnancies, multiple stressors, and depression.[13] With minimal life experience and preparation, they face the adult challenges of providing financial support, protection, love, nutrition, and other needs for a completely dependent child. The added stress of parenting a newborn may have adverse psychological consequences for both the mother and the infant. Children raised by adolescent mothers have an increased risk for abuse and a variety of developmental problems, such as poor intellectual and socioemotional functioning, poorer cognitive abilities, and difficulties in personal and social relationships.[14]

C. Treatment

Several studies have examined the effects of educational and support programs to improve maternal and child outcomes in adolescent-parent families. One study in mothers 17 years or younger showed that an educational intervention on family planning and health compared with standard well-baby care was effective for reducing the number of unplanned repeat pregnancies and increased the proportion of fully immunized children.[15] Another study in teenage mothers showed that postnatal educational home visits by nurse midwives compared with no home visits (only routine postnatal care) increased mothers' knowledge of contraception and effective use of contraception.[16] A study evaluating the effects of an intergenerational program for first-time adolescent parents reported that teenage mothers whose own mothers participated in a Teenage-Mothers-Grandmothers program were less likely to drop out of school and had significantly better self-esteem.[17] This study implies that the inclusion of mothers of parenting adolescents in postpartum support programs may be beneficial.

Adolescent mothers are more likely to live in conditions of socioeconomic deprivation, and lack of education in many teenage mothers has implications on the long-term ability to improve their socioeconomic status.[18] Therefore, interventions to reduce the incidence of unplanned and unwanted adolescent pregnancies may be beneficial for improving the long-term socioeconomic conditions for teenage mothers and their children.

Management of adolescent mothers may also include early screening for child abuse risk. Research in adolescent parents suggests that early prediction of child abuse potential is possible using several risk factors (e.g., maternal knowledge and expectancies about child development). Early prediction is important because children between 3 months and 3 years of age have a greater risk for abuse.[19]

In conclusion, some evidence supports the use of educational interventions on family planning and health for teenage mothers. The inclusion of mothers of parenting adolescents in postpartum support programs may have positive effects. In the postpartum period, screening for child abuse potential may be important, especially in adolescent mothers with multiple stressors who lack strong support networks.

III. INTIMATE PARTNER VIOLENCE

It is estimated that 1.5% to 17% of all pregnant women experience some type of abuse. Of those women who experienced abuse during pregnancy, 95% reported that the violence increased in the postpartum period. Other factors besides prenatal abuse that are associated with postpartum abuse include delayed (e.g., third trimester) initiation of prenatal care and alcohol or drug abuse by the mother or her partner.[20] Violence is also more likely with unplanned or adolescent pregnancies, but all women regardless of socioeconomic status, ethnicity, or marital status are at risk for violence.[21] Nearly half of men who assault their partners will also abuse their children, and children who witness violence have increased rates of anxiety and aggressive behavior.[22]

Some debate exists about the effectiveness of routine screening for violence in pregnancy and the postpartum period. However, a recent evidence-based consensus statement on intimate partner violence suggests that there is little evidence of harm and some evidence that asking about abuse increases the rate of safety behaviors and decreases actual episodes of assault.[21] Most women will not disclose spontaneously but will do so when asked directly. Qualitative studies suggest that the relationship with the care provider is as important as the questions that are asked. Simple short questions that are specific are more useful than general questions about abuse.[21] The American College of Obstetricians and Gynecologists recommends that physicians screen all women, including those in the postpartum period, for domestic violence.[23]

REFERENCES

1. Federal Interagency Forum on Child and Family Statistics: *America's children: key national indicators of well-being,* Washington, DC, 2000, U.S. Government Printing Office.
2. Statistics Canada: *2001 Census consultation guide: fertility recent trends,* http://www.statcan.ca/english/freepub/92-125-GIE/html/fer.htm. Accessed July 2005.
3. Sword W, Watt S: Learning needs of postpartum women: does socioeconomic status matter? *Birth* 32(2):86-92, 2005.

4. Lutenbacher M, Hall LA: The effects of maternal psychosocial factors on parenting attitudes of low-income, single mothers with young children, *Nurs Res* 47(1):25-34, 1998.

5. Ogunsiji O, Wilkes L: Managing family life while studying: single mothers' lived experience of being students in a nursing program, *Contemp Nurse* 18:108-123, 2005.

6. Peden AR, Rayens MK, Hall LA et al: Negative thinking and the mental health of low-income single mothers, *J Nurs Scholar* 36:337-344, 2004.

7. Hall LA, Gurley DN, Sachs B et al: Psychosocial predictors of maternal depressive symptoms, parenting attitudes, and child behavior in single-parent families, *Nurse Res* 40:214-220, 1991.

8. Sedlak AJ, Broadhurst DD: *The Third National Incidence Study of Child Abuse and Neglect (NIS-3)*, Washington, DC, 1996, National Clearinghouse on Child Abuse and Neglect Information.

9. Fraser JA, Armstrong KL, Morris JP et al: Home visiting intervention for vulnerable families with newborns: follow-up results of a randomized controlled trial, *Child Abuse Negl* 11:1399-1429, 2000.

10. Forgatch MS, DeGarmo DS: Parenting through change: an effective prevention program for single mothers, *J Consult Clin Psychol* 67:711-724, 1999.

11. Allan Guttmacher Institute: *U.S. teenage pregnancy statistics. overall trends, trends by race and ethnicity and state-by-state information*, New York, 2004.

12. Dryburg H: *Teenage pregnancy. Health reports*, vol 12, no. 1, Statistics Canada: catalogue 82-003. Available at: http://www.statcan.ca/english/kits/preg/preg3.htm. Accessed July 2005.

13. Birkeland R, Thompson JK, Phares V: Adolescent motherhood and postpartum depression, *J Clin Child Adolesc Psychol* 34:292-300, 2005.

14. Dukewich TL, Borkowski JG, Whitman TL: A longitudinal analysis of maternal abuse potential and developmental delays in children of adolescent mothers, *Child Abuse Negl* 23: 405-420, 1999.

15. O' Sullivan AL, Jacobsen BS: A randomized trial of a health care program for first-time adolescent mothers and their infants, *Nurs Res* 41:210-215, 1992.

16. Quinlivan JA, Box H, Evans SF: Postnatal home visits in teenage mothers: a randomized controlled trial, *Lancet* 361: 893-900, 2003.

17. Roye CF, Balk SJ: Evaluation of an intergenerational program for pregnant and parenting adolescents, *Matern Child Nurs J* 24(1):32-40, 1996.

18. Botting B, Rosato M, Wood R: Teenage mothers and the health of their children, *Popul Trends* 93:19-28, 1998.

19. Azar ST, Wolfe DA: Child abuse and neglect. In Mash EJ, Barkley RA, editors: *Treatment of childhood disorders*, New York, 1989, Guilford Press.

20. Wilson LM, Reid AJ, Midmer DK et al: Antenatal psychosocial risk factors associated with adverse postpartum family outcomes, *CMAJ* 154(6):785-799, 1996.

21. Cherniak D, Grant L, Mason R et al: Intimate partner violence consensus statement, *J Obstet Gynaecol Can* 27(4):365-388, 2005.

22. Kernic MA, Wolf ME, Holt VL et al: Behavioral problems among children whose mothers are abused by an intimate partner, *Child Abuse Negl* 27(11):1231-1246, 2003.

23. ACOG: *Screening tools: domestic violence*, Washington, DC, 2004.

Section F Return to Work

With the dramatic increase in female labor force participation since the 1960s, employment has become the norm for new mothers in many Western countries. In the United States, 54% of mothers with infants were employed in 2003.[1]

I. MATERNITY/PARENTAL LEAVE

Data from three separate postpartum studies have shown that longer maternity leaves (e.g., more than 6 weeks,[2] 15 weeks,[3] or 24 weeks[4]) are associated with better maternal mental health. Even before this research, though, the need for a period of leave from work after childbirth had been widely recognized. In 1919, the International Labor Organization (ILO) stipulated that all women working in industry and commerce should be entitled to a maternity leave of 12 weeks (in two equal parts preceding and following childbirth) plus a cash benefit that would equal at least two thirds of their earnings. The second convention, adopted in 1952, extended the 12-week leave to 14 weeks at full wages. By the late 1980s, the ILO reported that more than 100 countries provided paid maternity leave, and the average length of maternity leave worldwide was 12 to 14 weeks. In 1992, the European Union (EU) issued a directive mandating a paid 14-week maternity leave as a health and safety measure, and in 1998, this directive was expanded to a 3-month paid *parental* leave. As a result, 129 of 158 countries reporting to the International Social Security Association in 1997 provided at least some paid maternity leave. In most of these countries, the benefit was 80% to 100% of wages, and in 57 of these countries, the cash benefit replaced the full wage. The average "basic" leave was 16 weeks, which typically included 6 to 8 weeks before birth and the rest after childbirth. Ten EU countries typically provide for a leave until the child is 2 or 3 years old. Seven countries provide a paid paternity leave, usually only a few days in duration (longer in Scandinavian countries). In addition, several countries offer supplementary unpaid parental leaves.[5] Canada allows for 15 weeks of maternity leave, or 35 weeks of parental leave to care for a newborn or adopted child. This parental benefit can be claimed by one parent or shared between two partners.[6]

In contrast with the relatively liberal parental benefits provided by most European countries, unpaid maternity-parental-family leaves are offered in

Australia, New Zealand, and the United States. U.S. parental leave, governed by the Family and Medical Leave Act (FMLA), is not only unpaid but is also brief and not applicable to a large sector of the workforce. Specifically, the FMLA provides for 12 weeks of job-protected, unpaid parental leave for mothers and fathers, meaning that the employee has a right to return to the same job or a job comparable in pay and responsibility. During the time of leave, the employer must also continue employer-provided group health insurance. Small businesses (those with <50 employees) are excluded, leaving 42% of employees uncovered by this act.[7] Employees who are covered often use accumulated paid vacation and personal leave time first, before enacting the FMLA unpaid leave.

Given the relatively brief unpaid maternity leave available to women in the United States, economic issues appear to be the strongest influence in determining when a woman returns to work. Among employed first-time mothers giving birth between 1991 and 1994, 42% returned to work by 3 months after birth, and 76% returned to work within the first year after childbirth.[8] Data from three U.S. studies showed that employed mothers take an average of 10 to 11 weeks of maternity leave after delivering a child.[2,3,9] In contrast, fathers tend to take only a few days leave, usually from sick, vacation, or discretionary days, rather than "parental leave" per se.[2] In the Wisconsin Maternity Leave and Health Study, the majority of women (66%) believed that their 11-week leaves were too short, but they did not take longer leaves because they could not afford to do so.[2]

Providers should encourage mothers to take the amount of leave necessary to promote optimal physical and mental health. For many women, this constitutes a leave period of 3 to 6 months or longer. Fathers may also be encouraged to take a period of leave from work after childbirth, although there are currently little if any data on health benefits related to paternal leave or recommend duration of leave. Businesses and policymakers should also consider ways to make parental benefits available to all employed members and to provide wage replacement during the time of leave.

II. BREASTFEEDING AFTER RETURN TO WORK

Because breastfeeding promotes infants' health, it is important to encourage continued breastfeeding after mothers return to work. However, maternal employment outside the home is recognized as a significant risk factor for early weaning, likely a result of many mothers not realizing that they can continue to breastfeed after they return to work or school[10] and businesses not actively addressing the needs of breastfeeding mothers. Surveys have found that only 22% of U.S. businesses report providing workplace provisions for lactation, whereas only 13% of employees report having lactation provisions.[11] Businesses and communities can promote continued breastfeeding after return to work through policy and mother-friendly work sites. For example, the state of Texas gives a mother the right to nurse her baby in any location that she is authorized to be. It also describes a mother-friendly work site as one that allows flexible work schedules that provide time for milk expression; access to a private location and to a clean, safe water supply; and access to hygienic storage areas (e.g., refrigerator), for storage of breast milk.[10]

Support for breastfeeding in the workplace is not only humane, but it may also reap economic benefits, as seen with the Los Angeles Department of Water and Power breastfeeding support program. This program saved nearly $5 for every $1 spent on breastfeeding support because of decreased employee absenteeism and health-care costs.[10] Continued breastfeeding may also be promoted by the mother's initial return to a part-time work schedule, if this is a feasible option for the mother and her company.

A mother who wishes to continue breastfeeding after returning to work should consider the following issues:

1. Develop breastfeeding plans.
   Mothers should discuss breastfeeding plans with their manager, including access to private location for pumping, access to a water supply (for cleaning the pump) and refrigerator (for storing breast milk), and time allowance for pumping. Potential sources of time include break or lunch times, flexible hours, and part-time work.
2. Find a daycare provider.
   Consider finding a daycare provider near work or one who will cooperate with breastfeeding plans.
3. Make sure that breastfeeding is well established before returning to work.
4. Practice expressing milk before returning to work.
5. Consult with a lactation consultant, if needed.
6. Breastfeed more frequently when at home to maintain milk supply.

III. INFANT DEVELOPMENT

Optimal leave for infant development has been controversial and conflicting in the psychological literature. Given the interrelationship between family members' health, parents' return to work after childbirth should be planned in a manner that optimizes both the parents' and infant's health. Parents whose return to work requires alternative childcare arrangements should be encouraged to work on these arrangements weeks to months before they will be enacted. These arrangements should ensure the safety and nurturing of the child, and parents should be comfortable with the arrangements they choose.

IV. SUMMARY

Given the physical, emotional, and social stresses that often accompany childbirth, both mothers and fathers are at risk for psychosocial problems after the birth of a child. Fortunately, excellent treatment (e.g., psychotropic medication and psychotherapy) exists for these disorders. Parents can reduce the stress of this period by soliciting support (this is especially true for high-risk groups, such as single and adolescent parents) and, for employed parents, carefully planning their return to work.

V. SOR A RECOMMENDATIONS

DIAGNOSIS	REFERENCES
Postpartum Depression Screening: *Postpartum women can be effectively screened for depression using any one of the following scales: BDI, the PDSS, the EPDS, and the CES-D.*	12
Treatment	
Postpartum Depression: *Pharmacotherapy and psychotherapy are equally effective treatments; there appears to be no benefit to combining the two treatment methods*	13, 14
PTSD: *Effective therapies in general populations include:*	
Pharmacotherapies (specifically SSRIs)	15
Individual and group trauma-focused CBT	16
Stress management	16

Panic Disorder:	17
Antidepressants improve panic symptoms and global functioning in general populations; SSRIs and TCAs are equally efficacious. *Benzodiazepines also help reduce panic severity but are most useful in improving depression and functioning when used in combination with other therapies.* *CBT has been found to be effective in reducing panic frequency and severity in select groups.*	
OCD: *SSRIs are effective treatment in general populations.*	18
Eating Disorders: *Effective treatments in general populations include:* *Combination of pharmacologic and psychological treatments is the most optimal treatment (SSRIs are first choice for drug treatment).* *Psychotherapy alone is superior to drug treatment alone, which is superior to placebo.*	19

REFERENCES

1. U.S. Bureau of Labor Force Statistics: *Labor force participation of mothers with infants in 2003. MLR: the editor's desk,* Washington, DC, 2004, U.S. Bureau of Labor Force Statistics.
2. Hyde JS, Essex MJ, Clark R et al: Parental leave: policy and research, *J Soc Issues* 52(3):91-109, 1996.
3. McGovern P, Dowd B, Gjerdignen D et al: Time off work and the postpartum health of employed women, *Med Care* 35(5):507-521, 1997.
4. Gjerdingen DK, Chaloner KM: The relationship of women's postpartum mental health to employment, childbirth, and social support, *J Fam Pract* 38(5):465-472, 1994.
5. Kamerman SB: From maternity to parental leave policies: women's health, employment, and child and family well-being, *J Am Med Womens Assoc* 55(2):96-99, 2000.
6. Government of Canada: *Human resources and skills development canada.* Available at: http://www.hrsdc.gc.ca/en/home. shtml. Accessed July 2005.
7. Cantor D, Waldfogel J, Kerwin J et al: *Balancing the needs of families and employers: family and medical leave surveys,* Washington, DC, 2000, U.S. Department of Labor.
8. Smith K, Downs B, O'Connell M: *Maternity leave and employment patterns: 1961-1995,* Washington, DC, November 2001, U.S. Census Bureau.
9. Gjerdingen DK, McGovern PM, Chaloner KM et al: Women's postpartum maternity benefits and work experience, *Fam Med* 27:592-598, 1995.
10. Neilsen J. Return to work: practical management of breastfeeding, *Clin Obstet Gynecol* 47(3):724-733, 2004.
11. Galtry J: The impact on breastfeeding of labour market policy and practice in Ireland, Sweden, and the USA, *Soc Sci Med* 57:167-177, 2003.

12. Gaynes BN, Gavin N, Meltzer-Brody S et al: Perinatal depression: prevalence, screening accuracy and screening outcomes. Evidence report/technology assessment no. 119. AHRQ Publication No. 05-E006-2. Rockville, MD, February 2005, Agency for Healthcare Research and Quality.

13. Appleby L, Warner R, Whitton A et al: A controlled study of fluoxetine and cognitive-behavioural counselling in the treatment of postnatal depression, *BMJ* 314:932-936, 1997.

14. Misri S, Reebye P, Corral M et al: The use of paroxetine and cognitive-behavioral therapy in postpartum depression and anxiety: a randomized controlled trial, *J Clin Psychiatry* 65(9):1236-1241, 2004.

15. Stein DJ, Seedat S, Van der Linden GJ et al: Selective serotonin reuptake inhibitors in the treatment of post-traumatic stress disorder: a meta-analysis of randomized controlled trials, *Int Clin Psychopharmacol* 15(suppl 2):S31-S39, 2000.

16. Bisson J, Andrew M: Psychological treatment of post-traumatic stress disorder (PTSD), *Cochrane Database Syst Rev* (3)CD003388, 2005.

17. Ham P, Waters DB, Oliver N: Treatment of panic disorder, *Am Fam Physician* 71:733-739, 2005.

18. Brandes M, Soares CN, Cohen LS: Postpartum onset obsessive-compulsive disorder: diagnosis and management, *Arch Womens Ment Health* 7(2):99-110, 2004.

19. Bellini M, Merli M: Current drug treatment of patients with bulimia nervosa and binge-eating disorder: selective serotonin reuptake inhibitors versus mood stabilizers, *Int J Psychiatry Clin Pract* 8(4):235-243, 2004.

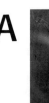

Interpretation of Summary Tables

In this third edition of *Family Medicine Obstetrics* we have incorporated evidence-based medicine recommendations at the end of most sections in this book. We have used the Strength of Recommendation Taxonomy (SORT) system that Ebell and colleagues[1] developed; this system uses a patient-centered approach to grade the medical literature. We have chosen to list only grade A recommendations and to limit these recommendations to those therapeutic or diagnostic interventions that improve the care for our patients.

The following process is used to arrive at a grade A recommendation:

"Is this a key recommendation for clinicians regarding diagnosis or treatment that merits a label?"
    If yes, then

"Is the recommendation based on *patient-oriented evidence* (i.e., an improvement in morbidity, mortality, symptoms, quality of life, or cost)?"
    If yes, then

"Is the recommendation based on expert opinion, bench research, a consensus guideline, usual practice, clinical experience, or a case series study?"
    If no, then

> *"Is the recommendation based on one of the following?"*
>
> • *Cochrane review with a clear recommendation*
>
> • *U.S. Preventive Services Task Force grade A recommendation*
>
> • *Clinical Evidence rating of Beneficial*
>
> • *Consistent findings from at least two good-quality randomized controlled trials or a systematic review/metaanalysis*
>
> • *Validated clinical decision rule in a relevant population*
>
> • *Consistent findings from at least two good-quality diagnostic cohort studies or systematic review/metaanalysis*

If yes, then Strength of Recommendation (SOR) = A

REFERENCE

1. Ebell MH, Siwek J, Weiss BD et al: Strength of Recommendation Taxonomy (SORT): a patient-centered approach to grading evidence in the medical literature, *Am Fam Physician* 69:549-557, 2004.

Adapted from *American Family Physician* "The Strength-of-Recommendation Taxonomy" feature found in the weekly edition of the journal.

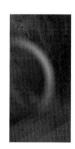

Analysis of Screening Tests

As with any screening test, risk scoring systems should be evaluated by their sensitivity, specificity, positive predictive value (PPV), negative predictive value (NPV), and reliability.

1. **Sensitivity and specificity:** The sensitivity of a test can be seen as the proportion of those individuals with a condition for whom the test is *positive*. Typically, screening tests such as newborn metabolic screens seek high sensitivity, possibly at the expense of specificity. Specificity is the proportion of those *without* the condition, in which the test is *negative*. Tests that determine definitive diagnosis (such as follow-up newborn metabolic testing) seek high specificity, also possibly at the expense of sensitivity.

2. **PPV and NPV:** PPV and NPV represent the likelihood a patient may or may not, respectively, develop a condition with a positive test. Predictive values are typically dependent on the incidence of a condition within a population, with greater incidence resulting in greater predictive values. Unfortunately, the manufacturer's information on sensitivity and specificity of a given test cannot be used to directly calculate the PPV or NPV for a given population. Maternal serum α-fetoprotein testing for fetal neural tube defects, for example, yields greater predictive values in Wales (where the test was developed), where there is a high incidence of fetal neural tube defects, than in the United States, where the incidence is lower. Pregnancy risk assessment can be expected to have greater predictive values, therefore, in a population that has a high incidence of poor pregnancy outcome than in a population that has a low incidence.

3. **Reliability:** Reliability is the consistency of the scoring instrument when applied more than once to the same individual. Reliability directly affects the quality of data used in risk calculation. Important determinants of reliability include not only the design of the instrument but also the clinical situation in which it is applied and the staff who apply it.

4. **Number needed to diagnose (NND):** The NND, a concept reviewed in an article in Bandolier, attempts to help quantify how many patients with a target condition must be tested to find one case. This allows comparison of the test without concerns about prevalence and allows the clinician to consider how prevalence in the test population will influence the results of the test. A perfect test would have a NND of 1.00, and most screening tests used in prenatal care have an NND between 1 and 1.5. The larger the NND, the more patients with the target condition will have to be tested to detect a single case. In the case below, for the DNA probe, the NND is 1.11; for other tests, using the sensitivity and specificity, the NND can be calculated by using the following formula:

$$NND = 1/[\text{Sensitivity} - (1 - \text{Specificity})]$$

ILLUSTRATION: CALCULATION OF SENSITIVITY, SPECIFICITY, POSITIVE PREDICTIVE VALUE, AND NEGATIVE PREDICTIVE VALUE

Following is the overall construction of a 2 × 2 table for a specific laboratory test:

Presence of Condition	Test Results	
	Positive	*Negative*
Present	True positive (TP)	False negative (FN)
Absent	False positive (FP)	True negative (TN)

With numbers placed in the above boxes for the true and false positive and negative, the sensitivity and specificity can be calculated as follows:

$$\text{Sensitivity} = TP/(TP + FN)$$
$$\text{Specificity} = TN/(TN + FP)$$

For example, the patient you are treating, based on her history, is part of a population with approximately 1% prevalence rate of chlamydia. When tested by a DNA probe with 95% sensitivity and 95% specificity, the initial 2×2 table for just the test would look like this:

"Generic"	Test Results	
Presence of Condition	**Positive**	**Negative**
Present	0.95	0.05
Absent	0.05	0.95

However, if the prevalence of the condition is low, the numbers above need to be modified to take this into account. For example, if the actual prevalence rate of chlamydia in this population is 1%, then the "absent" row needs to be 99 times larger to reflect the actual prevalence in the population. Once the prevalence is factored into the table, the NPV and PPV of the test can be calculated as follows:

Prevalence = 1%	Test Results	
Presence of Condition	**Positive**	**Negative**
Present	0.95	0.05
Absent	0.05 * 99 = 4.95	0.95 * 99 = 94.05

$$PPV = TP/(TP + FP), \text{ or}$$
$$PPV = 0.95/(0.95 + 4.95) = 0.161, \text{ or } 16.1\%$$

$$NPV = TN/(TN + FN), \text{ or}$$
$$NPV = 94.05/(94.05 + 0.05) = 0.9995, \text{ or } 99.95\%$$

Note that the interpretation of this is that a positive DNA probe for chlamydia in a patient from a population with a prevalence rate of 1% has a PPV (i.e., predicts the presence of the infection) of 16%. In other words, *five of six positive results on the DNA probe in this population do not accurately predict the presence of the disease.* The clinician, in applying the test result to the patient, would need to know this to select a test with a better PPV, which (in the case of infections) is often a culture.

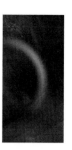

Immunization during Pregnancy

Live Virus Vaccines

Immunobiologic Agent	Risk from Disease to Pregnant Woman	Risk from Disease to Fetus or Neonate	Type of Immunizing Agent	Risk from Immunizing Agent to Fetus	Indications for Immunization during Pregnancy	Dose Schedule	Comments
Measles	Significant morbidity, low mortality; not altered by pregnancy	Significant increase in abortion rate; may cause malformations	Live attenuated virus vaccine	None confirmed	Contraindicated (see immunoglobulins)	Single dose SC, preferably as measles-mumps-rubella*	Vaccination of susceptible women should be part of postpartum care. Breastfeeding is not a contraindication.
Mumps	Low morbidity and mortality; not altered by pregnancy	Possible increased rate of abortion in first trimester	Live attenuated virus vaccine	None confirmed	Contraindicated	Single dose SC, preferably as measles-mumps-rubella	Vaccination of susceptible women should be part of postpartum care.
Poliomyelitis	No increased incidence in pregnancy, but may be more severe if it does occur	Anoxic fetal damage reported; 50% mortality rate in neonatal disease	Live attenuated virus (oral polio vaccine) and enhanced-potency inactivated virus vaccine†	None confirmed	Not routinely recommended for women in the United States, except women at increased risk for exposure	Primary: Two doses of enhanced-potency inactivated virus SC at 4- to 8-week intervals and a third dose 6-12 months after the second dose *Immediate protection:* One-dose oral polio vaccine (in outbreak setting)	Vaccination indicated for susceptible pregnant women traveling in endemic areas or in other high-risk situations.
Rubella	Low morbidity and mortality; not altered by pregnancy	High rate of abortion and congenital rubella syndrome	Live attenuated virus vaccine	None confirmed	Contraindicated, but congenital rubella syndrome has never been described after vaccine	Single dose SC, preferably as measles-mumps-rubella	Teratogenicity of vaccine is theoretic, not confirmed to date; vaccination of susceptible women should be part of postpartum care.

	Risk from disease to pregnant woman	Risk from disease to fetus or neonate	Type of immunizing agent	Risk from immunizing agent to fetus	Indications for immunization during pregnancy	Dose schedule	Comments
Yellow fever	Significant morbidity and mortality; not altered by pregnancy	Unknown	Live attenuated virus vaccine	Unknown	Contraindicated except if exposure is unavoidable	Single dose SC	Postponement of travel is preferable to vaccination, if possible.
Varicella	Possible increase in severe pneumonia	Can cause congenital varicella in 2% of fetuses infected during the second trimester	Live attenuated virus vaccine	None confirmed	Contraindicated, but no adverse outcomes reported if given in pregnancy	Two doses needed with second dose given 4-8 weeks after first dose; should be strongly encouraged	Teratogenicity of vaccine is theoretic, outcomes reported weeks 4-8 not confirmed to date. Vaccination of susceptible women should be considered postpartum.
Other							
Influenza	Increase in morbidity and mortality during epidemic of new antigenic strain	Possible increased abortion rate; no malformations confirmed	Inactivated virus vaccine	None confirmed	All women who are pregnant in the second and third trimester during the flu season (October-March); women at high risk for pulmonary complications regardless of trimester	One dose IM every year	—
Rabies	Near 100% fatality rate; not altered by pregnancy	Determined by maternal disease	Killed virus vaccine	Unknown	Indications for prophylaxis not altered by pregnancy; each case considered individually	Public health authorities to be consulted for indications, dosage, and route of administration	—

*Two doses necessary for adequate vaccination of students entering institutions of higher education, newly hired medical personnel, and international travelers.
†Inactivated polio vaccine recommended for nonimmunized adults at increased risk.

Continued

Immunobiologic Agent	Risk from Disease to Pregnant Woman	Risk from Disease to Fetus or Neonate	Type of Immunizing Agent	Risk from Immunizing Agent to Fetus	Indications for Immunization during Pregnancy	Dose Schedule	Comments
Hepatitis B	Possible increased severity during the third trimester	Possible increase in abortion rate and preterm birth; neonatal hepatitis can occur; high risk of newborn carrier state	Purified surface antigen produced by recombinant technology	None reported	Preexposure and postexposure for women at risk for infection	Three-dose series IM at 0, 1, and 6 months	Used with hepatitis B immunoglobulin for some exposures; exposed newborn needs birth dose vaccination and immunoglobulin as soon as possible. All infants should receive birth dose vaccine.
Hepatitis A	No increased risk during pregnancy	—	Inactivated virus	None reported	Preexposure and postexposure for women at high risk for infection; international travelers	Two-dose schedule 6 months apart	—
Inactivated Bacterial Vaccines							
Pneumococcus	No increased risk during pregnancy; no increase in severity of disease	Unknown, but depends on maternal illness	Polyvalent polysaccharide vaccine	None reported	Recommended for women with asplenia; metabolic, renal, cardiac, and pulmonary diseases; smokers; immunosuppressed indications not altered by pregnancy	In adults, one SC or IM dose only; consider repeat dose in 6 years for women at high risk	—
Meningococcus	Significant morbidity and mortality; not altered by pregnancy	Unknown, but depends on maternal illness	Quadrivalent polysaccharide vaccine	None reported	Indications not altered by pregnancy; vaccination recommended in unusual outbreak situations	One SC dose; public health authorities consulted	—

	Risk from disease to pregnant woman	Risk from disease to fetus or neonate	Type of vaccine	Risk from vaccine to fetus	Indications for vaccination during pregnancy	Dose schedule	Comments
Typhoid	Significant morbidity and mortality; not altered by pregnancy	Unknown	Killed or live attenuated oral bacterial vaccine	None confirmed	Not recommended routinely except for close, continued exposure or travel to endemic areas	Killed. *Primary:* Two injections SC at least 4 weeks apart. *Booster:* Single dose SC or ID (depending on type of product) *Booster:* Schedule not yet determined	Oral vaccine is preferred.
Anthrax	Significant morbidity and mortality; not altered by pregnancy	Unknown, but depends on maternal illness	Preparation from cell-free filtrate of *B. anthracis;* no dead or live bacteria	None confirmed	Not routinely recommended unless women work directly with *B. anthracis,* imported animal hides, potentially infected animals in high-incidence areas (not United States) or military personnel deployed to high-risk exposure areas	Six-dose primary vaccination SC, then annual booster vaccination	Teratogenicity of vaccine is theoretical.
Toxoids Tetanus-diphtheria	Severe morbidity; tetanus mortality rate 30%; diphtheria mortality rate 10%; unaltered by pregnancy	Neonatal tetanus mortality rate 60%	Combined tetanus-diphtheria toxoids preferred; adult tetanus-diphtheria formulation	None confirmed	Lack of primary series, or no booster within past 10 years; or consider tetanus, diphtheria, and pertussis immediately after delivery	*Primary:* Two doses IM at 1- to 2-month interval with a third dose 6-12 months after the second dose *Booster:* Single dose IM every 10 years after completion of primary series	All women should receive a dose of tetanus, diphtheria, and pertussis (Adacel) in the immediate postpartum period; may be given during pregnancy if there is a pertussis outbreak.

Continued

Specific Immunoglobulins

Immunobiologic Agent	Risk from Disease to Pregnant Woman	Risk from Disease to Fetus or Neonate	Type of Immunizing Agent	Risk from Immunizing Agent to Fetus	Indications for Immunization during Pregnancy	Dose Schedule	Comments
Hepatitis B	Possible increased severity during third trimester	Possible increase in abortion rate and preterm birth; neonatal hepatitis can occur; high risk of carriage in newborn	Hepatitis B immunoglobulin	None reported	Postexposure prophylaxis	Depends on exposure; consult Immunization Practices Advisory Committee recommendations (IM)	Usually given with hepatitis B virus vaccine; exposed newborn needs immediate postexposure prophylaxis.
Rabies	Near 100% fatality rate; not altered by pregnancy	Determined by maternal disease	Rabies immunoglobulin	None reported	Postexposure prophylaxis	Half dose at injury site, half dose in deltoid	Used in conjunction with rabies killed virus vaccine.
Tetanus	Severe morbidity; mortality rate 60%	Neonatal tetanus mortality rate 60%	Tetanus immunoglobulin	None reported	Postexposure prophylaxis	One dose IM	Used in conjunction with tetanus toxoid.
Varicella	Possible increase in severe varicella pneumonia	Can cause congenital varicella with increased mortality in neonatal period; very rarely causes congenital defects	Varicella zoster immunoglobulin (obtained from the American Red Cross)	None reported	Should be considered for healthy pregnant women exposed to varicella to protect against maternal, not congenital, infection	One dose IM within 96 hours of exposure	Indicated also for newborns of women who developed varicella within 4 days before delivery or 2 days after delivery; approximately 90-95% of adults are immune to varicella; not indicated for prevention of congenital varicella.

Standard Immunoglobulins

| Hepatitis A | Possible increased severity during third trimester | Probable increase in abortion rate and preterm birth; possible transmission to neonate at delivery if woman is incubating the virus or is acutely ill at that time | Standard immunoglobulin | None reported | Postexposure prophylaxis, but hepatitis A virus vaccine should be used with hepatitis A immunoglobulin | 0.02 ml/kg IM in one dose of immunoglobulin | Immunoglobulin should be given as soon as possible and within 2 weeks of exposure; infants born to women who are incubating the virus or are acutely ill at delivery should receive one dose of 0.5 ml as soon as possible after birth. |

Data from Atkinson WL, Pickering LK, Schwartz B et al: General recommendations on immunization. Recommendations of the Advisory Committee on Immunization Practices (ACIP) and the American Academy of Family Physicians (AAFP), Centers for Disease Control and Prevention, *MMWR Recomm Rep* 51(RR-2):1-35, 2002. Available at: http://www.cdc.gov/mmwr/preview/mmwrhtml/rr5102a1.htm. Retrieved October 11, 2002.
ID, Intradermally; IM, intramuscularly; PO, orally; and SC, subcutaneously.

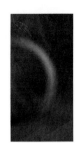

Measuring Clinical Effectiveness by Calculating the Number Needed to Treat

A clinical outcome that has a confidence interval that excludes unity (an odds ratio of 1) is statistically significant at the level indicated (90%, 95%, etc.). If the intervention being studied results in a decrease in the incidence of an adverse clinical outcome, the odds ratio/relative risk and associated confidence interval of that intervention will be less than unity (odds ratio of 1). Conversely, if the confidence interval is greater than and excludes unity, the intervention results in a statistically significant worsening of the designated clinical outcome.[1]

There is, however, a difference between an intervention that is statistically significant and one that is clinically significant. An epidemiologic tool can be used to demonstrate clinical utility or effectiveness. This tool is the *number needed to treat* (NNT) or, in some cases, the *number needed to harm* (NNH).[2]

Measurements such as odds ratios and relative risks and their associated confidence intervals are used to demonstrate statistical significance. For example, an odds ratio of 0.5 with a confidence interval of 0.30 to 0.70 indicates that the intervention results in a *relative* decrease in the odds of experiencing the clinical outcome of 50%. The formula for calculating an odds ratio is experimental event rate (EER)/control event rate (CER) = EER/CER. If the 95% confidence interval is that listed above, then the clinician would know with 95% certainty that, at best, there would be a *relative* decrease in the odds of an adverse outcome of 70% and at worst a 30% *relative* decrease in the odds of an adverse outcome. This type of statistical improvement may, at times, lead the clinician to overestimate its clinical effectiveness. The following example illustrates this point.

Intervention A compared with control B results in a decrease in the adverse outcome from an incidence of 5 per 10,000 to 2.5 per 10,000.

Example 1:

Experimental Event Rate	Control Event Rate
2.5/10,000 = 0.00025	5.0/10,000 = 0.00050

Odds ratio = EER/CER = 0.5

Take an intervention with the same odds ratio but with a clinical condition whose incidence is much greater.

Example 2:

Experimental Event Rate	Control Event Rate
25/100 = 0.25	50/100 = 0.50

Odds ratio = EER/CER = 0.5

Both of these interventions result in the same odds ratio. To determine which intervention will result in increased clinical significance, the clinician needs to calculate the *absolute risk reduction* (ARR) that occurs with a given treatment intervention. The formula for this is CER − EER = ARR. The ARR can be calculated as follows using the above examples:

Example 1: CER (0.00050) − EER (0.00025)
= 0.00025 or a 0.025% ARR

Example 2: CER (0.50) − EER (0.25)
= 0.25 or a 25% ARR

Although both of these interventions result in the same odds ratio, there is a 1000-fold improvement in the clinical effectiveness in example 2. The utility of calculating the ARR lies in its direct translation to the NNT. The NNT refers to the number of patients who will require a given intervention to prevent a given adverse clinical outcome. The formula for NNT is simply the inverse of the ARR, or 1/ARR. The NNT can be calculated as follows using the above examples:

Example 1: NNT = 1/ARR = 1/0.00025 = 4000

Four thousand patients would require the intervention to prevent *one* adverse outcome.

Example 2: NNT = 1/ARR = 1/0.25 = 4

Four patients would require the intervention to prevent *one* adverse outcome.

Similarly, when a given intervention results in a statistical increase in an adverse outcome, the absolute risk increase (ARI) can be calculated using the formula: CER − EER = ARI. The NNH refers to the number of patients receiving the intervention that results in one adverse outcome; thus, it is the inverse of ARI, or 1/ARI.

Throughout this textbook we have attempted to identify the ARR/ARI and NNT/NNH of interventions so that the clinician can decide whether the clinical benefit of a given intervention justifies the costs and potential risks to patients.

REFERENCES

1. McQuay HJ, Moore RA: Using numerical results from systematic reviews in clinical practice, *Ann Intern Med* 126:712-720, 1997.
2. Zapletal E, Lemaitre D, Menard J et al: The number needed to treat: a clinically useful nomogram in its proper context, *BMJ* 312:426-429, 1996.

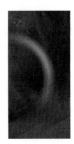

Drugs for Common Conditions in Pregnancy

Kent Petrie, MD

Conditions	Caution/Avoid	Acceptable	Comments
Vitamins and nutritionals	Alcohol Caffeine Saccharin Excessive vitamin A	Prenatal multivitamins Aspartame (Nutrasweet) Sucralose (Splenda)	Moderate caffeine use (5-6 mg/kg/day) is considered safe by most authorities. Saccharin has not been shown to be teratogenic in humans, but second-generation animal studies show increased incidence of bladder tumors. Vitamin A at doses greater than U.S. RDA (8000 IU/day) has been associated with craniofacial, CNS, and cardiac defects.
Coughs and colds	Phenylpropanol-amine Phenylephrine Pseudoephedrine Iodide preparations	Dextromethorphan Guaifenesin Codeine (caution near term) Hydrocodone (caution near term)	Rare malformations have been reported with the sympathomimetic amines phenylpropanolamine (now off market) and phenylephrine. Reports in 1992 of gastroschisis after first-trimester exposure to pseudoephedrine have not been confirmed by epidemiologic studies but warrant caution. Narcotic cough suppressant use near term may cause neonatal withdrawal. Chick embryo studies suggesting teratogenicity of dextromethorphan have not been confirmed in subsequent studies, and it is currently considered safe. Prolonged exposure to iodides may cause fetal hypothyroidism and goiter.

Conditions	Caution/Avoid	Acceptable	Comments
Allergic rhinitis	Brompheniramine	Chlorpheniramine Diphenhydramine Triprolidine Loratadine (Claritin/Clarinex) Cetirizine (Zyrtec) Astemizole (Hismanal) Fexofenadine (Allegra) Nasal steroids Nasal cromolyn	Antihistamines are generally considered safe. Case reports do exist for malformations associated with brompheniramine use. Long-term studies are limited on newer antihistamines. As a class, antihistamines are not considered teratogenic. The use of antihistamines in the last 2 weeks of pregnancy has been associated with an increased risk for retinopathy in premature infants.
Asthma	Zileuton (Zyflo)	Inhaled bronchodilators Epinephrine (subcutaneous) Theophylline/aminophylline Terbutaline (Brethine) Cromolyn (Intal) Leukotriene receptor antagonists Inhaled corticosteroids Prednisone/prednisolone	Pregnancy need not change the drug regimen for asthma. Among the newest class of drugs, leukotriene receptor antagonists, zafirlukast (Accolate) and montelukast sodium (Singulair) are listed as FDA category B and appear safe in pregnancy. Zyflo has been linked to fetal loss and cleft palate in animal studies, and is best avoided.
Nausea and vomiting Motion sickness	Scopolamine (transdermal) (avoid at term)	Meclizine (Bonine, Antivert) Dimenhydrinate (Dramamine) Doxylamine (Unisom) Phosphorated carbo solution (Emetrol) Trimethobenzamide (Tigan) Pyridoxine (vitamin B_6) Prochlorperazine (Compazine) Promethazine (Phenergan) Metoclopramide (Reglan) Ondansetron (Zofran)	Antihistamines and phenothiazines at usual doses are considered safe. Because of reports of CNS symptoms in nonpregnant adults taking high doses of pyridoxine, vitamin B_6 doses should not exceed 75 mg/day during pregnancy. Neonatal effects may occur with use of the anticholinergic scopolamine at term.
Acid peptic disorders	Misoprostol (Cytotec)	Antacids ± simethicone H2 Antagonists Sucralfate (Carafate) Proton pump inhibitors (Omeprazole, Lansoprazole, etc.)	Misoprostol has been used increasingly at term for labor induction, but should be otherwise avoided. H. pylori infection may be treated during pregnancy with proton pump inhibitors and antibiotics (see later) but not Pepto Bismol. Proton pump inhibitors appear safe as a class.

Continued

Conditions	Caution/Avoid	Acceptable	Comments
Constipation	Aloe vera laxatives	Psyllium (Metamucil) Senna (Ex-Lax, Sennocot) Docusate (Colace, Surfak) Bisacodyl (Dulcolax) Lactulose Polyethylene glycol (MiraLax) Cascara sagrada Milk of magnesia	Aloe vera laxatives have been associated with fetal meconium passage.
Diarrhea/ inflammatory bowel disease/ irritable bowel syndrome	Bismuth subsalicylate (Pepto Bismol)	Kaolin/Pectin Diphenoxylate (Lomotil) Loperamide (Imodium) Sulfasalazine (Azulfidine) Mesalamine (Rowasa, Asacol, etc.) Alosetron (Lotronex) Tegaserod (Zelnorm)	Bismuth in bismuth subsalicylate may bind to fetal bone. Prolonged chronic use of kaolin/pectin may cause maternal iron deficiency. Avoid sulfasalazine at term because of risk for neonatal jaundice. Newer drugs for irritable bowel syndrome, alosetron and tegaserod, are classified category B in pregnancy.
Headache (tension) and analgesia	Aspirin (caution near term) Tramadol (Ultram)	Acetaminophen NSAIDs (caution near term) Codeine and other narcotics (caution near term)	Avoid narcotics near term because of potential neonatal withdrawal. Avoid aspirin and NSAIDs near term because of constriction of the fetal ductus arteriosus and risk for persistent pulmonary hypertension in the newborn. NSAIDs near term also inhibit labor and prolong pregnancy. Low-dose aspirin may be used in special circumstances in pregnancy, but full-dose aspirin is listed as category D in the third trimester. Animal studies of tramadol have suggested embryo and fetal toxicity, and neonatal withdrawal has been reported in newborns of chronic users.
Headache, migraine	Ergotamines Topiramate (Topamax)	Triptans Butalbital (caution at term) Isometheptene/ dichloralphenazone (Midrin)	Avoid ergotamines because of their uterine stimulation properties. Triptans have not been associated with increased malformations. Data are accumulating to evaluate other side effects. Babituate combination drugs can cause neonatal withdrawal when used at high doses at term. Prophylactic medications for migraine (β-blockers, TCAs, and calcium channel blockers) may be used (see other categories). Animal studies of topiramate have suggested teratogenicity.

Conditions	Caution/Avoid	Acceptable	Comments
Depression/ psychotro- pics/ sleep aids	SSRIs Bupropion (Wellbutrin) Lithium Benzodiazepines Meprobamate (Miltown) Haloperidol (Haldol) Chlorpromazine (Thorazine) Risperidone (Risperdal) Olanzapine (Zyprexa) Quetiapine (Seroquel) Ramelteon (Rozerem)	TCAs Chloral hydrate Duloxetine (Cymbalta) Venlafaxine (Effexor) Nefazodone (Serzone) Buspirone (BuSpar) Trazodone (Desyrel) Mirtazapine (Remeron) Zolpidem (Ambien) Zaleplon (Sonata) Eszopiclone (Lunesta)	Despite their listing as category D by the FDA, TCAs have not been consistently shown to cause malformations after first-trimester exposure and are considered safe by most authorities. SSRIs have shown no teratogenic effects. Recent reports showing increased risk for persistent pulmonary hypertension in newborns exposed in second half of pregnancy warrant caution as a class. Bupropion has been linked to teratogenic effects in animal studies. Neonatal withdrawal (agitation and tachy-cardia) have been reported with all classes of antidepressants (TCAs, SSRIs, and norepinephrine reuptake inhibitors) and warrant close observation of the newborn. Early reports of the association of diazepam with oral clefts have not been confirmed. Concern still exists with benzodiazepines and the newer nonbenzodiazepine sleep aids about neonatal withdrawal when used near term. Ramelteon has been associated with decreased testosterone and cortisol levels and increased prolactin levels, and is classified category C. Among antipsychotic agents, the older haloperidol is preferred if necessary.
Hypertension and cardiovas- cular disease	ACE inhibitors Angiotensin II re- ceptor blockers Diuretics Reserpine HMG-CoA reductase inhibitors	Methyldopa Hydralazine β-Blockers (caution near term) Labetalol (caution near term) Calcium channel blockers Prazosin (Minipress) Clonidine (Catapres) Digoxin Nitroglycerin	ACE inhibitors and ARBs may cause fetal re-nal failure and oligohydramnios. ACE inhibitors have more recently been linked to cardiac and CNS defects with first-trimester fetal exposure. β-Blockers and combined α/β-blockers may cause IUGR. Neonates exposed to these drugs should be observed for 48 hours for bradycardia, hypotension, and hypoglycemia. Diuretics may decrease maternal plasma volume when administered in the second and third trimester. Reserpine near term can cause nasal dis-charge and newborn respiratory distress. Case reports of fetal malformations associ-ated with in utero exposure to the HMG-CoA reductase inhibitor, lovastatin, war-rant avoidance of this class of drugs during pregnancy.

Continued

Conditions	Caution/Avoid	Acceptable	Comments
Thrombophlebitis/anticoagulation	Warfarin (Coumadin) Streptokinase/ Urokinase	Heparin Low-molecular-weight heparins Alteplase, Reteplase (t-PA)	Warfarin teratogenicity includes skeletal and CNS defects and Dandy-Walker syndrome (cystic expansion of the fourth ventricle with hydrocephalus). Small amounts of streptokinase cross the placenta. Heparin and low-molecular-weight heparin do not cross the placenta. Experience is limited, but t-PA appears safe if the maternal condition warrants.
Epilepsy	Phenytoin (Dilantin) Phenobarbital Valproic acid (Depakene) Carbamazepine (Tegretol) Oxcarbazepine (Trileptal) Topiramate (Topamax) Trimethadione Lamotrigine (Lamictal) Gabapentin (Neurontin)	Ethosuximide (Zarontin)	Carbamazepine has long been considered the least teratogenic of the older anticonvulsants, but it is associated with both major and minor malformations. Although animal studies have not shown teratogenicity with lamotrigine, gabapentin, and oxcarbazepine, few human studies involving these newer agents exist and caution is advised. Animal studies of topiramate have suggested teratogenicity. Ethosuximide appears to have the lowest teratogenic potential. Because of the association of neural tube defects with fetal exposure to most all anticonvulsants, folic acid supplementation (4 mg/day) before conception and in the first trimester is recommended.
Hormonal medications	Oral contraceptives Medroxyprogesterone (Depo Provera) Androgenic steroids Danocrine (Danazol) Clomiphene (Clomid) Tamoxifen (Nolvadex) Raloxifene (Evista)	Prednisone Prednisolone Parenteral corticosteroids	Patients can be reassured about inadvertent first-trimester exposure to oral contraceptives, medroxyprogesterone, and clomiphene. Metaanalyses of existing data show no relation between exposure and malformations in general and genital malformations in particular.
Diabetes	Oral sulfonylureas Acarbose (Precose) Miglitol (Glyset) Repaglinide (Prandin) Pioglitazone (Actos) Rosiglitazone (Avandia)	Insulin Glyburide Metformin (Glucophage)	The known risk for hypoglycemia with the sulfonylureas and the presumed risk with newer oral agents make insulin the drug of choice for the treatment of diabetes in pregnancy. Newer studies suggest that glyburide is safe and effective in treating selected patients with gestational diabetes. Human data, beginning with studies of its use in polycystic ovary syndrome, are confirming safety of metformin in pregnancy, though reports of newborn hypoglycemia and hyperviscosity warrant caution at term.

Conditions	Caution/Avoid	Acceptable	Comments
Thyroid medications	Radioactive iodine Propylthiouracil (PTU) Methimazole (Tapazole)	Thyroxine T_4 (Synthroid) Triiodothyronine T_3 (Cytomel) β-Blockers	Propylthiouracil is preferred over methimazole because of the association of methimazole with aplasia cutis of the fetal scalp. β-Blockers may be used for symptomatic hyperthyroidism.
Bacterial infections	Tetracyclines Erythromycin estolate (Ilosone) Quinolones (Cipro, etc.) Aminoglycosides Nalidixic acid Clarithromycin (Biaxin) Sulfonamides (avoid near term) Trimethoprim (avoid first trimester) Nitrofurantoin (avoid near term) Chloramphenicol (avoid at term)	Penicillins ± clavulanate ± sulbactam Erythromycin base Vancomycin Azithromycin (Zithromax) Telithromycin (Ketek) Cephalosporins Loracarbef (Lorabid) Meropenem (Merrem) Clindamycin (Cleocin) Metronidazole (Flagyl)	Tetracycline chelates to developing teeth after the fifth month of pregnancy causing intense yellow staining. Aminoglycosides are potentially ototoxic to the developing fetus. Gentamicin may be used with careful monitoring of serum levels. Quinolone fetal arthropathy in animal studies has prompted warnings in pregnancy, but human data suggest low risk. Erythromycin estolate is associated with maternal hepatotoxicity. Animal teratogenicity data have warranted caution with clarithromycin use despite FDA category C listing. Azithromycin is preferred (category B). Trimethoprim is a folic acid antagonist and should be avoided before conception and in the first trimester of pregnancy. Sulfonamides at term can cause fetal hemolytic anemia and neonatal jaundice. Nitrofurantoin at term may cause hemolytic anemia in the rare fetus with G6PD deficiency. Oral metronidazole, previously considered teratogenic and carcinogenic in the first trimester, is now believed to be safe in all trimesters. Chloramphenicol at term has been associated with newborn cardiovascular collapse (gray baby syndrome).
Viral infections	Ribavirin Interferon-α	Acyclovir (Zovirax) Amantadine (Symmetrel) Rimantadine (Flumadine) Zidovudine (AZT) Zanamivir (Relenza) Oseltamivir (Tamiflu)	Ribavirin, teratogenic in animal studies, has been demonstrated to be safe in several human case reports. Interferon should be avoided until further human data are available. No adverse outcomes have been reported with newer antiherpetic agents (famciclovir, valacyclovir), but some authorities prefer acyclovir because of the quantity of data available. Animal data suggest low risk for the newer antiinfluenza drugs, inhaled zanamivir and oral oseltamivir.

Continued

Conditions	Caution/Avoid	Acceptable	Comments
Fungal infections	Griseofulvin Fluconazole (Diflucan) (caution first trimester) Ketoconazole (Nizoral) (caution first trimester) Itraconazole (Sporanox) (caution first trimester) Terbinafine (Lamisil) (caution first trimester)	Nystatin (Mycostatin) Miconazole (Monistat) Clotrimazole (Lotrimin) Terconazole (Terazol)	Griseofulvin is contraindicated in pregnancy based on animal data. Systemic triazole and imidazole antifungal therapy in the first trimester may induce fetal malformations. Fluconazole at daily doses of 400 mg/day in the first trimester is teratogenic. Single low doses (150 mg) appear to be low risk, but the CDC recommends using only topical vaginal antifungal agents during pregnancy. All topical antifungal creams are considered safe.
Tuberculosis infections Smoking deterrents	Streptomycin Pyrazinamide Nicotine (FDA category D)	Isoniazid (INH) Paraaminosalicylic acid (PAS) Rifampin (Rifadin) Ethambutol (Myambutol)	Streptomycin ototoxicity warrants avoidance in pregnancy. Other standard antituberculosis drugs may be given alone or in combination. Lack of clinical studies warrants caution with use of pyrazinamide. Intermediate-release nicotine preps (gum, spray, inhaler) are recommended over continuous release (patches) for smoking cessation programs in pregnancy. Ideally, smoking cessation should be accomplished before pregnancy, but benefits during pregnancy often outweigh risks in heavy smokers.
Parasitic infections	Lindane (Kwell) Primaquine Quinine Doxycycline	Permethrin (Nix, Elimite) Pyrethrins with piperonyl butoxide (RID, etc.) Pyrantel pamoate (Antiminth) Chloroquine Hydroxychloroquine Quinacrine Mefloquine (Lariam) (caution first trimester) Atovaquone/proguanil (Malarone) Crotamiton (Eurax) Metronidazole (Flagyl) Furazolidone (Furoxone) (avoid at term) Mebendazole (Vermox)	The potential neurotoxicity of lindane warrants avoidance in pregnancy. Pyrethrin with piperonyl butoxide is considered the drug of choice for lice and permethrin the drug of choice for scabies. Primaquine and furazolidone may cause hemolytic anemia in the rare fetus with G6PD deficiency. Quinine teratogenicity has been reported. Tetracycline chelates to developing teeth after the fifth month of pregnancy causing intense yellow staining. Concern exists about mefloquine fetal toxicity in the first trimester. The newer antimalarial, atovaquone/proguanil (Malarone), is preferred over mefloquine in chloroquine-resistant areas. Oral metronidazole, previously considered teratogenic and carcinogenic in the first trimester, is now believed to be safe in all trimesters.

Conditions	Caution/Avoid	Acceptable	Comments
Dermatologic agents	Isotretinoin (Accutane) Etretinate (Tegison) Podophyllum Podofilox (Condylox) Imiquimod (Aldara)	Topical tretinoin (Retin-A, Differin) Topical antibiotics Topical antifungals Topical steroids Immunomodulators (Elidel, Protopic) Calcipotriene (Dovonex) Benzoyl peroxide Hydroquinone bleaching agents	Isotretinoin and etretinate are potent teratogens. Topical retinoids are minimally absorbed and appear safe. ACOG recommends cryotherapy for genital warts in pregnancy and considers the use of topical agents contraindicated. Small doses of most topical dermatologic agents are safe during pregnancy.
Vaccines	*Contraindicated:* Live-attenuated virus vaccines: Measles Mumps Rubella Varicella Yellow fever Oral poliovirus	*Recommended routinely:* Tetanus/diphtheria toxoid Inactivated influenza virus *Recommended for epidemic or endemic exposure:* Inactivated bacterial vaccines: Pneumococcus polysaccharide Meningococcus polysaccharide Typhoid, plague, cholera Inactivated virus vaccines: Hepatitis A and B Inactivated poliovirus Rabies, Japanese encephalitis	Pregnancy has long been considered a contraindication to vaccination with live virus vaccines because of the theoretical risk that these viruses could cross the placenta and infect the fetus. Large population studies, however, have never confirmed an increase occurrence of adverse events or congenital anomalies in the fetus after accidental exposure. Such exposure should not be considered a reason to recommend interruption of pregnancy. Yellow fever may be given if exposure is unavoidable. Vaccines in development for use in pregnancy include GBS, HSV, and HIV.

ACE, Angiotensin-converting enzyme; ACOG, American College of Obstetricians and Gynecologists; ARB, angiotensin receptor blocker; CDC, Centers for Disease Control and Prevention; CNS, central nervous system; FDA, Federal Drug Administration; G6PD, glucose-6-phosphate dehydrogenase; GBS, group B streptococcus; HIV, human immunodeficiency virus; HMG-CoA, 3-hydroxy-3-methylglutaryl coenzyme A; HSV, herpes simplex virus; NSAIDs, nonsteroidal antiinflammatory drugs; RDA, Recommended Daily Allowance; SSRI, selective serotonin reuptake inhibitor; TCA, tricyclic antidepressant; t-PA, tissue plasminogen activator.

Index

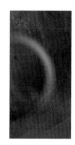

Page numbers followed by f refer to figure, t refer to table, b refer to box.

A

AAFP. *See* American Academy of Family
    Physicians
AAP. *See* American Academy of Pediatrics
AAS. *See* Abuse assessment screen
AASLD. *See* American Association for the Study
    of Liver Diseases
Abdominal pain
    causative factors, 89–90
    complication during first trimester, 130
    diagnostic testing, 307
    and gastrointestinal illness, 306–310
    in pregnancy, 307
    in second/third trimester, 90
    treatment of, 90
Abnormal labor progress, composite curves
    of, 385f
Abnormal maternal pelvis, 436
Abnormal maternal serum, screening, 196
Abnormal placentation
    and hysterectomy, 171
    incidence of, 480
Abnormal test, accuracy of, 339
ABO or Rh incompatibility, isoimmune hemo-
    lytic disease, 600
Abortion
    diabetes with, 25
    iatrogenic termination of pregnancy, 383
    spontaneous, 113, 383
Abruption
    assessment for, 527
    on bleeding, 167
    clinical diagnosis, 527
    with cocaine, 480
    conditions with, 167
    an echolucent retroplacental clot, 528f
    Grade 1, 167
    Grade 2, 167
    Grade 3, 167
    with hypertensive disorders, 480
    sonographic findings of, 527
Abruptio placenta, 167–168
    clinical presentation of, 167
    complications of, 168
    diagnosis of, 168
    incidence of, 167
    with placenta previa, 166
    risk factors, 167
Abstinence, risks and benefits of, 111

Abuse
    alcohol area of, in pregnant women, 112
    during pregnancy, risk factor for LBW, 109
Abuse assessment screen (AAS), for use in
    pregnancy, 104t
Academy of Breastfeeding Medicine, 82
ACE. *See* Angiotensin-converting enzyme
    inhibitors
ACE inhibitors, and angiotensin II receptor
    antagonists, 222
Acetaminophen
    to alleviate pain, 93
    to decrease pain, 591
    safe analgesic for pregnancy, 90
Acetazolamide, 239
Acetylcholinesterase level, for open NTDs, 198
ACIP. *See* Advisory Committee on Immunization
    Practice
ACMG. *See* American College of Medical
    Genetics
ACOG. *See* American College of Obstetricians
    and Gynecologists
ACOG and American Society of Anesthesiolo-
    gists, 398
ACOG guidelines, for oxytocin, 451
ACOG Task Force on Cesarean Delivery Rates,
    403
Acquired human immunodeficiency virus (HIV),
    11, 208, 545, 588, 625, 642
Acquired immune deficiency syndrome (AIDS),
    17, 289, 642
Acrocyanosis, 573
ACT. *See* Aviation Crew Training
Activated partial thromboplastin time (aPTT),
    217, 496
Active management of labor (AML), 393, 435
    evidence to support, 440–441
    goal of, 393
    key elements of, 393
Active management of third stage of labor
    (AMTSL), 482
Active prophylaxis, of postpartum atony and
    hemorrhage, 432–433
Acupressure, 87
    at Neiguan, or p6, 87
    during pregnancy, 52
Acupuncture, 52
    and chinese medicine, 52
    classic, 52

Acupuncture *(Continued)*
    complications of, 52
    overview of, 52
    during pregnancy, 52
    use of, 449
Acupuncture points, common, in maternity
    care, 53f
Acupuncture point spleen 4 (s4), 53
Acute asthma exacerbation
    management of, 206
    treatment of, 206
Acute bilirubin encephalopathy, 600
Acute chorioamnionitis, risk factors for, 471t
Acute conditions, develop during pregnancy, 44
Acute fatty liver, of pregnancy, 309–310
Acute hepatic disorders, in pregnancy, 309–310
Acute hepatitis B, treatment of, 282
Acute infection, incidence of, 35
Acute influenza, diagnosis of, 209
Acute neurologic conditions, 321–323
Acute ovarian vein thrombosis, 638
Acute pyelonephritis, 242, 293
Acute rubella infection
    during early pregnancy, 296
    maculopapular rash in, 295
Acute tubular necrosis, 478
Acute venous thromboembolism, during labor,
    496
Acute venous thrombotic event, treatment of,
    225
Acyclovir prophylaxis, 276
Acyclovir resistance, 608
Adacel, vaccine, for adolescents and adults, 48
ADA. *See* American Diabetes Association
ADA, on nutrition counseling, 156
Addison disease, 273
Adenosine, for acute termination of maternal
    supraventricular tachycardia, 218
Adequate anesthesia, 536
Admission monitor test strip, 412
Adolescent mothers, 658–659
    epidemiology, 658
    risks to child and, 658–659
    treatment, 659
Adolescent pregnancy, 71–72
    associated with, 108t
    contributing factors to, 107
    importance of, 107
    increased risks for, 108

Adolescent pregnancy *(Continued)*
　interventions, 107–112
　　developmental concerns, 108
　　historical perspective/incidence of, 107–108
　　management principles, 108–112
Adult respiratory distress syndrome (ARDS), 478
Advanced Cardiac Life Support Program, 315
Advanced Life Support and Obstetrics (ALSO), for EFM interpretation, 455
Advanced Life Support and Obstetrics course, 539
Adverse pregnancy outcome, cause of, 28
Advisory Committee for Immunization Practices, recommend influenza vaccine for pregnant women, 208
Advisory Committee on Immunization Practice (ACIP), 48, 280
AEDs. *See* Antiepileptic drugs
AFE. *See* Amniotic fluid embolism
Affective disorders, 330–335
AFI. *See* Amniotic fluid index
AFP. *See* α-fetoprotein
AFP level, increased, 196
Agency for Healthcare Research and Quality (AHRQ), 170
Agoraphobia, treatment of, 337
AHRQ. *See* Agency for Healthcare Research and Quality
AIDS. *See* Acquired immune deficiency syndrome
Airbags, 315
Airway obstruction, 585
AIUGR
　definition of, 182
　fetal complications of, 180
Alanine transaminases (ALT) and AST, 282
Albumin and γ-glutamyl transpeptidase levels, 307
Albumin levels, in pregnancy, 241
Albuterol, 205
Alcohol, abuse of, during pregnancy, 116–118
　adverse perinatal outcomes, 116–117
　diagnostic options, 117–118
　long-term sequelae, 117
　perinatal associations, 116
　prevalence of, 116
　treatment of, 118
Alcohol and caffeine, 71
Alcohol consumption, cause of, during pregnancy, 14
Allergy immunotherapy, during pregnancy, 204
Allis clamps, 564
α-blockers, 207
α-fetoprotein (AFP), 193
　with hCG and uE3, 196
　human chorionic gonadotropin and unconjugated estriol, combination of, 41
α-thalassemia, 228
ALPHA. *See* Antenatal psychosocial health assessment
ALSO. *See* Advanced Life Support and Obstetrics
Aluminum-containing antacids, 88
Amantadine and rimantadine, 209
Ambulation and positions, in labor, 395–397
　with epidural analgesia, 397
　history and traditions, 395
　physiologic effects of the supine position in, 395
Amenorrhea, symptoms of early pregnancy, 22

American Academy of Family Physicians (AAFP), 170, 288
　on breastfeeding policy statement, 631
　on VBAC, 177
American Academy of Pediatrics (AAP), 576
American Association for the Study of Liver Diseases (AASLD), 285
American College of Medical Genetics (ACMG), on counselling, 38
American College of Nurse-Midwives, 288
　on VBAC, 177–178
　on women monitored with continuous electronic fetal monitoring, 176
American College of Obstetricians and Gynecologists (ACOG), 112, 208, 268, 384, 412, 439, 454, 523, 576, 636
　guidelines, for exercise during pregnancy and postpartum period, 95, 96t
　on nonmedical use of ultrasound, 24
　on obstetric practice, 463
　practice bulletin, on GDM, 153
　recommendations, on VBAC, 176–177
American Diabetes Association (ADA), 248
　risk assessment for clinical characteristics with GDM, 152
American Heart Association, 581
American Institute of Ultrasound, 24, 523
American Medical Association, 288
American Society for Colposcopy and Cervical Pathology, 279
American Thoracic Society, guideline for CAP, 209
Amiodarone
　with congenital anomalies, 218
　with fetal and neonatal hypothyroidism, 218
　with fetal bradycardia, 218
AML. *See* Active management of labor
Amniocentesis, 197–198
　for advanced maternal age, 39
　for diagnostic purposes, 473
　during third trimester of pregnancy, 555–559
　fetal risks, 559
　with karyotype, 191
　maternal risks, 559
　preparation for, 558
　procedure for, 558–559
　to reduce amniotic fluid volume, 191
Amnioinfusion, 533–534
　complications of, 462, 533
　contraindications, 533
　effectiveness of, 587
　equipment, 533
　indications, 533
　and intrauterine pressure catheter, 532–534
　outcomes of, 462
　procedure, 533–534
　technique of, 461
　variable decelerations resolved after, 459f
Amnionicity and chorionicity, 162
Amniotic fluid, 556
　aspiration of, 558
　for chromosomes, 198
　circulation of, 189
　disorders of, 189–191
　from maternal plasma, 189
　monitoring for decreased, 341
　physiology of, 189
Amniotic fluid α-fetoprotein (AFP), and amniotic fluid acetylcholinesterase, 40
Amniotic fluid assessment, 524

Amniotic fluid bilirubin, in Rh isoimmunized pregnancy, 557
Amniotic fluid embolism (AFE), 312, 480, 495, 497
　diagnosis, 497
　epidemiology, 497
　management, 497
　pathophysiology, 497
　presentation of, 497
　prevention, 497
Amniotic fluid glucose, 557
Amniotic fluid index (AFI), 189, 342, 527
　NST and, 157
　with PPROM, 341
　reflects oligohydramnios, 373
　technique for, 524
　use of, 527
Amniotic fluid tests correlation, with positive amniotic fluid culture, 557t
Amniotic fluid volume, 342
Amniotic fluid white blood cell, counting, 557
Amniotic membranes, rupture of, 603
Amniotic membrane stripping, in prostaglandin production, 449
Amniotomy, 392
　after diagnosing labor, 393
　benefits and risks of, 449
　an intervention, 439
Amoxicillin, 260
　and clavulanate, for macrolide allergic patients, 209
Amphetamines, area of substance abuse in pregnant women, 112
Ampicillin, 267
　advantage of covering enterococcal infections, 473
　and erythromycin, 373
　and gentamicin, 267
　and sulbactam, 209
Amsel criteria, 270, 271t
AMTSL. *See* Active management of third stage of labor
Anaerobic gram-negative bacilli, 619
Anal sphincter and rectal mucosa, 546f
Anal sphincter complex, 543, 544f
Anal sphincter lacerations
　epidemiology of, 543
　risk for, 543
Anembryonic pregnancy, 144
Anemia
　common causes of, 227
　during pregnancy, 13–14, 227
　prevention of, 164
Anesthesia
　choice of, 561–562
　epidural, 215
　local, 547
　and local preparation, use of, 558
　for newborn circumcision, risks and benefits of, 591t
　types of, 561–562
　use of, 513
Aneuploidy, screening and invasive testing for, 197
Angiotensin-converting enzyme (ACE) inhibitors, 221
Angiotensin II receptor antagonists, 221
Antenatal fetal surveillance, initiation of, 341
Antenatal interventions, for prevention of preterm delivery, 356–358

Antenatal perineal massage, in labor, 426
Antenatal prophylaxis, 224–225
Antenatal psychosocial health assessment (ALPHA), 103
Antenatal testing
    to assess post-term pregnancy, 339
    with biophysical profiles, 221
    conditions for, 340
    for fetal surveillance, 339–351
    indications for, 340
    with nonstress tests, 221
    overview of, 339–341
    pregnancy-related conditions, 340
    with preterm premature rupture of membranes, 341
    types of, 341–347
        nonstress test, 341–343
        technique and interpretation, 342
    use of screening instrument, 339–340
        negative predictive value, 339–340
        positive predictive value, 339
        sensitivity, 339
        specificity, 339
    for women, 157
Antepartum care guidelines, 249–250, 291
Antepartum fetal assessment, 157
Antepartum management, strategies for, 168
Antepartum monitoring, 184
Anterior perineal trauma, with morbidity, 424
Anterior pituitary ischemia, 486
Anterior shoulder
    adduction of, 468f
    delivery of, 418f
Antibiotic prophylaxis, 215
    for early pregnancy failure, 146
    use of, 146
Antibiotics, 365, 552
    classified as, 258
    guidelines for, in pregnancy, 258–259
    for short courses, 233
    unsafe for use in pregnancy, 258
    use of, to prevent infection of newborn, 36
Antibiotic therapy
    to prolong pregnancy, 373
    use of, 473
Antibiotic treatment, 605
Anticoagulants, 639
    consensus guidelines for, 218t
    preconception exposure to, 223
    during pregnancy, 224
Antidepressants, 336
    safety information on, 333t
Anti-D immunoglobulin, 148
Antiemetic medication, for treatment of acute headaches, 238
Antiepileptic drugs (AEDs), 234, 334
    long-term effects of, 237
    metabolism of, 235, 236t
Antigen detection, using swab sample, 37
Antihistamine
    and vitamin B_6, 87
    in first trimester, 87
Antihypertensive medicines
    after delivery, 222
    treatment with, during pregnancy, 220–221
Antimicrobial therapy, in management of preterm premature rupture of membranes, 373t

Anti-phospholipid antibodies (APLAs), 224, 256
    autoimmune disorders, 216
    disseminated intravascular coagulation, 230
    management of, 256
    screening for, 256
Antipseudomonal penicillin, with macrolide, 209
Antiretroviral drugs, clinical scenarios and recommendations for use of, 290t
Antithrombin deficiency, inherited disorder, 224
Antithyroid drugs, 636
Antiviral therapy, for varicella pneumonia, 298
Anxiety disorders, 336–338
    generalized, 337
Aorta, coarctation of, 216
Aortic dissection, diagnose, 216
Aortic stenosis, 215
Apgar scores, 96, 417, 420, 572, 581
    determination of infant, 573t
    friends and family, 110t
    for mechanical ventilation, 472
    reduction in low, 406
APLAs. See Anti-phospholipid antibodies
Appendicitis, in pregnancy, 307–308
    clinical findings, 307
    differential diagnosis, 308
    perinatal outcomes, 307
    treatment of, 308
Appetite spurts, 631
APS. See Anti-phospholipid antibody syndrome
Apt test, modified, 476
aPTT. See Activated partial thromboplastin time
Aqueous penicillin G, 267
Arachidonic acid, conversion of, to active metabolites, 364
ARDS. See Adult respiratory distress syndrome
Arias–Stella reaction, 138
AROM. See Artificial rupture of membranes
Arrhythmias
    medications and therapies, 218
    prevention of, 218
Arterial blood supply, to myometrium, 565
Arterial thromboembolic disease, risk for, 213
Artificial rupture of membranes (AROM), 506
Artificial sweeteners, 31
ASB. See Asymptomatic bacteriuria
ASCUS. See Atypical squamous cells of undetermined significance
ASD. See Atrial septal defect
Aspartame, artificial sweeteners, 31
Aspartate, 282
Assess gestational age, 577f
Assisted vaginal delivery, 534–542
    anesthesia and analgesia, 534
    developmental outcomes of, 541
    with forceps or vacuum extraction, 534
    indications for, 534–535
    malposition, 535
    maternal exhaustion, 534
    nonreassuring fetal heart tones, 535
    prerequisites for, 535–536
    prolonged second stage of labor, 534
    prophylactic antibiotics after, 541
Asthma, 121
    cardinal feature of, 203
    chronic respiratory disease, 202
    clinical features and diagnosis of, 203–204
    course of, 202
    effect of pregnancy on, 202
    epidemiology, pathogenesis, and interaction with pregnancy, 202–203

Asthma (Continued)
    lung disease, 209
    management of, 204–207
    pathophysiology of, 202
    with pregnancy complications, 202
    presentation of, 203
    surveillance during pregnancy, 204
Asthma medications, during pregnancy, 205
Asymptomatic bacteriuria (ASB), 267, 292, 353
    diagnosis of, 35t, 293
    epidemiology of, 292–293
    pathogenesis of, 293
    on pregnant women, 39
    risk factors for, 292
    treatment of, 39, 294, 353
Asymptomatic BV, screening and treatment of, 271
Asynclitism, 387–388
    anterior, 388
Atenolol
    with IUGR, 221
    with thiazide diuretics, 221
Atopic eruption, of pregnancy, 319–320
    causative factors, 320
    clinical course, 320
    incidence of, 320
    key features, 319
Atrial fibrillation, 215
Atrial septal defect (ASD), 213, 215
Atypical antipsychotics, 334
Atypical squamous cells of undetermined significance (ASCUS), 326
Auscultate heart and lungs, 576
Australian carbohydrate intolerance, in Pregnancy Trial Group, 155
Autoimmune conditions, 254–257
Autopsy, option of, 379
Autosomal recessive disorders, 193
Autosomal trisomy, in live births, 192
Aviation Crew Training (ACT), for air crews, 2
Azathioprine, and 6-mercaptopurine, 233
Azithromycin, 260
    category B drug, 259
    and erythromycin, 209
    oral antibiotics, 37

B

B vitamin folic acid, periconceptual use of, 25
B vitamins, 70
Bacilli Calmette–Guérin, virus in, 47
Back counterpressure, manual pressure to low back, 58
Back pain, during pregnancy, 58
Bacterial pneumonia, 209
Bacterial vaginosis (BV), 270–272, 353, 357
    causative agent of, 472
    criteria for diagnosis of, 357
    diagnosis of, 270–271
    epidemiology of, 270
    history of, 270
    recommended regimens for, 271t
    screening of, 370
    treatment of, 271
Bacteriuria, diagnosis of asymptomatic, 35t
Bag and mask ventilation, 583
Balloon valvotomy, 215
Baseline measurements, 369
Baseline tachycardia, 458f

BDI. *See* Beck depression inventory
Beck depression inventory (BDI), 330, 647
Beclomethasone, antiinflammatory medication, 205
Bell's palsy, 322
Bendectin (pyridoxine), 45
Benign intracranial hypertension, 239
Benzathine penicillin, 215
Benzodiazepines, 336
Beriberi, autoimmune disorders, 216
β_2-agonist bronchodilators, 205
β_2-glycoprotein, phospholipid-binding proteins, 256
β-adrenergic agents, with antiinflammatory agents, 203
β-blockers
  for control of symptoms, 245
  to control tachycardia, 215
  and thiazide diuretics, 221
β-hCG *See* β-subunit of human chorionic gonadotropin
β-lactam, 209, 262
Betamethasone, in conjunction with β-sympathomimetic agents, 365
β-mimetic tocolytics, 362
β-subunit of human chorionic gonadotropin (β-hCG), 192
β-sympathomimetic agents, 215
β-sympathomimetic drugs
  and betamethasone, 238
  and nifedipine, 168
  use of, 362
β-thalassemia, 229
Bilirubin assessment, predischarge, 597
Bilirubin encephalopathy, chronic form of, 600
Bilirubin metabolism, aspects of, 595
Bimanual palpation, of uterine, 23
Bimanual pelvic examination, to diagnose ectopic pregnancy, 132
Biometric measurements, to assess gestational age and fetal weight, 60
Biophysical profile (BPP), 251, 339
  for evidence of fetal hypoxemia, 344–345
  indications and contraindications of, 345
  modified, 251, 345–346
    indications and contraindications, 345
    test administration/interpretation, 345
    use of, 345–346
  test administration, 345
  test interpretation, 345
  use of, 527
Biopsy, safe and accurate in pregnancy, 326
Bipolar disorder, 332–335
  electroconvulsive therapy, 334
  I and II, diagnosis of, 332–333
  nonpharmacologic treatment, 333
  pharmacologic treatment, 333
  and pregnancy, 332
  treatment of, in pregnancy, 334
Birth control options and birth planning, 159
Birth crisis, 375–381
  impact on families, 375–377
    caregiver reactions, 377
    extended family, 377
    maternal reactions, 375–376
    paternal reactions, 376
    siblings, 376–377
  medical management, 377
  preparation for, 375

Birth crisis *(Continued)*
  psychological management, 377–381
    available resources, 379
    conveying information, 377–379
    coping, 379–380
    discharge planning, 380
    examination, 379
    provider reactions, 380–381
    timing, location, and participants, 377
Birth rates
  to adolescents, 107
  for unmarried and married women, 107t
Birth weight
  and gestational age, 368
  predictor of neonatal outcome, 352
Bishop's cervical, modified, 384
Bishop's scores, 384
  calculating, 384t, 447t
Bladder drainage, 566
Bladder flap, develop, 563
Bladder injury, 566
Bleeding
  assessment of, 62
  disorders, 229–230
  during first trimester, 132
Blighted ovum, 144
Blood clots, 525
Blood cultures, 638
  from umbilical catheter, 604
Blood flow, during pregnancy, 97
Blood glucose
  checked with bedside monitor, 158
  monitoring, 155
  recommended by ADA, 155
  serum measures of, to check hypoglycemia, 158
Blood levels, for vitamins and minerals, 68
Blood loss
  with combined previa and abruption, 166
  estimating, 479
Blood pressure (BP), 216
  accurate measurement, 220t
  alterations in, 476
  determining diastolic, 29
  and heart rate, increase, cause premature delivery, 118
  an insensitive estimate of blood volume in pregnancy, 477
  measurement of, 29
  medication of, 494
  monitoring, 29
  normal, in pregnancy, 476
Blood transfusion, 16
Blood type, Rh, and antibody, screening of, 38
Blood urea nitrogen (BUN), 220
Bloody fluid, 556
Blue cohosh tincture, 56
B-lynch suture procedure, 565
BMI. *See* Body mass index
Body, delivery of, 418
Body mass index (BMI), 66
  and glucose intolerance, 152
Bonding and family adaptation, 612–614
  background, 612–613
  bonding after birth, 613–614
  prenatal bonding, 613
Bonding theory, 612–613
Booster dose, of diphtheria-tetanus, 47
Booster series, completion of, 47–48
Boric acid capsules, 274

Bottle-feeding, 611–612
  routines, 611
Bowel and bladder function, 616
Bowel injury, 566
BP. *See* Blood pressure
BPP. *See* Biophysical profile
Brachial plexus injury, 466
  risk for, 187
Bradycardia, occurs during ECV procedure, 518
Brandt–Andrews delivery
  cephalad shearing motion, 431
  of placenta, 431f
Breast abscess, with lactation mastitis, 634
Breast assessment, 625–626
  anatomic variants, 626
  examination, 625
  inverted nipples, 626
  surgeries, 625
Breast cancer, protection against, 624
Breast changes, in pregnancy, 92–93
  causative factors, 92–93
  treatment of, 93
Breast engorgement, 629
Breast examination, in diagnosing occult breast disease, 30
Breastfeeding, 111, 233, 283, 609–611, 623–632
  advantages and disadvantages of, 601
  after return to work, 661
  assessment of, 627
  benefits of, 80, 624–625
  contraceptive choices for, 640–643
  develop, 661
  discontinuing, 601
  encouraging, 80–84
  as infant feeding paradigm, 624
  for infants, 609–610
  influence of health-care system, 623–624
  as optimal nutrition and immunologic protection for infants, 79
  positions, 628f
  postpartum venous thrombotic event and anticoagulant use in, 226
  precautions, 610
  prevalence, 610
  pumping and storing breast milk, 610
  to reduce incidence of early-onset sepsis, 606
  routines, 610
  statistics of, 79–80
  support for, 82–84
  vitamin and mineral supplements for, 610–611
Breastfeeding-associated jaundice, 598
Breastfeeding promotion, 79–84
  future directions, 84
  role of family physicians, 84
Breast milk, caloric needs for, 72
Breast milk jaundice, 598, 630
Breast stimulation and cohosh tea, 449
Breast tenderness, symptoms of early pregnancy, 22
Breath, shortness of, 90–91
  causative factors, 90
  treatment of, 90–91
Breech delivery, 545
Breech presentation, 510–515
  diagnosis, 510
    complete breech, 510
    frank breech, 510
    incomplete or footling breech, 510
  epidemiology, 510
    incidence, 510
    predisposing factors, 510

Breech presentation *(Continued)*
incidence of, 500–501
management, 510–515
antenatal management, 510–511
complete breech, 511f
frank breech, 511f
incomplete breech, 511f
intrapartum management, 511–512
natural history, 510
associated fetal/neonatal conditions, 510
effect on perinatal morbidity/mortality, 510
spontaneous conversion from breech to
vertex, 510
Bronchial hyperactivity, 202
Brow presentation, 504–505
cause of, 504
diagnosis of, 504
abdominal palpation, 504
ultrasound versus X-ray diagnosis, 504
vaginal examination, 504
management, 504–505
Budesonide, antiinflammatory medication, 205
Bulbocavernosus repair, 548
BUN. *See* Blood urea nitrogen
Bupivacaine (Sensorcaine), 403
Bupropion
during breastfeeding, 124
use of, 124
Burping
expels air swallowed during feeding, 616
and vomiting, 616
Butoconazole, 273
BV. *See* Bacterial vaginosis

C
Caffeine, affect on fetus, 31
CAGE questionnaire, 117t
Calcium
for chronic hypertension, 222
for developing fetal skeleton, 70
during lactation, 72
and magnesium-based antacids, 88, 90
for reversal of magnesium toxicity, 364
supplementation of, 494
Calcium channel blockers, 364
dosage, 364
efficacy, 364
mechanism of action, 364
prolong pregnancy, 364
side effects, 364
CAM. *See* Complementary and Alternative
Medicine
Canadian perineal massage trial, 414
Candida albicans and *Klebsiella pneumonia,* 442
Candida glabrata, 273
Candida tropicalis, 273
Candida vulvovaginitis, 273–274
diagnosis of, 273
effect on perinatal outcome, 273
epidemiology of, 273
management of, 273–274
natural history, 273
CAP. *See* Community Acquired Pneumonia
CAP, guidelines for, 210
Caput succedaneum swelling, 388
Caput swelling, 388
Carbamazepine, 334
antiepileptic medications, 25

Carbamazepine *(Continued)*
with craniofacial defects, 334
drugs with hypothyroidism, 246
use of, 228
Carbohydrates
for normal energy production, 67
restricting, 156
sources of, 67
Carbon monoxide, across placenta, 28
Carboprost (Hemabate), 484
Cardiovascular conditions, 213–218
with maternal/fetal mortality, 214t
with subacute bacterial endocarditis prophy-
laxis, 214t
Carpal tunnel syndrome, 321–322
differential diagnosis, 321
epidemiology and history, 321
treatment of, 322
Catheter-obtained urine analysis, 360
Caulophyllum thalictroides, 56
CBC. *See* Complete Blood Cell Count
CBT. *See* Cognitive behavioral therapy
CDC. *See* Centers for Disease Control and
Prevention
Cefazolin, 267
Ceftriaxone
β-lactam, 209
with macrolide, 209
Center for Epidemiological Studies Depression
Scale (CES-D), 647
CenteringPregnancy®, 127
essential elements of, 128t
Centers for Disease Control and Prevention
(CDC), 36, 102, 209, 260, 357, 606
and ACOG, 288
guideline, on treatment of TB, 211
on HIV screening for pregnant women, 17
screening recommendations, impact of, 269
on tracked breastfeeding rates, 80
on tuberculosis, 16
website, safety of immunization, 47
Central nervous system (CNS)
abnormalities of, 223
developing, 208
Cephalic flexion, maintained by pressure, 515f
Cephalopelvic disproportion (CPD), 507
clinical diagnosis of, 436
diagnosis of, 436, 509
Cephalosporin allergy, 262
Cerebral artery, use of Doppler study of middle,
347
Cervical cerclage, reduce risk for delivery, 167
Cervical cytology, in pregnancy, 323–327
changes on, 325
clinical features of, 324–325
clinical prevention, 327
diagnosis of, 325–327
epidemiology and risk factors, 323
ethnic factors, 324
pathogenesis of, 324
prevention of, 325
Cervical dysplasia
identification of, 324
in pregnancy, 324
Cervical insufficiency, after LEEP, 28
Cervical intraepithelial neoplasia (CIN), 324
Cervical length
assessment of, to predict preterm birth, 62–63
normal, sonogram of, 360f
Cervical mucous, 325

Cervical ripening
and labor-induction agents, 448t
prostaglandins and, 447–449
Cervical spine injury, 466
Cervical trauma, common sources of, 367
Cervix
condition and appearance of, 132
dilation of, 383
effacement of, 383–384
transvaginal image of, 525f
trauma to, 367
ultrasound examination of, 355
CES-D. *See* Center for Epidemiological Studies
Depression Scale
Cesarean delivery, 560–569
fetal indications, 561
indications for, 560–561
instruments used during, 562
maternal indications, 560–561
overview and incidence, 560
risk for, 350
on subsequent pregnancies, 171–172
techniques of, 561–565
Cesarean delivery rate, 441
Cesarean section, indication for, 276
Cessation, motivation for, 122
CF. *See* Cystic fibrosis
Chadwick's sign, in early pregnancy,
23, 325
Change model, stages of, in pregnant women,
122f
CHB. *See* Complete Heart Block
Chemotherapeutic agents, 26
Chest compressions, 583–584
Childbirth education class, components
of, 77t
Childbirth, parenting, and newborn care, educational preparation for, 73–77
components of, 75–77
current trends, 73–74
research, 74–75
role of family medicine physicians, 77
Childbirth preparation, suggestions for incorporation of, 76t
Childhood illness, impact on, 121
Chinese medicine, acupuncture and, 52–54
Chiropractic
and manipulative medicine, 57–58
and osteopathy, 57
Chlamydia, 259–261
detection in early pregnancy, 36
diagnosis of, 259–260
effects on perinatal outcome, 259
epidemiology of, 259
natural history, 259
nonviral sexually transmitted disease,
17, 36–37
treatment of, 259, 260–261
Chlamydia cervicitis, differential diagnosis of,
259
Chlamydia testing, 260
Chlamydia trachomatis, 37
common bacterial sexually transmitted
disease, 259
Chloramphenicol, 258
Cholecystitis, complications of, 309
Cholelithiasis
and cholecystitis, 309
epidemiology of, 309
options for treatment, 309

Chorioamnionitis, 471–475
  diagnosis, 472–473
    amniotic fluid analysis, 473
    clinical presentation, 472–473
    differential diagnosis, 473
    laboratory findings, 473
    in preterm premature rupture of membranes, 556–557
  epidemiology
    preterm labor, 471
    term pregnancy, 471–472
  incidence of, 474
  management, 473–474
    choice of antibiotic agents, 473–474
    monitoring maternal condition, 474
    neonatal management, 474
    timing of antibiotic therapy, 473
  and oligohydramnios, 341
  pathophysiology
    microbiology, 472
    perinatal effects, 472
  predictors of, 471t
  prevention of, 474–475
  suspected, 555
  in term pregnancy, 472
  and umbilical cord compression, 371
Chorionicity and amnionicity, 162
  in gestation, 163
Chorionic sac, 134, 134f, 163
  transvaginal scan of "empty", 137f
Chorionic villi, as tiny, frondlike structures, 138
Chorionic villus sampling (CVS), 39, 198–199
  for advanced maternal age, 39
  and amniocentesis, comparison of, 39t
Chromosomal abnormality, 192
  age-specific rates of, 40t
  assessment for, 63–64
Chromosomal aneuploidy, 192, 198
  risk for, 192
Chronic airway inflammation, 202
Chronic anticoagulation with vitamin K antagonists, 223
Chronic autoimmune thyroiditis, 246
Chronic debilitating diseases, 15
Chronic hepatitis
  development of, 282
  prevalence of, 283
  risk for development of, after HBV infection, 281
Chronic hypertension, 219–222
  BP in woman with, 220
  cause of, 219
  clinical course and prevention of, 222
  diagnosis of, 220
  epidemiology and pathogenesis, 219
  timing of delivery, 221
  treatment of, 220–222
    with hydralazine, 221
    with IV labetalol, 221
Chronic posttraumatic stress disorder, 376
Chronic pyelonephritis, 241
Chronic renal conditions, 241–242
Chronic renal failure, 210
  effects of, 241
Chronic steroids, 206
CIN. See Cervical intraepithelial neoplasia
CIN grade 1 (CIN 1), 324
Circumcisions
  with Gomco or Mogen clamps, 593
  with mogen clamp, 593

Circumcisions (Continued)
  with Plastibell device, 593
Citta, unusual food cravings, 72
Clamp techniques, 592
Clavicle fracture, on anterior fetal shoulder, 469
Cleft lip and palate, 13
Clindamycin, 260, 267, 357
  prevention of, 261
Clinician behavior, interventions to change, 7t
Clotrimazole, 273
Clozapine (Clozaril), 334
CMV. See Cytomegalovirus
CNS. See Central nervous system
Coagulation disorders, 480–481, 485
Coagulopathy, 223, 230, 480
Coarctation, causes of secondary hypertension, 219
COC. See Combined oral contraceptives
Cocaine
  areas of substance abuse in pregnant women, 112
  chronic use of, 113
  prevalence rate of, 113
Cocaine-abusing pregnant patient, risk for, 115
Cocaine alkaloid, 113
Cocaine hydrochloride, 113
Cocaine, with preterm delivery, 14
Cognitive behavioral therapy (CBT), 331, 648
Colostrum, 629
Combined oral contraceptives (COC), 641
Combined spinal epidural (CSE) analgesia, 403
  advantage of, 403
Community Acquired Pneumonia (CAP), 208
Comorbid mental health disorders, 113
Complementary and Alternative Medicine (CAM), 51
  categories of, 51–52
Complete Blood Cell Count (CBC), 208
Complete Heart Block (CHB), congenital, 256
Concomitant thyroid disease, 86
Condylomata acuminate, 278
Congenital anomalies, 25
  cause of perinatal mortality in diabetes, 249
Congenital disseminated varicella, 298
Congenital hearing loss, prevalence of, 580
Congenital heart disease, risk for, in fetus, 216
Congenital malformations, causes of, 44
Congenital rubella syndrome (CRS), 38, 295
  eradication of, 50
  management guidelines, 296
  prenatal outcome, 296
  prevention of, 296
  risk for, 50
Congenital syphilis, 35, 263
  case definition, 264t
  diagnosis of, 265
  in fetal or perinatal death, 36
  phases of, 263
Congenital varicella, risk for, 16
Congestive heart failure, 209
  and myocardial ischemia, 362
  risk for, during pregnancy, 213
  serious cardiovascular side effect, 362
Conjoined twins, diagnosis of, 524
Constipation, 88–89, 616
  causative factors, 88
  treatment of, 88
Continuous Quality Improvement (CQI) techniques, 369

Contraction Stress Test (CST), 339, 343–344
  administration of, 343
  contraindications, 343
  equivocal, 343
  indications, 343
  interpretation, 343
  negative, 343
  positive, 343–344
    management of, 343–344
  use of, 344
Cooley's anemia, 229
Coombs' test, 598
Cord presentation, assessment of, 526
Correct latch/milk transfer, signs of, 625t
Corticosteroids
  effects of, on fetal maturation, 365f
  before preterm delivery, 366t
  in respiratory distress syndrome, 373
  for symptomatic reduction, 255
Coumadin, to effect anticoagulation, 217
CPD. See Cephalopelvic disproportion
CQI. See Continuous Quality Improvement techniques
CQI Plan/Do/Study/Act (PDSA) model, 369
Crack, 113
Crack and cocaine abuse, in pregnancy, 113–115
  adverse neonatal outcomes, 113–114
  adverse obstetric outcomes, 113
  adverse postneonatal outcomes, 114
  diagnostic options, 114
  ethical and medicolegal concerns, 114
  pharmacology, 114
  prevalence in groups at increased risk, 113
  treatment of, 115
"Cradle Cap", treatment of, 615
C-reactive protein (CRP), 373, 473–474, 604
Crigler-Najjar syndrome, 598
CRL. See Crown rump length
Crohn's disease, 232–233, 610
  adverse perinatal outcomes, 232
  fertility, 232
Cromolyn, safest drug, 91
Cromolyn sodium and leukotriene receptor antagonists, 205
Cromolyn versus inhaled corticosteroids, 205
Crowning, 387, 414
Crown rump length (CRL), 134f
CRP. See C-reactive protein
CRS. See Congenital rubella syndrome
Crying, 616
Cryoprecipitate, 485
Cryotherapy, with liquid nitrogen, 279
CSE. See Combined spinal epidural
CST. See Contraction Stress Test
CTRF. See Cystic fibrosis transmembrane regulator
C. trachomatis, 261
Cue-based feeding, 83
Culdocentesis, 138
Culture- and risk factor–based approach, 268
Culture test, 276
  screening test for ASB, 35
  standard for detection of chlamydia, 37
Cushing disease, causes of secondary hypertension, 219, 273
CVS. See Chorionic villus sampling
Cyanotic congenital heart disease, 216
Cyclosporine
  for extraintestinal manifestations, 233

Cyclosporine *(Continued)*
in severe, steroid-resistant ulcerative colitis, 233
Cystic fibrosis (CF), 193
autosomal recessive genetic disease, 38
carrier rates of, 38t
chronic debilitating diseases, 15
screening of, 38
Cystic fibrosis transmembrane regulator (CTFR) gene, 194
Cystitis and pyelonephritis, 132
Cytogenetic analysis, requirement of, 39
Cytogenetic testing, diagnostic accuracy of, by amniocentesis, 198
Cytomegalovirus (CMV), 299–301
diagnosis of, 300
epidemiology of, 299
evidence of, 288
herpes virus, 299
natural history, 299–300
prevention of, 300–301
treatment guidelines, 300
Cytoxan, on pregnancy, 12

D
D&C. *See* Dilatation and curettage
Daily allowances, recommended, 69t
Dane particle, 281
Data collection tools, 369
D-dimer, predictive value for venous thrombo-embolism in pregnancy, 496
Deafness, sequela of congenital rubella syndrome, 16
Deaver retractor, in visualizing anal sphincter complex, 547
Debendox (Bendectin), 87
Decidual cells, with cytoplasm, 325
Deep perineal laceration, repair of, 548
Deep venous thrombosis (DVT), 224
women with history of, 225
Dehydration, evidence of, 599
Delivery, 538
in "all-fours" position, 469t
manual techniques for, of infant, 428
in water, 415
Delivery room equipment, preparation of, 581t
Delivery sites, alternatives in, 393–394
Demand feeding, 83
Dental problems, 92
causative factors, 92
treatment of, 92
Depot medroxyprogesterone acetate (DMPA), 252, 641
Depression
diagnosis of, 330–331
epidemiology and natural history of, 330
incidence of, 330
nonpharmacologic treatment, 331
pharmacologic treatment, 331–332
prenatal intervention, 370
Depressive disorders, treatment for, in pregnancy, 334–335
Depressive episode, criteria for major, 646t
Dermatoses, of pregnancy, 317–321
background, 317
specific dermatoses, 317
DES. *See* Diethylstilbestrol

Diabetes, 71
with abortion, 25
antenatal treatment, 248–251
chronic medical problems, 24
classification of, 152
clinical features, 247–248
with congenital anomalies, 25
with decreased fertility, 25
diagnosis of, 248
dietary management, 250
epidemiology of, 246–247
glycemic control with, 10
and hypertension, 365
introduction, 246–247
pathogenesis of, 247
in pregnancy, 12
risk for, 159
type 1, 247
type 2, 247–248
white classification for, 248t
Diabetes mellitus (DM), 242, 273
type 1, 246
Diabetic nephropathy, 242
Diagnosis codes, 552
Diagonal conjugate measurement, estimation of, 390f
Diagonal conjugate, vaginal examination to determine, 390f
Diamine swab test, 271
Diamnionic, monochorionic (DiMo) pregnancy, 162
DIC. *See* Disseminated intravascular coagulation
Dichorionic, diamnionic (DiDi) twin gestation, 162
Dichorionic pregnancy
premature birth in, 162
ultrasound features of, 163
Dicloxacillin and cephalexin, 634
DiDi. *See* Dichorionic, diamnionic twin gestation
Diet, 156
and nutrition, during pregnancy, 31
Diethylstilbestrol (DES)
example of long latency period, 44
utero exposure to, 367
Digoxin, 218
in atrial fibrillation, 215
Dilatation and curettage (D&C), 145
for early pregnancy failure, 144
treatment for, 145
DiMo. *See* Diamnionic, monochorionic pregnancy
Diphenhydramine (Benadryl), 87
Diphtheria-tetanus, 47–48
Dipstick tests
for leukocyte esterase or nitrites, 40
screening test for ASB, 35
"discriminatory zone", 139
Disseminated intravascular coagulation (DIC), 163
Distal branch block, 591
Diuretics (acetazolamide), 323
Dizziness and syncope, 91
causative factors, 91
treatment of, 91
DM. See Diabetes mellitus
DMPA. *See* Depot medroxyprogesterone acetate
DNA PCR test, 276
Domestic violence, prenatal intervention, 370
Donor milk, use of, 630
Dopamine, depletion of, 113

Doppler assessment, of pregnancies, 184
Doppler testing, in management of abruptio, 168
Dorsal penile nerve block (DPNB), 589
Dorsal recumbency, for vaginal examinations, 396f
Dot-blot hybridization, 300
Double-stranded DNA virus, 281
Douching
bulb syringe for, 93
for leukorrhea, 93
Doula model, 406–407
Down syndrome, 28, 39
detection of, 41
multiple marker testing for, 40–41
sensitivity and specificity for screening tests for, 195t
Doxylamine, for treatment of morning sickness, 45
DPNB. *See* Dorsal penile nerve block
DPNB technique, 591
DR C BRAVADO, 455
Drug exposure, in early pregnancy, 43
Drugs and volume expansion, 585
Drug screening, 370
Drugs, for neonatal resuscitation, 585
Drug therapy, during pregnancy for chronic conditions, 43
Dual amnionic sac, 163
DVT. *See* Deep venous thrombosis
Dyspareunia, therapeutic ultrasound to treat, 425–426
Dystocia, 436
causes of, 435–436
diagnosis of, 435
factors associated with, 436–437
in nulliparous patient, 435–441
prevention of, 437–438
analgesia, 438
antenatal education, 437
diagnosis of labor, 437
intermittent monitoring during labor, 438
maternal support during labor, 437
persistent occiput posterior position, 438
position changes during labor, 437–438
role of hydration, 438
severe, 469
treatment, 439–440
cephalopelvic disproportion, 440
prolonged latent phase, 439
stage one management, 439–440
stage two management, 440
Dystocia, in nulliparous patient, 441
Dysuria, during pregnancy, 33

E
Early latent syphilis, 263
Early-onset infections, causes of, 603
Early pregnancy, symptoms of, 22
Eating disorders, 652–653
clinical course, 653
epidemiology and risk factors, 652
features/diagnosis, 653
treatment, 653
ECC. *See* Endocervical curettage
Eclamptic seizures, 493
ECT. See Electroconvulsive Therapy
Ectopic pregnancy, management of, 136, 140–143
conservative surgical treatment, 141
controversies in treatment of, 143

Ectopic pregnancy, management of *(Continued)*
coronal transvaginal scan of, 137f
diagnosis of, 144–145
efficacy of various forms of treatment for, 142
expectant management, 142
fertility after treatment for, 143
long-term consideration, 141
medical management, 141–142
open surgical treatment, 141
options for, 141t
short-term consideration, 141
treatment of, 145–148
Ectopic pregnancy, predictive of risk for, 137t
ECV. *See* External cephalic version
Edema and varicose veins, 91–92
causative factors of, 91
treatment of, 92
Edinburgh Postnatal Depression Scale (EPDS), 647, 647t
Efavirenz and hydroxyurea, 288
EFM. *See* Electronic fetal monitoring
EIA. *See* Enzyme-linked immunoassay
Elastic bands (sea-bands), 87
Elective Repeat Cesarean Delivery (ERCD), 169
Electroconvulsive Therapy (ECT), 334
Electronic fetal heart rate, monitoring protocols, 454–459
"high-risk" patient, 454
interpretation, 455
"low-risk" patient, 454
Electronic fetal monitoring (EFM)
to assess fetal wellbeing during labor, 454
continuous, 410–411
during active labor, 176
background, 410
versus IA, 410
indications for, 411
in low-risk populations, 411
medicolegal considerations, 411
risks of, 411
as screening test, 411
study results, 410–411
use of, 410
in low-risk women in labor, 436
without fetal scalp blood sampling, 392
Elliot forceps, 537
Embryo, as fetal pole, 134, 135f
Embryonic cardiac activity, 135
Embryopathy, 223
EMLA cream, 591
Empty bladder, 536
Endocervical curettage (ECC), 326
Endocervical glands, 325
Endocrine conditions, 243–252
diagnosis and treatment, 244
epidemiology, 243
Endocrine, response and metabolism, 98
Endometritis, 619
influence of cesarean section on, 620t
risk for, 472
Endometrium, ultrasound of, 139
Endomyometritis, 619
Endomyoparametritis, 619
Endotracheal intubation, 584
End-tidal carbon monoxide, 598
Endurance exercise, course of labor after, during pregnancy, 97t
Enemas, in early labor, 392
Energy, during pregnancy, 66
Enoxaparin and dalteparin, 224

Enzyme-linked immunoassay (EIA), 37, 260
EOGBS infections, case fatality rate for, 266
EPDS. *See* Edinburgh Postnatal Depression Scale
Epidural analgesia, 401, 603
adverse effects of, 403
avoidance of, 427
discontinuation of, for second-stage labor, 420–421
effects of, on labor and maternal and infant outcomes, 402t
use of, 420–421, 427
Epidural anesthesia, 230–231, 368, 427, 561
method of analgesia during labor, 207
use of, 176
Epidural block
effects of, 401
risks of, 401
Epidural drugs, changes in, 403
Epilepsy
chronic medical problems, 24
in pregnancy, 13
risks for infertility, in women, 25
Episiotomies and lacerations, definitions and classification of, 543–545
Episiotomy
common risk factor for hematoma, 480
concurrent use of, 428
cut before delivery of fetal head, 467
indications for, 545
median versus mediolateral, 427–428
mediolateral, 545
midline, 543
rates of, 543
relative contraindications to, 545
restrictive versus liberal use of, 427
and risk for severe perineal trauma, 427
routine use of, 543
types of, 543–545
use of, 368, 428
in vaginal birth, 427
Erb's palsy, 188, 466
ERCD. *See* Elective Repeat Cesarean Delivery
ERCD, reasons for choosing, 174
Ergot alkaloids, 238
Error rates, for processes with multiple steps, 3t
Errors, methods to mitigate effects of, 4
Erythrocyte sedimentation rates, as early markers of infection, 473
Erythromycin, 260
Erythromycin, oral antibiotics, 37, 267
Escherichia coli, 602, 619, 621
Escherichia coli food poison, 31
Essential thrombocythemia (ET), 231
Estimated fetal weight (EFW), 157, 528
ET. *See* Essential thrombocythemia
Ethambutol, drugs for use during pregnancy, 211
Etonogestrel (Implanon), 641
Euglycemia
during labor to prevent neonatal hypoglycemia, 158
maintenance of, during labor, 251
Evidence-based health care, to improve patient safety, 2
Excess fetal weight, use of ultrasound to determine, 528
Exchange transfusion, 600
goal of, 600
Exercises
avoid, during pregnancy, 100t
benefits of, during pregnancy, 96–97

Exercises *(Continued)*
contraindications to, during pregnancy, 95–96
goal of, 98
guide to, 99t
and pregnancy, 31–32, 95–100
Expectant management versus active induction of labor, 371
External cephalic version (ECV), 506, 516–520
complications of, 519
fetal and maternal complications, 519
reversion to breech, 519
contraindications to, 518
diagnosis, 516
effect on perinatal outcomes, 516
cost-effectiveness of external cephalic version versus cesarean delivery, 516
maternal morbidity and mortality with cesarean delivery, 516
morbidity associated with breech presentation, 516
incidence of breech, 516
management after attempted, 519
natural history, 516
conditions associated with breech presentation, 516
congenital anomalies, 516
performing an, 518–519
predicting success of, 517
success rates, 517
tocolysis, 517
scoring system for, 517
successful, 519
unsuccessful, 519
use of anesthesia with, 517

F
Face presentation, 502–504
diagnosis of, 503
abdominal palpation, 503
management, 503–504
radiologic examination, 503
vaginal examination, 503
management of, 502
Factor V Leiden, 224
Failure mode and effects analysis (FMEA), 3
proactive analysis, 4
False-positive results, causes of, 556
Family and Medical Leave Act (FMLA), 661
Family-centered maternity care, 74
Family physician, role of, 560
Family planning, 11, 624
FAS. *See* Fetal alcohol syndrome
Fascia, divide, 563
Fatality rate, 603
Father, role of, 111
Fatigue, symptoms of early pregnancy, 22
FDA. *See* Federal Drug Administration
FDA Drug Classification System, 45
Federal Drug Administration (FDA)
on first fetal pulse oximeter, 462
on STAN S31 fetal heart monitoring, 463
Feeding, signs for successful, 625t
Fentanyl citrate (Sublimaze), 404
Fern testing and pH testing, 314
Fetal abnormalities
clinical screening options, 194–198
detected with screening strategies, 192
diagnosis of, 198–199

Fetal abnormalities *(Continued)*
    epidemiology of, 192–194
    possible indicators of, 192–200
    screening, 194–197
    treatment of, 199–200
    use of ultrasound for, 193
Fetal acidosis, 235
Fetal alcohol syndrome (FAS), 28, 116
    appearance of, 117f
    cause of preventable mental retardation, 14
    principal features of, 117t
    risk for, 28
Fetal anatomic anomalies, chromosomal aneu-
        ploidies, 195
Fetal anatomic survey, 60
Fetal and neonatal outcomes, 172
Fetal aneuploidy, 198
    screening for, 63
Fetal anomalies, evaluation, 191
Fetal anticonvulsant syndrome, 237
Fetal biometry, 526
Fetal blood, presence of, 476
Fetal bowel obstruction, 196
Fetal cells
    and DNA/RNA, 193
    in maternal circulation, 199
Fetal death and GDM, association of, 152
Fetal demise, prevention of, 340t
Fetal distress, 455
Fetal Doppler technology, uses of, in maternity
        care, 347
Fetal electrocardiography, monitoring, 463
Fetal fibronectin test, 355
Fetal growth
    abnormal, 180
    antenatal surveillance of, 164
    importance of accurate assessment of, 180
    monitored during pregnancy, 184
Fetal head
    delivery of, by modified Ritgen maneuver,
        416f
    estimation of descent of, 388f
Fetal heart rate (FHR), 391, 460f
    accelerations, frequency of, 341
    auscultation of, 31
    decelerations, 342
    by Doppler, 133
    frequency of, 341
    intermittent auscultation of, 412
    interpretation, nomenclature for, 456t, 458t
    during labor, 177
    moderate baseline, 458f
    monitoring, 439
    patterns, reassuring versus nonreassuring,
        461t
Fetal heart tones
    auscultation of, 34
    fundal height and, 30–31
    nonreassuring, 545
    on side of small parts, 503
Fetal hyperglycemia, with metabolic rate, in third
        trimester, 151
Fetal hyperthyroidism, 245
Fetal injury, common clinical problems for, 4
Fetal intolerance, of labor, 454
Fetal lung maturity, 556
    assessing, 555
    testing for, 371
Fetal macrosomia, 62, 186, 436
    efforts to identify, 466

Fetal malformations, with medication, 13
Fetal membranes, rupture of, 371
Fetal monitoring, effects on, 338
Fetal movement
    history of, 344
    sign of fetal well-being, 33–34
    testing regimens, 344
Fetal movement counting, 344
    evidence to support use of, 344
Fetal occiput, use of pressure on, 421
Fetal oxygen saturation
    advantages, 463
    disadvantages, 463
    interpretation of, 463
Fetal pulse oximetry, reassuring, 460f
Fetal scalp pH sampling, 462
    contraindications for, 462
    indications for, 462
Fetal scalp stimulation, testing, 462
Fetal scalp trauma, 541
Fetal stress, evidence of, 96
Fetal surveillance and timing of delivery, 184
Fetal syphilis, prenatal diagnosis of, 264
Fetal tracing, 343
Fetal varicella embryopathy, 297
Fetal weight
    estimation of, 526
    special precautions for estimating, in labor, 513
Fetal well-being, antenatal assessment of, 63, 221,
        251, 527
Fetomaternal hemorrhage, 312
Fetuses, growth restriction in, is asymmetric, 180
Fetus with vertex, 503f
FEV$_1$. *See* Forced expiratory volume in 1 second
Fever, significance of, in infancy, 617
FHR. *See* Fetal heart rate
FHR auscultation, as primary method of fetal
        monitoring in labor, 412
FHR baseline variability, definition of, 455
FHR classification systems, 455
FHR variability, definition of, 455
Fingernail hypoplasia, 334
Finnish nephrosis, 196
First month of life, 572–617
First-trimester complications, 130–150
    diagnosis of, 130–139
        clinical features, 130–132
        epidemiology and risk factors, 130
        pathogenesis, 130
    an enlarged uterus, 186
    risk factors or causes for, 131t
First-trimester pregnancy, causes for, 130
First-trimester pregnancy loss
    management of, 144
    risk factors or causes for, 131t
First-trimester screening, 195
FISH. *See* Fluorescence in situ hybridization
Five-aminosalicylic acid medications, 233
Fluid replacement, with colloid or blood prod-
        ucts, 477
Fluorescence in situ hybridization (FISH), 199
Fluorescent treponemal antibody absorption
        (FTA-ABS), 264
FMEA. *See* Failure mode and effects analysis
FMLA. See Family and Medical Leave Act
Foam stability index, 556
Folate antagonist, use of, 228
Folate deficiency, 13, 227–228
Folate supplementation, for neural tube
        defects, 70

Foley catheter balloon, 566
Foley catheter protocols, 449
Foley catheters, 568
    for cervical ripening, 178, 449
    to empty bladder and monitor urine output,
        482
Folic acid, 70, 199
    absorption, 235
    reduce neural tube defects, 10, 25
Food and Drug Administration Classification
        of Drugs, in pregnancy, 45–46, 45t
Food-borne diseases, 31
Forced expiratory volume in 1 second (FEV$_1$),
        204
Force field, on guideline implementation, 8f
Forceps
    classification of, 536
    definitions, 536
    insertion of, 537
    procedure for, 537–539
    rotation of, 541
    versus vacuum, 541
Forceps-assisted vaginal delivery, 509
Formula sample diaper bags, distribution of, 83
Fourth-degree laceration, with extension, 546f
Free fluid, transabdominal scan showing, behind
        uterus in ectopic pregnancy, 138f
Friedman curve, 385
Friends and family Apgar scoring system, 109
FTA-ABS. *See* Fluorescent treponemal antibody
        absorption
Fulminant hepatitis, inflammation of liver, 310
Funneling, of lower uterine segment, 526
Fussy infants, 630–631

G
Galactosemia, or hereditary lactose deficiency,
        611
γ-linoleic acid, 56
Gardnerella vaginalis
    and mycoplasma hominis, 353
    and PROM, 442
Gaskin maneuver, 468
Gastroenteritis, with oral hydration, 309
Gastroesophageal reflux, evaluate and treat
        for, 205
Gastrointestinal conditions, 232–234
Gastroschisis, ventral defects, 196
Gauge needle, to inject lidocaine, 146f
GBS. *See* Group B streptococcus
GBS, maternal colonization with, 602
GCT. *See* Glucose challenge test
GDM. *See* Gestational diabetes mellitus
Gelpi retractor, 547f, 549
General anesthesia, 561
Genetic abnormalities, risk for, of fetus, 39
Genetic amniocentesis, 196
Genetic syndromes, chromosomal aneuploidies,
        195
Genital tract infection, 259
Genital tract trauma, 480
Gentamicin, cause ototoxicity in fetus, 258
Gentian violet, 274
Gestational age
    assessment, 61
    calculating, 135
    effect of
        on antenatal testing, 340–341

Gestational age *(Continued)*
    on diagnostic criteria, 340–341
    on NST interpretation, 341
  estimation of, 573
  fetal weight and, 526
Gestational diabetes
  aggressive treatment of, 188
  common obstetric condition, 159
  risk factors for, 152
Gestational diabetes mellitus (GDM), 97,
    151–160
  β-cell dysfunction of, 151
  classification of, 152
  complications of, 152
  consultation and referral of, 158–159
  diagnosed by blood glucose, 154
  diagnosis of, 152–154
  epidemiology of, 151–152
  fetal effects of, 151
    with fetal hypoglycemia, 151
    with fetal macrosomia, 151
    with hyperbilirubinemia, 151
    with hypertension, 151
  incidence of, 151
  long-term consequences and patient educa-
    tion, 159
  method of screening, 153
  pathophysiology of, 151
  prevention of, 154–155
  recurrence rates of, 152
  risk for development of type 2 diabetes, 159
  screening for, 152
  with shoulder dystocia, 151
  timing of screening, 153
  treatment of, 155, 155–158
  with type 2 diabetes, 151
Gestational hypertension, 220
Gestational sac, 134f, 163
Gestational thrombocytopenia, cause of thrombocytopenia, 229
Gilbert syndrome, 595, 598
Ginger, efficacy of, 54
Ginger therapy, for nausea and vomiting during
  pregnancy, 86
Glans oozes, 615
Glargine (Lantus), 157, 250
Glomerular disease, types of, 242
Glomerulonephritis, 242
Glucocorticoids, for fetal lung maturation,
  365–366
  dosage, 365
  efficacy, 365
  mechanism, 365
  side effects, 365
Glucocorticoid therapy, prophylactic inhaled, 205
Glucose-6-phosphate dehydrogenase level, 598
Glucose challenge test (GCT), 153
  comparison of differing cutoff values for, 153t
Glucose tolerance test (GTT), 153
Glyburide
  versus insulin, 156
  second-generation sulfonylurea, 156
  for treatment of GDM, 156
Glycemic control
  evaluation of, during periconception, 249
  in women with diabetes, 10
Glycemic index, reducing, 156
Gomco base plate, 593
Gomco technique, 592
Gonadotrophic medication, use of, 162

Gonococcal ophthalmia neonatorum, 262
Gonorrhea, 261–262
  cause of PID, 17
  diagnosis of, 261–262
  effects on perinatal outcome, 262
  epidemiology of, 261
  natural history, 261
  syphilis, chlamydia and, 357
Gonorrheal infection, management guidelines
  for, 262
Gram-positive aerobic cocci, 619
Gram's stain, 557
  and culture, 555
Graves' disease, 244, 636
  risk for development of, 318
Gray baby syndrome, 258
Group B streptococcus (GBS), 266–269, 294, 357,
    443, 462, 602
  diagnosis, 267
  effects on perinatal outcome, 266–267
  epidemiology of, 266
  management of, 267–269
  natural history, 266
  risk factors, 266
Group B streptococcus prophylaxis, 373
Group B streptococcus vaccine, development
  of, 269
Group prenatal care, 127
Growth charts, for biometric measurements of
  fetus, 182
Growth discordance, diagnosed during ultrasound examination, 163
GTT. *See* Glucose tolerance test
Gum hypertrophy and bleeding, during pregnancy, 92

H

H&E. *See* Hematoxylin and eosin
Haemophilus influenzae and *Moraxella catarrha-
lis,* bacterial agents, 208
Handheld Doppler
  for fetal heartbeat, 133
  use of, 133f
Hand hygiene, source of postnatal infections, 606
Hands-on method, 416, 421
Hands poised method, 416
Hashimoto disease, 246
HBeAg. *See* Hepatitis B e antigen
HBIG. *See* Hepatitis B immunoglobulin
HBsAg. *See* Hepatitis B surface antigen
HBsAg test report, 579
HBV. *See* Hepatitis B virus
HBV screening, guidelines for, 283
hCG. *See* Human chorionic gonadotrophin
hCG levels, during early pregnancy, 139
hCG testing, clinical utility of, 139
HCV. *See* Hepatitis C virus
Headaches, 91
  causative factors, 91
  treatment of, 91
Head, delivery of, 415–417
Health-care providers, 378
Health Insurance Portability and Accountability
  Act (HIPAA), 128
Healthy term infant, care of, at birth,
  572–573
  Apgar scoring, 572
  disposition, 573

Healthy term infant, care of, at birth *(Continued)*
  initial assessment, 572–573
  initial steps, 572
Hearing loss, 300
  risk factors for, 580
Hearing screening, 580
Heartburn, 88
  causative factors, 88
  treatment of, 88
Heart disease, structural, 213–218
  cardiovascular changes in pregnancy, 213
  general approach, 213
  specific diagnoses, 215–218
Heart rate
  assessment of, 572
  during decreased vagal tone, 97
Heavy metals, affecting fetal neurological development, 26
Hegar's sign, softening of cervical and uterine
  tissue, 72
HELLP syndrome, 310, 493
  coagulopathy from, 480
  treatment of, 229
Hematologic conditions, in pregnancy, 227–231
Hematomas, cause pain and hemodynamic
  effects, 481
Hematoxylin and eosin (H&E), 317
Hemoglobin A1c concentration, to monitor
  nongestational diabetes, 155
Hemoglobin Bart's disease, 229
Hemoglobin H disease, 229
Hemoglobinopathy, 13
  actions for, 13
  disorders, 228
  screening of, 38
Hemolytic uremic syndrome, and fatty liver, 230
Hemorrhage, as result of lacerations, 466
Hemorrhoids, 89
  causative factors, 89
  treatment of, 89
Hep B. *See* Hepatitis B vaccine
Heparin
  and aspirin, 224
  dosage of, 217, 226t
  record of use in pregnancy, 217
  use of, during labor, 226
Hepatitis A
  history of, 48
  indications for vaccination, 49
  during pregnancy, 49
  safety of, 49
Hepatitis B
  causes of, 15
  as STD, 15
Hepatitis B e antigen (HBeAg), 281
Hepatitis B immunization, 578–579
Hepatitis B immunoglobulin (HBIG), 578
Hepatitis B infection
  during pregnancy, 48
  risk factors for, 36
Hepatitis B surface antigen (HBsAg), 35–36, 578
  presence of, 36
Hepatitis B vaccine (Hep B), 578
  adverse effects of, 579
  for infants by maternal hepatitis B surface
    antigen status, 579t
Hepatitis B virus (HBV), 281–284, 578
  acute, 282
  clinical course and features, 281–282
  diagnosis of, 282

Hepatitis B virus (HBV) *(Continued)*
    epidemiology of, 281
    pathogenesis of, 281
    prevention of, 283–284
    series of, 579
    treatment of, 282–283
Hepatitis C virus (HCV), 284
    clinical features of, 285
    epidemiology of, 284–285
    management, 286
    pathogenesis of, 285
    in pregnancy, 284–286
    prevention of, 285–286
    transmitted by contaminated blood, 16
    treatment of, 285
Hepatosplenomegaly, 300
Herbal/homeopathic uterotonics, use of, 177
Herbal medicines
    applications of, 54
    forms of, 54
    overview of, 54
Herbal remedies, safety of, in pregnancy,
        55t–56t
Herbal therapy, 399
Heroin, during pregnancy, 15
Herpes, risk for fetus and newborn child, 18
Herpes simplex virus (HSV), 462, 607–608
    clinical features, 607
    diagnosis, 607–608
    epidemiology, 607
    prevention, 608
    risk factors, 607
    treatment, 608
    type 2, 275–277
        diagnosis of, 276
        effects on perinatal outcome, 276
        epidemiology of, 275
        history of, 275
        primary genital, 276
        recurrent genital, 276
Herpes zoster, in infancy, 298
HgA1c (hemoglobin A1c), 25
    target for, 25
High-dose oxytocin, 452
High-grade squamous intraepithelial lesions
        (HSIL), 279
High-reliability organizations, characteristics
        of, 4–6
High reliability organizations theory, 2
H. influenzae and *Staphylococcus aureus,* 208
Hip squeeze, 58
HIPAA. *See* Health Insurance Portability and
        Accountability Act
Histamine 2 receptor antagonists, with nizati-
        dine, 88
HIV. *See* Human immunodeficiency virus
HIV infection, antepartum screening for, 288
HIV testing, for pregnant women, 37
HLAs. *See* Human leukocyte antigens
HMBANA. *See* Human Milk Banking
        Association of North America
Homeopathy
    applications of, in maternity care, 57
    overview of, 57
Home uterine activity monitor, 357
HOOP (hands on or poised) trial, 416, 421
Hospital settings, incorporating continuous labor
        support in, 408
Hospital staffing, controversies regarding, 176
HPV. *See* Human papillomavirus

HSIL. *See* High-grade squamous intraepithelial
        lesions
HSV. *See* Herpes simplex virus
Human chorionic gonadotrophin (hCG), 23,
        133, 243
Human error rates, sample, in complex medical
        system, 3t
Human factors, role on errors, 4
Human immunodeficiency virus (HIV), 37, 208,
        273, 287–292, 625
    assessment of disease stage, 288
    diagnosis of, 288
    epidemiology of, 287
    pathogenesis of, 287–288
    pregnant women infected with, 37
    prevention of opportunistic infections,
        289–291
    risk factors for, 37
    sexually transmitted infections, 17
    treatment of, 288–289
Human insulin, 250
Human leukocyte antigens (HLAs), 233
Human Milk Banking Association of North
        America (HMBANA), 84, 630
Human milk, use of, 79
Human papillomavirus (HPV), 277–280
    clinical features, 278
    diagnosis of, 278–279
    epidemiology of, 278
    pathogenesis of, 278
    prevalence of, 278
    prevention of, 280
    risk factors of, 278
    role of, 324
    treatment of, 279–280
Hutchinson's teeth, 264
Hydatidiform mole, 137
Hydralazine, 493
Hydrotherapy, 399
    RCT of, 399
Hydroureter and hydronephrosis, 293
Hyperaldosteronism, causes of secondary hyper-
        tension, 219
Hyperbilirubinemia, 630
    cause of, 630
    complications of, 600–601
    and polycythemia, 158
Hypercoagulability, pregnancy-associated, 213
Hyperemesis, 72
Hypertension
    definition of, 491
    incidence of, 241
    in pregnancy, 12
    pseudotumor cerebri or benign intracranial,
        322–323
    pulmonary, 218t
    treatment of, 183
Hypertensive disorders, 167
    of pregnancy, 183
    symptoms of, 34
Hypertensive nephropathy, serum creatinine
        and urinalysis to detect, 222
Hyperthyroidism, in pregnancy, 244–245
    clinical features and laboratory evaluation,
        244
    treatment of, 244
Hyperuricemia and proteinuria, 12
Hypnosis, for managing labor pain, 399
Hypoglycemics, oral and pregnancy, 251
Hypotension, regional anesthesia cause, 215

Hypothyroidism
    cause of, 246
    diagnosis of, 246
    fetal and neonatal concerns, 246
    in pregnancy, 245–246
        clinical features and laboratory evaluation,
        245
    treatment of, 244, 246
Hysterectomy, with uterine rupture, 171

I

IAP. *See* Intrapartum antibiotic prophylaxis
IAS. *See* Internal anal sphincter
Iatrogenic prematurity, 182
IBCLC. *See* International Board Certified
        Lactation Consultant
IBLCE. *See* International Board of Lactation
        Consultant Examiners
ICP. *See* Intrahepatic cholestasis of pregnancy
ICSI. *See* Institute for Clinical Systems
        Improvement
ICV. *See* Internal cephalic version
Idiopathic hypertrophic subaortic stenosis
        (IHSS), 216
Idiopathic thrombocytopenia purpura (ITP),
        229
IDSA. *See* Infectious Diseases Society of America
IHSS. *See* Idiopathic hypertrophic subaortic
        stenosis
Intrauterine Growth Restriction (IUGR), 166
    asymmetric, 61–62
    diagnosis of, 341
    high-risk conditions, 345
    maternal complications, 180–181
    risk factors for, 180, 217
    symmetric, 61
Illicit drugs
    during pregnancy, 29
    use of, 29
ILO. *See* International Labor Organization
Immediate cesarean delivery, indications for,
        476
Immune-mediated thrombocytopenia, 229
Immune response phase, 282
Immune tolerant phase, 281
Immunization, 25–26
    benefits of, 47
    determination of, 298
    with diphtheria, 26
    testing for, for rubella, 38
    with tetanus, 26
Immunomodulators, 233
Imperatives, prescribing, during pregnancy, 44
Improvement, opportunities for, 5t
Inaccurate dating, role on occurrence of post-
        term pregnancies, 349
Inaccurate gestational age
    with IUGR, 40
    with multiple gestation, 40
Inactivated influenza virus
    and diphtheria toxoid, 25
    and tetanus, 25
Inactivated polio vaccine (IPV), 50
Incompetent cervix, 366–367
    diagnosis of, 367
        preconception, 367
        prenatal, 367
    epidemiology of, 366–367

Incompetent cervix *(Continued)*
   management of, 367
   pathophysiology of, 367
   treatment of, 367
Incompetent cervix, incidence of, 366
Indomethacin
   agent for tocolysis, 167
   effect on clotting, 168
Indomethacin (Indocin), 191
Induction of labor, 445–452
   preventive labor indications, 446
   relative contraindications to, 446
   standard fetal indications, 446
   standard maternal indications, 446
Infant development, 662
Infant feeding and nutrition, 609–612
Infant formula, preparation and storage of, 611
Infections
   evaluation and management of, in newborn,
      602–608
   in pregnancy, 258–306
   rapid tests for, 555
Infectious Diseases Society of America (IDSA)
      practice guideline, 208, 288
Infertility, risks for, in women, 25
Inflammatory bowel disease, 232–233
Influenza
   an annual seasonal infection, 48
   effect of, 209
Influenza vaccine
   from inactivated viruses, 26
   during influenza season, 204
Inhaled β-agonists, for acute symptoms, 205
Inhaled corticosteroids, doses of, 206t
INH, drugs for use during pregnancy, 211
Inhibin-A (INH-A), fourth serum marker, 193
INR. *See* International Normalized Ratio
Institute for Clinical Systems Improvement
      (ICSI), on blood pressure, 29
Institute of Medicine, on current health-care
      system, 1
Insulin
   analogs, 250
   critical growth hormone, 247
   subcutaneous or continuous infusion for, 158
Insulin aspart (Novolog), 157, 250
Insulin lispro (Humalog), 157, 250
Insulin resistance, after delivery, 158
Insulin therapy
   with fasting glucose, 155
   for gestational diabetes, 157
   goals and management of, 250–251
Interleukin-8 (IL-8), 604
Internal anal sphincter (IAS), 543
   disruption of, 553f
Internal cephalic version (ICV), 506
International Board Certified Lactation Consul-
      tant (IBCLC), 82, 631
International Board of Lactation Consultant
      Examiners (IBLCE), 631
International Classification of Disease,
      552
   ninth revision, 552
International Labor Organization (ILO), 660
International Lactation Consultant Association,
      on breastfeeding, 631
International Normalized Ratio (INR), 476
International Reference Preparation (IRP), 139
International Social Security Association, 660
Interpersonal therapy (IPT), 331

Interventions
   benefit of, for psychosocial problems, 103
   to change clinician behavior, 7t
Intimate partner violence, 103
Intradermal injections, 400f
Intradermal sterile water injections, 399
Intrahepatic cholestasis, of pregnancy, 320–321
   incidence of, 320
   key features, 320
   treatment of, 320–321
Intrahepatic cholestasis of pregnancy (ICP), 309
Intrapartum antibiotic prophylaxis (IAP),
      602, 606
Intrapartum bleeding, 475–479
   initial evaluation, 475–476
   history, 475–476
   management, 476
   maternal stabilization, 476
Intrapartum care, 291
Intrapartum complications, 454–499
Intrapartum fetal heart rate, monitoring,
      409–413
Intrapartum fetal pulse oximetry, continuous,
      462–463
Intrapartum insulin and intravenous fluid drip,
      sample, 158t
Intrapartum management, 251–252
Intrapartum pain management, 398–404
Intrapartum perineal massage, in labor, 426–427
Intrapartum procedures, 523–571
   use of ultrasound for, 528
Intrapartum prophylaxis, with intravenous
      penicillin, 268
Intrapartum resuscitation techniques, use of, 463
Intrapartum surveillance techniques, evidence to
      support use of, 463
Intrathecal narcotics
   actions of, 403
   for labor analgesia, 403
   side effects of, 404
Intraumbilical vein injection, use of,
      of oxytocin, 489
Intrauterine and extrauterine pregnancy, 137
Intrauterine device (IUD), 112, 147, 642
Intrauterine fetal demise (IUFD), 162
   management of second- or third-trimester, 164
Intrauterine fetal resuscitation, 459
Intrauterine fetal transfusions, 306
Intrauterine findings, scan showing vague, 134f
Intrauterine growth restriction, 300, 352
   ability to predict, 183
   biometric evaluation, 182
   clinical diagnosis, 182
   diagnosis of, 181–182
   long-term sequelae of, 181–182
   management of, 183–184
   prevention of, 183
   risk factors for, 180
   screening for, 182–183
Intrauterine growth restriction (IUGR), 13, 40,
      61, 68, 113, 121, 159, 181t, 205, 340, 454
   causes of, 164
Intrauterine infections, 180
Intrauterine pregnancy
   transabdominal transverse image of 91/
      2-week, 136f
   transvaginal ultrasound confirming, 23
Intrauterine pressure catheter, 532
   complications, 532
   contraindications, 532

Intrauterine pressure catheter *(Continued)*
   equipment, 532
   indications, 532
   placement technique, 532
Intravenous immunoglobulin, 600
Intravenous immunoglobulin (IVIG), 230, 498
Inverted uterus, 481
Iodides, drugs, with hypothyroidism, 246
Iowa trumpet, 531f
Ipswich Childbirth Study, 425
IPT. *See* Interpersonal therapy
IPV. *See* Inactivated polio vaccine
Iron, 611
Iron deficiency anemia, 13, 227
   severe anemia, 227
   treatment, 227
Iron-rich foods, 69
IRP. *See* International Reference Preparation
Isolated oligohydramnios, 190
   management of, 190
Isolated term oligohydramnios, 190
Isosorbide mononitrate, use of, 449
Isotretinoin (Accutane), 45
ITP. *See* Idiopathic thrombocytopenia purpura
IUD. *See* Intrauterine device
IUFD. *See* Intrauterine fetal demise
IUGR. *See* Intrauterine growth restriction
IV dextrose, for low blood sugar infant, 158
IVIG. *See* Intravenous immunoglobulin

J
Jarisch–Herxheimer reaction, 265
Jasmine flowers, in suppression of lactation, 56
Jaundice, with breastfeeding, 598–599
JCAHO. *See* Joint Commission on Accreditation
      of Health Care Organizations
Jehovah's witnesses, 481
Joel-Cohen method, of cesarean delivery, 564
Johnson method, 485
Joint Commission on Accreditation of Health
      Care Organizations (JCAHO), 3
J-shaped pelvic curve, 540

K
Karyotyping, amniocentesis for, 196
Kegel exercises, 568
Kernicterus, 600
   incidence of, 600
Kernicterus, causing CNS damage, 594
Kielland/Barton forceps, 507
Kleihauer–Betke (K–B) test, 168, 191, 313, 476
KOH. *See* Potassium hydroxide
Knee counterpressure, 58
Korotkoff 5 sound, for determining diastolic
      blood pressure, 29

L
Labetalol, as first-line antihypertensive medicine
      in pregnancy, 221
Labor
   advantages of position change in, 397
   ambulation in, 396–397
   benefits of continuous support in, 407–408
   cardinal movements of, 386

Labor *(Continued)*
  classic definition of, 383
  false, 383
  first stage of
    active phase, 385
    latent phase, 385
  induction and augmentation of, 56, 173, 175–176
  induction and future possibilities, 451–452
  management of, 382–434
  mechanism of, in left occiput anterior position, 387f
  physiologic cause of, 383
  second stage of, 386
  support in, 406–409
  third stage of, 386
  true, 383
Labor abnormalities, management of, 435–453
Labor and delivery management, 207
Labor induction, 449
  advances in cervical ripening and, 451
  alternative medicine, 449
  amniotic membrane stripping, 449
  amniotomy, 449–450
  Foley catheters with other methods, 450
  issues related to, 446–447
  prostaglandins, 450–451
  protocols for, 451
Labor management, 239
  Ps of, 390
Labor monitoring algorithm, 464f
Labor pain symposium, nature and management of, 402
Labor support, for adolescent patient, 111
Lacerations, repair of, in birth canal, 433–434
  classification, 545
  first-degree, 433
  fourth-degree, 433
  second-degree, 433
  third-degree, 433
Lactational Amenorrhea Method (LAM), 640
Lactose intolerance, a dose-dependent phenomenon, 72
Lactovegetarians, 71
LAM. *See* Lactational Amenorrhea Method
Lamaze and Bradley methods, in prenatal education, 398
Lamellar body counts, 556
Lamotrigine, 334
  use of, 334
Laparoscopic salpingostomy
  for removing ectopic pregnancy, 142
  in treating ectopic pregnancy, 142
Large-for-dates pregnancy, 186–188
  causative factors of, 186
    inaccurate dates, 186
    inaccurate measurement, 186
    molar pregnancy, 186
    multiple gestation, 186
    obesity, 186
    polyhydramnios, 186
    short stature, 186
    uterine leiomyomata, 186
  epidemiology and risk factors, 187
  workup of, 186
Large-for-gestational age, 186
Last menstrual period (LMP), 23, 348
  for calculating delivery date, 23

Latent tuberculosis infection (LTBI), risk factors for, 210
  as asymptomatic, 211
  treatment of, 211
  response to, 211
Latex condoms, use of, 280
LBW. *See* Low-birth-weight
Lead contamination, preventing, 611
Lead, in lead-based paint, 18
Lecithin/sphingomyelin ratio, 555
LEEP, cervical insufficiency after, 28
Left occiput posterior (LOP), 508
Leg cramps, treatments for, in pregnancy, 90
Legionella pneumophila, atypical organisms, 208
Leopold maneuvers, 501, 502f
Leukocyte esterase, rapid test for, 557
Leukocytosis, as white blood count, 473
Leukorrhea, 93
  causative factors, 93
  treatment of, 93
Leukotriene receptor antagonists, 205
LI 4 (Hegu), acupuncture points, 54
Lidocaine
  and bupivacaine, 547
  and prilocaine, 591
  safe in pregnancy, 218
Lidocaine gel application, 401
Lidocaine (Xylocaine), 403
Ligase chain reaction technology, for NAATs, 37
Linea nigra, 92
Lipid-soluble narcotics (fentanyl and sufentanil), 404
Listeriosis
  food-borne diseases, 31
  with preterm delivery, 31
Lithium, 333
  with hypothyroidism, 246
Liver disease, 209
LMP. *See* Last menstrual period
LMWH. *See* Low-molecular-weight heparin
Local anesthesia, 562
  with lidocaine, 558
Long-term renal function, effect of pregnancy on, 242
LOP. *See* Left occiput posterior
Low Apgar scores, 410
Low-birth-weight (LBW), 120, 203, 259
  increased rate of, 113
  and preterm labor, 102
Low-dose aspirin, 494
Lower genital tract trauma, risk for, 480
Lower genitourinary infection, 353
Lower uterine segment and cervix, assessment of, 526–527
Low-grade squamous intraepithelial lesions (LSILs), 279
Low-molecular-weight heparin (LMWH), 217, 218t, 496
LSILs. *See* Low-grade squamous intraepithelial lesions
LTBI. *See* Latent tuberculosis infection
Lumbar puncture, 474, 604
Lung disease, 209
Lung maturity, testing methods and interpretation, 555–556
Lupus nephritis, pregnant and nonpregnant women with, 242
Lupus-related renal disease, 242

M
Macrolides, 259
Macrosomia, 186–188
  clinical recommendations, 188
  diagnosis of, 187
  history of, 187
  an indicator of poor diabetic control, 250
  management of suspected fetal, 187–188
  natural history, 186–187
  risk factors for, 187
  screening for, 188
  ultrasound diagnosis of, 62, 187, 528
Magnesium sulfate, 215, 363–364, 477, 493
  adverse drug effects, 364
  agent for tocolysis, 167
  and calcium channel blockers, 207
  dosage, 364
  efficacy, 363–364
  hemodynamic effects of, 168
  mechanism of action, 363
  metabolism, 363
  placebo-controlled studies of, 363
  for tocolytic treatment, 461
  use of, 493
Magnesium toxicity, 364, 493
Magnetic resonance imaging
  method for diagnosis of DVT, 225
  use of, 307
Malpresentation and malpositions, 500–522
  diagnosis, 500–501
    abdominal palpation, 501
    auscultation, 501
    diagnostic ultrasonography, 501
    vaginal examination, 501
    X-ray examination, 501
  incidence, 500–501
    breech presentation, 500–501
    brow presentation, 500
    face presentation, 500
    transverse lie, 500
Manipulative therapy, 58
  applications of, 58
Manual vacuum aspirator (MVA), 145
  versus electric vacuum aspiration, 146
  with suction cannulae, 146f
MAP. *See* Mean arterial pressure
Marfan syndrome, 213
  for aortic dissection, 215
Marijuana and cocaine, 29
Marital adjustment, 655
  clinical course, 656
  treatment, 656
MAS. *See* Meconium aspiration syndrome
Mask of pregnancy, 92
Massive maternal injuries, 312
Mastitis, 633–635
  clinical presentation, 634
  definition and incidence, 633
  pathophysiology, 633–634
  treatment, 634
Mastitis, infection of breast tissue, 629
Maternal adjustment, 645–653
Maternal alcohol, cause for birth defects and mental retardation, 28
Maternal and Fetal Medicine Units (MFMU), 170
Maternal blood flow, 312
Maternal diabetes, 187
  laboratory evaluation for, 191
Maternal fever, predictors of infection, 472

Maternal group B streptococcal infection, 353
Maternal hydration, with oral water, 190
Maternal hyperthyroidism, 245
Maternal injury, minor, 312
Maternal morbidity, cause of, 479
Maternal mortality, 170
  cause of, 495
Maternal obesity, for cesarean delivery, 14
Maternal pelvimetry, techniques to assess, 513
Maternal position, at birth, 428
Maternal rubella serology, 38
Maternal serum AFP (MSAFP), 193
Maternal serum α-fetoprotein (MSAFP), 40, 162
Maternal serum quadruple screen, 193
Maternal serum screening, second-trimester,
  63, 196
Maternal serum triple screen (MSTS), 193
Maternal smoking, adverse effects of, 120
Maternal subclinical hypothyroidism, general
  screening for, 244
Maternal uterus and adnexa, evaluation of, 60
Maternity care
  CAM and applications in, 52–58
  complementary and alternative medicine in,
    51–58
  improving safety and quality in, 1–9
    characteristics of high-reliability organiza-
      tions, 4–6
    clinical process improvement, 6–7
    improving patient safety, 1–2
    strategies to improve, 2–4
Maternity/parental leave, 660–661
Mauriceau-Smellie-Veit maneuver, 514, 545
MBPP. See Modified biophysical profile
MCA. See Middle cerebral artery
MCV. See Mean cell volume
McRoberts maneuver, 467
Mean arterial pressure (MAP), with antihyper-
  tensive agents, 183
Mean cell volume (MCV), 193
Measles infection, during pregnancy, 50
Measles, mumps, and rubella (MMR), 47
  history of, 50
Meclizine (Antivert), 87
Meconium aspiration syndrome (MAS), 181,
  585, 630
Meconium-stained amniotic fluid (MSAF), 584,
  585, 587
  background and epidemiology, 585
  evaluating, 196
  intrapartum management for, 587
  management of, 587
  recognition and characterization of, 587
Meconium staining, during labor or delivery, 417
Medicaid Managed Care (MMC), 105
Medicaid programs, for maternity care, 105
Medical contraindications
  absolute, 95–96
  relative, 96
Medications
  classification of, 44–46
  during pregnancy, 46
  with teratogenic risk, 45t
Medicine practice domains, complementary
  and alternative, 51t
Megaloblastic anemia, 227–228
Meningococcal infection
  cause of bacterial meningitis, 49
  history of, 49
  safety in pregnancy, 49

Menses, irregular, an atypical LMP, 23
Menstrual age, of pregnancy, 134
Meralgia paresthetica (MP), 322
Mercury, 18, 31
Metabolic syndrome and insulin resistance, 181
Metformin
  in first trimester, 251
  with polycystic ovarian syndrome, 156
Methamphetamine abuse, during pregnancy, 118
Methamphetamines, 112
  effect of, 118
  use of, 118
Methotrexate
  and aminopterin, 228
  folic acid antagonist, 141
  use of, 141
Methyldopa, 221
  for treatment of chronic hypertension in
    pregnancy, 221
Methylergonovine (Methergine), 215, 291, 484,
  565
Metoclopramide (Reglan), 87
Metoprolol and pindolol, 215, 238
Metronidazole, 258, 357
  and ciprofloxacin, 233
MFMU. See Maternal and Fetal Medicine Units
MHA. See Microhemagglutination
Miconazole, 273
Microcephaly and optic atrophy, 113
Microhemagglutination (MHA), 264
Midazolam, 291
Middle cerebral artery (MCA), 347
Migraine headache, 238
  treatment of, 238
Military aviation, estimates on "human factors", 4
Milk composition, 629
Miscarriage
  management of, 144–148
  risk for, 130, 148
"Misgav Ladach" cesarean technique, 564
Misoprostol, 484, 619
  administer, 565
  contraindications to, 147
  prescription for, 147t
  prostaglandin E_1 analog, 146
  role in prevention of PPH, 482
Missed abortion, 145
Mitral stenosis, 215
  and aortic stenosis, 213
Mitral valve prolapse, 216
MMC. See Medicaid Managed Care
MMR. See Measles, mumps, and rubella
MMT. See Multiple marker testing
Modified biophysical profile (MBPP), 342
  negative predictive value of, 346
  positive predictive value, of, 346, 346t
Modified Ritgen maneuver, 538
Molding process, in contracted pelvis, 388
MoMo. See Monoamnionic, monochorionic
  pregnancy
Monoamnionic, monochorionic (MoMo)
  pregnancy, 162
Monochorionic pregnancy, complications from,
  162–163
Monozygous twins, after fertilization, 162
Mood disorders, 334
Morphine sulfate (Duramorph), 404
Mothers survey, results of nationwide listening
  to, 74t
Moxibustion, use of, 511

MP. See Meralgia paresthetica
MSAF. See Meconium-stained amniotic fluid
MSAFP. See Maternal serum AFP
MSTS. See Maternal serum triple screen
Multiple-dose methotrexate therapy, 142
Multiple gestation, 72, 161–168
  and adverse outcomes, 161–162
  clinical findings, 162
  common presentations, 162
  detection of, 161
  diagnosis of, 163
  discordant growth in, 162
  discovered by ultrasound, 186
  incidental diagnosis, 162
  management of, 163–164
  risk factor for, 161, 162
  variations of, 162
Multiple-gestation pregnancies, in screening, 197
Multiple marker testing (MMT), 41
  use of, 41
Multiple pregnancy, 519–520
Multiple sclerosis, 238
Multiple tests, use of, 556
Multivariate analysis, predictive factors in, 174
Mumps, and rubella, 296
MVA. See Manual vacuum aspirator
Myasthenia gravis, 238–239
  medications, 238–239
Myasthenic crisis, 238
Mycobacterium tuberculosis, 210
Mycoplasma pneumoniae and chlamydia pneu-
  moniae, atypical agents, 208
Myosin, affinity of, 362

N
NAATs. See Nucleic acid amplification tests
Naegele's rule, 23
NAEPP. See National Asthma Education and
  Prevention Program Expert Panel Report
Nalbuphine (Nubain), 404
Naloxone hydrochloride, 585
Naloxone (Narcan), 404
Naltrexone (ReVia), 404
Narcotic pain control, 399–400
Nasal congestion, 91
  causative factors, 91
  treatment of, 91
Nasal corticosteroids, for allergic rhinitis, 91
Nasooropharynx, with DeLee suction device, 417
National Asthma Education and Prevention Pro-
  gram (NAEPP) Expert Panel Report, 204
  expert panel statement, 207
National Center for Complementary and Alter-
  native Medicine (NCCAM), 51
National Collaborative Perinatal project, 71
National Health and Nutrition Examination
  Surveys (NHANES), 275
National Health Information Survey, comple-
  mentary and alternative medicine therapy
  included in, 52t
National High Blood Pressure Education Pro-
  gram (NHBPEP), 221
National Institute for Health and Clinical Excel-
  lence guideline, 176
National Institute of Child Health and Human
  Development (NICHD), 170, 615
National Institute of Health and Clinical Excel-
  lence, on vaginal birth, 178

National Institute of Mental Health prospective data, 332
National Institutes of Health (NIH), 285
    consensus development conference on cesarean childbirth, 169
    on counselling, 38
    for interpretation of EFM, 455
    for ultrasonography in pregnancy, 60t
National Survey on Drug Use and Health (NSDUH), 116
Natural Family Planning (NFP), 640
Nausea and vomiting, 54, 57, 86–88
    causative factors, 86
    in early pregnancy, 72
    prevalence and epidemiology, 86
    treatment of, 86–87
Nausea gravidarum, for diagnosing pregnancy, 23
Nausea, symptoms of early pregnancy, 22
NCCAM. See National Center for Complementary and Alternative Medicine
Needle tip, as bright echo, 558f
Negative Predictive Value (NPV), 618
Neiguan point, 53
Neisseria gonorrhea infection, 261
Neonatal alloimmune thrombocytopenia, 230
Neonatal asphyxia, 466
Neonatal circumcision, 588–594
    analgesia, 589–592
    epidemiology, 589
    risks, benefits, and informed consent, 589
Neonatal complications, 181
Neonatal grunting, effects on, 418
Neonatal herpes, management during pregnancy to prevent, 276–277
Neonatal infections
    bacterial causes, 603
    clinical features, 603–604
    diagnosis, 604
    pathogenesis, 603
    presumptive tests for predicting, 605t
    prevention, 606–607
    risk for, 83
    treatment, 604–606
Neonatal injury, common clinical problems for, 4
Neonatal intensive care unit (NICU), 155, 438
Neonatal jaundice, 594–601
    diagnosis, 596–597
        history, 596
        physical examination, 596–597
    epidemiology, 595
    pathogenesis, 595–596
        breastfeeding-associated jaundice, 595–596
        pathologic jaundice, 596
        physiologic jaundice, 595
        true breast milk jaundice, 596
    risk factors, 595
        ethnicity, 595
        gestational age, 595
Neonatal lupus, dermatologic and hematologic manifestations of, 256
Neonatal myasthenia
    of neonates, 239
    in premature infant, 239
Neonatal outcomes, adverse, in multiple gestation, 161–162
Neonatal resuscitation, 580–588
    medications for, 586t
Neonatal Resuscitation Program (NRP), 581
Neonatal sepsis, clinical signs of, 603

Neonate, general care of, 615
Nephrolithiasis, 308
    diagnosis of, 308
    management of, 308
    presentation of, 308
Nephrotic syndrome, 241–242
    diagnosis of, 241
Neural tube defects (NTDs), 193
Neurologic conditions, 234–239
Newborn circumcision
    common techniques for, 592f
    risks and benefits of, 590t
Newborn physical examinations, common and uncommon deviations from normal on, 574t
Newborns, preventive health measures for, 576–579
Newman score, 517t
New York Academy of Medicine, 402
New York Heart Association classification I or II, 213
NFP. See Natural family planning
NHANES. See National Health and Nutrition Examination Surveys
NHBPEP. See National High Blood Pressure Education Program
NICHD. See National Institute of Child Health and Human Development
Nicotine delivery systems, use of, in pregnancy, 123–124
NICU. See Neonatal intensive care unit
Nifedipine, 364
    agent for tocolysis, 167
    and hydralazine, 221
NIH. See National Institutes of Health
Nipple shields, 626b
Nipple stimulation, for ovarian suppression, 640
Nitrazine paper, 371
Nitrazine test, 391
Nitrazine, with bloody show and cervical mucus, 391
Nizatidine, during lactation, 88
NND. See Number needed to diagnose
NNT. See Number needed to treat
Non-GBS pathogens, incidence of, 602
Nonimmune hydrops fetalis, cause of, 305
Nonpregnancy-related conditions, during first trimester, 132
Nonreactive nonstress test, management of, 342–343
Nonreassuring fetal heart rate patterns
    assess and manage cause of, 459
    management of, 459–462
Nonreassuring fetal heart rate tracings, 459–461
Non-reassuring fetal status, 455
Nonsteroidal antiinflammatory agents, 255
Nonstress test (NST), 339, 492
    administration of, 342
    and amniotic fluid index, 157
    antenatal fetal surveillance, 159
    criteria for reactive or normal, 342
    evidence to support use of, 343
    improving diagnostic accuracy, 342
    indications and contraindications, 342
    use of, as screening test, 340t
Nontreponemal test, 36
Nonviable fetus and abruption, 478
Norepinephrine and epinephrine, 314
Normal accidents theory, 1
    premise of, 2

Normal delivery and birthing positions, 413–419
    maneuvers of, 415–418
    positioning for, 414–415
    preparation for, 413–414
Normal fetal surveillance tests, reassurance of, 340t
Normal FHR baseline, presence of, 455
Normal infant bowel movements, 616
Normal labor, 383–394
    causes of, 383
    definitions of, 383
    onset of, 383
    stages of, 383–393
        bishop's scores, 384
        care in, 389–391
        dilation, 383
        effacement, 383–384
        labor interventions, 391–393
        phases of, 384–386
Normal newborn, management of, 572–580
Nosebleeds, reduced or prevented by application of petroleum jelly, 91
Nothing by mouth (NPO), 391
NPO. See Nothing by mouth
NPV. See Negative Predictive Value
NRP. See Neonatal Resuscitation Program
NSDUH. See National Survey on Drug Use and Health
NST. See Nonstress test
NTDs. See Neural tube defects
Nuchal cord
    assessment for, 525
    presence of, 525
Nucleic acid amplification tests (NAATs), 37
    sensitivity of, 37
Nugent method, 271
Nulliparas and multiparas, 422
Number needed to diagnose (NND)
    definition of, 35
    use of, 35
Number needed to treat (NNT), concept of, 35
Nutrition, in pregnancy and lactation, 66–73
    conditions requiring dietary management, 71–72
    nutritional status, 66–71
    requirements for, 72–73
Nystatin cream, 273

O

Obesity, and gestational weight gain, 188
Obsessive-compulsive disorder (OCD), 336–337, 651–652
    clinical features/diagnosis, 652
    epidemiology and risk factors, 652
    treatment, 652
Obstetric contraindications
    absolute, 95
    relative, 96
Obstetric palsy, 322
    at-risk patients, 322
    footdrop palsy, 322
    pathophysiology of, 322
Obstetric ultrasound examinations, clinical standards for, 60–61
OCD. See Obsessive-compulsive disorder
Occiput anterior, 387, 538f
Occiput posterior, 387

Occiput posterior position, 507–509
  definition, causes, and effects, 507–508
    effects on perinatal outcome, 507–508
    epidemiology, 507
    natural history, 507
  diagnosis, 508
  management, 508–509
    delivery from an occiput posterior position, 508–509
    maneuvers to correct an occiput posterior position, 508
Odds ratios, 315t
Office library, in complementary and alternative medicine, 58t
Ogita test, 476
Olanzapine, 334
Oligohydramnios, 189–190, 349
  with abnormal fetal heart rate, 341
  in first and second trimesters, 189
  and polyhydramnios, 189–191
  prognosis of, 189
Omphalocele, ventral defects, 196
Ondansetron, serotonin receptor antagonist, 87
Open glottis, with closed glottis, 421
Open surgical approach, for treating ectopic pregnancy, 142
Operative vaginal delivery, 545
Opiates, abuse of, during pregnancy, 115–116
  associated perinatal effects, 115–116
  diagnostic options, 116
  long-term sequelae, 116
  pathophysiology of, 115
  prevalence of, 115
  screening options for, 116
  treatment of, 116
Opiates, substance abuse in pregnant women, 112
Optical density, 556
  of amniotic fluid, 556
  for assessment of bilirubin in Rh isoimmunization, 559
Optic atrophy, 223
"opt-out" approach, 288
Oral antihypertensive medicines, choice of, during pregnancy, 221
Oral dextrose, for low blood sugar infant, 158
Oral hypoglycemic agents, 157
Oral medications, use of, 251
Oral penicillin V, 215
Oral vitamin K, 578
Organic solvents, 18
Organizational change, phases of, 7
Oropharyngeal suction, 417
Overweight women, 68
Oxygenated blood, redistribution of, 190
Oxytocic agents, 485
Oxytocics, use of, 490
Oxytocin, 291, 451, 484, 618
  administer, 565
  as bolus injection, 215
  versus conservative, 443
  drug of choice for prevention of hemorrhage, 482
  induction of labor with, 178
  versus prostaglandin, 443
  release of, 82–83
  during second-stage labor, 535
  use of, 392, 440
Oxytocin augmentation, 439
  use of, 437
Oxytocin protocols, 439t

P
PACTG. See Pediatric AIDS clinical trials group
Pain
  methods for management of, in labor, 421
  during second stage of labor, 530
Pain control techniques, pharmacologic, 399–404
Pain management, options for, 589–591
Pain relief, in labor, 54
Pajot's maneuver, 538
Panic attacks, 336–337
  nonpharmacologic treatment, 336
  pharmacologic treatment, 336–337
Panic disorder, 652
  clinical course, 652
  clinical features/diagnosis, 652
  epidemiology, 652
  treatment, 652
PAPP-A. See Pregnancy-associated plasma protein A
PAPP-A and β-hCG, 195
Pap smears/human papillomavirus test, 325–326
Paracervical block, 530
  complications, 530
  contraindications, 530
  indications, 530
  technique, 530
  technique of administering, 401
Parenteral opioids, for labor pain, 400t
Parenting and family issues, preparation for, 78–79
  hospital care and counseling, 79
  prenatal counseling, 78
Partogram score
  assigning second-stage, 422t
  second stage with initial second-stage, for nulliparas, 422t
Partogram, use of, 422
Parvovirus B19, 305–306
  clinical features, 305
  diagnosis of, 305–306
  epidemiology of, 305
  pathogenesis of, 305
  prevention of, 306
  single stranded DNA virus, 305
  treatment of, 306
Paternal adjustment, 654–655
  clinical features, 654–655
  diagnosis, 654
  epidemiology/risk factors, 654
  treatment, 654–655
Pathogenesis, 194
Pathogens, cervical cultures for, 165
Pathologic jaundice, causes of, 596t
Patient and family education, 66–101
Patient health questionnaire-9, 647
PCR. See Polymerase chain reaction
PDSA. See Plan-Do-Study-Act cycle
PDSS. See Postpartum depression screening scale
Peak expiratory flow (PEF), 204
Peak expiratory flow rate (PFR), 204
Pediatric AIDS clinical trials group (PACTG), 289t
PEF. See Peak expiratory flow
PEG. See Polyethylene glycol
Pelvic adequacy, evaluation of, 388–389
Pelvic/back and leg pain, 90
  causative factors, 90
  treatment of, 90

Pelvic examination
  for detecting abnormalities of reproductive tract, 30
  for screening STD, 30
Pelvic fluid, analysis of, 138
Pelvic inflammatory disease (PID), 17, 259
Pelvic kidney, 242
Pelvic masses, presence of, 133
Pelvimetry, prognostic value of, in cephalic presentations, 30
Pelvis
  blood and amniotic fluid from, 564
  engagement in, 392
Pemphigoid gestationis, 317, 319f
  clinical course, 317
  pathophysiology, 317
  treatment/management of, 318
Penicillin
  allergic to, 265
  with β-lactamase inhibitor, 209
  during early pregnancy, 35
Penis/circumcision care, 615
Pennington clamps, 564
PEOPLE (Pushing Early or Pushing Late with Epidural) study, to reduce second-stage cesarean birth, 417
PEP. See Polymorphic eruption of pregnancy
Peptic ulcer disease, 233–234
  frequency of, 233
Percutaneous umbilical artery, diagnosis by, 230
Perimortem cesarean delivery, 315
Perinatal mortality, 349
  estimation of, 170
Perinatal units, characteristics of high-reliability, 5
Perineal and pelvic floor anatomy, 543
Perineal damage, prevention and treatment of, 428
Perineal healing, 640
Perineal laceration or episiotomy, overlapping repair of, 551f
Perineal skin, repair of, 548–549
Perineal tear, repair of, 433f
Perineal trauma, concern for, 542
Perineum trauma, management of, 423–430
  clinical course and prevention, 426–428
  diagnosis of, 424
  epidemiology, 424
    factors associated with increased, 424
    factors associated with lower rates of, 424
    incidence, 424
    wide variation in episiotomy rates, 424
  episiotomy, 424
  treatment of, 424–426
    method of repair of, 425
    suturing versus nonsuturing of, 424
    type of suture material for, 425
Periodontal disease, 370
  assessment for, 370
  treatment of, 357
Periodontitis, in pregnancy, 29
Peripartum cardiomyopathy
  diagnosis of, 216
  incidence of, 216
Permanent urinary diversion, 242
PFR. See Peak expiratory flow rate
Pharmacologic therapy, risks of, 205
Phenylalanine, product of aspartame, 31

Phenytoin, 334
    antiepileptic medications, 25
    drugs with hypothyroidism, 246
Pheochromocytoma, causes of secondary hypertension, 219
Phosphatidyl glycerol, 555–556
    appearance of, 555–556
    presence of, 555–556
    testing for, 555–556
Phototherapy, 599–600
    guidelines for, 599f
    types of, 599
Pica, compulsive eating of nonnutritive substances, 72
PID. *See* Pelvic inflammatory disease
PISA/clock repair, 551f
Placenta
    active third-stage management of, 432
    entrapped, 488
    evaluation, 524–525
    examination of, 432
    manual removal of, 432, 432f, 490
    retained and invasive placenta, 480
Placenta accrete
    risk factors for, 489t
    suspected, 490
Placental abruption, 121, 312, 477
    associated symptoms, 477
    bleeding characteristics, 477
    cause of fetal death in trauma, 312
    with chronic hypertension, 221
    with cocaine, 113
    incidence of, 221
    management of, 478–479
    ultrasound examination, 477
Placental cells, 39
Placenta previa, 166–167, 477–478
    abdominal ultrasound, 477
    anterior, 524
    clinical evaluation, 477
    clinical presentation of, 166
    complications of, 166
    diagnosis of, 166
    effects of prematurity, 477
    incidence of, 166
    management strategies of, 166
    posterior, 524
    risk factors for, 166
    transperineal or transvaginal ultrasound, 477
Plan-Do-Study-Act (PDSA) cycle, 6, 369–370
Plastibell device, 592
Platelet transfusions, in presence of active bleeding, 229
Pneumococcal infection
    administration of, 49
    current vaccine, 49
    history of, 49
    indication for vaccine, 49
Pneumocystis carinii, trimethoprim-sulfamethoxazole for, 289
Pneumonia, 208
    causative organisms of, 208
    complications of, 208
    diagnosis of, 208–209
    epidemiology and risk factors, 207–209
    an inflammation of bronchioles and alveoli, 207–210
    microbiology and clinical features, 208
    in pregnancy, 295

Pneumonia *(Continued)*
    prevention of, 209–210
    treatment of, 209
Pneumothorax, and acute tubular necrosis, 86
Podofilox, purified derivative of podophyllin, 279
Podophyllin, an antimitotic agent, 279
Podophyllin resin, 279
Poliomyelitis
    history of, 50
    indications for use, 50
    vaccination during pregnancy, 50
Poliovirus, an enterovirus, 50
Polycystic kidney disease, 242
Polyethylene glycol (PEG), 88
Polyglactin suture (Vicryl Rapide), 548
Polyglactin (Vicryl), 548, 550
Polyhydramnios, 190
    causes of, 190
    indicator of poor control, 250
    maternal effect of, 191
    treatments for, 191
Polymerase chain reaction (PCR), 260
    for NAATs, 37
Polymorphic eruption of pregnancy (PEP), 317, 319
    causative factors, 319
    clinical presentation, 319
    incidence of, 319
    key features, 319
    pathophysiology, 319
    treatment, 319
POPs. *See* Progestin-only pills
Positive predictive value (PPV), 618
Positive-pressure ventilation, delivering, 583
Postdates, 348
Posterior arm
    delivery of, 468
    to relieve shoulder dystocia, 468
Posterior fornix, appearance of, 132
Posterior shoulder, abduction of, 468f
Posterior superior iliac spine (PSIS), 400f
Postoperative blood replacement, criteria for, 566
Postoperative care and order writing, general principles of, 566–567
Postoperative care, differential diagnosis of, 566
Postpartum anal incontinence, 552–553
Postpartum contraception, 639–643
Postpartum depression, 645–650
    clinical features, 646–647
    diagnosis and screening, 647–648
    epidemiology, 645
    management recommendations, 648–650
    pathogenesis, 646
    prevention of, 650
    risk factors, 645
Postpartum depression screening scale (PDSS), 647
Postpartum endometritis, 619–622
    causes of, 619–620
    definition and epidemiology, 619
    diagnosis, 621
    prevention of, 621–622
    risk factors, 620–621
    treatment, 622
Postpartum hemorrhage (PPH), 479–486, 481
    causes of, 481
    clinical course, 486
    definitions of, 479
    delayed, 618–619
        definition, 618

Postpartum hemorrhage (PPH) *(Continued)*
    diagnosis, 618
    treatment, 618–619
    diagnosing and treating, 483f
    diagnosis/clinical features, 481
    diagnosis-specific approach to treatment, 484–486
    epidemiology, risk factors, and pathogenesis, cause-specific features, 479
    general epidemiology and risk factors, 479
    prevention, 481–482
    risk for, 485
    treatment, 482–486
Postpartum perineal pain
    therapeutic ultrasound to treat, 425–426
    topical anesthetics to treat, 425
Postpartum psychosis, 650–651
    clinical course, 651
    clinical features, 650
    epidemiology/risk factors, 650
    treatment, 651
Postpartum relapse, risk factors for, 124
Postpartum thyroiditis, 635–636
    clinical features, 635
    diagnosis, 635–636
    epidemiology/risk factors, 635
    pathogenesis, 635
    pitfalls and controversies, 636
    treatment, 636
Postterm pregnancy, management of, 339–351
    clinical course and prevention, 350
    clinical features, 349
        fetal complications, 349
        maternal complications, 349
    epidemiology and risk factors, 348–349
    pathogenesis, 349
Posttraumatic stress disorder (PTSD), 651–652
    clinical features/diagnosis, 651
    criteria for, 651
    epidemiology and risk factors, 651
    treatment, 651
Potassium hydroxide (KOH), 166
    with blood specimen, 476
Potassium iodide and dexamethasone, 245
PPH. *See* Postpartum hemorrhage
PPROM. *See* Preterm premature rupture of membranes
PPV. *See* Positive predictive value
PRAMS. *See* Pregnancy Risk Assessment Monitoring System
Preconception care, 10–20
    alcohol, 14
    cocaine, 14–15
    components of, 10
    family planning, 11
    genetics, 15
    health care for women, 10
    heroin, 15
    infectious diseases, 15–18
    medical conditions, 12–14
    mental health and perinatal outcomes, 19
    nutrition, 14
    parental social behavior, 14
    preconception risk assessment, 11
    pregnancy readiness, 11
    prenatal care and ongoing primary care, 11
    psychological risk, 18
    rationale for, 10
    tobacco, 14
    toxicities, 18

Preconception health promotion, 10–11
Preconception intervention, impact of, 10
Preconceptual screening, with hemoglobino-
    pathy, 38
Predelivery, 481
Prednisone
    treatment with, 230
    for use in pregnancy, 233
Preeclampsia, 220
    development of, 220
    incidence of, 28, 241
    monitoring for superimposed, 221
    multiorgan disease, 491
    superimposed, 221
Preeclampsia and eclampsia, 491–494
    diagnosis, 491–492
    epidemiology and pathogenesis, 491
        associated risk factors, 491
        causative factors, 491
    treatment, 492–494
        antepartum surveillance, 492
        HELLP syndrome, 493–494
        hypertension, 492–493
        mild preeclampsia, 492
        postpartum care, 494
        prevention, 494
        seizure prophylaxis, 493
        severe preeclampsia, 492
        timing of delivery, 492
Pregestational diabetes, classification of, 248t
Pregnancy
    adolescent, 71–72
    cardiovascular changes in, 214t
    chronic medical conditions in, 202–257
    commonly encountered medical problems in,
        258–329
    complications of, 151–201
    diagnosis and dating of, 22–24
        background, 22
        signs and symptoms of, 22–23
    diagnostic ultrasound in, 59–64
        common indications, 59–60
    exercise and, 31–32, 95–100
    heroin during, 15
    hypertensive disorders of, 34
    immunizations in, 47–51
    medical emergencies in, 495–498
    medications in, 43–46
        history, 43
    periodontitis in, 29
    physiologic adaptations to, 97–98
    physiologic changes and common discomforts
        of, 86–93
    physiology of, 72
    screening in, 34–41
    sexual intercourse during, 32
    treatment of psychiatric disorders in,
        330–338
Pregnancy-associated plasma protein A
    (PAPP-A), 192
Pregnancy dating, 180, 250
Pregnancy failure, early, 144–145
    anembryonic pregnancy, 144
    complete abortion, 144
    embryonic demise, 144
    incomplete abortion, 144
Pregnancy interventions, 102–129
Pregnancy, monitoring progress of, 33–34
    health promotion activities, 34
    laboratory testing, 34

Pregnancy, monitoring progress of (Continued)
    ongoing risk assessment, 33
    physical examination, 34
Pregnancy readiness, preconception promotion
    of, 11
Pregnancy-related conditions, during first
    trimester, 132
Pregnancy Risk Assessment Monitoring System
    (PRAMS), 102
Pregnancy tests, based on monoclonal antibody
    with hCG, 23
Pregnant women
    diet of, 66
    groups of, 25
    protein supplement for, 31
Preload, 213
Premature birth, in dichorionic pregnancy, 162
Premature labor, risk for, 238
Premature/low-birth-weight infants, prevention
    of, 369
Prematurity
    cause of perinatal mortality and morbidity,
        166
    complications of, 352
Prenatal care
    content of, 21–65
    federal funding for, 105
    history of, 21–22
    initial assessment, 28–32
    risk factors for inadequate, 22
Prenatal education, effect of, 398
Prenatal pediatric visit, 78–79
Prenatal psychosocial profile measures, 103
Prenatal social environment inventory, deter-
    mines stress in women's lives, 103
Prenatal Substance Abuse Treatment programs,
    components of, 115
Prenatal visits
    documentation of care, 27
    preconception care, 24–27
    schedule of, 26–27
    topics in preconception care, 25–26
Prepregnancy weight
    maternal, 187
    normal, 68
Preterm birth
    with oral betamimetics, 164
    prevention of, 161, 164
    risk for, 239
Preterm delivery (PTD)
    accurate assessment of risk for, 352
    clinical indicators and risk for, 353t
    DDS ratios for, 352
    high risk for, 357
    incidence of, 357
    management of, 368
        anesthesia, 368
        diagnosis of fetal asphyxia, 368
        fetal surveillance, 368
        maternal transfer, 368
        route and method of delivery, 368
    psychosocial interventions for prevention
        of, 356
        activity restriction, 356
        antenatal education, 356
        lifestyle modification, 356
        nutritional support, 356
        psychosocial support, 356
        regular nursing contact, 356
        sexual activity, 356

Preterm delivery (PTD) (Continued)
    risk factors for, 352–355, 354t
        demographic and historical risk factors,
            352–353
        establishment of risk, 353–355
        maternal infection, 353
Preterm labor (PTL), 239, 383, 471
    assessment of, 526
    common signs of, 33
    and delivery, increased risk for, 276
    diagnosis of, 356, 358–361
        distinguishing false from true labor, 360
            serial examinations, 360
            single-dose terbutaline, 360
    evaluation of, flow diagram of, 359f
    fetal prognosis, 361
    initial evaluation of symptomatic patient,
        358–360
        establish integrity of fetal membranes, 358
        fetal fibronectin, 360
        infectious disease surveillance, 360
        serial digital cervical examinations, 360
        ultrasound examination, 360
        urinalysis, 360
    management of pain in, 368
    and PPROM, association with, 266
    scoring system for, 33
Preterm labor, pharmacologic management of,
    361–366
    β-sympathomimetics, 362–363
        adverse drug effects, 362
        dosage and monitoring of therapy, 362
        efficacy, 362
        mechanism of action, 362
        metabolism, 362
    laboratory studies, 362
    tocolysis, contraindications to, 361
Preterm labor risk assessment, 354t
Preterm premature rupture of membranes
    (PPROM), 260, 341, 352, 371–373, 472
    definition of, 371
    diagnosis and initial assessment, 371
    epidemiology, 371
    on gestation, 372f
    management of, 371–373
    natural history, 371
    risk factors for, 371
    ultrasound evaluation of, 371
Primigravida, cervical effacement and dilation
    in, 384f
Procedure codes, 552
Prochlorperazine (Compazine), 87
Progestational agent versus placebo, in women,
    357f
Progesterone testing, quantitative serum, 139
Progesterone, use of, 370
Progestin-only pills (POPs), 640
Prolonged pregnancy, 383
Promethazine (Phenergan), 87
Prophylactic amnioinfusion, 533
Prophylactic bed rest, use of, 356
Prophylactic cesarean, 466–467
Prophylaxis, with β-blockers, 238
Prostaglandin F$_2$α, 207
Prostaglandins
    for cervical ripening, 177
    role in processes of cervical ripening, 364
    types of, 447
    use of, 450

Prostaglandins *(Continued)*
  use of, for cervical ripening, 176
Prostaglandin synthetase inhibitors, 364–365
  adverse drug effects, 364
  dosage, 365
  efficacy, 364
  mechanism, 364
  treatment of PTL, 364
Prosthetic heart valves, 225
Proteins
  in colostrum, 80
  for fetal growth, 67
  increased maternal blood, 67
Proteinuria
  hyperuricemia and, 12
  and uric acid, 12
Prothrombin gene mutation, 180
Pruritic skin diseases, algorithm for differential
    diagnosis of, in pregnancy, 318f
Pruritic urticarial papules and plaques of preg-
    nancy (PUPPP), 317, 320f
Pseudogestational sac, on ectopic pregnancy,
    136
Pseudotumor cerebri, 239
PSIS. *See* Posterior superior iliac spine
Psychoprophylaxis, 398
  history of, 398
  nonpharmacologic pain control techniques,
    399
Psychosocial interventions, 102–105
  identification of, 103
  interventions, 103–105
  psychosocial indicators and adverse perinatal
    outcomes, 102–103
Psychotherapy, with mild-to-moderate depres-
    sion, 331
PTD. *See* Preterm delivery
PTL. *See* Preterm labor
PTSD. *See* Posttraumatic stress disorder
Pudendal and paracervical blocks, 529–532
Pudendal block, 401, 531–532
  complications, 531
  contraindications, 531
  indications, 531
  technique, 531–532
Puerperal infection, common cause of, 622
Pulmonary problems, in pregnancy,
    202–212
  asthma, 202–207
  pneumonia, 207–210
  tuberculosis, 210–212
PUPPP. *See* Pruritic urticarial papules and
    plaques of pregnancy
Pushing, method of, during second stage,
    428
Pyelonephritis
  clinical signs of, 293
  treatment for, 294
Pyridoxine
  with doxylamine, 86
  in pregnancy, 56
  without doxylamine, 86

Q
Quad test, 41
Quality improvement program, design/
    implementation, 369–370
Quinolones, 258, 262

R
Radioisotope studies, method for diagnosis of
    DVT, 225
Radiopaque contrast agents, 84
RADIUS. *See* Routine antenatal diagnostic imag-
    ing with ultrasound study
Randomized controlled trial (RCT), 66, 260, 343,
    363, 382, 436, 462, 508, 530, 587, 618, 648
  with abnormal glucose tolerance, 155
  comparing theophylline, 206
  of low-dose aspirin, 164
Ranitidine and metoclopramide, 205
Rapid plasma regain (RPR), 36, 264
  and VDRL tests, 36
Rapid strep tests, 267
RCA. *See* Root cause analysis
RCT. *See* Randomized controlled trial
Recombinant factor VIIa, hemostatic drugs,
    482
Rectal mucosa and internal anal sphincter,
    549f
Red blood cell, risk for neonatal hyperbilirubi-
    nemia, 151
Reflux symptoms, during pregnancy, 88
Regional analgesia, 401–404
Regional anesthesia, 536
  use of, 437
Relapse rates, during pregnancy, 238
Relaxation techniques, 399
Renal disease, 241–242
  end-stage
    dialysis, 241
    transplant recipients, 241
Renal function, evaluation of, 220
Ropivacaine (Naropin), 403
Repetitive variable decelerations, severe, 459f
REPRORISK system, for medication during
    pregnancy, 46
Research and process improvement, difference in
    measurement between, 6t
Respiratory distress syndrome, 158, 181, 362, 373
Respiratory system, changes in, during preg-
    nancy, 203t
Resuscitation
  anticipation, 581
  assemble team, 581
  of depressed infant, 581–585
  overview of, in delivery room, 582f
  preparation for, 580–581
  unsuccessful, 585
Retained placenta, 481, 488–490
  diagnosis and treatment, 489–490
  epidemiology, 488
  pathogenesis and clinical features, 488–489
  prevention, 490
Rheumatic fever prophylaxis, 215
Rheumatic heart disease, 213
Rheumatoid arthritis, 254–255
  intrapartum management, 255
  natural history in pregnancy, 254–255
  use of medications, 255
Rh immunoglobulin, 314–316
Rh isoimmunization, 555
Rh status, with first-trimester abortion, 148
Rhythm method, 643
Richardson retractor, 564
Rickets, 630
Rifampin, drugs for use during pregnancy, 211
Risk assessment, guidelines for, 11
Risk factor–alone approach, 268

Ritgen maneuver
  deliver fetal head, 421
  modified, 416
Robin syndrome, 585
Room humidifier, use of, 91
Root cause analysis (RCA), 3
Routine admission test strip, evidence for, 412
Routine antenatal diagnostic imaging with
    ultrasound (RADIUS) study, 63
  criticisms of, 63
Royal College of Obstetricians and Gynaecolo-
    gists, on vaginal birth, 178
RPR. *See* Rapid plasma regain
Rubella, 16, 295–296
  epidemiology of, 295
  history of, 295–296
Rubella immunity, prenatal screening for, 50
Rubella infection, common childhood illness, 50
Rubin II maneuver, 468
Rubin's maneuver, 468f
Rutosides, mixture of natural or semisynthetic
    flavonoids, 92

S
Saline amnioinfusion, 461–462
  contraindications, 461
  indication for, 461
SBE. *See* Subacute bacterial endocarditis
Schizophrenia, 337–338
  diagnosis of, 338
  effect of, 338
  treatment of, 338
Scleroderma and systemic sclerosis, 256–257
Screening
  in first trimester, 192
  goal of, 194
  instruments, 118
  for IUGR, 182
  in pregnancy and predictive value, 34–41
  risk factors justify, 286t
  strategies of, 194
  for thrombophilic disorders, 231
  in women at high risk, 182–183
  in women at low risk, 182
Screening tests, criteria for, during pregnancy,
    34–35
Seat belt, for pregnant women, 32, 311
Secondary hypertension, cause of, 219
Second-degree laceration, with preservation, 546f
Second-stage labor, management of, 419–423
  background and definitions, 419
  duration of, 419–420
    background, 419–420
    evidence, 420
  duration of risk factors for, 420
  with epidural, 420–421
  episiotomy, 421
  oxytocin augmentation in, 422
  perineal pain, 421
  perineum, 421–422
  positions of, 420
  pushing techniques, 421
  use of partogram, 422
Second-trimester ultrasound, 198
Second twin, version of, 519–520
Seizure disorders, 234–238
  clinical background, 234
  preconception assessment and planning, 235

Seizure disorders (*Continued*)
   preconception counseling with, 13
Seizure prophylaxis, duration of therapy, 493
Seizures
   effects of pregnancy on, 235
   medications, 237
Selective serotonin reuptake inhibitors (SSRIs), 331
   use of, 334
Septic pelvic thrombophlebitis, 637–639
   clinical features, 638
   diagnosis, 638
   epidemiology and risk factors, 637
   incidence, 637
   pathogenesis, 637
   risk factors, 637
   treatment, 639
Septic shock, 497–498
   diagnosis, 497–498
   epidemiology, 497
   management, 498
   pathophysiology, 497
   prevention, 498
Serologic test, 276
Serotonergic symptom scores, comparisons of, 332
Serotonin nor-adrenaline reuptake inhibitors (SNRIs), 336
Serum α fetoprotein, screening of, 40
Serum bicarbonate levels, 312
Serum hCG testing, 139
   on posttreatment days, 142
Serum hormone test, 133, 139
Serum liver function tests, 211
Serum markers, 604
Serum radioimmunoassay test, for detecting hCG concentrations, 23
Severe hyperbilirubinemia, risk factors for development of, 595t
Severity, classified by ultrasound, 190
Sexual intercourse, during pregnancy, 32
Sexually transmitted disease (STD)
   incidence of, 108
   prevention of, 11
   screening of, 370
   and urinary tract infections, 113
SGA. See Small-for-gestational age
Sheehan syndrome, 486
Shortened cervix, sonogram of, 360f
Shoulder dystocia, 465–470, 545
   antepartum risk factors for, 465t
   and brachial plexus injury, 157
   complications associated with, 466
      maternal, 466
      neonatal, 466
   diagnosis, 466
   epidemiology, 465
      definition, 465
      incidence, 465
   incidence of, 188, 536
   intrapartum risk factors for, 465t
   management of delivery, 467–469
   prevention of, 466–467
   relative risk for, 249
   risk factors, 465
      antepartum, 465
      intrapartum, 465
   of vaginal deliveries, 157
Shoulder presentation, 505
Shoulder rotation, 468

Shoulders, delivery of, 417–418
Sibling adjustment, 657
Siblings, preparation of, for birth, 76–77
Sickle cell
   and hemoglobinopathies, 193
   and thalassemia, 228
Sickle cell anemia
   chronic debilitating diseases, 15
   screening for, 38
Sickle cell disease, 13, 228
   postsplenectomy state, 209
Sickle cell trait, 228
Sickle hemoglobin, 228
SIDS. See Sudden infant death syndrome
Silicone, from collection tubes, 556
Simpson forceps, 537, 537f
Sims' position for birth, 414
Single kidney, 242
Single-parent families, 657–658
   epidemiology, 657
   risks to single parent and child, 657–658
   treatment, 658
Sinusitis, evaluate and treat for, 205
SIUGR, diagnosed using serial ultrasound scans, 182
Sjögren syndrome, 256
Skin and hair changes, 92
   causative factors, 92
   treatment of, 92
Skin incision, perform, 563–564
SLE. See Systemic lupus erythematosus
Sleeping, 615–616
   patterns, 615
   position, 615–616
Small for-dates pregnancy, 179–184
   causative factors of, 180
   clinical issue of, 179
   intrauterine growth restriction, 180–182
Small-for-gestational age (SGA), 180
Smoking
   assessment for, 370
   cause, for low-birth-weight baby, 14
   cause of adverse pregnancy outcome, 28
   fetal effects of, 14
   during late pregnancy, 29
   maternal complications of, 14
   in pregnancy, 120–125
      cessation programs, 122–124
      epidemiology of, 120
      magnitude of, 120–122
   secondary exposure associations, 14
Smoking cessation
   pharmacologic approach to, 123–124
   postpartum, 124–125
   resources for, 123t
SNRIs. See Serotonin nor-adrenaline reuptake inhibitors
Society of Obstetricians and Gynecologists of Canada (SOGC), 178, 268, 347, 412, 454
SOGC. See Society of Obstetricians and Gynecologists of Canada
Sore nipples, 627–628
Soy-based formulas, 611
Spinal anesthesia
   and epidural anesthesia, 561
   for operative procedures, 403
   technique of, 561–562
Spinal headaches, 566
Spiral computed tomography, method for diagnosis of DVT, 225

Spiramycin, treatment for toxoplasmosis, 303
Spitting, 616
Splenda, artificial sweetener, 31
Spontaneous rupture of membranes (SROM), 506
Spontaneous vaginal delivery (SVD), 503, 508
SROM. See Spontaneous rupture of membranes
SSRIs. See Selective serotonin reuptake inhibitors
Standard screening test, for CF, 194
Staphylococcus aureus, 620
STD. See Sexually transmitted disease
Sterile gloves, use of, 391
Stool softeners, 539
Stop exercising, signals to, during pregnancy, 100t
Storing formula, 611
Streptococcus agalactiae, 621
Streptococcus pneumoniae, 208
   cause of pneumonia, meningitis, and bacteremia, 49
Streptococcus pyogenes, 621
Striae gravidarum, over abdomen, breasts, and hips, 92
"Stuck" twin, diagnosis of, 524
Subacute bacterial endocarditis (SBE), 214
   prophylaxis, 216t
   protocol for, 214t
Substance abuse, in pregnancy, 112–119
Sudden infant death syndrome (SIDS), 114, 615
   risk for, 114
Sufentanil citrate (Sufenta), 404
Sulfasalazine and mesalazine, 233
Sulfonamides, risk for kernicterus, 258
Sulprostone, synthetic prostaglandin E$_2$, 489
Suprapubic pressure, 467–468
Suspected intrauterine growth restriction, treatment options for, 183
Suture, type of, 550
SVD. See Spontaneous vaginal delivery
"Swiss Cheese Model of Accidents", 1
Symphysiotomy, for delivery of shoulder dystocia, 469
Syphilis, 36, 263–265
   diagnosis of, 264–265
   effects on perinatal outcome, 263–264
   epidemiology of, 263
   incidence/prevalence of, 263
   latent, 263
   natural history, 263
   prevention of, 265
   primary, 263
   secondary, 263
   sexually transmitted infections, 17
   testing of, on pregnant women, 36
   treatment of, 265
   WHO on, 18
Systemic lupus erythematosus (SLE), 230, 255–256
   natural history, 255
   neonatal lupus, 255–256
   in pregnancy, 12–13
   use of medications, 255

T
T$_3$. See Triiodothyronine
T-ACE questionnaire, 118t
T-ACE, screening instruments, 118
Tachycardia
   and hypotension, 481
   with valvular obstructive lesions, 214

Tap test, 556
Tay–Sachs disease
    chromosomal abnormalities and genetic
        disorders, 199
    chronic debilitating diseases, 15
TB. *See* Tuberculosis
TB infection, risk factors for, 210
TBG. *See* Thyroxine-binding globulin
TCAs. *See* Tricyclic antidepressants
Tenderness, presence of, 133
TENS. *See* Transcutaneous electrical nerve
    stimulation
Teratogen, 44
    broadened definition of, 44
Teratogenicity, 338
Teratogens, 44
    methods of identifying, 44–45
Terbutaline
    agent for tocolysis, 167
    and ritodrine, 362
    tocolysis, 461
    for tocolytic treatment, 461
Terconazole, 273
Term breech trial, 511
Term pregnancy, 383
Term PROM, 442–445
    clinical features and diagnosis of, 442
    epidemiology and risk factors, 442
    treatment of, 442
Test-of-cure (TOC) culture, 260
Tetanus series, in pregnant women, 26
Tetracycline derivatives, 259–260
Tetralogy of Fallot, 213
T. gondii, an obligate intracellular protozoan, 301
T. gondii prophylaxis, trimethoprim-
    sulfamethoxazole for, 289
Thalassemia, 13, 193, 228–229
    chronic debilitating diseases, 15
Thalidomide
    an antianxiety and antinausea agent, 43
    classic teratogens, 44
Theophylline therapy, 206
Thiamine deficiency, 611
Thioamides, 246
Thioamide therapy, goal of, 245
Third- and fourth-degree lacerations, repair
    of, 549
Third-stage labor, management of, 430–434
    assisted placental separation, 431–432
    delivery of placenta, 431–432
    spontaneous placental separation, 431
Third-trimester amniocentesis, indications for,
    555
Threatened abortion, with bleeding, 144
Three-dimensional ultrasound, on abnormal
    pregnancy, 199
Three-hour oral glucose tolerance tests, criteria
    for abnormal result, in pregnant women,
    154t
Thrombocythemia, essential, 231
Thrombocytopenia, 229–230
    causes of, 230
Thromboembolic disease, 231
    and chronic anticoagulation, 223–226
Thrombophilic disease, history of, 223–224
Thrombophilic disorders, 231
Thyroid disease, in pregnancy, 243
Thyroiditis, common postpartum problem, 159
Thyroid-releasing hormone (TRH), 243
Thyroid-stimulating hormone (TSH), 243, 635

Thyroxine-binding globulin (TBG), 243
Tight control, defined, 248
Tioconazole, 273
Tissue hypoperfusion, sensitive indicators of, 312
Tobacco and alcohol, 194
TOC. *See* Test-of-cure culture
Tocolysis
    administration and dosage of, 363t
    agent for, 167
    contraindications to, 361t
Tocolytic treatment
    indication for, 459
    methods of, 461
TOLAC
    benefits of, 170
    risks of, 170
    selection of, 175
Toluene, solvents, 26
Topical anesthesia, 591
TORCH. *See* Toxoplasmosis, other, rubella,
    cytomegalovirus and herpes), intrauterine
    infections
Total daily insulin, 250
Total serum bilirubin (TSB), 594, 597–598, 599f
Towne vaccine, 301
Toxicology screening, use of, during pregnancy,
    118
Toxoplasma gondii infection, treatment of, 303t
Toxoplasmosis, 301–304
    clinical features of, 302
    diagnosis of, 302
    epidemiology of, 301
    pathogenesis of, 301–302
    prevention of, 304
    treatment of, 303
Toxoplasmosis, other, rubella, cytomegalovirus
    and herpes, intrauterine infections
    (TORCH), 180
Traction, with pulling motion, 538
Transcutaneous bilirubin, 597
Transcutaneous electrical nerve stimulation
    (TENS), 399
Transfusion, need for, 171
Transfusion syndrome, characteristics of, 162
Transient fetal bradycardia, 530
Transvaginal ultrasound, for confirming intra-
    uterine pregnancy, 23
Transverse arrest, 506–507
    definitions and causes, 506
    management, 506–507
        change in maternal position, 506
        digital rotation, 506
        forceps-assisted delivery, 507
        manual rotation, 506–507
        use of oxytocin, 507
        vacuum-assisted delivery, 507
Transverse lie, 505–506
    diagnosis of, 505–506
        abdominal palpation, 505
        radiologic examination, 506
        vaginal examination, 505
    management, 506
        external version, 506
        labor and delivery management, 506
Trauma, in pregnancy, 311–316
    clinical course and prevention, 315
    clinical features of, 312–313
    diagnosis of, 313–314
        abdominal pain/tenderness, 314
        airway, 313

Trauma, in pregnancy *(Continued)*
        breathing, 313
        circulation, 313
        coagulation studies, 314
        disability, 313
        electronic monitoring to detect maternal/
            fetal injury, 313–314
        exposure, 313
        placental abruption, 313
        vaginal examination, 314
    domestic violence, 311–312
    epidemiology and risk factors, 311–312
    pathogenesis of, 312
    treatment of, 314–316
        aspiration, 314
        duration of monitoring, 315
        fluid resuscitation, 314
        tocolysis, 315
        vena cava compression, 314
Trauma patient, physiologic effects of pregnancy
    related to evaluation of, 313t
Treponemal tests, 264
Treponema pallidum spirochete, 263
TRH. *See* Thyroid-releasing hormone
Trial of labor
    factors associated with, after cesarean,
        173–174
    harms and benefits of, 170–171
    influence of maternal preferences on, after
        cesarean, 174–175
    management of, after cesarean, 175–176
    obstetric and historical factors associated
        with, after cesarean, 173
Trichomonas vaginalis, 274–275
    diagnosis of, 274
    effect on perinatal outcome, 274
    epidemiology of, 274
    history of, 274
    management of, 274
Tricyclic antidepressants (TCAs), 331, 648
Triiodothyronine (T$_3$), 243
Trimethoprim, folate antagonist, 258
Triple screen test, 41
Triple test, for trisomy 21, 196
Trisomy 13, chromosomal aneuploidies,
    192, 195
Trisomy, 192
    chromosomal aneuploidies, 192, 195
    with decreased analytes, 196
Trisomy, 21, 39, 192, 194
    age-specific rates of, 40t
    chromosomal aneuploidies, 198
    incidence of, 510
    with low AFP, 196
    during second trimester, 194
    second-trimester screening for, 198
Trophotropism, concept of, 166
TSB. *See* Total serum bilirubin
TSB levels, effect on, in infants, 599
TSH. *See* Thyroid-stimulating hormone
Tuberculosis (TB), 210–212
    clinical course and prevention of, 211
    clinical features of, 211
    diagnosis of, 211
    epidemiology and risk factors, 210
    infectious disease killer, 16–17
    pathogenesis of, 210–211
    during pregnancy, 16, 211
    treatment of, 211
Tuboovarian abscess, 132

Turbidity, of amniotic fluid, 556
Turner syndrome
    chromosomal aneuploidies, 195
    with cystic hygroma, 196
T. vaginalis infection, in pregnancy, 274
Twin gestation, 521–522
    choice of route of delivery, 522
        clinical considerations, 522
        presenting fetus breech, 522
    diagnosis of, 523
    presentation of, 521
Twin intrauterine pregnancy, 137
Twin labor
    management of, 521–522
        fetal heart rate monitoring, 521
        monoamniotic, 522
        planning for the newborns, 521
        ultrasound, 521
        use of oxytocin, 521
Twin pregnancy, diagnosis of, 162–163
Twin-twin transfusion syndrome, 162–163
    growth discordance, 163
    pathophysiology, 162
    sonographic findings, 163
    treatment of, 163
Two-dimensional ultrasound, for suspected ovarian torsion, 307
Type 2 diabetes, fasting blood sugar concentrations during pregnancy develop, 159

U
UFH. *See* Unfractionated heparin
UDCA. *See* Ursodeoxycholic acid
Ulcerative colitis, 232
    adverse perinatal outcomes, 232
    fertility, 232
Ultrasound
    for diagnosis of first-trimester pregnancy, 133
    to follow cervical status, 367
    method of assessing gestational age, 61
    terminology and abbreviations used in diagnostic, 64t
    use of, 24
Ultrasound, in labor and delivery, 523–529
    applications, 523
        fetal presentation, 523
        multiple gestation, 523–524
Umbilical artery Doppler velocimetry, 346–347
    evidence to support the use of, 346–347
    indications and contraindications, 346
    test administration and interpretation, 346
Umbilical cord traction, 489
Unbleeding and cramping, on dose of misoprostol, 147
Unconjugated serum bilirubin, 597
Underweight women, 68
Unfractionated heparin (UFH), 217, 218t, 496
Unipolar depression, 330–332
Ureaplasma cultured, discovery of, 472
Urinary frequency and incontinence, 89
    causative factors, 89
    treatment of, 89
Urinary incontinence, during pregnancy, 89
Urinary sediment, microscopic evaluation of, 40
Urinary tract infections, 238, 239
Urination, frequency of, 616
Urine, acidification of, with vitamin C, 239
Urine and blood pregnancy test, 130

Urine antigen testing, 604
    with latex agglutination, 604
Urine culture, 239
    for asymptomatic bacteriuria, 39–40
    baseline, 370
Urine tests
    to detect Chlamydia trachomatis, 37
    diagnostic accuracy of, 37
Ursodeoxycholic acid (UDCA), 309
U.S. Food and Drug Administration Pregnancy Labeling System, proposed, 46t
U.S. National Asthma Education Program Working Group, on asthma, 205
U.S. Preventative Services Task Force (USPSTF), 36, 277
    evidence for efficacy of interventions, 104
    on screening gestational age, 152
USPSTF. *See* U.S. Preventative Services Task Force
Uterine activity, to initiate softening of cervix, 384
Uterine and cervical pain, 421
Uterine anomalies, and leiomyomata, 167
Uterine atony, 479, 484
    soft or boggy uterus on palpation, 481
Uterine contractions, 397
    FHR recorded after, 454
    insufficient, 488
    with low-dose oxytocin infusion, 343
    in PTD, 366
Uterine curette, invention of, 145
Uterine drainage, compress uterus, 564
Uterine evacuation, 145
Uterine fibroids, undergo torsion or degeneration, 89
Uterine hemorrhage, 565–566
Uterine hyperstimulation, 343
Uterine relaxation, for entrapped placenta, 489–490
Uterine rupture, 170, 312, 481, 485, 561
    factors associated with, 170t
    with fetal mortality, 313
    risk for, 28
Uterine segment, assessment of lower, in managing vaginal birth after cesarean, 525–526
Uterus
    and cervix, transabdominal scan of, 136f
    close, 564
    coronal transvaginal scan of, containing dead embryo, 137f
    open, 563
    protective environment for fetus, 43
    transabdominal transverse scan of, containing 23-mm echogenic area, 136f
    transvaginal scan of, containing chorionic sac, 136f
    transvaginal scan of, pseudo sac in ectopic pregnancy, 138f
    transverse scan of, containing echoes of hydatidiform mole, 138f

V
Vaccines
    avoided in pregnancy, 51
    indicated in pregnancy, 47–49, 50
Vacuum, 541
Vacuum application
    advantages of, 539

Vacuum application (*Continued*)
    contraindications to, 539
    disadvantages of, 539
    procedure, 539–540
Vacuum-assisted vaginal delivery, 509
Vacuum cup, correct position of, 540f
Vacuum extraction, 368, 539–541
Vaginal amniotic fluid, to assess fetal lung maturity, 371
Vaginal birth after cesarean (VBAC), 169–178, 521
    contraindications for, 177
    epidemiology of, 169
    risks and benefits of trial of labor, 169–172
    use of consent forms for, 177
Vaginal birth
    ACOG 1999 practice guideline on, 176
    factors associated with, after cesarean section, 174t
Vaginal birth, risks and benefits of, 178
Vaginal bleeding
    absence of, 314
    causes of, 165
    complication during first trimester, 130
    diagnostic approach, 165–166
    differential diagnosis of, 476–477
    major causes of, 166–168
    management of, 477–479
    during pregnancy, 33
    in second and third trimesters, 165–168
    speculum examination, 165–166
Vaginal breech delivery
    factors favorable for, 512
    factors unfavorable for, 512–513
    technique of, 513–515
Vaginal delivery
    demographic factors associated with, after cesarean, 173
    prognosis for, 389
    in women with prior cesarean birth, 172–173
Vaginal dimensions, changes in, 325
Vaginal mucosa
    closing, 547–548
    repair of, 547
Vaginal pool specimens, testing from, 556
Vaginal speculum examination, 132
Valium, for noneclamptic status epilepticus, 237
Valproic acid, 334
    antiepileptic medications, 25
    fetal levels of, 334
    use of, 228
Valsalva pushing, 417
Valvular heart disease, 217
Valvuloplasty, 215
Vancomycin, 267
Varicella, contagious disease, 16
Varicella vaccine
    history of, 49
    maternal exposure during pregnancy, 49–50
    use of, 50
    during pregnancy, 50
Varicella zoster, 297–299
    effects on perinatal outcome, 297–298
    epidemiology of, 297
    history of, 297
    management guidelines, 298
    prevention of, 298–299
Varicella zoster immunoglobulin (VZIG), 49, 298
    new form of, 298
VariZIG, 298

VAS. *See* Vibroacoustic stimulation
Vasa previa, fetal hemorrhage, 476
Vasopressors, use of, 314
VBAC. *See* Vaginal birth after cesarean
VDRL. *See* Venereal Disease Research Laboratory
Vegetarianism, 71
Venereal Disease Research Laboratory (VDRL), 36, 264
Venography, method for diagnosis of DVT, 225
Venous Doppler, method for diagnosis of DVT, 225
Venous pressure, in pelvis, 91
Venous thromboembolism, 495–497
    anticoagulation for, 496
    diagnosis, 496
    epidemiology, 495
    management, 496
    pathophysiology, 495–496
    prevention, 497
Venous thrombotic events (VTEs)
    and/or receiving long-term anticoagulation, 224–225
    diagnosis of, 225
    intrapartum and emergency management of, 226
    with risk factor, 224
    with thrombophilia, 223
    and thrombophilia, 224
Ventricular septal defect, 213
Ventriculomegaly, 300
Verapamil, to treat maternal supraventricular tachycardia, 218
Vernix or meconium, 391
Vertex crowns, 540f
Vertical transmission
    estimates of, 285
    risk factors, 286t
Very-low-birth-weight (VLBW), 161
Vibrio parahemolyticus, in oysters and sushi, 31
Vibroacoustic stimulation (VAS), 342, 462
Viral neuraminidase enzyme, 209
Viral pneumonia, caused by multiple organisms, 208
Vitamin and mineral, 68–71
Vitamin B$_6$ (pyridoxine), 56

Vitamin B$_{12}$ deficiency, 228, 630
Vitamin C, 70
Vitamin D, 70, 610
Vitamin K, 610
    to prevent clotting defects in newborn, 237
Vitamin K deficiency bleeding (VKDB), 576
    classic, 577
    incidence, 576
    laboratory findings in, 577
    late, 577
    risk factors, 576
    treatment, 577
    types of, 576
Vitamin K deficiency coagulopathy, 237
Vitamin K prophylaxis, 576
Vitamins and minerals, 72, 611–612
Vitamin toxicity, 70
VKDB. *See* Vitamin K deficiency bleeding
VLBW. *See* Very-low-birth-weight
Von Willebrand disease, 230
VTEs. *See* Venous thrombotic events
Vulvovaginal candidiasis, treatment of, 273
VZIG. See Varicella zoster immunoglobulin

W
Warfarin
    as category D, 217
    cause an anticoagulant effect in fetus, 223
    efficacy in preventing valvular thromboses, 217
    first-trimester exposure to, 223
    vitamin K antagonists, 223
Warm compresses, during second stage of labor, 427
Warming formula, 611
Waste-anesthetic gas, reduce fertility, 26
Water aerobics, to diminish pregnancy-related low back pain, 90
Water, immersion in, during delivery, 415
Water-soluble narcotics, 404
Weaning, cause of, 627
Weight gain
    caloric needs and, 67–68

Weight gain *(Continued)*
    components of, in normal pregnancy, 68t
    patterns, nonstandard, 68
    during pregnancy, 67, 67t, 71, 187
    range of, in pregnancy, 29, 30t
    recommendations for, 68
Whiff test, 271
WHO. *See* World Health Organization
WIC. *See* Women, Infants and Children
Wigand-Martin maneuver, 514
Wisconsin Maternity Leave and Health Study, 661
Women, Infants and Children (WIC), 66, 105, 568
    supplemental nutrition program for, 80
Woods screw maneuver, 468f
World Health Organization (WHO), 227, 479, 627
    examined role of calcium supplementation, 494
    on normal birth, 382
Worst-case analysis, 389

X
Xiphoid, 92
Xylene, solvents, 26

Y
Yolk sac, 134, 135f
    and chorionic sac wall, 134, 135f
    visibility of, 134f

Z
Zanamivir, administered in inhaled form, 209
Zavanelli maneuver, 469
Zero station, diagnosis, 388f
Zung depression scale, 330
Zygosity, 162